Science Press Springer-Verlag

Research on Acupuncture, Moxibustion, and Acupuncture Anesthesia

Editor in Chief
Zhang Xiangtong (H.T. Chang)

With 518 Figures, 12 Color Photographs and 327 Tables

Science Press, Beijing
Springer-Verlag
Berlin Heidelberg New York Tokyo

Responsible Editor Lou Pengxun

Published by Science Press, Beijing

Distribution rights throughout the world, excluding The People's Republic of China, granted to Springer-Verlag Berlin Heidelberg New York Tokyo

ISBN 3-540-10901-3 Springer-Verlag Berlin Heidelberg New York Tokyo
ISBN 0-387-10901-3 Springer-Verlag New York Heidelberg Berlin Tokyo

Printed in Hong Kong

Printing and binding: C & C Joint Printing Co., (H.K.) Ltd.
2131/3140-543210

Science Press Book No. 4243-55

PREFACE

Acupuncture and moxibustion in China have a long history dating back to ancient times. In years B. C. stone needles were used to treat ailments. For centuries the Chinese people have been using acupuncture and moxibustion in their practice of combating diseases. They have by summing-up their experiences, carried forward and developed the methods and theories of acupuncture and moxibustion and the points for the application of these techniques. In 1958 medical workers in our country discovered acupuncture anesthesia on the basis of the therapeutic and analgesic effects of acupuncture and moxibustion. Since then the study of acupuncture and moxibustion by integrating clinical practice with fundamental research and combining traditional Chinese medicine with western medicine has led to a new way of development and fully demonstrated their scientific basis. China now has a large number of trained workers for clinical and theoretical research of acupuncture and moxibustion, and by their research on the principle of acupuncture anesthesia, a new field in science is being explored, and some new techniques in medical science are being popularized. We have, to a certain degree, mastered clinically the law and mechanism of acupuncture anesthesia, especially its analgesic effect. At the same time we have advanced the scientific researches of acupuncture in neurophysiology, neurochemistry and neuropharmacology. In promoting the study of acupuncture and moxibustion, channels and collaterals, the work of systematizing our heritage of traditional Chinese medicine has made a promising step forward.

A national symposium on acupuncture and moxibustion and acupuncture anesthesia was held in Beijing from the 1st to the 5th June, 1979. More than 200 representatives from the whole country attended it and made reports on the results of their researches on acupuncture and moxibustion and acupuncture anesthesia. These reports were highly praised by the more than 100 scientists from abroad, participating in the enthusiastic discussion of them. They all wished to be able to see at an early date the full texts of the articles read at the meeting, and the domestic scientists also desired that a collection of selected papers be published as soon as possible, so as to promote the exchange of knowledge and to raise scientific researches to a higher level. For this reason, we have first selected a part of the articles for publication to meet the request of our readers.

In this selection there are 119 articles. The first one written by Qian Xinzhong, Minister of Public Health, gives a systematic and general account of the advances in acupuncture, moxibustion and acupuncture anesthesia. The rest of the articles are divided into four parts:

I. Research on the mechanisms of acupuncture, moxibustion and acupuncture anesthesia;
II. Research on channel-collaterals and points;
III. Clinical research on acupuncture and moxibustion;
IV. Clinical research on acupuncture anesthesia.

Under the guiding policy of "let a hundred flowers blossom and a hundred schools of thought contend", we have selected papers that are representative of a good cross section of the different views presented at the meeting. We believe that it is both impossible and unnecessary to force people to conform to a single view and that an objective evaluation can be obtained only through much work and free and thorough discussion.

Acupuncture, moxibustion and acupuncture anesthesia are originated in China and are an invaluable medical heritage of our country. However, since ancient times they have been among the cultural things that China has exchanged and cooperated with other countries. Therefore, acupuncture, moxibustion and acupuncture anesthesia have now become the common wealth of all mankind and an interesting subject for researches by medical workers throughout the world. It is our duty to continue this exchange and cooperation begun by our ancestors. We hope that the present selection may make some contribution toward the realization of this object.

Thanks are due to all who have helped us in the compilation of this selection.

The Editors

CONTENTS

Preface . . . .
Progress in Scientific Research on Acupuncture, Moxibustion and Acupuncture Anesthesia by Integrating Traditional Chinese and Western Medicine
Qian Xinzhong . . . .

PART I RESEARCH ON THE MECHANISMS OF ACUPUNCTURE, MOXIBUSTION AND ACUPUNCTURE ANESTHESIA

(1)

Interaction in Thalamus of Afferent Impulses from Acupuncture Point and Site of Pain
Zhang Xiangtong (H.T. Chang) 21
Participation of Descending Inhibition in Acupuncture Analgesia
Shen E 31
Inhibitory Action of Electroacupuncture on Dorsal Horn Neurons of the Spinal Cord
Wu Jianping, Xing Jianghuai, Xing Baoren, Lu Jingen, Chen Yuchu 39
Observations on Operant Conditioning and Single Unit Activity of the Prefrontal Cortex of Rhesus Monkeys During Acupuncture
Liu Jinlong, Qi Dailin, Han Xiangwen, Hou Gangxing, Zhou Huiju, Jin Wenlong, Wang Zuoqing, Yang Congguo, Liu Zuozhou 50
Analgesic Effects of Several Modes of Electroacupuncture in Monkeys and Their Reversal by Naloxone
Huang Ye, Wang Qingwei, Zheng Jinze, Li Derong, Xie Guoyang 60
Relationship Between Nucleus Raphe Magnus and Higher Brain Regions in Inhibition of Viscero-Somatic Reflexes
Du Huanji, Zhao Yanfang 70
Effect of Stimulation of Midbrain Raphe Nuclei on Discharges of Nociceptive Neurons in Nucleus Parafascicularis of Thalamus and its Significance in Acupuncture Analgesia
Zhang Guilin, Wei Jinbo, Zhou Lingbao, Lin Yaomin, Luo Zhengliang, Zhou Lanxian, Zhang Zuchen 82
Effect of Electroacupuncture and Some Exogenous Monoamines on Unit Discharges of the Dorsal Nucleus Raphe
Department of Biophysics, Department of Physiology, Beijing Medical College 93
Influence of Electro-Stimulation of Nucleus Raphe Magnus and Locus Caeruleus on the Analgesic Effect of Acupuncture in the Spinal Trigeminal Nucleus
Zhong Guogan, Liu Minzhi, Jiang Yan, Liu Xiang, Wang Shao, Liu Suping 98
Effects of Electro-Stimulation and Electroacupuncture of Midbrain Raphe on Neurons in the Head of Caudate Nucleus in Conscious and Unrestrained Rabbits
Sun Gongduo, Li Xuming, Yang Kongshun, Cheng Shaojie, Du Xiujie 106

Effects of Acupuncture, Brain-Stimulation and Analgesics on the Groaning Response Elicited by Tegmental Stimulation in Cats
Zhu Henian, Lin Baocheng, Zhu Yuanxiang, Song Chaoyou, Wu Chongren 117
Effects of Electroacupuncture and Exogenous Transmitters Applied Microiontophoretically on Pain Discharges in Mesencephalic Reticular Formation
Huang Chengjun, Zhang Zidong, Liu Zuoyan, Tu Zongpin, Xiao Hongmei 127
Inhibition of Evoked Discharges of Posterior Nuclear Group of Thalamus Induced by Stimulation of Central Grey Matter, Caudate Nucleus and Electroacupuncture in Waking Rabbits
Zhao Zhiqi, Shao Dianhua, Yang Zhenquan 138
Role of Caudate Nucleus in Acupuncture Analgesia
He Lianfang, Xu Shaofen, Jiang Chengchuan 146
Effect of Acupuncture on Nociceptive Discharges of Cingulate Gyrus neurons
Sun Xinde, Zhou Shaoci, Xu Junmei, Zhang Senfu 158
Preliminary Observations on the Changes in Slow Potentials of Cerebral Cortex Induced by Acupuncture and "Pain"
Wang Boyang, Yang Boyi, Jiang Deming 170
Role of Cerebral Cortex in Acupuncture Analgesia
Cooperative Research Group for Brain in Acupuncture Analgesia, Beijing 177
Effect of Cord Dorsum Stimulation on EEG and Behavior in Unrestrained Rabbits
Shen Kefei, Ho Shufang, Wang Peifen 185
The Role of the Bulbar Reticular Formation in Inhibition of Visceral Pain by Acupuncture
Huang Zhongsun, Jin Shuran, Zhou Baohe, Fei Ruwei, Zhang Neng, Fan Weizheng, Sun Anping, Wang Dili 195
Research on Mechanism of Acupuncture Anti-Visceralgia—I. An Experimental Observation on Integration in Medulla Oblongata
The 1st Department of Physiology, Institute of Acupuncture and Moxibustion, Academy of Traditional Chinese Medicine 205
Research on Mechanism of Acupuncture Anti-Visceralgia—II. Effect of Morphine Antagonist on Electroacupuncture Anti-visceralgia
The 1st Department of Physiology, Institute of Acupuncture and Moxibustion, Academy of Traditional Chinese Medicine 217
Relationship Between Cerebral Cortex and Acupuncture Inhibition of Visceral Pain
Chen Peixi, Chen Zhuhua, Weng Jiwei, Ren Huifang, Zhang Jinmei, Zhang Jinghang, Feng Jianqiang. 227

(2)

Role of Central Neurotransmitters in Acupuncture Analgesia
Han Jisheng, Tang Jian, Ren Minfeng, Zhou Zhongfu, Fan Shaoguang, Qiu Xuecai

. . . . 241
Endorphin and Acupuncture Analgesia
Zhang Anzhong, Pan Xiaoping, Xu Shaofen, Cheng Jieshi, Mo Wanying 256
Enkephalin Involvement in Acupuncture Analgesia–Radioimmunoassay
Zou Gang, Yi Qingcheng, Wu Shixiang, Lu Yixin, Wang Fansheng, Yu Yuegui, Ji Xinquan, Zhang Zuxuan, Zhao Dandan 267
Effect of Intracerebral Microinjection of Naloxone on Acupuncture and Morphine-analgesia in the Rabbit
Zhou Zhongfu, Du Mingyi, Wu Wenying, Jiang Ying, Han Jisheng. 279
Effects of Naloxone on Analgesia Produced by Different Strengths of Electroacupuncture
Zhang Anzhong, Zeng Dayun, Zhang Lingmei, Cheng Jieshi, Ye Zhijun, Ou Shupei 296
Effect of Morphine Tolerance on Acupuncture Analgesia
Zhang Anzhong, Xu Shaofen, Zhang Lingmei, Zeng Dayun 303
Central 5-Hydroxytryptamine, Opiate-like Substances and Acupuncture Analgesia
Han Jisheng, Tang Jian, Fan Shaoguang, Ren Minfeng, Zhou Zhongfu, Zhang Wanqin, Liang Xinan 309
Role of Brain Serotonergic and Catecholaminergic Systems in Acupuncture Analgesia
Jin Guozhang, Zhang Zhende, Yu Leiping, Han Yifan, Xu Jian, Feng Jie, Pan Jiancui 317
Effect of Microinjection of Noradrenaline into Hypothalamus of Acupuncture Analgesia
Pan Jiancui, Zhang Shengmei. 332
Role of Cholinergic Nerves in Electroacupuncture Analgesia—Influence of Acetylcholine, Eserine, Neostigmine and Hemicholinum on Electroacupuncture Analgesia
Guan Xinmin, Yu Bi, Wang Caiyuan Liu Xiaochun. 341
Action of Sympathetic Nerve and Its Mediator in Mechanism of Acupuncture Anesthesia
Yan Huijin, Xu Chengtao, Chen Mengqin, Liu Bochun, Chen Houlan, Cai Liangwan Xu Caimin, Li Huizhen, Wei Yue, Fu Guanying 352
Study of Role of Humoral Factors in Central Action of Acupuncture Analgesia
Chen Mengqin, Zheng Yongfang, Xue Zuohong, Wen Yunyi, Nie Zaimin, Zhang Baozhen 360
Common Basis of Electroacupuncture Analgesia and Morphine Analgesia
Zhang Zuxuan, Zhang Yuanzhen, Yu Qixiang, Li Chunbao, Chen Rongsan. 372
Role of Histamine in Acupuncture Analgesia
Lu Zusun, Cheng Jun. 379
Substance P: Its Analgesic Effect and Influence on Caudate Neutronal Activity in Conscious Rabbits
Zhang Chongli, Sun Gongduo, Yan Huijin, Yang Kongshun, Ye Liangqin, Li Xuming, Xie Yikuan, Cheng Shaojie, Wang Hong, Zhao Bingshun, Jiang Yanjia, He Guoliang. 388

Possible Role of Hypothalamus-Pituitary-Adrenal System in Acupuncture Analgesia
Liu Xuegao, Yang Zijiang, Li Qinzhang, Huang Yiming, Xu Hao, Xiao Changqi, Liang Zhixi 397
Relationship of Lip-Acupuncture Analgesia with Pituitary-Adrenocortical System
Miao Ming, Liu Huici, Gao Aili, Huang Weiqiu, Xu Bin, Yin Qizhang 408
Study of Effect of Acupuncture on Experimental Deep and Referred Pains
Zhou Shaoci, Weng Enqi, Ye Qiang, Wang Hua, Kang Yanping 414

(3)

Study of Receptors of Needling Sensation at Somatic Acupuncture Points
Hou Zonglian (C.L. Hou) 428
Effect of Electroacupuncture at Point "Zusanli" on Activity of Muscle Mechanoreceptors and Afferent Fibres in Cats
Tan Depei, Zhang Shujie, Mao Jianping 437
Some Observations on Receptive Structures in Certain Acupuncture Points and Their Afferent Pathways conducting "Needling Sensations" in Human Beings
Lin Wenzhu, Xu Minghai, Wang Zhiyu, Dai Jingdian, Chen Guomei, Shen Jingyan 443
Composition of Afferent Fibers at Point "Zusanli" in Relation to Acupuncture Analgesia—A Functional Morphological Investigation
Lu Guowei, Xie Jingqiang, Yang Jin, Wang Yongning, Wang Qilin 453
Analysis of Afferent Fibers Transmitting Needling Signals of Acupoint
Lu Guowei, Zhao Guoshun, Liang Rongzhao, Wang Yongning, Xing Weichang, Shi Guang 466
An Analytical Study of the Afferent Fibers for impulses of Acupuncture Analgesia
Chen Longshun, Tang Jingshi, Fan Li, Wang Kemo, Yan Jianqun 478
The Area (Sensitive Area) of the Production of Traction Pain of Stomach, Its Area of Origin and Afferent Pathway
Yu Pin, Li Zhennian, Zhang Kun, Li Guizhen, Lu Yongli, Jiang Shuxue 490
Electron Microscopic and Fluorohistochemical Observations of Nerves in Human Stomach Wall Removed During Operations Under Acupuncture Anesthesia
Yu Yi, Pang Junyun, Guo Yanru 504
Somatotopic Projection of the Raphe Nuclei to Spinal Dorsal Horn in the Cat —A Horseradish Peroxidase Study
Ju Gong, Shu Siyun 516
Influence of Electroacupuncture on Ultrastructure of Synapses in Medial Region of Rat Thalamus
Ai Minkang, Wu Zhongjing, Li Tongping 529
Effect of Pain on Ultrastructure of Intermediate Lobe of Pituitary
Yuan Dexia, Huang Shansheng, Ying Guohua, Li Xiangyin, Fu Zhiliang 539

The Relation between Acupuncture Anesthesia and Neurotransmitters and Enzymes of Locus Coeruleus and Raphe Nucleus
Ge Zi, Huang Weimin, Wang Zhiying, Song Wancheng 558
Effects of Electroacupuncture on Cell-mediated Immunity in Human Body
Wu Jinglan, Zong Anmin, Chai Xinmei, Cai Dehua, Ren Zhichun, Luo Huimin, Kao peiwen, Hu Zuofang 568

PART II RESEARCH ON CHANNEL-COLLATERALS AND POINTS

Adrenergic Nerve Fibers—The Chief Factor Affecting Changes of Electric Resistance of Rabbit Pinna in Experimental Peptic Ulcer
Research Laboratory of the Mechanisms of Acupuncture Anesthesia, Morphology Group, Beijing Medical College 577
Experimental Study of the Afferent Pathway in Formation of Low-Resistance Points on the Auriculae of Rabbit
Yin Huizhen, Zhou Shaoci, You Guofen 588
Morphological Study of Sensations Produced by Needling Different Points
Pan Chaochong, Zhao Aifeng 597
Relative Regularity between Jingluo Points and Spinal Segmental Innervation
Yang Feng, Ren Shizhen 618
Relations Between Channels and Lymphatic System
Gong Qihua, Cao Jiren 628
An Observation on Phenomenon of Propagated Sensation Along the Channels
Academy of Traditional Chinese Medicine, the PLA Hospital. No. 262 and the People's Hospital of Jishan County of Shanxi Province 638
Studies of Phenomenon of Blocking Activities of Channels and Collaterals
Research Group of Acupuncture Anesthesia, Institute of Medicine and Pharmacology of Fujian Province, et al 653
The Phenomenon of Propagated Sensation Along Channels (PSC) and the Cerebral Cortex
Xue Chongcheng 668
Study of Objective Parameters in Phenomenon of Propagated Sensation Along Channels
Wu Sihong, Sheng Lingling, Gu Peikun, Yang Hongying, Tie Shuangyu 684
Propagated Sensation Along Channels (PSC) Induced by Stimulation of Ear Points
Research Group of Acupuncture Anesthesia and Channels, Guangxi College of Traditional Chinese Medicine 692
Phenomenon of Propagated Sensation Along the Channels Induced by Limitation of Spontaneous Conscious Activity (Entering Quiescent Condition)
Wang Buxiong, Cui Lihua, Chu Weizhong 703
Preliminary Study of Excitation of Propagated Sensation Along Channels
Zhang Jin, Liu Wancheng, Wang Tong, Cheng Keming, Yu Shuzhuang, Zhang Ruxin

. . . . 711

Studies of Phenomenon of Latent Propagated Sensation Along the Channels: I. The Discovery of a Latent PSC and Preliminary Study of Its Skin Electrical Conductance
Zhu Zongxiang, Yan Zhiqiang, Yu Shuzhuang, Zhang Ruxin, Wang Juyi, Liu Yiming, Hao Jinkai, Zhang Xuliang, Yu Shuling, He Qingnian, Meng Zhaowei 721

Studies of Phenomenon of Latent Propagated Sensation Along the Channels: II. Investigation of the Lines of LSPC in the 12 Main Channels
Yu Shuzhuang, Zhang Min, An Suqi, Yang Shuying, Zhang Shuyuan, Zhu Zongxiang, He Qingnian 729

Preliminary Investigation of Phenomenon of Sensory Conduction Along the Channels in Patients with Poliomyelitic Sequelae
Sheng Lingling, Wu Sihong, Gu Peikun, Tie Shuangyu, Yang Hongying 736

Preliminary Observations on Propagated Sensation Along Channels (SPC) in 102 Cases of Spinal Cord Transection
Fu Zhaoming, Li Boning, Xiao Zhijiang 740

Studies of Relation Between Propagated Sensation Along Channels and Effectiveness of Clinical Acupuncture Analgesia
Cooperative Group in Research of PSC, Fujian Province 745

Existence of Channel System as Evidenced by 93 Cases of Skin Diseases Appearing along the Channels
Li Dingzhong 754

Algesthesia and Paresthesia Propagated Along the Channels (Report of 80 Cases)
Liu Chengzhong 772

PART III CLINICAL RESEARCH ON ACUPUNCTURE AND MOXIBUSTION

Research on the Origin and Development of Chinese Acupuncture and Moxibustion
Wang Xuetai 783

Acupuncture in Combination with X-Ray Examination for Diagnosis of Gastrointestinal Diseases
Zhang Fachu, Li Shuchin, Wang Siaoya, Ying Ruchun, Qu Chunshui, Ying Chaoti, Xie Ruiling, Ching Shaoqi 800

Studies of Version by Moxibustion on Zhiyin Points
Cooperative Research Group of Moxibustion Version of Jiangxi Province 810

Olinical Investigation of Treating Patients with Acute Bacillary Dysentery by Acupuncture
Qiu Maoliang, Sheng Canruo, Li Naiying, Wang Junmei, Wang Jinsheng, Xu Bingqing, Lu Zhenchu, Deng Guogang, Zhang Wanwen 820

Experimental Study of Acupuncture Treatment of Acute Bacillary Dysentery: Role of Humoral Immune Mechanism
Xu Bingqing, Lu Zhenchu, Deng Guogang, Zhang Wanwen, Li Naiying, Wang Junmei, Qiu Maoliang, Sheng Chuanruo, Wang Jinsheng, Wu Defu 829

Clinical Research on Acupuncture Treatment of Malaria
Group of Acupuncture Treatment on Malaria, Institute of Acupuncture and Moxibustion, Academy of Traditional Chinese Medicine 837

Acupuncture Treatment of 209 Cases of Cerebral Thrombosis and Observation of Effect on Rheoencephalogram and Electromyogram
Department of Neurology and Department of Physiological Research No. 2, Institute of Acupuncture and Moxibustion, Academy of Traditional Chinese Medicine 845

Electroacupuncture and Magnesium Sulfate Administration for Cholelithiasis: Clinical Investigation of 522 Cases and Preliminary Consideration of Features of Stone-excretion
Zhao Shiduo, Song Xieen, Pan Guishan, Lin Zhihua, Wang Shanmin, Wang Laixiu, Sun Huafeng 851

Clinical Observation of Effect of Acupuncture on Angina Pectoris
Liu Fuzai, Li Jinglin, Liu Guizhi, Wang Yizhong, Chi Huichang Gao Benqi, Meng Jinghi, Liu Ruiting, Xu Huiren 861

Effect of Acupuncture on Experimental Acute Myocardial Infarction
Yang Youmi, Liu Ruiting, Meng Jingbi, Li Lianda, Gao Xiuzi, Wang Pingping 876

Study of Effect of Acupuncture on Blood Pressure Regulatory System
Huang Bingxian, Pan Hua, Xiang Manjun, Yang Minggang, Yu Zhanjiu, Wu Yulan 883

Analysis of Therapeutic Effect of Acupuncture in 66 Cases of Gastroptosis
Gastroptosis Treatment Group, Radiological Department, Institute of Acupuncture and Moxibustion and Academy of Traditional Chinese Medicine 892

Clinical Observation of Acupuncture Treatment of Acute Perforation of Peptic Ulcer
Zhuang Ding, Wang Yuanchao, Yang Xiuzhen, Tian Zaishan, Liu Yingyun, Yuan Heping, Li Donghua 898

Effect of Needling "Zusanli" on Gastrointestinal Function and Analysis of Its Afferent Pathway
Zhuang Ding, Gao Huihe, Yang Xiuzhen, Wang Yuanchao, Zai Shixing, Lin Yinli, Wang Wensu, Chen Xiaomei, Li Zhonghua, Shen Mingbao, Yu Lili, Jiang Songlin, Yu Bin, Li Fenglian, Jin Guilian, Gong Qihua, Ouyang Zirong, Fan Li, Hua Xingbang, Zhang Wanwen, Qiu Yongchao, Gong Yanhua, Zhu Lingying 910

Investigation of Mechanism of Acupuncture Treatment of Perforated Peptic Ulcer
Huang Guanqing, Tang Meilai, Wang Kaizhi, Liu Shihua 919

Observation of the Effects of Acupuncture Therapy on Vesicle and Anal Incontinence Caused by Congenital Spina Bifida Over the Lumbosacral Region
Research Group on Vesical and Anal Incontinence, First Hosptal, Bethune Medical College 923
The Induction of Labor by Electroacupuncture Stimulation—Analysis of 771 cases
Zhu Renlie, Gao Xiuhui, Zhou Yulian, Yu Jin 930
Acupuncture Treatment of Peripheral Facial Paralysis
Yang Zhaomin, Wang Juming, Hu Ningqi 938
Acupuncture of "Xiangyang" Point in Treatment of Central Serous Chorioretinopathy—Analysis of 600 Cases
Department of Ophthalmology, First Hospital, Zhejiang Medical College 945
Observation of Sensorineural Deafness Treated with Acupuncture
Audiological Research Group, Bethune Medical College and Deaf-mutism Research Group, Unit 81112, PLA 951

PART IV CLINICAL RESEARCH ON ACUPUNCTURE ANESTHESIA

Acupuncture Anesthesia in Neurosurgery
National Cooperative Group of Acupuncture Anesthesia for Neurosurgery 961
Laryngectomy under Acupuncture Anesthesia (Report of 430 Cases)
Huang Henian 973
Acupuncture Anesthesia in 1,965 Cases of Maxillary Sinusotomy
National Cooperative Group of Acupuncture Anesthesia for Radical Simusotomy. 978
Clinical Analysis and Preliminary Experimental Observations of 1,802 Cases of ORO-Maxillo-Facial Operations Under Acupuncture Anesthesia
Qiu Weiliu, Lin Guochu, Yuan Wenhua, Liu Shixun, Ha Qi, Fan Baohua, Chen Shaodong, Liu Yugui, Shen Jiannan, Ma Guizhen, Lu Juying 983
Summary of 9,375 Cases of Thyroidectomy Under Acupuncture Anesthesia
National Cooperative Group for Acupuncture Anethesia in Thyroidectomy 993
Operative Treatment of Hyperthyroidism Under Acupuncture Anesthesia
Zhu Yu, Yang Baoheng, Wang Xiuhua, Luo Laikui, Zhuang Liding 999
Clinical Studies of Acupuncture Anesthesia for Lung Resection
Department of Acupuncture Anesthesia, Beijing Tuberculosis Research Institute 1008
Clinical Study of 1,067 Cases of Pulmonary Resection Under Acupuncture Anesthesia
Shanghai, First Tuberculosis Hospital and Shanghai Institute of Acupuncture and Moxibustion 1015
Clinical Observation of Acupuncture Anesthesia for Open Heart Operations Under Extracorporeal Circulation With Related Physiological and Biochemical Changes—A Report of 230 Cases

Third People's Hospital of Shanghai Second Medical College and Acupuncture Research Laboratory of Shanghai Second Medical College 1021
Acupuncture Anesthesia in Mitral Commissurotomy for Severe mitral stenosis
Shanghai Chest Hospital 1031
Regulatory Function of Acupuncture in Subtotal Gastrectomy Under Acupuncture Anesthesia
Zhou Shu, Lou Ailin, Zhou Lu, Luo Qingdao, Zhou Longwu, Zheng Chaoqiang, Cui Suying, Cheng Lanying, Chen Yuzhen, Xu Rongkun, Zheng Xiaozhao 1038
Clinical Evaluation of Acupuncture Anesthesia in Subtotal Gastrectomy and a Study of Type-classification Based on Differentiation of Syndrome in Traditional Chinese Medicine
Zhang Guangzheng, Ye Qiang, Xiang Limin, Wu Chuande, Zhu Meimei, Gu Yanqing, Xue Lunxian, Zhou Shaoci, Weng Enqi, Dai Yongzhen, Mao Liang, Yang Zhen, Zhang Meili, Ke Xuefan 1053
Observation of Visceral Dragging-Pain-Reaction During Subtotal Gastrectomy
Chen Peixi, Pan Wenzheng, Zhang Ming, Weng Jiwei, Feng Jianjiang 1065
Preoperative Comprehensive Forecast of the Effectiveness of Acupuncture Anesthesia in Subtotal Gastrectomy for Peptic Ulcer
Acupuncture Anesthesia Coordinating Group for Gastrectomy, Beijing Medical College 1076
Clinical Analysis of 1,000 Cases of Cesarean Section Under Acupuncture Anesthesia
The Research Group of Acupuncture Anesthesia for Cesarean Section, Beijing Obstetrics and Gynecology Hospital 1080
Investigation of Electro-Needling of Jizhong Point in Abdominal Total Hysterectomy
Xu Zhengyi, Xue Biru, He Shufang, Zheng Zehui, ... 1091
Clinical Study of Abdominal Tuboligation Under Acupuncture Anesthesia
National Cooperative Group of Acupuncture Anesthesia for Abdominal Tuboligation. 1099
An Analysis of Different Methods of Anesthesia for Prostatectomy
Zhuang Xinliang, Qu Guilian, Chen Shoulin, Zhang Lingdi 1105
Clinical Experience in Acupuncture Anesthesia for Cervical Spine Operation Through Anterior Approach
Wang Kuan, Ma Lihua, Dong Fangchun, Zhang Tancheng 1111
Acupuncture Anesthesia Using Yeping Point for Upper Extremity Operations—A Report on 72 Cases
Lei Yunshan, Li Baoxiang, Wang Dongsheng. 1116
On the Proposed Mechanism of Analgesic Effect of Acupuncture Anesthesia in Lateral Meniscectomy
Guo Bangfu, Yao Zhiyin, Zhang Qingcai, Shen Lei, Wang Liujiang 1123
Relationship Between Effect of Acupuncture Analgesia and Sympathetic Functional Activity

Cao Xiaoding, Mo Huanying, Su Qingfen, Li Kaiqiao, Li Shengchang, Xu Cixiong. 1129

On Relationship of Individual Difference and Effectiveness of Acupuncture Anesthesia
Department of Acupuncture Anesthesia, Beijing Institute of Tuberculosis 1139

Comprehensive Preoperation Forecast of Effectiveness of Acupuncture Anesthesia and Screening of Variations
National Cooperative Group of Preoperation Forecast of Effectiveness of Acupuncture Anesthesia 1145

Experimental Study of Screening of Stimulation Parameters of Electric Needling in Acupuncture Anesthesia
Shi Minsheng, Zhang Jian, Cong Yinbin, Liu Runqi, Li Baoqin, Jia Zhiping 1157

Study of Role of Psychological Factors in Acupuncture Anesthesia
Xu Shulian, Song Weizhen, Guo Nianfeng, Sun Changhua, Wu Zhenyun. 1163

PROGRESS IN SCIENTIFIC RESEARCH ON ACUPUNCTURE, MOXIBUSTION AND ACUPUNCTURE ANESTHESIA BY INTEGRATING TRADITIONAL CHINESE AND WESTERN MEDICINE

Qian Xinzhong

Medicine is a branch of science developed by man engaged in a constant struggle with nature. It may be said that since the appearance of mankind on earth, there has been medical activity. This points to the fact that people of all countries have their own heritage of traditional medicine, which has contributed to the multiplication of their own nations.

Traditional Chinese medicine and pharmacology are the outcome of the struggle of the Chinese people with diseases. Its history goes back to time immemorial. Longstanding practice has resulted in a rich store of clinical experience and theoretical knowledge. More than 2,000 years ago, traditional Chinese medicine formed for itself an independent system guiding clinical practice. Acupuncture and moxibustion constitute an important part of this system.

According to ancient Chinese literature, early in the primitive society, needling (bian) and moxibustion were employed to treat diseases. The stone needles then in use are the predecessors of modern acupuncture needles. The stone needles discovered by our archaeologists in recent years[1] are similar in shape to the sharp and round needles of the "nine needles" described in *Neijing* (Canon of Medicine)[2]. The appearance of this kind of stone needle can be traced as far back as the New Stone Age, about 10,000-4,000 years ago.

By the time of the Spring and Autumn Period and the Warring States (770-221 B.C.), the theory of Jingluo (channels and collaterals) had been established. The ancient classic *Huangdi Neijing* gives a systematic illustration of the points of the channels and collaterals as well as the theory and methods of acupuncture and moxibustion, thus laying down the theoretical foundation of this therapy with the theory of channels and collaterals as its core. Between the years 256-260 A.D. the book *Zhen-jiu Jiayijing,* a classic on acupuncture and moxibustion, came out. It is the earliest and most complete book of acupuncture and moxibustion so far preserved.

---

(1) Primitive stone needle used in acupuncture therapy in ancient China. The *Suwen* of *Neijing* says, "The needling stone cures the disease externally", "It (disease) is indicated for treatment with the needle stone".

(2) *Huangdi Neijing,* for short, *Neijing,* is the oldest Chinese medical classic still available. It is thought to be written in the era of the Warring States, a stock taking of the medical progress achieved during and before that period. The work consists of two distinct books, *Suwen* (Plain Questions) and *Lingshu* (Mystical Gate), each in nine volumes.

From the third century to the end of the nineteenth, new developments were made in Chinese acupuncture and moxibustion. On the one hand, the number of acupuncture points used to treat diseases was greatly increased. In addition to the 361 original channel points, several hundred new ones were discovered. In classification there appeared the "points of the fourteen channels." On the other hand, through the summing-up of practice were found many vital points such as Wushu, Shumu, Sizong and the 12 points used by Madanyang. More obvious is the variation of the modes of needling. The use of filiform needles was a significant development, as was modification of the method of moxibustion. The theory of acupuncture and moxibustion was continuously enriched and raised to a higher level. Acupuncture and moxibustion education also had new development. As of the seventh century, a professional training course in acupuncture and moxibustion was established in the Imperial Medical Bureau, staffed by acupuncture professors, assistants, teachers, aides and students (*Old Tang Annals, Official Repertory*). In the fourth century, Yancetu the Chart, showing locations of the acupuncture points, appeared. The ninth century ushered in the blockprinted edition of books of acupuncture and moxibustion. The printed wall chart illustrating acupuncture points made its appearance as of the seventeenth century.

In 1882, acupuncture and moxibustion faculties in the Imperial Medical College were disbanded by the Qing Dynasty which held these medical arts in contempt. In 1840, with the invasion of China by the imperialists in the wake of the Opium War, western medicine was introduced into China, shoving the traditional Chinese medicine into the background. On top of this, under the reign of the Guomindang government, orders were issued to forbid the practice of traditional medicine. In consequence its development was set back. However, being simple, effective and rooted in the masses, the practice of acupuncture and moxibustion still prevailed among the people.

The Chinese Communist Party has always shown great concern for the development of traditional Chinese medicine. Early in the years before liberation, treatment by combined traditional Chinese and western medicine, training of acupuncturists, and publication of acupuncture and moxibustion books were encouraged in the old liberated areas. This was warmly welcomed by the masses.

Since the founding of New China, still greater attention has been paid to the therapy of acupuncture and moxibustion, leading to its further development. Articles on acupuncture and moxibustion published in the newspapers and magazines from 1949 to 1977 amounted to as many as 8,000. In the same period various acupuncture and moxibustion training classes were run and a large number of acupuncture and moxibustion books were compiled and published. On the basis of the several hundred points already in use, many new ones have been discovered in practice, and new methods of acupuncture and moxibustion created. Methods of acupuncture comprise in the main: needling with filiform needles, electro-needling, auricular needling, scalp needling, heat needling, needling with long awl-like needles, warming needling, scratching, needle lifting, skin needling, point injection of a small amount of drugs, needle retention, point intradermal embedding of needle, point ligation, point ultraviolet light radiation, point iontophoresis, point laser stimulation, point ultra-sound stimulation, point magnetotherapy, etc. The methods of moxibustion include warming with combustible moxa cones and sticks, cauterization with combustible moxa cones, indirect moxibustion with moxa cones, moxibustion with warmed bamboo tubes, electric moxibustion, and moxibustion with various drugs. The advent of these new points and new techniques has played a very important role in widening the scope of application of acupuncture and moxibustion as well as in improving the results of the therapy. Clinically, acupuncture and moxibustion have already been used to treat about 300 different diseases, with good or very good results in 100 or so.

CLINICAL OBSERVATIONS OF ACUPUNCTURE AND MOXIBUSTION

Of the papers received at this meeting, nearly 100 are clinical reports. The following is an outline of the contents of these papers.

Acupuncture in treatment of coronary heart diseases. Many units and areas in our country have carried out observations on acupuncture therapy of coronary heart diseases. For the 600 cases and more reported at this meeting, the marked effectiveness rate was 47%, effectiveness rate was 89%, and nitroglycerin discontinuation-reduction rate was 93%. Based on meticulous observations, some clinicians claimed that acupuncture is effective in relieving the symptoms of coronary heart disease as well as in eliminating angina pectoris. Electrocardiograms taken by these authors of more than 500 cases of coronary heart diseases before and after acupuncture therapy gave an effectiveness rate of 53%. Observations and analyses made by certain units by means of electrocardiography, ultra-sound cardiography, measurement of the cardiac output and cerebral hemadromography, showed that acupuncture could improve coronary circulation, left heart function and cerebral circulation.

Acupuncture for acute bacillary dysentery. Acupuncture is found to have a good effect on acute bacillary dysentery. One of the papers submitted at this meeting reports 645 cases treated by this technique. Of these, 478 were Flexner's dysentery; 121, Sonne dysentery; 10, dysentery caused by *Shigella boydii;* and 36, dysentery caused by *Shigella schmitzii.* Judging by the clinical symptoms and signs and the results of stool culture, 92% of the cases were cured within 10 days. Follow-up of 268 cases 6 months after treatment revealed a relapse of 33. Studies were also made by the authors of patients' serum protein electrophoresis, total plasma complement content, immune globulin content, bactericidal ability of plasma, specific antibody titer, stool SIgA content, serum bacterolytic enzyme and phagocytic power of the hepatic reticuloendothelial system. They are of the opinion that the therapeutic effect of acupuncture in acute bacillary dysentery is related to the increase of body immunity following acupuncture needling.

Acupuncture for cholelithiasis. Acupuncture has a definite effect on gallstones. Some authors treated cholelithiasis by electroacupuncture and oral administration of magnesium sulfate. Of 522 cases so treated, the expulsion rate was 35% for the stable type, 89% for the acute type, and 50% for the shock type, the total expulsion rate being 78%. Stone expulsion began 1-5 days after treatment in 360 cases (69%). The expulsion rate for the controls receiving magnesium sulfate only was 20.5%. This procedure is readily accepted by the patients, because with its use operation can be obviated in some of them.

Still some workers treated acute icteric virus hepatitis by acupuncture. Based on the results of 212 cases so treated, they pointed out that with acupuncture the icterus index can be rapidly restored and that the longterm effect is fairly good.

Our doctors have also shown interest in correcting abnormal position of the fetus by moxibustion. Of 2,069 cases of various abnormal positions of fetuses in the 29th-40th weeks of pregnancy, 1,869 were corrected by moxibustion, a correction rate of 90%. Of these, 86% had 1-4 moxibustion treatments and 14% 5-10. Studies after treatment on the respiration, pulse, blood pressure, vascular reaction, skin temperature, differential blood count, endocrinic change, and animal experiments (rabbit uterus activity curves) led the authors to believe that the mechanism of moxibustion of the Zhiyin point in correcting abnormal fetal position may lie in increasing the activity of the uterus and movements of the fetus. Acupuncture is effective in inducing labor and in the treatment of cervical erosion. As already reported at this meeting, the success rate was as high as 72% for the 771 cases undergoing induced labor by electroacupuncture. So far no untoward effects have been observed in mother and fetus. Of 1,010 cases of cervical erosion treated by acupuncture, 630 improved and 100 did not respond. The effectiveness rate for the cases of first and second degree erosion was 92%, and for those of the third degree, 75%, the total effectiveness rate being 90%.

A certain degree of therapeutic effect of acupuncture was also observed in sequelae of infantile paralysis, peripheral facial nerve paralysis, hemiplegia and traumatic paraplegia. For some 1,900 cases of peripheral facial nerve paralysis treated by acupuncture, the cure rate ranged between 50–70%, the effectiveness rate exceeding 90%. Electrical stimulation examination of a portion of these patients showed that the therapeutic effect was most marked in cases without degeneration, less so in those with partial degeneration, and poor in cases with complete degeneration. Based on the electromyograms the authors believed that after needling, most of the patients with complete or partial loss of facial muscular innervation on the affected side accompanied by lowered excitability may be benefited by acupuncture with reinnervation of the muscle fibers and regeneration of the damaged nerve.

Acupuncture has, in addition, varying degrees of effect on diseases of the eye, ear, nose, laryngopharynx and mouth cavity, such as acute keratitis, acute rhinitis, otitis media, stomatitis, acute tonsillitis and certain diseases of the fundus of the eye. Of the 403 cases of old central retinochoroid diseases reported at this meeting, the cure rate and marked effectiveness rate were 61% and 7% respectively, the total effectiveness rate being 97%. Follow-up studies demonstrated the stable long-term therapeutic effect in most cases.

Much work has been done by the Chinese medical workers in treating deafness and deaf-mutism, too. Their long-standing observations led to a better understanding of this problem. Otorhinolaryngologic examination and audiometric determinations showed that the effectiveness rate for those cases, in which the causes of the disease were clear, was deafness, 30% deaf-mutism, 20%. The authors pointed out that the effect was better in patients with sudden deafness of short duration due to reversible lesions, senile deafness and traumatic deafness. While in those with long-term and irreversible juvenile deafness or deafness due to typhoid, influenza and measles, the results were poor. Acupuncture was found to have little effect against congenital deaf-mutism or deaf-mutism due to febrile and infectious diseases. No improvement was observed after needling in patients suffering from complete loss of hearing and vestibular function.

Furthermore, acupuncture has a comparatively good antiphlogistic and analgesic effect. This has long been known to our doctors and used by them to treat a variety of inflammations and pains. At this meeting, the results of more than 900 cases of different inflammations treated by acupuncture have been reported. Of these, 366 were infections due to contaminated gynecologic and obstetric surgery. Before treatment, all the cases had a body temperature above 38°C and a total W.B.C. count of 10,000-30,000/mm³. After treatment, the temperature dropped rapidly and returned to normal within 2-3 days in most cases. Besides, it was noted that needling has a regulative action on the total W.B.C. count.

From the above it can be seen that acupuncture and moxibustion are fairly effective in the treatment of many diseases. Their action on the human body varies. According to ancient medical classics, they cure diseases mainly by means of adjusting the relationship between Yang and Yin, promoting the communication between the channels and collaterals, regulating the vital energy (qi) and blood, boosting positive factors and eliminating negative ones. From the viewpoint of modern medicine, the principal action of acupuncture and moxibustion is to regulate the function of the human body and increase its resistance (enhancing immunity and the antiphlogistic, analgesic, antispastic, antishock and antiparalytic ability of the body). Therefore, further exploration, study and application of these techniques are of high significance to the protection of people's health as well as to the development of medicine itself.

CLINICAL STUDY OF ACUPUNCTURE ANESTHESIA

Acupuncture anesthesia is a great discovery made by the broad masses of Chinese medical personnel on the basis of acupuncture analgesia. Originally, its discovery was prompted by the finding that stimulation of acupuncture points could relieve pain of the wound left by operation on the tonsil under local anesthesia. Guided by this discovery, acupuncture was put to trial in tonsillectomy as an anesthetic measure with success. Later its use was gradually widened to cover from minor and simple operations to major and difficult ones. As a result of more than 20 years' extensive clinical practice, we now have a clearer knowledge of this procedure, its indications and the principles governing its clinical application. It may be said that the value of acupuncture anesthesia as an anesthetic measure has already been firmly established.

1. The scope of clinical application. More than 2,000,000 cases have been operated on in China under acupuncture anesthesia. Mass learning of this procedure in the early years once led to its application in more than 100 different types of operations, minor and major. Its effect is comparatively stable in 20-30 kinds of ordinary operations. Generally speaking, the operative rate for acupuncture anesthesia is around 20%. In certain operations it may reach 70–80%, and in some others it may be used routinely. Its use in thyroid, maxillary sinus, glaucoma and abdominal tubal ligation operations has been popularized. It is thought to be more effective in head, neck and chest surgery. Acupuncture anesthesia has been used as the routine by a few units with rather satisfactory results in operations such as cesarean section, subtotal gastrectomy, splenectomy, total laryngectomy and operation on the cervical vertebra through the anterior approach. Some hospitals employ it as the method of choice for craniocerebral surgery, prostatectomy, meniscectomy and lobectomy. Since 1972, acupuncture anesthesia has also been used in open heart surgery undertaken under extracorporeal circulation with satisfactory results. From the papers received at this meeting, some examples of indications for acupuncture anesthesia are given below according to the sites of operation.

As shown in a report, the fine to excellent rate for 4,466 cases of craniocerebral surgery was 76.6%. Indications for acupuncture anesthesia included various tumors of the cerebral hemisphere, cerebellum, pons, cerebellar horn and sella turcica, vascular anomalies and brain abscess. Contraindications to acupuncture anesthesia included coma, deaf-mutism, mental disturbances in uncooperative individuals, deeply-seated and widespread lesions requiring lowering of the temperature and pressure. The authors were of the opinion that acupuncture anesthesia is best suited to operations on the anterior and posterior cranial fossae, and recommended it to be used routinely.

Acupuncture anesthesia can be used for many operations on the eyes, ears, nose, laryngopharynx and mouth cavity. In some hospitals the fine to excellent rate for thyroid operation under acupuncture anesthesia was above 80%. Patients with hyperthyroidism may also be selected as candidates for this form of anesthesia, provided that it is well prepared preoperatively and that unsatisfactory control of the basal metabolism rate, a recent history of crisis and complications of atrial fibrillation and heart failure can be ruled out.

Acupuncture anesthesia is often employed for dilation of mitral stenosis, the fine to excellent rate being around 70%. Papers submitted at this meeting reported the use of acupuncture anesthesia in a total of more than 350 cases of open heart surgery using extracorporeal circulation, mainly for repair of interventricular septal defect, the fine to excellent rate being also around 70%. The use of this form of anesthesia has eliminated to some extent the untoward effects of anesthetics on the myocardium. Heart surgery for less complicated lesions may be performed with acupuncture anesthesia as one of the methods of choice.

Pneumonectomy is an operation that was carried out under acupuncture anesthesia earlier in our country. To be reported at this meeting are more than 2,000 such cases, the fine to excellent rate being roughly 80%. With strict control of the patient's respiration, acupuncture anesthesia may be employed for pneumonectomy. Its superiority is especially apparent in patients suffering from severe pulmonary tuberculosis, with very poor function of the lung, and unable to undergo general anesthesia. It is used but rarely in operations for removal of tumors of the lung, because the lesions are themselves rather complicated.

More difficulties are encountered in the use of acupuncture anesthesia for subtotal gastrectomy. In order to improve its effect in this operation, our doctors have carried out special studies. At well-equipped units, the fine to excellent rate for this operation exceeds 80%, otherwise it is only around 60%. For appendectomy, the corresponding figure is 60-70%.

The effect of acupuncture anesthesia in cesarean section is fairly stable. For a total of more than 2,000 cases reported at this meeting the fine to excellent rates all exceeded 80%. It is found that with this form of anesthesia, maternal physiological disturbances seldom occur, the functions of maternal respiration and circulation are stable and bleeding is minimal, thus ensuring the supply of blood and oxygen for the fetus as well as the safety of the mother and the infant. It is not only indicated in ordinary cases undergoing cesarean section but also in those who are suffering from toxemia of pregnancy and anemia.

With the extensive practice of family planning in our country, large numbers of abdominal tubal ligations are done under acupuncture anesthesia. As shown in a report of 23,554 cases operated upon under acupuncture anesthesia, the fine to excellent rate was 85.8%. Other papers also gave it in excess of 80%. The advantages of acupuncture anesthesia for this type of operation lie in that it is simple easy to perform, safe and conducive to quick recovery.

In urinary surgery, for example, in prostatectomy, since the patients are in general older in age and are often suffering from diseases of the cardiovascular system, acupuncture anesthesia is more practicable than other anesthetic procedures. In bone surgery, such as lateral meniscectomy and cervical vertebral operation through the anterior approach, the effect of acupuncture anesthesia appears to be stable, too.

Some authors reported that acupuncture anesthesia plus basal anesthesia constitutes a desirable procedure for upper abdominal operation in children, and suggested that patients with severe trauma, hemorrhagic shock, and critical illness are also indicated for acupuncture anesthesia.

2. Principles governing the clinical application of acupuncture anesthesia. In recent years, with a view to improving the effect of acupuncture anesthesia, units throughout the country have worked in concert to study the principle and practice of acupuncture anesthesia by looking for more effective points; improving the methods of needling, surgical techniques and instrumentation; varying the stimulation parameters; judicious use of adjuvants and enhancing the accuracy of preoperative forecast so as to increase the adaptability of the patient to operation. Through repeated practice, they have made much headway in this aspect. Briefly, it is as follows.

(1) Methods of needling. The number of points needed for an operation has been greatly reduced. Take pneumonectomy and gastrectomy for instance; the number of needles required to effect anesthesia in these operations has gradually been decreased from the past several dozen to today's 1-6. Point selection is in general made in two ways. One is to select points following the theory of channels and collaterals as illustrated in traditional Chinese medicine, and the other according to the neuroanatomicophysiological theory in modern medicine. The former consists in selecting points along the channels according to the manifestations of disease and in areas nearer to locations of pain. The latter includes selection of points along the same nerve (needling somewhere lateral to the incision site or needling directly the nerve stem which innervates the field of operation), along the proximal and distal spinal cord segments, and needling of the cavum epidurale of the spinal cord. Stimulation is given manually, by electricity or by point injection of drug solutions (or sterile water). Currently, electrostimulation is most frequently performed. Studies have also been made on such problems as the length of induction period and parameters for effective and proper needling including the pattern, frequency and amplitude of the pulse. The various methods of acupuncture anesthesia evolved on the basis of different point selection and stimulation meet a variety of requirements. For example, scalp acupuncture anesthesia is particularly suited to operations for extensive and deep burns.

(2) Pretesting. It is considered important to estimate, on the basis of both clinical and laboratory findings, the effectiveness of acupuncture anesthesia before operation, in order to select suitable cases and improve the anesthetic effect by necessary measures. It has been found that apart from the nature of the disease and severity of the lesion, factors closely related to the effectiveness of acupuncture anesthesia include patient pain threshold, tactile sensation, finger plethysmography, clinical classification based on the principles of traditional Chinese medicine, and various psychologic factors. Generally, the results of anesthesia are good in patients in whom the pain threshold is high or can be elevated by needling; the tactile sensation threshold rises after needling; the amplitude of finger pulse waves increases

or is not much decreased after a definite amount of pain stimulation; and diagnosis by the principles of traditional Chinese medicine shows the disease belonging to the type of Yangxu (lack of positive factors). Psychological factors such as emotional state of the patient have an influence on the effect of anesthesia but not a decisive one.

(3) Adjuvants. Acupuncture anesthesia has not yet been improved to such a level that it can ensure complete painlessness. Therefore, as with many other forms of anesthesia, the judicious use of certain adjuvants to increase its analgesic action is justifiable. In the early period, the adjuvants most frequently employed in acupuncture anesthesia were central nervous system sedatives and analgesics such as dolantin, phenergan, phenobarbital and wintermin. Local anesthetics included novocaine, xylocaine, dicaine and anticholinergic agents such as atropine. With the advances in research on the mechanism of acupuncture analgesia, some nonanalgesics were also used to influence the transmitters of CNS, as were certain other approaches. Now in clinical use are haloperidol, phenytoin sodium, aspirin, acetazolamide, etc., all showing some definite effect. The methods commonly practiced are: (a) needling given alone, as in abdominal tubal ligation; (b) needling used mainly but supported with certain drugs, depending on patient's condition and the operation to be performed (most operations can be done under this form of anesthesia); (c) drugs mainly employed but supported by needling to help to regulate and stabilize the function of the body and facilitate the performance of operation. These, of course, require further investigation.

3. Evaluation. As is seen from the above, we have already had a preliminary understanding of the indications for and the principles governing clinical practice of acupuncture anesthesia. To sum up, acupuncture anesthesia has the following characteristics:

(1) Patients remain in a conscious state throughout the operation. All mental, sensory and motor functions are kept normal except for the pain sensation which becomes dull. In these circumstances, the patient usually can cooperate well with the operating surgeon. For instance, in operations on acoustic neuroma, it is possible to raise the intact rate of the facial nerve; in cutting the trigeminal nerve root, it is possible to have it done more accurately; in thyroid surgery, it is possible to avoid injury to the recurrent laryngeal nerve. Furthermore, kept in a conscious state, patients can speak themselves to help the surgeons improve manipulation and operate more safely, accurately, gently and rapidly. It may be said that nearly all operations that are carried out with acupuncture anesthesia have been modified in techniques as well as in procedure. Take, for instance, cesarean section. In the past, it usually took several hours; now under acupuncture anesthesia it can be performed in but 20 minutes or so.

(2) Little or no anesthetic is needed, thereby precluding the possibility of postoperative drug sideeffects apart from anesthetic accidents. In patients who are hypersensitive to anesthetics, critically ill, weak and suffering from dysfunction of the heart, lung, liver and kidney, or in shock, acupuncture anesthesia provides a wide margin of safety for the patient both during and after operation. As is well known, the surgery for tumor of the acoustic nerve is rather difficult. Some units had made a comparison between acupuncture anesthesia and other forms of anesthesia in this operation. One of the papers by these units reported that out of 333 cases done under general anesthesia, 35 were complicated by pneumonia, whereas of 311 cases carried out in the same period under acupuncture anesthesia, only 9 had this complication. Another paper reported that of 50 cases operated upon under drug anesthesia, 5% had lung infection and damage to the brain stem, and 2% died of severe com-

plications, whereas of another 50 cases having the operation under acupuncture anesthesia none developed any of these disorders. Of 155 cases of open heart surgery using extracorporeal circulation and acupuncture anesthesia, 5 developed respiratory complications as against 11 out of 60 cases operated on under general anesthesia.

(3) Postoperative pain is mild, and generally there are no such reactions as nausea and vomiting. Both food intake and physical activity can be resumed early. Another effect of needling is to mobilize and enhance anti-disease factors in the human body, thus hastening postoperative rehabilitation. Some authors compared the changes in immune reaction in patients having pneumonectomy under general anesthesia and those receiving the operation under acupuncture anesthesia. They found that the phagocytic power of mobilized white blood cells and transformation of lymphocytes were inhibited in the general anesthesia series, but not in the series of acupuncture anesthesia. A similar phenomenon was noted in patients having tubal ligation under acupuncture anesthesia.

(4) No sophisticated instruments are needed and manipulation is simple and easy to master. Its use is suited to the countryside and mountainous areas, the construction sites, the frontier regions and various emergency conditions.

Problems remaining to be solved in acupuncture anesthesia are: incomplete analgesia, incomplete control of visceral reaction, and unsatisfactory muscle relaxation. These are the disadvantages of acupuncture anesthesia compared with other forms of anesthesia. However, their existence by no means depreciates the value of acupuncture anesthesia as a useful anesthetic procedure under specific conditions. All these deficiencies can be overcome, as previously stated, by strict observation of the clinical principles, careful selection of cases, modification of techniques and adoption of supplementary measures. In short, acupuncture anesthesia is not a substitute for other forms of anesthesia but a new addition to the armamentarium of anesthesiology. The combination of acupuncture anesthesia with surgical operation means a significant development of acupuncture itself. On the one hand it demands surgery to modify and improve its operative techniques, on the other it calls for further theoretical research, giving an impetus to the investigation of the mechanism of analgesia and of the physiology of pain.

MECHANISMS OF ACUPUNCTURE, MOXIBUSTION AND ACUPUNCTURE ANESTHESIA

Popularization of acupuncture-moxibustion therapy and extensive use of acupuncture anesthesia have led to a nationwide multidisciplinary coordination in the research on the mechanism of these techniques. Academically, there exist two different views, the neurohumoral and the channel-collateral view. The latter will be discussed separately; here I would like to discuss the progress achieved in the field of neuro-humoral research.

1. Action of acupuncture on the body. In light of the indications for acupuncture therapy revealed thus far, it is presumed that acupuncture acts in two ways, i.e., to regulate the functions of the various systems of the body and to strengthen its resistance against disease. A large amount of experimental work reported at this meeting has further confirmed this mode of action of acupuncture.

In animal experiments, needling certain points may regulate the function of the respiratory, digestive, circulatory, urinary, endocrine, nervous and energy metabolism systems. The regulatory effect of acupuncture on the cardiovascular system, for example, is quite marked. As shown by the results of experiments in dogs, needling the points Neiguan, Renzhong, Chengjiang, etc. may greatly increase the stability of the blood pressure regulating system. In experimental hemorrhagic shock, needling Renzhong demonstrated an apparent antishock effect, attended with a marked fall in mortality and diminution in the amount of blood transfusion needed to restore the blood pressure to normal. Hemodynamic studies showed that the cardiac output and the blood flow in the kidneys and small intestines of acupuncture treated animals were more stable compared with those of the controls.

Acupuncture has an effect on the function of many endocrine glands. As noted in animal experiments it may lead to an increase in the release of pituitary adrenocorticotropin and in the secretion of corticoid and adrenal medullary substance. Also observed in animals after repeated needling were morphological changes associated with the increase of thyroid function.

Tests made prior to operation under acupuncture anesthesia indicated that changes in the function of the autonomic nerve in the induction period were related in some degree to the results of anesthesia. In those patients in whom needling lowered the function of the sympathetic nerve the results were mostly better, suggesting that needling is capable of regulating the function of the autonomous nervous system.

There are also reports of the effects of needling on immunity. In laboratory observations, both the E-rosette test and lymphocyte transformation test indicated that electrical stimulation markedly enhanced the immunological functions of human blood cells. Similar results were observed in animals. Furthermore, animal experiments showed that moxibustion could increase the phagocytic activity of the giant phagocytes and the antibody titer in the blood. Some laboratories reported that after needling the content of sulfohydryl in tissues, which is closely related to the defensive mechanism, was increased.

The various actions of acupuncture and moxibustion on the body are interrelated. Regularization of function leads to increase of the body resistance, while strengthening of the body resistance is itself a reflection of function regulation. The clinical effect of acupuncture and moxibustion therapy is all the more realized by their various actions on the body. For instance, the antiphlogistic effect of needling is none other than a comprehensive expression of the influence of needling on the autonomic nervous system, local circulation, cellular immunity and endocrine glands.

2. Mechanism of the analgesic action of acupuncture. As shown by a large amount of clinical practice, needling possesses a very good analgesic effect. In recent years scientific workers in all parts of the country have carried out a series of human and animal experiments on this subject. Through these experiments and by means of various pain-causing or traumatic factors and different pain threshold determination criteria, they found that acupuncture can raise skin pain threshold in man as well as in animals. They also made a series of studies on the conditions for and the laws governing the change in pain threshold. Some laboratories took, in addition, the activity and conditioned reflex of monkeys as an criterion in their study, because the completion of these reactions requires participation of the higher centers of the nervous system which renders the animal as a model more similar to humans in pain sensation than any other models. In the monkey models the analgesic action of acupuncture has been further confirmed.

In recent years, more rapid advances have been made in the study of the analgesic action and mechanism of acupuncture. This is also an important topic for discussion at this meeting. From the hundreds of papers we have received it seems clear that a preliminary understanding has already been attained of the mechanism of the analgesic action of acupuncture.

(1) The role of the nervous system in analgesia by acupuncture.

(a) The action of the peripheral nerves. To needle directly the nerves that transmit the pain sensation, or to needle the pain-originating sites (the so-called electroacupuncture of the same nerve), may lead not only to blocking of the pathways of the pain fibers of this nerve, but also to inhibition of the reaction of the dorsal horn cells in the spinal cord to traumatic stimulation. This method has already been extensively used clinically, e.g., cross needling and needling beside the incision site, with good results in relieving epidermal pain. The peripheral nerve serves as an afferent nerve for the transmission of needling signals, but according to the study of some of our laboratories, types II, III and IV fibers probably also play a role.

(b) The action of the central nervous system. Extensive electrophysiological studies carried out by our scientific workers in all parts of the country revealed the process of participation of the various levels of the central nervous system such as the spinal cord, brain stem, thalamus, caudate nucleus and cortex in the relief of pain by acupuncture.

Our scientists found that needling stimulation may lead to postsynaptic inhibition in the dorsal horn. They also noted that the signal of needling ascends from the spinal ventrolateral fasciculus to the medulla oblongata to activate the medial reticular formation, then descends along the dorsolateral fasciculus, giving rise to depolarization of the endings of the finer afferent fibers of the spinal cord, resulting in presynaptic inhibition, and partially blocking the afferent impulse of the fine fibers.

The role of the brain stem in acupuncture analgesia has also received our scientists' attention. It is found that the activity of the pain sensory neurons of the midbrain reticular formation can be inhibited by electrical stimulation. Electroacupuncture of the nucleus of raphe not only can raise animal pain threshold, but also can markedly increase the analgesic effect of needling. Destroying the locus caeruleus may apparently enhance the analgesic action of electroacupuncture, while stimulating it weakens the inhibitory effect of electroacupuncture. Combined laboratory studies showed that the surrounding gray matter of the aqueduct of the midbrain, the medial giant cell nucleus of the reticular formation of the brain stem and the group of nuclei of raphe may discharge impulses upon receiving the signal of needling, descending to inhibit the neuronal activity of transmitting pain signals via the dorsal horn in the spinal cord, and ascending to inhibit the release of electricity by the pain-sensitive cells of the parafascicular nucleus of the thalamus. These structures of the brain stem themselves are in turn subject to the control of such higher centers as accumben nucleus, septal region, and habenular body.

Some scientists are of the opinion that, so far as the thalamus is concerned, the parafasicular nucleus is an important station for transmission of pain signals. The needling signal may exert an inhibitory influence on the thalamus through the higher centers such as the caudate nucleus and cortex and through the lower centers such as the nucleus of raphe.

Quite a few papers submitted to this meeting reported on observation of the caudate nucleus. Stimulating this nucleus may raise the level of animal pain threshold, thereby strengthening the analgesic action of electroacupuncture. Destroying it will lead to weakening of its analgesic effect. It was observed in clinical practice that stimulation of the caudate nucleus could relieve severe pain caused by cancer in its late stage.

There are also data on the role played by the lateral lemniscus and cerebral cortex in acupuncture analgesia.

To sum up, after entering the central nervous system the pain signals have to travel a long way to reach the cerebrum, wherein the dorsal horn of the spinal cord and the parafascicular nucleus of the thalamus are probably two key centers, transmitting and receiving pain sensation. On the other hand, some centers in the central nervous system, when excited, can inhibit the transmission and reception of pain signals. These centers include the caudate nucleus, gray matter surrounding the aqueduct of midbrain, nuclei of raphe and their descending pathways. The signal of needling passes through the spinal cord to enter the brain, then, after undergoing complicated regulation, most probably causing excitation of this intrinsic analgesic system, ascends to inhibit the parafascicular nucleus and descends to inhibit the dorsal horn, displaying the effect of analgesia.

(2) The action of the transmitter of the central nervous system in analgesia by acupuncture. The role of the transmitter in analgesia is also discussed in many reports received at this meeting. The increase or decrease of 5-hydroxytryptamine content in animal brain may respectively enhance or weaken the analgesic effect of acupuncture. The action of catecholamine is contrary to this. Blocking with drugs the receptor of catecholamine transmitter increases the action of acupuncture, while receptor stimulants weaken its analgesic action. Blocking the synthesis of acetylcholine in the brain or blocking the cholinergic receptor may lead to lowering of the analgesic effect of acupuncture.

In recent years, discovery of the endogenous morphine-like substance has stimulated research and the assumption of the presence of an intrinsic anti-pain mechanism in the nervous system. The relationship between this endogenous morphine-like substance and analgesia of acupuncture has aroused much interest of the scientific workers. In a short period of 2-3 years, our scientists succeeded in working out the methods of isolation, extraction and determination of this substance, as well as in synthesizing artificially the highly active enkephalin and its derivatives. Experiments in both man and animal showed that the analgesic effect of acupuncture could be partially antagonized by the morphine antagonist, naloxone. With acupuncture analgesia, the content of endorphin was markedly increased in animal brain and was found to be closely related to the analgesic effect. Delaying degradation of enkephalin may greatly prolong the analgesic effect of acupuncture. Clinically, under acupuncture analgesia, the content of endorphin in human spinal fluid is markedly increased.

In action, the nervous system and the transmitters cooperate with each other instead of being isolated from each other. For example, while the signal of needling increases the content of the morphine-like substance in the brain, it acts on the gray matter surrounding the aqueduct of the midbrain and then stimulates the nuclei of raphe and releases 5-hydroxytryptamine through the descending fibers to inhibit the dorsal horn of the spinal cord.

(3) The role of other factors in acupuncture analgesia. Determination by the skin blister method of the blood exudated from the wound in patients operated on under acupuncture anesthesia revealed that in those patients in whom the effect of anesthesia was good, the pain-causing action was comparatively weak. According to the reports of some units, acupuncture may lower the concentration of potassium ion, histamine and bradykinin in the peripheral blood. The pain-causing action of these substances is well known.

The use of aspirin enhances the analgesic action of acupuncture, signifying the possibility of participation of prostaglandin in the mechanism of acupuncture analgesia.

Does the psychological factor play a role in acupuncture analgesia? This is an interesting question to scientists both at home and abroad. According to some of our scientific workers, pseudo-needling and verbal hinting or visual and auditory hinting may produce in patients tested a psychological effect of needling which raises the pain threshold and pain tolerance threshold. Contrarily, verbal hinting of "pain" lowers the pain threshold. Whether the subjects to be tested are mentally prepared for the pain stimulation or not has also a definite effect on the pain sensation. This explains that psychological factors do play a part in acupuncture analgesia and therefore deserve attention in clinical practice. On the other hand, placebo has no effect on pain and pain tolerance threshold both before and after acupuncture. The level of sensitiveness to skin sense hinting and the degree of trust in the surgeon are also not apparently related to the results of acupuncture anesthesia. We have also a few papers introducing the use of acupuncture anesthesia in veterinary medicine. These all speak eloquently for the fact that psychological factors do not play a decisive role in acupuncture anesthesia.

In short, the research achievements of various medical groups throughout the country have already provided us with a broad framework of the mechanism of acupuncture analgesia. Acupuncture analgesia is a complicated dynamic process that under needling stimulation of the body a series of changes occur, extending from the periphery to various levels of the CNS, involving many factors such as the nerves and the humors, and the causation and relief of pain. Of course, there are still many problems remaining to be elucidated.

STUDY OF THE THEORY OF CHANNELS AND COLLATERALS

The theory of channels and collaterals forms the theoretical basis of acupuncture-moxibustion therapy. It is a problem involving every aspect of the study of the mechanisms of acupuncture, moxibustion and acupuncture anesthesia. Judging by the treatises submitted at this meeting, in recent years the study of the channel-collateral theory in brief has been centered on: the phenomenon of sensation transmission along the channels; the action of needling on the pathway of transmission; the relation between the visceral organs and the body surface; and the morphologic basis of the channels and collaterals.

1. Sensation propagation along the channels. When stimulation is applied to the points of the channels, a sensation of soreness, numbness, distension and burning is transmitted along the course of channels and collaterals. This phenomenon is called "sensation propagation along the channels." Records depicting findings similar to this phenomenon are found in ancient Chinese medical literature. Recent reports on this finding appeared first in China early in the fifties. Since 1972, medical units of more than 20 provinces, municipalities and autonomous regions have carried out a series of investigations into this phenomenon, using uniform methods and standards. It was found that it appears in people of various nationalities, of all ages, in both sexes, and in different health conditions. An analysis of the results of investigation on 63,228 subjects produced an incidence of 12-24%. It was also noted that the pathway seen in the phenomenon is basically the same as described in ancient classics. It is dual transmission, advances at a slower rate, and can be blocked by the application of a slight pressure. When reaching a corresponding organ, it gives rise to change in function of that organ. Change sometimes also occurs in the analgesia threshold along the pathway of transmission. When the sensation is transmitted to the diseased region, the symptoms often improve. The nature of sensation transmission along the course of channels remains obscure. Similarly reported is the development of skin and sensory diseases along the course of the channels.

2. The action of acupuncture on transmission pathway. According to traditional Chinese medicine, needling acts through the channels and collaterals. Hence the study of action of needling on the pathway of transmission constitutes part of the research on the channels and collaterals. The transmission pathway of acupuncture analgesic action has already been discussed in some detail. Other problems much studied include the effect of needling Zusanli on the gastrointestinal tract; the effect of needling Neiguan on correcting cardiac arrhythmia;. and the effect of needling Renzhong or Suliao on elevating blood pressure. A large number of laboratory studies showed that when the involved factor, the nerve or the body fluid, is blocked, destroyed or removed, the effect of acupuncture will become correspondingly weakened or disappear entirely. This confirms the presumption that acupuncture mainly acts through the nerves and body fluid. However, the possibility of participation of some other factors than the nerves and body fluid is mentioned by some authors, too.

3. Relationship between the visceral organs and the body surface. The channels connect internally with the viscera, and externally with the extremities. Needling points over the body surface along the course of the channel can cure diseases of the visceral organs. On the other hand, pathology of the visceral organs can also affect the body surface through the channels, as manifested, for instance, by the appearance of points of tenderness, sensitivity and low electric resistance on the body surface (including local organs such as the auricle). The investigation of the influence of pathology of the visceral organs on the body surface also provides for an approach to the study of the channels and collaterals. Some units found in animal experiments that there exists a certain relationship between the stomach and the auricle. For example, when the stomach is diseased or when it is stimulated, the low electric resistance points on the auricle will increase in number. It was found that the sympathetic nerve of the auricle and the vagus nerve of the stomach both take part in this process. Obviously, this further points to the specific relationship between the viscera and the body surface, being in part the substantial basis of the channel-collateral theory.

4. Morphological basis of the channels and collaterals. The formation of the concept of channels and collaterals should have its anatomical basis. In view of the fact that channels and collaterals are the lines which connect the acupuncture points and that each acupuncture point has its relative specificity, as shown by clinical and laboratory observations, our scientific workers had from the fifties to the sixties made extensive studies on the acupuncture points on cadavers, anatomically and histologically. Through these investigations they found the existence of a definite relationship between the points and the lines connecting them with the peripheral nerves and blood vessels. They also noted that the distribution of the channel points is related to segmental innervation. At the needling sensation points were seen mostly the endings of nerves, next the vessels.

In the course of an operation under acupuncture anesthesia, some doctors have observed that stimulating the nerve often causes a sensation of numbness; stimulating the blood vessel, a sensation of pain; and stimulating the muscle, tendon or periosteum, a sensation of soreness and distension.

Some other workers studied needling sensation points by histochemical methods and low skin electric resistance points by means of microradiography. Studies were also made by some authors of the channels and collaterals with regard to their relation to the autonomic nerves and to the lymphatic system.

Apart from the above four subjects, the nature of the vital energy of the channels is also being studied. The discovery of ancient books on moxibustion in the Mawangdui tombs of the Western Han Dynasty in 1974 has also given an impetus to research into ancient Chinese medical literature on the theory of channels and collaterals in recent years.

SUMMARIZE EXPERIENCE AND CONTINUE TO ADVANCE

In the past two decades, we have made considerable progress in the scientific study of acupuncture, moxibustion and acupuncture anesthesia by integrating traditional Chinese medicine with western medicine. Man's recognition of the objective world will never come to an end. We are confident that the study of acupuncture, moxibustion and acupuncture anesthesia will continue in depth. To sum up the past and look forward to the future, I would like to express a few opinions on the scientific research in this field:

1. Traditional Chinese medicine is the accumulation of the experience of the toiling masses of the Chinese people in their long-standing struggle against diseases and the crystallization of their wisdom. Chairman Mao spoke highly of it as "a great treasury" of medicine.

In the history of mankind there once appeared many ancient cultures such as the Egyptian, Babylonian, Greek, Roman, Indian and Chinese cultures. All these brilliant ancient cultures left a rich heritage of medical as well as pharmacological records. Of these, some have been discarded, others have been partly preserved, and still others have been inherited and further developed, prevailing among the people as traditional medicine. It can be said today that as a result of more than several thousand years of practice, we have inherited part of our ancient culture. We have a vast accumulation of ancient medical literature and adequate resources in medicinal herbs. In short, traditional Chinese medicine is characterized by the following three features:

(1) Practicability. Traditional Chinese medicine and pharmacology had not only contributed in the past to the fertility and prosperity of the Chinese nation, but today still plays an important role in the protection of the health of our people. It is a medical and pharmacological system formed as a result of continuous development and experience.

(2) Theoretical basis. Since the publication of *Neijing* about 2,000 years ago, traditional Chinese medicine has formed a systematic theory on anatomy, physiology and pathology as well as on the development, diagnosis and treatment of disease. Since this theory was first originated in practice and has since been continually substantiated and enriched by it, so it can in turn effectively guide practice.

(3) Popularity. China is a multinational country. To the creation of Chinese medicine

and pharmacology, all Chinese nationalities have made their contributions. Traditional Chinese medicine is simple and easy to practice. It has long taken root in the people and has long been introduced into other countries where it has been well received by the people. Through the exchange of experience with other countries, traditional Chinese medicine has in turn assimilated the experience of other medical systems and has thus enriched itself continually.

Traditional Chinese medicine has survived over 2,000 years of feudal rule, nearly 100 years of semi-feudal and semicolonial rule, and especially the suppression of the reactionary rule of the Guomindang. Today under the leadership of the Chinese Communist Party and guided by the policy of integration of traditional Chinese medicine with western medicine laid down for us by Chairman Mao and Premier Zhou, both Chinese medicine and Chinese pharmacology will certainly flourish in the future and make new contributions towards the modernization of our medical science.

2. The systematization of Chinese medicine and pharmacology should be done under the guidance of the principle of dialectical materialism and should follow the road of integration of traditional Chinese medicine with western medicine. In this respect the study of the mechanism of acupuncture analgesia has set for us an excellent example. Early in the seventies, guided by the idea of the unity of opposites and modern knowledge of neurophysiology, some of our scientific workers put forward the conception that in the human body there exists the contradiction of " dolorific factors and analgesic factors"; that in the nervous sytems there exist two different sets of structures with two different functions which cause and control pain respectively; and that in the humoral system there also exist both these substances. The essence of acupuncture analgesia lies in using needling to mobilize the analgesic factors and to activate the analgesic functions of the body at different levels, and to promote transformation of pain into painlessness. This idea has effectively boosted the study of the mechanism of acupuncture analgesia and has been confirmed and substantiated by the results of studies carried out thereafter.

The sorting out and studying of our traditional medical heritage demands an earnest attitude and the spirit of "seeking truth from facts" on the part of our scientific workers. In the clinical use of acupuncture, moxibustion and acupuncture anesthesia, there are some therapeutic effects that can be explained by modern scientific knowledge and theory; there are others that can only be explained in part; and there are still others that cannot yet be explained. Towards the last, the adoption of a careful attitude is especially imperative. Under no pretext should they be lightly given up as nonexistent because for the time being we still do not understand them. The study of the clinical application and theory of acupuncture anesthesia should be continued on an even larger scale. We should continue to make our efforts to explore, study and raise to a still higher level the traditional Chinese medicine by means of modern scientific methods and theories. Research on the integration of traditional Chinese medicine with western medicine should be thoroughly planned, with proper control, reliable and objective standards, careful and accurate observations and complete and detailed records. All data and materials pertaining to this research should be subjected to statistical treatment and scientific analysis so that they fulfill all the requirements of a scientific experiment. The adoption of various approaches and methods should be encouraged. As already shown in the clinical application of acupuncture anesthesia, the adoption of different methods of needling is conducive to its betterment and further development. Different academic views ought to complement and, not repel, each other. As, for instance, in the investigation of the mechanism of acupuncture anesthesia we have the neurohumoral view and the channel-collateral view existing side by side.

3. To speed up the integration of traditional Chinese medicine with western medicine, attention should be paid to the creation and training of a force of key personnel. In recent years in acupuncture anesthesia we have already formed such a force. Today, in addition to the barefoot doctors, worker doctors and neighborhood doctors who treat the most commonly seen diseases by acupuncture and moxibustion in cities as well as in the countryside, there is a relatively large number of professional acupuncturists and acupuncture anesthetists engaged in clinical and laboratory work. Of these, some have attained a higher level of expertise. Besides, doctors trained in traditional and western medicines and those specialized in other branches of medicine also can use acupuncture and moxibustion to treat diseases in their respective fields that indicate for this therapy. In the study of the mechanism of acupuncture anesthesia, we already have a trained researcher force. With the growth of this force, some new disciplines have been established such as pain physiology, synaptophysiology, etc. Some new techniques pertaining to basic medical science such as the microelectrode technique and isotope technique have been popularized. All these have promoted the study of physiology, neurochemistry and neuropharmacology, and have given an impetus to research into the theory of acupuncture, moxibustion and channels and collaterals. Nevertheless, this force is far from being adequate to meet the needs of our work, especially when the technical level is taken into account. Today, the most urgent task lying before us is to build a higher expertise force of acupuncture, moxibustion and acupuncture anesthesia doctors. Acupuncture and moxibustion clinicians should be given the opportunity to receive advanced training. Schools of traditional Chinese medicine, should, if possible, restore old or set up new faculties of acupuncture and moxibustion, or run acupuncture schools for the training of senior and junior acupuncture and moxibustion professional workers. The force engaged in theoretical research on the mechanism of acupuncture anesthesia should also be strengthened. The improvement of this specialty may be combined with the development of physiology, physiochemistry, pharmacology and certain marginal disciplines, or with the establishment of various specialized research institutes.

4. Science and technology in the 20th century are changing with each passing day. In these circumstances, to adopt a closed door policy is bound to end up in backwardness. We have in the past established national or regional professional coordinating groups to carry on socialist coordination in acupuncture, moxibustion and acupuncture anesthesia research. These groups often exchange experiences among themselves, holding lectures and discussions. Beginning from 1959, more than ten national academic conferences on acupuncture, moxibustion, acupuncture anesthesia and the theory of channels-collaterals have been held. This conference is the largest one ever held. Apart from publishing scientific research papers in the press and periodicals, we also are issuing a specialized journal, the *Journal of Acupuncture Anesthesia,* as a medium for wider exchange of knowledge and experience in this field.

Acupuncture-moxibustion therapy, including acupuncture anesthesia, has already drawn the attention of the academic circles of many countries and become a research subject of interest. So far as we know, countries and regions or territories which are now employing or which have used acupuncture anesthesia number well over 30. The number of countries us ing acupuncture and moxibustion to treat various diseases is even greater. Roughly speaking, about 24 countries and regions have establishd acupuncture associations or societies. International conferences devoted to the subject of acupuncture and moxibustion are being held almost every year. Journals dealing specifically with the science of acupuncture and moxibustion and the theory of channels and collaterals amount to 24, containing quite a number of papers of high quality. Many foreign countries are also engaged in research on the mechanism of acupuncture and moxibustion and that of acupuncture anesthesia. The advent of acupuncture anesthesia has aroused people's interest in the physiology of pain. The International Pain Research set up thereafter has scientists as its members from more than 50 countries and territories. It has convened two international meetings since its establishment. Among the scientific research papers read at these meetings, some are of value in clarifying the mechanism of acupuncture anesthesia, acupuncture and moxibustion, others are helpful the search for new analgesic methods and drugs. All these are worthy of attention and learning.

Science and technology is the common treasure-house of all mankind. The development and advancement of acupuncture and moxibustion in traditional Chinese medicine, an ancient and yet fresh branch, should therefore draw on the efforts of scientific workers all over the world. Hence the importance of international exchange of experience and cooperation should be emphasized. This is also the reason why we have this time so many foreign scientists enthusiastically accepting our invitation to attend this meeting. Since time immemorial, acupuncture and moxibustion have been an important part of cultural exchange between the Chinese people and the peoples of many other countries. Let us continue and develop further this exchange and cooperation started by our ancestors long ago! Our meeting symbolizes a good beginning in this respect. The foreign scientists attending our meeting presented many very good papers on their experience in clinical practice and research. We should learn from our friends as a pupil, learn from the peoples of all other countries, cooperate with our foreign colleagues, and do our share in strengthening the friendly ties between all peoples of the world in continuously improving acupuncture therapy, and in raising the level of medical science as a whole.

Unite and look ahead! Unite for the four modernizations! Unite for still greater victories!

PART I
RESEARCH ON THE MECHANISMS OF ACUPUNCTURE, MOXIBUSTION AND ACUPUNCTURE ANESTHESIA

PART I
RESEARCHE ON THE MECHANISMS OF ACUPUNCTURE, MOXIBUSTION AND ACUPUNCTURE ANESTHESIA
(1)

INTERACTION IN THALAMUS OF AFFERENT IMPULSES FROM ACUPUNCTURE POINT AND SITE OF PAIN

Zhang Xiangtong (H.T.Chang)
(Shanghai Institute of Physiology, Academia Sinica)

As we have stated repeatedly, the analgesic effect of acupuncture is essentially the result of interaction, in the central nervous system, between the afferent impulses from the region of pain and the afferent impulses from the point of acupuncture[1,2,3]. From experimental evidence it appears that the processes of integration of the nociceptive impulses and the non-nociceptive impulses and their significance are apparently different at different levels of the central nervous system. The inhibition of the pain reflex actions is thought to occur mainly in the spinal cord[4]; whereas the inhibition of pain perception and the modulation of autonomic function and affective behavior are mainly in the higher centers. Again, the processes of interaction between the nociceptive and the non-nociceptive impulses from the regions innervated by nerves from the same or adjacent spinal segments are thought to take place both in the spinal cord and in the higher centers, while those between the impulses from distant regions probably occur only in the higher centers including the reticular formation and the intralaminar nuclei of the thalamus.

In view of the fact that pain perception is a conscious process in which the afferent messages must be processed in the thalamus before being sent to the cerebral cortex, the thalamus is considered an important structure related to the mechanism of acupuncture analgesia.

In order to refresh our memory of neuroanatomy it may be pertinent to present here in Fig. 1, a sketch of the thalamus which was made from a cross-section of the cat thalamus at the level of the Meynert tract. At this level two important structures, the parafascicular nucleus (Pf) and the centromedian nucleus (CM) can be identified in the medial part of the thalamus. The term "CM-Pf complex" has often been used in recent literature to designate the combinution of these structures. But we are inclined to regard them as two separate entities, since the centromedian nucleus as a distinct nucleus does not exist, or exists in a very primordial condition, in lower mammals. From the phylogenetical point of view the parafascicular nucleus is an old structure which can be identified in almost all forms of lower mammals, while the centromedian nucleus seems to be present only in higher animals and tends to become more and more developed both in size and in cell organization in the ascending scale of phylogenetical evolution. For instance, the centromedian nucleus is of about the same size as, or slightly bigger than, the parafascicular nucleus in cat, but in the human brain the centromedian nucleus is many times as big as the nucleus parafascicularis. This differential development in structure undoubtedly reflects a differentiation in the

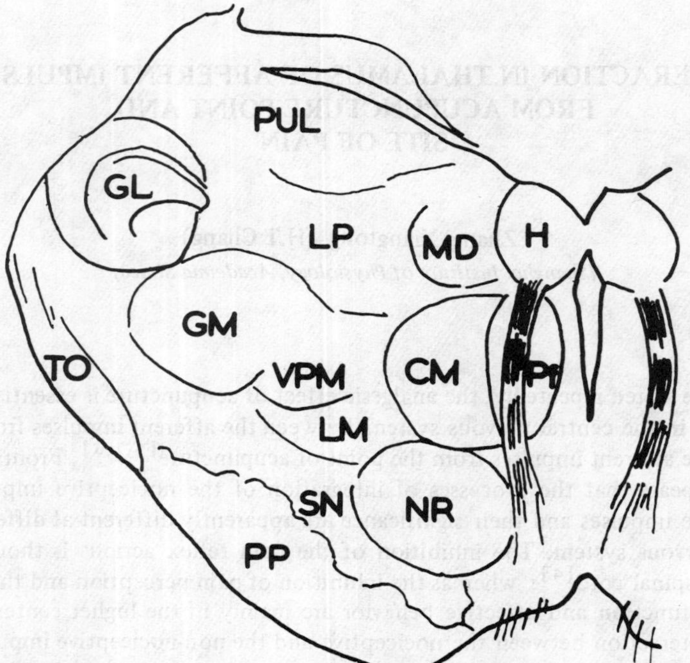

Fig. 1 Schemiatic drawing of the cross-section of cat thalamus at the level of fasciculus habenulo-interpeduncularis, showing the relative position of the centromedian nucleus (CM) and the parafascicular nucleus (Pf).

functions of these two nuclei during the long history of evolution.

It has been demonstrated that a large number of unmyelinated fibers in the spinothalamic tract are projected directly to the parafascicular nucleus, but not to the centromedian nucleus. On the other hand, the centromedian nucleus receives abundant fibers from the bulbar reticular formation while the parafascicular nucleus does not. Therefore we have reason to assume that Pf is essentially a pain receiving center and CM a center mainly for modulation of pain impulses in the thalamus. It is probably through the CM that the afferent impulses from the acupuncture point exert their inhibitory action on pain.

To test the validity of this hypothesis it is necessary to demonstrate (1) that the neurons in the parafascicular nucleus can respond to a nocuous stimulus, and (2) that such response can be modified by acupuncture needling or other innocuous stimuli. In all of our experiments, the electrical discharges of single parafascicular neuron were recorded with traditional glass capillary microelectrodes in animals immobilized with neuromuscular blocking agents. The typical response of a parafascicular neuron to a nocuous stimulus are shown in Fig. 2. The records were taken from a Pf neuron in the rat, showing the discharges of a neuron in response to forceful pinching of the tail with a pair of strong forceps. The nociceptive discharges, as distingvished from the non-nociceptive discharges, are characterized by the

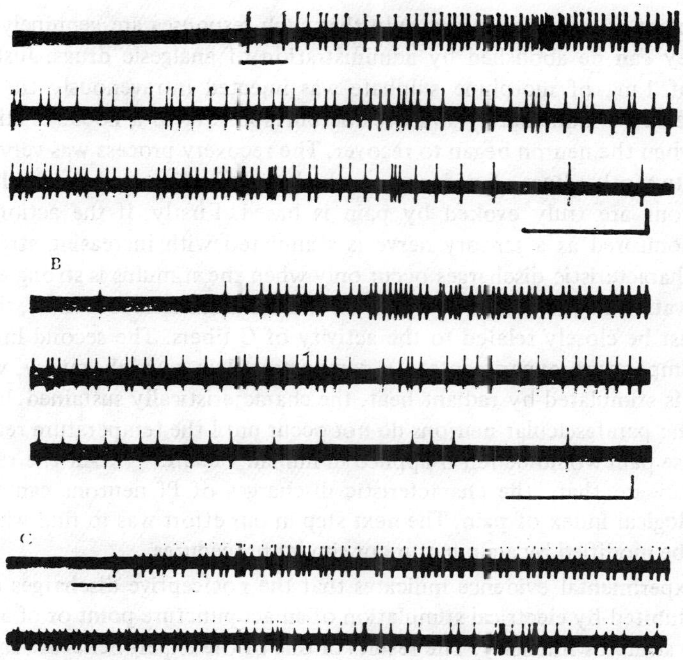

Fig. 2 Electrical discharges of a single parafascicular neuron of albino rat in response to forceful pinch of the tail with a pair of strong forceps. The three tracings in each set of record are continuous recordings. *a, b* and *c* are responses of the same neuron to nocuous stimuli applied to the tail three times in succession, showing no sign of adaptation as exhibited by their similarity both in frequency and in duration of sustained after-discharges in all the three records. Horizontal bar below each record indicates duration of tail pinching. Calibration: 1 sec, 4 mV. (From H.-T. Chang, 1973)

following four features: (1) the long and variable latent period ranging from 80 to 500 msec., (2) sustained post-discharges sometimes lasting longer than 10 seconds, the exact duration of which seems to vary with the stimulus strength, (3) no sign of adaptation as often observed in responses to innocuous stimulation and (4) it can be readily abolished by analgesic agents such as morphine. The three recordings a, b, and c in this figure are the neuronal discharges produced by successive pinches of the tail, and the durations of the sustained discharges by closely repeated assaults inflicted upon the tail are 13, 14 and 17 seconds respectively. There is not the slightest sign of adaptation or attenuation in frequency and duration of these responses. Similar results were obtained in other experiments in which strong electrical stimulation of the sciatic nerve was used instead of pinching of the tail[1].

Although the electrical responses of Pf neurons to nocuous stimuli or strong electrical stimulation of a sensory nerve show all the characteristics of pain, the evidence seems to still be insufficient to assert unequivocally that such responses are genuinely produced by pain unless they can be abolished by administration of analgesic drugs. Just as expected, after a dose of 1 mg of morphine sulphate was injected intravenously the same neuron stopped its discharges immediately and became unresponsive to a nocuous stimulus until 7 minutes later when the neuron began to recover. The recovery process was very slow.

There are two other lines of evidence on which the assertion that the discharges of parafascicular neurons are truly evoked by pain is based. Firstly, if the action potential of the nerve is monitored as a sensory nerve is stimulated with increasing strength one will find that the characteristic discharges occur only when the stimulus is strong enough to produce the C elevation in the action potential of the nerve stimulated. Hence, the response of Pf neurons must be closely related to the activity of C fibers. The second line of evidence comes from temperature experiments. As demonstrated in our laboratory, when the foot pad of the rat is stimulated by radiant heat, the characteristically sustained, high-frequency discharges of the parafascicular neurons do not occur until the temperature reaches 45°C, at which an intense pain would be felt if applied in human beings[5]. All the results of these experiments indicate that the characteristic discharges of Pf neurons can be taken as a reliable physiological index of pain. The next step in our effort was to find whether these Pf discharges can be modified by acupuncture or similar procedures.

Further experimental evidence indicates that the nociceptive discharges of the Pf neurons can be inhibited by electrical stimulation of an acupuncture point or of a sensory nerve with moderate stimulus intensity. The results of one of the experiments are shown in Fig. 3. It is seen from this figure that the sustained responses of a Pf neuron to a nocuous stimulus appeared much less intense with the addition of the background stimulation of the sciatic nerve than without it. Records a and b in this figure are the responses of a Pf neuron to the repeated pinches of the tail with a pair of strong forceps. Record c is the nociceptive dis-

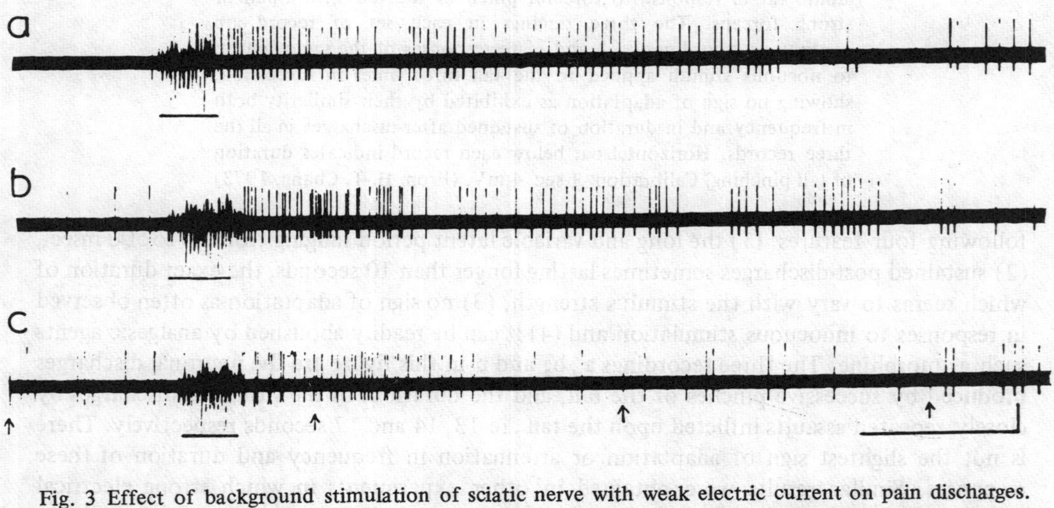

Fig. 3 Effect of background stimulation of sciatic nerve with weak electric current on pain discharges. Records *a* and *b* are responses of a Pf neuron to natural pain stimulus (pinch of tail) and *c*, response of the same neuron to pain stimulus delivered during the course of continuous stimulation of sciatic nerve with single pulses (pulse width, 0.5 msec., intensity, 1.6V) Arrows indicate moments when stimulating pulses were applied to the sciatic nerve. (From H.-T. Chang, 1973)

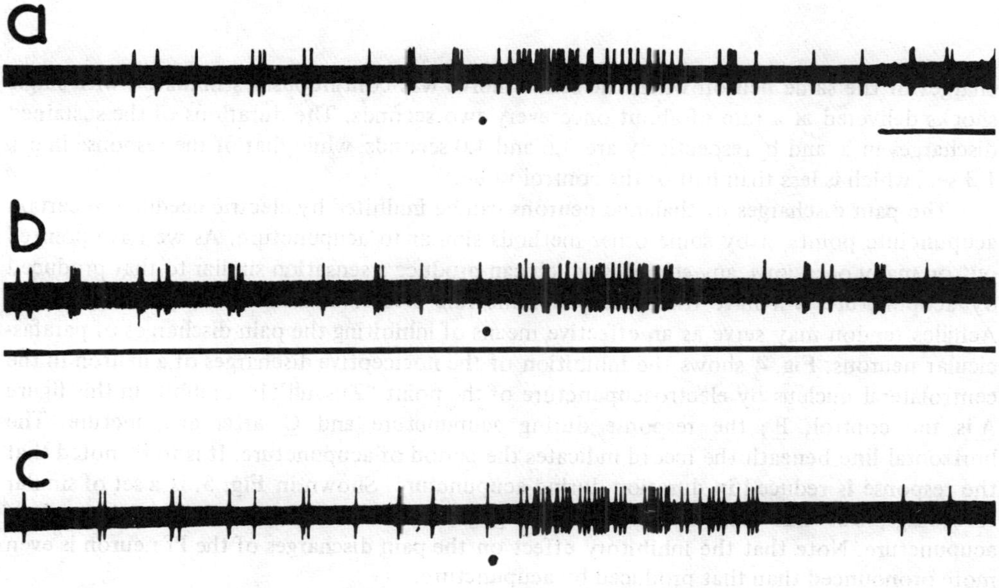

Fig. 4 Inhibitory effect of electric needling of acupuncture point "Tsu-san-li" on the nociceptive discharges of a CL neuron in cat, *a*, response to a brief burst of stimulating pulses applied to peroneal nerve (Pulse width 0.7 msec., intensity, 25v.), *b*, response of the same neuron during electro-acupuncture, *c*, pain discharges after acupuncture. Records *a*, *b* and *c* are continuous recordings. Note the reduction of response duration in *b*. The line beneath the recordings indicates the period of electro-acupuncture. Time 1 sec. (From H.-T. Chang, 1973)

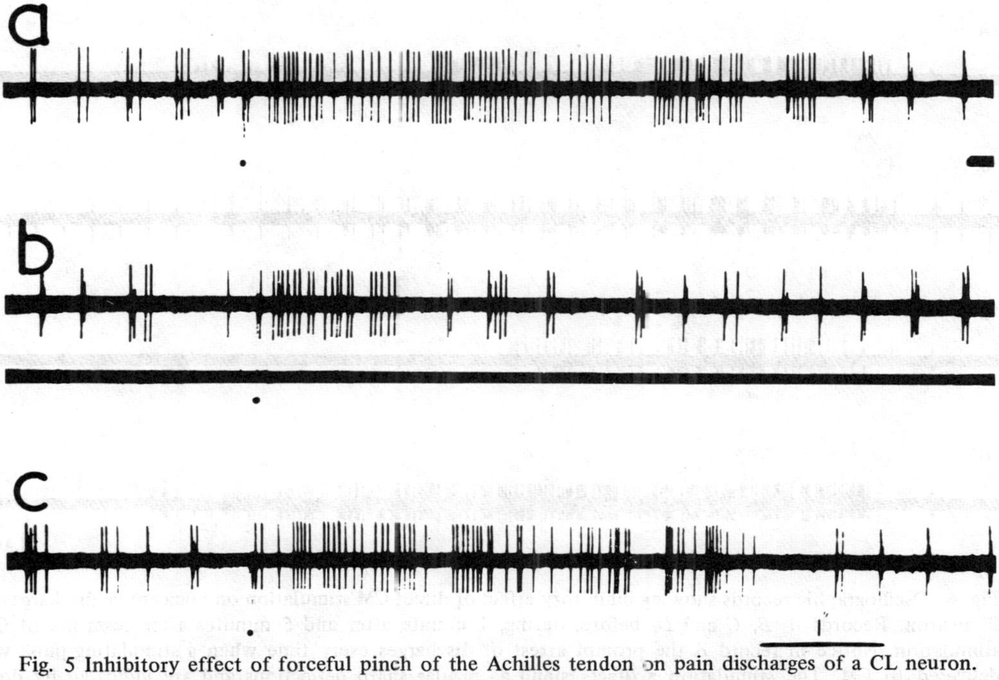

Fig. 5 Inhibitory effect of forceful pinch of the Achilles tendon on pain discharges of a CL neuron. *a*, response to a brief burst of stimulating pulses applied to the peroneal nerve (pulse width, 0.7 msec., intensity, 25v.), *b*, pain discharges during pinch of tendon, *c*, after cessation of pinch. Note the marked reduction in duration of pain discharges. The line beneath recordings *a* and *b* indicates the period of pinch. Time, 1 sec. (From H.-T. Chang, 1973)

charges of the same neuron when the sciatic nerve was continuously stimulated with single shocks delivered at a rate of about once every two seconds. The durations of the sustained discharges in a and b respectively are 3.6 and 4.0 seconds, while that of the response in c is 1.3 sec. which is less than half of the control value.

The pain discharges of thalamic neurons can be inhibited by electric needling of certain acupuncture points or by some other methods similar to acupuncture. As we have pointed out on many occasions, any stimulus which can produce a sensation similar to that produced by acupuncture will have the same pain-inhibiting effect. Thus, forceful pinching of the Achilles tendon may serve as an effective means of inhibiting the pain discharges of parafascicular neurons. Fig. 4 shows the inhibition of the nociceptive discharges of a neuron in the centrolateral nucleus by electroacupuncture of the point "Zusanli" in a rabbit. In this figure A is the control, B, the response during acupuncture and C after acupuncture. The horizontal line beneath the record indicates the period of acupuncture. It is to be noted that the response is reduced in duration during acupuncture. Shown in Fig. 5. is a set of similar recordings, but this time a foreful pinching of the Achilles tendon is used instead of acupuncture. Note that the inhibitory effect on the pain discharges of the Pf neuron is even more pronounced than that produced by acupuncture.

As demonstrated elsewhere, the centromedian nucleus receives a large amount of ascending fibers from the bulbar reticular formation which has been known as an important medullary center for convergence of heterosensory impulses including those under the effect of acupuncture. It has been established that electrical stimulation of an acupuncture point can evoke potentials both in the bulbar reticular formation and in the centromedian nucleus

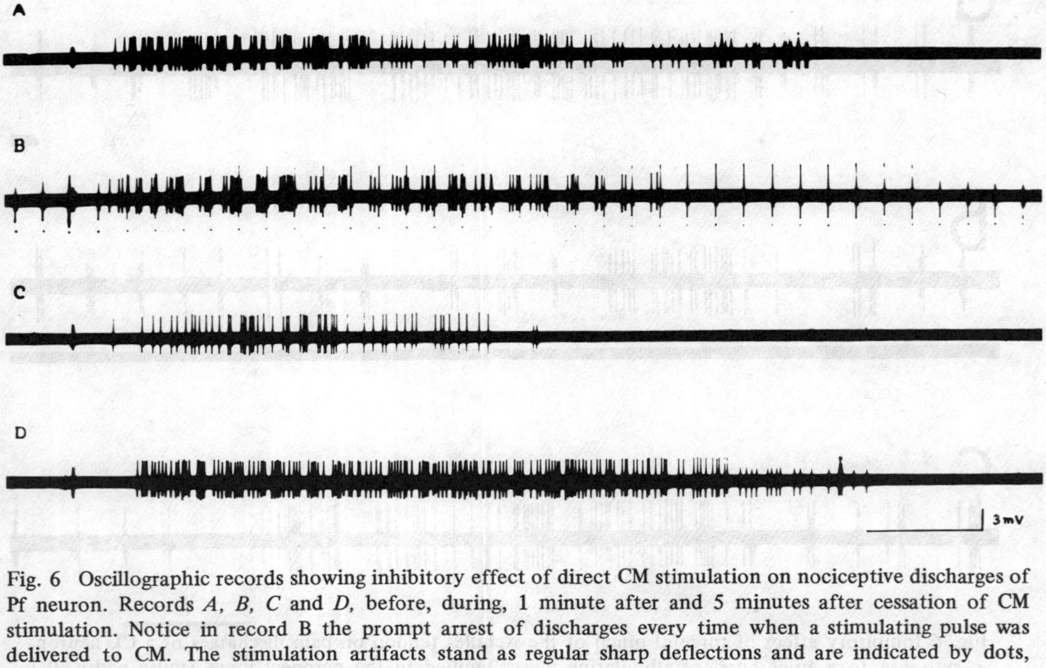

Fig. 6 Oscillographic records showing inhibitory effect of direct CM stimulation on nociceptive discharges of Pf neuron. Records *A, B, C* and *D,* before, during, 1 minute after and 5 minutes after cessation of CM stimulation. Notice in record B the prompt arrest of discharges every time when a stimulating pulse was delivered to CM. The stimulation artifacts stand as regular sharp deflections and are indicated by dots, Calibration: 1 sec, 3 mV. (From F. S. Lo et al, 1978)

and that slimulation of the bulbar reticular formation can inhibit the long latency of neuronal discharges in the region of nuclei parafascicularis and centralis lateralis[6]. It is thus assumed that the inhibitory effect of acupuncture on the nociceptive discharges of the parafascicular neurons is achieved through the action of centromedian neurons. If that is the case, it should be possible to inhibit the nociceptive discharges of parafascicular neurons by direct stimulation of the centromedian nucleus. The results of an experiment of this kind are presented in Fig. 6 in which A is the control showing the nociceptive discharges of a parafascicular neuron, B, the nociceptive discharges of the same neuron during a 4/sec stimulation of the contromedian nucleus, C and D, show results one minute and five minutes after cessation of CM stimulation,. It can be seen here that both the discharge duration and the number of spikes are decreased on CM stimulation[7].

Close examination of the oscillographic recordings reveals that the high frequency discharges were readily arrested almost every time when a stimulating pulse was delivered to the CM. The duration of the arrest following each pulse ranged from 100 to 170 msec with a mean of 136 msec. In the experiment in which these recordings were made, the frequency of CM stimulation was set at 4 per second. As can be seen here,each stimulating pulse produced a complete arrest of the Pf discharges for a period of about 136 msec or a duration of about 544 msec in every second. This means that about half of the discharges were inhibited. From this it may be inferred that increase in rate of CM stimulation from 4 to 8 per second would result in a complete inhibition of the discharges. Although the theoretical forecast has not been completely substantiated by experiment, the degree of inhibition was definitely increased. The result of one of our experiments is presented in Fig. 7, in which A is the control, B, the nociceptive discharges of a Pf neuron during 4.5/sec stimulation of the CM, C, 7.5/sec stimulation and D, 60/sec stimulation. The degree of inhibition was evidently higher when the stimulus frequency was set at 7.5/sec than at 4.5/sec.

During an analysis of the inhibitory effect of direct CM stimulation on the nociceptive discharges of Pf neurons, it was noticed that the inhibition of the Pf discharges appeared not to be immediate, but at a delay of about 15–20 msec following the delivery of the stimulating pulse. In consideration of the close spatial relation between the two nuclei, the long duration of the latent period would be inexplicable unless it is assumed that a circuit of long neuronal chain is involved in the elaboration and transmission of the inhibitory effect of CM excitation. We are inclined to think that such a circuit may consist of many forebrain structures in which the caudate nucleus is probably an important link.

So far, we have described the inhibitory effect of direct CM stimulation on parafascicular discharges. One may wonder whether the CM neurons could be activated by stimulation of an acupuncture point or a peripheral nerve. And, if they could, what the differential effect of stimulation at different frequencies would be. An *ad hoc* experiment showed that certain CM neurons could readily be activated by stimulation of an acupuncture point or electrical stimulation of the deep radial nerve. The results are presented in Fig. 8. In each recording the lower line shows the discharges of the CM neuron and the upper line is the spike density distribution histogram. In this figure, A shows the spontaneous discharges of a CM neuron, B, the increased activity of the neuron during electrical stimulation at a frequency of 8/sec and C, the increased activity of the same neuron at 4/sec stimulation. In these records it is clearly shown that both 8/sec and 4/sec stimulation of the deep radial nerve were effective for activation of the CM neurons, while the 60/sec stimulation was

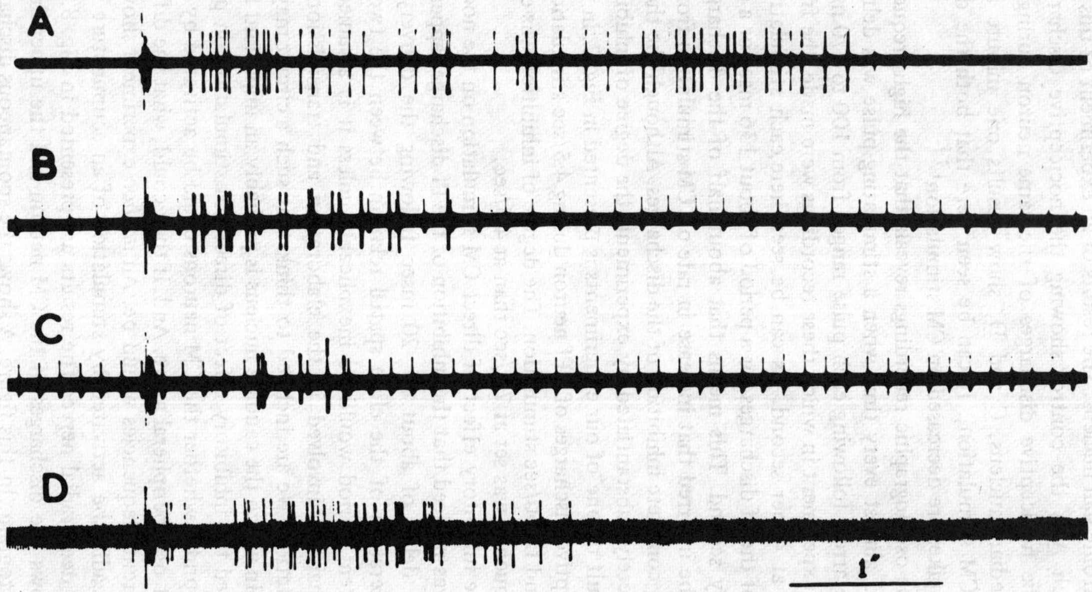

Fig. 7 Comparison of inhibitory effects on nociceptive discharges of Pf neuron, of different frequencies of CM stimulation. A. Control. Discharges of a Pf neuron in response to strong electrical stimulation of Contralateral sural nerve. B, C and D, mociceptive discharges of the same Pf neuron as appeared during the course of continuous direct stimulation of the centromedian nucleus with electrical pulses delivered at frequencies of 4/sec, 8/sec. and 60/sec respectively.

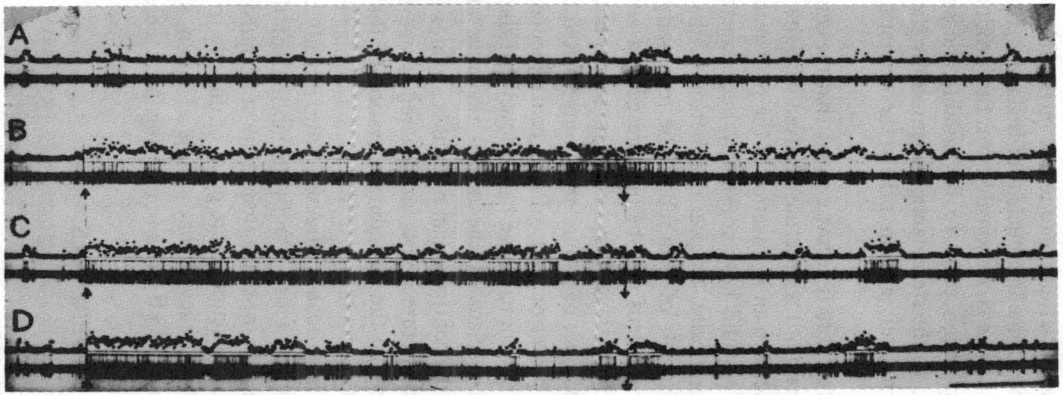

Fig. 8 Responses of a CM neuron to stimulation of the deep branch of homolateral radial nerve with electrical pulses at different frequencies (pulse width 0.15 msec., intensity 3.9V). In each record the lower tracing shows oscillographic recording of spike discharge and the upper tracing, spike density histogram of the discharges taken at a bin of 1 minute. The upward-and downward-pointed arrows indicate respectively the onset and termination of stimulation. *A*, spontaneous firing of the CM neuron. *B*, *C* and *D*, discharges of the same CM neuron to stimulation of deep branch of radial nerve at frequencies 8/sec., 4/sec. and 60/sec respectively. The firing rate of the neuron is the highest in B, and the lowest in D. Time, 10 sec. (From Luo Feisun and Yuan Junsu, unpublished.)

apparently not so effective. This agrees remarkably well with the results of direct CM stimulation. In both cases the 4/sec and 8/sec stimulation is better than the 60/sec stimulation. Therefore We have ample reason to recommend the low frequency stimulation in acupuncture for analgesia purposes, especially when a remote acupuncture point is used.

In view of the fact that numerous patients suffering from intractable pain are in urgent need of proper management in clinics, an understanding of the processes of interaction between the nociceptive and non-nociceptive impulses in the thalamus is imperative. There have been many reports in recent years about attempts to relieve intractable pain by making lesions stereotactically localized in the centromedian nucleus of thalamus. This was done on the assumption that the centromedian nucleus is responsible for the production of pain. The results of this kind of surgical operation seem to be variable and sometimes even disappointing. In some patients subjected to the stereotactic thalamotomy the pain might be temporarily relieved but only to return later, and in others the operation was plainly ineffective.

From the experimental data presented here it seems evident that the centromedian nucleus is not a center for production of pain but a structure involved with the modulation of pain. Destruction of this nucleus would lead to an aggravation of the pain because of the loss of the pain-suppressing influence, which would have constantly been exerted on the pain sensitive neurons in the thalamus. Theoretically, surgical destruction of the centromedian nucleus cannot bring about the desired result of pain relief. The temporary relief of pain following the lesion in the centromedian nucleus may be interpreted as a result of inadvertent interruption of the afferent pain fibers traversing the centromedian nucleus, since, as mentioned earlier in this report, a large number of pain-related unmyelinated fibers from the spinothalamic tract pass through the posterior part of the centromedian nucleus and terminate in the parafascicular nucleus. In summary, we have shown that the parafascicular nucleus and probably the centrolateral nucleus in the medial thalamus are centers for receiving nociceptive impulses, and that the centromedian nucleus is a center for modulation of pain. Afferent impulses from the acupuncture points are believed to exert an inhibitory effect on the parafascicular neurons through the preceding activation of the centromedian nucleus. The inhibition of the nociceptive discharges of the parafascicular neurons by the activity of the centromedian neurons is probably affected both directly and through a forebrain neuronal circuit. To produce the most effective inhibition of the nociceptive discharges of the parafascicular neurons, the optimal frequency of stimulation is about 8 pulses per second, whether it is applied to an acupuncture point or directly to the centromedian nucleus. On theoretical grounds it is believed that a surgical lesion, stereotactically placed in the centromedian nucleus, can not be effective in relieving intractable pain.

REFERENCES

[1] CHANG, H.-T.: *Scientia Sinica,* **16**:25, 1973.

[2] CHANG, H,-T.: *Scientia Sinica,* **21**:829, 1978.

[3] CHANG, H.-T.: *Chinese Med. J.,***92**:7, 1979.

[4] WU, C. P., CHAO, C. C. and WEI, J. Y. *Scientia Sinica,* **17**:688, 1974.

[5] 张香桐等：针刺麻醉临床和原理研究资料选编第 167 页，上海人民出版社，1977。

[6] SHEN, K. F. and HO, S. F.: *Scientia Sinica,* **20**:475. 1977.

[7] LO, F. S. *Scientia Sinica,* **21**:534, 1978.

PARTICIPATION OF DESCENDING INHIBITION IN ACUPUNCTURE ANALGESIA

Shen E

(Shanghai Institute of Physiology, Academia Sinica)

It has been shown recently in the works of many authors that acupuncture activates some brain structures and thereby modulates the sensory inflow of pain. The descending inhibitory system seems to play an important role in this mechanism.

It has been known since the time of Sherrington that the flexor reflex is enhanced after spinal transection. This implies that there is the presence of an everlasting tonic with a descending influence from supraspinal structures. Evidence has accumulated in recent years indicating that such a descending inhibitory system is indeed at work in modulating the transmission of pain impulses in the spinal cord, especially from recent studies on the mechanism of morphine analgesia, brain stimulation- produced analgesia and acupuncture analgesia[1,2].

Hu et al. first demonstrated in 1972 that the diminution of the pain reaction of a rabbit by electrical stimulation of the spinal cord was mediated by descending inhibition[3]. An increase in the irritability of the unilateral skin area below the level of ipsilateral section of the dorsal quadrant of the spinal cord was shown by violent struggle and vocalization when the skin in the related area was lightly pinched. Such exaggerated reactions could no longer be inhibited by electrical stimulation of the spinal cord.

At first, we were interested in how to relax the contracted abdominal muscles during abdominal operation under acupuncture anaesthesia. Experimental study on animal models showed that contraction of the abdominal muscles elicited by stimulation of the splanchnic nerve of a waking rabbit was inhibited effectively by electrical stimulation of a nerve or acupuncture points in the lower limb[4]. The same phenomenon could also be observed in the unanaesthetized, immobolized cat which was more convenient for analysis of the neural pathways. The reflex discharges in intercostal nerve innervating the abdominal muscle were recorded in the immobilized cat instead of using EMG in the rabbit. It was thought that the inhibitory effect of electro-acupuncture could probably be accomplished at the spinal level since the response under study was a spinal reflex and the acupuncture points were on the lower limb. However, complete transection of spinal cord at the cervical or higher thoracic level resulted in a marked diminution of the inhibitory effect of electro-acupuncture accompanied by an enhancement of the viscerosomatic reflex (VSR), which was considered to be a sign of release from tonic descending control[5].

In order to determine the location of the descending spinal pathway, various sections were made at T_{1-3} level. It was found that section of the dorsal columns, ventral funiculi, or medial part of the grey matter affects neither the viscerosomatic retlex nor the inhibitory effect of electroacupuncture. The crucial site lies in a region in the vicinity of the dorsal horn of the dorsolateral funiculi. Bilateral section of these regions resulted in the most effective release of the VSR and the diminution of the inhibitory effect (Fig. 1)[5]. This phenomenon was not due to spinal shock since such sections did not alter the blood pressure or the monosynaptic reflex. From the constriction status of the pupils, the normal blood pressure level and the low intensity of electro-acupuncture employed, stress is not considered to be a serious problem.

There are two possibilities: (1) the tonic descending impulses are necessary for the inhibition, i.e., the inhibitory effect is due to the convergence of the tonic descending impulses and the acupuncture signals on to the reflex arc; (2) the acupuncture signals ascend first to the brain to activate some supraspinal structures which in turn send back the descending impulses to inhibit the spinal reflex. It was found that bilateral section of the ventrolateral funiculi at high thoracic level did not augment the VSR but abolished the inhibitory effect of hind limb acupuncture. Therefore, it seemed reasonable to assume that the ascending pathway for acupuncture signals might travel through these funiculi. Since afferent input from the forelimb enters the spinal cord above the level of the section, needling of the forelimb affords an opportunity to solve this problem. It is interesting to note that the

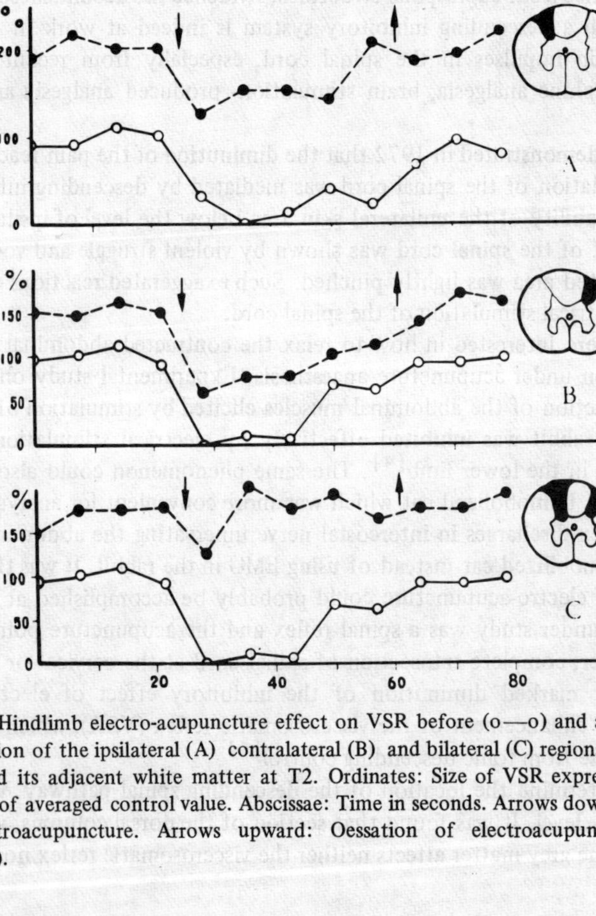

Fig. 1 Hindlimb electro-acupuncture effect on VSR before (o—o) and after (● ...... ●) destruction of the ipsilateral (A) contralateral (B) and bilateral (C) regions of the dorsal horn and its adjacent white matter at T2. Ordinates: Size of VSR expressed as a percentage of averaged control value. Abscissae: Time in seconds. Arrows downward: Onset of electroacupuncture. Arrows upward: Oessation of electroacupuncture. (From Ref.[5]).

inhibitory effect of the forelimb electro-acupuncture persisted after the sectioning of the ventrolateral funiculi as shown in Fig. 2[5]. Hence the activation of some supraspinal structure through the acupuncture signals by way of the ventrolateral funiculi is necessary for the inhibitory effect, and the tonic descending inhibitory impulses are insufficient for the acupuncture effect.

Subsequently, the central localization of the origin of the descending inhibitory impulses involved in this effect was studied. When an intercollicular transection was made, the viscerosomatic reflex was more or less depressed. The inhibitory effect of electroacupuncture, however, was not seriously affected except that it was common to observe a shortening of the after-inhibition of electroacupuncture. It was evident that the main supraspinal structure concerned with the inhibitory effect must be situated in the brain stem below the intercollicular level[5]. Various sections and lesions were then made in our laboratory. It was found that the most important structure to use to produce this effect lies in the bulbar medial reticular formation including the posterior group of the raphe nuclei[6].

Next the question of whether the inhibitory effect under observation affects nociceptive transmission arose. The viscerosomatic reflex did not appear until the A-delta fibers in the splanchnic nerve were excited. When a short train of pulses at this strength was delivered to the splanchnic nerve, it was found that the blood pressure was elevated and the pupils dilated. In the chronic animal, the stimulation of the splanchnic nerve by means of imbedded electrodes with a short train of pulses having just enough strength to elicit contraction of abdominal muscles, provoked vocalization and violent movents in the cat. Such a stimulus can therefore be regarded as nociceptive in nature. However, there remains

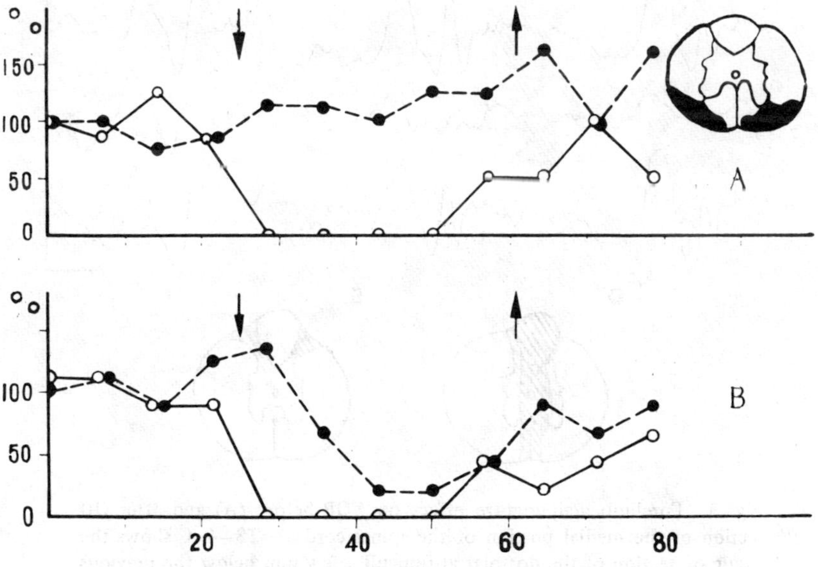

Fig. 2 Hindlimb (A) and forelimb (B) electro-acupuncture effect on VSR before (o—o) and after (• ...... •) destruction of bilateral ventrolateral funiculi at T2 in the same animal. Conventions as in Fig. 1 (From Ref.[5]).

the possibility that the descending inhibitory impulses elicited by acupuncture exert their effect only on the motorneuron or certain premotor interneurons involved in the reflex but have nothing to do with the ascending transmission of nociceptive impulses. In order to clarify this point, a splanchnically evoked potential was recorded from the orbital cortex. It was found that the evoked orbital potential (EOP) occurred only when the A-delta fibers in the splanchnic nerve were excited and that it could be inhibited by electro-acupuncture of either limb. To our surprise, the inhibitory effect on the evoked potential was almost abolished by sectioning of the dorsolateral funiculi at high spinal level as shown in Fig. 3. The inhibitory effect of forelimb acupuncture was found to persist after vertical sectioning which extended from the dorsal columns through the central grey to the ventral funiculi at the level of T_{3-4}. However, the inhibitory effect diminished markedly if sections of the bilateral dorsolateral funiculi were made a few mm below the level of the previous lesion[7]. Destruction of the region of the bulbar raphe nuclei resulted in almost the same diminution of the acupuncture effect on EOP[7]. In another series of experiments, inhibition of the EOP was produced by direct stimulation of the nucleus raphe magnus. This kind of inhibitory effect was also nearly a eliminated after sectioning of the dorsolateral funiculi at T_{3-4}[8]. It is obvious that the descending inhibitory impulses originating from bulbar medial reticular formation are able to block, at least partially, the ascending transmission of visceral A-delta afferent impulses. Recently G. L. Zhang et al., have observed that the

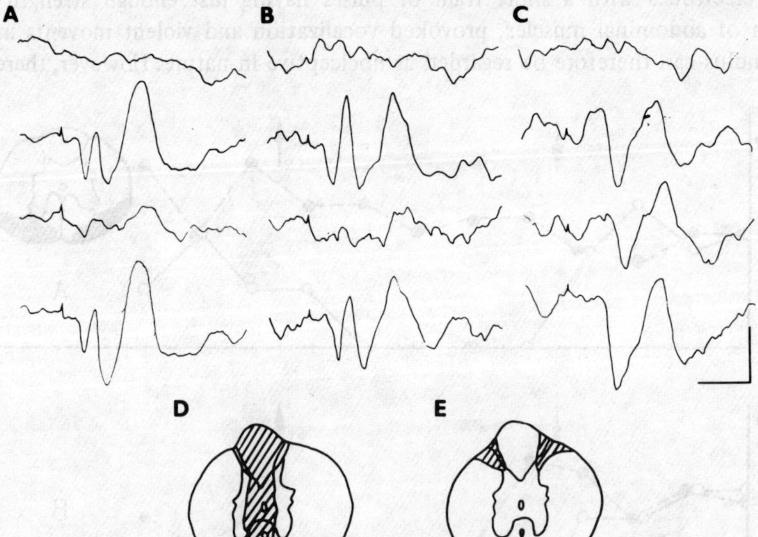

Fig. 3 Forelimb acupuncture effect on EOP before (A) and after (B) section of the medial portion of the spinal cord at T3–4. C shows the result of section of the dorsolatral funiculi a few mm below the previous section in the same cat. In each series the traces from upper to lower are averaged spontaneous brain waves, averaged EOP before, during and 10 minutes after electro-acupuncture. Calibration: 30μV, 20 msec. D and E show the lesion. (From Ref.[7]).

diminution of the inhibitory effect of acupuncture on the unit discharges of the neurones in the nucleus parafasicularis of thalamus is in response to the noxious stimulation of hindlimb following sectioning of the dorsal half of the spinal cord[9]. It is sufficiewt to say that both the visceral nociceptive transmission and the somatic nociceptive transmission are subject to modulation by the descending inhibitory impulses induced by acupuncture.

The fonction of the neurotransmitter system involved in electro-acupuncture on the viscerosomatic reflex has been investigated. In some preliminary acute experiments we injected 3μg of p-chlorophenylalanine into the lateral ventricle of the cat. It was noted that the VSR was released from tonic descending inhibition and the inhibitory effect of acupuncture was slightly diminished, 1–3 hours after injection[10]. Injection of 200–300μg of 5-HT into the lateral ventricle enhanced the inhibitory effect slightly but significantly[10]. In another

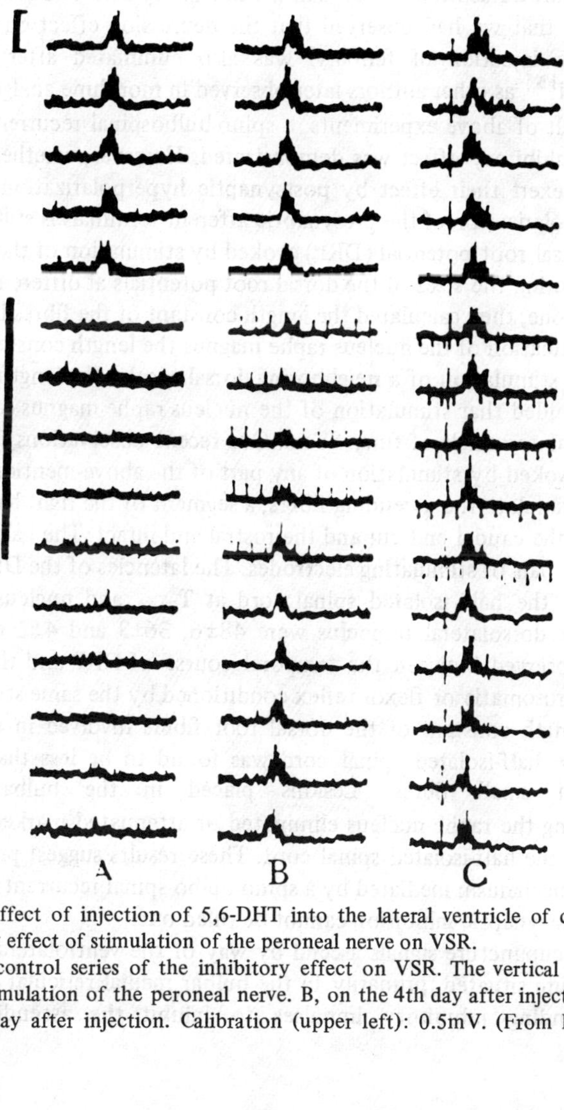

Fig. 4 Effect of injection of 5,6-DHT into the lateral ventricle of cat on the inhibitory effect of stimulation of the peroneal nerve on VSR.

A, a control series of the inhibitory effect on VSR. The vertical bar shows during stimulation of the peroneal nerve. B, on the 4th day after injection. C, on the 8th day after injection. Calibration (upper left): 0.5mV. (From Ref.[11]).

series of experiments a dose of 500–1000μg of 5,6-dihydroxytryptamine was injected into the lateral ventricle. The animals were kept alive for several days and then the inhibitory effect was precisely tested. To quantify the acupuncture stimulation, the common peroneal nerve was stimulated instead of the acupuncture points and action potentials in the same nerve were monitored. The strength of stimulation was adjusted to allow only groups I+II of nerve fibers to be excited. It can be seen from Fig 4 that the inhibitory effect is diminished on the 4th and 8th days after injection[11]. The same is true when 80–100μg of the drug were injected into the region of the nucleus raphe magnus[11]. Intraperitoneal injection of p-chloroamphetamine (5mg/kg) markedly diminished the inhibitory effect 4–24 hours after injection[11]. Recently Dong and Jiang observed that the fluorescence of 5-HT neurones in the nucleus raphe magnus increased and that of the NA terminal in this region decreased during acupuncture analgesia in rats[12]. Therefore, as in morphine analgesia, 5-HT seems to be an important neurotransmitter involved in the inhibitory effect of acupuncture. It should be mentioned here that we had observed that the depression effect on the viscerosomatic reflex by systemic injection of fentanyl was also eliminated after sectioning of the dorsolateral funiculi[5] as other authors later observed in morphine analgesia[2].

From the result of above experiments, a spino-bulbospinal recurrent circuit underlying the acupuncture inhibitory effect was demonstrated. However, whether the descending inhibitory impulses exert their effect by postsynaptic hyperpolarization of the dorsal horn neurons or by depolarization of the presynaptic afferent terminals is still unknown. Proudfit et al. recorded dorsal root potential (DRP) evoked by stimulation of the nucleus raphe magnus[13]. By measuring the sizes of the dorsal root potentials at different distances from the dorsal root entry zone, they calculated the length constant of the fibres involved in the DRP. In the case of stimulation of the nucleus raphe magnus the length constant was about 3 mm, and in the case of stimulation of a neighboring dorsal rootlet the length constant was about 8 mm. They concluded that stimulation of the nucleus raphe magnus caused depolarization of primary afferent terminals of finer fibers. Our recent observations show that DRPs (T_{11} or L_6) could be evoked by stimulation of any part of the above-mentioned recurrent circuit (Fig.5)[14]. To stimulate the ascending fibers, a segment of the right half of a thoracic cord was isolated with the caudal end cut and the rostral end intact. The half isolated spinal cord was then put on a pair of stimulating electrodes. The latencies of the DRPs (left L_6) evoked by stimulation of the half isolated spinal cord at T_{2-4} and nucleus raphe magnus and surface of the left dorsolateral funiculus were 48±6, 36±3 and 4±2 msec respectively. A correlation was observed between the temporal course of DRP and that of the inhibitory phase of the viscerosomatic or flexor reflex conditioned by the same stimulus which evoked the DRP. The length constant of the dorsal root fibers involved in the DRP evoked by stimulation of the half-isolated spinal cord was found to be less than 3 mm, indicating depolarization of small fibres. Lesions placed in the bulbar medial reticular formation including the raphe nucleus eliminated or attenuated markedly the DRP evoked by stimulation of the half-isolated spinal cord. These results suggest probable participation of a presynaptic mechanism mediated by a spino-bulbo-spinal recurrent circuit, although the possibility of a postsynaptic inhibition cannot be ruled out.

To sum up, acupuncture signals ascend by way of the ventrolateral funiculi, activate a supraspinal structure situated, primarily in the bulbar medial reticular formation, and then accentuate descending inhibitory impulses to inhibit the ascending transmission of

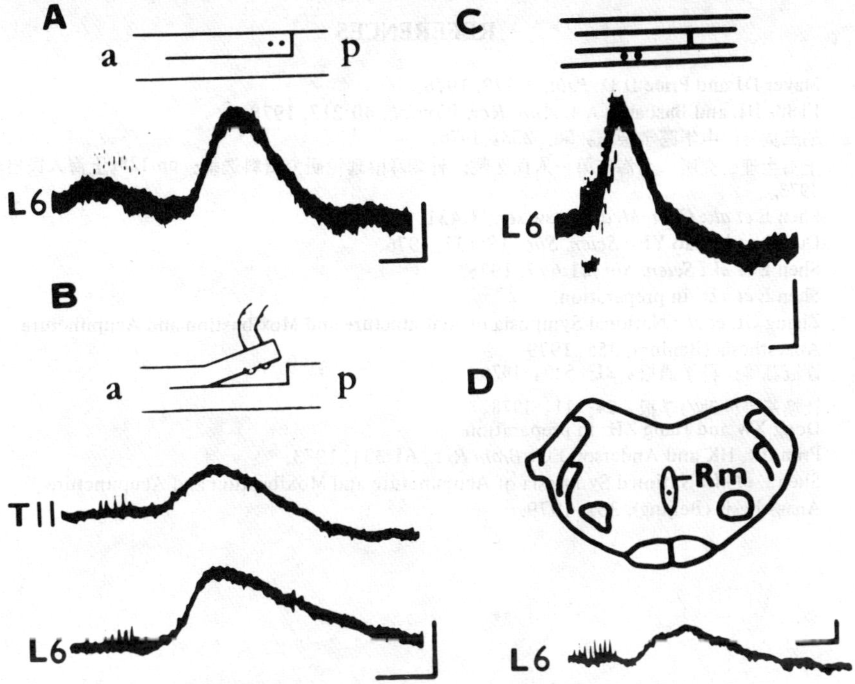

Fig. 5 A. DRP(L_6) elicited by stimulation of the ventrolateral funiculi. An L-shaped incision was made at T_{2-4}, the two spots show the points of insertion of stimulating electrodes. a:anterior, p: posterior.

B. DRPs (T_{11} and L_6) elicited by stimulation of the half isolated spinal cord at T_{2-4}.

C. DRP(L_6) elicited by stimulation of the surface of the dorsolateral funiculi. The dorsal columns caudal to the stimulating points were cut.

D. DRP(L_6) elicited by stimulation of the nucleus raphe magnus. Calibration in A, B, C, D: 100μV, 25 msec. (Unpublished).

nociceptive afferent impulses. Presynaptic mechanism may be an important component in the descending inhibition. 5-HT seems to be an essential neurotransmitter involved in this effect. What is new in our work is that the descending inhibition we observed is induced by peripheral stimulation such as acupuncture instead of stimulation of brain structures. This mechanism may work in daily physiological activities since the inhibition can be obtained even when only group I+group II fibres in the nerve were excited.

REFERENCES

[1] Mayer DJ and Price D D: *Pain,* **2**:379, 1976.

[2] Fields HL and Basbaum A I: *Ann, Rev. Physiol.,* **40**:217, 1978.

[3] 胡三觉等：中华医学杂志，**56**：238，1976。

[4] 上海生理研究所　上海市第一人民医院：针刺麻醉理论研究资料选编：pp.128，上海人民出版社，1973。

[5] Shen E *et al.*: *Chin. Med.J., new ser.,* **1**:431, 1975.

[6] Du HJ and Chao YF : *Scien. Sin.,* **19**:137, 1976.

[7] Shen E *et al.*: *Scien. Sin.,***21**:677, 1978.

[8] Shen E *et al.*: in preparation.

[9] Zhang GL *et al.*: National Symposia of Acupuncture and Moxibustion and Acupuncture Anaesthesia (Beijing), 355, 1979

[10] 许冠荪等：科学通报，**21**：549，1976。

[11] 杜焕基等：动物学报，**24**：11，1978。

[12] Dong XW and Jiang ZH: in preparation

[13] Proudfit, HK and Anderson EG: *Brain Res.,* **61**:331, 1973.

[14] Shen E *et al.*: National Symposia of Acupuncture and Moxibustion and Acupuncture Anaesthesia (Beijing), 362, 1979.

INHIBITORY ACTION OF ELECTROACUPUNCTURE ON DORSAL HORN NEURONS OF THE SPINAL CORD

Wu Jianping, Xing Jianghuai, Xing Baoren
Lu Jingen , Chen Yuchu
(Shanghai Institute of Physiology, Academia Sinica)

I. INTRODUCTION

In our previous study[1] it was demonstrated that, in spinal cats, repetitive electrical stimulation in the frequency of 100 Hz applied to afferent nerves or acupuncture points, or manual needling of the points, inhibited the responses of dorsolateral funiculus fibers to noxious stimulus. The duration of the inhibitory effect was relatively short, lasting generally not more than several dozen seconds. However, in chloralose-anesthetized cats, as reported by Pomeranz in 1977[2], the response of the dorsal horn neurons induced by noxious stimulus could be continuously inhibited by electroacupuncture of 4 Hz delivered to the acupuncture points. The inhibition emerged 10–15 minutes after the onset of electroacupuncture and persisted till 10–30 minutes after its cessation. In view of this discrepancy, the present study was undertaken to re-examine the inhibitory action of electro-acupuncture of different frequencies on dorsal horn neurons and, at the same time, the membrane potential changes of these neurons during the inhibition was also observed in order to elucidate the mechanism of the inhibition.

II. METHODS

Experiments were performed on 25 cats. After the trachea and the external cervical vein were canulated under ether anaesthesia, chloralose (65mg/Kg) was injected intravenously and the ether was removed. The lumbar region of the spinal cord was exposed by a laminectomy. Hair of the left hind limb, distal to ankle joint, was clipped for applying the radiant heat stimulus. The fixation of the animal was the same as described in the previous paper[1].

The unit discharges of dorsal horn neurons were recorded with a glass microelectrode, having a tip of a diameter of about 2μ after being broken under the microscope. The microelectrode was filled a using presssure with 2 M of potassium citrate.

During the experiments, the dorsal part of L_7-S_1 spinal segments was explored with microelectrode while the left hind limb was lightly palpated to locate the receptive fields of dorsal horn neurons. Once a neuron responded to palpation, its receptive field was pinched moderately with a pair of forceps. If a persisting pinch induced sustained discharges, the receptive field was finally tested with radiant heat stimulus. The source of the radiant heat was a 50 W film projector bulb. At a distance of 1 cm in front of the bulb was fixed a thermistor which, being in close contact with the skin during heating, was employed to measure the skin temperature and thus to automatically control the intensity of the heat so that the skin temperature was maintained at 54°C or 58°C. The duration of the radiant heat stimulus was 10 seconds. The typical skin temperature change produced by radiant heat stimulus is shown in Fig. 1, L. It was measured with a thermocouple placed on the skin. It should can be noted that, except for the first or second or so, the skin temperature was principally kept stable at 54°C. The heat stimulus was applied once every 4 minutes in order to avoid sensitization of the receptors by too frequent stimulation. After taking three successive responses to heat stimulus as a control, electroacupuncture was applied to left Huantiao and Futu points by means of acupuncture needles. In some experiments the Zusanli and Sanyinjiao, or Yangling and Futu points or to ipsilateral hamstring nerve were used. The effectiveness of stimulating different acupuncture points has not been systematically compared. The duration of electroacupuncture was generally 15–20 minutes, except for those experiments where the membrane potential change was observed. The frequency of electroacupuncture was usually 5 Hz, but sometimes 100 Hz was also used for comparison. The current intensity was generally below 3 mA. After electroacupuncture, three responses to heat stimulus were taken again as a control.

In some experiments, the spinal cord was transected at C_1 or at the lower thoracic level. In these experiments, the effect of electroacupuncture on the responses of the range of wide dynamic dorsal horn neurons to strong electric stimulation of the sural nerve was observed.

The body temperature of the animals was kept between 36–38°C. The blood pressure was routinely monitored by means of a canula inserted into the carotid artery. All the data were collected when the mean blood pressure was above 80 mm Hg. Great variations in blood pressure often indicated the need for a supplementary dose of chloralose. During microelectrode recording the animal was paralyzed with gallamine triethiodide and kept alive by means of artificial respiration. Bilateral artificial pneumothorax was also performed.

All the responses were recorded with a 4 channel data recorder, the frequency response being 0–2 KC. After the experiments the data were processed with a digital computer or were photographed.

III. RESULTS

(I) The Inhibitory Action of Long-standing Electroacupuncture

Complete data were recorded from 19 dorsal horn neurons in 14 cats. According to the readings on the micromanipulator, the depths of their location from the dorsal surface of the spinal cord were 1093–1939μ, with 11 neurons being deeper than 1500μ. All neurons had relatively wide receptive fields. They responded to hair bending; moderate pinch of the skin with forceps inducing sustained firings; and radiant heat stimulus of 54°C or 58°C eliciting long lasting high frequency discharges. All these resdonses suggest that the neurons were of the lamina V type.

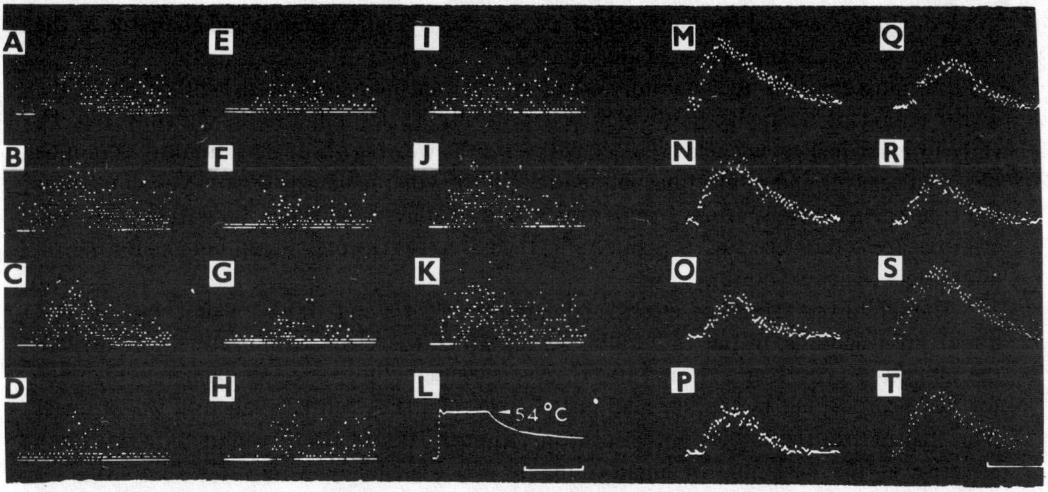

Fig. 1 Inhibitory effect of electroacupuncture on the response of dorsal horn neurons to noxious stimuli in chloralose-anaesthetized cat. Record A-K were taken from a dorsal horn neuron which was markedly inhibited by electroacupuncture, M-T, another neuron moderately inhibited. All records were sequential pulse density histogram of the unit discharges. The whole sweep contains 256 points, each represents 100 msec. The ordinate represents the density of discharges in each 100 msec. The radiant heat stimulus, lasting 10 seconds, was applied at 1.5 sec following the onset of each sweep. All records were successively taken with intervals of 4 minutes. A–C: three successive control responses to radiant heat stimuli. D–G: responses during 5 Hz electroacupuncture at Huantiao and Futu points, intensity 0.8 mA. H–K: four responses after the cessation of acupuncture. The responses were markedly inhibited during acupuncture and recovered in about 10 minutes after the acupuncture (Record J). M, N: control responses of another neuron. O–R: responses during electroacupuncture (Huantiao and Futu points, 2 mA). S, T: responses after acupuncture. The responses were moderately inhibited during acupuncture and recovered immediately on cessation of acupuncture. Time mark: 10 seconds.
Record L was a typical example of skin temperature change produced by radiant heat stimulus.

With a radiant heat stimulus of 10 seconds, the discharge rate of most neurons increased at the beginning of the stimulus. About half of the neurons reached their summit and then declined shortly before the end of the stimulus (Fig. 1, M, N and S, T), while other neurons usually reached the peak at the end of the stimulus (Fig. 1, A–C and J, K). The discharge frequency of most neurons returned to the control level in 15 seconds following the stimulus. When the repetition rate of the heat stimulus was once every 4 minutes, the responses of the dorsal horn neurons were fairly stable.

The inhibitory action of electro-acupuncture in the frequency of 5 Hz (0.7–2.8 mA, except those used for 3 neurons) was tested on 19 neurons. Marked inhibition was demonstrated in 6 neurons (31.6 %), the responses being reduced to less than one third of the control. Eight neurons (42.1 %) were moderately inhibited and 3 neurons lightly inhibited. In these cases the amplitudes of the responses were reduced to about half and a little more than two thirds of the control value respectively. No significant effect was found with 2 neurons (10.5 %). In other words, 73.7 % of the neurons were markedly or moderately inhibited by electro-acupuncture. A–K and M–T in Fig. 1 are two series of records showing the marked and moderate inhibitory effect of electroacupuncture on two dorsal horn neurons respectively. It can be seen that during the 15 minutes electro-acupuncture the number of spike discharges evoked by radiant heat stimulus was greatly reduced and the peak of the response was significantly lowered and delayed.

For most neurons, the inhibitory effect of electroacupuncture persisted throughout the whole period of its application which was generally 15–20 minutes (as shown in Fig. 1). Only in individual cases could a tendency toward the wearing off of the inhibitory action be observed near the end of electroacupuncture. On the other hand, the response of all neurons but one, recovered from inhibition immediately following cessation of the electroacupuncture (see Fig. 1, S and A–K; the latter was the only exception manifesting an after-effect of acupuncture).

The inhibitory effects of electroacupuncture of 5 Hz and 100 Hz were compared in 4 dorsal horn neurons. In the 15 minutes during which the electroacupuncture was applied, the inhibitory effects of 5 Hz and 100 Hz electroacupuncture were approximately the same for two neurons, but in another neuron the effect of 5 Hz electroacupuncture was stronger than that of 100 Hz. In yet another neuron, although 100 Hz electroacupuncture was more effective at the beginning of application, its effect gradually wore off with continuous stimulation so that the response had already largely recovered 15 minutes after application (Fig. 2, D–G). This kind of "adaptation" to acupuncture stimulus seemed to be more pronounced in spinal cats. In three spinal cats, 4 wide dynamic range dorsal horn neurons which responded to a single strong electric stimulus to sural nerve with two bursts of discharges were observed. In three out of the four neurons the inhibitory effect of electro-acupuncture of 100 Hz frequency wore off in one minute after the onset of stimulation, and the response completely recovered or even became enhanced. In the other neuron, the effect was also attenuated in one minute after electro-acupuncture. On the other hand, the inhibitory effect of 5Hz electroacupuncture proved to be very long-lasting. In Fig. 2 it is shown that the inhibitory effect of 5 Hz electroacupuncture persisted throughout the period of continuous stimulation (K–O), whereas that of 100 Hz electroacupuncture disappeared almost completely in only 30 seconds (Fig. 2, P–T).

In order to evaluate the possible role played by the descending inhibitory pathways in the mechanism of inhibition elicited by electroacupuncture, the following observations were made in two neurons. After the demonstration of the inhibitory effect of electroacupuncture, the descending inhibitory pathways were reversibly blocked by putting cubes of frozen saline on the exposed lower thoracic spinal cord. Then the effect of electroacupuncture was studied again. After blocking, while both the spontaneous discharges and the responses to radiant heat stimulus of these two neurons were markedly enhanced which indicated that the blocking was effective, the inhibitory effects of electroacupuncture were diminished. But in another neuron, transection of the dorsal half of the thoracic spinal cord did not exert any significant influence on the inhibitory effect of acupuncture.

(II) The Membrane Potential Changes Produced by Electroacupuncture

In the present study it was observed with extracellular recordings that a single electroacupuncture stimulus usually elicited evoked discharges of a dorsal horn neuron followed by an inhibitory period during which the neuronal discharges were depressed. In order to observe the membrane potential changes of dorsal horn neurons induced by electroacupuncture, intracellular recordings were made from 11 lamina V type dorsal horn

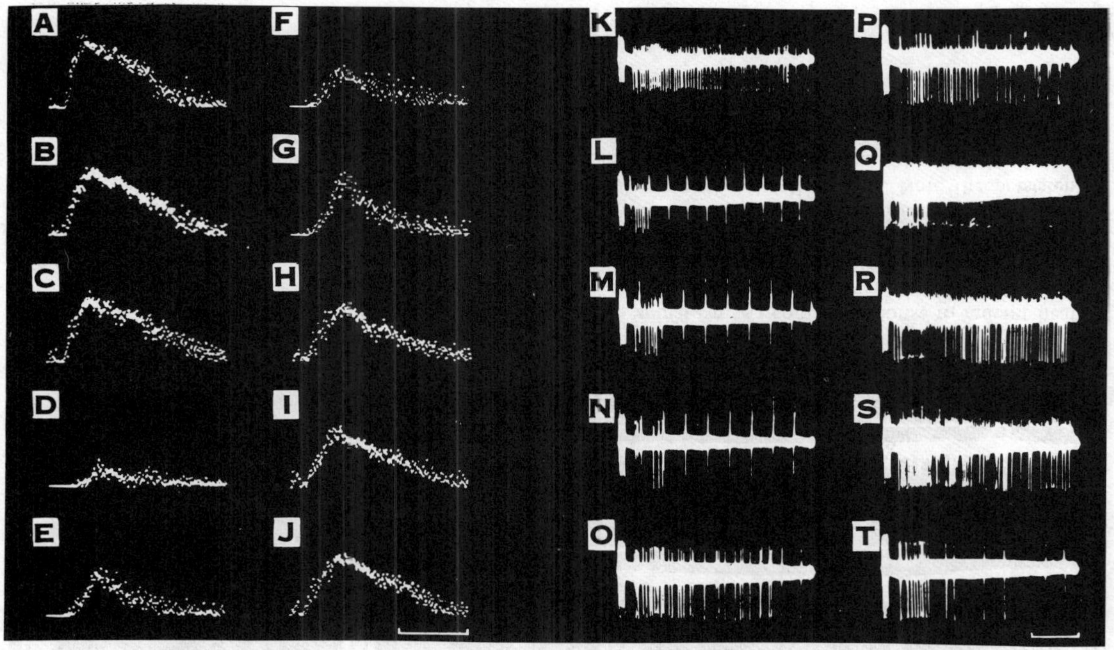

Fig. 2 Comparison of inhibitory effects induced by 100 Hz and 5 Hz electroacupuncture. Records A–J were recorded from a neuron in an anaesthetized cat, all conditions except for the frequency of electroacupuncture were the same as in Fig. 1, A–C: control responses. D–G: responses during electroacupuncture of 100 Hz (Huantiao and Futu points, 1.9 mA). In D the response was markedly inhibited, but the inhibition wore off rapidly (E–G). H–J: control responses after acupuncture. Time mark: 10 seconds. Records K–T were taken from another neuron in a spinal cat. K: control response to a strong electric shock applied to sural nerve. L was the response just at the beginning of 5 Hz electroacupuncture (Huantiao, Futu points, 3.6 mA), M, 5 minutes and N, 15 minutes later respectively. O: control response after acupuncture. The responses during acupuncture were markedly inhibited. Records P–T were the responses of the same neuron in another series of observation. P: control, Q: 5 seconds after the onset of 100 Hz electroacupuncture (Huantiao, Futu points, 3.6 mA). R, S:30 and 70 seconds later respectively. T: control response after the end of acupuncture. Notice that the responses in R and S were enhanced. The response after acupuncture was somewhat depressed (cf. P with T). Time mark: 0.5 second.

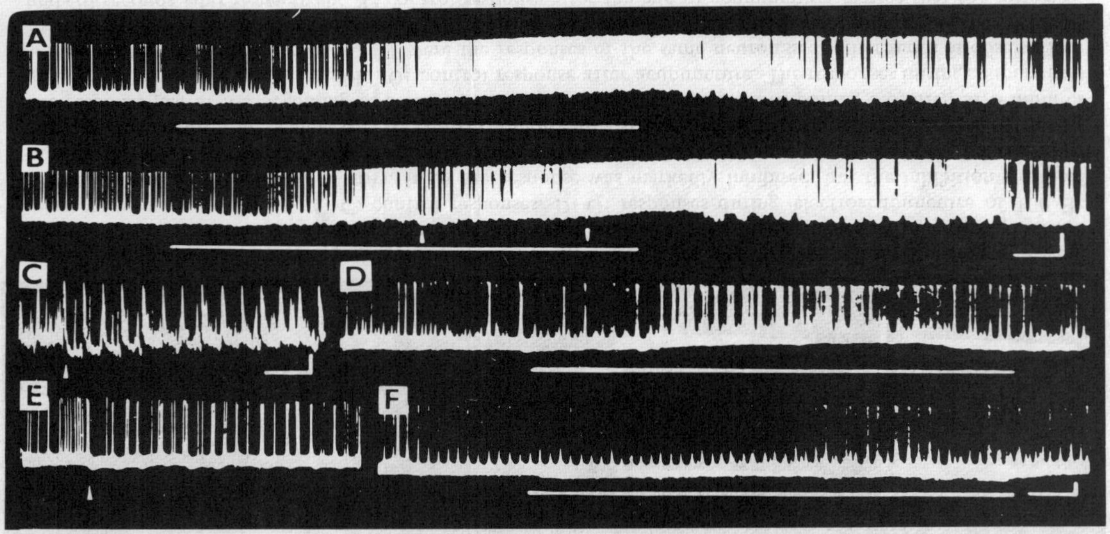

Fig. 3 The relation between the inhibitory effect of electroacupuncture and membrane potential changes. Records A–C were intracellular recordings from a neuron in a spinal cat. A: control response to radiant heat; B: short period of 5 Hz electroacupuncture, indicated by arrows, was applied to Huantiao and Futu points (4.6 mA) during the late part of the response. C: amplification of a part of record B, shwoing each electro-acupuncture pulse elicited spike discharges followed by IPSP and inhibition of discharges. Time mark and calibration: 1 second, 20 mV, for A and B; 0.5 second, 5 mV for C. D–F were recorded intracellularly from another neuron in a chloralose-anaesthetized cat. D: control response to radiant heat. Note the persistent depolarization of membrane and the increase of discharges. The arrow in E indicates the onset of electro-acupuncture (Huantiao and Futu points, 2 mA) which produced hyperpolarization. F: the response induced by radiant heat on the background of 5 Hz electro-acupuncture. Time mark: 1 second, calibration: 10 mV. The lines underlying Records A, B, D, F indicate the periods of radiant heat stimulus.

neurons, among which, 4 were recorded from spinal cats and 7 from chloralose-anesthetized cats. The membrane potential recorded ranged from 20 to 60 mV. The response to radiant heat stimulus and the inhibitory effect of electroacupuncture were studied in each neuron. In all these neurons, a single electric pulse applied to the acupuncture points invariably elicited a transient excitatory postsynaptic potential (EPSP), often associated with spike discharges, and this was followed by a long lasting inhibitory postsynaptic potential (IPSP). The amplitude of the IPSP sometimes reached nearly 10 mV, during which, the spontaneous as well as the evoked neuronal discharges were effectively inhibited. The records in Fig. 3, A–C were taken from a neuron in a spinal cat. The electroacupuncture elicited an IPSP accompanied by the inhibition of spike discharges (B and C). Records D–F were from another neuron recorded from an anaesthetized cat. Record D was the control response to radiant heat stimulus. The membrane in D was markedly depolarized with an increase of spike discharges. A single electric pulse to the acupuncture points elicited a long duration IPSP (Fig, 3. E. Fig. 4, E is the averaged record of the same IPSP). Electroacupuncture of 5 Hz produced a persistent hyperpolarization of the membrane and on this background the long lasting depolarizing change of the membrane seen in control response (Record D) induced by heat stimulus could no longer be observed and the number of evoked spike discharges was also greatly diminished (Fig. 3, F). In some experiments, the membrane potential changes elicited by electroacupuncture were averaged by a computer. Fig. 4 shows the averaged records obtained from 4 dorsal horn neurons. Records A, B and C, D were from two neurons recorded in spinal cats, in which the durations of IPSP evoked by 2 Hz electro-acupuncture stimulus were 95 msec and 52 msec respectively. Records E and F

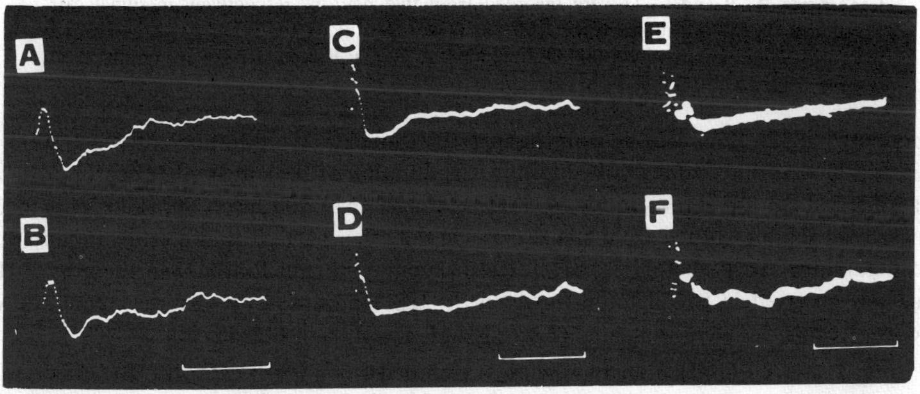

Fig. 4 Averaged records of the membrane potential changes evoked by electroacupuncture. A, B and C, D were recorded from two neurons respectively in spinal cats and were evoked by electroacupuncture at Huantiao and Futu points. The intensity of electroacupuncture: 5.9 mA for A, B and 1.9 mA for C, D. Frequency: 2 Hz for A and C and 5 Hz for B and D. Note the durations of IPSP evoked by 5 Hz electroacupuncture were longer than by 2 Hz. E, F were recorded from two neurons in chloraloseanaesthetized cats and evoked by 2 Hz electro-acupuncture at Huantiao and Futu points (intensity: 2 mA). All records were the average of 25 responses. The duration of the sweep:256 msec for A–D, 512 msec for E and F. Note the durations of IPSP in E, F were longer than in A–D. Time mark: 100 msec for A–D, 200 msec for E and F.

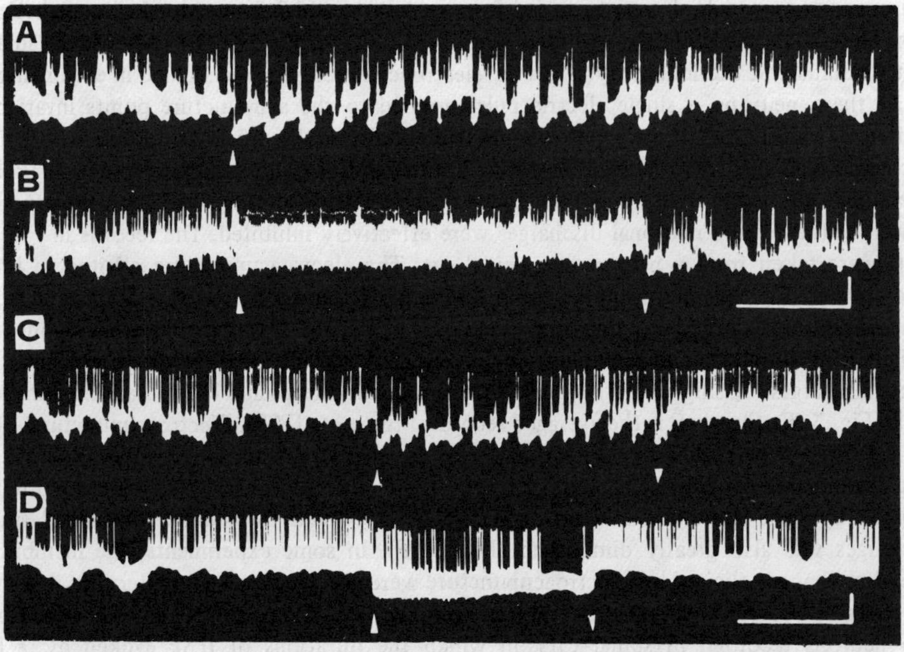

Fig. 5 The membrane potential changes evoked by electroacupuncture of different frequencies. A, B and C, D were recorded from two neurons respectively in spinal cats. Frequency of electroacupuncture: 5 Hz for A and C, 100 Hz for B and D. Intensity: 1.9 mA for A, B and 1.7 mA for C and D. Acupuncture points: Huantiao and Futu points for all records.

represented IPSPs from two neurons in anaesthetized cats, the durations of which were as long as 390 msec and 340 msec. In addition, the duration of IPSP in another neuron from an anaesthetized cat not shown in Fig. 4 was also longer than 400 msec. All these were much longer than those recorded from spinal cats. On the other hand, it is interesting to note that the duration of IPSP elicited by 5Hz electroacupuncture was longer than those by 2 Hz. This was observed in two neurons in which the IPSPs produced by electroacupuncture of the two frequencies were compared (Records A, C and B, D of Fig. 4).

Fig. 5 shows records from two neurons recorded from spinal cats with the effects of 5 Hz and 100 Hz electroacupuncture on the membrane potential compared. With the frequency of 5 Hz, each stimulus elicited a large IPSP and caused inhibition of the spike discharges (Records A and C). The 100 Hz electroacupuncture only induced a transient hyperpolarizing change in one neuron (Record B). This was obviously due to the inability of the neuronal pathway responsible for the production of IPSP to follow such a high frequency stimulus; while in another neuron, it could evoke, in a short period, a large persisting hyperpolarization of the membrane and produce inhibition of the spike discharges (Record D).

IV. DISCUSSION

The present study demonstrated that in cats lightly anaesthetized with chloralose, electrical stimulation of the acupuncture points effectively attenuated the response of lamina V type dorsal horn neurons to radiant heat. This inhibition was characterized by rapid onset, and by having no significant attenuation throughout the period of electroacupuncture and no detectable after-effects. These results were different from those of Pomeranz and his colleagues[2], where, according to these authors, a long latency and also a long after-effect of the inhibition were observed. We have never seen in our experiments any enhancement of inhibition resulting from long continuous application of electroacupuncture, nor have we observed significant after-effects after the cessation of acupuncture except in the one case mentioned above. The intensity and frequency of acupuncture used in the present study were comparable with those used in the Pomeranz study. Only the acupuncture points stimulated and the noxious stimuli were different in the two studies. The discrepancies might well be related to these factors.

The segmental interaction between the afferent impulses of electroacupuncture and radiant heat stimulus obviously plays an important role in the mechanism of inhibition revealed in the present study, because (1) the inhibition could also be demonstrated in spinal cats; (2) the cold block of the spinal cord or the transection of the dorsal half of the spinal cord did not completely eliminate the inhibitory effect. On the other hand, the possibility of indirect inhibition of dorsal horn neurons through the activation of descending inhibitory centers by electroacupuncture cannot be excluded. Though the relevent data are too limited to draw any definite conclusion, the following evidence still strongly indicates the possible involvement of the descending inhibition. (1) The inhibitory effect of electroacupuncture was reduced after the cold block of the spinal cord. (2) The adaptation to the 100 Hz electroacupuncture was more prominent in spinal cats. (3) The duration of IPSP evoked by electroacupuncture was shorter in spinal cats than in anaesthetized animals. Therefore, we are inclined to believe that in chloralose anaesthetized cats both segmental interaction and descending inhibition are involved in the mechanism. Pomeranz *et al*.,[2] claimed that no inhibitory effect of acupuncture could be seen in spinal cats, and postulated from this and their other observations that the inhibition may be related to the release of morphine-like substances from the pituitary gland. The inhibitory action of acupuncture observed in the present study, however, did not have a long latent period on after-effect, so it seems unlikely that the humoral factors play any major role in the inhibition.

In our previous study[1] it was observed that the duration of inhibition of electroacupuncture on the response of the spinocervical tract fibers was fairly short. The same phenomenon was also observed in intact and unanaesthetized cats (unpublished data). In all these experiments the frequency of electroacupuncture was 100 Hz. The results of the present study show that 3 out of 4 neurons observed in spinal cats were inhibited for only several dozen seconds with continuous electroacupuncture stimulation at the same frequency. In anaesthetized cats there was also marked adaptation, although its development was much slower than in spinal animals. The inhibitory effect of 5 Hz electroacupuncture was fairly persistent in both spinal or anaesthetized cats. In this respect the results of Lo *et al.*,[3] showing that electroacupuncture of 4–8Hz had stronger inhibitory effect than that of 60Hz on pain discharges of neurons in parafascicular nucleus of thalamus and Huang's conclusion of the superiority in analgesic effect of 2 Hz electroacupuncture over the 100 Hz one[4] are in accordance with what was observed in the present study.

In some of the 11 neurons from which intracellular recordings were made the membrane potential was relatively low, indicating that the neurons had been damaged during penetration. The data on these neurons, however, were also included, since the main tocos of this study was the IPSPs evoked by electroacupuncture and the depolarization of the membrane facilitates the detection of IPSPs.

Electroacupuncture elicited IPSPs in all 11 neurons. The IPSPs always appeared following an EPSP so that their latent period was difficult to determine, though most likely they were postsynaptic in nature. Hongo *et al.*,[5,6] has described polysynaptic long duration EPSPs and IPSPs in spinocervical neurons and interneurons which were elicited by the flexion reflex afferents (FRA). In addition, it was already known that stimulation of acupuncture points activated a large number of FRA[7].Thus it seems to be reasonable to postulate that the IPSPs evoked by electroacupuncture were probably mediated by FRA. The amplitude of these IPSPs sometimes reached 10 mV or even more, during which the initiation of spike discharges was prevented. When the electroacupuncture was delivered in 5 Hz or 10 Hz frequency, particularly in anaesthetized animals in which the duration of IPSP was very long, the evoked IPSPs often superimposed on to one another, forming a persisting hyperpolarizing change of the membrane accompanied by a profound inhibition of spike discharges. However, when the frequency was high, for example 100 Hz, the synaptic transmission in the polysynaptic pathway would be rapidly blocked by continuous stimulation. As a result of this, the IPSP could no longer be elicited and the inhibitory effect deteriorated rapidly except at the very beginning of stimulation. This phenomenon was particularly pronounced in spinal cats. Therefore, the inhibitory effect of electro-acupuncture observed with extracellular recordings may well be accounted for by postsynaptic inhibition of the dorsal horn neurons. This, however, does not necessarily mean that presynaptic inhibition do not take any part in the mechanism. Further study is certainly needed for clarification of this problem.

V. SUMMARY

The inhibitory effect of relatively long period electroacupuncture on the response of dorsal horn neurons to noxious heat stimuli was investigated in the chloralose-anaesthetized cat.

In the period of electroacupuncture of 15–20 minutes (5 Hz,<3 mA) applied to acupuncture points on the ipsilateral hind limb, the response of lamina V type dorsal horn neurons to noxious heat stimuli was continuously inhibited. About 74% of the neurons had the responses reduced to less than half of the control value. The inhibitory effect went pari passu with the progress of acupuncture stimulation, and underwent no significant change throughout the course of stimulation.

The intracellular recordings demonstrated that single pulse stimulation of the acupuncture points evoked an EPSP-IPSP sequence in dorsal horn neurons. The IPSP, being possibly polysynaptic in nature and having a long duration and a relatively large amplitude, could effectively inhibit the spike discharges elicited by noxious stimuli. Thus the inhibitory effect of electroacupuncture seemed to be closely related to the IPSP it produced in dorsal horn neurons.

In contrast to the long lasting stable inhibitory effect of 5 Hz electroacupuncture, the effect of 100 Hz stimulus tended to decrease gradually with time if the duration of application was prolonged. This adaptation phenomenon was particularly prominent in spinal cats. There were also preliminary data suggesting the involvement of both the segmental interaction and descending inhibition in the mechanism of inhibition produced by acupuncture stimuli.

REFERENCES

[1] Wu Chien-ping *et al.*: *Scientia Sinica*, **5**: 526, 1974.
[2] Pomeranz B *et al.*: *Exp. Neurol.*, **54**: 172, 1977.
[3] Lo Fu-sun *et al.*: in preparation.
[4] Huan Ye *et al.*: in preparation.
[5] Hongo T *et al.*: *Exp. Brain Res.*, **1**: 338, 1968.
[6] Hongo T *et al.*: *J. Physiol.*, **199**: 569, 1968.
[7] Wei Jen-Yü *et al.*: *Kexue Tongbao*, **4**: 184, 1973.

OBSERVATIONS ON OPERANT CONDITIONING AND SINGLE UNIT ACTIVITY OF THE PREFRONTAL CORTEX OF RHESUS MONKEYS DURING ACUPUNCTURE

Liu Jinlong*, Qi Dailin**, Han Xiangwen*,
Hou Gangxing***, Zhou Hui ju**, Jin Wenlong*,
Wang Zuoqing***, Yang Congguo***, Liu Zuozhou***
*(*Department of Physiology, Guangxi Medical College, Nanning)*
*(**Department of Physiology, Guiyang Medical College, Guiyang)*
*(***Department of Physiology, Third Medical College of PLA, Chongqing)*

The sensation of pain is an extremely complex process. It is not only related to the intensity of noxious stimulation, but is also influenced by other factors, such as the shift of attention, change of mental state, past experience with pain, etc. Operation under acupuncture anaesthesia is performed with the patient completely consciousness, so he is naturally affected by psychological factors. In fact acupuncture analgesia in the human body is mainly a sort of physiological effect, some recent investigations have suggested[1]. The mechanism by which psychological has yet factors work in acupuncture analgesia to be clarified, and so requires further investigations.

It is known that the prefrontal cortex is closely related to psychological activities and has, at the same time, some influence on the sensation of pain. Prefrontal lobotomy had at one time, been used clinically as a last resort to relieve intractable pain. After such an operation, although the pain does not disappear, nor is the threshold elevated, the patient would no longer feel the suffering coused by pain. It has been called the state of pain without suffering. This post operation effect was suggested to be the result of distraction and impairment of the ability to form appreciable emotional responses[2]. Therefore, it is not unreasonable to investigate whether the prefrontal cortex plays a role in the mechanism of acupuncture analgesia. In order to study this problem, experiments were made on conscious, movable monkeys by observing defensive operant conditioned reflexes evoked by noxious stimulation as an indication of pain. At the same time, unit activity was recorded from the prefrontal cortex to compare the behavioral observations with electro-physiological investigation.

I. METHODS

Twelve adolescent rhesus monkeys (Macaca mulatta), weighing from 3.5–5 kg were used.

1. Training of monkeys. The animal was seated in a restraining chair. A wick electrode moistened with saturated potassium chloride was placed on the distal third of the tail.

Noxious stimulation was produced by a 57–9D stimulator, from which direct current of graduated intensity increments beginning from zero intensity was delivered to the wick electrode. On the right side of the chair, there was a lever connected to the stimulator via a switch. If the monkey made a pull at the lever to turn on the switch, the stimulus intensity would immediately drop to zero, and simultaneously, an electric pulse would be delivered to the lower channel of a 2-trace oscillograph and a L_{323} 2-channel tape recorder to record the lever-pulling action. It usually required about 1–3 weeks' training for the monkey to form conditioned response.

2. Surgery. All animals underwent aseptic surgery under Nembutal anaesthesia (25–40 mg/kg intravenously). The scalp was incised and the skull over the dorsolateral prefrontal cortex was exposed. A hole approximately 5 mm in diameter was made in the bone that the dura mater was left intact. A pedestal was implanted over the hole and cemented to both the skull and anchoring stainless steel screws with dental acrylic resin.

3. Recording. Recording sessions started 7–10 days after the operation. A MWT-1 micromanipulator was mounted on the implanted pedestal. A tungsten microelectrode with a tip 1–3μm in diameter was inserted through the intact dura into the prefrontal cortex. The signal from the microelectrode was led into a JSD-731 AC amplifier via a FET-input and a negative capacity-compensated preamplifier. It was monitored on the upper trace of the oscillograph. The output of the amplifier was also recorded on the upper channel of the 2-channel tape recorder. All data were analysed from the taped records by a TQ-19 computer to obtain sequtential spike intensity histograms. The analogue output of the computer was plotted on a TZ6 plotter.

4. Testing procedures:

(1) When a prefrontal unit was isolated, the spontaneous unit discharges were recorded for 4–5 minutes;

(2) Graded DC current, single electric pulse (10 msec pulse duration, 30–40V) and a brief train of pulses (10 pulses at 10 Hz, 20–30V lasting for 1 sec) were applied to the wick electrode at the tail 4–5 times each, and the unit activity and the threshold of the conditioned response were recorded;

(3) Electroacupuncture with frequencies of 8–12 Hz was applied to Zusanli points bilaterally for 10–25 minutes, during which steps (1) and (2) were repeated;

(4) 5–10 minutes after cesstion of the electroacupuncture, steps (1) and (2) were repeated again.

II. RESULTS

1. The influence of acupuncture on operant conditioning. Before acupuncture, the stability of the threshold of the operant conditioned response was observed. Noxious stimulation was applied to the monkey's tail 4–5 times every five minutes. The mean value of these four or five trials was taken as the pain threshold of this five-minute period. It was found that during a period of 60–90 minutes, the variation of the pain threshold was not more than 25% of the mean value. When electroacupuncture was applied to Zusanli points bilaterally, the pain threshold rose gradually in 10–15 minutes. After cessation of the acupuncture, the pain threshold usually returned to its original value within 5–10 minutes.

A total of 47 tests was carried out, and the pain threshold was elevated 41.2% during acupuncture, ranging from 4.9–102.6%.

2. The influence of acupuncture on prefrontal unit activity:

(1) Observations on the spontaneous unit activity: The activity of 111 neurons in the pre-arcuate, post-arcuate, and principal sulcus areas was recorded (Fig.1). All these neurons

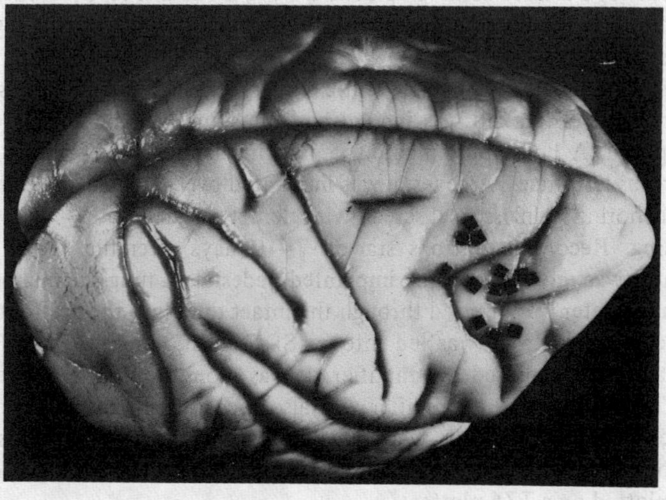

Fig. 1 Photograph of monkey's brain showing sites of electrode penetration on prefrontal cortical surface(black square).

had the property of spontaneous discharge, but wide differences existed between their rates: some neurons only made disconnected impulses at irregular intervals of several seconds, whereas others discharged at frequencies as high as 72 Hz. Of the 77 neurons located in the pre-arcuate and the principal sulcus areas, 8 (10.3%) made discharges at mean rates more than 10 Hz and 6 (7.8%) at mean rates lower than 1 Hz. The majority (81.9%) of them, however, made discharges at mean rates ranging from 1–10 Hz. Most of the neurons (82.4%) showed irregular isolated impulses, while the rest (17.6%) made discharges in bursts of 2–20 impulses at rates as high as from 600–800 Hz. Of the 34 neurons located in the post-arcuate area, 5 (14.6%) had discharge mean rates lower than 1 Hz, 25 (73.6%) discharged at mean rates ranging from 1–10 Hz, and 4 (11.8%) discharged in bursts. It seemed that there was no distinct difference in the types of spontaneous discharges between the pre- and post-arcuate areas. Still the neurons which were located in the same electrode track and were only several scores of microns apart may show wide varieties of discharge rates (Fig.2).

(2) The influence of noxious stimulation on unit activity.

(i) Effect of graded DC current applied to tail. 40 prefrontal neurons were studied during operant conditioning. Under the influence of noxious stimulation, most of the neurons (52.5%) increased their discharge rates greatly, and 6 of them increased 100–1000 per cent. Only 10 (25%) decreased their discharge rates. In some cases, diphasic responses, viz. a brief period of decrease in discharge rate followed by a long-term increment, or a brief increase followed by a long-term decrement, were observed. It was found that all

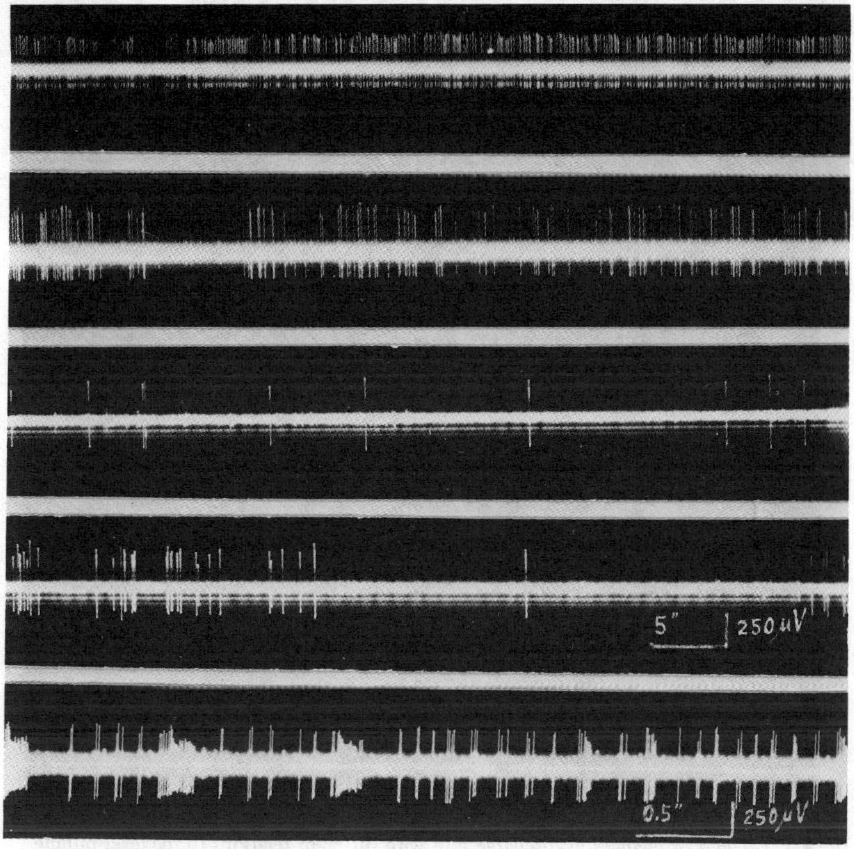

Fig. 2 Spontaneous discharges recorded from five prefrontal neurons located in the same electrode only several tens of microns apart.

the responses, including excitatory, inhibitory and diphasic, could last for a long period, from several seconds to scores of seconds. As to the relationship between changes in discharge rate and lever-pulling action, a wide variety of spike activity patterns existed in different neurons. As shown in Fig. 3, some neurons decreased or increased their discharge rate prior to the leverpulling action, while others failed to respond until the action started.

(ii) Effects of single and train stimulations. In order to study the temporal relationship between noxious stimulus and change in unit activity, a single electric pulse and/or a brief train of pulses were used in some cases. Of the 32 neurons examined, 11 increased their discharge rate in response to noxious stimulation, 9 decreased it, while that of the remaining 12 remained unchanged. Some of the neurons also showed diphasic responses. It was interesting to note that almost all the responses obtained, including excitatory, inhibitory, and diphasic responses, were mainly long-duration changes in the basic discharging rate rather than shortduration phasic reactions.

(3) Effect of electro-acupuncture.

(i) Effect on the spontaneous neurons discharge. In most neurons, the spontaneous

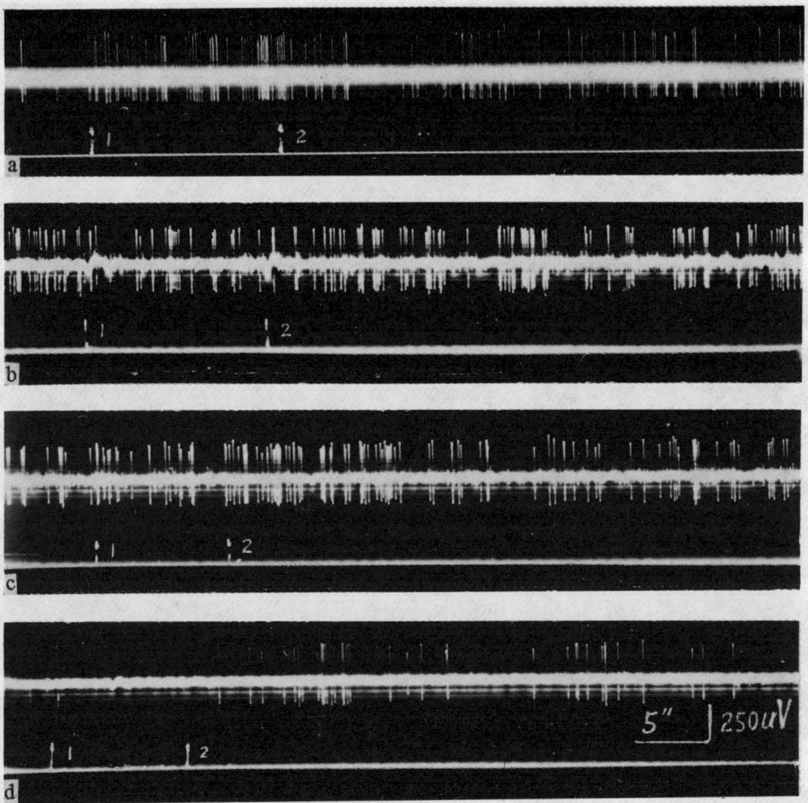

Fig. 3 Types of changes in discharge rate with different relations to the lever-pulling action in different neurons during operant conditioning;

a. firing rate increased prior to lever-pulling action,

b. firing rate decreased prior to lever-pulling action,

c. firing rate increased after lever-pulling action,

d. firing rate decreased prior to and increased after lever-pulling action;

upper turacings: unit discharges;
lower tracings: onset of stepwise direct current stimulation (1), and lever-pulling action (2) respectively.

dischargeing rate increased during electroacupuncture. Of 19 neurons tested, 11 (57.8%) increased from 50 to 800% of their original value, and 6 of them increasd to more than 100–800%. Only 4 of them decreased their discharge rate. It was discovered that there was no relationship between the effect induced by electroacupuncture stimulation and the level of the background spontaneous discharge rate of the neuron prior to the application of electro-acupuncture.

(ii) Effect on nociceptive response. As shown in Fig. 4, although the spontaneous discharge increased during electroacupuncture in most of the neurons tested, the discharge rate soon drop down, when a noxious stimulus was applied. In 55.6% of the neurons, it decreased to 1/2–1/10 of their original values. In only 26.9% of the neurons did it increased. Under the influence of electroacupuncture, the effect of noxious stimulation was weakened or even reversed. As shown in Fig. 4, an excitatory response was induced before electro-acupuncture, but the response disappeared 20 minutes after the aplication of acupuncture. An enhancement of the response was found only in rare cases.

As to the relationship between the changes in discharge rate of neurons and the elevation of the pain threshold, consistency was found only in certain cases, and all the rest showed no consistency. In addition, no difference in the effect of electro-acupuncture between the trained monkeys and the controls was found.

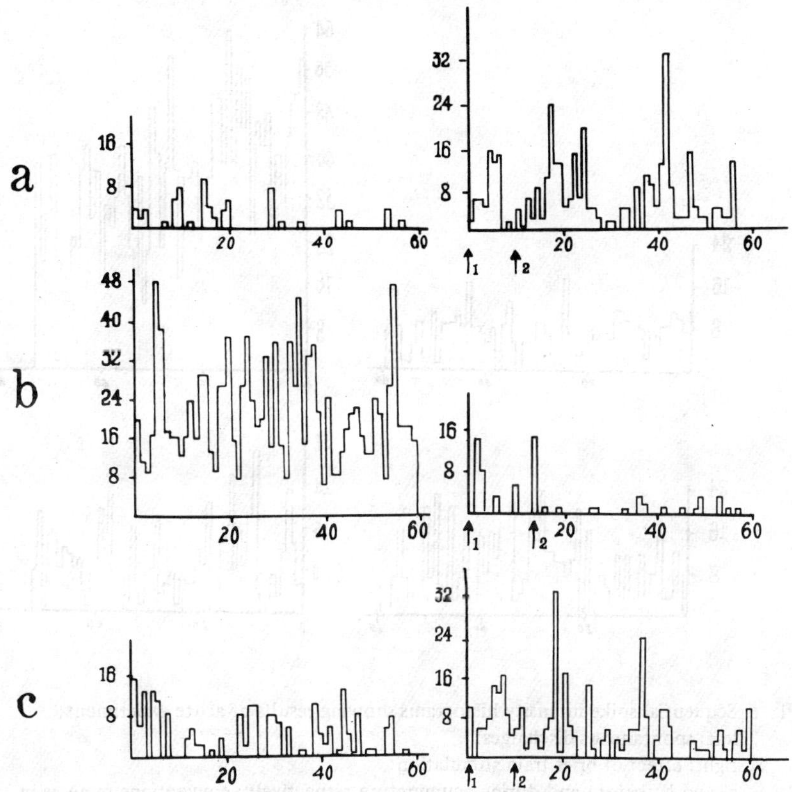

Fig. 4 Sequential spike intensity histograms showing influence of electroacupuncture on prefrontal unit activity;
left: spontaneous discharges;
right: effect of stepwise direct current stimulation;
a, b, and c: before, during and after electro-acupuncture, respectively;
each histogram constructed by four consecutive sweeps of 60 sec duration, with a bin width of one sec;
ordinate: number of impulses per second;
abscessa: time scales, 1 sec;
arrow 1: onset of stimulation;
arrow 2: lever-pulling action.

(4) Acute experiments: In order to determine whether the responses mentioned above were secondary to muscular activity, 25 neurons were isolated under acute conditions. The animals were paralyzed by Flaxedil administered intravenously, and experiments were carried out under artificial respiration. Most of the neurons examined, discharged solitary impulses at irregular intervals, and 15 fired in bursts. The results obtained were similar to those of the chronic experiments. As shown in Fig. 5, the discharge rate was increased in response to noxious stimulation, and during electroacupuncture spontaneous discharges were increased while nociceptive ones were significantly inhibited.

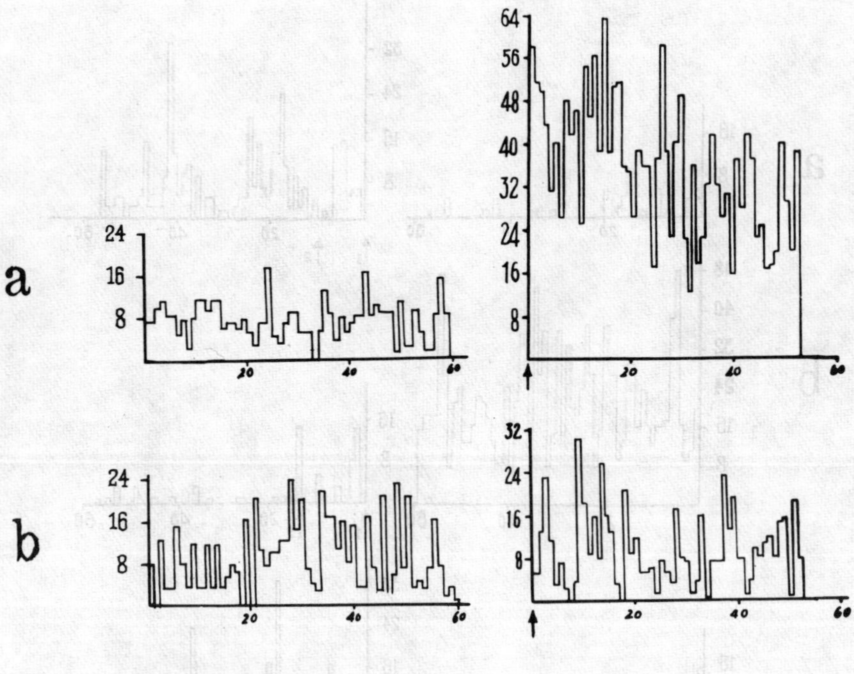

Fig. 5 Sequential spike intensity histograms showing results of acute experiment;
left: spontaneous discharges;
right: effect of brief train stimulation:
a, and b: before and during acupuncture respectively; conventions same as in previous figure.

3. Effect of Dolantin: When a small dose of Dolantin (0.5–2mg/kg I.M.) was given to a monkey, its pain threshold started to rise in 5–10 minutes, reaching its peak in 15–25 minutes, and then returned to its original level in about 40–90 minutes. The effect of Dolantin on prefrontal unit activity was studied in 5 monkeys. An increment of the spontaneous discharge rate and the inhibitory effect on nociceptive response were found in some cases after the administration of Dolantin. In rare cases, the effect of noxious stimulation was reversed.

III. DISCUSSION

At present, no physiologist has found a specific stimulus which can produce pain without any other sensation. Therefore, it is of great importance to establish reliable animal models for pain research. The results of the present study show that operant conditioning of the monkey can be used as an indication of pain for the study of acupuncture analgesia[3,4] because: (1) the threshold is comparatively stable; (2) higher nerve centers are involved in the response; and (3) the time course of the alterations in threshold induced by acupuncture is quite similar to that observed in patients in the clinic. During electro-acupuncture, the threshold rises gradually after a period of induction (about 10–30 minutes), and returns to its original level after cessation of acupuncture. It is reasonable to suggest that the operant conditioned response may be more reliable for reflecting actual pain sensation.

The results of electrophysiologicl experiments of this study show that the prefrontal unit activity is affected by noxious stimulation and acupuncture, because (1) in most neurons, spontaneous discharges are significantly increased under the influence of noxious stimulation; (2) during acupuncture, the spontaneous discharge rate also increases significantly in the vast majority of the prefrontal neurons, but their responses to noxious stimulation are weakened or even reversed.

It was reported that evoked potentials elicited by somatic stimulation were recorded in the pre- and post-arcuate areas of the prefrontal cortex in rhesus monkeys under acute conditions[5,6]; and that the dorsolateral prefrontal cortex was involved in processing kinesthetic information[7] and kinesthetic discrimination[8]. During delayed alternation performance in monkeys, some of the neurons located in the periprincipal region increased or decreased their discharge rate in response to the lever-pressing action. Such neurons were thought to be motor neurons in nature and might be related to the initiation or execution of the lever-pressing action[9]. So, it is reasonable to question whether the unit activity alterations observed in the present study are related to or induced by, muscle contractions. The data obtained show, however, that (1) there is no change in the discharge rate when the animal pulls the lever spontaneously in the absence of noxious stimulation; (2) in untrained animals, the change in unit activity can be evoked by noxious stimulation without lever-pulling actions, and (3) the effects of noxious stimulation and electroacupuncture still exist after the animal has been paralyzed by Flaxedil. Therefore, it seems that these changes are neither secondary to muscular activities nor directly related to the initiation or execution of voluntary movement. This interpretation is in accord ance with results reported recently[10].

On the other hand, the unit activity alteration induced by noxious stimulation is probably not a specific pain reaction, because in some cases no parallel correlations can be found in changes between the unit activity and the pain threshold. When the pain threshold has been elevated markedly by electro-acupuncture or Dolantin, changes in unit activity can still be produced by noxious stimulation. Besides, some other characteristics of the changes in unit activity, such as adaptation, long lasting reaction time (over several scores of seconds) etc. also indicate that these changes may not be directly related to pain.

It is widely accepted that the dorsolateral prefrontal cortex is not directly involved in sensory and motor control, but that it plays an important role in psychological activities, such as learning, short-term memory, attention, emotion, etc[11]. As mentioned above, the fact that there exists a wide diversity of spike activity patterns in different neurons in relation to the lever-pulling action, indicates that these neurons may have different physiological functions. It was reported that during delayed-response performance in monkeys a variety of changes in discharge rate could be found in different neurons and in different periods of the session. Prefrontal neurons were hence classified into six basic types according to the firing-frequency variations related to the principal periods of delayed-response trials (cue, delay, and response periods)[12]. Similar results were also reported by other authors[13,14,15,16]. Therefore, the unit activity alterations induced by noxious stimulation in the present study are probably related to psychological activities, which would account for the difference between the effect produced by graded DC current during operant conditioning and that produced by single and train stimulations. This is because, in the former condition, noxious stimulation will not stop until the animal actively pulls the lever demonstrating that psychological factors, especially learning, memory, attention desire, etc. are involved. According to the data obtained showing that electroacupuncture can increase the spontaneous discharge rate of prefrontal neurons and weaken or even reverse their responses to noxious stimulation, we suggest that the dorsolateral prefrontal cortex may play a role in the psychological aspect of the analgesic effect of acupuncture.

IV. SUMMARY

Experiments were carried out on 12 conscious and movable adolescent monkeys (Macaca mulatta). The animals, in a restraining chairs were trained to pull a lever to escape noxious electrical stimulation of the tail. The single unit activity was simultaneously recorded with a tungsten microelectrode in the dorsolateral prefrontal cortex. A total of 111 neurons were recorded in the pre-arcuate, post-arcuate and principal sulcus areas. Spontaneously active neurons were found in all the cortical areas explored, but their discharge rates varied widely. Under the influence of noxious stimulation, most of the neurons increased their discharge rate greatly. In some cases, diphasic responses, i.e. a brief period of decrease in the firing rate followed by a long-term increment, or a brief increase followed by a long-term decrement, could be seen. As to the relation between the changes of discharge rate and the action of lever-pulling, a wide diversity of spike activity patterns existed in different neurons; some decreasd or increased their discharge rate prior to the lever-pulling action and others failed to respond until the action had started. During acupuncture, the lever-pulling threshold, which was used as an indicator of pain, was increased within 10–30 minutes; the spontaneous discharge rate was also increased in most neurons, but it was not related to the level of back-ground activity. At the same time, the effect of noxious stimulation was also weakened or even reversed. Nevertheless, the change in the discharge frequency and the elevation of lever-pulling threshold sometimes showed no consistency. Similar results were also obtained from two rhesus monkeys paralyzed by Flaxedil under acute conditions. After administering Dolantin, both the threshold of operant avoidance and the spontaneous discharge frequency increased, and the response of some neurons to noxious stimulation was weakened or reversed. It was suggested that the dorsolateral prefrontal cortex may play a role in the psychological aspect of the analgesic effect of acupuncture.

REFERENCES

[1] 江振裕等：动物学报，24：1，1978。

[2] White, J.C. and Sweet, W.H.: Pain and Neurosurgeon: A Forty Year Experience, Charlos Thomas, Springfield, Illinois, 1969.

[3] Sandrew, B.B.: *Fed. Proc.*, **36**:561, 1977.

[4] 黄 晔等：中华医学杂志，**4**：193，1978。

[5] Bignall, K.E. and Imbert, M.: *EEG. Clin. Neurophysiol.*, **26**:206, 1969.

[6] Бамуеь, А.С. Лиротоь, А.А. и Орлоь, А.А. Неирофизиолотия 9:437. 1977.

[7] Manning, F.J.: *Brain Res.*, **149**:77, 1978.

[8] Mishkin, M. *et al.*: *Ibid.*, **130**:163, 1977.

[9] Kubota, K. and Niki, H.: *J. Neurophysiol.*, **34**:337, 1971.

[10] Sakai, M.: *Brain Res.*, **147**:377, 1978.

[11] Brutkowski, S.: *Physiol. Rev.*, **45**;721, 1965.

[12] Fuster, J.M.: *J. Neurophysiol.*, **36**:61, 1973.

[13] Kubota, K. *et al.*: *Ibid.*, **37**:1197, 1974.

[14] Niki, H.: *Brain Res.*, **68**: 197, 1974.

[15] Sakai, M.: *Ibid.*, 81:297, 1974.

[16] Niki, H. and Watanabe, M.: *Ibid.*, **105**:79, 1976.

ANALGESIC EFFECTS OF SEVERAL MODES OF ELECTROACUPUNCTURE IN MONKEYS AND THEIR REVERSAL BY NALOXONE

Huang Ye, Wang Qingwei, Zheng Jinze,
Li Derong, Xie Guoyang

(Shanghai Brain Research Institute, Academia Sinica)

Previously we have established a model of operant lever-pressing responses evoked by nociceptive stimuli in rhesus monkey (Macaca mulatta), on which the analgesic effects of distant and adjacent segmental electroacupuncture and their time course were observed and compared. Recently we have shown that the analgesic effects of adjacent and distant segmental electroacupuncture would be partially or entirely blocked by injection of naloxone, a morphine-receptor blocking agent. This suggested that the electroacupuncture might activate a pain-inhibiting system which released endogenous morphine-like substances to inhibit the pain sensation and, in the case of distant segmental electroacupuncture, that this system might play an even more important role. The aim of the present study is to compare the analgesic effect of electroacupuncture at a homo-segmental point with that at distant and adjacent segmental points, in order to test the reversal action of naloxone on the analgesic effect of homo-segmental electroacupuncture. This study will also discuss the possible mechanisms involved in various modes of electroacupuncture analgesia.

I. METHODS

18 monkeys weighing 4–8 kg were used in the present investigation. In the case of adjacent segmental and homo-segmental analgesia, the nociceptive stimulus was applied to the medial surface of the forearm which is innervated by the medial cutaneous nerve and in the case of distant segmental analgesia, to the skin area of the lower extremity innervated by the saphenous nerve. After the operant conditioning reflexes to nociceptive stimuli were established, the response time was usually about the same whether the nociceptive stimulus was delivered to the upper or the lower extremity. In order to prevent tolerance of electroacupuncture, intervals of 7–10 days were allowed between experimental sessions. Details of the experimental methods of adjacent and distant segmental electroacupuncture analgesia were described in previous articles[1,2]. The homo-segmental electroacupuncture was delivered through a pair of stainless steel needles of 1 cm long, insulated along the tips and inserted into the skin. One needle was directed perpendicularly to the medial cutaneous

nerve and the other was inserted 1 cm away. The criteria for the correct location of the needles were as follows: (1) Electrical stimulation through the needles significantly prolonged the response time. (2) The response was immediately resumed on cessation of electro-acupuncture. A "Pe-Hong" electronic stimulator was used for electro-acupuncture. The stimulation frequency was 80 Hz and the current intensity was adjusted between 2–8 mA. The experimental procedure was similar to that of adjacent segment electro-acupuncture.

II. RESULT

1. Measurement of the pain response time in monkeys. In order to acquire stable response times, we took the threshold current intensity plus 0.5 mA as the intensity of pain-testing stimulus. This varied slightly from animal to animal but was generally about 1.5 mA. The response time was fairly stable during experimental sessions. The mean values in 18 monkeys during 21 experimental sessions lasting from 2.5 to 5 hours each were 0.8–0.92 sec as shown in Fig. 1.

The variation of the response time was independent of the duration of experimental sessions. For many animals it was less than 0.2 seconds during the whole experimental session. Only in certain animals was it slightly longer; still it did not exceed 1 sec. These results seem to be similar to those obtained from the monkey behaviour experiments by Sandrew[3].

2. Effect of electro-acupuncture and injection of Fentanyl on the response time. Electro-acupuncture of appropriate intensity had an analgesic effect. During the application of electro-acupuncture, 9 out of 10 monkeys showed a lengthening of the response time of up to 15 sec. In addition to lengthening the response time, the lever-pressing action became slower and its strength weaker. But in the same animal the analgesic effect of electro-acupuncture might vary greatly from time to time. As soon as a stable operant conditioning response had been established in a monkey, it could differentiate definitely the nociceptive stimulus from the stimulation of electro-acupuncture. Within certain intensity ranges of electro-acupuncture, the animals were usually quiet, neither lifting legs nor pressing the lever. However, if the intensity of electro-acupuncture was suddenly raised to an unbearable level, the monkey would press the bar repeatedly and even struggle violently.

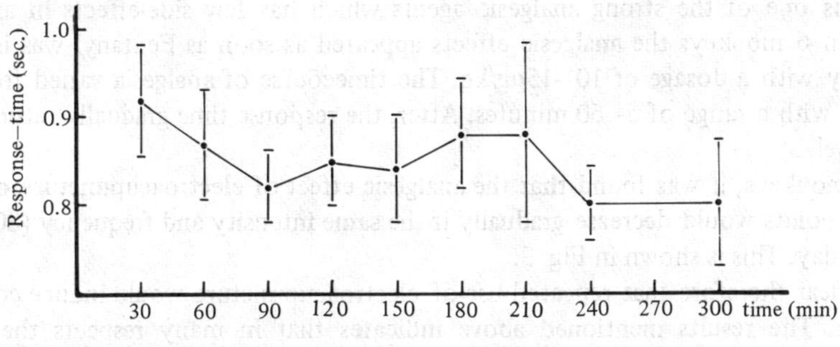

Fig. 1 The range of variation of response-time in experimental sessions.

When that happened, the intensity was immediately lowered. Usually the appropriate intensity of electroacupuncture for bringing about satisfactory analgesic effect would cause some excitation in the first 2–5 minutes of application. This was shown by frequent random lever-pressing and even some struggling. Then, along with adaptation to the intensity of electroacupuncture , analgesia gradually manifested itselt. In addition, both 2 Hz and 80 Hz electroacupunctures would have significantly sedative effects, such as decreasing random lever-pressing activity, slowing down and deepening respiration, and the closing of eyes. With the advance of time, the animal would become sleepy and drowsy. However, as soon as the electroacupuncture stopped, the animal would immediately recover as shown by EEG changes (see Fig. 2).

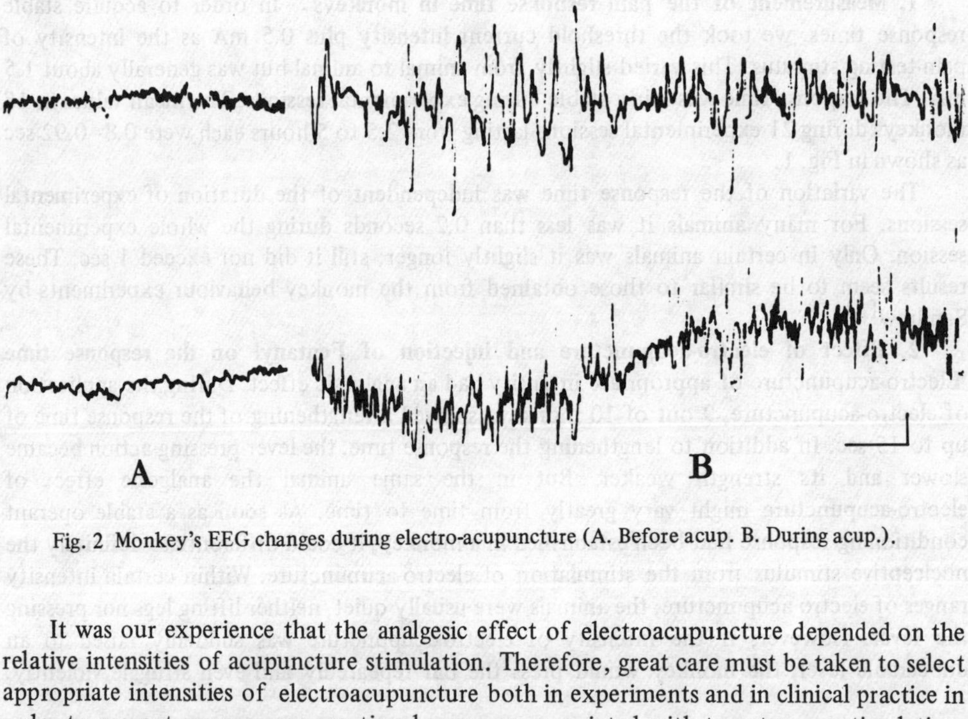

Fig. 2 Monkey's EEG changes during electro-acupuncture (A. Before acup. B. During acup.).

It was our experience that the analgesic effect of electroacupuncture depended on the relative intensities of acupuncture stimulation. Therefore, great care must be taken to select appropriate intensities of electroacupuncture both in experiments and in clinical practice in order to prevent unnecessary emotional responses associated with too strong a stimulation. Fentanyl is one of the strong analgesic agents which has few side-effects in animals. As observed in 6 monkeys the analgesic effects appeared as soon as Fentanyl was injected intravenously with a dosage of 10–15μg/kg. The timecourse of analgesia varied from animal to animal, with a range of 5–60 minutes. After, the response time gradually returned to the control level.

In 5 monkeys, it was found that the analgesic effect of electroacupuncture of adjacent segmental points would decrease gradually if the same intensity and frequency (80 Hz) were used everyday. This is shown in Fig. 3.

It is clear therefore that repeated use of electroacupuncture would induce conspicuous adaptation. The results mentioned above indicates that in many respects the effect of electroacupuncture is very similar to that of morphine-like substances.

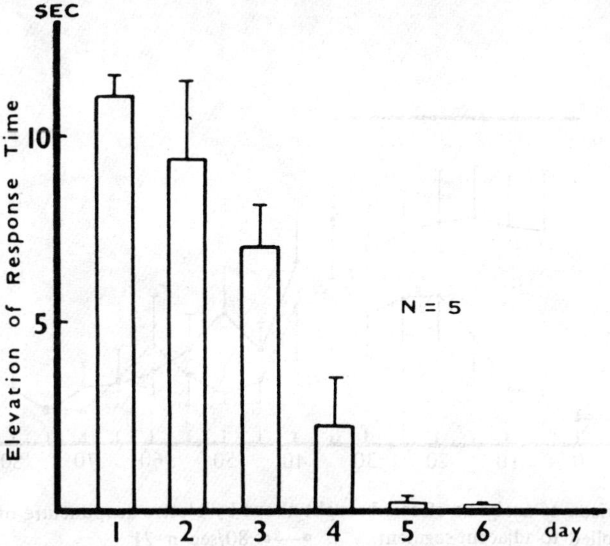

Fig. 3 Electro-acupuncture tolerance.

Table 1. Comparison of Analgesic Effects of Electroacupuncture with Two Frequencies on Adjacent and Distant Pain Sources

No. of Animals	No. of Expt.	Freq. of Electro-acup. & Site of Pain Source		Analgesic Effect	P Value
7	14	Adjacent Segment	2/sec	2.48 ± 0.85sec	< 0.01
			80/sec	6.96 ± 1.08 sec	
6	10	Distant Segment	2/sec	4.39 ± 1.40 sec	< 0.05
			80/sec	2.16 ± 0.76 sec	
7	9	2/sec	Distant Segment	4.22 ± 1.36 sec	< 0.05
			Adjacent Segment	1.80 ± 0.75 sec	
7	9	80/sec	Distant Segment	1.41 ± 0.70 sec	< 0.05
			Adjacent Segment	4.41 ± 1.60 sec	

Analgesic Effect= (Pain Response-time During Electroacupuncture) – (Pain Response-time in Control Period).

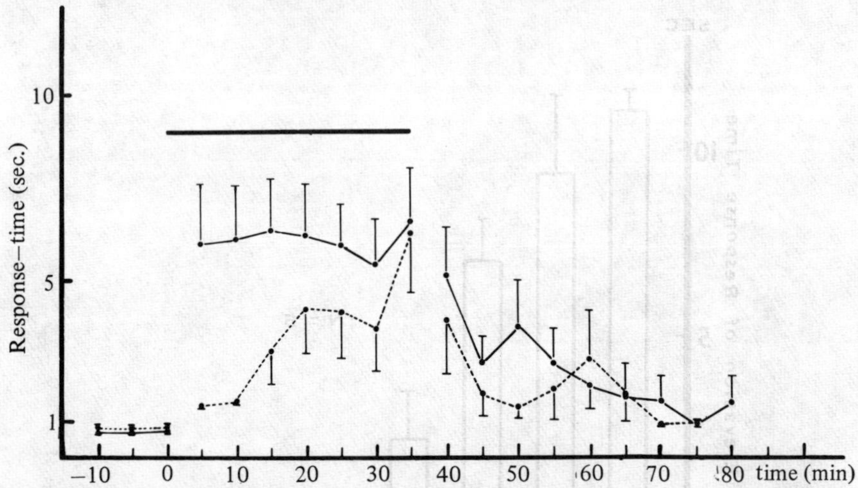

Fig. 4 Comparison of analgesic effects brought about by electro-acupuncture of two different frequencies applied to adjacent segment. •—• 80/sec n=21 •.....• 2/sec n=15 — acup.

3. Analgesic effects of adjacent- and distant-segmental electro-acupunctures with different frequencies

(1) Comparison of analgesic effects: For the purpose of comparison, the experiments were carried out in two groups: In the first group only the frequency of electroacupuncture was changed, with the site of nociceptive stimulation kept constant, and in the second group only the sites of nociceptive stimulation changed with the frequency of electroacupuncture fixed. The results obtained, shown in Table 1, indicate that the analgesic effect of electroacupuncture is dependent on the segmental relationship of the site of nociceptive stimulation with respect to that of acupuncture stimulus. Under our experimental conditions, an adequate frequency for adjacent-segmental electroacupuncture was found to be 80 Hz and that for distant-segmental electroacupuncture was 2 Hz. The results also indicate that with the frequency of 2 Hz, the analgesic effect of distal segmental electro-acupuncture was stronger than that of an adjacent one, while with the frequency of 80 Hz, the effect of the latter was stronger.

(2) Comparison of the timecourse of analgesia: Electroacupuncture of an adjacent-segmental point at 80 Hz for 5 min increased response time to 5.88–1.60 sec (M.±S.E.) as compared with 0.6 sec for the control (Fig. 4).

The increased response time remained at this level throughout the 15 minutes period of electroacupuncture. In 5 experiments the response time even exceeded 15 sec. After cessation of electroacupuncture, the response time began to be reduced and returned to about one half of the maximum value within 10 minutes. The aftereffect lasted for about 40 minutes. In 11 out of 15 experiments the response time showed no change whatsoever after 5 minutes of electroacupuncture at 2 Hz. 10 minutes later it began to rise gradually to the mean value of 4.10 ± 1.27 sec, then it tended to decrease. At 35 minutes, however, it rose again to 6.19 ± 1.68 sec. The aftereffect also lasted about 40 minutes.

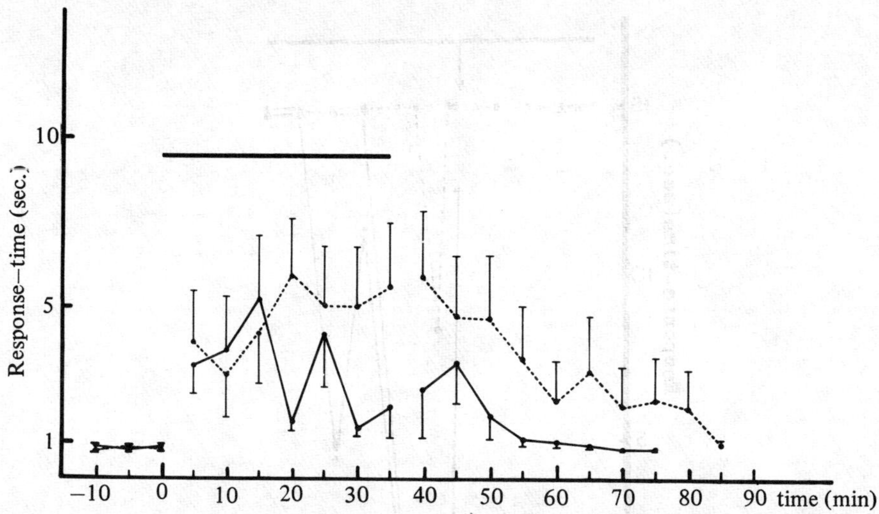

Fig. 5 Comparison of analegesic effects brought by electro-acupuncture of two different frequencies applied to distant segment.
●—● 80/sec n=10
●.....● 2/sec n=12 — acup.

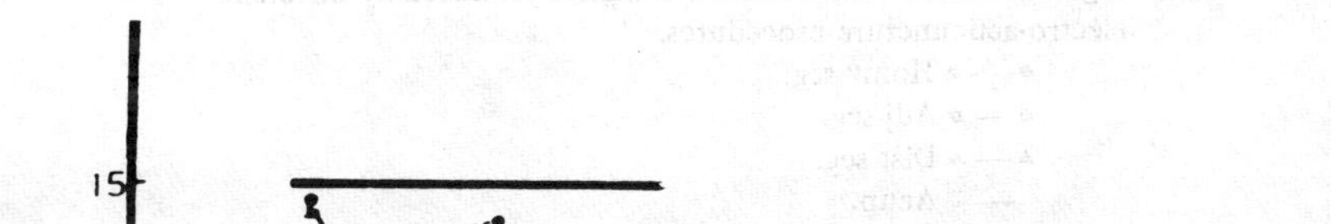

Fig. 6 Comparison of analgesic effect of electro-acupuncture applied to home-, adjacent and distant segments. ●.....● Homv-seg — Adj. seg. ▲—▲ Dist. seg. — acup.

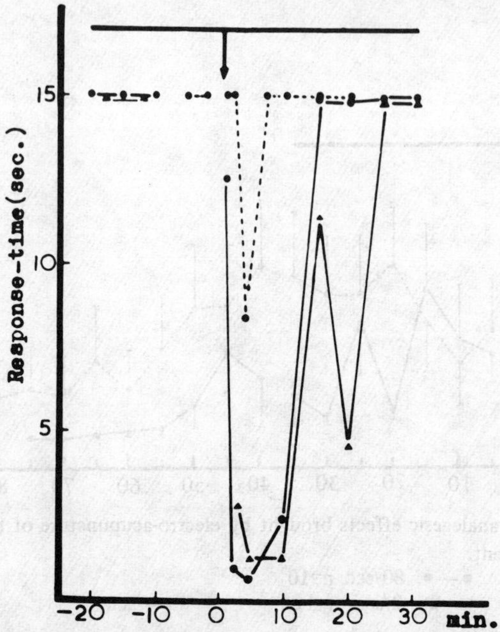

Fig. 7 Effects of naloxone on analgesia produced by different electro-acupuncture procedures,

●- - - ● Homv seg.
●—● Adj seg.
▲—▲ Dist seg.
—— Acup.
↓ Naloxone

After 5 minutes of distant segmental electroacupuncture at 80 Hz, in 8 out of 10 experiments the response time was lengthened having a mean value of 3.28 ±0.82 sec. After 15 minutes it rose to 5.31±1.82 sec and decreased rapidly afterwards. Its aftereffect lasted for about 20 minutes. On the other hand, after 5 minutes of distant segmental electroacupuncture at 2 Hz, the response time in 10 out of 12 experiments was increased, with a mean value of 3.97±1.48 sec. After 20 minutes it attained to a new height (5.99±1.63 sec). 50 minutes after the end of electro-acupuncture, the response time gradually returned to its control level (Fig. 5.)

As mentioned previously, the analgesic effect of electroacupuncture applied to a given point was closely related to both the site of pain with respect to the point and the frequency of electroacupuncture. In both adjacent- and distant-segmental electroacupuncture at 80Hz, stimulation for 5 minutes was sufficient to bring about a certain analgesic effect which could be maintained for a certain period. On the other hand, in the case of distant segmental electroacupuncture at 2 Hz, an induction period of 20 minutes was necessary to bring about a satisfactory analgesic effect, and the aftereffect would last longer than that of the electroacupuncture at 80 Hz with the same intensity. These data may be of valve to the study of the mechanism of acupuncture analgesia as well as to the proper selection of different modes of electroacupuncture in clinical practice.

4. Analgesic effect of homo-segmental electroacupuncture and its timecourse. Since the distribution of monkey's cutaneous nerves varies individually, for homo-segmental electroacupuncture the position of the medial cutaneous nerve of the forearm must be carefully identified first. As soon as it was correctly located and stimulated, the response time immediately and notably lengthened. In general, the intensity of electroacupuncture was adjusted within the range of 2–8 mA. With optimal intensity, the analgesic effect of homo-segmental electroacupuncture at 80 Hz was greater than that of adjacent- and distant-segmental ones and almost no induction period was necessary. However, the analgesic effect tended to decrease gradually with the lapse of time owing probably to adaptation. Fig.6 shows the differences in analgesic effects and their time course among the same, adjacent- and distant-segmental electroacupuncture with the same frequency and optimal (bearable to the animal) intensity. It appears that different modes of stimulation produced different degrees of analgesic effects with different underlying mechanisms.

5. Effect of naloxone on homo-segmental electroacupuncture analgesia. 13 experiments were carried out on seven monkeys. An analgesic effect which made the response time longer than 15 sec was produced by electroacupuncture of appropriate intensity at 80 Hz. Then a dose of naloxone (0.05–0.1mg/kg) was injected intravenously. Three experiments showed no reversal of analgesia and the other 10 experiments showed a partial reversal which was less than that found in analgesia by adjacent segmental electroacupuncture. The timecourse of reversal was also shorter than that in the adjacent-segmental test on the same animal. Fig.7 shows the degree and timecourse of the reversal of homo-, adjacent- and distant-segmental electroacupuncture analgesia by equal doses of naloxone, of these, the reversal of distant segmental analgesia was the greatest in degree and the longest in duration, while that of homo-segmental analgesia was the least and the shortest.

III. DISCUSSION

We have established an operant conditioning reflex model in monkeys for nocuous stimulation which we think is method close to natural conditions. In fact, what is presented here in this paper is fairly similar to what we have observed in the clinic about the rules of electro-acupuncture analgesia. Furthermore, results obtained from this model also agree with those from acute animal experiments, i.e. that pain in any part of the body may be more effectively inhibited by stimulation of a nerve which belongs to the same segment as the nerve innervating the area of pain[6].

Previously we have found hyperalgesia caused by naloxone in this model[2]. In this respect, results reported by various authors did not seem to agree with one another, This probably happened because after injections of naloxone some authors did not make pain-tests in time and follow carefully the time course of variation of pain response, or because under normal conditions the endorphine system was in a resting state and the endogenous morphine-like substances were insufficient.

Stimulation of the same, adjacent- and distant-segmental points with electroacupuncture of appropriate intensities produces analgesic effects with different timecourse and aftereffects. For homo-segmental electroacupuncture analgesia, almost no induction period is needed. But for distant-segmental electroacupuncture analgesia, an induction period of about 20 min is generally indispensable. Duration of the aftereffects also differs from one to another. Furthermore, the reversals of the same, adjacent- and distant-segmental analgesia in a given animal by naloxone of the same dosage are different both in degree and in timecourse. Hence mechanisms involved in the same and distant segmental analgesia might not be the same In addition the quantities of released endogenous morphine-like substances and the amounts of receptors and the patterns of nervous circuits involved in each case may not be the same. It was reported[2] that the endorphine system seemed more important in analgesia by distant segmental electro-acupuncture of 2 Hz. We have found that the reversal of the homo-segmental electroacupuncture analgesia by naloxone seems rather weak, a fact probably due to the lack of enkephalinergic fibers among the primary afferent nerve fibers[7] and to the poor activation of the endorphine system when the homo-segmental nerve is stimulated. Nevertheless, the reversal of the analgesia of long duration homo-segmental electroacupuncture by naloxone is more significant. Such analgesia also has certain aftereffects. These facts suggest that long duration stimulation of homo-segmental nerves may activate the endorphine system to some degree.

In addition, we have found, unexpectedly, that for a few animals (monkeys Nos. 1 and 3) which had received electroacupuncture for a long time, a very small dose of naloxone (0.05mg/kg) was sufficient to give rise to significant and long-lasting reversals. It seems that repeated experiments with nociceptive stimuli and electroacupuncture made the experimental environment itself a conditioning stimulus for releasing endogenous morphine-like substances. Under such circumstances, the endogenous morphine-like substances released may be more than normal, so a half dosage of naloxone should be sufficient to reverse the analgesia. Therefore it seems to us from the present experiments that the activation of endorphine system depends on the mode of electroacupuncture and perhaps also on the environment.

IV. SUMMARY

Operant lever-pressing responses evoked by nociceptive stimuli were established in rhesus monkeys (Macaca mulatta). The degree and the duration of the analgesic effect of electro-acupuncture at two different frequencies were taken as criteria to assess the relative effectiveness of analgesia of adjacent-, distant- and homo-segmental electroacupuncture. In the case of the stimulation of a distant-segmental point, a better effect was achieved with lower frequency (2 Hz) after an induction period of 20 minutes. The aftereffect lasted for half an hour after the termination of electroacupuncture. However, the case of stimulation of the adjacent-segmental point with the higher frequency (80 Hz) had apparently better analgesic effects, although its aftereffect was less pronounced than that in the distant segmental case. If stimulating pulses of 80 Hz were delivered directly to the cutaneous nerve innervating the skin area where nociceptive stimuli were applied, the analgesic effect was even more pronounced than that in the adjacent-segmental case. Such effect emerged almost immediately, without any period of induction, and no aftereffect could be observed.

After an intravenous injection of 0.05–0.1mg/kg naloxone, the analgesic effect of electroacupuncture was reversed. The reversal of the analgesic effect of homo-segmental electroacupuncture appeared less significant than that of the distant and adjacent segmental electroacupuncture. The result also shows that electroacupuncture can produce effects similar in many respects to morphine-like substances, such as analgesia, sedation, tolerance and synchronization in EEG. Therefore it is suggested that endogenous morphine-like substances may play an important role in the process of acupuncture analgesia especially when the distant- and adjacent-segmental acupuncture points are used. For analgesia by homo-segmental electroacupuncture, this may not be so important since the reversal of analgesia by naloxone in this case was not significant.

REFERENCES

[1] 上海生理研究所针麻组：针刺麻醉，**1**：106，1978。

[2] 黄　晔等：中华医学杂志，(**4**)：193，1978。

[3] Sandrew BB *et al.*: *Arch. Int. Pharmacodyn.*, **231**:274, 1978.

[4] 上海市第一人民医院等：中华外科杂志，(**1**)：19，1977。

[5] 上海生理研究所第二研究室针麻组：中华医学杂志，(**5**)：340，1975。

[6] 吴建屏等：中国科学 (**5**)：526，1974。

[7] Lars Terenius: *Toxicol.*, **18**: 189, 1978.

RELATIONSHIP BETWEEN NUCLEUS RAPHE MAGNUS AND HIGHER BRAIN REGIONS IN INHIBITION OF VISCERO-SOMATIC REFLEXES

Du Huanji , Zhao Yanfang

(Shanghai Brain Research Institute, Academia Sinica)

I. INTRODUCTION

It was shown in early work that electroacupuncture had an obvious inhibitory effect on visceral nociceptive reactions of cats[1] and that the supraspinal neural structures were necessary for this effect[2–4]. The results also showed that lesion in the nucleus raphe magnus (Rm) and its adjacent medial reticular formation of the medulla oblongata could almost completely eliminate the inhibitory effect of electroacupuncture on the viscero-somatic reflex (VSR), while lesions in other raphe nuclei could not[3]. The analgesic effects of acupuncture were also significantly reduced following electrolytic lesions of Rm or microinjection of 5, 6-dihydroxytryptamine into Rm[5].

It was further found that electrical stimulation of Rm and its adjacent ventrolateral reticular formation had inhibitory effect on VSR and other visceral nociceptive reactions, and that the inhibitory effects caused by both brain stimulation and electroacupuncture disappeared after bilateral sectioning of the dorsolateral funiculi[6]. It was thus inferred that the Rm might take an active part in the modulation of nociceptive inputs in the spinal cord[3–6]. In addition, available evidence indicates that a number of higher regions of the brain, such as the periaqueductal grey[7], the central tegmental tract[8], the nucleus centrum medianum[9], the head of caudate nucleus[10–12] and the nucleus accumbens[13], are also involved in the acupunctural analgesia. On the other hand, some neural structures (e.g. the locus coeruleus) are regarded as antagonistic to acupunctural analgesia[14–15]. The aim of the present investigation is to find out the functional relationship between Rm and the other brain regions in the process of acupuncture analgesia.

II. METHODS

Experiments were performed on cats. Surgical procedures were done under ether anaesthesia. The animals were immobilized with Flaxedil and maintained on artificial respiration. Observation was started four hours after removal of ether (in detail see [1,16]).

The central end of the splanchnic nerve was stimulated by a train of electric pulses (0.2 msec, 20–25 Hz, 5 sec) and the repetitive VSR were elicited and recorded from the ipsilateral 11th intercostal nerve. The intensity of stimulus was supramaximal, generally over 5 volts. In addition to the VSR, the stimuli elicited a pressor reflex and a galvanic skin reflex (decrease in skin resistance). All these physiological events were recorded on a pen-writing polygraph. These reflexes were usually regarded as visceral nociceptive reactions[1,6]. Since both the ascending visceral nociceptive inputs and the VSR can be inhibited in the same manner by electroacupuncture[17], it seems relevant to regard the changes in VSR as a reflection of the central transmission of the visceral nociceptive messages.

The ipsilateral points Yanglingchuan and Fengshi were selected for electroacupuncture. Repetitive pulses (0.2 msec, 100 Hz, 10 sec) delivered to the common peroneal nerve were also used to mimic electroacupuncture. The optimal intensity was determined by the activation of low threshold group III (or A-delta) afferent fibres, and the action potential of the nerve was monitored simultaneously on an oscilloscope[18].

In the experiment of brain stimulation, the cat's head was routinely mounted onto a stereotaxic apparatus and the nuclei of the brain were identified according to an available cat's atlas. A concentric electrode, consisting of an outer tube of 0.5 mm diameter and an inner wire of 0.1 mm diameter which except for the tip was insulated, was used for brainstem and diencephalon stimulation. A bipolar electrode consisting of two insulated needles (0.32 mm diameter) separated by 1 mm was used for telencephalon stimulation. The parameters of stimuli were as follows: pulse width, 0.2 msec; frequency, 100 Hz; train duration, 10 sec. The brain stimulation was given 5 sec before the splanchnic stimulation. The intensity varied in the range of 0.1–2.0 mA according to the brain regions stimulated (see below). The stimulated sites were marked by Prussian blue reaction method for histological examination. The extent of the brain and the spinal lesions was also examined histologically. Further details of methodology have been described in a previous paper[6].

III. RESULTS

(I) Inhibitory effect of brain stimulation on VSR

We have systematically stimulated the brainstem and extensive areas in the forebrain to observe the effect on VSR.

1. General features of effects of brain stimulation on VSR

(1) The nature of the effect on VSR produced by brain stimulation was mostly inhibitory. Sometimes, the inhibition of the VSR was accompanied by inhibition of pressor reflex and/or galvanic skin reflex[6,19,20]. However, when some regions in the telencephalon were stimulated, a facilitatory effect on the VSR (sometimes also the other two reflexes) could be seen[20].

(2) Generally speaking, the more rostral the stimulation site, the higher the threshold for production of the inhibitory effect. For example, the threshold in Rm was generally lower than 0.1 mA, in the periaqueductal grey 0.15–0.2 mA, in the nucleus centrum medianum 0.2–0.3 mA and in the telencephalon, mostly over 1.0 mA.

(3) Under the present conditions, the inhibition of VSR elicited by stimulation of the lower brainstem, especially the Rm, occurred rapidly and also disappeared rapidly after the stimulus ceased. On the contrary, the inhibition elicited by stimulation of the higher brain

regions, especially the thalamus and telencephalon, appeared to be a very slow process both in development and decay stages.

(4) The inhibitory effect of brain stimulation and that of acupuncture were found to be able to potentiate each other[6]. This same effect was produced by brain stimulation and morphine, and by acupuncture and morphine.

2. Inhibitory effect of different raphe nuclei. For the purpose of comparison, the intensity of stimulus for raphe nuclei was kept in a range of 0.1–0.2 mA. The inhibitory effects of stimulation of different raphe nuclei were found to be very different. Rm stimulation showed the strongest inhibitory effect. However, the inhibitory effects of the nucleus raphe palladus, nucleus linealis rostralis and intermedialis, nucleus raphe obscurus, nucleus raphe centralis superior and nucleus raphe pontis decreased progressively in that order. No inhibitory effect could be observed in stimulation of the nucleus raphe dorsalis (see Fig. 1A and B).

3 Distribution of inhibition sites in various brain regions. Owing to the great variation of the threshold in different brain regions, we had to use different stimulus intensity for different brain regions to map the distribution of the inhibition points. The results, as shown in Fig. 1A, B, and C, were obtained from experiments in which stimulus strengths of 0.1–0.2 mA, 0.15–0.3 mA and 1–2 mA were used respectively. The inhibitory effects were classified according to the degree of reduction in amplitude of the VSR caused by brain stimulation. Details of the classification have been given elsewhere[6]. According to the distribution of the strong and moderate inhibition points in the brain, three kinds of inhibition areas can be identified:

(1) Dense area: Rm, the tractus tegmentalis centralis, the septum and nucleus accumbens.

(2) Less dense area: The medial part of medullary reticular formation, the nucleus raphe palladus, the midbrain reticular formation, the lateral part of the periaqueductal grey, the ventral part of the nucleus centrum medianum, the area preoptica-hypothalami, the head of the nucleus caudatus and the capsula interna.

(3) Scattered area: The lateral part of medullary reticular formation, the pontic reticular formation, the midbrain raphe nuclei (except the nucleus raphe dorsalis), the ventral tegmental nucleus of Tsai, the nucleus ruber, the rostral portion of the gyrus cinguli, the nucleus amygdala.

Therefore, judging from the distribution of the inhibition site and the threshold for inhibition, we find that the Rm is apparently the structure which is most directly involved in the inhibitory effect in the brain regions explored. The tractus tegmentalis centralis and its adjacent periaqueductal grey are effective regions for inhibition of VSR in the upper brainstem. The septum, the nucleus accumbens, the capsula interna and the head of the nucleus caudatus are relatively effective regions in the telencephalon.

(II) Effect of lesion in Rm on inhibition of VSR produced by brain stimulation

In early experiments, we noticed that the inhibitory effects of midbrain stimulation on the VSR were greatly decreased following a Rm lesion. It was then assumed that the diminution of the inhibitory effect following the Rm lesion was probably due to interruption of the

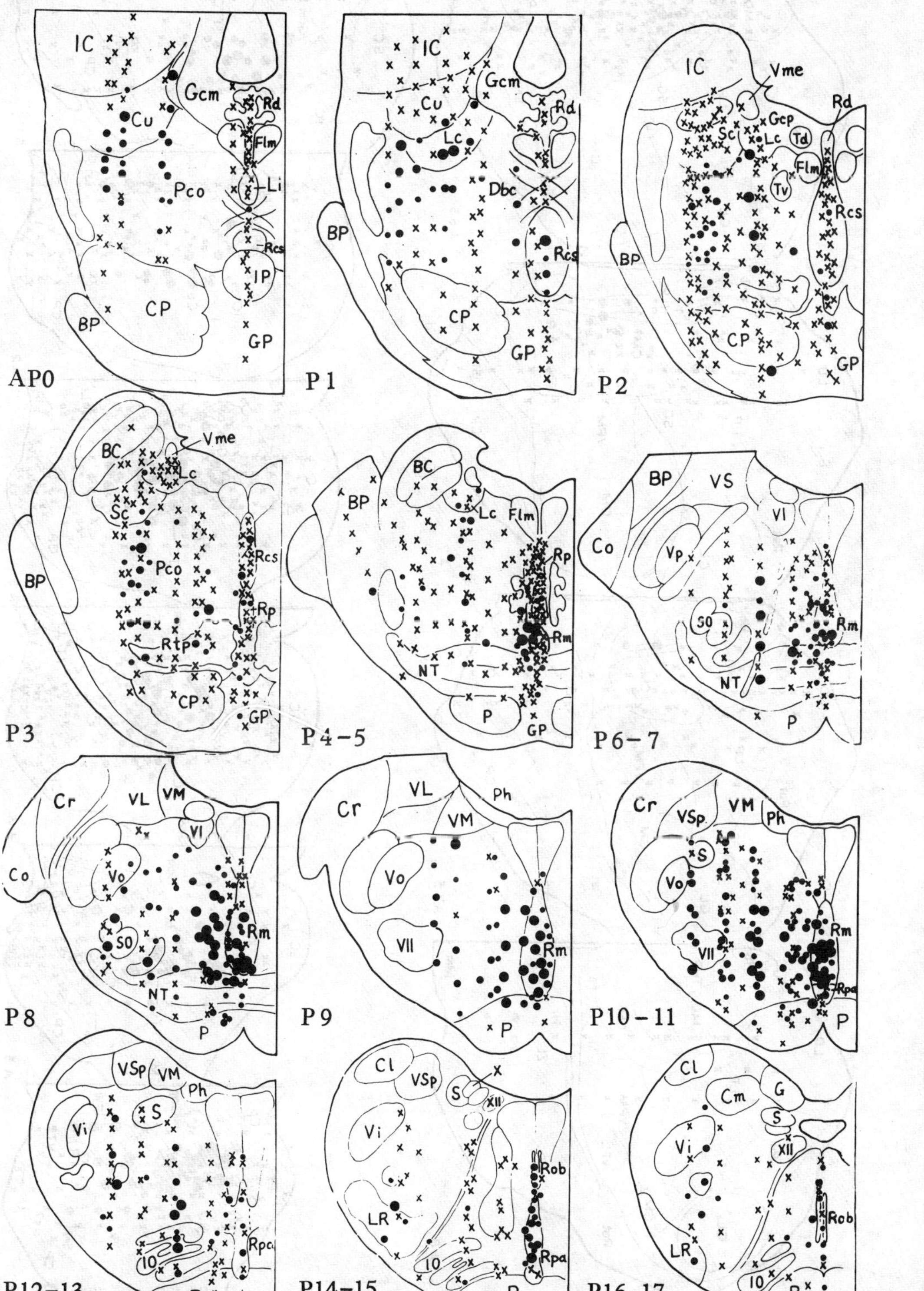
AP0
IC
Cu
Gcm
Rd
Flm
Li
Pco
Rcs
IP
CP
BP
GP
P1
Lc
Dbc
P2
Vme
Gcp
Sc
Td
Tv
P3
BC
Rtp
Rp
P4-5
NT
Rm
P
P6-7
VS
VI
Vp
Co
SO
P8
Cr
VL
VM
Vo
P9
Ph
VII
P10-11
VSp
S
Rpa
P12-13
Vi
10
P14-15
Cl
X
XII
LR
Rob
P16-17
Cm
G

A

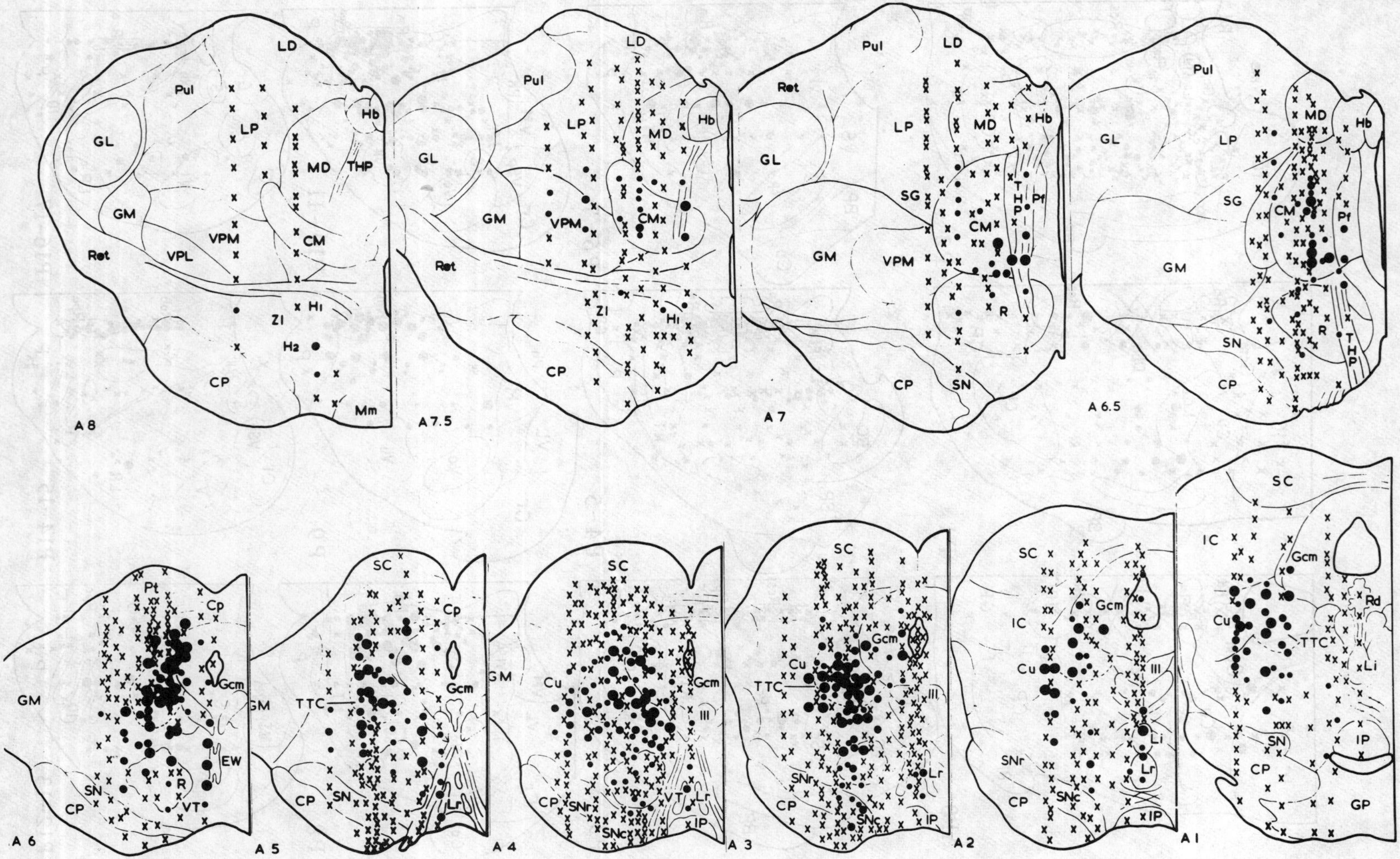
A 8
LD
Pul
LP
GL
MD
THP
Hb
GM
VPM
CM
Ret
VPL
H1
ZI
H2
CP
Mm
A 7.5
LD
Pul
LP
MD
Hb
GL
GM
CMx
VPM
Ret
ZI
H1
CP
A 7
Pul
LD
Ret
LP
MD
Hb
GL
SG
THP
Pf
CM
GM
VPM
R
CP
SN
A 6.5
Pul
MD
Hb
GL
LP
SG
CM
Pf
GM
R
SN
THP
CP
A 6
Pt
Cp
Gcm
GM
EW
SN
R
CP
VT
A 5
SC
Cp
Gcm
GM
TTC
CP
SN
Lr
A 4
SC
GM
Cu
Gcm
III
CP
SNr
VT
Lr
SNc
IP
A 3
SC
Gcm
Cu
TTC
III
SNr
Lr
CP
SNc
IP
A 2
SC
Gcm
IC
Cu
III
Li
SNr
Lr
CP
SNc
IP
A 1
SC
IC
Gcm
Rd
Cu
TTC
Li
SN
IP
CP
GP

B

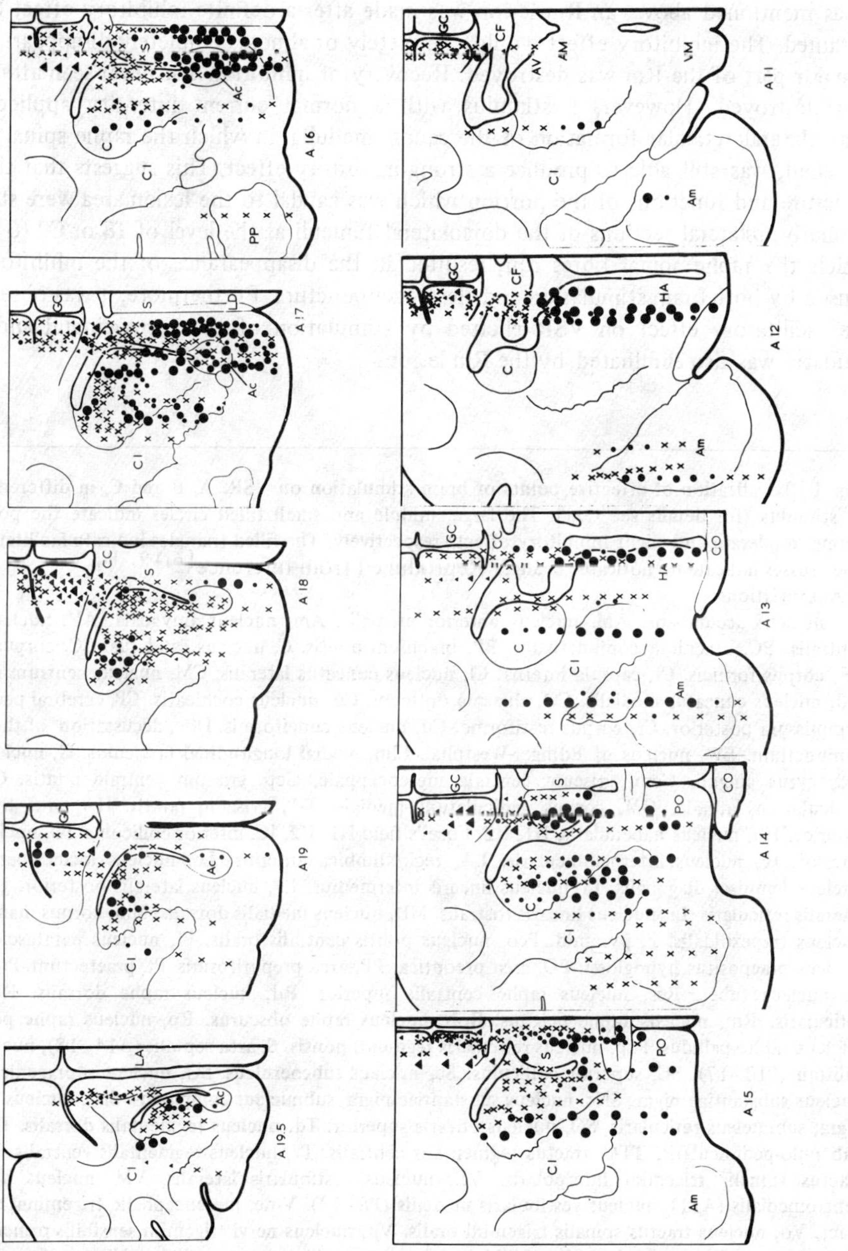
A 16
A 17
A 18
A 19
A 19.5
A 11
A 12
A 13
A 14
A 15
GC
CF
AV
AM
VM
Am
Ac
CI
PP
S
LD
HA
CC
CO
PO
LA

C

descending pathway from the midbrain. In the present study, we found the same phenomenon in all the regions explored.

In a total of 45 cases, in which the stimulation sites were distributed in most of the areas mentioned above, an Rm lesion was made after a definite inhibitory effect had been obtained. The inhibitory effect would completely or almost completely disappear affer a major part of the Rm was destroyed. Recovery of inhibition was never seen after the Rm was destroyed. However, a stimulus with a normal current intensity applied to the ventrolateral reticular formation of the caudal medulla, in which the raphe spinal pathway travelled, was still able to produce a strong inhibitory effect. This suggests that the neural structure and function of the portion which was caudal to the lesion area were still intact. Similarly, bilateral sections of the dorsolateral funiculi at the level of T8 or C2 (6 cases), in which the raphe spinal fibres run, resulted in the disappearance of the inhibitory effect caused by both brain stimulation and electroacupuncture. Furthermore, it was observed that the facilitatory effect on VSR elicited by stimulation of the gyrus cinguli and nucleus caudatus was also eliminated by the Rm lesion.

Fig. 1 Localization of effective points of brain stimulation on VSR. A, B and C, in different intensity of stimulus (for details see text). The large, middle and small filled circles indicate the points giving strong, moderate and slight inhibitory effects respectively. The filled triangles indicate facilitatory effect. The crosses indicate no noticable change. Reproduced from reference[6,19,20].

Abbreviations:

Ac, nucleus accumbens. AM, nucleus anterior medialis. Am, nucleus amygdala. AV, nucleus anterior ventralis. BC, brachium conjunctivum. BP, brachium pontis. C, nucleus caudatus. CC, corpus callosum. CF, corpus fornicis. CI, capsula interna. Cl, nucleus cuneatus lateralis. CM, nucleus centrum medianum. Cm, nucleus cuneatus medialis. CO, chiasma opticum. Co, nucleus cochlearis. CP, cerebral peduncle. Cp, commissura posterior. Cr, corpus restiforme. Cu, nucleus cuneiformis. Dbc, decussation of the brachium conjunctium. EW, nucleus of Edinger-Westphal. Flm, medial longitudinal fasciculus. G, nucleus gracilis. GC, gyrus cinguli. Gcm, griseum centrale mesencephale. Gcp, griseum centrale pontis. GL, corpus geniculatum laterale. GM, corpus geniculatum mediale. GP, griseum pontis. HA, area hypothalami anterior. Hb, nucleus habenularis. H1, H2, Forel's field H1, H2. IC, inferior colliculus. IO, nucleus olivaris inferior. IP, nucleus interpeduncularis. LA, regio limbica anterior. Lc, nucleus locus coeruleus. LD, nucleus lemnisci diagonalis. Li, nucleus linearis intermedius. LP, nucleus lateralis posterior. LR, nucleus lateralis reticularis. Lr, nucleus linearis rostralis. MD, nucleus medialis dorsalis. Mm, corpus mamillare. NT, nucleus trapezoidalis. P, pyramid. Pco, nucleus pontis centralis oralis. Pf, nucleus parafascicularis. Ph, nucleus praepositus hypoglossi, PO, area preoptica. PP, area prepyriformis. Pt, praetectum. Pul, pulvinar. R, nucleus ruber. Rcs, nucleus raphe centralis superior. Rd, nucleus raphe dorsalis. Ret, nucleus reticularis. Rm, nucleus raphe magnus. Rob, nucleus raphe obscurus. Rp, nucleus raphe pontis. Rpa, nucleus raphe pallidus. Rtp, nucleus reticularis tegmenti pontis. S, area septalis (A14–18), nucleus tractus solitraii (P10–17). SC, superior colliculus. Sc, nucleus subcoeruleus. SG, nucleus suprageniculatus. SN, nucleus substantiae nigra. SNc, nucleus substantiae nigra, subnucleus compactus. SNr, nucleus substantiae nigra, subnucleus reticularis. SO, nucleus olivaris superior. Td, nucleus tegmentalis dorsalis. THP, tractus habenulo-peduncularis. TTC, tractus tegmentalis centralis. Tv, nucleus tegmentalis ventralis. Vi, nucleus tractus spinalis trigemini interpolaris. VL, nucleus vestibularis lateralis. VM, nucleus hypothalami ventromedialis (A11), nucleus vestibularis medialis (P8–13). Vme, mesencephalic trigeminal nucleus and tract. Vo, nucleus tractus spinalis trigemini oralis. Vp, nucleus nervi trigemini sensibilis principalis. VPL, nucleus ventralis posterolateralis. VPM, nucleus ventralis posteromedialis. VS, nucleus vestibularis superior. Vsp, nucleus vestibularis spinalis. VT, ventral tegmental nucleus of Tsai. ZI, zona incerta. III, nucleus nervi oculomotorius, VI, nucleus nervi abducentis. VII, nucleus nervi facialis. X, nucleus nervi vagi dorsalis motorius. XII, nucleus nervi hypoglossi.

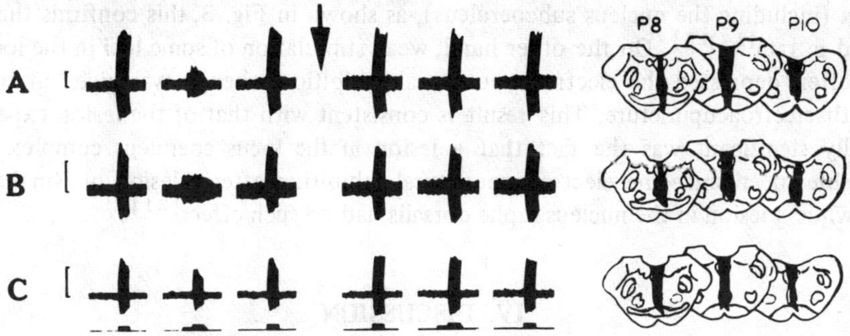

Fig. 2 Effect of Rm lesion on inhibition of VSR produced by brain stimulation. Records of the repetitive VSR. Each of them consists of about 125 single VSR. The inhibitory effects caused by stimulation of the griseum centrale mesencephali (A), tractus tegmentalis centralis (B) and nucleus linearis rostralis (C) disappear completely after Rm lesion (arrow), their respective extent being shown on the right. Narrow filled column on the baseline is the marker of the splanchnic stimuli (5 sec), and the wide one, that of the brain stimuli (10 sec). Calibration, 100 μV.

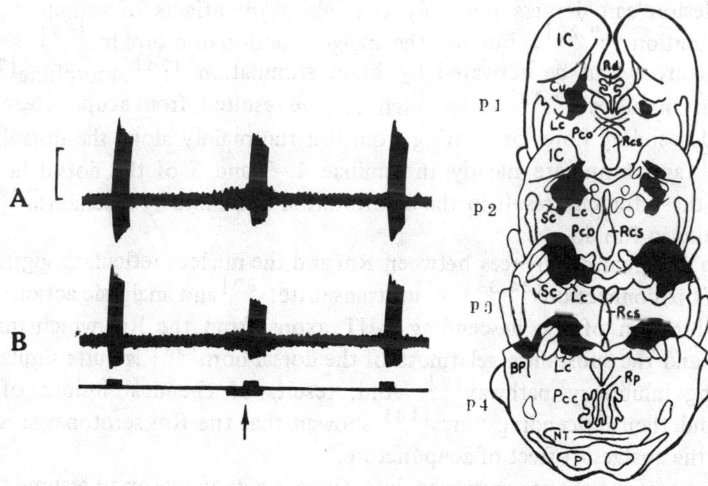

Fig. 3 Effect of locus coeruleus complex lesion on electroacupunctural inhibition of VSR.

VSR records are the same as in Fig. 2. A, control. B, after lesion. Extent of the lesion is shown in the diagrams. The filled column pointed by the arrow indicates the duration of electroacupuncture.

(III) Tonic depression of locus coeruleus on Rm

In acute experiments on cat we have observed that the inhibitory effect of electroacupuncture on the VSR was enhanced after the destruction of the locus coeruleus complex (including the nucleus subcoeruleus), as shown in Fig. 3, this confirms the results observed in rats[14,15]. On the other hand, weak stimulation of some loci in the locus coeruleus often depressed the electroacupunctural inhibition when it was given in combination with electroacupuncture. This result is consistent with that of the lesion experiment. Especially significant was the fact that a lesion in the locus coeruleus complex was no longer able to enhance the electroacupunctural inhibition after a lesion in Rm had been made, while a lesion in the nucleus raphe dorsalis had no such effect[21].

IV. DISCUSSION

1. Rm and analgesia

Since we suggested that the Rm might be the essential central link in the process of pain modula on by acupuncture[3], numerou findings have been emerging, and many authors have reached similar condlusion[22–25]. These data can be summed up as follows.

(A) In various species of animals including the rat[25], rabbit[26], cat[6,27] and monkey[28], stimulation of Rm has been shown to reduce different nociceptive reactions and to suppress selectively or preferentially the nociceptive activities of neurons in the dorsal horn[29–31]

(B) Rm lesion can depress not only the inhibitory effects of acupuncture[4,5,26] and brain stimulation [19,20], but also the analgesic action of morphine[25].

(C) Rm neurons can be activated by brain stimulation [24], morphine[24,32] and somatic afferent impulses[32,33] which might also be resulted, from acupuncture.

(D) The descending fibres originating from Rm run mainly along the dorsolateral funiculi[29,34,35] and terminate mostly in laminae 1–3 and 5 of the dorsal horn[34,35]. Sectioning of these funiculi result in the deterioration of inhibitory mechanism[4,6,34,36], much like lesions in Rm do.

(E) There are great differences between Rm and the nucleus reticularis gigantocellularis in respect to fibre connection[34,35], neurotransmitter[37] and analgesic action[5,24,25].

(F) The location of the descending 5-HT axons from the Rm which innervate the marginal area and the substantia gelatinosa of the dorsal horn[38] is quite similar to that of the descending inhibitory pathway[2].. And, results of chemical lesions of Rm 5-HT neurons[5] and their descending fibres[18] showed that the Rm serotonergic system may play a role in the analgesic effect of acupuncture.

On the basis of the above-mentioned data, there is a good reason to assume that the Rm is probably a structure derived from the medial reticular formation. One of important functions of Rm is modulating the nociceptive inputs at the spinal cord level. It seems likely that the acupuncture, brain stimulation and opioid analgesics exert their analgesic effect more or less through this Rm serotonergic system.

2. Relationship between higher brain regions and Rm.

In this respect, there are three points worthy of comment.

(A) It has been known that acupuncture can regulate the nociceptive discharges of neurons in the medial thalamus[39] and the midbrain reticular formation[26]. Does Rm affect the integration of pain in the higher brain region? It was reported that Rm stimulation can increase, and Rm lesion can decrease the acupunctural inhibitory effect on nociceptive responses.This was regarded as an involvement of Rm in the ascending pathway of pain[26].

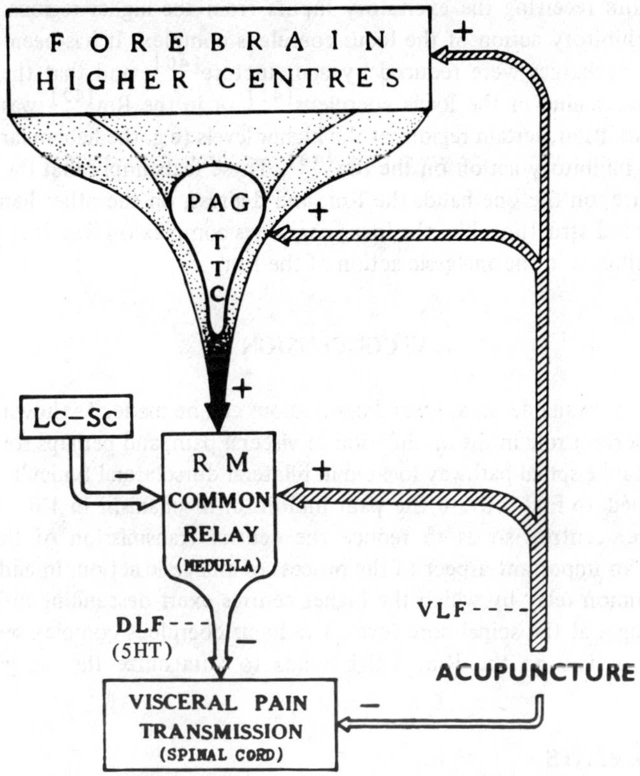

Fig. 4 Schematic diagram of possible role of Rm in inhibition of visceral pain transmission.

DLF, dorsolateral funiculi. Lc-Sc, locus coeruleus complex. PAG, periaqueductal grey. RM, region of nucleus raphe magnus. TTC, area of central tegmental tract. VLF, ventrolateral funiculi. 5-HT, 5-hydroxytryptaminergic fibres. Plus indicates excitation; minus, inhibition.

However, the possibility that it is only a consequence of the descending inhibition exerted by Rm can not be ruled out.

(B) Our findings on brain stimulation have suggested the existence of descending inhibitory effects from higher brain regions. In the light of the characteristics of the inhibitory effects of brain stimulation (see above), it is reasonable to assume that the efferent pathway from the higher regions may consist of polysynaptic loops. Considering the fact that following the Rm lesion the inhibitory effect on VSR produced by different brain regions disappeared, we conclude that the descending impulses from the higher brain regions activated by acupuncture and other influences may converge directly or indirectly in Rm, the final common relay in the medulla (Fig. 4), so as to modulate the nociceptive inputs in the spinal cord.

(C) Apart from receiving the excitatory inputs from the higher regions, the Rm is at least under an inhibitory action of the locus coeruleus complex. It has been reported that the spontaneous discharges were reduced by acupuncture[40], and that the fluorescent intensity of noradrenaline in the locus coeruleus[41] or in the Rm[42] was decreased to some degree. In addition, certain regions at the higher levels (e.g. the habenular nucleus) also seem to exert an inhibitory action on the Rm[43]. These facts imply that the acupunctural inputs may activate, on the one hand, the Rm, and depress, on the other hand, the inhibitory action of neural structures like the locus coeruleus complex on Rm. It appears that the latter effect contributes to the analgesic action of the Rm.

V. CONCLUSION

On the basis of available data, several conclusions can be made. As shown in Fig. 4, Rm may play an important role in the modulation of visceral pain, and perhaps somatic pain, via the serotonergic raphe-spinal pathway located in bilateral dorsolateral funiculi. Acupunctural inputs are assumed to first activate the pain inhibition mechanism in Rm, and secondly, to activate higher centres, so as to reduce the central transmission of the nociceptive impulses. This is an important aspect of the process of analgesic action. In addition, the Rm may act as a common relay by which the higher centres exert descending influence on the nociceptive messages at the spinal cord level. The locus coeruleus complex seems to exert a tonic inhibitory action on the Rm, which tends to antagonize the analgesic effect of acupuncture.

ACKNOWLEDGEMENTS

We wish to thank Mr. R. K. Zheng for technique asistance, and Mr. F. Y. Yang and Miss H. J. Xu for making histological sections.

REFERENCES

[1] 杜焕基等：新医药学杂志 (4)：25—28，1975。
[2] 沈 锷等：中华医学杂志 **54**：628—633，1974。
[3] Du, H.J. and Chao, Y.F.: *Scientia Sinica*, **19**:137–148, 1976.
[4] 杜焕基,赵燕芳：科学通报 **23**：442—446，1978。
[5] Chiang, C.Y. *et al.*: *Chinese Med. J.*, **92**:129–136, 1979.
[6] 杜焕基等：生理学报 **30**：1—9，1978。
[7] 许冠荪等：科学通报 **20**：234—237，1975。
[8] 魏仁榆等：科学通报 **19**：520—524，1974。
[9] 罗蒻荪等：中国科学 **21**：456—464，1978。
[10] 上海生理研究所第二研究室针麻组：中华医学杂志 **55**：340—342，1975。
[11] 上海第一医学院生理学教研组：中华医学杂志 **55**：336—339，1975。
[12] 张德星等：生理学报 **30**：21—28、1978。
[13] 张德星等：生理学报 **30**：95—97，1978。
[14] 陕西省中医研究所针麻原理研究室：陕西新医药 (1)：66—68，1976。
[15] 张德星等：科学通报 **23**：117—121，1978。
[16] 杜焕基等：科学通报 **19**：277—280，1974。
[17] Shen, E. *et al.*: *Scientia Sinica*, **21**:677–685, 1978.
[18] 杜焕基等：动物学报 **24**：11—20，1978。
[19] Du, H.J. *et al.*: *Kexue Tongbao*, **25**:964–969, 1980.

[20] 杜焕基,赵燕芳: 科学通报 **26**: 122—125,1981。
[21] 杜焕基,赵燕芳: 生理学报 **31**: 153—161, 1979。
[22] Mayer, D.J. and Price, D.D.: *Pain,* **2**:379–404, 1976.
[23] Fields, H.L. and Basbaum, A.I.: *Ann.Rev.Physiol.,* **40**:217–248, 1978.
[24] Oleson, T.D. *et al.*: *Pain,* **4**:211–230. 1978.
[25] Proudfit, H.K. and Anderson,E.G.: *Brain Res.,* **98**:612–618, 1975.
[26] 广西医学院针麻研究小组: 动物学报 **24**: 29—40, 1978。
[27] Oliveras,J.L. *et al: Pain,* **1**:139–145, 1975.
[28] Willis,W.D. *et al.*: *J.Neurophysiol.,* **40**:968–981, 1977.
[29] Fields,H.L. *et al.*: *Brain Res.,* **126**:441–453, 1977.
[30] Guilbaud,G. *et al.*: *Brain Res.,* **126**:355–360, 1977.
[31] Belcher,G. *et al.*: *Brain Res.,* **151**:307–321, 1978.
[32] Anderson,S.D. *et al.*: *Brain Res.,* **123**:363–368, 1977.
[33] Moolenaar,G.M. *et al.*: *Exp.Neurol.,* **53**:304–313, 1976.
[34] Basbaum,A.I. *et al.*: *Proc.Natl.Acad. Sci. (USA),* **73**:4685–4688, 1976.
[35] Basbaum,A.I. *et al.*: *J. comp.Neurol.,* **178**:209–244, 1978.
[36] Basbaum,A.I. *et al.*: *Pain,* **3**:43–56, 1977.
[37] Dahlström,A. *et al.*: *Acta Physiol.Scand.* **62**:suppl.232, 1964.
[38] Oliveras,J.L. *et al.*: *Brain Res.,* **138**:393–406, 1977.
[39] Chang,H.T.: *Scientia Sinica,* **21**:829–846, 1978.
[40] 陕西省中医研究所针麻原理研究室: 陕西新医药 (1): 62—64, 1977。
[41] 董新文等: 生物化学与生物物理学报 **10**: 119—125, 1978。
[42] 董新文,蒋芝华: 生理学报 **33**: 24—29, 1981。
[43] 王　绍等: 全国针灸麻醉学术讨论会论文摘要(二), 北京, 29—30, 1979。

EFFECT OF STIMULATION OF MIDBRAIN RAPHE NUCLEI ON DISCHARGES OF NOCICEPTIVE NEURONS IN NUCLEUS PARAFASCICULARIS OF THALAMUS AND ITS SIGNIFICANCE IN ACUPUNCTURE ANALGESIA

Zhang Guilin, Wei Jinbo, Zhou Lingbao,
Lin Yaomin, Luo Zhengliang, Zhou Lanxian,
Zhang Zuchen
(Hubei Medical College)

From the large amount of experimental data in recent years[1–9] it becomes evident that brain 5–hydroxytryptamine (5–HT) and raphe nuclei may play an important role in acupuncture analgesia, but the site on which the raphe nuclei exert their action and the route by which the acupuncture analgesia is induced still remain to be determined.

Morphological studies have demonstrated that the midbrain raphe nuclei (MRN) project mainly to the diencephalon and telencephalon including nucleus parafascicularis (PF), and that axons of the medullary raphe nuclei project mainly to the spinal cord[10–13]. The latter may be involved in the descending inhibition evoked by acupuncture[14]. Recently some investigators[15–17] reported that the nucleus raphe magnus might modulate the pain messages at the spinal level. However, Zhang[18] believes that the integration of pain takes place mainly in the thalamus.

The purpose of the present investigation is to observe the effect of stimulation of MRN on the transmission of pain impulses in the thalamus and to ascertain if there is an ascending modulatory action of the raphe nuclei. Such a study may help us understand the mechanism of acupuncture analgesia.

I. METHODS

1. Experimental animals and operations. Eighty-three rabbits weighing 2.0–2.8kg each were used. The operations were performed under the action of a mixture of 10% urethane and 1% chloralose given intravenously in a dosage of 5ml/kg. The operations included tracheotomy and insertion of a cannula for artificial respiration, opening of the fourth ventricle for drainage of the cerebrospinal fluid, and exposure of the cerebral cortex and the peroneal nerve. The incisions were infiltrated with 2% procaine. After the operations had been completed, the opening in the skull was sealed with agar. An appropriate volume of 10% glucose saline was infused through the auricular vein.

The dorsal half of the spinal cord at the level between T_{3-4} was transected in thirty rabbits. The extent of transection was identified macroscopically after the experiments.

Observations began 5–6 hours after anesthetization. The animals were immobilized with d-tubocurarine and artificial respiration was carried out to keep the animals awake but in a paralyzed state.

2. Peripheral stimulation. A pair or a train of electric pulses, 0.5 msec in width, 100Hz, 30–50 msec in train duration and 30–70V in intensity (unloaded), was applied through an isolator to the contralateral peroneal nerve as noxious stimulus. Pinching of the skin with a pair of forceps was used as natural nocuous stimulus. Hair displacement and rotation of joints were employed as innocuous stimuli in order to observe their influence upon the unit discharges.

3. Central stimulation. According to the brain atlas of rabbit[19], a concentric electrode was inserted stereotaxically (AP_{9-10}, L or $R_{0.0}$ and $H_{-4.5-6.0}$) to stimulate the MRN. The electric shocks consisted of square wave pulses, 2 msec in width, 10 Hz in frequency and 6V in intensity[20]. The stimulation usually continued for 10–20 minutes.

The unit discharges of PF were examined from time to time during the raphe stimulation. When it changed significantly, the raphe stimulation was stopped to observe the course of restoration.

With the completion of the experimental observations, the stimulation site was marked with the tip of the electrode by means of the Prussian blue reaction and then checked histologically. Fig.1 is a cross-section of the midbrain of the rabbit showing the position of the stimulating electrode situated in the raphe area of the midbrain.

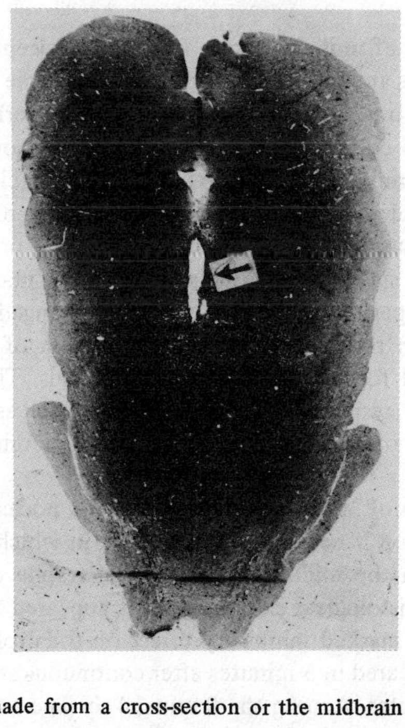

Fig. 1 Diagram made from a cross-section or the midbrain of rabbit. The tip of the stimulating electrode was marked by passing an anodal current (1 ma, 30 sec) to the elcctrode. The arrow indicated the raphe area of the midbrain.

4. Electroacupuncture stimulation. A pair of acupuncture needles were inserted into the acupuncture points Hegu of the forelimb. The output of model G6805 stimulator was connected to the needles delivering continuous waves at a frequency of 140 cycles/minute with an intensity of 4–7 V. The duration of electroacupuncture was 5–20 minutes.

5. Intraventricular injection. A cannula made from an injection needle with an outer diameter of 0.5 mm was inserted into the lateral ventricle at coordinates[21] A_1, L_3 and H_5. A dose of 100μg/200μl of (pH 4.35) 5–Hydroxytryptamine creatinine sulphate dissolved in saline was injected slowly with a microinjector via the cannula into the lateral ventricle in 2–4 minutes. At the end of the experiment, 0.2ml of blue-ink was injected to determine the extent of perfusion.

6. Recording and analysis of unit discharge. Glass microelectrodes filled with 3*M* KCl were used for recording the unit discharges in the PF. The diameter of the tip of microelectrode was about 1 μ, with a resistance of 7–20 megaohms. The microelectrode was introduced stereotaxically to the region of PF according to the atlas of rabbit brain (P_5, L or $R_{1.2-1.7}$ and H_{+1-2}). The unit discharges recorded by the microelectrodes were displayed on an oscillograph after amplification. The amplified potentials were also recorded on the magnetic tape and played back later for further analysis with Model TQ–19 (A) medical data processor.

II. RESULTS

1. General observations of unit discharges from the nociceptive neurons in PF. When a train of 3 electric pulses was applied to the peroneal nerve, some neurons in the PF responded with specific patterns of unit discharges similar to those described before[18]. Prolonged discharges of these neurons could be induced by natural nocuous stimuli such as pinching with forceps. Most of the units were found to be responsive exclusively to nocuous stimulation. These units were regarded as nociceptive neurons. A few of them were also responsive to innocuous stimulation such as hair displacement. In the present study the units that showed a response to both strong electric pulse and natural nocuous stimuli were selected for observation. The latent period of the evoked response ranged generally from 160 to 500 msec, with the longest even reaching 1 sec. After cessation of the stimulation, sustained after-discharges often lasted for several to over ten seconds. There were also a few units that presented an inhibitory response to noxious stimuli, such as a decrease in frequency or even temporary suspension of spontaneous discharges. Sometimes this inhibitory response might last several seconds.

2. Effect of stimulation of MRN on discharges of the nociceptive neurons in PF. The effect of stimulating MRN on 9 neurons was observed, in which the location of the tip of the stimulating electrode in the midbrain raphe nuclei (raphe dorsalis, raphe centralis superior) was identified by histological examination. It appeared that electric stimulation of the MRN brought about a marked inhibitory effect on the evoked nociceptive discharges. In eight units the effect appeared in 5 minutes after continuous stimulation of the MRN, and in the ninth one in 10 minutes. Among the 9 units, 4 showed complete inhibition, 5 partial inhibition. Complete inhibition was characterized by disappearance of evoked discharges and by temporary suspension or decrease in frequency of spontaneous discharges. Partial inhibition was manifested by lengthening in latency, shortening in burst, lowering in frequency, decreasing in the total number of spikes of the evoked response and decreasing in frequency of spontaneous discharges. After termination of the midbrain raphe stimulation, two kinds of aftereffects were observed in the course of recovery. Six units showed a sustained after-effect of inhibitory action, but the other 3 units presented a rebound phenomenon, i.e., a brief period of inhibitory effect followed by a facilitatory effect. Fig.2 shows the inhibitory effect of electric stimulation of MRN on the nociceptive discharges of a PF neuron.

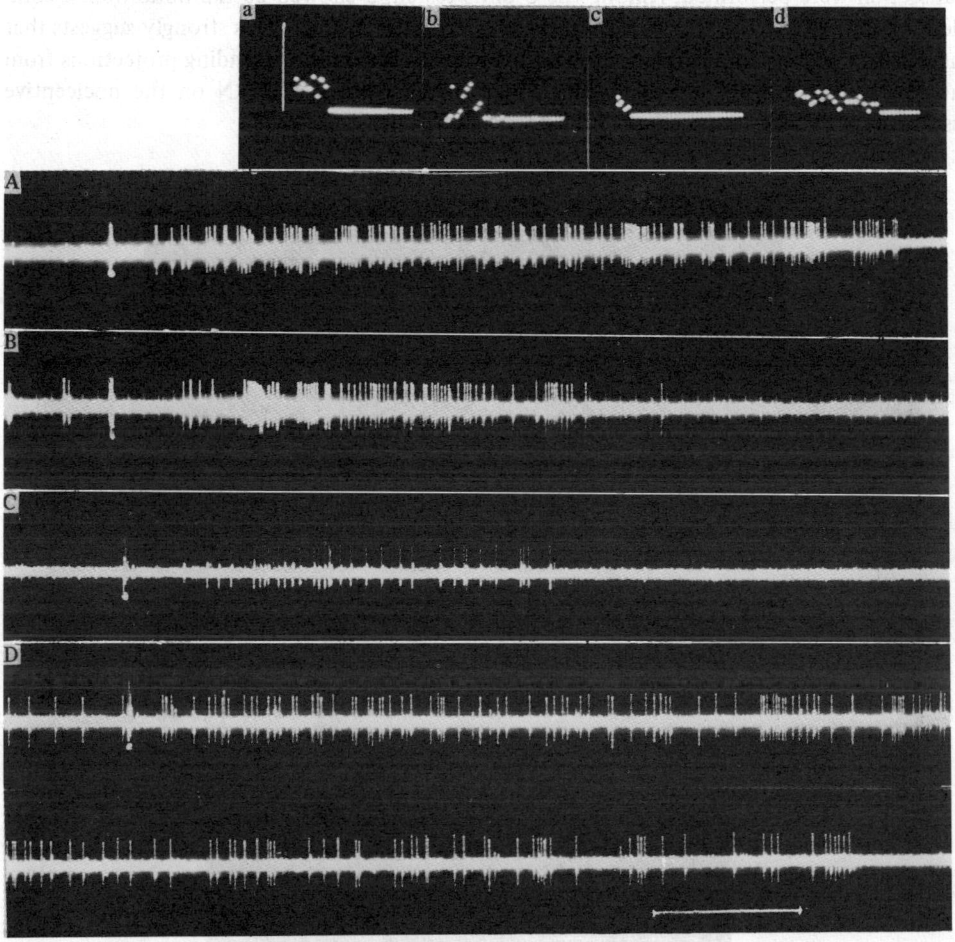

Fig. 2 Inhibitory effect of electric stimulation of MRN on the nociceptive discharges of a PF neuron. A. response to a train of electric pulses applied to the contralateral peroneal nerve. B. and C. nociceptive discharges after stimulation of MRN for 5 and 10 minutes respectively. Pulses of low amplitude are artifacts of stimuli. D. nociceptive discharges 3 minutes after cessation of the stimulation of raphe nuclei. Time: 1 sec. Small white points indicate the artifacts of stimuli. a, b, c and d are sequential spike density histograms obtained from the corresponding discharges of A, B, C and D respectively. Time at each address: 500 msec. The value of both X and y is 32.

3. Effect of stimulation of MRN on the nociceptive discharges in PF after transection of the dorsal half of the spinal cord. The dorsal half of the spinal cord was transected in thirty rabbits in order to interrupt the descending inhibitory pathway in the spinal cord[22]. The effect of stimulating the MRN on 8 units were studied in such preparations. A marked inhibitory effect on nociceptive discharges in PF was demonstrated just as if no transection were performed. Among the 8 units tested, 5 showed partial inhibition, 2 complete inhibition and the remaining 1 showed a facilitatory effect. This strongly suggests that the inhibitory effect on PF neurons is probably mediated by the ascending projections from the MRN. Fig. 3 shows the inhibitory effect of stimulation of MRN on the nociceptive discharges in PF after transection of the dorsal half of the spinal cord.

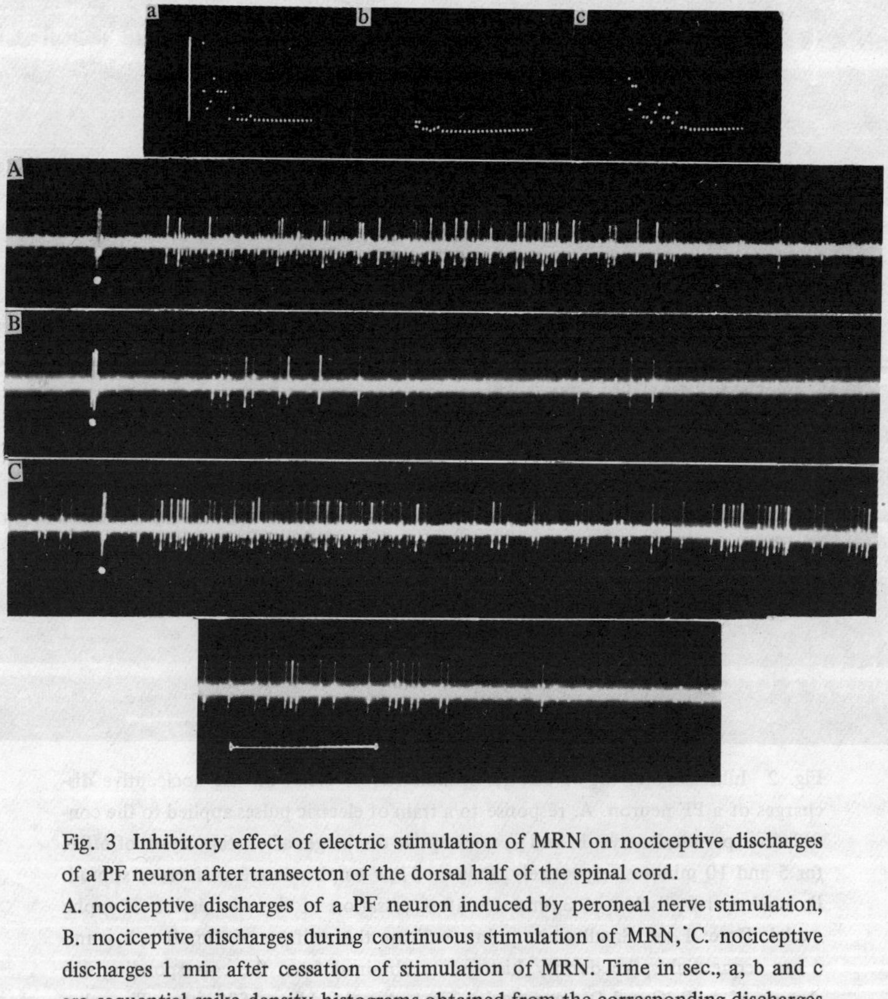

Fig. 3 Inhibitory effect of electric stimulation of MRN on nociceptive discharges of a PF neuron after transecton of the dorsal half of the spinal cord.
A. nociceptive discharges of a PF neuron induced by peroneal nerve stimulation, B. nociceptive discharges during continuous stimulation of MRN, C. nociceptive discharges 1 min after cessation of stimulation of MRN. Time in sec., a, b and c are sequential spike density histograms obtained from the corresponding discharges of A, B and C respectively. Time for each address 500 mesc.

4. Effect of intraventricular injection of 5–HT on the nociceptive discharges of PF neurons. 5 units were observed. All showed an excitatory response to noxious stimuli. One to three minutes after intraventricular injection of 100 μg of 5–HT a marked inhibitory effect was observed. Three units showed partial and 2 units showed complete inhibition. Fig. 4 shows the inhibitory effect that appeared 90 seconds after intraventricular injection of 5–HT and ended within 8 minutes. This inhibitory action was analogous to that produced by midbrain raphe stimulation mentioned above. No similar effect on nociceptive discharges by intraventricular injection of an equal volume of saline was observed in the 5 units used as controls.

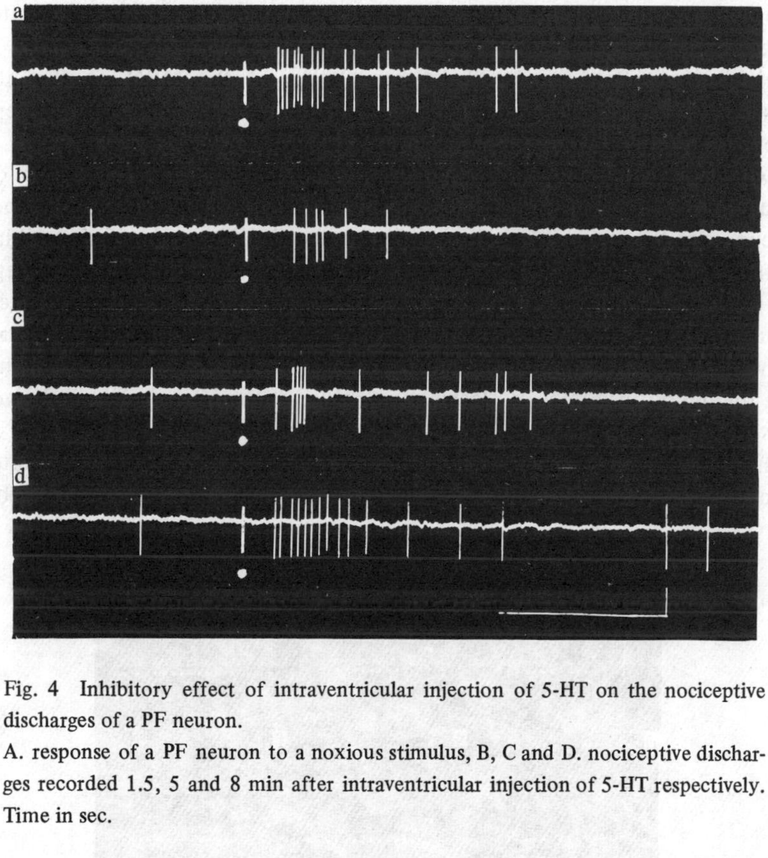

Fig. 4 Inhibitory effect of intraventricular injection of 5-HT on the nociceptive discharges of a PF neuron.
A. response of a PF neuron to a noxious stimulus, B, C and D. nociceptive discharges recorded 1.5, 5 and 8 min after intraventricular injection of 5-HT respectively. Time in sec.

5. Influence of stimulation of MRN and intraventricular injection of 5–HT on the spontaneous rhythmic discharges of the non-nociceptive neurons in PF. The effects of MRN stimulation on four non-nociceptive neurons were studied for comparison. The frequency of spontaneous discharge was found to be lowered as soon as stimulation of MRN was started and the effect lasted for several to over ten seconds, then the discharge frequency fluctuated during continuous stimulation of MRN. After termination of the MRN stimulation no aftereffect on spontaneous discharge was observed. Another 6 non-nociceptive units were observed after intraventricular injection of 5–HT. Four of them showed a temporary decrease in frequency and the other 2 showed no effect. The difference between responses of nociceptive and non-nociceptive neurons to MRN stimulation and intraventricular injection of 5–HT indicates that the former is more sensitive to 5–HT and thus more liable to prolonged inhibition.

6. Effect of stimulation of regions beyond the MRN on the nociceptive discharge in PF. The effect of stimulation of nucleus reticularis tegmenti of the midbrain on the nociceptive discharges in PF was proved to be similar to that of MRN stimulation in the seven units investigated. Among these, 4 were partially inhibited, 2 completely inhibited and the remaining 1 showed no effect. Two of them presented rebound phenomena in the recovery course. In another 19 units, the effects on the nociceptive discharges varied with the site of stimulation. For example, stimulation of interpeduncular nucleus (4 units) elicited no effect, while that of the medial lemniscus (2 units) showed a facilitatory effect.

The inhibitory effect produced by stimulation of the MRN on the nociceptive discharges in PF as observed in the present investigation is consistent with the reports that stimulation of these areas would induce significant analgesic effect[23–25].

7. Effect of electroacupuncture on the nociceptive discharges in PF. The effect of electroacupuncture on the nociceptive discharges in PF was also investigated. Among the 11 nociceptive neurons in PF tested by electroacupuncture at the Hegu point, 6 showed inhibitory, 2 facilitatory, and 3 no effect. These results were also in accord with those reported by others[18,26]. In the majority of cases, a partial inhibition was observed after electroacupuncture for 5 minutes. After cessation of electroacupuncture, a remarkable aftereffect was seen which lasted for about 8 minutes. Fig.5 is the sequential spike density histograms indicating the inhibitory effect of electroacupuncture at the Hegu point on the nociceptive discharges of a PF neuron.

Among the other 9 nociceptive neurons in PF tested by electroacupuncture at the Hegu point after transection of the dorsal half of the spinal cord, 7 showed inhibitory and

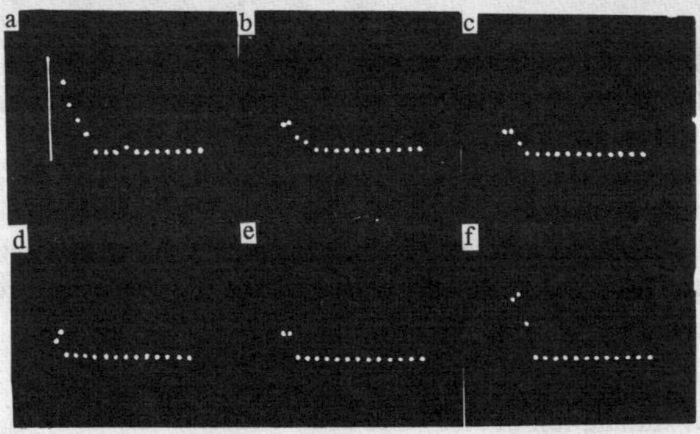

Fig. 5 Sequential spike density histograms indicating the inhibitory effect of electroacupuncture of the Hegupoint on the nociceptive discharges of a PF neuron. a. response to electrical stimulation of the peroneal nerve, b. nociceptive discharges during electroacupuncture, c, d, e and f. nociceptive discharges recorded 1, 3, 5 and 8 minutes after cessation of electroacupuncture respectively. Time: 1 sec/address. The value of both x and y is 32.

2 facilitatory effect. The units showing inhibitory effect were partially inhibited by electroacupuncture for 5 minutes. However, it showed a tendency of recovery when electroacupuncture continued. After cessation of electroacupuncture, the aftereffect was weaker than that in intact animals, and may have even disappeared (Fig.6).

It seems evident that after transection of the dorsal half of the spinal cord, the inhibitory effect of electroacupuncture on the nociceptive discharges in PF was significantly affected. This suggests that the descending inhibitory action on the spinal cord may play an important role in the process of acupuncture analgesia.

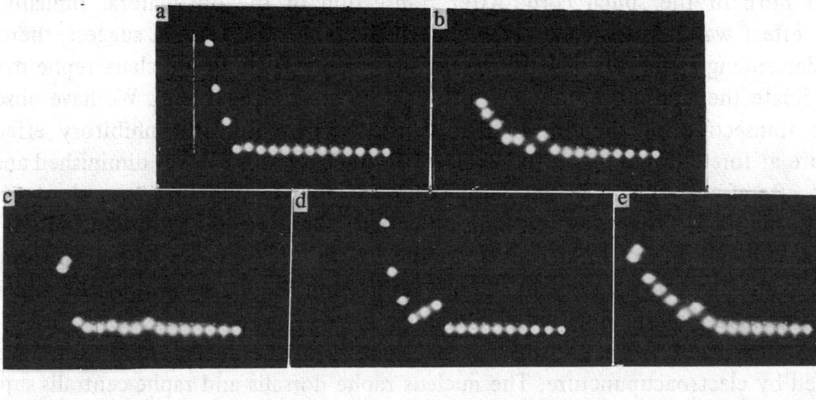

Fig. 6 Sequential spike density histograms indicating the effect of electro-acupuncture of the Hegu point on the nociceptive discharges of a PF neuron after transection of the dorsal half of the spinal cord. a. response to electrical stimulation of the peroneal nerve. b. c and d: nociceptive discharges at 5, 10 and 15 minutes after the onset of electroacupuncture respectively, e. nociceptive discharges 1 min after cessation of electrcupuncture. Time: 1 sec/address. The value of both x and y is 32.

III. DISCUSSION

Brain serotonergic neurons are concentrated mainly in the raphe nucleus. Some investigations demonstrated that damages or suppression of the functional activities of brain serotonergic neurons could attenuate the analgesic effect of acupuncture[1–6], whereas activation or strengthening of the functional activities of these neurons could potentiate it[5,9,23,24,]. Assay of 5–HT in the brain during acupuncture disclosed that either the 5–HT content in the thalamus, medulla, and raphe nuclei area was increased or the release of brain 5–HT was accelerated[7,8,27] These investigations strongly suggested that the raphe nucleus and the brain 5–HT were most intimately related with acupuncture analgesia.

However, the axons of neurons of raphe nuclei project extensively to most areas of the central nervous system. How they participate in the mechanisms of acupuncture analgesia deserues further investigation.

Some studies demonstrated that the inhibitory effect of acupuncture on the viscero-somatic reflex needed the participation of descending inhibition originating from some supraspinal structure[28]. In the experiments with cat damage of the medullary raphe nuclei and the adjacent area diminished the acupuncture effect significantly[14]. This suggested that the medullary raphe nuclei might be involved in the descending modulation during acupuncture. Hu et al[22] demonstrated that electrical stimulation of the spinal cord of rabbits caused analgesia which was mediated by a descending inhibitory system located in the dorsolateral funiculi of the spinal cord. Lately it has been shown[15–17] that stimulation of nucleus raphe magnus suppressed the neuronal response to noxious stimuli in the dorsal horn of the spinal cord. After transection of the dorsolateral funiculi, this inhibitory effect was diminished or even abolished[15,17]. This would suggest, therefore, that the descending inhibitory system originating mainly from the nucleus rephe magnus could modulate the transmission of pain information at the spinal level. We have observed that after transection of the dorsal half of the spinal cord, the inhibitory effect of acupuncture at forelimb points on the nociceptive discharges in PF was diminished and the inhibitory aftereffect following the termination of the acupuncture was shortened or completely nullified. Thes results indicated that the descending inhibition via the dorsolateral funiculi might influence the transmission of the pain impulses from the periphery to the thalamus and might thus be involved in the mechanism of the inhibitory effect of acupuncture on the nociceptive discharges in PF.

On the other hand, it was shown[29] that neurons of the nucleus raphe dorsalis could be activated by electroacupuncture. The nucleus raphe dorsalis and raphe centralis superior are the main origins of the ascending serotonergic system, projecting widely to regions of the forebrain including the parafascicular nucleus. Our investigation demonstrated that after transection of the dorsal half of the spinal cord, the inhibitory effect of stimulation of MRN on the nociceptive discharges in PF still persisted. Thus, it is most probable that the MRN can be activated by electroacupuncture and this in turn can modulate the pain impulses in the thalamus via ascending projections. Relevant data also showed that there are inhibitory serotonergic pathways that originate from the MRN to the hippocampus or amygdala. Thus, the ascending inhibitory action of the MRN is being disclosed gradually.

Since the neurons in the raphe nuclei were proved to be serotonergic neurons by means of fluorescence histochemistry[10], many investigations have shown that stimulation of the raphe nuclei can induce the release of brain 5–HT or changes of its metabolism[20,32,33]. In the present investigation, a similar inhibitory effect on nociceptive discharges in PF was evoked by stimulation of MRN or by intraventricular injection of 5–HT. Thus, the inhibitory effect of stimulation of the MRN may be related to the release of 5–HT from serotonergic neurons. Recently it was reported that there was a high concentration of enkephalins in midbrain raphe nucleus. The opiate antagonist naloxone strongly reduced analgesia induced by stimulation of the nucleus raphe magnus in the cat[35].

Thus it seems probable that more than one kind of substance may be released from the raphe nucleus when it is activated, and these substances may all be involved in the mechanism of analgesia.

The raphe nucleus is a part of the brain stem reticular formation. There are reciprocal connections between the raphe and adjacent reticular formation[11,12,36,37] which also projects to the parafascicular nucleus[38]. These connections form one part of the substrate for reciprocal raphe-reticular interaction. These experimental data provide an explanation for the results obtained in the present investigation that a similar inhibitory effect on nociceptive discharges in PF could be elicited by stimulation of the nucleus reticularis tegmenti of the midbrain and by stimulation of the MRN. Therefore, the nucleus reticularis tegmenti may also play some role in the modulation of the pain impulses in the thalamus.

IV. SUMMARY

To investigate the role of the midbrain raphe nuclei in acupuncture analgesia, experiments were performed in rabbits immobilized with d-tubocurarine and subsequently kept conscious under artificial respiration. The electrical activities of the neurons in the nucleus parafascicularis of the thalamus were recorded by KCl-filled glass microelectrodes. The results obtained were as follows:

(1) The electrical stimulation of the midbrain raphe nuclei had a marked inhibitory effect upon discharges of the nociceptive neurons in the PF. After termination of the midbrain raphe stimulation, some neurons showed aftereffect of the inhibitory action, but some of them presented a rebound phenomenon. Similar results were obtained by stimulating the nucleus reticularis tegmenti of the midbrain and by intraventricular injection of 5–hydroxytryptamine. The inhibitory effect persisted after transection of the dorsal half of the spinal cord (at T_{3-4}). This strongly suggested that the inhibitory effect might be mediated by the ascending projections from the midbrain raphe nuclei.

(2) The nociceptive discharges of PF neurons could also be inhibited by electroacupuncture of the Hegu point. After the dorsal half of spinal cord was cut, the inhibitory effect due to the electroacupuncture was diminished and the aftereffect either markedly shortened or entirely gone. These results indicated that the descending inhibition via the dorsolateral funiculi upon the transmission of the pain impulses from the periphery to the thalamus was also involved in the mechanism of acupuncture.

REFERENCES

[1] 陕西省中医研究所针麻原理研究室：陕西新医药，(5)：59，1975。

[2] 江振裕等：中华医学杂志，**57** (10)：611，1977。

[3] 易庆成等：科学通报，**22** (1)：43，1977。

[4] 北京医学院基础部针麻原理研究组：科学通报，**20** (10)：483，1975。

[5] 北京医学院基础部针麻原理研究组生理组：新医药学杂志，(**3**)：37，1976。

[6] 中医研究院针灸经络研究所生化组：新医药学杂志，(**3**)：35，1976。

[7] 湖南医学院针麻原理研究组：中华医学杂志，(**8**)：478，1973。

[8] 易庆成等：中国科学，(1)：83，1977。

[9] 北京医学院基础部针麻原理研究组生理组：科学通报，**20**(11)：532，1975。

[10] Dahlström A. *et al*: *Acta. physiol. Scand.*, **62**, (Suppl 232) 1, 1964.

[11] Brodal, A. *et al.*: J. *comp. neurol.*, **114**:239, 1960.

[12] Bobillier, P. *et al.*: *Brain Res.*, **85**:205, 1975.

[13] Bobillier, P. *et al.*: *Brain Res.*, **113**:449, 1976.

[14] 杜焕基等：中国科学 (6)：631，1975。
[15] Fields, H. L. *et al.*: *Brain Res.*, **126**:441. 1977.
[16] Guilhaud, G *et al.*: *Brain Res.*, **126**:355. 1977.
[17] Willis, W. D. *et al.*: *J. Neurophysiol.*, **40**(4): 968, 1977.
[18] 张香桐：中国科学，(1)：28，1973。
[19] J.布瑞希等：电生理学方法，上海科学技术出版社，1963。
[20] Aghajanian, G. K. *et al.*: *Science.*, **156**:402, 1967.
[21] Sawyer, C. H. *et al.*: *J. comp, neurol.*, **101**:801, 1954.
[22] 胡三觉等：中华医学杂志，**56**：238，1976。
[23] 陕西省中医研究所针麻原理研究室：陕西新医药，(6)：59，1977。
[24] 湖北医学院针麻研究组：针刺麻醉，(1)：59，1978。
[25] Mayer, D. J. *et al.*: *Brain Res.*, 68:73, 1974.
[26] 上海生理研究所：中华医学杂志，**53**：131，1973。
[27] 叶惟泠等：科学通报，**22**(8)：367，1977。
[28] 沈　锷等：中华医学杂志，**54**：628，1974。
[29] 北京医学院基础部针麻原理研究组电生理组：针麻原理研究资料汇编，103页，1977。
[30] Segal. M.. *Brain* Res., 94:115, 1975.
[31] Wang, R. Y. *et al.*: *Brain Res.*, 120:85, 1977.
[32] Ashkenazi, R. *et al.*: *J. Physiol.*, 223:255, 1972.
[33] Holman, R. B. *et al.*: *J. Physiol.*, 223:243, 1972.
[34] Hong, J. S. *et al.*: *Brain Res.*, 134: 383, 1977.
[35] Oliveras, J. L. *et al.*: *Brain Res.*, **120: 221, 1977.**
[36] Taber–Pierce, E. *et al.*: *Brain Res.*, **107**:137, 1976.
[37] Brodal, A. *et al.*: *J. comp. neurol.*, **114**:261, 1960.
[38] Nauta, J. H. *et al.*: Reticular formation of the brain, p3, J. & A. Churchill LTD Press, 1958.

EFFECT OF ELECTRO ACUPUNCTURE AND SOME EXOGENOUS MONOAMINES ON UNIT DISCHARGES OF THE DORSAL NUCLEUS RAPHE

Department of Biophysics, Department of
Physiology, Beijing Medical College

In recent years, a number of researchers have demonstrated that serotenin (5-HT) in the brain and the raphe nuclei (5-HT containing neurons) are closely related with acupuncture analgesia. In this paper the effects of electroacupuncture and some monoamines on the unit discharge of the dorsal raphe nucleus (DRN) are investigated.

I. THE EFFECTS OF ELECTROACUPUNCTURE AND NOCICEPTIVE STIMULATION ON THE UNIT DISCHARGES OF RAT DRN.

Methods: Male rate weighing 200–400 g were operated on under chloral hydrate anaesthesia (400 mg/kg), paralysed with an intraperitoneal injection of tubocurarine (1–2 mg/kg), and subsequently kept alive by artificial respiration.

Unit discharges were recorded extracellularly with a glass microelectrode filled with 2M KC1 and 0.4M $K_3Fe(CN)_6$ (tip diameter 1–2μm and tip resistance 5–20 MΩ). The stereotaxic coordinates of DRN were deterained according to König's atlas[1]. In order to aviod the sagittal sinus, the microelectrode was inserted into the brain tissue with an inclination angle of 15 to the left. The unit discharges were displayed through a microelectrode amplifer on a double-beam oscilloscope. The experimental results were recorded on magnetic tapes and processed by a Japanese Model ATAC-501-10 computer.

The electroacupuncture stimulations were carried out with pulses (frequency 8 cycles/sec, width 1.5 msec, loaded voltage about 2V and duration 3–10 minutes) on the points corresponding to human acupuncture points Zusanli and Sanyinjiao. Noxious stimulation was applied to the tail of the rat by means of two needles with a train of five pulses (wave width 1 msec, frequency 200 cycles/sec, intensity 24–40V). The exact site of the tip of the microelectrode was marked by the Prussian blue method in one neuron of each experiment[2].

All experimental data were analyzed statistically. The changes in the firing rate were considered statistically significant only when the mean values of the changes in firing rates were over twice the standard error of the spontaneous dischage (i.e. $P<0.05$).

Results: Spontaneous discharges of 75 units were recorded on 42 male rats.

1. Spontaneous discharge in DRN: It was characteristically slow and regular with a mean value of about 1.5 spikes/sec and 200 μV–2mV in amplitude. This is basically similar to the results reported in other literature[3, 4].

2. The effect of electroacupuncture on discharges of DRN: Twenty-seven units were observed. There were four types of units responding to electroacupuncture: excitation (15units), inhibition (4 units), biphasic responses comsisting of an excitation followed by an inhibition (1 unit) and no effect (7 units).

The mean value of spontaneous firing of 15 excitatory units was 1.3±0.2 spikes/sec. using the frequency of spontaneous firing as 100%, the firing rate during electroacupuncture stimulation was increased to 220±13% (P<0.001), the increment being 120% on the average.

It was shown that the firing rate of most units in DRN increased markedly during electro-acupuncture stimulation. After the cessation of needling, the firing rate returned gradually to its original level. At the momemt of cessation, the firing rate was 122±16%; 5 minutes after cessation of needling it became 136±18%; and 10 minutes after cessation, it was 155 ± 23% (P<0.05) (Fig. 1). After cessation of needling the firing rate of most units fluctuated markedly, which was very much like the oscillatory phenomenon observed in other regulative processes[5].

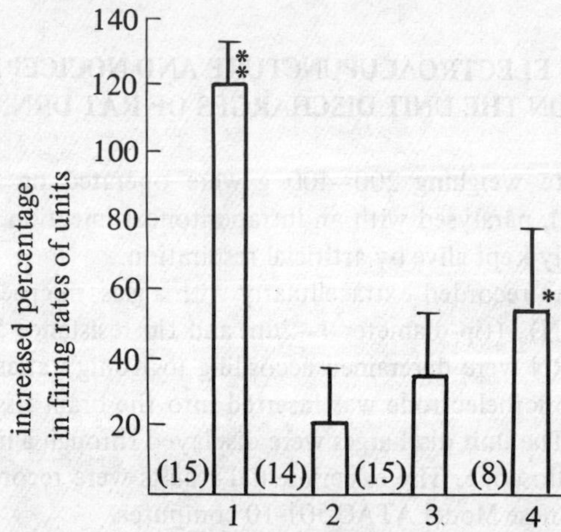

Fig. 1 Changes in firing rates in the excited units of DRN by electro-needling.
Ordinate: Increased percentage in firing rates of units.
Abscissa: 1. electro-needling
2. cessating of needling
3. 5 min post-needling
4. 10 min post-needling
Note: the values in parenthesis are number of units and bars are standard errors.
*P<0.05
**P<0.001

3. The effect of nociceptive stimulation on discharges of DRN: This effect was observed in 31 units. There were three types of units; those responding to noxious stimulation excitation (6 units), those showing inhibition (4 units) and those with no effect (21 units).

In the 6 units excited by noxious stimulations, the increment of the frequency was 155% on the average. In the 4 units inhibited by noxious stimulation, the mean value of decrement was 42%.

Discussion:

(1) The effect of electroacupuncture on the functional activities of DRN:

It was reported that the efficacy of electroacupuncture analgesia was decreased greatly after destruction of DRN[6,7] or intranuclear injection of 5,6-dihydroxytryptamine[7]. On the other hand, the animal's pain threshold was enhanced by electrical stimulation of DRN and the effect of acupuncture analgesia was increased significantly by the same stimulation[8]. Biochemical studies showed that in rats, 5-HT and its main metabolite,— 5-hydroxyindoleacetic acid, mcasured in the area of raphe nuclei increased markedly during acupuncture analgesia, this suggests that 5-HT turnover was raised by electro-needling[9]. It was found that during electroacupuncture, the anabolism and catabolism of 5HT were both enhanced[10]. The present results indicate that during electroacupuncture, the discharges of most units in DRN were enhanced. Bramwell reported that the firing rate of the neurons in raphe nuclei might be taken as an index of 5-HT turnover in the brain[11]. Thus the present results are in accord ance with the view that the 5-HT in the brain is involved in acupuncture analgesia.

(2) The possible route of the action of DRN in the process of acupuncture analgesia.

According to the present experimental results, of the 14 units of DRN observed, only 2 units show convergence of electro-needling and nociceptive signals. Therefore, the direct interaction between two signals in the same unit of DRN does not seem to be an important mechanism in acupuncture analgesia.

Axons from DRN and median raphe project to many areas of the telencephalon and diencephalon, for example, hypothalamus, basal ganglion, limbic system, cerebral cortex and the intralaminar nuclei of thalamus.

Descending fibers from the raphe nuclei of the caudal portion of the brainstem descend along the fasciculus spinalis anterior and lateralis to the anterior, lateral and posterior horns of the spinal cord[2,12,13,14]. Electro-physiological studies demonstrated that electrical stimulation of DRN had a marked inhibitory effect on nociceptive discharges of rabbit parafascicular nucleus (pf)[15]. The inhibitory effect of electro-needling on rat cortical potential evoked by tooth pulp stimulation was markedly depressed after local lesions of DRN[16]. The responses of dorsal horn interneurons in lamina V of the spinal cord to noxious stimulus were depressed by stimulation of cat DRN[17]. It is thus suggested that the role played by the DRN in acupuncture analgesia is to exert inhibitory influence through the ascending and descending pathways on the neural structures related to pain.

II. THE EFFECTS OF MICROIONTOPHORESIS OF 5-HT AND NORADRENALINE (NE) ON THE UNIT DISCHARGES OF RAT DRN AND THEIR RELATIONS TO THE EFFECTS OF ELECTRO-NEEDLING.

Methods: 25 adult rats each weighing 240–310 g were used. Three barrel microelectrodes were filled with (1) 2M KCl and 0.4M $K_3Fe(CN)_6$ (tip resistance below 30MΩ), (2) serotonin creatinine sulphate (0.05M, pH 4–5). and (3) noradrenaline bitartrate (0.12M, pH 4–5) respectively. The ejecting current was 40–60 nA and the retaining current was 10 nA. The duration of ejection was commonly 45–60 sec.

Results:

1. The effects of microiontophoresis of 5-HT and NE on unit discharges in DRN: 5-HT was applied electrophoretically to 34 units. Twenty-one units were depressed, 9 units were excited and 4 units were without effect. NE was given electrophoretically to 23 units, of which 13 units were depressed, 8 units were excited and 2 units showed no effect. To make a comparison between the two groups of neurons administered 5-HT and NE respectively, there were more depressed units in the former group, in which the depression was also deeper and lasted longer. In the group administered NE, the activity of the cell recovered markedly 2 min after ejection.

2. The effect of microiontophoresis of 5-HT on units excitatory and nonexcitatory to electro-needling.

In the units stimulated by electro-needling 14 units were depressed. Only one unit was stimulated by 5-HT. However, in the non-excitatory units, 5 units were depressed, 8 units were excited by 5-HT and 4 units showed no effect. Paired T-test done between the excitatory and non-excitatory units showed $P<0.01$, indicating that the effects of the iontophoresis of 5-HT on the units stimulated by electro-needling were mostly depressive.

3. The effect of microiontophoresis of NE on units excitatory and non-excitatory to electro-needling.

Twenty units were injected electrophoretically with NE. In the ten units stimulated by electro-needling, 7 units were inhibited and 3 were stimulated by NE. In the ten nonexcitatory units, 5 units were inhibited, 4 were excited and one was unaffected. A paired T-test was made between excitatory and non-excitatory units with $P>0.05$, indicating that there was no significant correlation between the effect of NE and electro-needling.

Discussion: Our present experimental results demonstrate that the effects of microiontophoresis of 5-HT on most neurons were depressive, though some were excitatory or nil. However, it was reported in other literature that all neurones showed inhibitory effect[18,19]. It might be that there exist two types of neurones in DRN, nevrons containing 5-HT and nevrons containing catecolamine (CA) [20], which would respond differently to microiontophoresis of 5-HT.

In the 15 DRN units stimulated by electro-needling, 14 units were depressed by micro-iontophorest of 5-HT. This phenomenon suggests that the units activated by electro-acupuncture were mainly nevrous containing 5-HT in DRN which played an important role in acupuncture analgesia. This is in accord ance with the results that the effect of acupuncture analgesia was enhanced by electrical stimulation of DRN or the raising of the levels of 5-HT in the brain. Histochemical studies indicate that terminals containing

NE projecting to DRN[15,20] possibly originated from locus coeruleus (LC), because these terminals disappeared after lesion of LC. Some pharmacological studies show that after selectively depleting CA in the brain by intracerebral injection of 6-OH DA, the terminals distributed in the DRN degenerated. Morgane points out that the discharges of neurons in the midbrain raphe (including DRN) were decreased by electrical stimulation of LC[21]. The action of NE-containing neurons and NE transmitter was thought to regulate the 5-HT containing neurons in DRN[22,23], and thereby to influence acupuncture analgesia[24].

III. CONCLUSION

1. During stimulation of acupuncture points, units in DRN showed excitation, inhibition, excitation-inhibition or no effect, with excitation as the leading effect.

2. During the period of microiontophoresis of 5-HT and NE, the discharges of most units in rat DRN were depressed. A comparison between the group given 5-HT and those given NE, showed that the former had more depressed units and was lower in the degree and longer in duration of the depression. It is considered that the two neurotransmitters, 5-HT and NE might play regulative roles in the functional activities of DRN.

3. Many more units were depressed by microiontophoresis of 5-HT in the units excited by electro-needling than in the units non-excitatory to acupuncture. It is suggested that it was mainly the 5-HT containing neurons in DRN that were activated by the electro-needling stimulation which played an important role in acupuncture analgesia.

REFERENCES

[1] Köning JFR and Klippel RA: *The Rat Brain,* 1963.

[2] Fuxe K and Jonsson G: *Adv. Biochem. Psychopharmacol.,* **10**:1, 1974.

[3] Aghajanian GK *et al*: *Science,* **169**:1100, 1970.

[4] Aghajanian GK *et al.*: *Brain Res,* **81**:364, 1974.

[5] Mittelstaedt H: Процессы Регулирования в Виологии, 1960.

[6] 陕西省中医研究所针麻原理研究室：陕西新医药，(5)：59，1975。

[7] 江振裕等：科学通报，22：41，1977。

[8] 陕西省中医研究所针麻原理研究室：陕西省中医研究所针麻原理研究资料选编(二)，第 19 页，1976。

[9] 中医研究院针灸经络研究所生化组：中医药研究参考，(2)：30，1976。

[10] 韩济生等：科学通报，24：278，331，1979。

[11] Branwell GJ: *Brain Res.,* 79:515, 1974.

[12] Dahlström A and Fuxe K: *Acta physiol. scand. suppl.,* **232**:1, 1964.

[13] Anden NE *et al.*: *Acta physiol. scand.* **67**:313, 1966.

[14] Ungerstedt U: *Acta. physiol. scand. Suppl.,* **367**:1, 1971.

[15] 湖北医学院基础部针麻研究组：湖北医学院科技通讯(针刺麻醉专辑)，(1)：33，1976。

[16] 陕西省中医研究所针麻原理研究室：陕西新医药，(4)：23，1976。

[17] Liebeskind JC: *Brain Res.,* **50**:441, 1973.

[18] Bramwell GJ and Gönye T: *Neuropharmacol.,* **15**:457, 1976.

[19] Aghajanian GK *et al.*: *Life sciences,* **11**(13): part 1, 615, 1972.

[20] Lindvall O *et al.*: *J. Comp. neurol.,* **154**:317, 1974.

[21] Morgane PJ *et al.*: *Anat. Rec.,* **178**:421, 1974.

[22] Svensson TH *et al.*: *The Pharmacologist,* **16**:244, 1974.

[23] Foote WE *et al.*: *Nature,* **222**: 567, 1969.

[24] Tong XW *et al.*: *Act Physiol. Sinica,* **31**:273, 1979.

INFLUENCE OF ELECTRO-STIMULATION OF NUCLEUS RAPHE MAGNUS AND LOCUS CAERULEUS ON THE ANALGESIC EFFECT OF ACUPUNCTURE IN THE SPINAL TRIGEMINAL NUCLEUS

Zhong Guogan, Liu Minzhi, Jiang Yan, Liu Xiang,
Wang Shao, Liu Suping
(Department of Physiology, Bethune Medical College)

I. INTRODUCTION

It was previously observed that electro-acupuncture of body points markedly depressed the reaction to noxious stimuli of the cells of the caudate subnucleus in the spinal trigeminal nucleus. It was further established by pharmacological methods that this depressive effect is mainly a presynaptic inhibition[1]. Many investigations in recent years have demonstrated that the nucleus raphe and locus caeruleus of the brain stem play an important role in acupuncture analgesia[2–6]. Basbaum et al. reported that the nucleus raphe and locus caeruleus might project fibers directly or indirectly to the spinal trigeminal nucleus[11–14]. Thus, it seems reasonable to assume that the transmission of painful impulses in the spinal trigeminal nucleus may be regulated by the nucleus raphe and locus caeruleus. The aim of the present work is to determine the relationship between these two nuclei and to assess the analgesic effect of acupuncture.

II. METHODS

The experimental methods were essentially the same as previously reported[1]. Experimental observations were made on paralyzed but conscious cats. Asingle square pulse above 20 V with a width of 0.5 msec was administered as a nocuous stimulus to the inferior alveolar nerve, while single square pulses of 2–10 V were given as electro-acupuncture stimulation to the "Jiache" acupoint. Evoked unit discharges were recorded by means of a glass microelectrode in the caudate subnucleus of the spinal trigeminal nucleus. The duration of the inhibitory effect of electro-acupuncture on pain-evoked discharges, i.e. time course of inhibition, or TCI, measured in msec was taken as the index of electro-acupuncture analgesia. TCI was determined by the delay of the stimulator in adjusting the interval between the electro-acupuncture stimulation and the pain stimulus. A train of repetitive pulses from the G5805 acupuncture anaesthesia apparatus was applied through concentric electrodes to the nucleus raphe magnus and locus caeruleus to observe the change in TCI before and after electro-stimulation. The parameters of central stimulation were 18–29 V in intensity, 2 hertz in frequency and 10 minutes in duration.

In some experiments LSD (100μg/kg body weight) was given intravenously 1–2 minutes before stimulation of nucleus raphe magnus to block 5-HT effect. In other experiments the effect of single square pulse stimulation of the nucleus raphe magnus and locus caeruleus on the pain-evoked discharges of the caudate subnucleus in the spinal trigeminal nucleus was observed.

The position-fixing coordinates of the nucleus raphe magnus and locus caeruleus were determined with reference to E.J. Taber[10], M. Sasa et al. [11,12] and the Atlas of R.T. Snider. The coordinates of the nucleus raphe magnus were $P_{5.0}$, L_o, and $H_{-8.5}$ and those of the locus caeruleus $P_{2.0}$, $L_{2.0}$ and $H_{3.0}$. A histological examination was made after each experiment to verify the location of the tips of the stimulating electrodes by using the Prussian blue reaction.

The physiological conditions of the experimental animals were maintained within the normal range during the experiments.

III. RESULTS

(I) Spontaneous fluctuation of TCI of electro-acupuncture.

Since TCI was taken as the index of the analgesic effect of electro-acupuncture, it was necessary to determine whether the TCI was stable or not under normal conditions.

The TCI of 18 pain-sensitive cells was repeatedly determined every 5' for 30'. The avevage value of TCI was 302 msec. The range of fluctuation was ± 50 msec except in 2 cases. Statistical analysis gave a value of –7.4 ± 18.2 (S.D.)% of the control value for the range of fluctuation. P>0.05 (T-test), indicating that the difference was insignificant.

(II) Effect of stimulation of the nucleus raphe magnus on TCI of electro-acupuncture.

In 14 cats the tips of the stimulating electrodes were located inside the nucleus raphe magnus. The results of stimulation 27 times in the 14 animals were as follows: TCI was prolonged in 22 cases, one of which is shown in Fig. 1; TCI was not changed in 4 cases; and in 1 case TCI was slightly shortened. The range of TCI in the above 27 cases was, before stimulation of the nucleus raphe magnus, 125–1200 msec. After stimulation it shifted to between 325 and 2000 msec. Statistical analysis of these 27 trial cases shows an average prolongation of TCI of 125 ± 166 (S.D.)%, the difference being a very significant (P<0.01) compared with the control group mentioned above.

The prolongation of the TCI of electro-acupuncture usually started 5–10 minutes after stimulation of the nucleus raphe magnus and reached its climax 6 to 25 minutes after the stimulation. It would then gradually return to the initial state.

In 4 cats the tips of the stimulating electrodes were found near the nucleus raphe magnus. Stimulation at these sites 9 times, showed no change of TCI in 8 cases and slight prolongation in 1 case. LSD, a 5-HT antagonist, was injected intravenously in 3 other cats in a dose of 100μg/kg before stimulation of the nucleus raphe magnus. No prolongation of TCI could be observed in all 5 experiments.

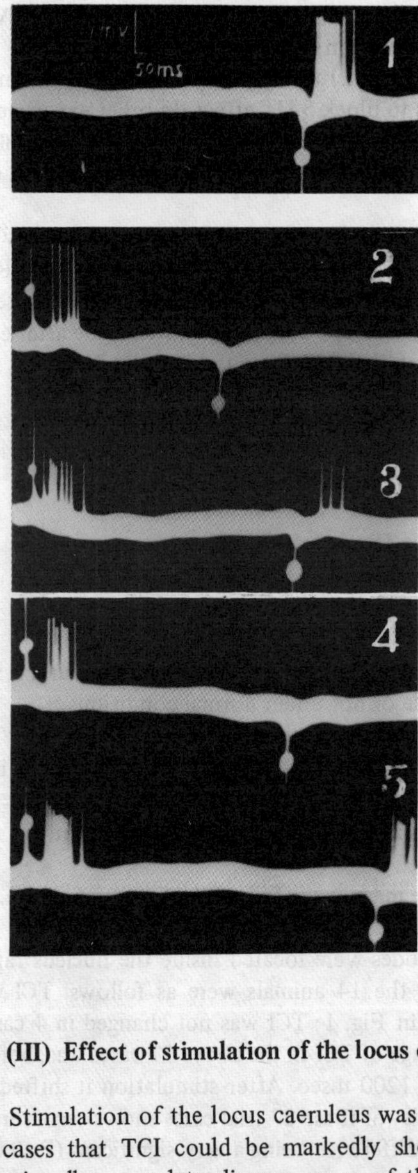

Fig. 1 Prolongation of TCI in the spinal trigeminal nucleus following stimulation of the nucleus raphe magnus.

(1) Pain-evoked discharges recorded in the spinal trigeminal nucleus elicited by stimulation of the inferior alveolar nerve.

(2)(3) Before stimulation of the nucleus raphe magnus, pain-evoked discharges were inhibited when the interval between electro-acupuncture and pain stimulus was 200 msec (2); they reappeared when the interval was increased to 300 msec (3).

(4)(5) After stimulation of the nucleus raphe magnus, pain-evoked discharges were inhibited when the interval between electroacupuncture and pain stimulus was 300 msec (4); they reappeared when the interval was prolonged to 400 msec (5). The small dots in the photographs represent electro-acupuncture artifact and large dots represent pain stimulation artifact (the same for the following figures).

(III) Effect of stimulation of the locus caeruleus on the TCI of electro-acupuncture.

Stimulation of the locus caeruleus was repeated 20 times on 12 cats. It was shown in all 20 cases that TCI could be markedly shortened by stimulation of the locus caeruleus. Occasionally, complete disappearance of the inhibitory effect of electro-acupuncture was observed. The range of TCI in the 20 cases was 100–925 msec before stimulation and 0–400 after stimulation. Statistical analysis of these data shows a mean shortening of 81.6 ± 25.6 (S.D.)% following stimulation of the locus caeruleus with the difference being very significant ($P<0.01$). One example is shown in Fig. 2.

The above effect usually appeared 5–10 minutes after stimulation of the locus caeruleus and subsided 30–60 minutes after cessation of stimulation.

When the stimulating electrodes were outside the mass of the locus caeruleus (3 cats) no changes in TCI could be observed even though the same intensity of electric stimulation was

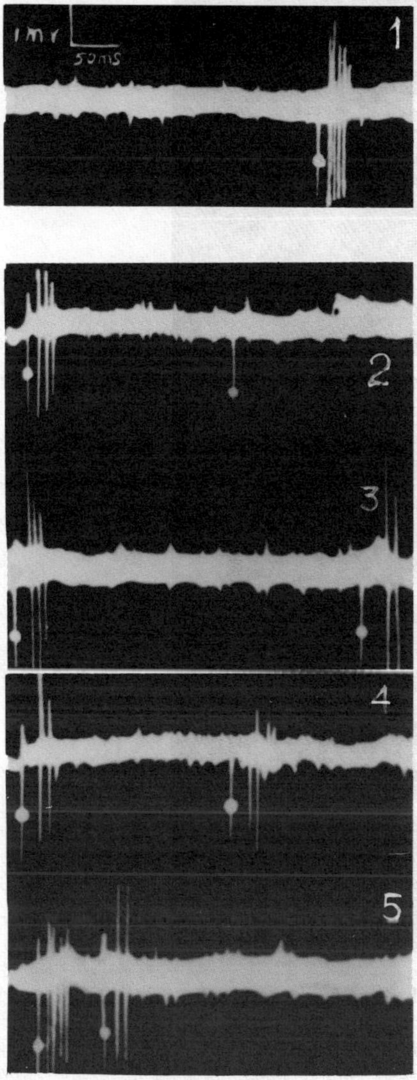

Fig. 2 Shortening of the TCI of electro-acupuncture in the spinal trigeminal nucleus following stimulation of the locus caeruleus.

(1) Evoked discharges in pain-sensitive neuron.

(2)(3) Before stimulation of locus caeruleus, pain-evoked discharges were inhibited when the interval between electro-acupuncture and pain stimulus was 250 msec (2); they reappeared when the interval was increased to 350 msec (3).

(4)(5(5) After stmulation of the locus caeruleus, pain-evoked discharges continued when the interval between electro-acupuncture and pain stimulus was either 250 msec (4) or 50 msec (5).

applied (5 trials). It was observed in cat No. 19 that when the stimulating electrode was inserted beyond the mass of the locus caeruleus, stimulation gave no change in TCI. As soon as the stimulating electrode was moved 0.5 mm dorsally to make the tip of the stimulating electrode lie in the locus caeruleus, stimulation under the same conditions as before resulted in the complete disappearance of the inhibitory effect of electro-acupuncture on pain-evoked discharges. Furthermore, it was demonstrated in another cat that stimulation of the locus caeruleus could shift TCI from 125 msec to 0 (i.e. complete disappearance of inhibitory effect), while the same stimulation was no longer effective after a direct current of 2 mA had been sent through the stimulating electrode for 30 sec to destroy the locus caeruleus.

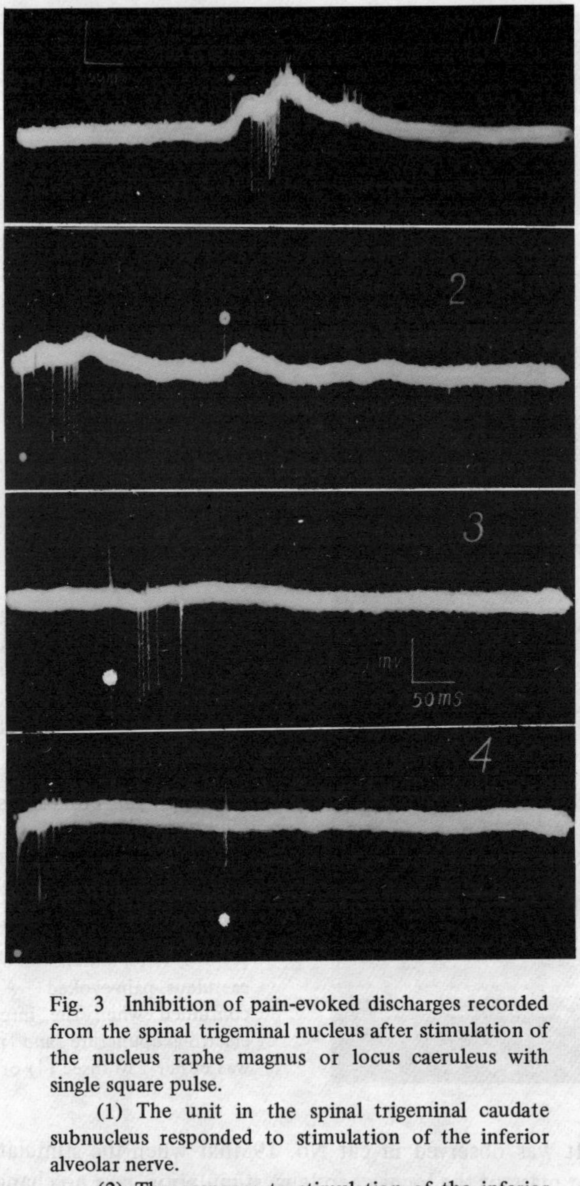

Fig. 3 Inhibition of pain-evoked discharges recorded from the spinal trigeminal nucleus after stimulation of the nucleus raphe magnus or locus caeruleus with single square pulse.

(1) The unit in the spinal trigeminal caudate subnucleus responded to stimulation of the inferior alveolar nerve.

(2) The response to stimulation of the inferior alveolar nerve was inhibited when the nucleus raphe magnus was stimulated 270 msec. prior to the pain stimulus.

(3) The unit in the spinal trigeminal caudate subnucleus responded to stimulation of the inferior alveolar nerve.

(4) The response to stimulation of the inferior alveolar nerve was inhibited when the nucleus locus caeruleus was stimulated in 270 msec. prior to the pain stimulus.

These results indicate that the shortening of TCI or the disappearance of inhibitory effect of acupuncture was definitely caused by stimulation of the locus caeruleus.

(IV) The effect of stimulation of the nucleus raphe magnus and locus caeruleus with single shock.

It was found that the spinal trigeminal caudate subnucleus reacted both to stimulation of the inferior alveolar nerve and to that of the nucleus raphe magnus or locus caeruleus. It was also found that the stimulation of nucleus raphe magnus or locus caeruleus can inhibit the responses of the spinal trigeminal nucleus to the inferior alveolar nerve (Fig. 3).

The nucleus raphe magnus or locus coeruleus was stimulated with single square pulses of 5–10 V and the inferior alveolar nerve with single square pulses of 20 V. A total of 36 such units in 18 cats were recorded in the spinal trigeminal caudate subnucleus, among which, 10 units reacted to stimulation of both the inferior alveolar nerve and the nucleus raphe magnus, and 26 units reacted to stimulation of both the inferior alveolar nerve and the locus caeruleus. When the nucleus raphe magnus was stimulated 100–300 msec. before the stimulation of the inferior alveolar nerve, pain-evoked discharges were completely inhibited in the 10 units (Fig. 3–2). When the locus caeruleus was stimulated 100–300 msec before the stimulation of the inferior alveolar nerve, complete inhibition of pain-evoked discharges was noted in 22 of the 26 units (Fig. 3–4) and partial inhibition occurred in the remaining 4, as shown in the decrease in frequency of the pain-evoked discharges.

IV. DISCUSSION

It was found that different effects were obtained when single or repetitive pulses were applied to the nucleus raphe magnus and locus caeruleus. When single shock was given, the inhibitory effect on responses of the spinal trigeminal caudate subnucleus to the stimulation of the inferior alveolar nerve was characterized by rapid onset and the absence of aftereffects. When repetitive pulses were used, the effect on the TCI of electro-acupuncture varied with the site of central stimulation, i.e. prolongation of TCI after stimulation of the nucleus raphe magnus and shortening of TCI after stimulation of the locus caeruleus. The repetitive pulse application was characterized by a slow onset, a latent period of 5–10 minutes, and a long aftereffect lasting more than 30 minutes.

The fact that stimulation of the nucleus raphe magnus or the locus caeruleus with single pulses could inhibit the pain-evoked discharges of the spinal trigeminal caudate subnucleus indicates that the nucleus raphe magnus or locus caeruleus may have a direct inhibitory effect on the transmission of pain impulses in the spinal trigeminal nucleus.

The effects elicited by stimulating the nucleus raphe magnus and locus caeruleus with single pulses are in accordance with the observations of Sasa[11,12]. However, we cannot as yet offer a satisfactory explanation for diverse effects produced by single and repetitive stimulations.

The abundant experimental evidence available in recent years indicates the possible existence of direct or indirect projection fibers from the nucleus raphe magnus and locus caeruleus to the spinal trigeminal nucleus[11–14]. We also observed short latency discharges in the spinal trigeminal caudate subnucleus evoked by stimulation of the nucleus raphe magnus or locus caeruleus, suggesting the existence of direct or indirect (through some intermediate neurons) projection from these two nuclei to the spinal trigeminal caudate subnucleus. It is possible that the above inhibitory effects produced by stimulation of the nucleus raphe magnus or locus caeruleus with single pulses might have been brought about through their descending projection fibers. Using Wall's antidromic action potential technique, Lovik observed that presynaptic inhibition might participate in the depression of the evoked discharges of the spinal trigeminal nucleus[13]. In our experiment, the existence of presynaptic inhibition should be taken into consideration, since the TCI of electro-acupuncture were as long as 100–300 msec.

The effect of prolongation or shortening of TCI in our experiments following stimulation by repetitive pulses of the nucleus raphe magnus and locus caeruleus respectively coincides with the experimental results obtained by other investigators using visceral-somatic reflexes as indices[7,8]. Based on the fact that these effects had a delayed onset and a prolonged aftereffect, and that there exist ascending projection fibers to the forebrain from both the nucleus raphe magnus and the locus caeruleus[9,15,16], it is reasonable to assume that their effects might be brought about by way of the projection fibers of these two nuclei to the forebrain. This would activate certain mediator systems including the enkephalin system. Since naloxone can reverse the analgesic effect produced by stimulation[7] of the nucleus raphe magnus and since a high density of opiate receptors are present in the spinal trigeminal caudate subnucleus[18], we are inclined to think that the endorphin system might also participate in this effect. The possibility that the descending systems from the nucleus raphe magnus and locus caeruleus might also be responsible for this effect does exist. But what is worth to noticng is that if the above effect is really brought about through the action of the descending systems, then it seems that it is not brought about simply through the descending projection fibers to the spinal trigeminal caudate subnucleus, but rather through some other more complicated nerve paths or mechanism.

V. CONCLUSIONS

1. Stimulation of the nucleus raphe magnus may yield two types of effects. One is the inhibition of pain-evoked discharges in the spinal trigeminal caudate subnucleus by stimulation of the nucleus raphe magnus with single pulse. This is characterized by a rapid onset and absence of aftereffects. The other is prolongation of TCI after stimulation of the nucleus raphe magnus by repetitive pulses. This is characterized by a slow onset and prolonged aftereffects.

2. Stimulation of the locus caeruleus may also produce two types of effects. One is inhibition of the pain-induced discharges in the spinal trigeminal caudate subnucleus by stimulation of the locus caeruleus with single pulse. This is characterized by a rapid onset and the absence of aftereffects. The other is the shortening of TCI after stimulation of the locus caeruleus with repetitive pulses. This is characterized by a slow onset and a prolonged aftereffects.

REFERENCES

[1] 吉林医科大学生理教研室　中国科学，(6): 615，1977。
[2] 江振裕等：科学通报，(1): 41，1977。
[3] 陕西中医研究所　针刺麻醉原理研究资料选编，(二) 19，1976。
[4] 陕西中医研究所　陕西新医药，(1) 66，1976。
[5] 张德星等：科学通报，(二) 117，1978。
[6] 杜焕基　赵燕芳：中国科学，(6) 631，1975。
[7] 杜焕基等：生理学报，30 (1): 1，1978。
[8] 杜焕基等：生理学报，31 (2): 154，1979。
[9] 北京医学院基础针麻原理研究组生理组：中枢神经介质概论，科学出版社　45—48，1977。
[10] Taber E. J.: *Comp. Neuro.*, **116**: 27, 1961.
[11] Sasa M. *et al.*: *Brain Res.*, **101** (2) : 199, 1976.
[12] Sasa M. *et al.*: *Brain Res.*, **55** (1) : 203, 1973.
[13] Lovick T. A. et al.: *Pain in the Trigeminal Region*, Elsevier/North-Holland Biomedical Press, 307, 1977.
[14] Basbaum A. I. *et al.*: *Proceedings Nat. Acad. Sci. U. S. A.* **73** (12) : 4685, 1976.
[15] Brodal A. *et al.*: *J. Comp. Neurol.*, **114**:239, 1960.
[16] Bobillier P. *et al.*: *Brain Res.*, **113**: 449, 1976.
[17] Oliveras *et al.*: *Brain Res.*, **120**:221, 1977.
[18] Atweh S. F. : *Brain Res.*, **124** : 53, 1977.

EFFECTS OF ELECTRO-STIMULATION AND ELECTROACUPUNCTURE OF MIDBRAIN RAPHE ON NEURONS IN THE HEAD OF CAUDATE NUCLEUS IN CONSCIOUS AND UNRESTRAINED RABBITS

Sun Gongduo, Li Xuming, Yang Kongshun ,*
Cheng Shaojie,* Du Xiujie

(Brain and Behavior laboratory, Department of Physiology, Guiyang Medical College)

It has been reproted that the spontaneous activities of the neurons in the head of the caudate nucleus of conscious and unrestrained rabbits may be modulated by electroacupuncture of the "Hegu" point in the form of either activation or inhibition[1]. In order to analyse the possible paths involved in the modulation of the caudate neurons, the effects of electroacupuncture and electro-stimulation of the midbrain raphe nuclei on the caudate neurons have been investigated.

I. METHOD

Experiments were carried out on thirty-two rabbits of both sexes weighing each about 2 kg. The unit activities in the head of the caudate nucleus of each of 95 units were recorded by chronic microelectrode techniques[2]. The recorded sites were within areas corresponding to the A_{2-4}, RL_{2-4} and H_{6-3} in Sawyer's atlas.

A bipolar stimulating electrode was implanted in the midbrain raphe nuclei P_{9-10}, $RL_{0-0.5}$, $H_{-(5-6)}$.

Parameters of the stimulation of the raphe were: square waves with frequency of 2–3 spikes/sec, wave width: 0.2–0.5 msec, intensity: 5–15 Volts. The stimulation lasted for 60–120 sec.

Parameters of the electroacupuncture were: the "Hegu" point stimulated by electroacupuncture unilaterally with the G-6805 electroacupuncture apparatus at a frequency of 2.8–3 spikes/sec. The intensity was adjusted so as to elicit a slight trembling of the extremities and the duration of stimulation was about 5 min.

The single unit discharge was recorded with a self-filled glass microelectrode[4,5]. An MWT-1 type microdriver was used to search for the neurons. The discharges were picked up by a negative capacitance compensated cathode follower preamplifier and then were displayed on one beam of a double oscillograph (SBR-1) to be photo graphed. An auditory monitor

* Guiyang Traditional Chinese Medical College.

was used routinely. The discharges were recorded by a tape recorder (602-A) and were selected strictly according to the previously determined criteria[1]. However, the ratio of signal-to-noise of all the discharges observed was more than 3:1. The wave form of the discharges was monitored with the help of the trigger of the oscillograph in order to make sure that the discharges were from the same neuron throughout the experiment.

At the end of each experiment an insulated stainless steel electrode with an uninsulated tip was inserted into the caudate nucleus and the raphe nuclei of the midbrain respectively. A DC current of 50–100μA was applied to the electrode for 15–30 sec. The stimulation and recorded sites were marked by the Prussian blue reaction method. The brain was cut into slices of 1 mm or sections of 20 μm thick for histological location.

The experimental data were analysed with a medical computer (TQ-19). The apparatus was used for statistical analysis was as follows: the signals of discharge led from the Y-pole of an oscilloscope to a Schmidt's trigger and a shaping circuit and fed into the negative pole of the oscilloscope to modulate the brightness were displayed as bright dots.

II. RESULTS

(I) Observation of spontaneous activities

The spontaneous activities of the neurons in the head of the caudate nucleus were observed. Among the 95 units observed there were 22 (23.2%) of high frequency (>10 spikes/sec), 70 (73.7%) of medium frequency (1–10 spikes/sec) and 3 (3.1%) of low frequency (<1 spike/sec). These data are similar to those in the previous report[1].

The head of the caudate nucleus was subdivided into three regions according to depth: a superficial region (H_{6-5}), an intermediate region (H_{5-4}) and a deep region (H_{4-3}). Fig. 1

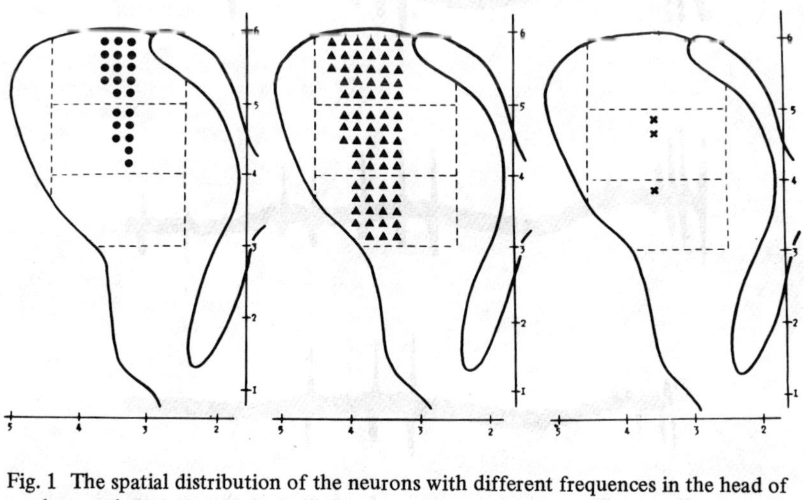

Fig. 1 The spatial distribution of the neurons with different frequences in the head of caudate nucleus.
• The high frequency neuron. ▲ The medium frequency neuron.
X The low frequency neuron. Each symbol represents a unit.

shows the spatial distribution of neurons with different firing frequencies. The high frequency ones were distributed mostly in the superficial region (14 out of 22 units, 63.6%), and were not found in the deep region. The medium frequency ones were distributed widely in the H_{6-3} region, with 28 units (40%) in the superficial region, 23 units (32.8%) in the intermediate region and 19 units (27.2%) in the deep region. Three low frequency neurons were found in the intermediate and deep regions.

(II) The effects of electro-stimulation of the midbrain raphe nuclei

The effects of single pulse or repeated pulse stimulation of the midbrain raphe nuclei on different neurons were observed.

1. The effect of single pulse stimulation. A single square wave pulse, 0.2 msec, 5–15 Volts, was sent through the midbrain raphe nuclei every 15 sec. No consistent response could be found in most of the neurons. However, there were 2 out of 64 units that showed definite evoked response. One of them is shown in Fig. 2.

2. The effect of repetitive pulse stimulation. The spontaneous activities of most of the 95 neurons observed could be modulated by repetitive pulse stimulation of the raphe nuclei. They could be classified into three types: excitatory, inhibitory and unaffected.

(1) Excitatory effect: There were 30 out of the 95 units that showed a marked excitatory effect (31.6%). The difference between the pulse numbers 5 min before and after the stimulation was significant ($P<0.05$).

It was found that by repetitive pulse stimulation of the midbrain raphe nuclei, the activity of the neurons of the caudate nucleus was enhanced, the discharge frequency was

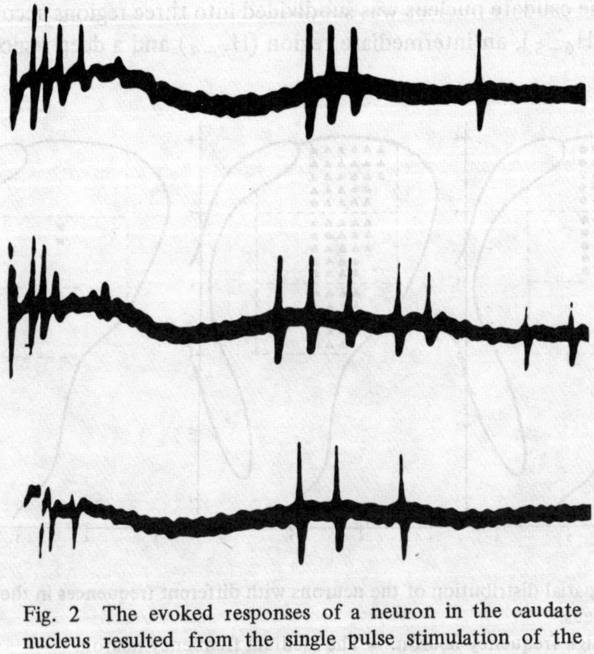

Fig. 2 The evoked responses of a neuron in the caudate nucleus resulted from the single pulse stimulation of the raphe nuclei. (unit 12-1-002).

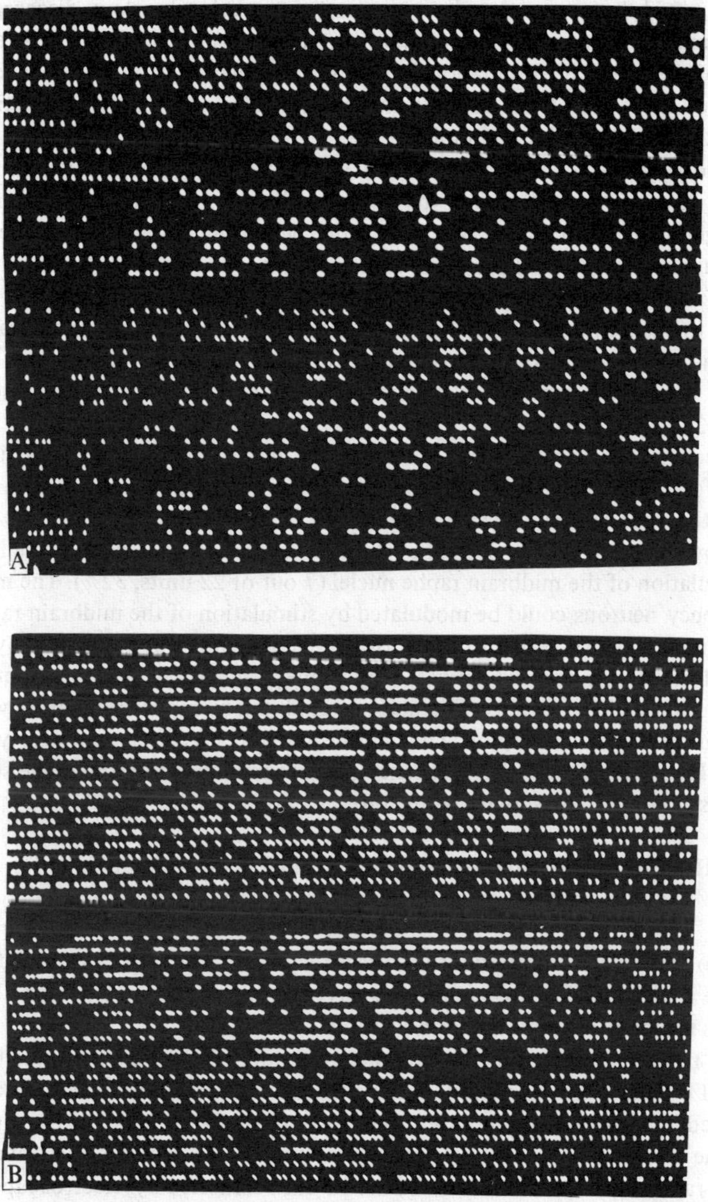

Fig. 3 The excitatory effect of repetitive pulses stimulation of midbrain raphe nuclei on a neuron in the caudate nucleus. (unit 26-2-003)

A. The spontaneous activity 4 min. before the stimulation.

B. The activity 4 min. after the stimulation. Each bright dot represents a single discharge.

increased, and rapid bursts appeared in contrast to previously slow discharges. After cessation of stimulation the firing rate of the neurons was still higher than before, showing the retention of the effect of stimulation. It seems that a new level of functional activity of some neurons of the head of the caudate nucleus was attained following repetitive pulse stimulation of the nuclei of midbrain raphe.

(2) Inhibitory effect: There were 30 out of the 95 units that showed an inhibitory effect (31.6%). The difference between the pulse numbers 5 min before and after the stimulation was significant ($P<0.05$). It was shown that when the stimulation of the midbrain raphe nuclei was repeated, the discharges of some neurons in the head of the caudate nucleus were gradually inhibited with their frequencies decreased. Sometimes the discharge frequencies decreased to such an extent that the discharges even ceased for up to several seconds. After the cessation of stimulation, the discharges of the neurons still remained inhibited, showing for a period the aftereffect of the stimulation. Fig. 4 shows the results of an experiment on 28–1–001 neuron.

(3) Unaffected units: There were 35 of the 95 units (36.8%) under experiment that showed no effect. The difference between the pulse numbers 5 min before and after stimulation of the midbrain raphe was not significant ($P>0.05$).

Fig. 5. shows that : (A) Only a small portion of the high frequency units could be modulated by stimulation of the midbrain raphe nuclei (7 out of 22 units, 32%). The majority of medium frequency neurons could be modulated by stimulation of the midbrain raphe nuclei (53 out of 70 units, 75.9%). None of the 3 low frequency units was modulated by the stimulation. (B) Most of the neurons activated by raphe stimulation were distributed in the superficial and intermediate regions. The neurons inhibited by raphe stimulation were mostly distributed in the superficial region. The neurons showing no effect were widely distributed throughout H_{6-3}. (C) Those high frequency neurons modulated by the raphe stimulation were mostly distributed in the superficial region.

(III) The relationship between the effect of electro-stimulation of the midbrain raphe nuclei and electroacupuncture

In order to make clear this relationship, the effect of repeated electro-stimulation of the midbrain raphe nuclei and electro-acupuncture was observed on the same neuron. The results of observations made on 30 units are given in Table 1.

Of the 30 neurons observed in the experiment, 9 units (30%) were activated by electroacupuncture, 11 units (36.7%) inhibited and 10 units (33.3%) unaffected. About 66.7% were modulated by electroacupuncture. The ratio is similar to that in the previous report[1]. Of the 9 units activated by electroacupuncture, 8 units could be activated by stimulation of the raphe nuclei as well. And of the 11 units inhibited by electroacupuncture, 7 units were also inhibited by stimulation of the raphe nuclei. Fig. 6 and Fig. 7 illustrate the results of two typical experiments.

Electroacupuncture could further activate the neurons which had already been activated by stimulation of the midbrain raphe nuclei. Likewise, the neurons which had been inhibited by stimulation of the midbrain raphe nuclei could be further inhibited by electroacupuncture.

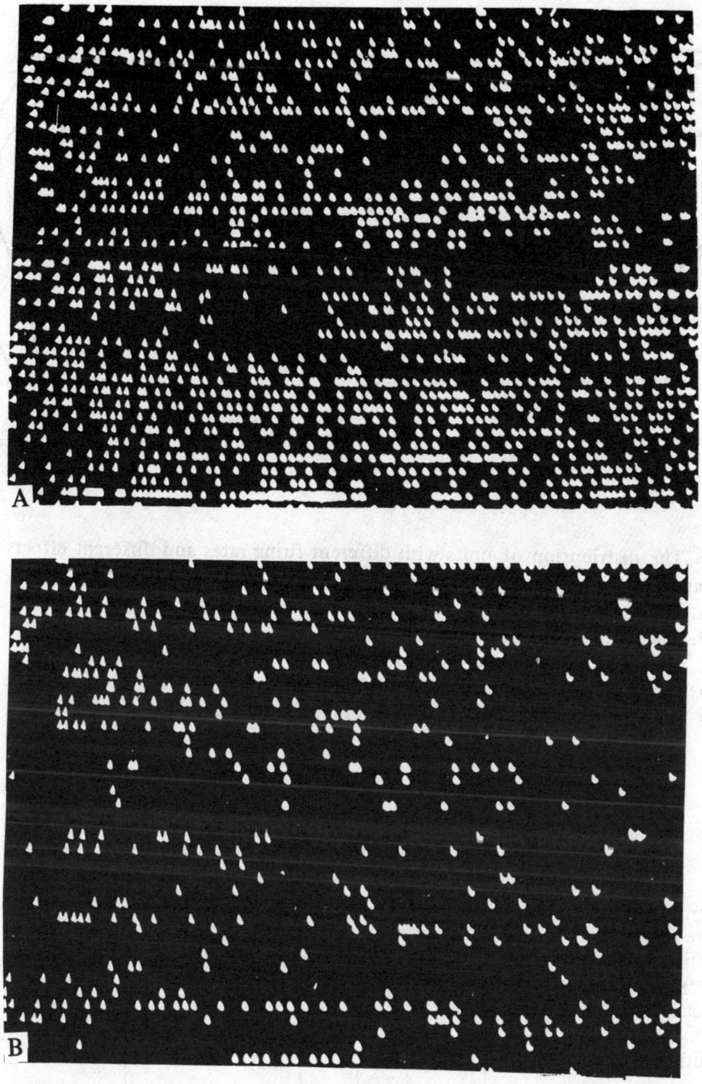

Fig. 4 The inhibitory effect of repetitive pulses stimulation of midbrain raphe nuclei on a neuron in the caudate nucleus. (unit 28-1-001)

A. The spontaneous activity 4 min. before the stimulation.

B. The activity 4 min. after the stimulation. Each bright dot represents a single discharge.

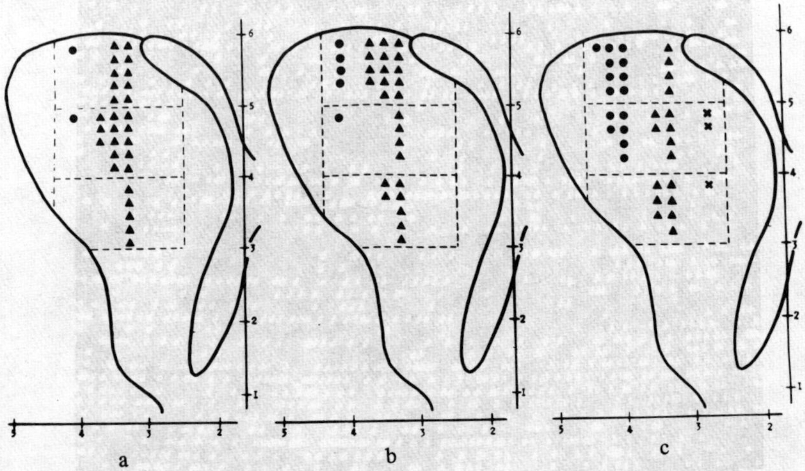

Fig. 5 The distribution of units with different firing rates and different effects of stimulation of the midbrain raphe nuclei.

A. The distribution of activated neurons.

B. The distribution of inhibited neurons.

C. The distribution of unaffected neurons.

• The high frequency unit. ▲ The medium frequency unit.

× The low frequency unit. Each symbol represents a unit.

Table 1. The effect of stimulation of midbrain raphe nuclei and electroacupuncture on the neurons in the caudate nucleus

The Effect of Electroacupuncture of 'Hegu' Point	The Effect of Stimulation of the Raphe		
	Activated	Inhibited	Unaffected
Activated	8	0	1
Inhibited	4	7	0
Unaffected	7	0	3
Total	19	7	4

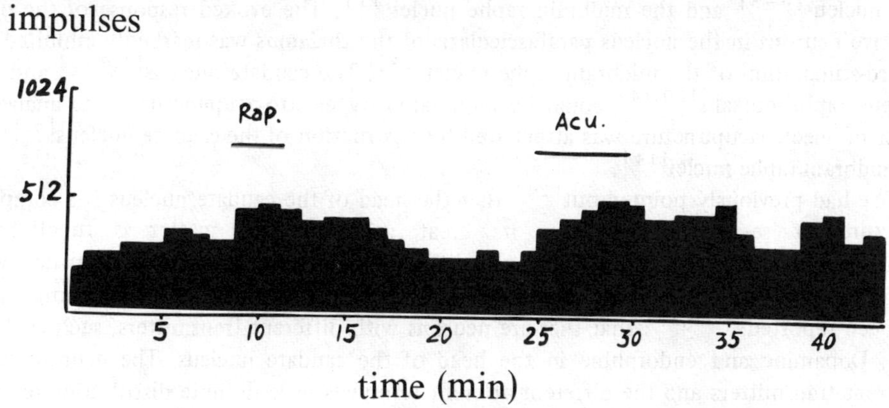

Fig. 6 The sequencial impulse density histogram showing excitatory effect. (unit 26-2-003) The horizontal bars represent the stimulations.

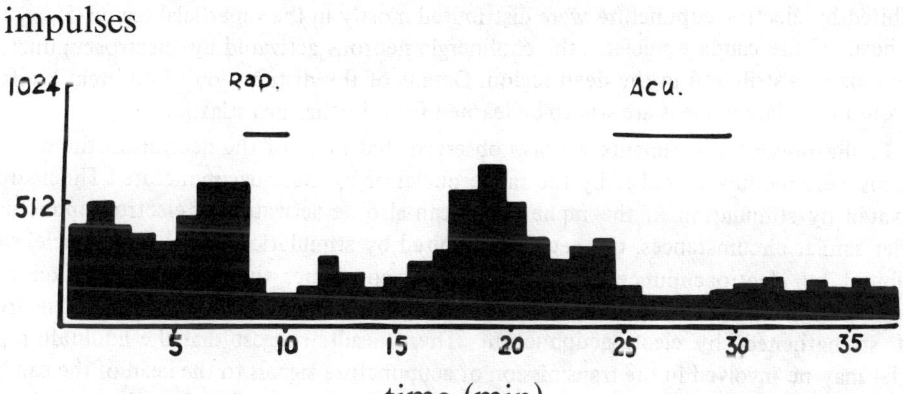

Fig. 7 The sequencial impulse density histogram showing inhibitory effect. (unit 28-1-001) The horizontal bars represent the stimulations.

III. DISCUSSION

In recent years, many authors have proved that the caudate nucleus[1,6–9] and raphe nuclei[10–14] are involved in the process of acupuncture analgesia. There is a close relationship between the midbrain raphe nuclei and the caudate nucleus. The data from morphological researches also show that the efferent fibres of the raphe nuclei of the midbrain project into the caudate nucleus[15–18] and vice versa[16–19]. When the raphe nuclei was stimulated, an evoked unit response could be recorded in the caudate nucleus[18–20]. The pain threshold was elevated by electroacupuncture,[6,7] electro-stimulation of the caudate nucleus[6-8] and the midbrain raphe nuclei[11]. The evoked response of the pain sensitive neurons in the nucleus parafascicularis of the thalamus was markedly inhibited by electro-stimulation of the midbrain raphe nuclei[23]. The caudate nucleus[1,6-9] and the nucleus raphe dorsalis[10,14] could be modulated by electro-acupuncture. The analgesic effect of electroacupuncture was attenuated by destruction of the caudate nucleus[6,7] or the midbrain raphe nuclei[11].

We had previously pointed out[24] that the head of the caudate nucleus is a complex structure. It seems unlikely that its great mass of grey matter is functionally homogeneous. It is composed of numerous different types of neurons. It is important that we find out whether there is any structural or functional differentiation in this complex. It has been reported[8,25,26] that ther are neurons with different transmitters, such as Ach, 5HT, Dopamine and endorphine in the head of the caudate nucleus. The neurons with different transmitters and the different afferent terminals have definite distribution regions in the caudate nucleus[8,15,25-28]. There is a functional distinction between the anterior and the posterior[27,29-31], and between the dorsal and the ventral parts in the caudate nucleus[7,32-34]. The present investigation suggests that there may be distinctly different distribution regions for the units, with different frequencies, in the head of the caudate nucleus of the conscious, unrestrained rabbit. It was reported[9] that serotonergic neurons inhibited by electro-acupuncture were distributed mostly in the superficial region (H_{6-5}) of the head of the caudate nucleus; the cholinergic neurons activated by electroacupuncture were mostly distributed in the deep region. Details of the distribution of different kinds of neurons in caudate nucleus are still to be learned from further investigations.

In the present experiments we also observed that most of the neurons in the caudate nucleus were modulated either by the raphe nuclei or by electroacupuncture . The neurons activated by stimulation of the raphe nuclei can also be activated by electroacupuncture . Under similar circumstances, the neurons inhibited by stimulation of the raphe nuclei were inhibited by electroacupuncture , too. At the same time, they all had a period with aftereffects. The effect of stimulation of the midbrain raphe nuclei on the caudate neurons was strengthened by electroacupuncture . These results suggest that the midbrain raphe nuclei may be involved in the transmission of acupuncture signals to the head of the caudate nucleus. The raphe region might play a role in the mechanism of the aftereffect of acupuncture analgesia, since the aftereffect of stimulation of the midbrain raphe nuclei on the caudate neurons was commonly observed. Although the majority of neurons of the head of the caudate nucleus could be modulated by repetitive pulse stimulation of the midbrain raphe nuclei, single pulse stimulation did not elicit any such reaction in most of them. The modulation of neurons in the caudate nucleus by stimulation of the midbrain raphe nuclei probably takes place through some multisynaptic pathways, such as the midbrain-substantia nigracaudate nucleus pathway[42-45], or the recurrent circuit of the forebrain as has been suggested by Prof. Zhang Xiangtong[38-40]. The details of multisynaptic pathways and their analgesic action in electro-acupuncture are still not clear and need further investigation.

IV. SUMMARY

1. A chronic microelectrode study of the unit discharge of the head of the caudate nucleus of conscious, unrestrained rabbits was carried out.

2. The activity of most neurons in the head of the caudate nucleus could be modulated by stimulation of the midbrain raphe nuclei, producing either activation or inhibition with a certain amount of aftereffect.

3. The units modulated by the raphe were mainly medium frequency neurons. The units inhibited by raphe stimulation were mostly located in the superficial region and those activated were in the intermediate and superficial regions.

4. Stimulations of the raphe and electro-acupuncture activated or inhibited most neurons in the caudate nucleus in the same direction.

It is postulated that during electro-acupuncture the midbrain raphe nuclei may act as a relay station in modulating the caudate nucleus, and thus, form a neuronal circuit to modulate the nociceptive transmission.

REFERENCES

[1] 孙公铎等：中华医学杂志 58：139，1978。
[2] 孙公铎等：科学通报 23：447，1978。
[3] McGinty DJ *et al.*: *Brain unit activity during behàvior,* p. 224, Spring Field, 1973.
[4] 孙公铎：贵阳医学院科研资料汇编(针麻原理研究专辑) 6-1，1977。
[5] Казанский ВВ:Физиол. Ж. СССР.59:965,1973.
[6] 上海生理研究所第二研究室针麻组：中华医学杂志 55：340，1975。
[7] 上海第一医学院生理学教研组：中华医学杂志 55：336，1975。
[8] 上海第一医学院华山医院针麻研究协作组：中华医学杂志 55：427，1975。
[9] 上海第一医学院基础医学部生理学教研组针麻研究组：中华医学杂志 58：135，1978。
[10] 陕西省中医研究所针麻原理研究组：陕西新医药 5：59，1975。
[11] 江振裕等：中华医学杂志 57：611，1977。
[12] 杜焕基等：生理学报 30：1，1978。
[13] 吴本阶等：科学通报 24：570，1979。
[14] 广西医学院针麻研究小组：动物学报 14：24，1978。
[15] 郑则慧等：生理学报 30：41，1978。
[16] 周敬修等：全国针灸针麻学术讨论会论文摘要(二)北京 第18页，1979。
[17] Geyer MA *et al.*: *Brain res.,***106**:241, 1976.
[18] Miller JJ *et al.*: *Brain res.,* **97**:113, 1975.
[19] Usunoff KG *et al.*: *Brain res.,* **74**:143, 1974.
[20] Alpe HR *et al.*: *Brain res.,* **122**:357, 1977.
[21] Mayer DJ *et al.*: *Science,* **194**:1351, 1971.
[22] Dliveras JL *et al.*: *Exp brain res.,* **30**:32, 1974.
[23] 湖北医学院基础部针麻研究组：针刺麻醉 1：59，1978。
[24] 孙公铎等：贵阳医学院科研资料汇编(针麻原理研究专辑) 1－14，1977。
[25] McLennan H *et al.*: *J. Physiol.* **187**:163, 1966.
[26] McLennan H *et al.*: *J. Physiol.* **189**:393, 1967.
[27] Ternaux JP *et al.*: *Brain res.,* **121**:311, 1977.
[28] Tassin JP *et al.*: *Brain res.,* **107**:291, 1976.
[29] 张德星等：生理学报 30：21，1978。
[30] 张德星等：全国针灸针麻学术讨论会论文摘要(二)北京 第15页，1979。
[31] Simon H *et al.*: *Breain res.,* **115**:215, 1976.
[32] Дрягин Юм Ж. Высш.Нерв. Деят.24:64,1974.
[33] Costall C *et al.*: *Breain res.,* **123**:89, 1977.
[34] Graybiel CW *et al.*: *Exp. brain res.,* **34**:189, 1979.
[35] 赵志奇等：全国针灸针麻学术讨论会论文摘要(二)北京 第19页，1979。
[36] Апьб-Фессар Д:Бюлл.Эксп. Мед.4:387,1978.

[37] 张香桐：中国科学 1：28，1973。
[38] 张香桐：中国科学 4：456，1978。
[39] 罗弗荪等：中国科学 4：465，1978。
[40] 张香桐：全国针灸针麻学术讨论会论文摘要(一)北京 第18页，1979。
[41] Jacobs BL *et al.*: *Brain res.,* **147**:147, 1978.
[42] Bobillie P *et al.*: *Brain res.,* **113**:449, 1976.
[43] Bunneg BS *et al.*: *Brain res.,* **117**:423, 1976.
[44] Dray A *et al.*: *Brain res.,* **151**:431, 1978.
[45] Davies J *et al.*: *Europ. J. Pharmacol.,* **51**:91, 1978.

EFFECTS OF ACUPUNCTURE, BRAIN-STIMULATION AND ANALGESICS ON THE GROANING RESPONSE ELICITED BY TEGMENTAL STIMULATION IN CATS

Zhu Henian, Lin Baocheng, Zhu Yuanxiang
Song Chaoyou, Wu Chongren
(Department of Physiology, Second Military Medical College, Shanghai, China)

In 1937[1] and 1952[2] we used the Horsley-Clarke stereotaxic apparatus to study the "groaning response" in cats. We found that, under light anesthesia, when a well-localized small area in the lateral tegmental region of the cat was stimulated, the groaning response as well as other autonomic responses such as the rise of blood pressure, a dilatation of the pupils, pilo-erection and other somatic movements could be obtained. We designated this area as the "groaning center" which was further studied in chronic experiments[3] with bipolar electrodes implanted in this area, and it was found that when this area was stimulated, it showed more vigorous responses stimulating pain and rage.

The purpose of our present study is to ascertain whether the groaning response induced by tegmental stimulation in cats is one of the manifestations of the pain response. If the groaning response could be proved to be a pain response, it would be very meaningful towards the studying of the problems of pain and acupuncture analgesia.

I. METHODS

34 cats weighing 2–3.5kg each were used for this experiment. They were either under pentobarbital sodium (35mg/kg) or 1% chloralose-10% urethane (4.5ml/kg) anesthesia. After the animal's head was fixed in our self-designed Kiangwan No. I stereotaxic apparatus, a small hole was drilled in the skull over the "groaning center", and a bipolar electrode (with tips separated at 0.4mm) was inserted into the lateral tegmental region corresponding approximately to Fr_2, LR_5, H_{-3}, in Jasper atlas[4] (Fig. 1).

The parameters of electric stimulation (square wave) for the "groaning center" and other brain areas such as the supraoptic nucleus area (SOA) and the caudate nucleus were: 4–12 volts; 90 pulses/sec. ; width 0.3 msec. Each stimulation lasted 10 or 15 seconds.

The electric needling apparatus used was G6805.

The groaning responses obtained from electric stimulation of the "groaning center" were recorded with the tape recorder and transformed into oscillographic records. We usually stimulated the "groaning center" once every 10 minutes. The latency, number and loudness of the groaning response were calculated from the oscillographic photographs. The

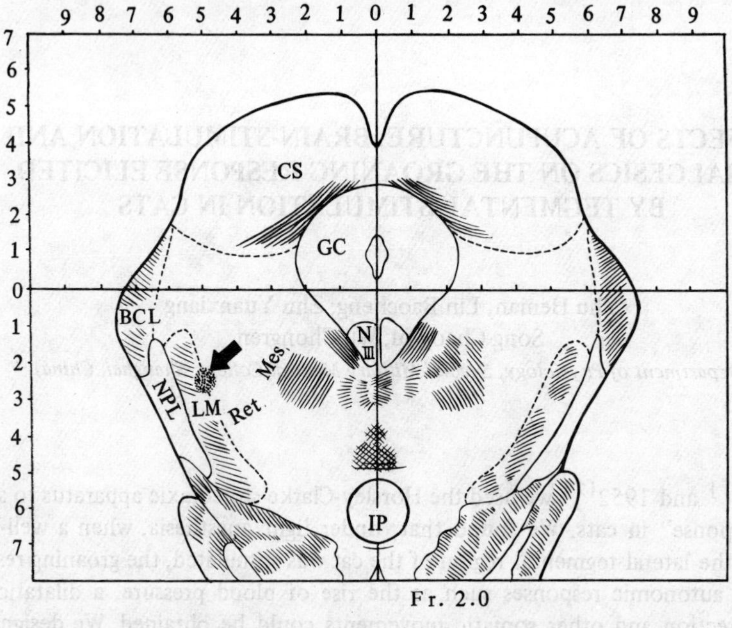

Fig. 1 The schematic diagram of location of the "groaning center". The arrow points to the "groaning center".
LM: lemniscus medialis; NPL: Nucleus paralemniscalis;
Ret. Mes.: Substantia retioularis mesencephalica;
BCI: Brachium colliculi inferioris;
CS: Colliculus superior; GC: Griseum centrale;
IP: Nucleus interpeduncularis.

sum of the maximum values of the loudness of groanings under the different experimental conditions was calculated and treated statistically with the + test.

Our experimental program was as follows:

1. To observe whether there will be any variation in the groaning response when the "groaning center" is stimulated at different time intervals.

2. To observe, during stimulation of the "groaning center", whether clamping the ear of the cat (pain stimulus) by toothed hemostat will enhance the groaning response or abate it.

3. To stimulate the "groaning center" and in the meantime to inject dolantin or morphine intravenously or locally into the center and to observe if these analgesics will depress the groaning response.

4. To observe whether the electric needling of certain acupoints such as "Hegu" or "Zusanli" will depress the groaning response.

5. To observe whether the stimulation of certain brain areas such as SOA or caudate nucleus will depress the groaning response.

II. RESULTS

1. The "groaning center" alone was stimulated in several animals as control experiments. The result was that, when the "groaning center" was stimulated once every 5 or 10 minutes for 2 hrs, the resulting groaning response was rather constant, with very little variation either in latency, number or loudness ($P>0.05$) (Fig. 2).

2. The effect of pain stimulation on groaning response

In six animals, we used toothed hemostats to clamp the ear as a pain stimulus and found that when the "groaning center" was stimulated with simultaneous clamping of the ear for 15 seconds, the groaning response was greatly enhanced, with an increase of 76% ($P<0.05$) as compared with that before clamping. 5 or 10 minutes after cessation of clamping we stimulated the "groaning center" alone, and although there was slight increase of the response, it was of no statistical significance (Fig. 3).

3. The effect of the injection of dolantin and morphine on groaning response

(1) The effect of the injection of dolantin (2mg/kg)

Experimental results of 7 cats showed that there was depression effect on the groaning response induced by tegmental stimulations, as shown by the increase of latency and also reduction in number and loudness of groanings (Fig. 4). 5 minutes after injection, the

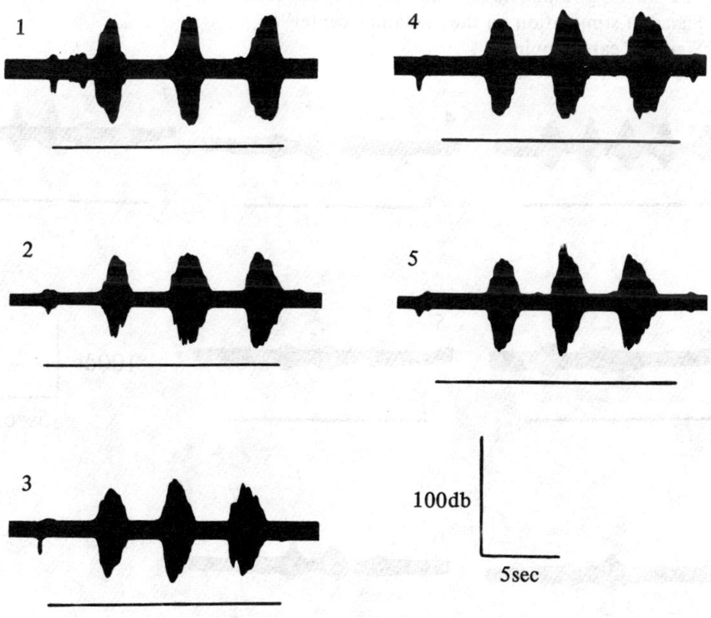

Fig. 2 Control experiments (Cat No. 13).
Stimulation of the groaning center once every 10' for 2 hrs.
1–5 The groaning responses of the 1st, 3rd, 6th, 9th and 12th stimulations respectively.
—— Signal of stimulation on the "groaning center"

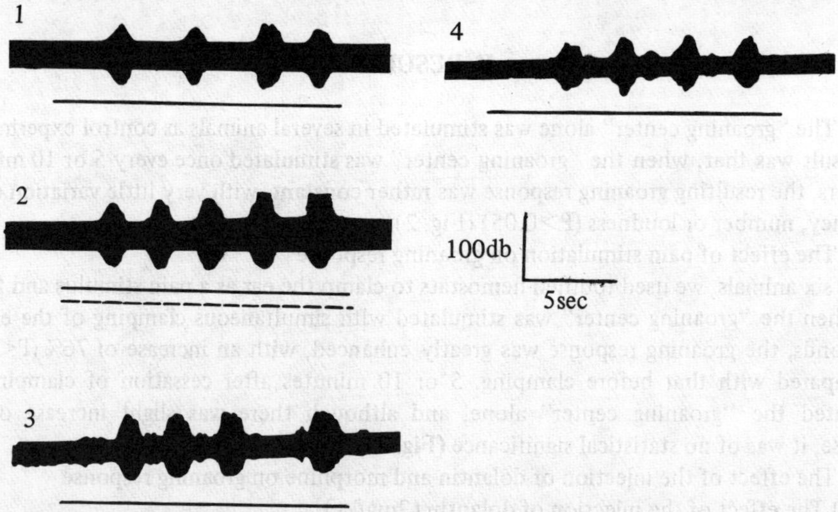

Fig. 3 The effect of pain stimulation by clamping the ear with teethed hemostat (Cat No. 14).

1 The groaning response before ear-clamping.
2 The groaning response produced by stimulation of the "groaning center" and clamping the ear simultaneously.
3–4 The groaning responses at 5' and 10' after ear-clamping.
—— Signal of stimulation on the "groaning center".
----- Signal of ear-clamping.

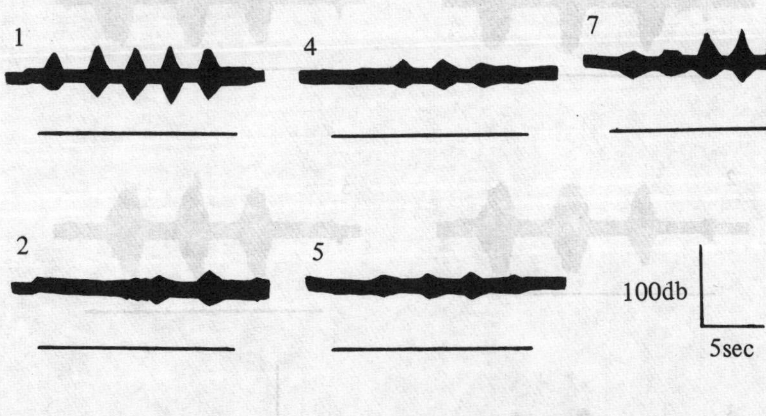

Fig. 4 The effect of intravenous injection of dolantin (2mg/kg) (Cat No. 5).

1 The groaning response before injecting dolantin.
2–7 The groaning responses at 5', 15', 25', 35', 60' and 90' after injecting dolantin respectively.
—— Signal of stimulation on the "groaning center".

depression effect was evident as the loudness of groanings diminished by 58% as compared with that of the preinjection response ($P<0.05$). 15 minutes after injection, the depression effect was more pronounced; when the reduction reached 70% ($P<0.01$), and then the groaning response showed gradual recovery. But a depression effect of 40% ($P<0.05$) still cxistcd one hour after injection.

(2) The effect of the injection of morphine

Injection of morphine intravenously (2mg/kg) also depressed the groaning response and was even more effective than that of dolantin (Fig. 5). 5 minutes after the injection of morphine, the loudness of groanings declined 99% ($P<0.01$). 15 and 25 minutes after the injection of the drug, the loudness of groanings declined to 96% and 79% respectively (both $P<0.01$), and then the depression effect diminished gradually. It was 90 minutes after the injection that the depression effect was no longer of any statistical significance.

In 4 cats, we used the microinjection method to inject morphine (10 $\mu g/5\mu l$) into the "groaning center" directly, which also showed a significant depression effect on groaning response very similar to that by intravenous injection (Fig. 6). And from 5 to 90 minutes after giving the drug, the groaning response declined all along by over 80% (5–60 minutes after injection, $P<0.01$; 90 minutes after injection, $P<0.05$).

We used saline for microinjection as controls, and it was shown that saline did not produce any apparent depression effect on the groaning response.

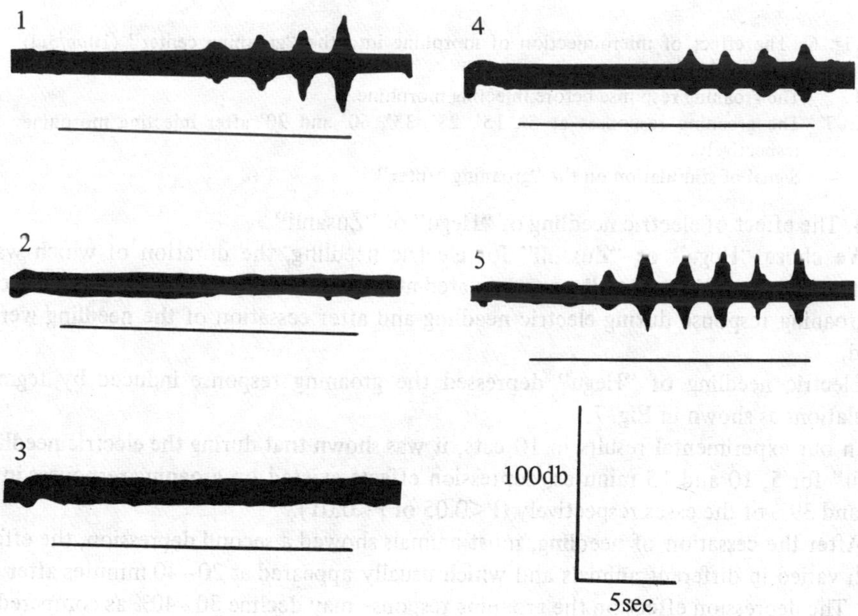

Fig. 5 The effect of intravenous injection of morphine (2mg/kg) (Cat No. 16)
1 The groaning response before injecting morphine
2–5 The groaning responses at 5', 15', 25' and 35' after injecting morphine respectively.
—— Signal of stimulation on the "groaning center".

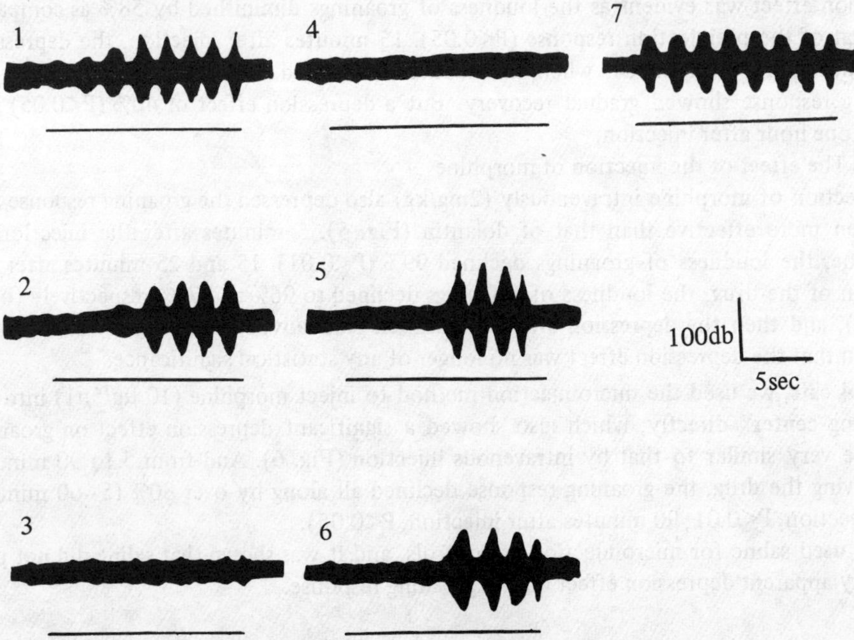

Fig. 6 The effect of microinjection of morphine into the "groaning center" (10μg/5μl) (Cat No. 31).

1 The groaning response before injecting morphine.

2–7 The groaning responses at 5', 15', 25', 35', 60' and 90' after injecting morphine respectively.

— Signal of stimulation on the "groaning center".

4. The effect of electric needling of "Hegu" or "Zusanli"

We chose "Hegu" or "Zusanli" for electric needling, the duration of which was 15 minutes. The "groaning center" was stimulated at 5 or 10 minute intervals and the effects on the groaning response during electric needling and after cessation of the needling were observed.

Electric needling of "Hegu" depressed the groaning response induced by tegmental stimulations as shown in Fig. 7.

In our experimental results in 10 cats, it was shown that during the electric needling of "Hegu" for 5, 10 and 15 minutes, depression effects existed on groaning responses in 27%, 33% and 39% of the cases respectively ($P<0.05$ or $P<0.01$).

After the cessation of needling, most animals showed a second depression, the effect of which varied in different animals and which usually appeared at 20–40 minutes after cessation. The depression effect on the groaning response may decline 30–40% as compared with that before needling ($P<0.05$ or $P<0.01$).

The effect of electric needling of "Zusanli" was similar to that of "Hegu".

5. The effect of stimulation of SOA and the caudate nucleus on the groaning response.

(1) The effect of stimulation of SOA

When we stimulated the SOA and the "groaning center" simultaneously for 15 seconds,

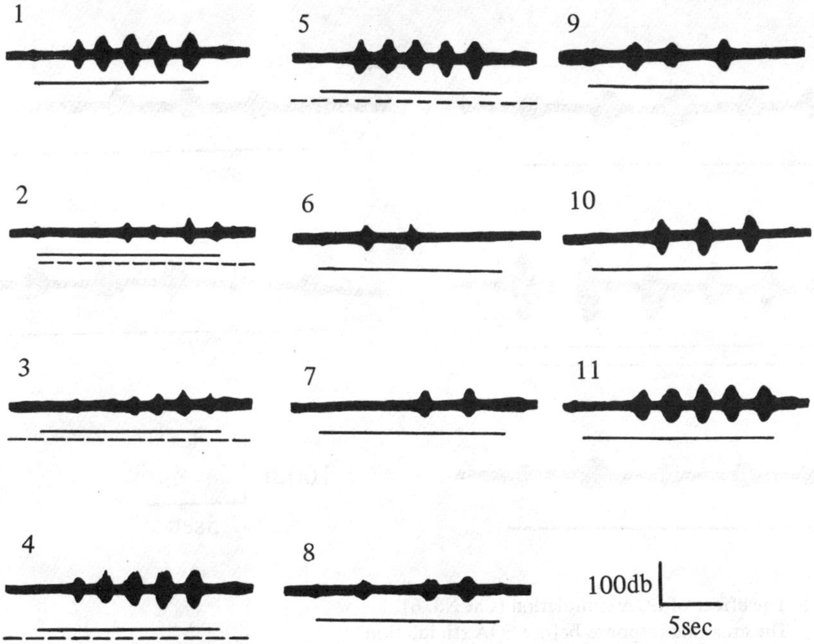

Fig. 7 The effect of electric needling of the acupoint "Hegu" (Cat No. 14).
1 The groaning response before electric needling
2 The groaning response produced by stimulating the " groaning center " and electric needling on "Hegu" simultaneously.
3–5 The groaning responses during electric needling on "Hegu" at 5', 10' and 15'.
6–11 The groaning responses at 5', 10', 20', 30', 40' and 60' after electric needling on "Hegu".
—— Signal of stimulation on the "groaning center".
----- Signal of electric needling on "Hegu'..

the groaning response was enhanced in some animals, and reduced in others. However, statistical treatment of the results in 7 cats did not show any significance.

10 and 20 minutes after the cessation of stimulation of SOA, we stimulated the "groaning center" alone, and in both cases the depression effect on the groaning response was present, especially at 10 minutes after the cessation. The depression effect was more marked and the groanings declined 35% ($P<0.01$) as compared with that before the stimulation of SOA. 20 minutes after the cessation of SOA stimulation, the depression effect on the groaning response was not significant (Fig. 8).

(2) The effect of stimulation of caudate nucleus

From the results found in 4 cats, it was shown that with the simultaneous stimulation of the "groaning center" and the caudate nucleus, the groaning response showed an immediate depression of 32% ($P<0.05$) as compared with the result obtained before the stimulation of the caudate. The duration of the depression effect of the caudate was rather short. In most animals, 10 minutes after the cessation of caudate stimulation, the groaning response was found to have recovered its prestimulation level (Fig. 9).

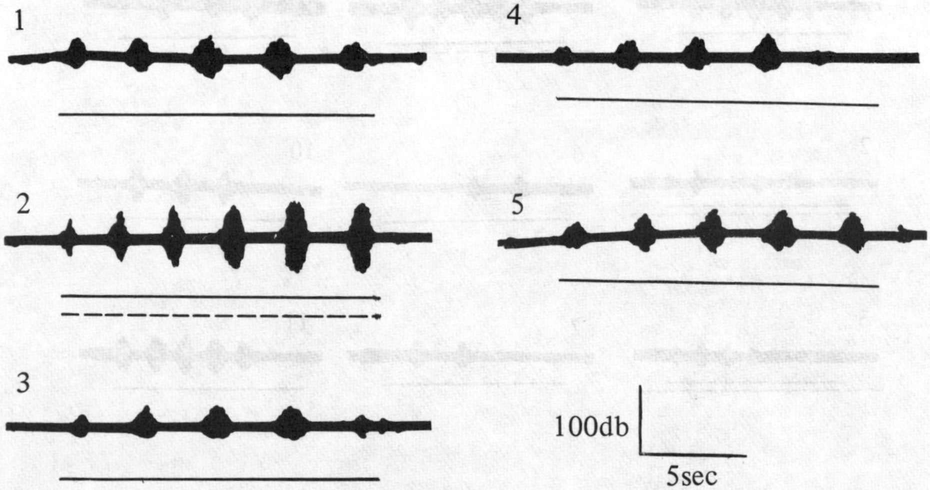

Fig. 8 The effect of SOA stimulation (Cat No. 6).
1 The groaning response before SOA stimulation.
2 The groaning response of simultaneous stimulation on both the "groaning center" and the SOA.
3–5 The groaning responses at 10', 20', and 30' after SOA stimulation.
—— Signal of stimulation on the "groaning center".
----- Signal of stimulation on SOA.

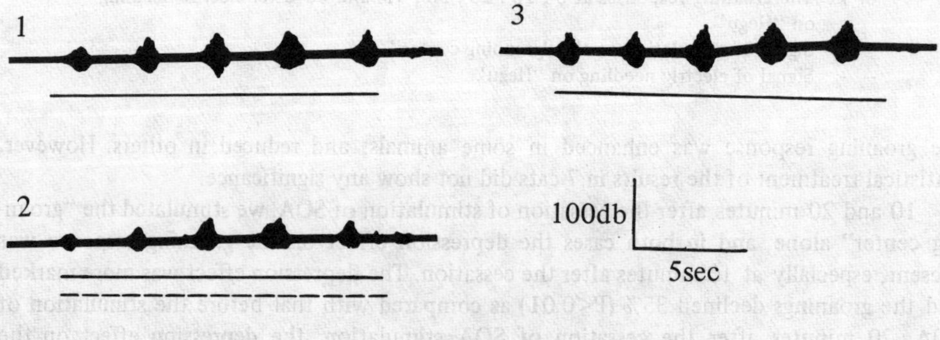

Fig. 9 The effect of caudate nucleus stimulation (Cat No. 6).
1 The groaning response before caudate nucleus stimulation
2 The groaning response of simultaneous stimulation on both "groaning center" and the caudate nucleus
3 The groaning response at 10' after stimulation on caudate nucleus
—— Signal of stimulation on the "groaning center"
----- Signal of stimulation on caudate nucleus

III. DISCUSSION

1. Our results have shown that when the "groaning center" alone is repeatedly stimulated at 5 or 10 minute intervals, the groaning responses obtained will be rather constant and steady during a period of 2 hours, which leads us to believe that the changes in groaning response under different experimental conditions are not due to functional fluctuations of the "groaning center".

2. Both intravenous injection of morphine or microinjection of this drug into the "groaning center" would produce a depression effect on the groaning response. Beechey[5] asserted that the action of morphine on cats is chiefly an analgesic but not a sedative effect, although some believe that sedatives generally have analgesic effect. It is quite possible that the action of morphine on the groaning response is not a sedative effect but is an analgesic effect on the "groaning center".

3. A large number of reports in our country have demonstrated that electric needling of acupoints would produce an analgesic effect. Our experimental results have shown that electric needling of "Hegu" would depress the groaning response, and this depression effect would occur both during needling and after the cessation of needling. In the former case the depression has been found more likely to be a nervous factor, and in the latter it was probably due to a humoral factor. In order to prove this view, it is necessary to collect data from chronic experiments. In contrast with electric needling (analgesic effect), clamping of the ear (pain stimulus) would enhance the groaning response (algesic effect). It seems that the "groaning center" not only can be depressed by analgesic information but also can be activated by algesic information.

4. Many papers have confirmed that stimulation of the caudate nucleus or the SOA would produce an analgesic effect[6–12]. We stimulated both areas in a series of our experiments and a depression effect of the groaning response was found to exist in both. In the case of caudate stimulation, the depression effect lasted only for a short duration, while with the stimulation of SOA, the depression effect lasted much longer and remained very marked within a period of 20 minutes after the cessation of the stimulation. We consider that this is probably due to the humoral effect of the SOA stimulation. Of course, it needs further experimentation to clarify this point.

IV. SUMMARY

By injecting appropriate amounts of analgesics such as morphine and dolantin, by electric needling of certain acupoints such as "Hegu" and "Zusanli" and by stimulation of certain areas in the central nervous system, all of them would depress the groaning response, and these results may be considered as analgesic effects to the "groaning center".

REFERENCES

[1] Loo, Y. T. and Chu, H. N. : *Chin. J. Physiol.*, **11**:301, 1937.
[2] 倪国壇，朱鶴年：生理学杂志，1：231，1952。

[3] 倪国壇等: 生理科学进展，4: 317，1962。
[4] Jasper, H. H. and Ajmone-Marsan, C.:"A Stereotaxic Atlas of the Diencephalon of the Cat", The National Research Council of Canada, Ottawa, 1954.
[5] McKenzie, T.S. and Beechey, N. K. : *Electroencephal. and Clin. Neurophysiol.*, **14**:501, 1962.
[6] Lin, B. C. *et al.*: In "National Symposia of Acupuncture and Moxibustion and Acupuncture Anaesthesia", Beijing, pp. 339–340, 1979.
[7] Lin, B. C. *et al.*: In "National Symposia of Acupuncture and Moxibustion and Acupuncture Anaesthesia", Beijing, pp. 338–339, 1979.
[8] Lin, B. C. *et al.*: In "National Symposia of Acupuncture and Moxibustion and Acupuncture Anaesthesia", Beijing, pp. 337–338, 1979.
[9] Schmidek, H. H. *et al.*: *J. Neurosurgery*, **35**:715, 1971.
[10] 上海第一医学院生理教研组: 中华医学杂志，55: 336，1975。
[11] 上海生理研究所第二研究室针麻组: 中华医学杂志，55: 340，1975。
[12] 上海第一医学院华山医院针麻研究协作组: 中华医学杂志，55: 427，1975。

EFFECTS OF ELECTROACUPUNCTURE AND EXOGENOUS TRANSMITTERS APPLIED MICROIONTOPHORETICALLY ON PAIN DISCHARGES IN MESENCEPHALIC RETICULAR FORMATION

Huang Chengjun, Zhang Zidong, Liu Zuoyan,
Tu Zongping, Xiao Hongmei
(Department of Physiology, Wuhan Medical College)

A number of investigations carried out in recent years have shown that during acupuncture analgesia, there are usually fluctuations in the level of noradrenaline (NA), 5-hydroxytryptamine (5-HT) and acetylcholine (ACh) in the brain while destruction or stimulation of the corresponding nuclei or alteration of the level of neurotransmitters in the CNS by pharmacological means may modify the pain threshold as well as the effect of acupuncture analgesia (AA)[1-6]. These results suggested that these neurotransmitters might be closely related to pain and analgesia and play an important role in the process of AA. But the details of the mechanism underlying AA are yet unknown.

Electrophysiological studies on the mechanism of AA have demonstrated that acupuncture has a significant inhibitory effect on pain discharges from neurons in the corresponding structures at different levels of the CNS[7-11]. In previous experiments we have noted that the discharge of pain-sensitive neurons to noxious stimuli in the mesencephalic reticular formation (MRF) could be inhibited by electroacupuncture and morphine[12]. The aim of the present investigation is to study the effect of NA, 5-HT and ACh applied iontophoretically with multibarrelled glass microelectrodes on the pain discharges of the neurons in MRF and to compare it with that of electroacupuncture.

I. METHODS

72 albino rats weighing 200–400 g each were used as experimental animals. Operations were performed under anesthesia with a mixture of 10% urethane and 1% chloralose (0.7 ml/100 g, i.p.). Experiments were started 5–6 hours after anesthesia. Each animal was then immobilized with d-tubocurarine (0.1–0.2 mg/100 g, i.p.) and maintained in a conscious state under artificial respiration.

According to Krieg's atlas of the rat brain[13], multibarrelled glass microelectrodes were inserted stereotaxically into the MRF in order to explore and record the unit discharges of pain-sensitive neurons. The range to be explored was similar to that in our previous studies, and the positions of the tips of the electrodes were verified by histological examination[12].

The diameters of the tips of three- and five-barrelled glass microelectrodes used were in the range of 3–8 and 5–12 microns respectively. The central barrel filled with 4 M sodium chloride solution was used as the recording electrode (with a direct current resistance of 2–16 megaohms). One of the side barrels was filled with 0.9% or 1 M sodium chloride solution and was used as control. As required by the experiments, the remaining barrels were filled separately with solutions of the following reagents: 0.1–0.4 M noradrenaline bitartrate (pH 4.1–4.4), saturated solution of 5-hydroxytryptamine creatinine sulfate (pH 3.6), 0.1–0.5 M acetylcholine chloride (pH 4.2–4.5), 0.4 M atropine sulfate (pH 4.1). These reagents were ejected by an anodal current of 50–100 nA. As a rule, the duration of iontophoresis was from 10 seconds to 1 minute, but in a few cases, it was prolonged to several minutes. During iontophoresis, both the spontaneous and pain discharges of the neuron were studied. A retaining current of 20 nA was used for all reagents.

The noxious stimuli used included electrical stimulation of an exposed nerve and natural stimuli. The sural or common peroneal nerve was stimulated for this purpose with a train of strong rectangular pulses (pulse width 0.5 msec, intensity 20–30v, 50Hz, for 100 msec, or 10Hz, 1000 msec). The toes or the tail of the animal were pinched with a pair of toothed forceps. Non-noxious stimuli included brushing the hairs of the feet and squeezing the calves.

The electroacupuncture points corresponded to bilateral "Zusanli" or "Hegu" points in man. The electroacupuncture stimulation was delivered with the Model G 6805 electro-needling apparatus. The frequency was 4/sec, and the intensity of stimulation was increased to such a level that weak twitching of the toes could be observed.

The unit discharges, picked up by the tip of the microelectrodes after being fed to a cathode follower, were amplified and displayed on an oscilloscope. The data were recorded simultaneously on a magnetic tape which could be played back later for further analysis and photographing.

II. RESULTS

One hundred and twelve neurons resp onsive to noxious stimuli with a specific pattern of discharge were recorded in MRF corresponding to the region $AP_{5.0-6.5}$, R or $L_{1.0-2.0}$, $H_{5.3-8.2}$. The response was characterized by a long latent period of more than 100 msec to an intense stimulation of the common peroneal nerve or sural nerve, an increased discharge frequency prolonged after discharges which lasted from several sec to more than 20 sec, and a lack of adaptation to frequent repetitive stimulation (Figs. 1–A, 2–A, B). This pattern of discharges is believed to be related to pain sensation, and hence the term pain discharges. Among the 112 neurons recorded, there were 89 which were responsive only to noxious stimuli, while the remaining 23 neurons were also responsive to non-noxious stimuli with weak and transient excitation.

1. The effect of electro-acupuncture on pain discharges from the neurons in MRF. The effects of electroacupuncture applied at points "Zusanli" or "Hegu" were examined on 50 pain-sensitive neurons. A significant inhibitory effect on the pain discharges of 41 neurons (82%) was observed. In a few neurons, the inhibitory effect was manifested by a total subsidence of discharges to noxious stimuli, but in most cases, it was manifested by a prolonged latent period, lowered frequency of discharge, shortened duration of discharge and decrease

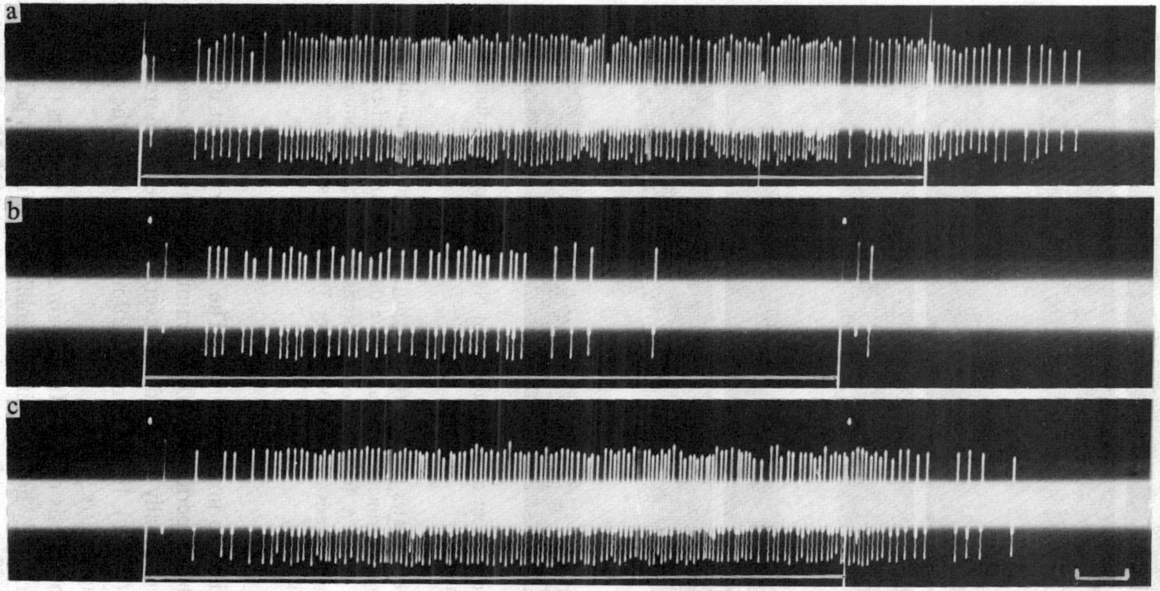

Fig. 1 Inhibitory effect of electroacupuncture on the pain discharges of a neuron in MRF horizontal line indicates noxious stimulus (pinching the toes); time, 1 sec.
A, before electroacupuncture. B, after 28 min bilateral electroacupuncture of Zusanli. C, 10 minutes after cessation of electro-acupuncture.

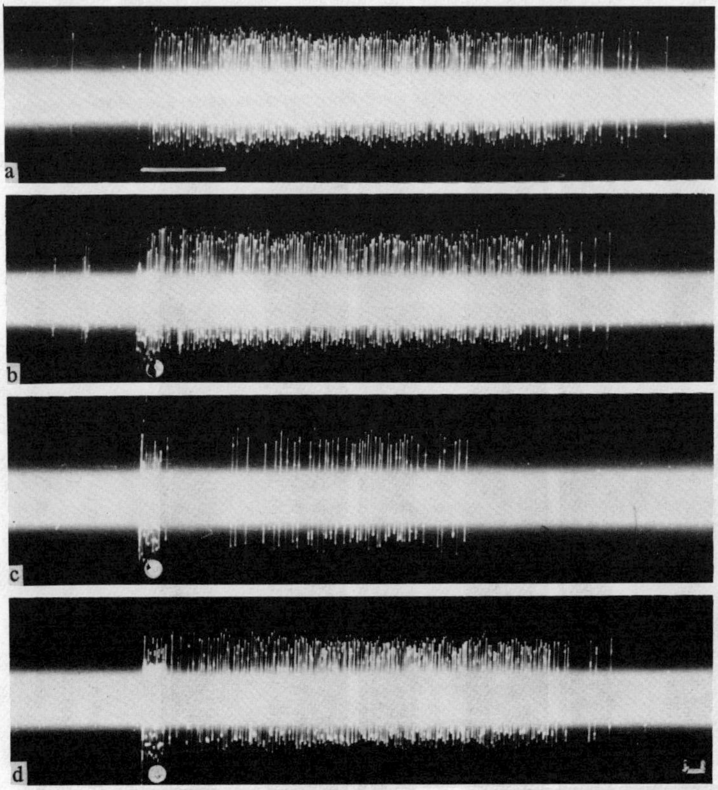

Fig. 2 Inhibitory effect of iontophoresis of NA on the pain discharges of a neuron in MRF

horizontal line indicates pinching the toes; dot shows electrical stimulation of common peroneal nerve (above the dot is the artifact of train stimuli); time 1 sec. A, B, before iontophoresis of NA. C, iontophoresis of sec. D, iontophoresis of Na^{+}, 100 nA for 1 minutes, stimulating the nerve at 31st sec.

in the total number of spikes to noxious stimuli. The inhibitory effect of electroacupuncture usually appeared after a period of 10–20 minutes. After the cessation of electroacupuncture, the aftereffect usually persisted for several minutes to more than 10 minutes, and in some, even longer (Fig. 1). In the remaining 9 neurons (18%), the pain discharge was not affected by electroacupuncture.

2. The effect of iontophoresis of NA. In 51 pain sensitive neurons tested, it was found that NA applied iontophoretically had a significant inhibitory effect on pain discharges in 38 neurons (74.5%) and no effect on the remaining 13 neurons (25.5%). The inhibition was complete only in a few instances but moderate in the majority of cases. The patterns of inhibition were similar to those of electro-acupuncture (Fig. 2). After cessation of iontophoresis of NA, the aftereffect may last from several seconds to two minutes or more. In the majority of cases, the spontaneous discharges of the tested neurons were inhibited during iontophoresis of NA with a latent period lasting from several seconds to more than 20 sec. The inhibitory effect on pain discharges and spontaneous discharges usually occurred in the same neurons. However, in a small number of neurons, though NA had no effect on spontaneous discharges, it nevertheless produced a significant inhibitory effect on pain discharges. It is worth while to point out that when the same ejecting current was applied through the control barrel to the neurons which could be inhibited by NA, no significant changes in spontaneous and pain discharges were observed, only a small number of neurons showed slight and transient decrease in spontaneous discharges which was significantly different from the inhibitory effect of NA applied iontophoretically to the same neurons (Fig. 2–D). No significant excitatory effect of NA on the discharge activity of the tested neurons was ever observed.

The effect of iontophoresis of NA and electro-acupuncture on pain discharges was studied on 28 pain-sensitive neurons. It was found that 19 neurons (67.9%) were inhibited both by electroacupuncture and NA; 5 (17.9%) were neither influenced by NA nor by electro-acupuncture; the pain discharges of the remaining 4 neurons (14.2%) were not influenced by NA but could be inhibited by electroacupuncture.

The effects of co-stimulation by NA and electro-acupuncture were studied on 8 neurons. NA was applied iontophoretically for 1 min at a certain stage during electroacupuncture, and the response to noxious stimulus was tested at the 31st sec of NA iontophoresis. It was observed in 6 neurons that the inhibitory effects on pain discharges were stronger under joint stimulation than electroacupuncture alone. These results suggest that NA is able to potentiate the inhibitory effect of electroacupuncture on pain discharges.

3. The effect of iontophoresis of 5–HT. 37 pain-sensitive neurons were examined. 5–HT when applied iontophoretically had a significant inhibitory effect on the pain discharges of 28 neurons (75.7%). The inhibition was complete in some neurons, but was partial in the majority of them. The patterns, characteristics and time course of the inhibitory effects of 5–HT were similar to those of NA and electroacupuncture (Fig. 3). In the remaining 9 neurons (24.3%), the pain discharges were not affected. 5–HT had also a profound inhibitory effect on spontaneous discharges in the majority of neurons examined. When the same ejecting current was passed through the control barrel, no inhibitory effects were observed. No obvious excitatory effect of 5–HT on the discharge activity has ever been noted in tested neurons.

A comparison was made between the effects of 5–HT and electroacupuncture on pain discharges in the same neurons. Among the 19 neurons tested, 15 (78.9%) were inhibited by both electroacupuncture and 5–HT, while 1 (5.3%) was not influenced by either of them. The remaining 3 (15.8%) were not influenced by 5–HT but could be inhibited by electroacupuncture.

The combined effect of 5–HT and electroacupuncture was tested in 9 neurons. It was observed that 5–HT could enhance the inhibitory effect of electroacupuncture in 7 of them.

4. The effect of iontophoresis of Ach. Among the 69 pain-sensitive neurons examined, 61 (88.4%) showed significant excitatory response to Ach, characterized by a latent period of 1–5 sec, an increase in frequency of spontaneous discharges, and a prolonged excitatory aftereffect lasting from several seconds to more than 10 sec after cessation of Ach iontophoresis (Figs. 4, 5). The excitatory response could be elicited without attenuation by

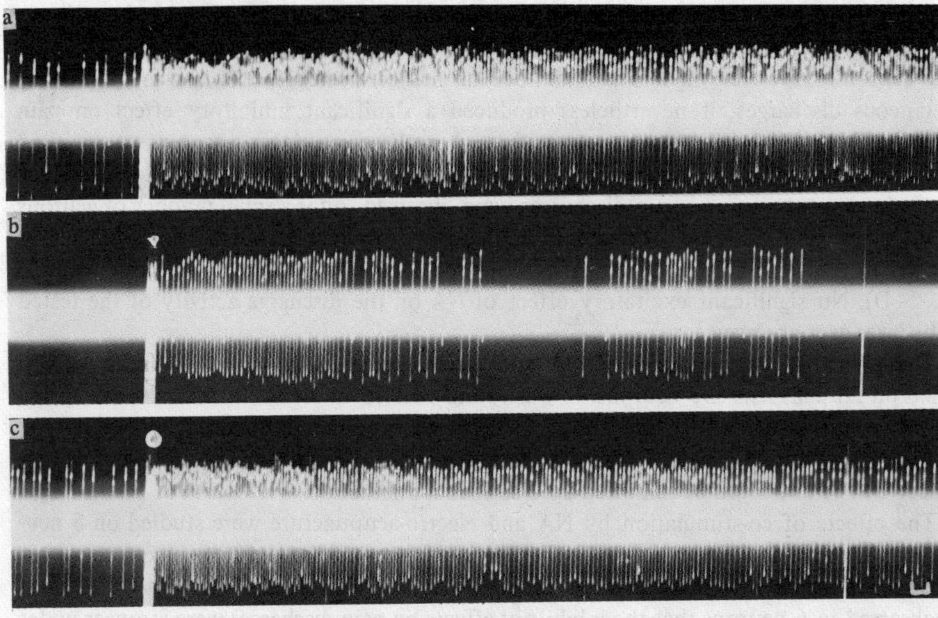

Fig. 3 Inhibitory effect of iontophoresis of 5-HT on the pain discharges of a neuron in MRF

dot indicates electrical stimulation of common peroneal nerve (below the dot is the artifact of train stimuli); time, 1 sec.
A, before iontophoresis of 5-HT. B, iontophoresis of 5-HT, 100 nA for 1 minutes, stimulating the nerve at 31st sec. C, iontophoresis of Na^+, 100 nA for 1 min, stimulating the nerve at 31st sec.

repeated application of Ach to the same neuron. No excitatory response of the neurons, however, was observed when the same ejecting current was conducted through the control barrel. The spontaneous discharges of the remaining 8 neurons (11.6%) were not affected by Ach.

The effects of Ach on the evoked pain discharges were examined in 23 neurons showing excitatory response to Ach. It was found that the pain discharges in 18 neurons (78.3%) could be distinctly augmented by the application of Ach (Figs. 4, 5), while the remaining 5 (21.7%) were not affected. An inhibitory effect of Ach on spontaneous and pain discharges of the neurons tested has never been observed.

Furthermore, the influence of atropine applied iontophoretically or intravenously (0.1 mg/100 g) on Ach effects and on pain discharges was studied in 9 pain-sensitive neurons. It was observed that the excitatory effect of Ach in all of the neurons tested could evidently be mitigated or nearly abolished by atropine. The pain discharges of 8 neurons were significantly weakened by atropine, while those of the remaining 1 were not affected. In another 7 neurons tested by the application of atropine Fig. 6, the pain discharges of 6 neurons were weakened significantly Fig. 7, while those of the remaining 1 were not affected.

The effect of electro-acupuncture on excitatory action of Ach and on pain discharges was investigated on the same neurons. Among the 14 pain-sensitive neurons tested, a significant inhibitory effect was observed in 10 neurons (71.4%) on both occasions on pain

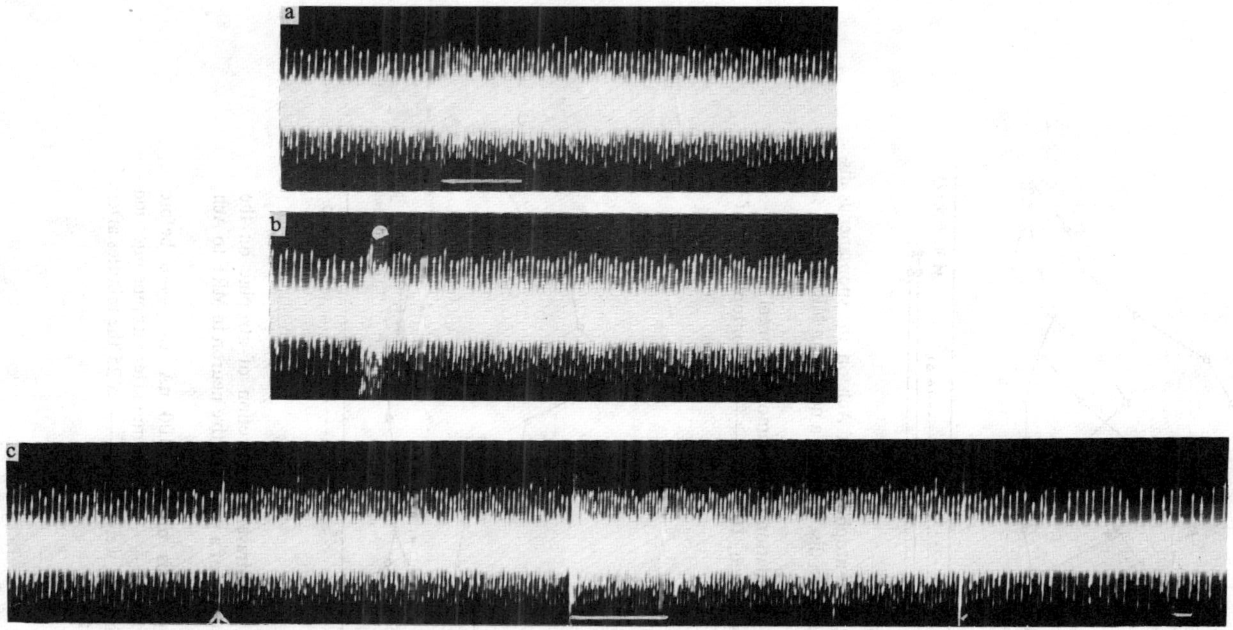

Fig. 4 Effect of iontophoresis of Ach on the spontaneous discharges and the pain discharges of a neuron in MRF

horizontal line indicates pinching the toes; dot shows electrical stimulation of common peroneal nerve (below the dot is the artifact of train stimuli); arrows show the initiation and termination of iontophoresis of Ach; time, 1 sec. A, B, before iontophoresis of Ach. C, iontophoresis of Ach, 100 nA for 40 sec, pinching the toes at 18the sec.

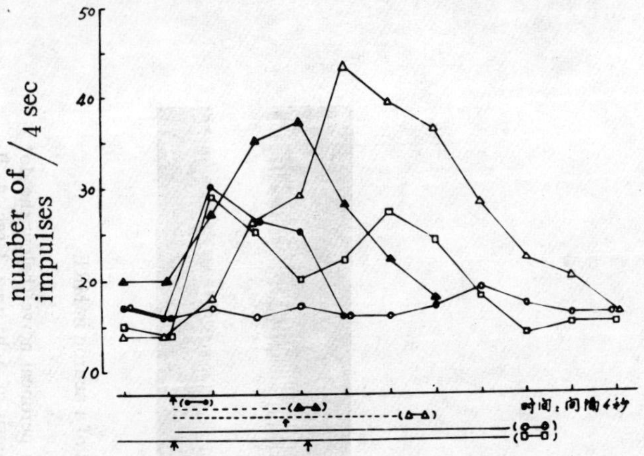

Fig. 5 Effect of iontophoresis of Ach on the spontaneous discharges and the pain discharges of a neuron in MRF

↑ electrical stimulation of common peroneal nerve.----- iontophoresis of Ach, 100 nA. ————iontophoresis of Na^+,

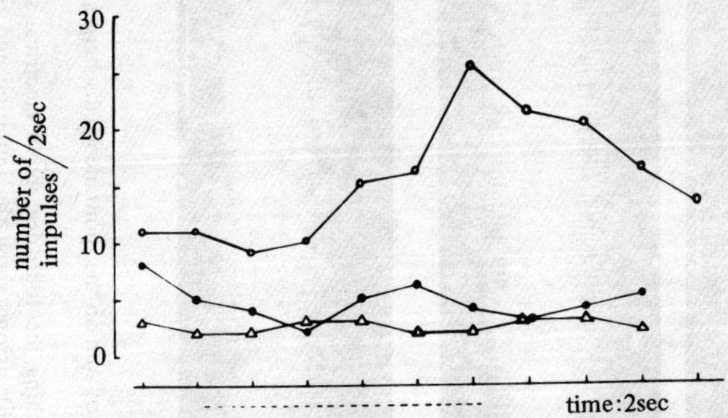

Fig. 6 Effect of intravenous injection of atropine on the excitatory response of a pain-sensitive neuron in MRF to Ach

-----iontophoresis of Ach, 100 nA. o———o before atropine injection. o———o 5th min after atropine injection (0.1 mg/100 g body weight). Δ———Δ 25 the minutes after atropine injection.

discharges only in 2 neurons (14.3%), and on excitatory effect of Ach only in the remaining 2 (14.3%). The inhibitory action of electroacupuncture on the excitatory effect of Ach usually persisted from a few minutes till more than 10 min after the cessation of electroacupuncture.

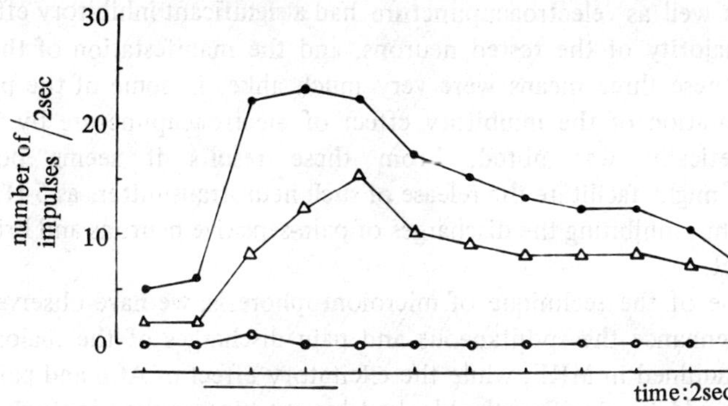

Fig. 7 Effect of intravenous injection of atropine on the pain discharges of a neuron in MRF

——pinching the toes. o——o before atropine injection. o——o 10th min after atropine injection (0.1 mg/100 g body weight). Δ——Δ 30th minutes after atropine injection.

III. DISCUSSION

Neurophysiological investigations demonstrated that a considerable amount of ascending fibers transmitting pain signals in the ventrolateral fasciculus of the spinal cord did not project directly to the thalamus, but made synaptic connections in the reticular formation of the brain stem. The neurons in the reticular formation receiving afferent fibers from ventrolateral fasciculus respond only to noxious stimulus or stimulation of Aδ and C fibers. The afferent inputs related to pain ascending from the spinal cord may relay in the reticular formation and thence to the medial nuclei of the thalamus[14–17]. Besides, additional evidence shows that the reticular formation of the brain stem includes not only important pathways for transmission of pain signals, but also serves as a center for the regulation and integration of pain sensation[18-24]. In our previous work and present study, we have verified that the pain-sensitive neurons in MRF can be inhibited by electroacupuncture and morphine. These results suggest that the neurons in MRF might have played an important role in the process of analgesia evoked by electroacupuncture.

A number of investigations have shown that central 5-HT and NA have a significant analgesic effect[1,25–28]. In this study we have noted in albino rats that 5-HT or NA applied iontophoretically has a significant inhibitory effect on spontaneous and pain discharges on the majority of pain-sensitive neurons in MRF. These results suggest that the analgesic effect of 5-HT and NA in CNS may be accomplished by their inhibitory effect on the discharge activity of pain-sensitive neurons in certain structures of the CNS.

There are a number of papers dealing with the effect of central 5-hydroxytryptaminergic nerve structures and 5-HT on AA[3,5,6]. From the reference material and information available, it seems that the relation between central NA and AA is rather complicated, and it is therefore difficult to draw an unequivocal conclusion at present[29–34]. We have demonstrated in albino rats that either 5-HT or NA applied iontophoretically as well as electroacupuncture had a significant inhibitory effect on pain discharges in the majority of the tested neurons, and the manifestation of the inhibitory effects elicited by these three means were very much alike. In some of the pain-sensitive neurons, an augmentation of the inhibitory effect of electroacupuncture by 5-HT or NA applied iontophoretically was noted. From these results it seems possible that electroacupuncture might facilitate the release of such neurotransmitters as 5-HT and NA at the level of MRF, thus inhibiting the discharges of pain-sensitive neurons and bringing about a pain-relieving effect.

Through the use of the technique of microiontophoresis, we have observed that ACh could significantly enhance the spontaneous and pain discharges of the majority of pain-sensitive neurons examined in MRF, while the excitatory effect of ACh and pain discharges from the neurons could be significantly blocked by atropine applied iontophoretically or intravenously. These results suggest that, as a neurotransmitter, Ach probably participates in the transmission of pain signals in MRF. Besides, electroacupuncture could inhibit the excitatory response of the pain-sensitive neurons evoked by iontophoresis of ACh. This suggests that electroacupuncture might have a post-synaptic inhibitory effect on pain-sensitive neurons in MRF.

A number of articles have reported the central analgesic effect of Ach and the participation of Ach in the process of AA[2,35]. In the present study, it was found that local iontophoretic application of Ach exhibited an excitatory instead of an inhibitory effect on the pain-sensitive neurons in MRF. The effect of ACh at cellular level was in contradiction to that in an intact animal. To clarify the discrepancy, further investigation is needed. Taking into account the intricacy in organization of and relation between the central analgesic structures and the nerve structures subserving pain, and the diversity of the corresponding transmitters, we are inclined to assume that ACh might be a neurotransmitter in certain links of analgesic structures in the brain, and might possibly participate in the process of AA, but it might also be an excitative or facilitative neurotransmitter of certain synapses in the path for the transmission of pain signals.

IV. ABSTRACT

The effects of noradrenaline, 5-hydroxytryptamine and acetylcholine applied iontophoretically through three-or five-barrelled glass microelectrodes on pain discharges of the pain-sensitive neurons in mesencephalic reticular formation (MRF) of albino rats were observed and compared with those of electroacupuncture.

1. Electro-acupuncture applied at bilateral "Zusanli" or "Hegu" points had a significant inhibitory effect on pain discharges in the majority of neurons examined.

2. NA and 5-HT applied iontophoretically exhibited likewise striking inhibitory effects on pain discharges and spontaneous discharges in the majority of neurons examined. It was further demonstrated that both NA and 5-HT could enhance the inhibitory effect of electro-acupuncture. From these results it seems possible that electro-acupuncture might have evoked a release of neurotransmitters such as NA and 5-HT at the level of MRF, inhibiting the discharges of the pain-sensitive neurons, and producing a pain-relieving effect.

3. Ach applied iontophoretically could strikingly enhance the spontaneous and pain discharges in the majority of neurons examined. The excitatory effect of Ach and pain dis-

charges from the neurons could be significantly blocked by atropine applied iontophoretically or intravenously. The results suggest that, as a neurotransmitter, Ach probably participates in the transmission of pain signals in MRF. Electroacupuncture could inhibit the excitatory effect of Ach. This suggests that electroacupuncture might have a post-synaptic inhibitory effect on pain-sensitive neurons in MRF.

REFERENCES

[1] 湖南医学院针麻原理研究组：针刺麻醉原理的探讨，411页，人民卫生出版社，1974。
[2] 北京医学院生理教研组：针刺麻醉原理的探讨，428页，人民卫生出版社，1974。
[3] 北京医学院基础部针麻原理研究组生理组：全国针刺麻醉研究资料选编，522页，上海人民出版社，1977。
[4] 陕西省中医研究所生理针麻组：陕西新医药，(6)：10，1974。
[5] 陕西省中医研究所针麻原理研究室：陕西新医药，(5)：59，1975。
[6] 陕西省中医研究所针麻原理研究室：陕西新医药，(5)：53，1975。
[7] 张香桐：中国科学，(1)：28，1973。
[8] 上海生理研究所：中华医学杂志，(3)：131，1973。
[9] 上海中医学院等：中华医学杂志，(3)：136，1973。
[10] 上海生理研究所针麻组：针刺麻醉原理的探讨，294页，人民卫生出版社，1974。
[11] 广西医学院针麻研究小组：全国针刺麻醉研究资料选编，407页，上海人民出版社，1977。
[12] 武汉医学院生理教研室：全国针刺麻醉研究资料选编，402页，上海人民出版社，1977。
[13] Bureš, J.et al（范世藩、汀振裕译）：电生理学方法，348页，上海科学技术出版社，1963。
[14] Bowsher, D: *Brain,* **80**:606, 1957.
[15] Casey, KL: *Amer. Scientist,* **61**:194, 1973.
[16] Mehler WR *et al.*: *Brain,* **83**:718, 1960.
[17] Collins, WF *et al.*: *J. Neurophysiol,* **23**:47, 1960.
[18] Lim.RKS: *Ann.Rev. Physiol.,* **32**:269, 1970.
[19] Pond, FJ *et al.*: *Brain Res.,* **120**:469, 1977.
[20] Kerr, DIB *et al.*: *Amer. J. Physiol.,* **183**:253, 1955.
[21] Kaelber, WW *et al.*: *Brain,* **90**:83, 1967.
[22] 广西医学院人体学教研组针麻研究小组：针刺麻醉原理的探讨，257页，人民卫生出版社，1974。
[23] 许冠荪等：科学通报，(5)：234，1975。
[24] Mayer, DJ *et al.*: *Science,* **174**:1351, 1971.
[25] 北京医学院基础部针麻原理研究组生理组：中枢神经介质概论，296页，科学出版社，1977。
[26] Chase, TN *et al.*: *Ann. Rev. Pharmacol.,* **(13)**:181, 1973.
[27] 同[25]，269页。
[28] Segal, M *et al.*: *Brain Res.,* **123**:369, 1977.
[29] 陕西省中医研究所针麻研究小组：针刺麻醉原理的探讨，394页，人民卫生出版社，1974。
[30] 韩济生等：生理学报，31 (1)：11，1979。
[31] 韩济生等：北京医学院学报，(4)：209，1978。
[32] 北京医学院基础部针麻原理研究组生理组：中华医学杂志，(3)：129，1978。
[33] 潘建粹等：全国针灸针麻学术讨论会论文摘要(二)，118页，北京，1979。
[34] 中国医学科学院分院二室针麻组：医药研究通讯，(1)：13，1975。
[35] 同[25]，259页。

INHIBITION OF EVOKED DISCHARGES OF POSTERIOR NUCLEAR GROUP OF THALAMUS INDUCED BY STIMULATION OF CENTRAL GREY MATTER, CAUDATE NUCLEUS AND ELECTROACUPUNCTURE IN WAKING RABBITS

Zhao Zhiqi, Shao Dianhua, Yang Zhenquan,
(Shanghai Institute of Physiology, Academia Sinica)

In our previous work with acute experiments, it has been found in cats that unit discharges in the spinocervical tract fibers evoked by nocuous stimulation can be inhibited by the electroacupuncture of certain points of the body[1]. It has been reported that afferent impulses from spinocervical tract fibers were transmitted at least partly to the posterior nuclear group of thalamus (PO) which may be concerned with the transmission of the messages of pain[2,3]. In order to study further the central mechanism of acupuncture analgesia, it is the attempt of the present study to find the correlation between the unit discharges of PO neurons and the animal behavioral responses elicited by nocuous stimulation in a waking animal and to observe the inhibitory effect of brain stimulation and electroacupuncture.

Experiments were performed in 12 adult rabbits. Surgical operations were carried out under Nembutal (40mg/kg) anesthesia. Stimulating electrodes and the base of the micro-driver were implanted according to Sawyer's stereotaxic altas of rabbit's brain. The center of the base of the micro-driver was located at the coordinates of PO (P_6, L_{L5}) and two pairs of stimulating electrodes made of 150 μm insulated stainless steel wire were implanted for stimulation of the head of caudate nucleus (A_5 , L_{L3} H_{+4}) and midbrain central grey matter (AP_0 , L_0 , H_{-1}) respectively. Observations were usually made three days after the operation.

During observation, the rabbit was in a restrained condition in a wooden box, but its head and trunk could still move a little. A MWT–I micro-driver[4] (made in China) was fixed on the base before experimental observation. The multi-unit discharges of PO neurons were recorded with a Tungsten microelectrode insulated with glass (tip diameter about 15μm). In a few experiments glass microelectrodes (tip diameter about 1μm) were used for recording the single unit discharges of PO neurons. A pair of stainless steel needles, insulated except for a part 1mm in length from the tip, were inserted into the tail for somatic stimulation. When single pulses of 1 msec width and 50V strength were applied to the tail, little behavioral responses were evoked apart from the movement of the tail. A short train of pulses (duration 30 msec, frequency 300Hz) delivered to the tail was used as nocuous stimulation which could elicit the animal's aversive behavioral responses, such as withdrawal of the limbs and movement of the trunk and head or even violent struggles. The strength of stimulation, varying from 20–25V, was usually so adjusted as to avoid the struggle of the animal. Throughout the period of observation, which usually lasted for several hours, the animal's aversive behavioral responses remained stable.

Unit discharges of PO neurons were fed to a field-effect transistor fixed on the micro-driver's base, amplified by a DC–AC amplifier in the conventional manner, displayed on a oscilloscope and recorded simultaneously with an FM data recorder. After the experiments, the data were first sent to a "Bioelectrical Pulse Slicer" which could select the impulses and eliminate the stimulation artifacts[5]. Selected impulses were then fed into a computer to be processed into a sequential spike density histogram. Meanwhile, the unit discharges selected by the "Bioelectrical Pulse Slicer" were also displayed on a monitoring oscilloscope for identification. The localization of the stimulating electrodes and the tips of recording microelectrodes were checked histologically.

1. Unit Responses of Posterior Nuclear Group of Thalamus (PO) to Nocuous Stimulation.

Unit discharges were all recorded from the Posterior Nuclear Group of Thalamus (PO) which is located in a region including the Suprageniculate Body (SG) and the Magnocellular division of the Medial Geniculate Body (MGm) or a region medial to it. Spontaneous discharges in this PO were in the form of separated single spikes when the animal was in an awake and quiescent state, and tended to be in burst formation while in the sleeping state. About one-third of the PO neurons responded to somatic sensory stimuli. Most of them showed characteristics of heterosensory and heterotopic convergence. They responded to various modes of sensory stimuli, including light electrical, light mechanical, nocuous, and acoustical stimuli (Fig.1), but no response to joint movement had been found. The receptive field of these PO units to somatic stimulation was wide and bilateral.

Particular attention was paid to those PO units which were responsive to nocuous stimuli. Fig.1d shows the multiunit discharges induced by single electric shock (50V) applied to the tail of the animal, which elicited no behavioral responses apart from the movement of the tail. When a train of electric pulses was given, long bursts (about several hundred milliseconds or more) of discharges with markedly increased frequency appeared (Fig.1e), while at the same time, distinct aversive behavioral responses of the animal were observed. These characteristics of the PO neurons to nocuous stimuli, as described above, were quite similar to those of the wide dynamic range units of spinal neurons[1]. 8 out of 11 units with long-burst discharges to nocuous stimuli were inhibited after intravenous injection of the analgesic Fentanyl (30μg/kg). Fig. 3-b shows the inhibitory process in one unit. Discharges from this kind of neuron could also be elicited by intraarterial injection of bradykinin[3]. But the long-burst discharges could not be evoked in these units by spontaneous or passive movement of the animal. It seems to suggest that the activity of these units is related with the transmission of the messages of pain.

The inhibitory effect of electrical stimulation of the ventrolateral portion of the central grey matter, the dorsomedial part of the head of the caudate nucleus, and acupuncture points on nociceptive discharges of PO neurons has been studied. The inhibitory effect of brain stimulation and electroacupuncture on aversive behavioral responses (withdrawal of limbs as well as the movement of the body and the head) were rated as "strong", when the aversive responses to all 3 trails of nocuous stimulation were greatly reduced or abolished, and as "weak" if the responses were only slightly reduced. In a part of the experiments, EMG was also taken to assess the degree of inhibitory effect.

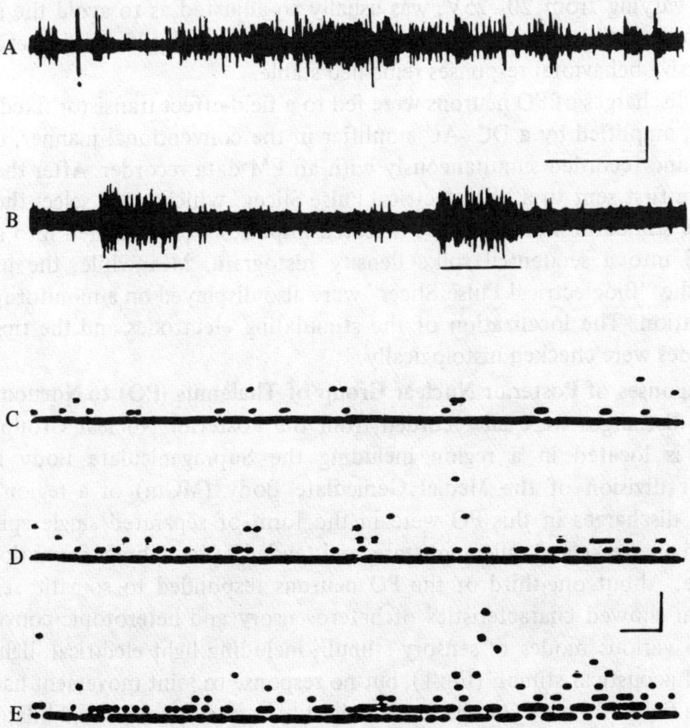

Fig. 1 Mulitunit discharges of PO neurons. A, response to electrical stimuli of tail (a train of square waves: duration 10 ms, frequency . 300 Hz, 25V) B, response to click stimuli (duration 240 ms, frequency 100 Hz). Calibration: 300 μV, 500ms. C–E, Sequential spike density histogram representing a computer cumulation of 3 consecutive samples of evoked discharges of a PO neuron by a train of square wave stimuli C, Spontaneous discharges, D, and E, response to single and a train of square waves respectively. Calibration: Abscissa 77 ms. Ordinate 1 impulses/5 ms.

2. Inhibitory Effect of Brain Stimulation. Nocuous electric stimuli were given to the animal's tail in 3 experiments with intervals of 20 seconds. Square wave pulses (width 0.1 msec, repetition rate 5–50 pulses/sec) were used for brain stimulation. The constant current intensity for stimulation of the central grey matter and caudate nucleus was 100–600 μA and 200–1000 μA, respectively.

(1) Electrical stimulation of Central Grey Matter (CG). Changes of nociceptive discharges of PO neurons and aversive behavioral responses during the course of brain stimulation were investigated on 9 rabbits. At the beginning of brain stimulation, the animal usually showed staring eyes, erection of ears, etc., as if it were an "alert" reaction. After a while, the animal became quiet, and aversive behavioral responses to nocuous stimulation at this moment were greatly inhibited, which significantly differs from those seen in the control experiments. The maximal inhibitory effect was usually seen 1–2 minutes after the termina-

tion of brain stimulation. And it was accompanied by an after-inhibition which might last for several minutes or longer.

Intimate correspondence in the development of inhibition and its recovery between unit discharges and behavioral responses was found in 19 out of 32 PO units activated by nocuous stimulation. Fig. 2 shows the sequential spike density histogram in one of these units, where marked inhibition on PO unit discharges, after-inhibition and recovery from inhibition can be noticed.

(2) Stimulation of the head of Caudate Nucleus (Cd) produced a strong inhibitory effect on the aversive behavioral responses elicited by nocuous stimulation. In these instances, nociceptive discharges in PO neurons were also markedly reduced. Fig. 3-a shows changes of discharges of a PO neuron during a stimulation of Caudate Nucleus. This unit was also inhibited by an injection of Fentanyl (Fig. 3-b).

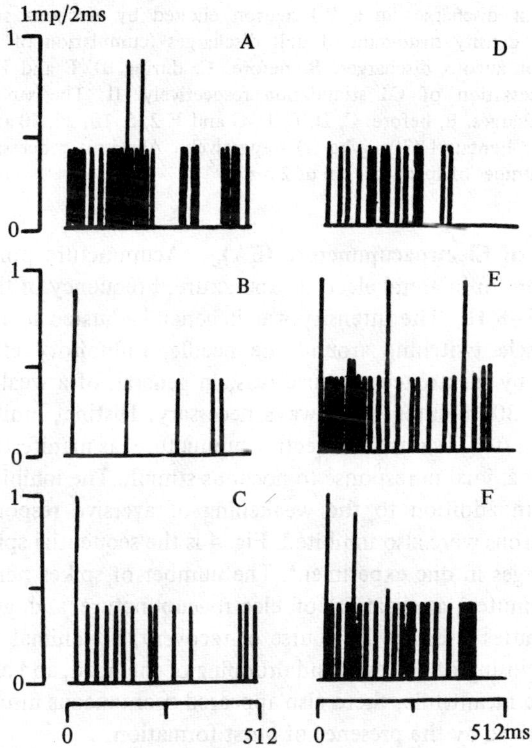

Fig. 2 Sequential spike density histogram respresenting a computer cumulation of 3 consecutive samples of evoked discharges of a PO neuron by a train of pulse stimuli. A, before. B, during. C, D, E and F respectively 1, 5, 10, and 20 minutes after cessation of stimulation of central grey matter (CG). Abscissa: processing time (512 ms), Ordinate: Number of spike in a bin of 2 ms.

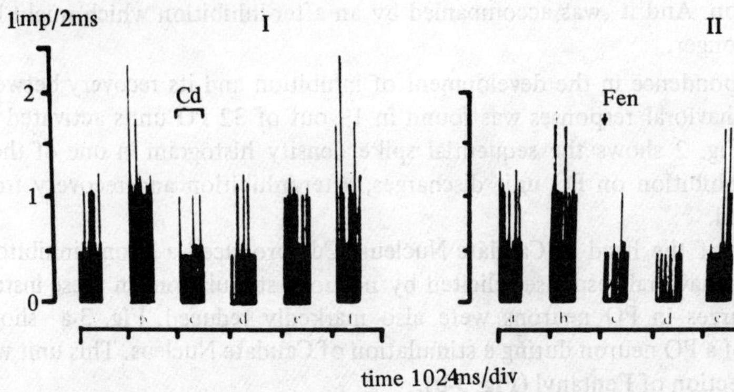

Fig. 3 Inhibitory effect of stimulation of Caudate Nucleus (Cd) and injection of Fentanyl on unit discharges in a PO neuron elicited by nocuous stimulation. I: Sequential spike density histogram of unit discharges (cumulation of 3 consecutive samples). A, spontaueous discharges. B, before. C, during. D, E and F 1, 5 and 10 minutes after cessation of Cd stimulation respectively. II: The same neuron. A, spontaneous discharges. B, before. C, D, E, F, G and F 2, 5, 10, 20, 40 and 50 minutes after injection of Fentanyl (30 μg/kg iv) respectively. Abscissa: processing time (512 ms). Ordinate: number of spike in a bin of 2 ms.

3.Inhibitory Effect of Electroacupuncture (EA). Acupuncture points "Huan Tiao" or "Bei Shu" were chosen for bilateral electroacupuncture. Frequency of the electric pulse used for stimulation was 5–8 Hz. The intensity was in general adjusted so as to be just sufficient to initiate local muscle twitching around the needle. Inihibitory effect on the aversive behavioral responses by electroacupuncture was, in general, of a weak type. An induction period of about 20–30 minutes was always necessary. Distinct inhibitory effect usually appeared 30 minutes after the onset of electroacupuncture, as manifested by a weakening of the movement of the animal in response to nocuous stimuli. The inhibitory effect might last for many minutes. In addition to the weakening of aversive responses, the nociceptive discharges of PO neurons were also inhibited. Fig. 4 is the sequential spike density histogram of PO neuron discharges in one experiment. The number of spikes per unit time decreased after the 20–30 minutes' application of electroacupuncture and gradually returned to control levels 50 minutes later. In the course of recovery, the animal often showed signs of drowsiness, such as closing of the eyes and drooping of the head, and almost no spontaneity in movements; in the meanwhile, there also appeared spontaneous discharges of PO neurons in a pattern characterized by the presence of burst formation.

Table 1 summarizes the relationship between the aversive behavioral response of the animal and unit discharges of 42 PO neurons. On brain stimulation or electroacupuncture, both the aversive behavioral responses to nocuous stimulation and the nociceptive discharges of PO neurons were inhibited. Among the three kinds of stimulation (CG, Cd, EA), the CG stimulation apparently produced the strongest inhibitory effect, the Cd stimulation ranked next and the EA the least. An interesting characteristic common to both brain stimulation and electroacupuncture was that after termination of stimulation, the evoked PO neuron discharges always recovered earlier than the aversive behavioral responses. These results indi-

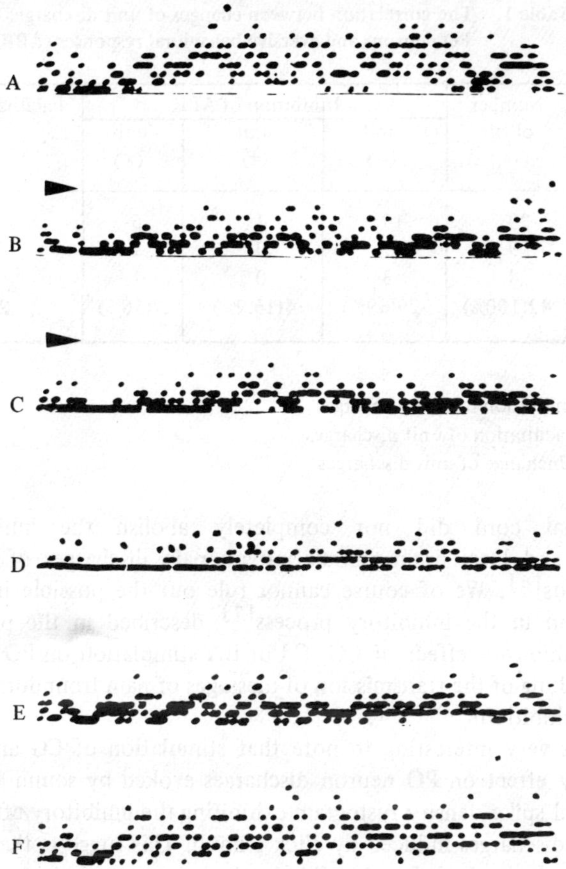

Fig. 4 Sequential spike density histogram recpresenting a computer cumulation of 3 consecutive samples of nociceptive discharges of a PO neuron. A, before. B and C, during 20 and 30 minutes of bilateral electro-acupuncture "Huan Tiao" point. D, E and F, 5, 30 and 50 minutes after the cessation of electroacupuncture respectively. Calibration: abscissa: 77 ms. ordinate: 1 impulses/5 ms.

cate that PO neurons may have taken part in the transmission of nocuous information, and that the pattern of discharges of PO neurons may reflect to a certain degree changes in pain sensations.

Since evoked field potentials could be recorded from PO when the CG and Cd were stimulated, it seems reasonable to believe that the inhibitory effect observed is a result of interaction between the afferent impulses from these structures and the impulses of nocuous stimuli in the Posterior Nuclear Group of the Thalamus. This possibility was strongly supported by the fact that in acute experiments, transection of the decending inhibitory path-

Table 1. The correlation between changes of unit discharges of PO neurons and aversive behavioral responses (ABR)

Site of stimul.	Number of site	Inhibition of ABR			Facilitation of ABR
		unit (–)	unit (+)	unit (X)	unit (+)
CG	29	19	4	5	1
CD	9	7	0	1	1
EA	4	3	0	1	0
Total	42(100%)	29(69%)	4(16.7%)	7(16%)	2(4.8%)

(–): Inhibition of unit discharges
(+): Facilitation of unit discharges
(X): Unchange of unit discharges

way in the spinal cord did not completely abolish the inhibitory effect of electroacupuncture and local brain stimulation on pain discharges of the Parafascicular Nucleus of Thalamus[6]. We of course cannot rule out the possible involvement of the descending inhibition in the inhibitory process[7] described in the present paper. It is possible that the inhibitorn effect of CG, Cd or EA stimulation on PO neurons is due, at least partly, to blocking of the transmission of messages of pain from dorsal horn neurons to PO by descending inhibition[8, 9, 10].

Besides, it is very interesting to note that stimulation of CG and Cd also exerted a marked inhibitory effect on PO neuron discharges evoked by sound and photic stimuli. Fig. 5 is a sequential spike density histogram exhibiting the inhibitory effect of CG stimulation on PO neuron discharges induced by click stimuli. This suggests that brain stimulation can modulate the transmission of various kinds of sensory signals instead of only the pain signals specifically.

Summary: Multi-unit activities evoked by nocuous stimuli were recorded from the Posterior Nuclear Group of Thalamus (PO) in unanesthetized, restrained rabbits. The unit activities recorded over that region showed heterosensory and heterotopic convergence. It was observed that PO neurons responded to both nocuous and non-nocuous somatic stimuli and sound stimuli, and had wide receptive fields in the different regions of the body.

There was a close relationship between the long-burst discharges of PO neurons and the aversive behavioral responses elicited by nocuous stimulation. Stimulation of the Central Grey matter of the midbrain (CG) or the head of Caudate Nucleus (Cd) electroacupuncture (EA) points could exert an inhibitory influence on the PO discharges, as well as on the aversive behavioral responses evoked by nocuous stimuli. The aftereffect of stimulation was common. An "induction period" was necessary for electroacupuncture to produce inhibition. The recovery of unit discharges from inhibition occurred earlier than the aversive behavioral changes. These results indicate that PO neurons may have taken part in the transmission of nocuous information, and that the changes in the pattern of PO neurons reflects in some degree the changes in pain sensations.

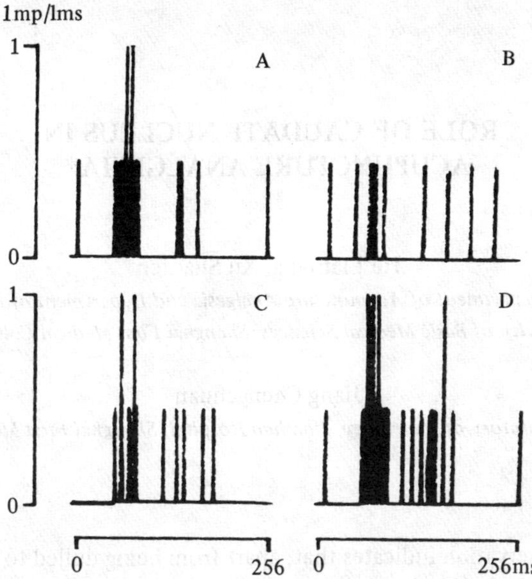

Fig. 5 Sequential spike density histograms indicate inhibitory effect of CG stimulation on discharges of a PO neuron evoked by click. A, before, B, during, C and D, 1 and 5 minutes after the cessation of CG stimulation. Abscissa: processing time (256ms), Ordinate: number of spikes in a bin of lms.

REFERENCES

[1] 吴建屏等：中国科学，**17** (5)：688，1974。(5): 688, 1974.

[2] Peggio, G.F. et al.: *Johns Hopk. Hosp. Bull.,* **106**: 266, 1960.

[3] Guilbaud, G.C. et al.: *Archiv. Ital. Biol.,* **115**:35, 1977.

[4] 孙公铎等：科学通报，**23**(7): 447, 1978.

[5] 陈俊强等：*A in Press*。

[6] 张桂林等：生理学报，**31**(3): 209, 1979.

[7] Shen, E. et al.: *Scientia Sinica,* **21**(5): 677, 1978.

[8] He, J.F. et al.: *National Symposia of Acupuncture and Moxibustion and Acupuncture Anesthesia,* p., 34, Beijing, 1979.

[9] Pomeranz, B. et al.: *Exp. Neurol.,* **64**: 327, 1979.

[10] Carstens, E.D. et al.: *J. Neurophysiol.,* **42**: 588, 1979.

ROLE OF CAUDATE NUCLEUS IN ACUPUNCTURE ANALGESIA*

He Lianfang, Xu Shaofen
(Research Department of Acupuncture Analgesia and Department of Physiology, Faculty of Basic Medical Sciences, Shanghai First Medical College)

Jiang Chengchuan
(Research Laboratory of Neurology, Huashan Hospital, Shanghai First Medical College)

Our previous observation indicates that, apart from being dulled to pain, patients undergoing surgery with acupuncture analgesia are fully conscious and normal in body functions as revealed by recordings of certain physiological indices[1]. Such a state implies that acupuncture may activate certain parts of the brain thus resulting in analgesia. It has been reported that the stimulation of the caudate nucleus is able to inhibit extralemniscal afferent activity and raise the pain threshold[2,3,4]. The question is whether the caudate nucleus plays a role in acupuncture analgesia. The present paper gives a brief account of our research work done on this subject in recent years.

I. CAUDATE NUCLEUS AND ELECTRO-ACUPUNCTURE ANALGESIA

(I) Analgesic Effect of Caudate Stimulation

1. Animal experiment[5]. Experiments were performed on rabbits. The animal with bipolar stimulating electrodes implanted chronically into the caudate nucleus was kept in a quiet state and the pain threshold of the ear skin was measured with a potassium ion electrophoretic dolorimeter at intervals of 3 minutes. As the pain threshold became quite stable, electrical stimulation with a frequency of 4–5 pulses/sec, a pulse duration of 0.5–1.0 msec and an intensity of 3.0–7.5 V or 100–200 μA was applied to the dorsal part of the head of the caudate nucleus 1 minute prior to the measurement of the pain threshold. The result was that the stimulation of the anterodorsal part of the head of the caudate nucleus (plane $A_2 - A_5$, according to Sawyer's atlas) was able to raise the pain threshold, giving an average elevation of 44.9% in 31 rabbits. Analysis of variance showed a highly significant difference ($P<0.001$) between the average of 3 determinations of pain threshold before and during caudate stimulation. Of the 3 rabbits in which the electrodes happened to be implanted into

* Summary of studies in this college.

the posterior part of the head of the caudate (plane A_1), stimulation produced elevation of the pain threshold in 1 rabbit, drop of the pain threshold in another and no effect in the third.

The results indicate that the stimulation of the anterodorsal part of the head of the caudate nucleus brings forth analgesia.

Under certain conditions, analgesia was gradually enhanced with each stimulation to reach a high level, fluctuate there and outlast the period of stimulation, manifesting a temporal summation and an aftereffect (Fig. 1).

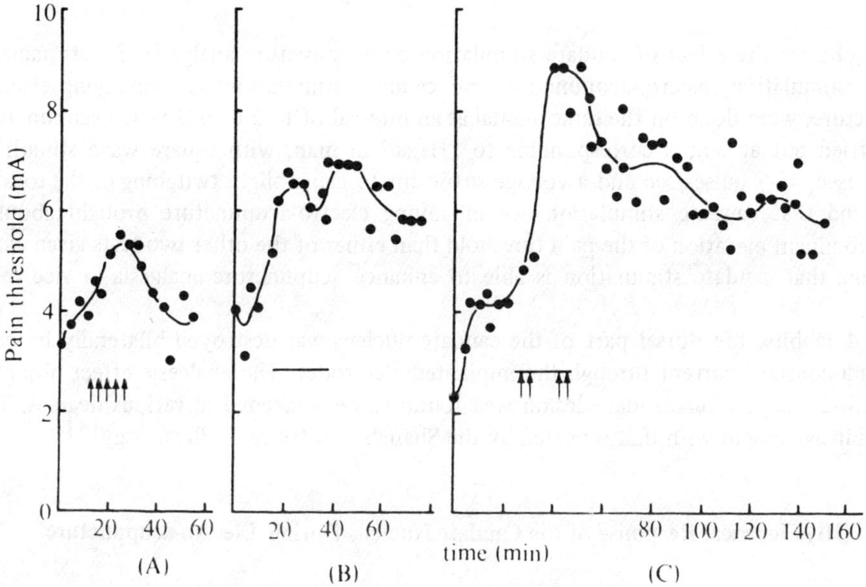

Fig. 1 Effect of caudate stimulation on electro-acupuncture analgesia
(A) Caudate stimulation
(B) Electro-acupuncture of "Hegu".
(C) Caudate stimulation accompanying electro-acupuncture
↑ Caudate stimulation
—— Electro-acupuncture

2. Clinical observation[6]. An implantation of electrodes into the head of the caudate nucleus was performed on 17 patients suffering from intractable pain due to late malignancies or phantom limb pain, to whom medication was found to be unsatisfactory. Biphasic waves, 3–5 pulses/sec in frequency and 1 mA in intensity, delivered from a G-6805 therapeutic machine were applied to the caudate for 20 minutes during a pain attack. It was found that the stimulation was able to relieve pain in the head, neck, trunk and limbs and its effect was quite satisfactory in most cases. Generally, analgesia became obvious 5 minutes after the onset of stimulation and lasted for several hours after its cessation. It seems that analgesia produced by caudate stimulation is similar to that by acupuncture of distal "points" in pain relief, tranquilization, phenomena of induction and aftereffect, and extensive effect on the body without clear segmental topography. Further observation revealed that both caudate stimulation and acupuncture brought forth elevation of the pain threshold, depression of somatosensory evoked potentials recorded over the scalp or from the centrum medianum of the thalamus, and depression of pain responses as expressed by alterations in galvanic skin activity, respiratory movement and vascular plethysmogram of the finger[7]. The similarities between caudate stimulation and acupuncture suggest a possible relationship between these two processes.

(II) Effect of Caudate Stimulation and Caudate Lesion on Electro-acupuncture Analgesia[5]

To observe the effect of caudate stimulation on acupuncture analgesia, 3 tests namely, caudate stimulation, electro-acupuncture and caudate stimulation accompanying electro-acupuncture, were done on the same animal at an interval of 1–2 days. Electro-acupuncture was carried out at points corresponding to "Hegu" in man, with square wave stimuli of 0.5–1 msec, 4–5 pulses/sec and a voltage sufficient to cause slight twitching of the toes. It was found that caudate stimulation accompanying electro-acupuncture brought about a more prominent elevation of the pain threshold than either of the other two tests given alone, indicating that caudate stimulation is able to enhance acupuncture analgesia or vice versa (Fig.1).

In 4 rabbits, the dorsal part of the caudate nucleus was destroyed bilaterally by conducting a constant current through the implanted electrodes. The analgesic effect observed within 4–20 days after caudate lesion was found to be weakened in various degrees. The result is in agreement with that reported by the Shanghai Institute of Physiology[8].

(III) Electrical Response of the Caudate Nucleus During Electro-acupuncture

1. Caudate potentials evoked by electrical stimulation of acupuncture points[5]. In acute experiment, potentials with a latency about 30–40 msec evoked by electrical stimulation of "Hegu" or "Susanli" point could be recorded from the same site of the head of the caudate nucleus, the source being located in the dorsal part. The caudate showed response to each stimulus applied to the acupuncture point, provided the frequency of stimulation was lower than 5 pulses/sec (Fig. 2). It is possible that low frequency of electro-acupuncture is optimal for the activation of the caudate nucleus.

2. Effect of electro-acupuncture on caudate neuronal activity[9]: Techniques of micro- and multimicro-pipettes and microiontophoresis were used to record the unit discharge for studying the effect of electro-acupuncture. Of the 110 spontaneously active units tested, 35 were activated by acupuncture, 43 were depressed (Figs. 3,4) and 32 insignificantly affected. Some units changed their activity at the onset of acupuncture, while others exhibited gradual excitation or depression several minutes later. The effect could persist for a certain length of time after withdrawal of acupuncture. Similar results obtained from chronic experiments on unrestrained rabbits have also been reported[10].

Of the 50 units tested by acetylcholine (ACh) microiontophoresis, 39 were found to be sensitive, most of which also responded to electro-acupuncture. Of the 77 units tested with serotonin (5-HT), 27 were sensitive, most of which also responded to electro-acupuncture. In

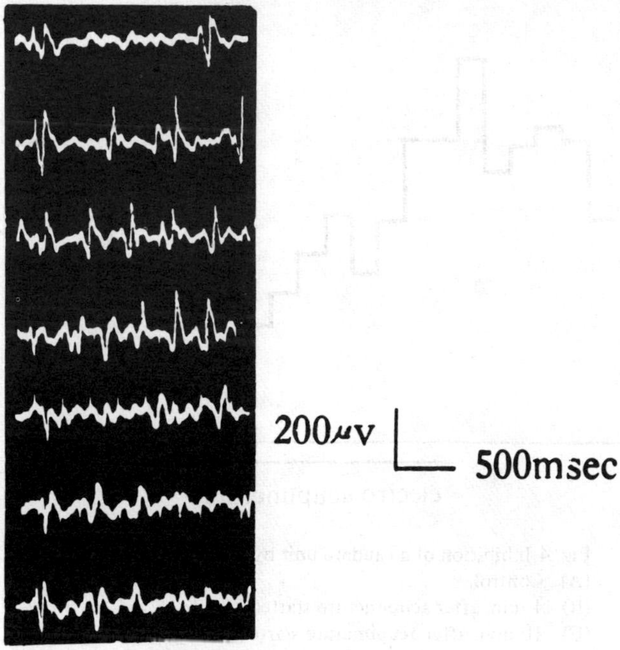

Fig. 2 Caudate potential evoked by electro-acupuncture Frequency of stimulation: 0.7, 2, 3, 4, 5 and 7 pulses/sec (from top to bottom).

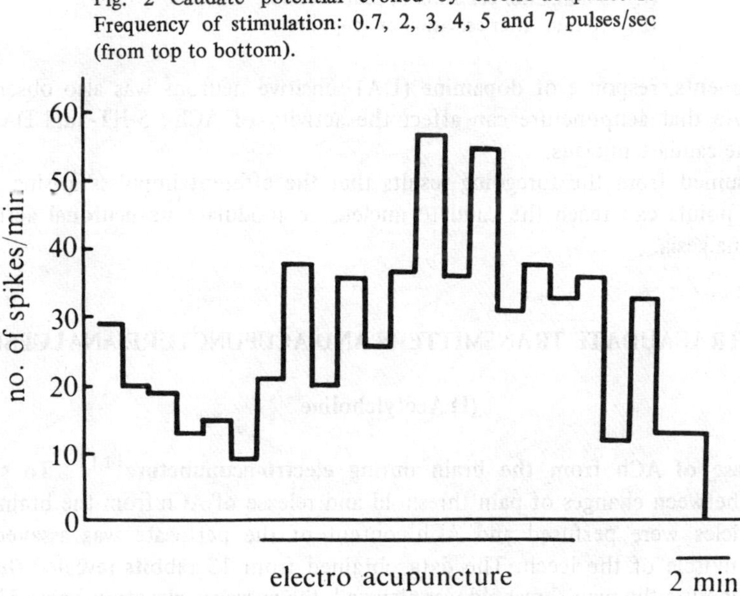

Fig. 3 Activation of a caudate unit by electro-acupuncture.
(A) Control.
(B) 5 min. after acupuncture started.
(C) 10 min. after acupuncture started.
(D) 5 min. after cessation of acupuncture.

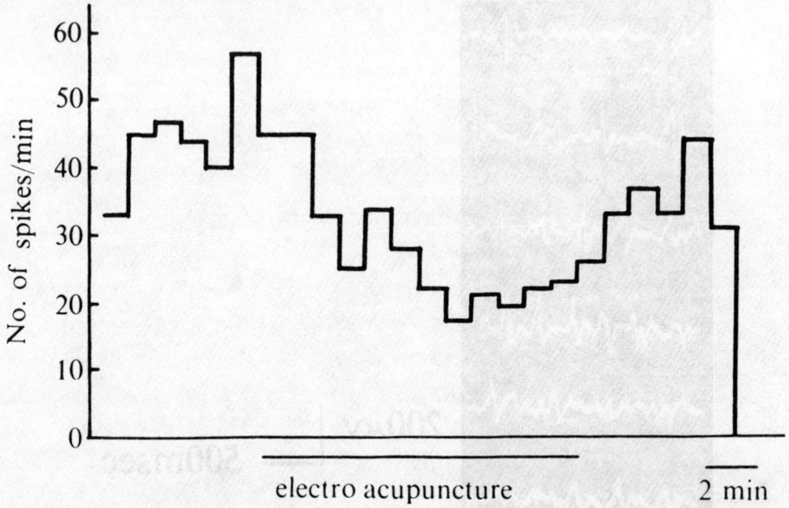

Fig. 4 Inhibition of a caudate unit by electro-acupuncture.
(A) Control.
(B) 4 min. after acupuncture started.
(C) 10 min. after acupuncture started.
(D) 20 min. after acupuncture started.
(E) 5 min. after cessation of acupuncture.
(F) 10 min. after cessation of acupuncture.

a few experiments, response of dopamine (DA) sensitive neurons was also observed. The results indicate that acupuncture can affect the activity of ACh-, 5-HT- and DA-sensitive neurons in the caudate nucleus.

It is assumed from the foregoing results that the afferent impulses arising from the acupuncture points can reach the caudate nucleus to modulate its neuronal activity thus resulting in analgesia.

II. INTRACAUDATE TRANSMITTERS AND ACUPUNCTURE ANALGESIA

(I) Acetylcholine

1. Release of ACh from the brain during electro-acupuncture[11]. To study the relationship between changes of pain threshold and release of ACh from the brain, rabbits' lateral ventricles were perfused and ACh content of the perfusate was assayed on the longitudinal muscle of the leech. The data obtained from 13 rabbits revealed that during electro-acupuncture the pain threshold was elevated, the average elevation being 72.8%, and the ACh content showed an increase too, which amounted to an average of 59.1%. The result was significantly different from that in the 6 control rabbits ($P<0.05$, $P<0.01$). Twenty minutes after cessation of acupuncture the pain threshold and ACh content were still at a relatively high level (Fig. 5).

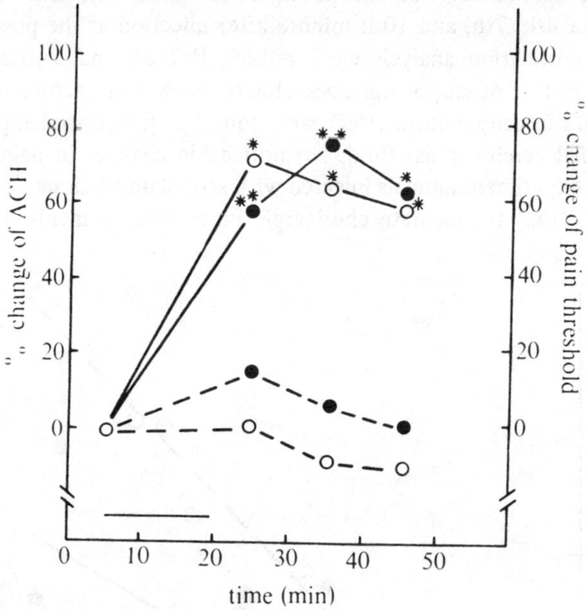

Fig. 5 Effect of electro-acupuncture on ACh content in lateral ventricular perfusate.
●—●% change of ACh in acupuncture group
●---●% change of ACh in control group
o—o% change of pain threshold in acupuncture group
o---o% change of pain threshold in control group
—— Electroacupuncture
*P<0.05 **P<0.01

It should be emphasized that there is an association between the elevation of pain threshold and the increase of ACh content in the perfusate. In 2 out of the 13 rabbits, acupuncture failed to raise the pain threshold and ACh did not increase either. On the contrary, in 11 rabbits with favorable acupuncture effects ACh increased simultaneously with the elevation of the pain threshold. Statistical analysis with X^2 test showed a high significance ($P=0.0013$). Since the head of the caudate is rich in ACh and lies lateral to the anterior horn of the lateral ventricle, the increase of ACh in lateral ventricular perfusate may be mainly due to the increased output of the caudate[12]. In clinical observation, it was found that Ach content increased as analgesia was brought on during acupuncture or caudate stimulation.

2. Effect of intracaudate microinjection of cholinergic blocker on electro-acupuncture analgesia[13]. To explore the role of the intracaudate ACh in acupuncture analgesia, micro-injection experiments were done on rabbits with permanent injection cannulae implanted into the head of the caudate. As the pain threshold rose markedly during acupuncture, scopolamine (60 μg in 2 μl artificial cerebrospinal fluid) was injected into both caudate nuclei in 17 rabbits. The result was that the rising pain threshold dropped significantly ($P<0.001$). Taking the average of 3 determinations of pain threshold at the 9th, 12th, and

15th minute during acupuncture as the pre-injection value (X), and the average of 3 determinations at the 4th, 7th, and 10th minute after injection as the post-injection value (Y), the results of correlation analysis were r=0.68, P<0.01 and Y=0.28+0.58X. Thus, intracaudate microinjection of scopolamine was able to block acupuncture analgesia (Fig. 6). No noticeable changes in acupuncture effect were found in the control experiment animals injected with artificial cerebrospinal fluid. No noticeable changes in pain threshold were found in the control experiment animals injected with scopolamine alone.

It seems possible that the caudate cholinergic mechanism is involved in acupuncture analgesia.

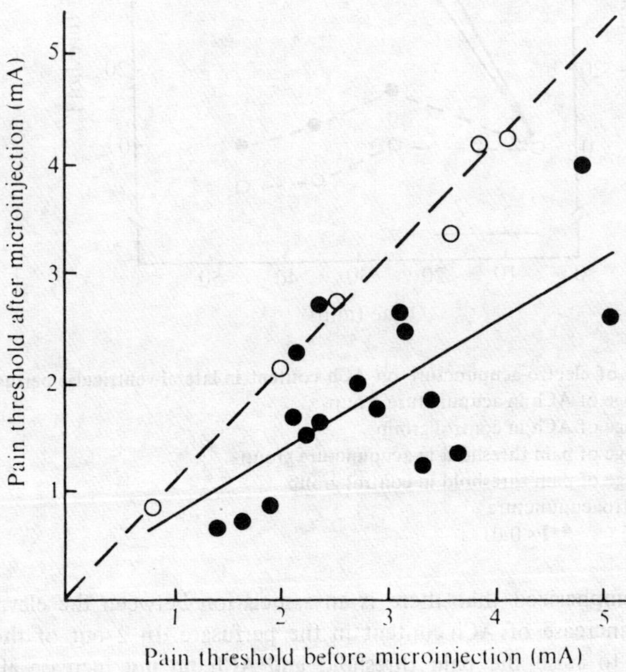

Fig. 6 Correlation of pain thresholds before and after microinjection in experiments of scopolamine and of art. CSF.
● Scopolamine r=0.68 (P<0.01) Y=0.28+0.58X
o Art CSF r=0.98 (P<0.001) Y=1.06

(II) Endorphin

1. Changes of cyclic 3′, 5′-adenosine monophosphate level in caudate perfusate during electro-acupuncture analgesia[14]. To examine the effect of acupuncture on cAMP content in caudate perfusate, techniques of pushpull perfusion and competitive protein binding analysis were used. It was found in 8 rabbits that the cAMP content decreased simultaneously with the elevation of the pain threshold, the average contents at the 20th and 30th minute during acupuncture being 62.7% and 62% of those measured before acupuncture (Fig. 7).

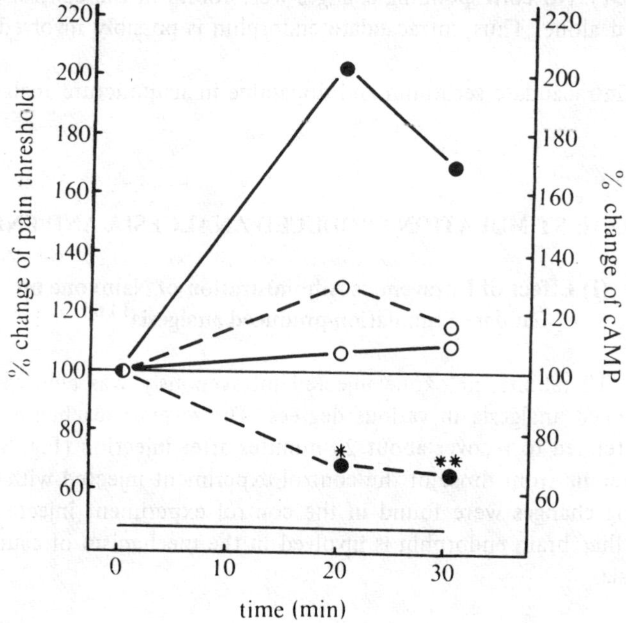

Fig. 7 Effect of electro-acupuncture on pain threshold and cAMP content in caudate perfusate.
●—●% change in pain threshold in acupuncture group
o—o% change in pain threshold in control group
●---●% change in cAMP in acupuncture group
o---o% change in cAMP in control group
—— Electro-acupuncture
*P<0.05 **P<0.01

The result was significantly different from that of the control experiment (P<0.01, P<0.05).

In another 6 rabbits, the effect of naloxone was examined. Pain threshold and cAMP content measured at the 20th minute during acupuncture were taken as control. Then naloxone, a morphine antagonist, (0.4 mg/kg body weight) was injected intravenously. Five minutes after injection, the pain threshold dropped and cAMP content increased, the average being 62.8% and 197.5% of the control value respectively, showing a significant reversal as compared with the control experiment (P<0.01, P<0.05).

Since endorphin can lower cAMP level in the tissue by inhibiting cyclase, and change in cAMP content in the caudate perfusate during acupuncture is reversed by naloxone, it is possible that there is a relationship between intracaudate endorphin and acupuncture effect.

2. Effect of intracaudate microinjection of naloxone on acupuncture analgesia[15]. To explore further the relationship between intracaudate endorphin and acupuncture analgesia, naloxone (3μg in 2μl normal saline) was injected into the head of the caudate nucleus in 11 rabbits during acupuncture. It was found that the rising pain threshold dropped, reaching a minimum at the 5th minute after injection, and then it tended to recover. The data showed a significant reversal of acupuncture effect as compared with the control experiment of saline injection (P< 0.01). No corresponding changes were found in the control experiment with naloxone injected alone. Thus, intracaudate endorphin is possibly involved in acupuncture analgesia.

The role of intracaudate serotonin and dopamine in acupuncture analgesia needs yet to be studied.

III. CAUDATE STIMULATION-PRODUCED ANALGESIA AND ENDORPHIN

(I) Effect of Intravenous Administration of Naloxone on Caudate Stimulation-produced analgesia[16]

In 9 out of 10 rabbits, naloxone injected intravenously was able to reverse caudate stimulation-produced analgesia in various degrees. The reversal reached a maximum at the 5th minute and tended to recover about 20 minutes after injection (Fig. 8). The data were significantly different from those of the control experiment injected with saline (P<0.01). No corresponding changes were found in the control experiment injected with naloxone alone. It seems that brain endorphin is involved in the mechanism of caudate stimulation-produced analgesia.

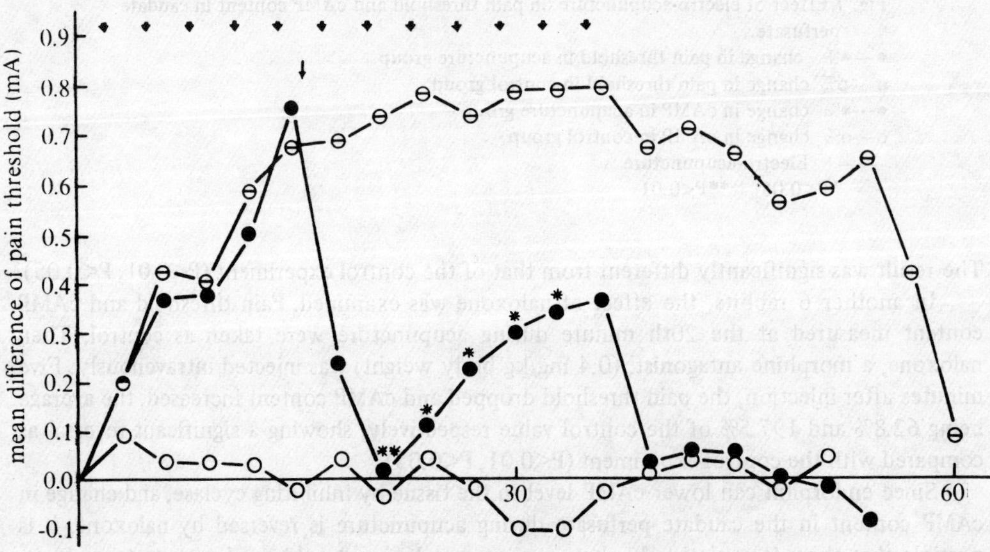

Fig. 8 Effect of nalxone on caudate stimulation produced analgesia.

↓ Caudate stimulation; ↓ Injection

● Naloxone experiment

θ Normal saline control experiment

o Naloxone control experiment

*P<0.05; **P<0.01

(II) Reversal of Caudate Stimulation-produced Analgesia by Naloxone Microinjection Into Central Grey[16]

To study whether caudate stimulation-produced analgesia is related to the central grey, microinjection experiments were done. In 9 rabbits naloxone (2 μg in 2μl saline) was injected into the central grey as the pain threshold rose markedly during caudate stimulation. As a result, the rising pain threshold dropped to reach a minimum at about the 6th minute and tended to recover about 18 minutes after injection. The data showed significant difference as compared with those of the control experiment injected with saline ($P<0.01$). No corresponding changes were found in the control experiment injected with naloxone alone. Since naloxone diffuses easily it may affect not only the central grey but also the nearby reticular formation.

The results suggest that caudate stimulation-produced analgesia may be related to the release of endorphin onto the opiate binding sites such as the central grey.

IV. DISCUSSION

1. Caudate nucleus is one of the structures mediating acupuncture analgesia in the central nervous system. It has been reported that the head of the caudate possesses an ability to inhibit the somatosensory response of the medial thalamus, the most effective region being in the dorsal part[3]. In the present paper, the dorsal part showed response to electrical stimulation of acupuncture points, and was effective, while being stimulated, in raising the pain threshold as expressed by inhibition of the defense reaction elicited by a noxious stimulus. It was found that stimulating the anterior part of the head of the caudate usually brought on good analgesic results, while stimulating the posterior part produced poor effects or even hyperanalgesia. The result is similar to the observation made on rats[17]. In line with the observation made in recording unitary response[18], we have found that the caudate could show evoked response to each stimulus applied to the acupuncture points only when low frequency was used. By applying stimulation of low frequency to the caudate, analgesia has been achieved both in laboratory experiments and clinical treatments. The analgesic effect of acupuncture was found to be synergic with that of caudate stimulation, and weakened either by destroying the dorsal part of the head of the caudate with constant current or by blocking its neurotransmitter mechanism with scopolamine or naloxone. Assumably, one of the central mechanisms in acupuncture analgesia is that the afferent impulses arising from the acupuncture point can reach the caudate to modulate its neuronal activity and activate its inhibitory function, thereby resulting in analgesia. Thus the caudate nucleus is one of the structures mediating acupuncture analgesia in the central nervous system.

2. Possible analgesic mechanism of the caudate nucleus during acupuncture: In the caudate nucleus, there exist numerous interneurons and various transmitters. Their complex interconnection and interaction are important in the regulation of nervous function. The fact that microinjection of cholinergic blocker into the caudate partially blocked electro-acupuncture analgesia indicates that caudate cholinergic activity may favor acupuncture analgesia. The caudate is abundant in DA, which inhibits the release of ACh in the presynaptic level and antagonizes the function of the latter[19]. Consistent with the observation is the fact that the dopaminergic activity of the anterior part of the head of the caudate is unfavorable to acupuncture analgesia[17]. The reversal of acupuncture effect on cAMP content in the caudate perfusate and on the pain threshold by naloxone suggests that acupuncture effect is related to the release of endorphin in the caudate. The caudate is rich in opiate receptors, part of which are at dopaminergic endings and may modulate DA release in an inhibitory fashion[20, 21]. It would thus appear that during acupuncture, these three transmitters interact with one another to facilitate the analgesic effect of the caudate. However, it has been reported that endorphin also exerts an inhibitory action on ACh release[20]. In addition, the caudate contains abundant 5-HT and γ- butyric acid (GABA) and the transmitter systems in the caudate are in a complicated interaction. Their role in acupuncture analgesia is worthy of further study.

To elucidate further the role of the caudate nucleus in acupuncture, it is necessary to explore the mechanism of caudate stimulation-produced analgesia. The reversal of acupuncture analgesia by naloxone microinjection into the caudate nucleus implies also the possible involvement of endorphin in analgesia produced by the caudate. This possibility is supported by the experimental results that naloxone administered either intravenously or by microinjection into the central grey could reverse analgesia produced by caudate stimulation. Since the head of the caudate lies lateral to the anterior horn of the lateral ventricle, it most likely releases endorphin to the cerebrospinal fluid which in turn acts on opiate receptors in the periventricular and periaqueductal grey. However, the existence of other links from the caudate to the central grey cannot be excluded.

Morphological studies have revealed that there are reciprocal interconnections between the caudate and the medial thalamus, nuclei raphe, and substantia nigra[22], suggesting their close functional correlation. The medial thalamus is considered to be important in the integration of pain sensation under the cerebral cortex, and the somatosensory response recorded from the centrum medianum, the parafascicularis and the centralis lateralis of the medial thalamus could be inhibited by caudate stimulation[2, 23]. The caudate might be a structure in a circuit, through which acupuncture exerts its inhibitory effect on pain discharge of the parafascicularis and centralis lateralis[24]. The raphe system is considered to be connected with the periventricular and periaqueductal grey[25, 26] and mediate opiate and stimulation-produced effect from midbrain sites[27] and acupuncture analgesia as well[28, 29]. The substantia nigra, aside from its motor function, has been found to be related to analgesia which could be reversed by naloxone[30]. These obser vations have raised the question whether the mechanism of analgesia produced by the caudate involves its functional connections with the raphe system and the substantial nigra. The problem needs further investigation.

The authors are indebted to Professor Xu Fengyan and Professor Yang Zaochen for their kind help and advice.

REFERENCES

[1] 曹小定等：针刺镇痛效果与交感机能活动的关系 本书第 页。

[2] Feltz, P. *et al.*: *J. Neurophysiol.*, **30**:55, 1967.

[3] Rogers, D. K. and McKenzie, J. S.: *Brain Res.*, **56**:345, 1973.

[4] Schemidek, H. H. *et al.*: *J. Neurosurg.*, **35**:715, 1971.

[5] 上海第一医学院生理学教研组：《中华医学杂志》 **55**：336，1975。

[6] 上海第一医学院华山医院针麻研究协作组《中华医学杂志》 **55**：427，1975。

[7] Jiang Chengchuan *et al.*: National Symposia of Acupuncture and Moxibustion and Acupuncture Anaesthesia, P. 331, Beijing, June 1–5, 1979.

[8] 上海生理研究所第二研究室针麻组《中华医学杂志》 **55**：340，1975。

[9] 上海第一医学院基础医学部生理学教研组针麻研究组：《中华医学杂志》 **58**：135，1978。

[10] 孙公铎等：《中华医学杂志》 **58**：139，1978。

[11] 许绍芬等：《科学通报》 **23**：572，1978。

[12] Portig, P. J. and Vogt, M.: *J. Physiol.*, **204**:687, 1969.

[13] 何莲芳等：《生理学报》 **31**：47，1979。

[14] 许绍芬等：上海第一医学院学报 **5**：21，1978。

[15] 何莲芳等：《上海第一医学院学报》 **7**：333，1980。

[16] 何莲芳等：《上海第一医学院学报》 1981，待发表。

[17] 张德星等：《生理学报》 30：21，1978。

[18] Sedgwick E. M. and Williams T D: *J. Physiol* **189**:281, 1967.

[19] Ladinsky H. *et al.*: *Brain Res* **84**:221, 1975.

[20] Pollard H. *et al.*: *Nature* **268**:745, 1977.

[21] Pollard H. *et al.*: *Brain Res* **151**:392, 1978.

[22] 周敬修等：待发表。

[23] McKenzie J. S. *et al.*: *Brain Res* **27**:382, 1971.

[24] 张香桐：《中国科学》 (1)：28，1973。

[25] 黄登凯等：待发表。

[26] Azmitia E. C. and Segal M.: *J. Comp Neurol* **179**:641, 1978.

[27] Fields H. L. and Andersom S. D.: *Pain* **5**:333, 1978.

[28] 陕西省中医研究所针麻原理研究室：《陕西新医药》 4：23，1976。

[29] 江振裕等：《科学通报》 22：43，1977。

[30] Segal M. and Sandberg D.: *Brain Res* **123**:369, 1977.

EFFECT OF ACUPUNCTURE ON NOCICEPTIVE DISCHARGES OF CINGULATE GYRUS NEURONS

Sun Xinde, Zhou Shaoci, Xu Junmei,
Zhang Senfu
(Research Laboratory of Brain Function, Department of Biology, East China Normal University)

As an important component of the limbic system, cingulate gyrus, its anterior part in particular, is correlated with the sensation of pain. It has been found possible by stimulating the anterior part of cingulate gyrus to raise the pain threshold of an animal[1] and to strengthen the analgesic effect of acupuncture markedly[2]. According to recent reports of Domesick (1969, 1970, 1972), cingulate gyrus is closely related anatomically to nucleus medialis dorsalis and nucleus lateralis ventralis of thalamus, to centrum tegmentum, to the reticular formation, and also to nucleus caudatus[5]. This, in a way, furnishes a neuro-anatomical basis for the belief that the anterior part of cingulate gyrus is possibly involved in the mechanism of acupuncture analgesia. But the real question to be answered is whether the signals of pain sensation and acupuncture can be transmitted to this region and how the two signals interact with each other there. The present article deals mainly with the observations on the influence of nocuous stimuli on the electrical activities of single neurons in the anterior part of cingulate gyrus and on the changes in such activities under the influence of acupuncture.

I. METHODS

76 adult rabbits and 42 albino rats were used for the experiments. For surgical operation, the animals were anesthetized either with a mixture of 10% urethane and 1% chloralose in a dosage of about 5 ml per kg (rabbits), or with ether (rats).

The following operations were performed: tracheotomy and insertion of a canula for artificial respiration, opening of the fourth ventricle to drain off the cerebro-spinal fluid, exposure of the cerebral regions concerned, and isolation of the peroneal nerve on one side. All the skin incisions were made after infiltration with 2% procaine.

After operations Flaxedil was injected intravenously in the rabbits and intraperitoneally in the rats in a dosage of about 5 mg per kg. Artificial respiration was given at the same time. Throughout the experiment, physiological saline containing 5% glucose was infused continuously.

Recording electrodes were inserted stereotaxically in the cingulate gyrus, according to the brain atlases of rabbit (Sawyer, C. et al. 1954) and albino rat (Krieg, W.G.S. 1946). The electrodes were of two kinds: One was a glass micro-electrode filled with 3M KCL, the resistance of which ranged from 10 to 20 megaohms. The other was a micro-electrode made of insulated stainless steel wire with a diameter of 0.2 mm. Electrical discharges of the neurons picked up by the micro-electrode were fed into a medical data computer (Type-TQ-19) to construct the sequential spike density histogram, and recorded with an X-Y plotter (Type-Lz3-104). The evoked potential was averaged from 120 to 200 sweeps by the TQ-19 medical data computer and displayed on an oscilloscope for photographic recording.

A train of 3 rectangular pulses of 100 Hz, 0.3 msec in width, 20–25v and 100–300μA in intensity applied to the peroneal nerve was used as the nocuous stimulus, which was strong enough to activate the C afferent fibres in the nerve. The electro-acupuncture was given to bilateral Zusanli points. The parameters of the pulses were 0.3 msec in width, 10V in intensity and 80 Hz in frequency.

In order to analyze the afferent pain pathway to cingulate gyrus, lesions were made in some central tracts and nuclei of thalamus by passing a direct current of about 200–300 μA in intensity and 60 sec in duration.

II. RESULTS

(I) Responses of Cingulate Neurons to Peripheral Nocuous Stimuli

In the anterior part of cingulate gyrus of rabbits, it was easy to find neurons which gave spontaneous discharges with a frequency of 4.45 ± 3.82 per second. Responses to nocuous stimuli were demonstrated in 193 neurons, which was 6.31% of the total number of neurons observed.

The neurons responsive to nocuous stimuli could be divided into two types. The frequency of the discharges of the type one neurons was increased by nocuous stimulation. The latent period of the response was far from being constant, varying generally from 100 to 500 msec, and occasionally it was as long as 2,000 msec. The response usually lasted for 3 to 10 seconds. Since the frequency of their spontaneous discharge was generally low, the increase in the frequency of discharge due to stimulation was considered to be very conspicuous (Fig. 1a). When other types of strong nocuous stimuli, such as pinching the tail or ear, or pricking the pad, were applied, the same effect was also observed. Light and innocuous stimuli, such as touching or gently stroking the fur or light pressure on the skin, generally failed to elicit any appreciable response. This type constituted 51.7% of all the neurons examined. Figure 2 is a diagram of the spatial distribution of neurons of this type in cingulate gyrus.

The frequency of discharge of type two neurons was decreased by nocuous stimulation. Neurons of this type in the anterior part of cingulate gyrus demonstrated either a temporary silence of electrical discharge or a decrease in its frequency in response to nocuous stimuli. The duration of silence in some cases was as long as 15 seconds, after which the discharge was gradually resumed (Fig. 1b). There are also cases in which the silence period discharge was rather short, being only 500–800 msec, and the restoration of discharge frequency was quite speedy (Fig. 1c). Natural nocuous stimuli might also cause a temporary cessation of electric discharge or a lowering of its frequency. It was observed that in certain cases a cor-

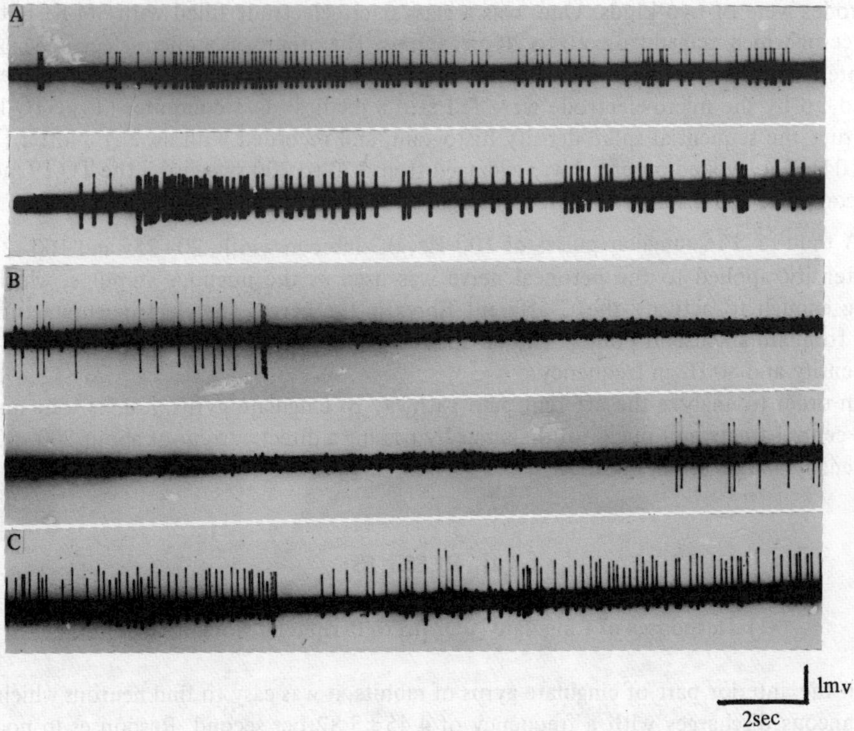

Fig. 1 The responses of cigulate gyrus units to the peripheral nocuous stimuli. A shows two recorders of angmentation of electrical discharges of two units caused by a strong electrical stimulation (a transient train of pulses, 20 v.) of pereneal nerve. B and C are recorders of responses of two units of Type-II, showing an inhibition of spontaneous discharges under the same stimulation.

relation existed between the duration of silence and the strength of the peripheral nocuous stimuli (Fig. 3).

Type two neurons constituted 48.7% of the 193 neurons responsive to nocuous stimulus. Fig. 2b shows their spatial distribution.

(II) The Effect of Morphine on the Response Caused by Nocuous Stimuli

After an intravenous injection of morphine hydrochloride (3 mg per Kg), the response of cingulate neurons to nocuous stimuli changed immediately and disappeared completely in 5 minutes. After 20 minutes, however, it gradually recovered. Figure 4 shows the response in a neuron before and after the morphine injection. Fig. 4a shows an inhibition of over one second caused by a stimulus of a short train of 5 pulses; 4b shows that one minute after the injection of morphine the duration of inhibition began to shorten. Fig. 4c shows complete abolishment of the inhibition 5 minutes after the injection. In Fig. 4d and 4e the response gradually recovers.

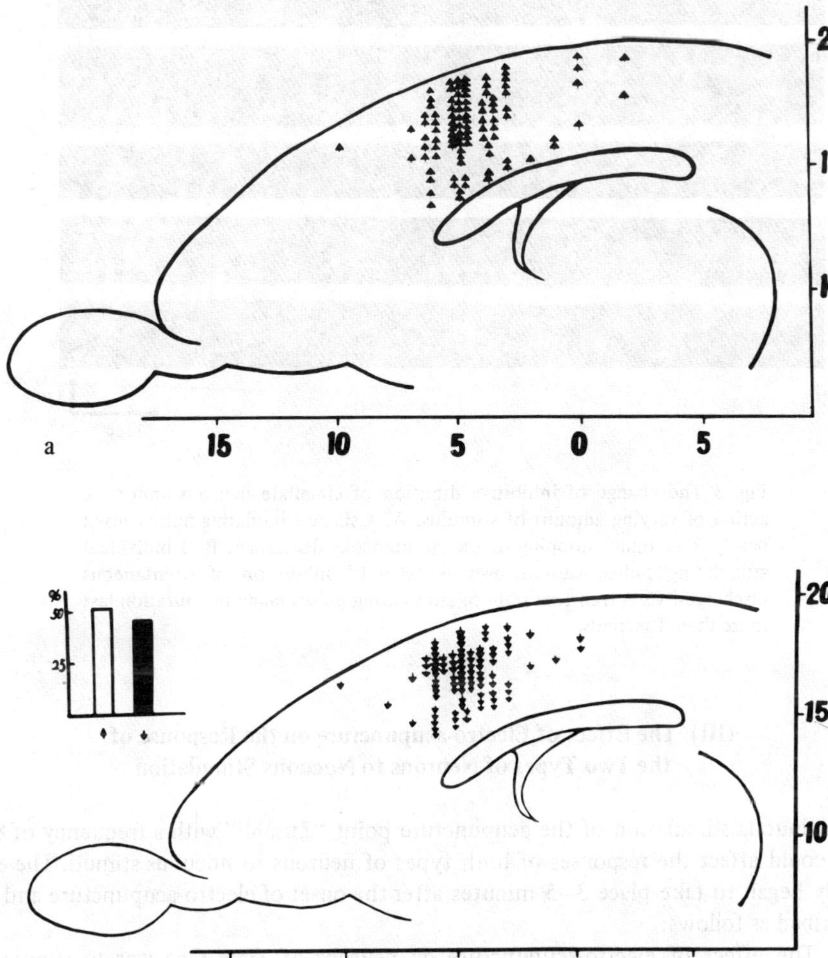

Fig. 2 The space distribution ot the neurons of two types in the anterior part of cingulate gyrus of the rabbits. The arrows pointing upward (A) represent neurons Type I, whereas those pointing downward (B) represent neurons Tupe II. The histogram shows the percentage of neurons of these two types.

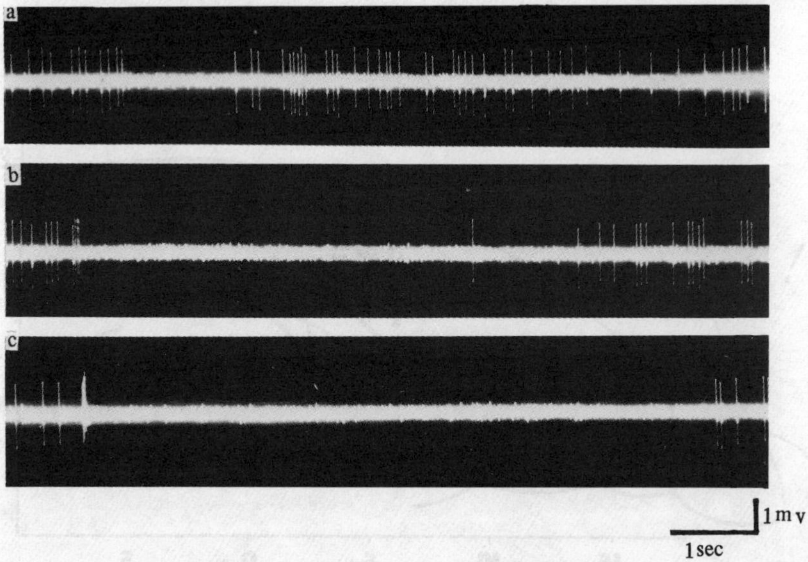

Fig. 3 The change of inhibitive duration of cingulate neurons under the action of varying amount of stimulus. A, A single stimulating pulse caused nearly 2 seconds' stopping of the spontaneous discharges. B, 3 individual stimulating pulses caused over 4 seconds' inhibition of spontaneous discharges. C, A transient train of stimulating pulses made the duration last more than 8 seconds.

(III) The Effect of Electro-acupuncture on the Response of the Two Types of Neurons to Nocuous Stimulation

Continuous stimulation of the acupuncture point "Zusanli" with a frequency of 80 per second could affect the responses of both types of neurons to nocuous stimuli. The effects generally began to take place 3–5 minutes after the onset of electro-acupuncture and could be described as follows:

(a) The effect of electro-acupuncture on neurons of Type One was to suppress the augmentation in the discharge elicited by nocuous stimuli. Figure 5a shows sequential spike density histograms indicating the effect of electro-acupuncture on the responses of a Type One neuron. It can be seen that the peak of augmentation caused by nocuous stimuli disappeared three minutes after the acupuncture had been applied, and after cessation of the needling the peak reappeared. In some units the effect was manifested as prolonging of the latency, shortening of the response duration, lowering of the discharge frequencies, etc.

(b) Electro-acupuncture eliminated the inhibition of Type Two neurons by nocuous stimuli or shortened its duration. Fig. 5b shows the behaviour of a Type Two unit whose discharge was temporarily inhibited by the nocuous stimulus but under the influence of acupuncture this inhibitory process was eliminated. After cessation of the needling the inhibition reappeared.

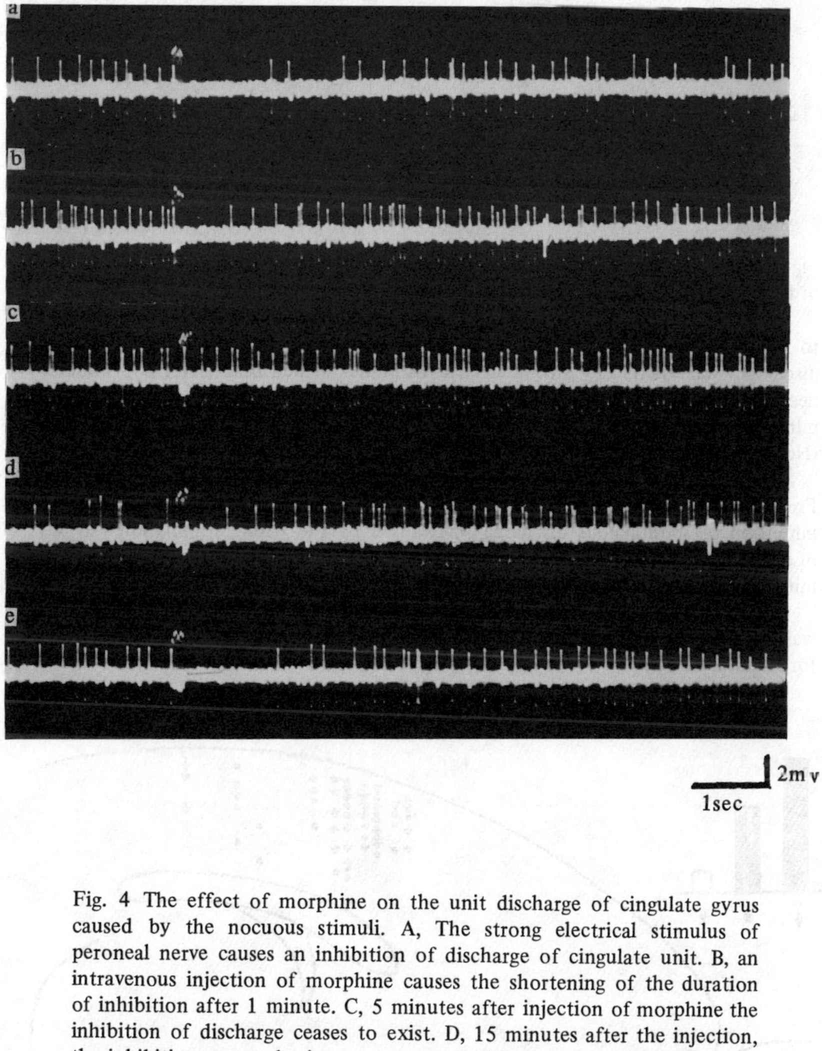

Fig. 4 The effect of morphine on the unit discharge of cingulate gyrus caused by the nocuous stimuli. A, The strong electrical stimulus of peroneal nerve causes an inhibition of discharge of cingulate unit. B, an intravenous injection of morphine causes the shortening of the duration of inhibition after 1 minute. C, 5 minutes after injection of morphine the inhibition of discharge ceases to exist. D, 15 minutes after the injection, the inhibitive process begins to reappear. E, 20 minutes after injection, the duration of inhibition recovers.

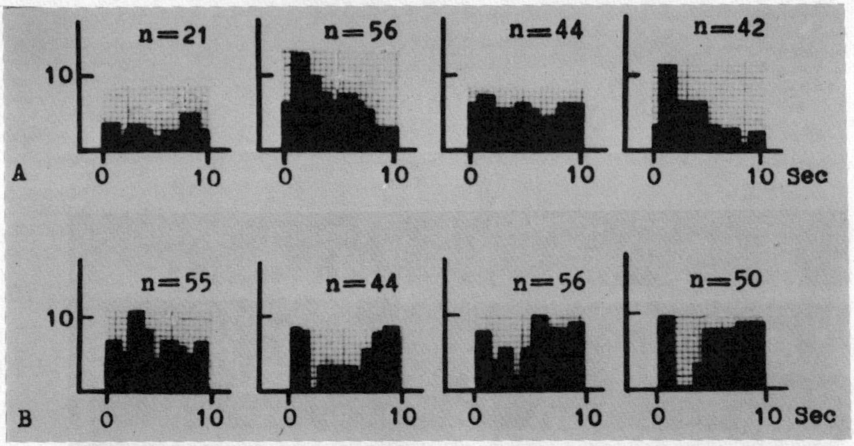

Fig. 5 The influence of electro-acupuncture on the electrical discharge of the neurons of two types, caused by the nocuous stimulus.

A. Effect of acupuncture on the response of neurons of Type One. From left side to right: 1. Histogram of spontaneous discharges density. 2. The augmentation of discharges was elicited by strong electrical stimulus of peroneal nerve. 3. 3 minutes needling depresses the discharge, caused by the stimulation of peroneal nerve. 4. 3 minutes after the stoppage of needling the augmentation of discharge recovers. (No. of experimental unit:94–2)

B. Effect of acupuncture on the response of cingulate neuron of Type Two. From left side to the right: 1. Histogram of discharges density of one neuron. 2, An inhibition of spontaneous discharge was caused by the strong stimulation (20 V.) of peroneal nerve. 3. The inhibition process was weakened by the needling. 4, 3 minutes after stoppage of the needling the inhibition of discharge recovered.

(Histograms of 10 seconds instantaneous frequency of single neuron discharges was constructed by the computer Type-TQ-19. Analysis time: 1 sec., Time delay for stimulus: 1sec.)

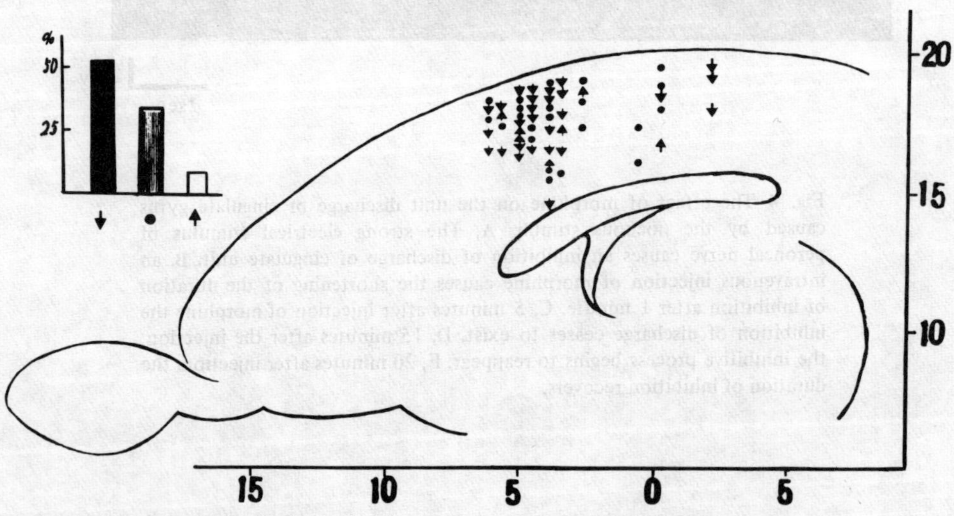

Fig. 6 The diagram shows the space distribution of the 65 cingulate neurons, on which the electro-acupuncture have had effects.

The arrows pointing downward represent neurons, on which the acupuncture has an inhibitive effect, whereas those pointing upward represent neurons, discharges of which have been facilitated by acupuncture. The spots represent neurons, on which the acupuncture has no effect. The histogram shows the percentage of these neurons in the anterior part of the cingulate gyrus.

The two phenomena just described seemed to show that electro-acupuncture produced a depressive effect on the nociceptive responses of these neurons.

However, in the case of a few Type One units, the effect of electro-acupuncture was a further increase in the firing rate of the nociceptive responses. Of the 65 units on which effects of needling were observed, 53.9% showed a depressive effect, 10.7% showed a facilitatory effect, and the remaining 35.4% failed to show any obvious change in electrical activities under the influence of electro-acupuncture.

These three kinds of neurons were intermingled irregularly in the cingulate gyrus as shown in Fig. 6.

III. DISCUSSION

1. In spite of the abundant investigations on the functions of the cingulate cortex, the response of the cingulate neurons to peripheral stimulation has not yet been studied adequately[9–13]. Previous work in this respect was largely concerned with the changes in the electrical activities of these neurons brought about by stimulation of the nerves of internal organs, especially the parasympathetic nerves. According to Bachman, et al. (1977), stimulation of the vagus nerve induced responses from 20% of cingulate neurons. Bachman and MacLean (1971) made observations on the waking squirrel monkey and concluded that light, sound and somatic stimulation could excite no response whatever from cingulate neurons. The present investigation revealed that it was possible to elicit marked changes in electrical activities of cingulate neurons by means of nocuous stimulation, including strong electric stimuli given to a peripheral nerve and natural nocuous stimuli as well. Responses could also be elicited in a number of units by certain natural stimuli, such as touching the whiskers, blowing the hair, pure tone or light clapping of hands. These phenomena shall be dealt with in a separate article.

Thus our experimental results seem to be in conflict with those of Bachman, et al.[15]. The discrepancy is possibly due to the difference in the animals used and in the conditions under which the investigations were carried out. The fact that Bachman worked with a much smaller number of units than we did may also be taken into account. In our work, only 6.31% of cingulate neurons responded significantly to external nocuous stimuli. Nevertheless, one thing is quite definite and that is, the afferent impulses of nocuous stimuli can affect the electric discharge of a portion of cingulate neurons, or in other words, pain-impulses can be transmitted to this region of the limbic system.

2. It is interesting to know how the pain-impulse is transmitted to this region. Working with 42 albino rats, we used a stainless steel electrode to record the evoked potential in the anterior part of cingulate gyrus elicited by stimulation of the peroneal nerve. The evoked potential generally included what we called the fast response which was a negative wave with a latency of 25–30 msec and an amplitude of 20–40 μV, and the slow response, a positive wave with a latency of over 50 msec and an amplitude of 20–40 μV. The slow response was quite variable and its timing was irregular. It should be emphasized that the slow response occurred only when the Aδ afferent fibers were excited (Fig. 7), and could be abolished by injection of morphine. Fig. 8 shows the evoked potential before and after an injection of morphine. It can be noticed that the response vanished 5 minutes after the injection and re-

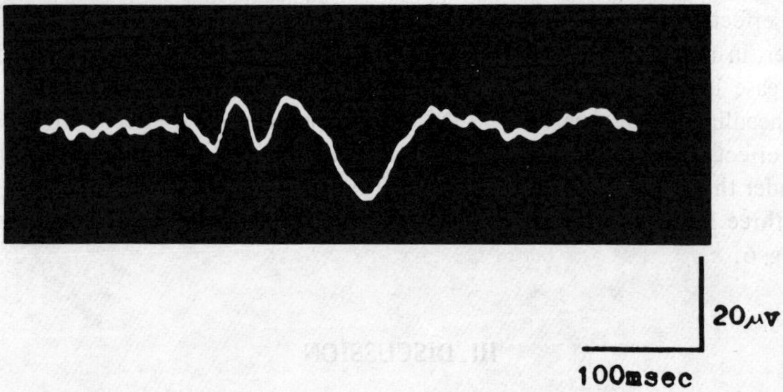

Fig. 7 Evoked potential of the anterior part of cingulate gyrus caused by the strong stimulation of the peroneal nerve. No. of animal; 78–36.

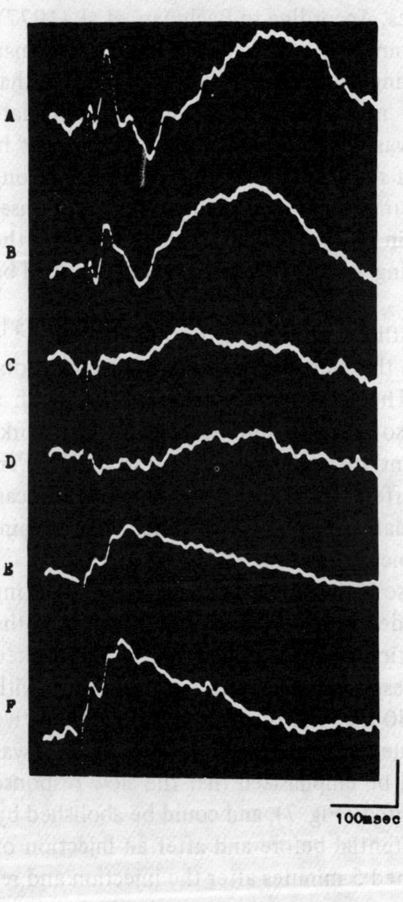

Fig. 8 The effect of morphine on the evoked potential caused by nocuous stimuli on the anterior part of cingulate gyrus. A, Before injection of morphine. B-F, 5 minutes, 10 minutes, 15 minutes, 50 minutes and 80 minutes after the injection.

covered gradually 30 minutes afterwards. Taking also into consideration the observations made on single neurons, it seems probable that this response is somehow related to pain. In order to define the pathway of these responses, sections or electrolytic lesions were made in the brain-stem and the cerebral-cortex (Fig. 9). No obvious change in response could be found after injuries to the medial forebrain bundle or after an incision made parallel with and lateral to the longitudinal sulcus on the surface of the cortex adjacent to the recording site. But the response was diminished or abolished after destruction of most part of the nuclei reticularis and nuclei anterior lateralis thalami (Fig. 10). This seems to indicate that the pain-impulses may be transmitted from the posterior thalamic nuclei to the anterior part of cingulate gyrus via nuclei anterior or nuclei reticularis.

3. Former investigations on cingulate gyrus dealt chiefly with its role in the function of internal organs and behaviour[9, 10, 11, 12, 13]. Since 1974 we have been studying the phenomenon that excitation of cingulate gyrus raised the pain threshold of animals and remarkably strengthened the analgesic effect of acupuncture. This effect was lost when the anterior part of cingulate gyrus was destroyed[1, 2]. Our experimental results indicate

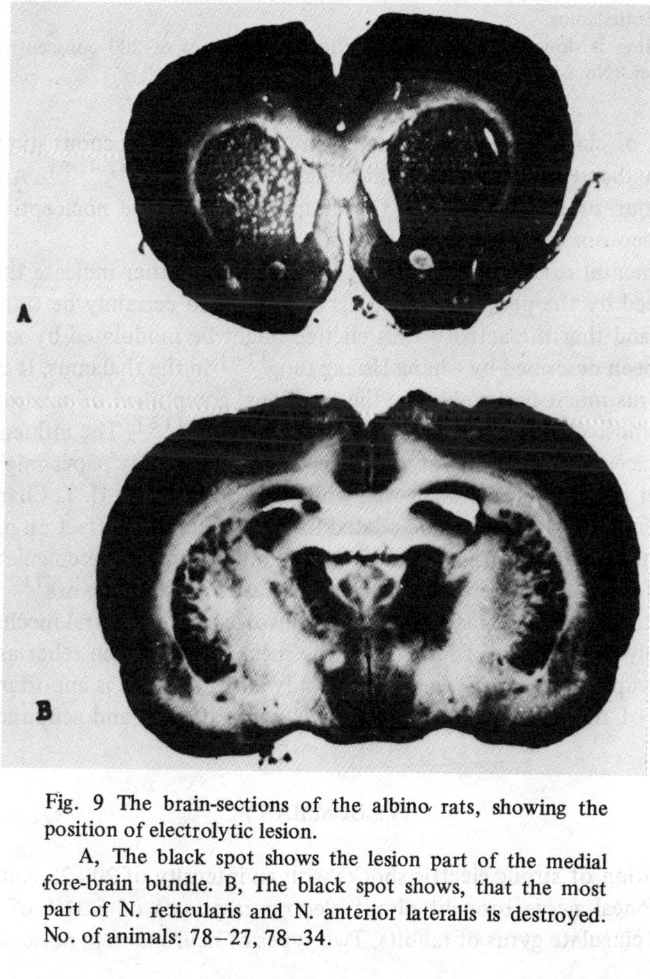

Fig. 9 The brain-sections of the albino rats, showing the position of electrolytic lesion.

A, The black spot shows the lesion part of the medial fore-brain bundle. B, The black spot shows, that the most part of N. reticularis and N. anterior lateralis is destroyed. No. of animals: 78–27, 78–34.

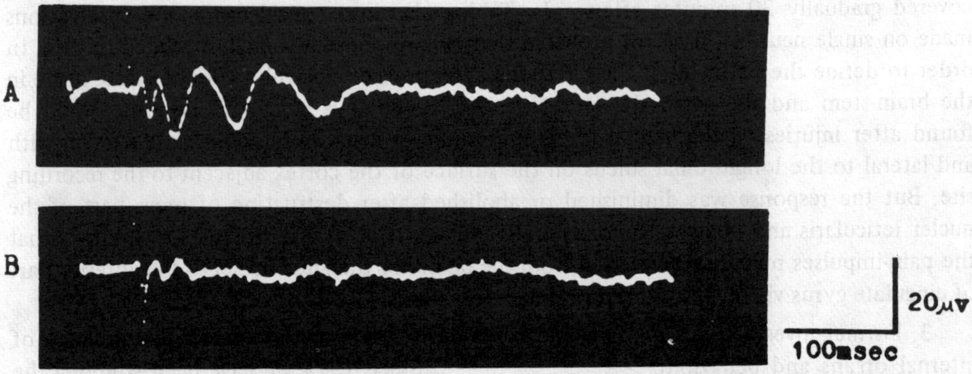

Fig. 10 The effect of electrolytic lesion of N. anterior lateralis thalamus and N. reticularis thalamus on the evoked potential of cingulate gyrus. A, Evoked potential caused by the stimulation of peroneal nerve. B, The evoked potential disappeared after the lesion of N. anterior lateralis thalamus and N. reticularis thalamus.

Each recording is done after the accumulation of responses of 200 consecutive sweeps by TQ–19 computer. (No. of animal: 78–34.)

that the activity of cingulate gyrus correlates directly with the nocuous stimulation. This is compatible with the recent neuroanatomical data of Domesick[3, 4, 5]. Another piece of evidence in favour of this concept is the disappearance of the nociceptive responses of cingulate gyrus neurons as a result of an injection of morphine.

The experimental results of the present investigation further indicate that the afferent impulses produced by the peripheral nocuous stimuli could certainly be transmitted to the cingulate gyrus and that the activity thus elicited might be modulated by acupuncture in a way which has been described by Chang Hsiang-tung[16] in the thalamus. It is probable that the cingulate gyrus might be involved in the emotional component of pain reaction which is the component most effectively suppressed by acupuncture[18]. The influence of acupuncture on the nociceptive response at this level as shown in this paper might underlie the emotional aspect of acupuncture analgesia, while that observed by H. T. Chang in the nuclei parafascicularis in the thalamus may be related to the acupuncture effect on pain perception. The afferent impulses of electro-acupuncture may impinge upon the cingulate neurons partially by way of the medial forebrain bundle as indicated in another work[17]. Therefore, it seems that the cingulate gyrus may be not only involved in the central mechanisms of pain, but also probably play an important role in the mechanism of pain relief as well as in the mechanism of acupuncture analgesia. Further study along this line is important in evaluating the importance of the limbic system in the mechanism of pain and acupuncture analgesia.

IV. SUMMARY

(1) Application of strong electric shocks with an intensity of 20–25 volts and 100–300 μA to the peroneal nerve brought about electric responses of 6.31% of neurons in the anterior part of cingulate gyrus of rabbits. Two types of neurons were noticed.

Type One constituted 51.7% of the 193 neurons observed and showed an increase in the frequency of discharge when a stimulus was given. Type Two comprised the remaining 48.3% which responded to the nocuous stimulus with a reduction or temporary cessation of the discharges. These two types of response were both eliminated after intravenous injection of morphine.

(2) A study was made on the effect of electro-acupuncture on 65 neurons which were responsive to peripheral nocuous stimuli. The parameters of the electro-acupuncture were 80 Hz in frequency, 10V in intensity and 0.3 msec in width. Continuous stimulation of point Zusanli for 3–5 minutes resulted in inhibition of activity of 53.9% of units. Electro-acupuncture lowered the frequency, shortened the duration or prolonged the latency of responses of Type One neurons. On the other hand, the inhibition of Type Two neurons by nocuous stimuli was eliminated or shortened under electro-acupuncture. Besides, electro-acupuncture facilitated the nociceptive response of 10.7% of units, and produced no effect at all on the remaining 35.4% of the neurons.

(3) The evoked potential of cingulate gyrus of 42 albino rats caused by strong electrical stimulation (20–25 V in intensity) of the peroneal nerve was reduced or abolished by electrolytic lesion of nuclei reticularis thalami and nuclei anterior lateralis thalami.

The results indicated that the anterior part of cingulate gyrus participates in the process of acupuncture analgesia. It is probable that the cingulate gyrus might be involved in the emotional aspect of acupuncture analgesia. The pain signals caused by peroneal stimulation may be transmitted to the anterior part of cingulate gyrus via brain stem and related nuclei of the thalamus, the nucleus anterior lateralis thalami or nucleus reticularis thalami in particular.

REFERENCES

[1] 上海师范大学生物系等单位：针刺麻醉资料汇编。上海针麻办公室编。1974年，第二册，48页。

[2] 殷慧镇、周绍慈、孙心德等：刺激和损毁扣带回对针刺镇痛效应的影响。上海师范大学学报，1：96，1979。

[3] Domesick, V. B.: *Brain Res.*, **12**:296, 1969.

[4] Domesick, V. B.: *Brain Res.* **20**:19, 1970.

[5] Domesick, V. B.: *Brain, Behavior and Evolution*, **6**:457, 1972.

[6] Sawyer, C. *et al.*: *J. Comp. Neurol.*, **101**:801, 1954.

[7] Krieg, W. G. S.: *J. Comp. Neurol.*, **84**:221 and **84**:277, 1946.

[8] König, J. F. R. & Klippel, R. A.: The rat brain, A stereo-taxic atlas of the forebrain and lower parts of the brain stem, The William & Wilkin Co. 1963.

[9] Gless, P. *et al.*: *J. Neurol.*, **13**:178, 1950.

[10] Kaada, B. R.: *Acta Physiol. Scand.*, **24**:83 (Suppl.), 1951.

[11] Kaada, B. R.: Handbook of Physiology, Sect. I, Neurophysiology, Vol. II, p.1345–1372, Amer. Physiol. Soc., Washington, D. C. 1960.

[12] Lewin, W. *et al.*: *J. Neurophysil.*, **23**:445, 1960.

[13] Talairach, J. *et al.*: *EEG & Clin. Neurophysiol.*, **34**:45, 1973.

[14] Bachman, D. S. *et al.*: *Brain Res.*, **130**:253, 1977.

[15] Bachman, D. S. *et al.*: *Int. J. Neurosci.*, **2**:109, 1971.

[16] Chang Hsiang-tung: *Scientia Sinica*, **16**:25, 1973.

[17] 殷慧镇、周绍慈、尤国芬：损毁内侧前脑束对针刺镇痛效应的影响。(待发表)。

[18] 蔡大衛等：电针刺激对人体痛感觉和情绪的影响。全国针灸针麻学术讨论会论文摘要，(二) 49页，1979。北京。

PRELIMINARY OBSERVATIONS ON THE CHANGES IN SLOW POTENTIALS OF CEREBRAL CORTEX INDUCED BY ACUPUNCTURE AND "PAIN"

Wang Boyang, Yang Boyi, Jiang Teming
(Fudan University, Shanghai)

In the field of research in the mechanism of acupuncture analgesia, a lot of studies have been done by means of electrophysiological methods on the fast events of the nervous system. Nevertheless, from the fact that acupuncture needs an inducing period and that it has an aftereffect, it is reasonable to assume that slow electrical events might exist also in the central nervous system during acupuncture. This report shows some preliminary observations in this respect.

I. METHODS

(I) Electrodes

Two kinds of non-polarized electrodes were used in our experiments.

(1) Silver / chloride. This was made according to Rowland[1] by coiling the silver wire (purity:99%, diameter: 0.2 mm) into a tight helix around a glass rod 2 mm in diameter, and then stretching the helix slightly to separate the individual coils from one another. Then the helix was chemically cleaned by immersion for a few minutes in ether for removal of greasy materials, and then in 1:1 dilution of concentrated HCl for removal of any extraneous iron or other contaminants. Then it was chloridized for 1 minute in dilute HCl (1:100 concentrated HCl) in a dark room, using another silver wire as cathode and a 6 V dry cell battery source (about 100mA). The electrode was then inserted into a 5mm glass tube 15mm long with its tapered end pre- packed with cotton yarn. The tube was packed with cotton wool and filled with normal saline. The upper end was sealed off with dental cement. A piece of red opaque plastic tubing was slipped over the glass tube in order to shield the interior from light.

(2) Calomels. These were reconstructed from calomels of "Lei Ci" type 222. The glass envelope was withdrawn, the cotton with KCl at the tip of the electrode (about 1/2–1/3) was pulled away and replaced by cotton soaked with normal saline.

Before these electrodes were used, the potential difference between one another was measured, and three of them (two for recording and one for reference) which were the most stable and had the least potential difference were selected for use.

(II) Operative Procedure

Experiments were carried out on the curarized rabbit maintained by artificial respiration.

There were four sites, 1 cm apart, for recording electrodes (0.5 cm from sutura coronalis and sutura sagittalis). The reference electrode was placed in the spongy bone just behind the orbit (to a depth of about 2 mm). Another site, 1 cm behind the posterior recording electrode, was for stimulation when necessary (Fig. 1).

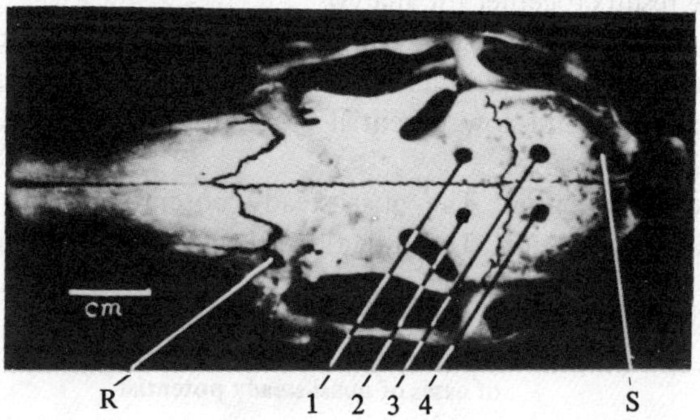

Fig. 1 Sites of electrode. 1, 2, 3, 4, for recording; R: for reference; S: for stimulation.

After the scalp was exposed and cleaned with H_2O_2, holes for fixing the electrodes were made in the skull with the dura remaining intact. The electrodes were then implanted, with the cotton yarn of the recording electrodes touching the dura, and fixed with dental cement.

Observation started 2–3 hours after operation in order to get physiological stability.

(III) Stimulation

Two kinds of needling were used in our experiments. One was hand manipulation at point "Zusanli", usually at the right hind leg; another was electrical needling, usually at points "Zusanli" and "Shangjuxu" of the right hind leg, sometimes at the point "Zusanli" on both sides. Electrical current was delivered from an electrical stimulator (BT-701) with pulse rate of about 180 c/min (at mark "3") and intensity of about 16–44 V (between marks "3" and "5"). The duration of stimulation was usually about 15 minutes.

We used two methods for "pain" stimulation: clamping the nasal septum by means of toothed forceps for 1–2 minutes, and smearing 75% alcohol in a cut on the buttock for 3–4 minutes.

(IV) Recording

The slow potentials of the cerebral cortex led by non-polarized electrode were amplified by a pre-amplifier through a low-pass filter, and displayed on the oscilloscope. The time constant of the whole amplifier system was about 6 seconds.

The camera used for recording was driven by a slow rotary machine. The film speed was fixed at 5 mm per minute.

II. RESULTS

The results from 26 rabbits showed that there was no significant difference in the response of slow potential between using Ag/AgCl (15 cases) and calomels (11 cases). Therefore, we put the results together for analysis.

There were a good many representations of the so-called "slow potential". For the purpose of the present study, three kinds of slow potential were recorded. They were the quasi-steady potential, the infra-slow potential oscillation (abbreviated to ISPO) and the spreading depression.

1. The quasi-steady potential: The quasi-steady potential shifted frequently during acupuncture or "pain" stimulation. The direction of change and the number of cases are listed in Table 1.

Table 1. The direction of shift and number of cases of quasi-steady potential

	Needling		"Pain"
	Electrical	Manipulative	Stimulation
Upward (positive)	15	12	2
Negligible	8	8	6
Downward (negative)	1	0	11
Total	24	20	19

It can be seen that, in most cases, the direction of potential change elicited by acupuncture is positive (upward), with the exception of only one which shifts in the negative (downward) direction.

The shift of quasi-steady potential was more significant in electrical needling than in manipulation. The time course of the potential change was very slow, and it did not maintain the higher level during the whole period of stimulation, but returned to the initial level gradually (Fig. 2 A). The amplitude of the shift varied with individuals, being usually about 200–400 μV and rarely exceeding 1 mV.

The quasi-steady potential shifted in a negative direction during "pain" stimulation. The time course of the potential change was also very slow, which was maintained in the 3–4 minutes during which period the " pain" stimulation persisted, and returned to the initial level as the stimulation was withdrawn (Fig. 2 B).

2. ISPO: The ISPO appeared in 15 of 26 cases in our experiments. The rhythm of ISPO was about 5–6 osc/min, with an amplitude of 0.1–0.2 mV (near to the "A" rhythm classified by Aladjalova[2]).

The number of cases with changes in amplitude of ISPO induced by acupuncture are

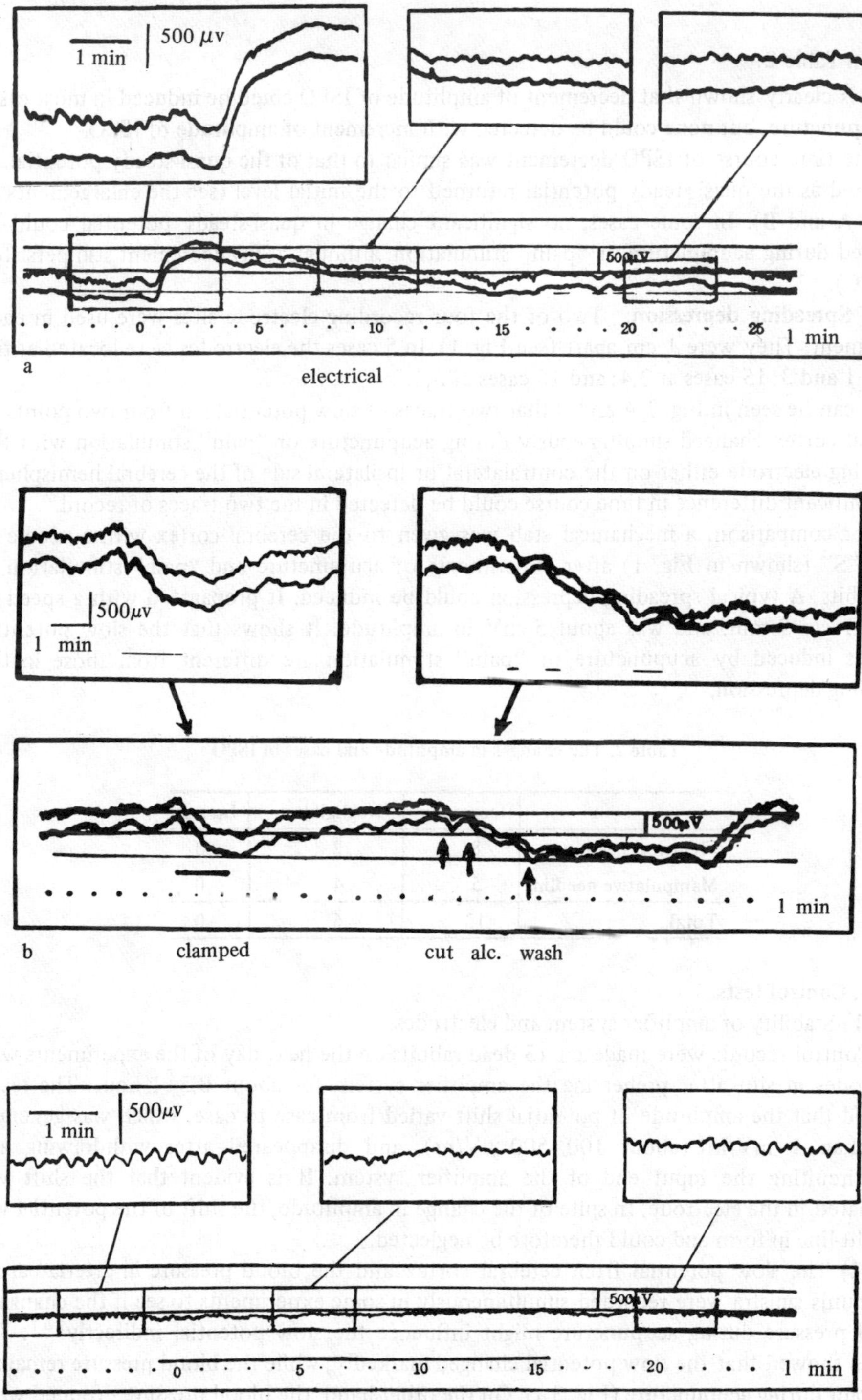

Fig. 2 Slow potential changed during acupuncture or "pain" stimulation. Positive is up. A Electrical needling. B. "pain" stimulation. C. Manipulative needling. The enlargements on upper rows show the ISPO in respective regions. Further explanation, see text.

listed in Table 2.

It is clearly shown that decrement of amplitude of ISPO could be induced in most cases by acupuncture, but none could be detected with increment of amplitude of ISPO.

The time course of ISPO decrement was similar to that of the quasi-steady potential. It recovered as the quasi-steady potential returned to the initial level (see the enlargements of Fig. 2 A and B). In some cases, no significant change in quasi-steady potential could be observed during acupuncture or "pain" stimulation, although ISPO decrement still persisted (Fig. 2C).

3. Spreading depression: Two of the four recording electrode sites were used in each experiment. They were 1 cm apart (see Fig. 1). In 5 cases the electrodes were located at the points 1 and 3; 15 cases at 2,4; and 16 cases at 3,4.

It can be seen in Fig. 2 A and B that two traces of slow potential led from two points of cerebral cortex changed simultaneously during acupuncture or "pain" stimulation with the recording electrode either on the contralateral or ipsilateral side of the cerebral hemisphere. No significant difference in time course could be detected in the two traces of record.

For comparison, a mechanical stab was given to the cerebral cortex with a needle at point "S" (shown in Fig. 1) after experiments of acupuncture and "pain" stimulation in 19 rabbits. A typical spreading depression could be induced. It propagated with a speed of about 1 cm/5 min. and was about 5 mV in amplitude. It shows that the slow potential changes induced by acupuncture or "pain" stimulation are different from those in the spreading depression.

Table 2. The changes in amplitude and cases of ISPO

	Decrease	Negligible	Increase
Electrical needling	8	2	0
Manipulative needling	5	4	0
Total	13	6	0

4. Control tests:

(1) Stability of amplifier system and electrodes.

Control records were made on 13 dead rabbits on the next day of the experiments with electrodes in situ after preheating the amplifier system for about 0.5–1 hour. The result showed that the amplitude of potential shift varied from case to case, which was generally less than 1 mV/hr (about 100–500 μV/hr), and disappeared after withdrawing and shortcircuiting the input end of the amplifier system. It is evident that the shift was originated in the electrode. In spite of the change in amplitude, the shift of the potential was straight-line in form and could therefore be neglected.

(2) The slow potential from cerebral cortex and the blood pressure in arteria carotis communis sinistra were recorded simultaneously in some experiments to see if the change in blood pressure during acupuncture might influence the slow potential indirectly[3]. The results showed that the slow potential changed markedly, while the blood pressure remained constant during acupuncture (Fig. 3A). On the other hand, the blood pressure dropped when the vagus nerve was pulled, while the slow potential remained relatively stable (Fig. 3 B). When the cerebral cortex was stimulated, the blood pressure rose, but the potential of a

cortical point 1 cm away from the stimulated point remained relatively stable, which, nevertheless, changed significantly about 5, minutes after stimulation (Fig. 3C). Thus it can be concluded that changes in slow potential are independent of the blood pressure.

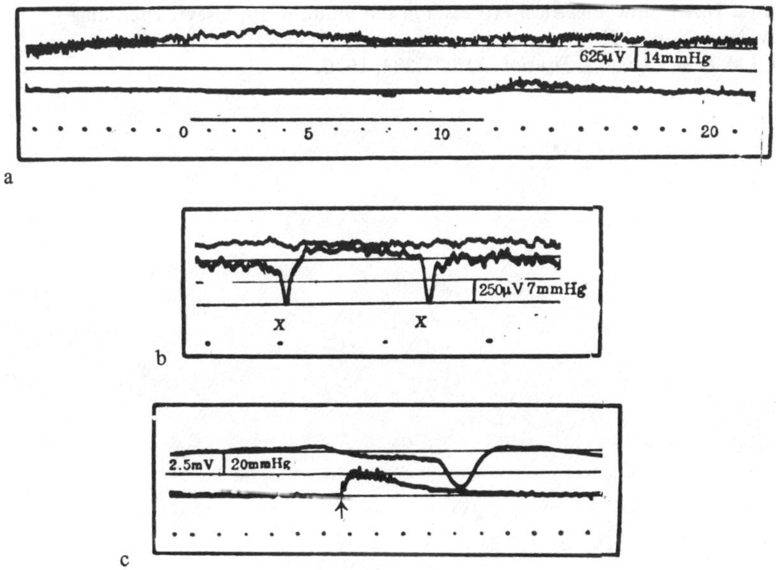

Fig. 3 Slow potential (upper trace, positive being up) and blood pressure (lower trace) recorded simultaneously for contrast. A. Manipulative needling. B. pull the vagus nerve. C. Cortex stimulation. Time is recorded in 1 minute intervals. Further discription, see text.

III. SUMMARY

The changes in slow potentials of the cerebral cortex induced by acupuncture and "pain" stimulation were recorded by non-polarized electrodes in 26 curarized rabbits.

1. The quasi-steady potential shifted in positive direction during acupuncture, but in negative direction during "pain" stimulation.
2. The amplitude of infra-slow potential oscillation decreased during acupuncture or "pain" stimulation.
3. No spreading depression could be detected when slow potential changes occurred.
4. These changes in slow potential are independent of alteration in blood pressure.

REFERENCES

[1] Rowland, V.: *Electroenceph. Clin. Neurophysiol.*, **13**(2):290, 1961.

[2] Aladjalova, N.A.: Slow Electrical Processes in the Brain, p. 19, Elsever Publishing Company, New York, 1964.

[3] Besson, J.M. *et al.*: *Amer. J. Physiol.*, **218**(1):284, 1970.

ROLE OF CEREBRAL CORTEX IN ACUPUNCTURE ANALGESIA

Cooperative Research Group for Brain in
Acupuncture Analgesia, Beijing*

It is well known that acupuncture anesthesia was developed from the clinical experience that pain in patients can be relieved by acupuncture. Then the mechanism of the analgesic action of acupuncture has been investigated ever since. It may be related with the central nervous system. We know human pain perception is a reflection to pain stimulation. The signal of any sensory perception, including that of pain of course, must reach the cerebral cortex before consciousness can be produced. Any functional change of the cerebral cortex may exert its influence on perception. Therefore, to investigate the role of cerebral cortex in acupuncture analgesia is one of the areas of studies on the mechanism of acupuncture anesthesia. Recently, research work in this area has become very active, because of the development in theoretical research and electronic technology. We think that this study may be helpful in understanding further the neurophysiology and the theory of the meridians.

Since as early as in 1909, when Cushing [1] reported that the patient complained of pain after electrical stimulation of the post-central gyrus, similar work has been done in many countries[2]. In order to relieve intractable pain, neurosurgeons have operated on patients to remove cerebral cortex or to stimulate and damage related groups of nuclei by means of stereotaxic surgery. Whether the cerebral cortex plays a role in the mechanism of analgesia, especially acupuncture analgesia, is a question that has given rise to much controversy. The purpose of this article is to investigate the role of cerebral cortex in acupuncture analgesia by means of evoked potential with pain rating under consciousness.

I. METHODS

Pain stimulation was applied on a middle finger with stimulator through an isolator (frequency 1 cps, duration 0.2–0.6 msec, unloaded voltage 105–275V). The intensity must be tolerable for the subject. The stimulating electrode was a pair of silver strips of $3 \times 35 mm^2$ each.

Cerebral evoked potential (CEP) was recorded at the contralateral scalp corresponding to the hand region of the somatosensory area. The reference electrode was placed in the center of the forehead. The signal of evoked potential was fed to the computer via

*The 1st Department of Physiology, Institute of Acupuncture, Academy of Traditional Chinese Medicine; Beijing Institute of Neurosurgery; Beijing Institute of Traditional Chinese Medicine; Beijing Second Medical College; Beijing University.

pre-amplifier to be averaged and was recorded by X–Y plotter.

"Neiguan" and "Jianshi" were stimulated by electro-acupuncture unilaterally (duration 0.2 msec, frequency 100 cps, 1–7V).

Subjects lay on bed comfortably, keeping the eyes closed and in conscious state. The electroencephalograph was monitored by an oscillograph. The results were treated by statistics.

II. RESULTS

(I) The relationship between CEP and pain perception

There has been a lot of research work on human perception with the evoked potential technique. Opinions differed as to whether the evoked potential could reflect pain sensation. From the following observations we consider that the CEP can serve as a non-specific index of pain perception.

1. Comparing cerebral potentials produced by non- pain and pain stimulation: This was carried out on 23 normal adults. We found that the pattern of potential evoked by non-pain stimulation was simple and the amplitude of wave P2 (latency about 200 msec, positive phase) was low. However, the waveform of potential evoked by pain stimulation was complex. The amplitude was high and the duration was wide. We found that the difference between the amplitudes of wave P2 of the non- pain and pain CEP was very significant statistically ($P < 0.001$) (Fig. 1).

So we suggested that the wave P2 was related to pain perception. In order that any effect of stimulating strength on this difference may be excluded, analysis of the component of CEP related to pain was performed.

2. Analyze the CEP related to pain by injecting fentanyl (or morphine) and ketamine : The CEP by pain stimulation were observed before and after intravenous injection of fentanyl (0.1 mg or morphine) and ketamine (50 mg). This was carried out on 24 general surgical patients. We found that the amplitude of the late component P2 was decreased after injection of either of these two drugs ($P<0.02$, $P < 0.05$) (Fig.2).

We also observed the influence of noxious stimulation on the late components (P2, N2) after administration of ketamine (20 mg/kg) or morphine (6–8 mg/kg). This was performed

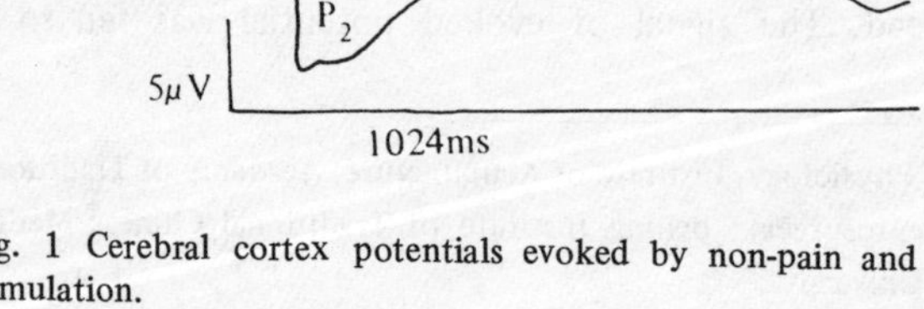

Fig. 1 Cerebral cortex potentials evoked by non-pain and pain stimulation.

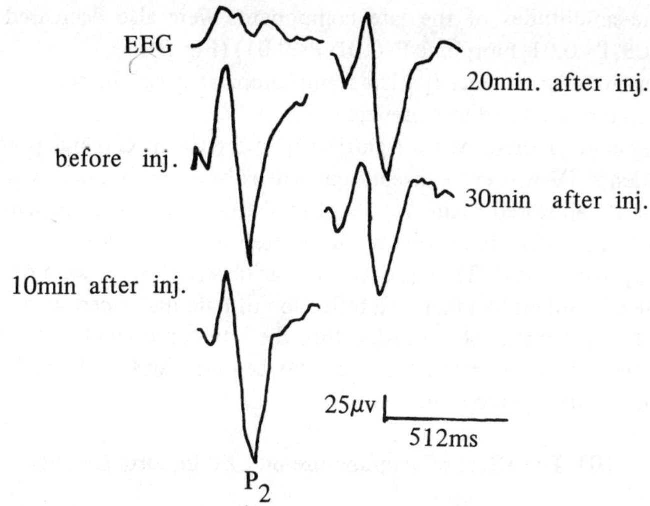

Fig. 2 Cerebral cortex evoked potential after administration of fentanyl (0.1 mg).

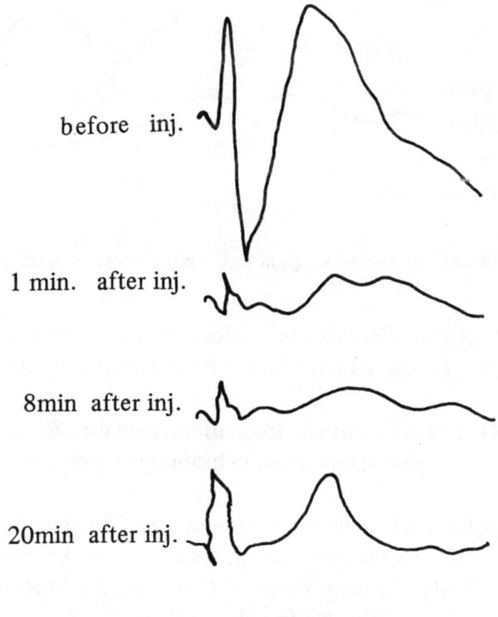

Fig. 3 Effect of ketamine on cerebral cortex potentials evoked by noxious stimulation (cat).

on 20 cats. The amplitudes of the late components were also decreased after injection (ketamine $P<0.05$, $P<0.01$; morphine $P=0.01$, $P<0.01$) (Fig. 3).

From the above experiments (patients and animals) it can be seen that the late component of CEP is closely related to pain perception.

3. In syringomyelia there was a significant difference in cerebral potentials on both sides. Some patients' P2 was even absent, and when they were treated with medicines and acupuncture, the P2 appeared again. We also found that some other patients lost their pain perception unilaterally after brain operation. Therefore, we could not record CEP at the contralateral scalp (or cortex). Though such cases as observed by us were only a few, we still consider that the CEP might be taken as a reflection of pain under certain circumstances.

From the above, it might be suggested that the late component of CEP (latency about 200 msec, positive phase) is related to pain perception, and CEP might be taken as a non-specific index of pain perception.

(II) The effect of acupuncture on CEP in normal adults

The amplitude of CEP was decreased during electro-acupuncture at "Neiguan" and "Jianshi" (15 cases) in which only P2 showed a significant difference (Fig. 4).

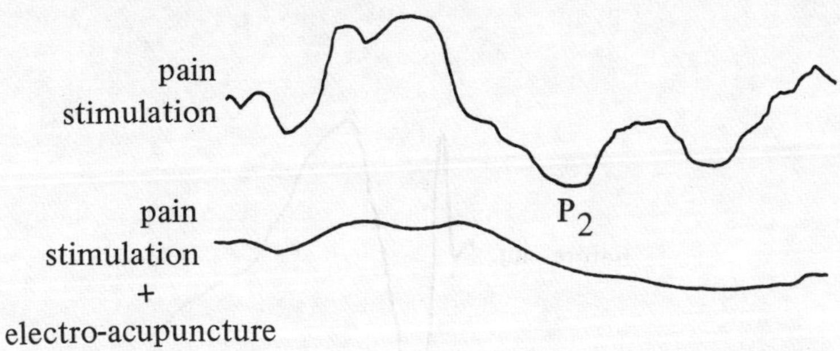

Fig. 4 Effect of electro-acupuncture on cerebral evoked potentials.

The depression of CEP was parallel to subjective sensation of reduced pain by needling (corresponding rate 89%). It seemed to indicate the effect of acupuncture analgesia.

(III) The effect of electro-acupuncture on CEP due to pain stimulation in brain operation.

On recording the CEP from scalp before operation (23 cases) or both scalp and cerebral cortex simultaneously after operation (8cases), we could see that the CEP patterns from the two sites were similar. Only the amplitude of CEP recorded directly from the cortex was higher than that from the scalp. Under the influence of acupuncture we observed a depression of CEP, but only the component P2 showed a significant difference ($P<0.001$) (Fig. 5). The depression of CEP was parallel to analgesia rating. Such results can be observed

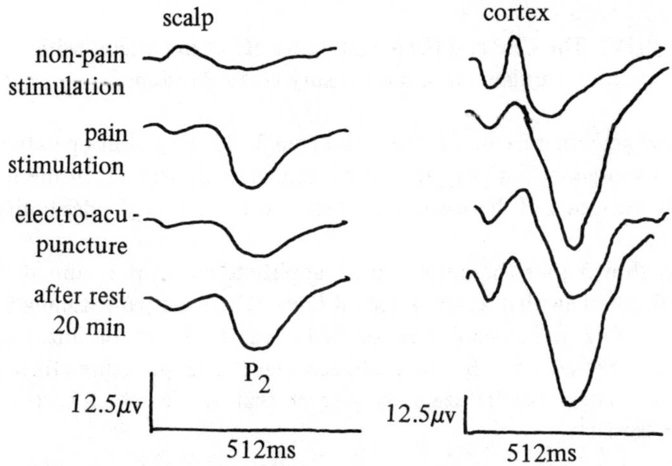

Fig. 5 Evoked potentials and acupuncture effect recorded from cerebral cortex and scalp simultaneously.

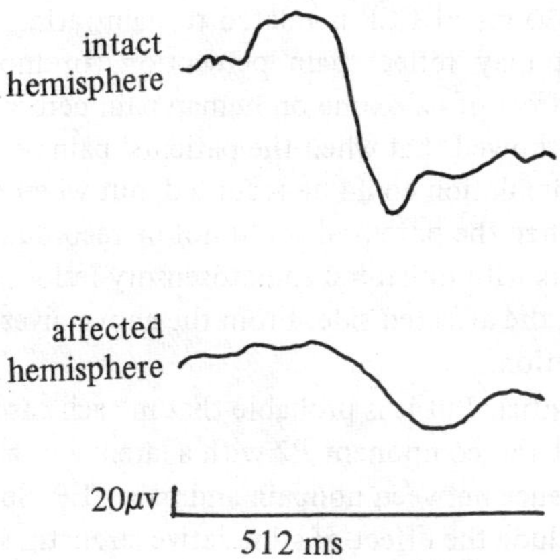

Fig. 6 Difference in evoked potentials between intact hemisphere and affected hemisphere in a patient with unilateral somatosensory cortical lesion.

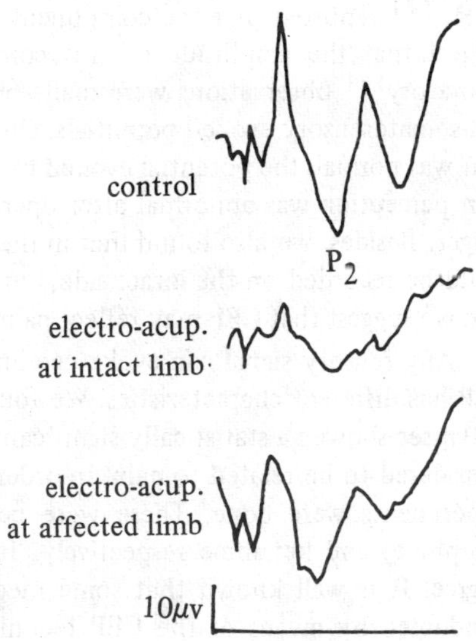

Fig. 7 Comparison between cerebral evoked potentials during electro-acupuncture of the intact and the affected limb.

both in healthy adults and in patients under brain operation.

(IV) The CEP and the acupuncture effect in patients with unilateral somatosensory cortical lesion.

The effect of acupuncture on CEP was observed 3–12 days after operation. It was made sure by the neurosurgeon that only the gray matter was destroyed. In these patients there appeared a difference in CEP between the intact and the affected sides both in latency and amplitude (Fig. 6).

It was also shown that the inhibition of amplitude by acupuncture at the intact limb was more significant than that at the affected limb. When the pain stimulation was applied to the affected limb(Fig. 7), the depression of P2 was 14.5% at the intact one. But it was only 4.3% at the affected limb. So we could see that the acupuncture effect at the affected limb was weaker. These results seem to suggest that the cerebral cortex is involved in acupuncture analgesia.

III. DISCUSSION

1. In this article we use the method of somatosensory evoked potential to investigate the role of the cerebral cortex in acupuncture analgesia. It is indicated that the CEP may be related to pain. However, there are different opinions about this. Chen, A. C. and Chapman, C. R. [3] reported that the component 175–260 ms of CEP is related to pain rating, and suggest that the amplitude of this component may reflect pain perception. In another laboratory[4] observations were made on the effect of naloxone on human pain perception and somatosensory evoked potentials. Our work showed that when the patients' pain perception was normal, the potential evoked by pain stimulation could be recorded, but when their pain perception was abnormal after operation, then the potential could not be recorded any longer. Besides, we also found that in the patients with unilateral somatosensory lesion, CEP could be recorded on the intact side, but not on the affected side. From the above investigation we suggest that CEP may reflect pain perception.

Any sensory signal can evoke cerebral potential. But it is probable that in each case the CEP has different characteristics. We found that the component P2 with a latency of about 200 msec showed a statistically significant difference between nonpain and pain CEP. So it is considered to be related to pain. In order to exclude the effect of stimulative strength, some experiments were done. These were performed on patients and cats using fentanyl (or morphine) and ketamine respectively. It is shown that the CEP reflects pain to a certain degree. It is well known that some medical research work on anesthesia and analgesia is conducted by means of the CEP technique[5]. Therefore, we consider that the CEP may be taken as a nonspecific index for pain perception both in clinical and experimental investigation of acupuncture analgesia.

2. Many reports have shown that the CEP is inhibited by acupuncture, its late component with long latency being especially significant[6]. We find that the amplitude of the late component is decreased during acupuncture at "Neiguan" and "Jianshi". This component is related to the nonspecific projective system, and also to pain perception. Besides, it is parallel to pain rating. Therefore, the evoked potential may be used as an index for the effect of acupuncture analgesia.

3. The relationship between the cerebral cortex and pain perception is an unsolved problem. There are different opinions about it. Many research workers report that the cerebral cortex is related to pain. When the post-central gyrus is stimulated, pain perception can be produced[7]; when the cortex is damaged, the pain threshold is elevated[8], or spontaneous pain[9] and oversensitivity[10] appear; when the cortex is stimulated, patients with chronic pain feel the pain, and after removing the cortex, the pain is relieved, etc. However, one paper reported that after removing the hemispheres, the pain threshold showed no change, and so it was suggested that the pain perception was localized in the thalamus[11]. Another work reported that pain perception could not be produced when the somatosensory cortex was stimulated. In our work we observed that pain was either decreased, or oversensitive, or showed no change in the patient with unilateral somatosensory cortical lesion. It is suggested that the cerebral cortex is essential for normal perception. We also noted that the CEP on the intact and the affected sides was different, and that the acupuncture effect on both sides was different, too. So there should be some relationship between cerebral cortex and pain perception. It is a fact, however, that the higher the level that is damaged in the pain pathway, the more variable the effect that follows, and one can hardly predict what result will happen. Therefore we can realize that it is a complex problem to find out the relationship between cerebral cortex and pain perception.

We know there are ascending and descending pathways between the cerebral cortex and subcortical structures. If the connections between the cerebral cortex and the thalamus are interrupted, patients will have an abnormal sensation or oversensitivity in pain perception. Hence some suggest that the main center of pain perception is situated in the thalamus. Actually both the cerebral cortex and the thalamus play a role in central integration of pain perception. There are a lot of clinical reports about treating central intractable pain by destroying certain groups of nuclei in the thalamus[12]. It is our aim to further investigate the exact role of the cerebral cortex in acupuncture analgesia, the relationship, both functional and structural, with certain thalamus nuclei, and the influence of functional changes on acupuncture analgesia. All these problems need to be studied further and their solution will be helpful in elucidating the mechanism of acupuncture analgesia and pain physiology.

Conclusion

The following conclusions are drawn from the present work:

1. The late component (latency about 200 ms) of CEP is related to pain perception.
2. The amplitude of the late component is inhibited by electrical acupuncture.
3. Cerebral cortex does play a role in the mechanism of acupuncture analgesia.

REFERENCES

[1] Cushing, H.: *Brain,* **32**: 44, 1909.

[2] Paul Gloes: Experimental Neurology, pp.237–255, Oxford, London, 1961.

[3] Chen, A. C. and Chapman, C. R.: Second World Congress on Pain of the International Association for the Study of Pain (Montreal, Canada), p.302, 1978.

[4] Buchsbum, M. S. : *Nature,* **270**(5638): 620, 1977.

[5] 上津原甲一等：脑と神经 24 (9): 1199，1972。

[6] 北京市中医研究所经络室：中医研究所资料选编，1977。

[7] Penfield, W. and Boldrely, E.: *Brain*, **60**: 389, 1937.

[8] Marschall, T.: *J. Neurol Neurosurgery Psychiat.*, **14**:187, 1951.

[9] Howard, L. Field. *et al.*: *Brain*, **97**: 169, 1974.

[10] Hamby, W. B.: *Arch Neurol Chicago*, **5**:528, 1961.

[11] 上海生理研究所二室针麻组：针刺麻醉临床和原理研究资料选编，上海人民出版社，P 156—199，1977。

[12] Hamby, F. J. and Hitchcock, E. R. : Acta Neurochirurgica Suppl. 24, Advance in Stereotactic and Functional Neurosurgery, 2. pp. 15–73,pp.219–235, Spring-Verlag Wein-New York, 1977.

EFFECT OF CORD DORSUM STIMULATION ON EEG AND BEHAVIOR IN UNRESTRAINED RABBITS

Shen Kefei, Ho Shufeng, Wang Peifen
(Shanghai Institute of Physiology, Academia Sinica)

I. INTRODUCTION

It has been reported clinically that satisfactory acupunctural analgesic results can be obtained in abdominal surgery by using the points Jizhong, Zhongshu, Mingmen and Yaoshu along the Dumai channel on the back of the body[1]. The remarkable effects were mainly muscular relaxation, hypalgesia and tranquility. Acording to the meridian atlas, Dumai channel passes along the midline of the back of the body as well as the head and face. Anatomically, the above-mentioned acupuncture points are located at the interspinal spaces of the lower back. It was emphasized by the acupuncturists that good electric needling effect was obtained only when the needle tip was inserted deep into the yellow ligament, adjacent to the epidural space.

In the present study an attempt was made to study in detail the electric needling effect of Dumai points on animals. The stimulating electrodes were implanted chronically on the lumbar vertebral lamina of rabbits. The effect of cord dorsum stimulation on electroencephalogram (EEG) and related behavior changes were observed under waking and unrestrained conditions. The result showed that EEG synchronization with behavioral signs of tranquility was manifested when the cord dorsum stimulation was moderate, and EEG desynchronization and hypotonia supervened when stimulation was intense. These results fitted in well with those of acupuncture needling of the lower back midline points for analgesia in abdominal surgery. It is therefore an ideal animal model for studying the mechanisms underlying acupuncture analgesia of Dumai points.

II. METHODS

The experiments were performed on 25 waking, unrestrained albino rabbits. Implantation of EEG recording electrodes on the skull and stimulating electrodes on vertebral lamina was carried out under sodium pentobarbital (35 mg/kg iv.). The recording of stimulating electrodes were stainless steel wire 0.4 mm in diameter. Three pairs of EEG recording electrodes were implanted on either side of the skull close to the anterior and posterior parts of sensori-motor areas and visual area. Each of the electrodes was connected to a transistor socket by thin plastic coated wire. Both the electrodes and sockets were fixed in place by dental cement. The eye movement was monitored by electrodes implanted in the frontal bone at the upper rim of the orbit. The electro-myogram (EMG) was recorded by insulated stainless steel wire 0.2mm in diameter with a bared anterior portion 5 mm in length. These wires were inserted percutaneously into the muscles (tibialis anterior, gastrocnemius, quadriceps, semi-membranous and nuchal muscles) when necessary.

The stimulating electrodes were implanted in the mid-dorsal part of 2nd lumbar vertebral lamina with one on each side of the base of vertebral spinous process approximate to the mid-dorsal portion of the spinal cord, or at a more lateral part of the lamina near the base of the transverse process approximate to the lateral or ventrolateral surface of the spinal cord. When unipolar stimulation was given the indifferent electrode used was a round silver plate of 1 cm in diameter which was embedded subcutaneously on the lower back near the site of incision. An extra pair of electrodes was implanted in 5 animals on the mid-dorsal portion of the lst sacral vertebral lamina to stimulate the cauda equina. Care should be taken in implantation of the stimulating electrodes that the bony lamina had to be trephined through, yet the tip of the electrode should not exceed the inner surface of the lamina. The electrodes were fixed in place with dental cement. To avoid the animal's gnawing the wires, all the wires were passed underneath the skin and made their exit at the posterior part of the neck.

The stimulating pulses were generated by a square wave stimulator (JSD-631) with an isolation unit. The pulse width of the square wave was 0.5 msec and the frequency used was either 100 Hz or 10 Hz. The intensity of current was monitored by an oscilloscope.

The experimental sessions started on the 4th day after operation. Electrophysiological recording and behavior observation were carried out while the rabbit was in a lighted soundproof cage (60 × 60 × 60cm). The room temperature was kept at 20°C.

The response time of defensive reflex of head jerk elicited by focusing radiant heat on the blackened snout was taken according to the method used by Chiang *et al.*[2].

III. RESULTS

(I) Effect of Cord Dorsum Stimulation on EEG and Behavior

When a repetitive stimulating current at 100 Hz was given with a gradually increasing strength to the dorsal part of the spinal cord of the rabbit, the EEG synchronization usually appeared in the neocortex after a short period of 2–3 minutes. The EEG was characterized by high voltage slow wave and burst of spindles. The rhythm was 5–7/sec with waxing and waning. The EEG synchronization was always bilateral and manifested particularly in the frontal and parietal leads (Fig. 1A).

The behaviour of the animal during EEG synchronization showed corresponding signs of tranquility. The animal lay down on the ground with the body stretched, ears drooping and eyes half shut. In the meantime the respiratory rate slowed down and the spontaneous EMG activities became greatly reduced (Fig. 2B).

The EEG synchronizing effect could be easily induced when the animal was in a state of relaxed wakefulness. When the animal was in an alert state such as hopping, searching and grooming, the EEG synchronization usually appeared with a long delay. Sometimes it was

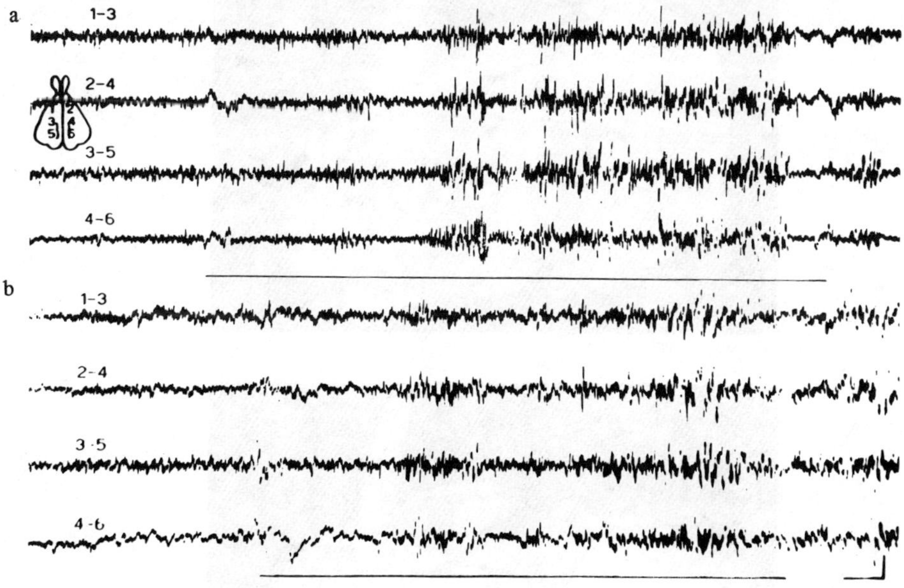

Fig. 1 EEG of rabbit during cord dorsum stimulation.

A. High frequency stimulation (100 Hz. 0.5 ms pulse width, 0.5 mA) applied through electrodes implanted on L2 vertebral lamina at cord dorsum. The line beneath EEG recordings indicates the period of cord dorsum stimulation EEG synchronization

B. Low frequency stimulation (10Hz, 0.5 ms pulse width, 1.0 mA) applied to the same site as in A. EEG occurs during and after cord stimulation. Calibration: 5 sec, 200μV.

necessary to increase the stimulating strength to chock the movement of the animal or to force the animal to assume a squatting position. As soon as the animal calmed down, EEG synchronization supervened. It was difficult to elicit the EEG synchronization when the animal was in a highly agitated state.

The EEG synchronization, once appeared, would last for a certain period of time even if the stimulation was stopped. Occassionally, it would shift into a REM sleep, a stage characterized by rapid eye movement, twitching of the vibrissae, facial muscle or one of the limbs, and EEG desynchronization. The EEG synchronization could be repeatedly induced by cord dorsum stimulation in a single experimental session without any sign of habituation. The more times it was stimulated, the easier the EEG synchronization could be induced.

(II) Stimulating Parameters and Effective Sites

The optimum stimulating current for EEG synchronization in cord dorsum stimulation varied from 0.4 to 0.8 mA. If the stimulating current applied was slightly beyond the optimum range, the induction period for EEG synchronization would be greatly prolonged. If the stimulating current was increased still further, desynchronization would occur. At the

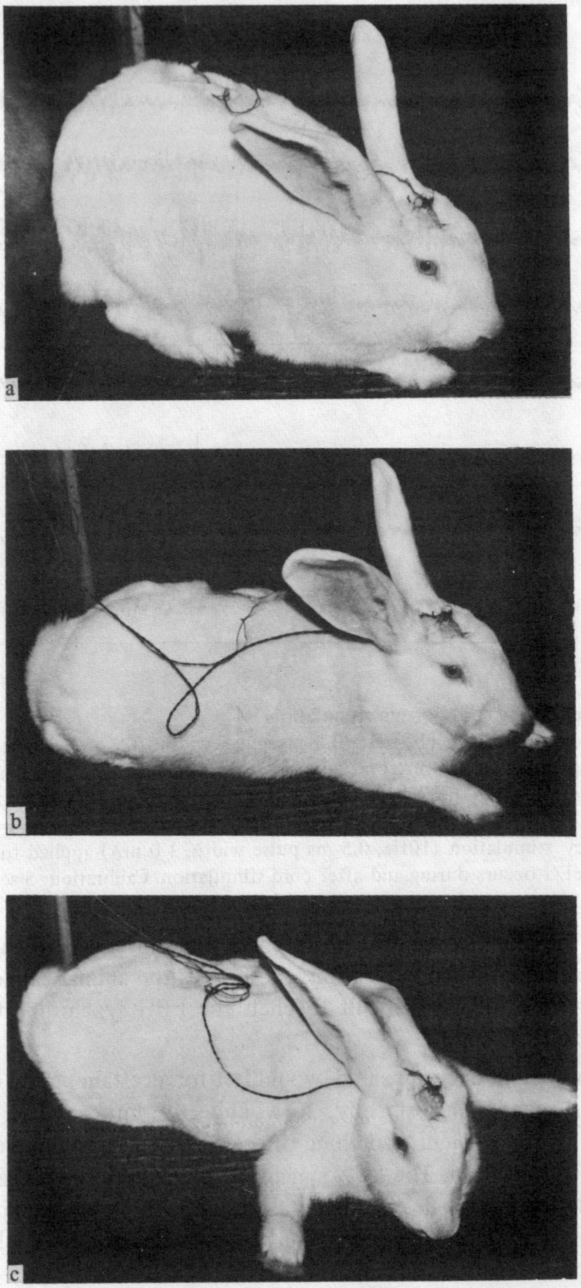

Fig. 2 Posture of rabbit before and after cord dorsum stimulation.

A. Control, animal in squatting position.
B. After moderate cord dorsum stimulation, (100 Hz, 0.5 ms pulse width, 0.4 mA)
C. After intense cord dorsum stimulation (100 Hz, 0.5 ms pulse width, 2.4 mA) the animal lay flat with the limbs, body and head all touching the ground.

same time the animal would move about or lick its lower limbs or perineal area suggest signs of hyperesthesia, and then an appropriate attenuation of the stimulating current woı impel the animal readily to a state of calmness with EEG synchronization.

The effective frequency of cord dorsum stimulation to induce EEG synchronization a behaviour tranquility included not only 100 Hz but also 10 Hz. The only difference betwe the two frequencies was that the lower frequency had a wider range of stimulating streng than the higher one. As shown in Fig. 1B, the same synchronizing effect of EEG can evoked when 10Hz stimulation was given to the dorsum of the spinal cord.

EEG synchronization and the related behavioral changes could be reproduced so lo as the stimulus strength and frequency are adequate regardless of the site of stimulation.

(III) Effect of Cauda Equina and Acupuncture Point Stimulation on EEG

Cauda equina was stimulated through the electrodes implanted on the lamina of the] sacral vertebra to see whether the same synchronizing effect could be obtained. The resı was positive. It can be seen from Fig. 3A and 3B that either frequency, 100Hz or 10Hz, effective. As soon as the EEG synchronization appeared, the animal entered into a tranqı state.

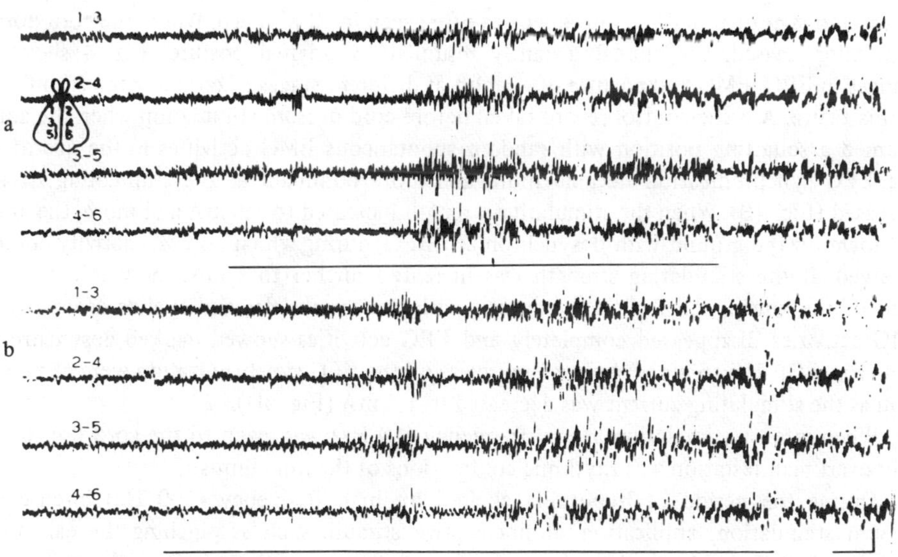

Fig. 3 EEG of a rabbit during cauda equina stimulation.

A. High frequency stimulation (100 Hz, 0.5 ms pulse width, 1.0 mA) applied through implanted electrodes at S1 vertebral lamina. EEG synchronization occurs during stimulation.

B. Low frequency stimulation (10 Hz, 0.5 ms pulse width, 1.5 mA) applied to the same site as in A. EEG synchronization occurs. Line beneath EEG recording indicates the period of cauda equina stimulation. Calibration: 5 sec, 200 μV.

For comparison, the effect of electro-needling on acupuncture points of the limbs and body was studied under the same experimental conditions. A pair of acupuncture needles were inserted into the points Zusanli and Shangjuxu at the proximal one third of the anterior tibial muscle, or Huatuogiaji located at the back of the body lateral to the vertebral spines. It was found that both the higher (100 Hz) and the lower frequencies (10Hz) were able to induce the EEG synchronization within 1–2 minutes, provided that the stimulating strength was adequate (1.5–2.0 mA). The characteristics of the EEG were similar to those in natural sleep (slow wave sleep) or cord dorsum stimulation. The EEG synchronization lasted for a certain period of time after the cessation of electric needling. Behaviorally, the animal lay down on the ground silently with the eyes half open.

(IV) Effect of Intense Stimulation of Cord Dorsum

When a strong stimulating current (100Hz, 2 mA) was given to the cord dorsum (the increase of current ought to be gradual) an entirely different result ensued. The tonus of the whole body after a brief period of restlessness quickly reduced to such an extent that the animal could no longer maintain its normal posture and collapsed on the ground (Fig. 2C). EMG recording on the neck or limb muscles revealed that the spontaneous muscle activities decreased to a minimum or disappeared entirely. EEG was characterized by desynchronization, i. e., high frequency low amplitude fast waves. At the same time electrooculogram showed no sign of rapid eye movement as often seen in REM Sleep. When the cord dorsum stimulation ceased, the animal instantly resumed its original posture. Fig. 4 shows the changes in EEG, EMG and posture of a rabbit at different stages of cord dorsum stimulation. In this figure, A is the control record taken before cord dorsum stimulation when the animal assumed a squatting position with random spontaneous EMG activities in the quadriceps. The EEG synchronization became more and more dominant as the stimulating strength increased (Fig. 4B). When the stimulating strength increased to 1.5 mA and more, the animal lay down on the ground with desynchronized EEG, during which no EMG activity could be observed. If the stimulating strength was increased further to 3 mA, the whole body and head of the animal fell flat on the ground with the ear auricles and eyelids drooping. The EMG activities disappeared completely and EEG activities showed marked desynchronization (Fig. 4C). The tonus of the neck muscles and the EEG synchronization were resumed as soon as the stimulating current was decreased to 1.5 mA (Fig. 4D).

When intense stimulation at low frequency (10 Hz) was given to the cord dorsum, the only overt manifestation was rhythmic contractions of the hind limbs.

During the period of hypotonia elicited by high frequency (100 Hz) intense cord dorsum stimulation, application of nociceptive stimuli, such as pinching the ear auricle, applying electric shocks to the skin of the foot or focusing radiant heat on the snout of the rabbit could no longer elicit the defensive flexor reflexes. A detailed study on the response time with the radiant heat method showed that the latency of the avoiding response was greatly lengthened. As shown in Fig. 5 the response time before stimulation is 3.4 ± 0.45 sec. It increased to 14.9 ± 2.14 sec after 10 minutes of cord stimulation. Among the 10 animals 6 had a latency longer than 20 sec, and the latency for the other 4 animals also increased to a certain extent. After cessation of cord dorsum stimulation, the response time recovered within 10 minutes (Fig. 5).

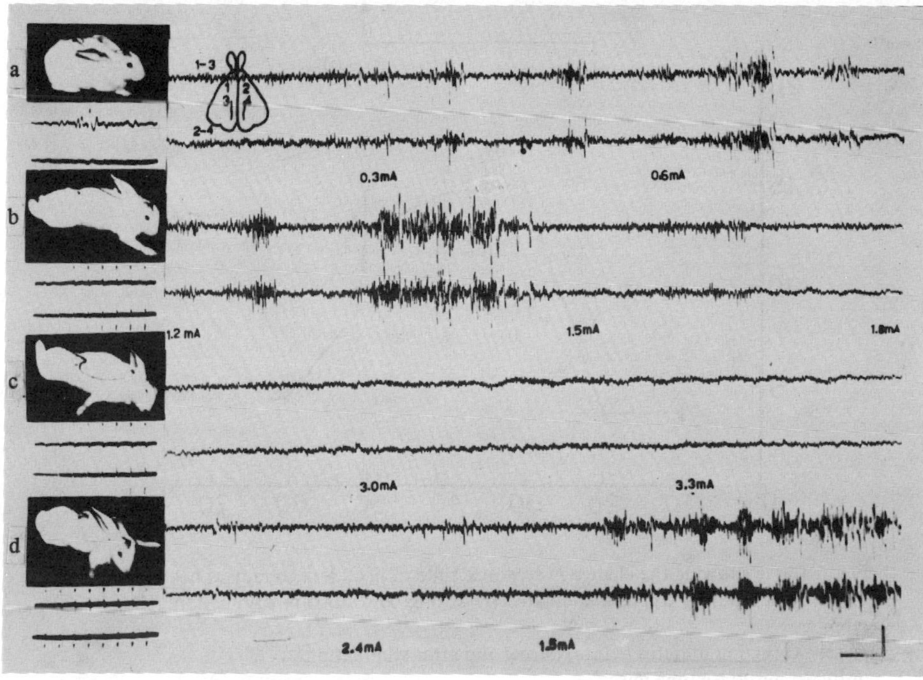

Fig. 4 Change of EEG, EMG and posture in rabbit during cord dorsum stimulation.

A. Weak stimulation applied at L_2, Before stimulation animal in squatting position with spontaneous activities in extensor muscle. After stimulation EEG synchronization prolongs.

B. With moderate stimulation, EEG synchronization becomes predominant. When stimulating current is increased to 1.5 mA, EEG desynchronization occurs. Animal lies on the ground with head still erect. EMG activity vanishes.

C. Strong stimulation, with EEG desynchronization and hypotonia. No EMG activities.

D. Decreasing the stimulating strength to 1.5 mA, EEG synchronization resumed. Erection of head, but no EMG activities in hind limbs.

A, B, C, and D are the serial records of a rabbit. EEG records are on the right, and EMG on the left where the upper lines were recorded from quadriceps muscle, lower lines from semimembranosus muscle.

Calibration for EEG: 5 sec, 200 μV

Calibration for EMG: interval between stimulating artifacts is 10 ms.

If the strength of cord dorsum stimulation was increased further, fibrillation of muscles in the lower back and hind limbs became evident. In response to every shock applied to the spinal cord, evoked muscle action potentials of 5–7 ms latency could be recorded from the corresponding muscles. The animal lay on the ground without any voluntary movement except deep respiration. When the cord stimulation stopped, the animal resumed its squatting posture instantaneously.

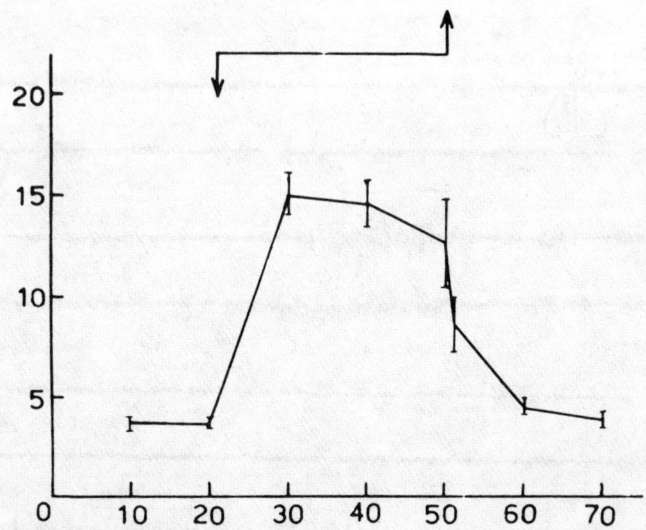

Fig. 5 Curve showing the change in response time of head jerk to radiant heat applied to the snout during hypotonia elicited by strong cord dorsum stimulation at L_2 in rabbits.
Abscissa: time in minutes before, during and after stimulation
ordinate: response time in sec.
no. of animals = 10, small vertical bar = standard error.

IV. DISCUSSION

One of the thorny problems in using the rabbit as an experimental animal in sleep research is the spontaneous recurrence of EEG synchronization, especially when the animal is kept in quiet and undisturbed surroundings. Furthermore, it is not easy to differentiate in the rabbit by behavioral signs between the state of relaxed wakefulness and that of drowsiness or light sleep, since these states are all manifested by quiescent squatting on the ground with eyes half open. We have even observed that the head of the rabbit was still kept in an upright position during the state of REM sleep. In view of the disadvantages mentioned above, the following criteria were employed to evaluate the efficacy of cord dorsum stimulation: (1) Before stimulation the animal was in an active waking state with constant orientating reflexes and grooming activities. After stimulation for a few minutes it squats on the ground and shifts to a tranquil state with eyes half open. (2) The EEG before stimulation contains only randomly dispersed slow wave or spindles, and after stimulation EEG synchronization develops within 3 minutes. (3) The synchronized tranquilizing effect should be induced in most trials by stimulus of optiamal parameters.

It should be pointed out here that cord dorsum stimulation did not always result in EEG synchronization. The possible factors responsible for this variability might be multiple, both intrinsic and extrinsic. Among the intrinsic factors involved, the excitatory state of the animal seemed to be of prime importance. It was not easy to induce the synchronizing effect when the animal was in a highly excited state such as moving around restlessly or sniffing everything encountered or grooming itself endlessly. Among the extrinsic factors high intensity noise and strong somatosensory stimuli including pinching the tail or pinna or brushing hair in inverted direction may be mentioned. These observations on animals may probably explain the reason for the absence of clinical report that patients who received dorsal column stimulation as a therapeutic measure to relieve their intractable pain had any experience of entering into a somnolent state during stimulation.

Abundant evidences in neurophysiological research indicate that EEG synchronization and related behavior changes could be induced by direct stimulation of various regions of the central nervous system. One of the common features of these central stimulations is that the stimulus frequency must be low, viz., 8/sec. Another outstanding feature is that weak stimuli result in synchronizing effect and strong stimuli, desynchronizing effect. It is therefore reasonable to assume that strong stimulation might have activated the thin fibers in the ascending sensory tract of the spinal cord which is known to be concerned with transmission of pain messages. It is probable that the ascending influence arising from the low threshold tract fibers may be related to the synchronized sleep center at higher levels of the central nervous system and those from the high threshold fibers to the desynchronized arousal center. It was suggested by Hodes that both cortically directed synchronizing and desynchronizing influences coexist in the cord. His hypothesis was based on the fact that injection of novocaine to one side of the spinal cord at C_1 level could induce bilateral electrocortical synchronization and desynchronization[7,8]. Pompeiano *et al.* reported that EEG synchronization could be elicited in cats when low threshold group II cutaneous fibers were activated by low rate stimulation; and EEG desynchronization and behavioral arousal could be elicited when high threshold group III cutaneous fibers were activated[9,10]. Electrophysiological evidence further indicated that group II cutaneous afferent fibers project mainly to the nuclei of bulbar and caudal part of pontile reticular formation including the gigantocellular nucleus, the function of which is to antagonize the activity of reticular activating system, while group III cutaneous afferent fibers project chiefly to the nuclei of pontile and mesencephalic reticular formation, which is part of the reticular activating system[11]. It is possible that groups II and III fibers entering the spinal cord may be functionally related to the tract fibers of low and high threshold respectively, through which the activities of synchronizing and desynchronizing centers are modulated. The action of cord dorsum stimulation is to activate the tract fibers artificially.

It has been verified recently in our laboratory under acute experimental conditions that intense stimulation of cord dorsum in cat does activate directly the dorsolateral funiculi and dorsal funiculi, and through the descending inhibitory influence of these fibers the afferent inflow was checked at the spinal level. From the above results it seemed reasonable to conclude that the EEG and EMG changes evoked by cord dorsum stimulation are essentially results of direct activation of the ascending and descending fiber tracts in the white matter of the spinal cord.

V. ABSTRACT

Cord dorsum stimulation was given through electrodes implanted in the dorsal lamina of the 2nd lumbar vertebra of 25 waking, unrestrained rabbits to mimic electro-acupuncture of Dumai points on the back of the body. It was found that cord dorsum stimulation at low intensity (0.4–0.8mA) for several minutes resulted in EEG synchronization accompanied by signs of tranquility and other behavior changes. In most cases EEG synchronization outlasted the cord dorsum stimulation for various lengths of time. The synchronizing effect could be easily produced no matter which part of the spinal cord was stimulated. These synchronizing effects were most readily observed when the animals were in a state of relaxed wakefulness. When the animal was in a state of agitation either spontaneous or induced by strong sensory stimulation, the synchronizing effect could not be obtained. The cauda equina was stimulated in 5 animals through the electrodes implanted on the dorsum of S_1 vertebral lamina. The EEG synchronization and tranquility could also be produced by stimulation of the region over the cauda equina at lower intensity. EEG desynchronization, hypotonia and absence of defensive responses to nocuous stimuli became manifest as the stimulating current of cord dorsum stimulation was increased to 2 mA or more. The possible mechanisms of EEG and behavior effects of cord dorsum stimulation were discussed.

REFERENCES

[1] Acupuncture Anesthesia Group, International Peace Maternity and Child Welfare Hospital, *et al.*: *Chinese Med. J.*, new series 4:481, 1978.

[2] Chiang Chen-Yü *et al.*: *Scientia Sinica*, **18**:651, 1975.

[3] Hess, W.R.: *Brain Mechanisms and Consciousness*, p.117, Springfield, 111. Thomas, 1954.

[4] Hess, Jr. R. *et al.*: *Electroencephal. clin. Neurophysiol.*, **5**:75, 1953.

[5] Magnes, J. *et al.*: *Arch. Ital. Biol.*, 99:33, 1961.

[6] Favale, E. *et al.*: *Arch. Ital. Biol.*, 99:1, 1961.

[7] Hodes, R.: *Electroencephal. Clin. Neurophysiol.*, **15**:651, 1963.

[8] Hodes, R.: *Arch. Ital. Biol.*, **102**:183, 1964.

[9] Giaquinto, S. *et al.*: *Arch. Ital. Biol.*, **101**, 131, 1963.

[10] Pompeiano, O. *et al.*: *Arch. Ital. Biol.*, **100**:343, 1962.

[11] Pompeiano, O. *et al.*: *Arch. Ital. Biol.*, **101**:552, 1963.

THE ROLE OF THE BULBAR RETICULAR FORMATION IN INHIBITION OF VISCERAL PAIN BY ACUPUNCTURE

Huang Zhongsun, Jin Shuran, Zhou Baohe,
Fei Ruwei, Zhang Neng, Fan Weizheng,
Sun Anping, Wang Dili
(Department of Physiology, Chongqing Medical College)

Abundant experimental evidences in recent years indicate that the analgesic effect of acupuncture is essentially the result of interaction between pain impulses and the afferent impulses from the acupuncture point at different levels of the central nervous system.

A few years ago, we reported that reflex discharges in splanchnic nerves and the inhibitory effect of acupuncture were remarkably diminished or abolished when a lesion was made in the upper part of the medulla oblongata[1]. It suggests that this part of the central nervous system plays an important role in the inhibitory influence of acupuncture on the visceral pain.

The present investigation was designed to study the electrophysiological characteristics of the neuronal activities in response to visceral painful stimuli in bulbar medial reticular formation, their peripheral afferent pathways, the bulbar projecting area of visceral painful stimuli and the inhibitory effect of acupuncture.

I. METHODS

The experiments were performed on 97 cats and 66 rabbits. The animals were anesthetized with a single dose of a mixture of 1% Chloralose and 20% Urethane at the beginning of surgical preparation and then immobilized with Flaxedil and ventilated artificially during observation.

Two kinds of noxious visceral stimuli were used:

(1) Stimulating the central cut end of the greater splanchnic nerve with single rectangular pulses (intensity 6–20 V, wave width 0.1 ms) or a brief train of rectangular pulses (6–20 V, 0.1 ms, duration of the train 100 ms, frequency 100 C/S).

(2) Pulling the body of the stomach with a force of 500 gm. for 5 seconds.

Tungsten microelectrodes (tip diameter 1–3μ, direct current resistance 10–25 MΩ) were used to record the unit activities from Nucleus Reticularis Gigantocellularis (RGC). The microelectrode was usually inserted at the points 3–4 mm. anterior to the obex, 1–1.5 mm. lateral to the midline. The depth of penetration was about 3–5 mm. beneath the surface of the medulla. In some animals, insulated stainless steel electrodes with bare tips (20–80μ) were used to record the evoked potentials from the medulla.

The potentials from the RGC were recorded in the store system of 14A-21 electromyograph and displayed simultaneously on an oscilloscope for monitoring purposes.

The arterial blood pressure was sometimes monitored, and was used as one of the indices of painful reaction.

Zusanli, Renzhong, Shangjizhong (T_8-T_9 interspinous space) points were selected as main points for electro-acupuncture.

At the end of some experiments, the location of the tips of the recording electrodes was identified by histological methods.

The details of the experimental procedures were described in preceding papers[2,3,4].

II. RESULTS

(I) RGC response to visceral painful stimulation

About 500 units in RGC area were observed, which responded differently to visceral stimuli. In 30% of the units (the frequency of the spontaneous discharges ranging from 10 to 20 impulse/sec.) an excitatory response was produced by stomach traction.

The excitatory effect, i.e., the increase of frequency of unit discharges, not only existed throughout the period of the stomach traction, but also lasted for several seconds after the stimulation had stopped (Fig. 1A). 12% of the cells of RGC showed an inhibitory effect. The rest of the cells were not affected by visceral stimulation.

Fig. 1B shows the excitating effect of electrical stimulation of the splanchnic nerve on an RGC neuron. The response to this kind of stimulation usually had a short latency and was much shorter in duration than that evoked by stomach traction.

The waveform of the evoked potentials recorded from the medulla in response to splanchnic nerve stimulation was biphasic (positive-negative). The evoked potential had a latency of about 10–30 ms and an amplitude of 200–400μV.

Both the single unit responses and the evoked potentials mentioned above could be reduced markedly by intravenous injection of morphine (3–5 mg/Kg. body wt.) in 30 out of 36 animals. The inhibitory effect of morphine appeared a few minutes after the intravenous injection, reached the maximum level usually after 20–30 minutes, then the effect declined gradually and disappeared in about 1 hr. (Fig. 2).

Besides, many RGC neurons could also be activated by somatic painful stimulation, such as forceful pinching of the skin of the hind limb, which was unbearable when applied to human subjects (Fig. 3).

(II) Analysis of the peripheral afferent pathways and the projection areas in the medulla of the visceral pain

It was found that the response of RGC neurons evoked by visceral painful stimuli was not significantly changed ($t=0.74$, $P>0.05$) after the bilateral vagi were cut just below the diaphragm or in the neck, but when the greater splanchnic nerves were blocked bilaterally with 1% procaine the response was significantly reduced ($t=2.55$, $P<0.05$).

In other experiments, when the parietal peritoneum was blocked with procaine, the

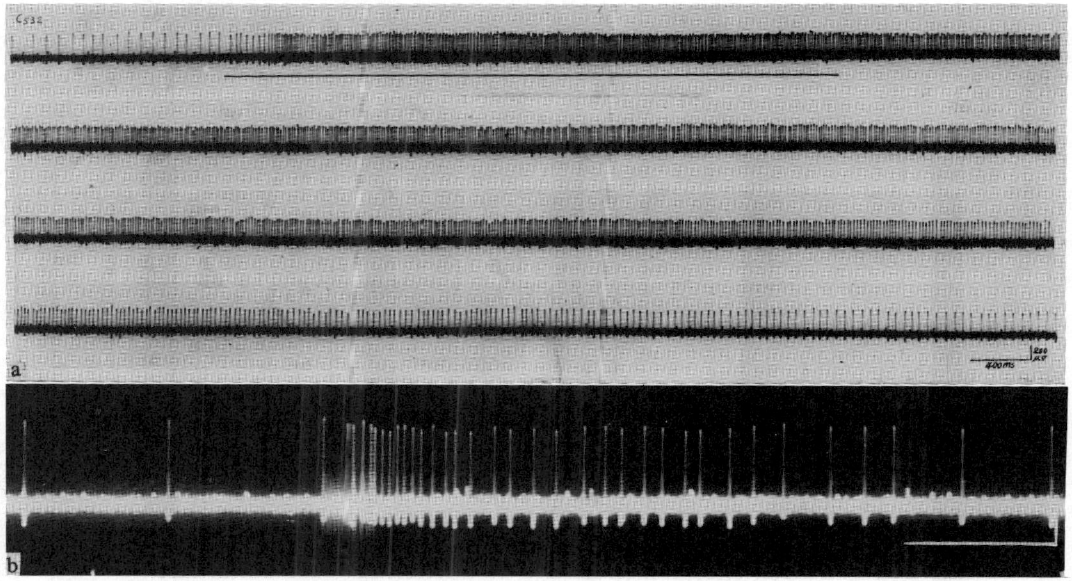

Fig. 1 The responses of an RGC neuron to two kinds of visceral stimuli.

A. The response to stomach traction, —indicating the period of stomach traction.

B. The response to electrical stimulation of the central cut end of splanchnic nerve (intensity 10 V, wave width 0.1 ms, train duration 100 ms, frequency 100 cps.)

Calibration: 200 μV 400 ms.

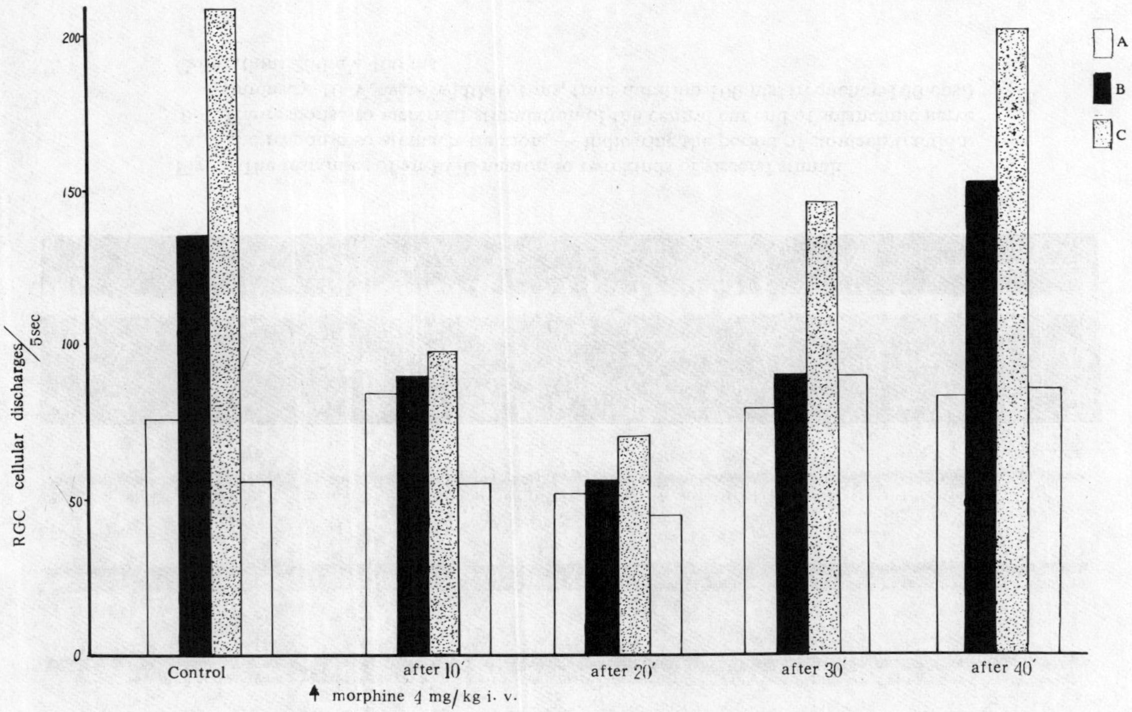

Fig. 2 The inhibitory effect of morphine on the responses of an RGC neuron to visceral and cutaneous stimuli.

A. Spontaneous discharges
B. Response to stimulation of greater splanchnic nerve
C. Response to forceful pinching of the skin.

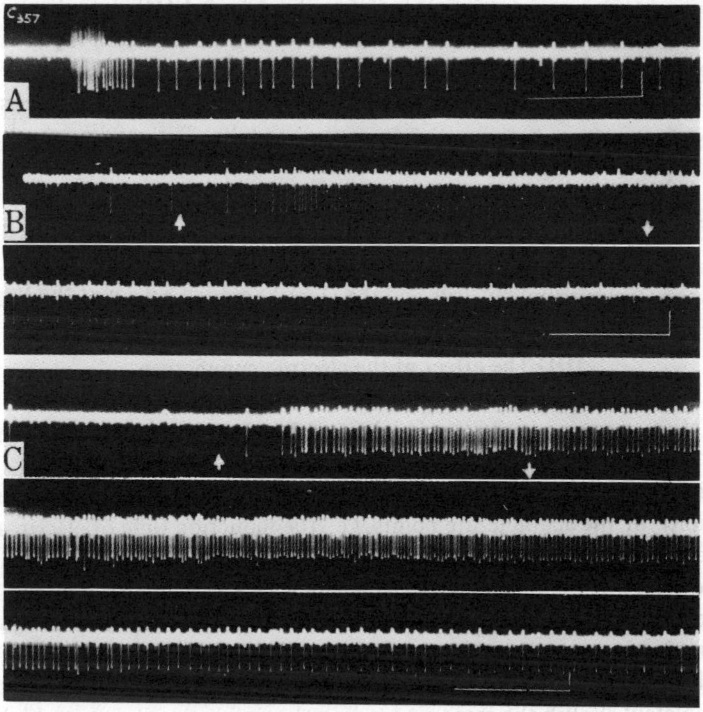

Fig. 3 The convergence of sensory impulses from various sources on an RGC neuron.
A. Response to stimulation of greater splanchnic nerve.
B. Response to traction of the stomach (↑ ↓).
C. Response to forceful pinching of the skin of the hind limb (↑ ↓).

Table 1. Discharges from 126 cells of different medullary areas elicited by visceral stimulation

Inductory area in bulbar medulla	No. of experiments	Stimulation of greater splanchnic n.							Traction of stomach						
		Total cells	Discharge increased		Discharge decreased		Discharge unchanged		Total cells	Discharge increased		Discharge decreased		Discharge unchanged	
			No. of cell	%	No. of cell	%	No. of cell	%		No. of cell	%	No. of cell	%	No. of cell	%
RGC	30	76	54	71.1	9	11.8	13	17.1	69	48	69.6	8	11.6	13	18.1
NC	14	47	3	6.4	13	27.6	31	66.0	50	31	62.0	7	14.0	12	24.0

RGC: Nucleus Reticularis Gigantocellularis NV: Nucleus of Vagus sensory area visceral pain reaction (as manifested by the abdominal EMG activities) was further decreased. So it seems that the somatic nerves innervating the parietal peritoneum were also involved in the mediation of visceral pain.

The next question was to find out to which part of the medulla the visceral pains projected. Totally 126 units were recorded from the medulla. The results are summarized in Table 1.

It was evident from Table 1 that the splanchnic nerve mainly projected to the RGC region while the afferent impulses evoked by stomach traction were transmitted both to the RGC region and the Nucleus of Vagus sensory area (NV), including the nucleus of the Solitary tract, the Commissural Nucleus and the Dorsal Sensory Nuclei of the Vagus.

(III) The effect of the electro-acupuncture

The excitatory response in RGC was inhibited by electro-acupuncture at Shangjizhong, Renzhong, or Zusanli points in 24 out of 30 animals.

To obtain a good analgesic effect of electro-acupuncture, two things must be noted besides the choice of the acupuncture points, i.e., the induction time of electro-acupuncture should not be shorter than 15–20 minutes and the stimulus intensity should be kept at 10–20 V. The effective frequency of electro-acupuncture varied with the pain indices used to study the effect. For example, the inhibitory effect on the medullary evoked potentials emerged when the frequency was 3–5 cps, but to inhibit the unit discharges of neurons, stimuli of high frequency (50–100 cps) were more effective. In general, electro-acupuncture could not completely abolish the response to visceral painful stimuli, but could decrease it to a certain extent (Fig. 4).

The aftereffect of electro-acupuncture generally lasted from only a few seconds to a few minutes, and only in a few cases was it longer than ten minutes.

It is interesting to note that electro-acupuncture itself often elicited evoked potentials as well as unit responses in the same region of the medulla or in the same neuron as the visceral stimuli did. This is shown in Fig. 5.

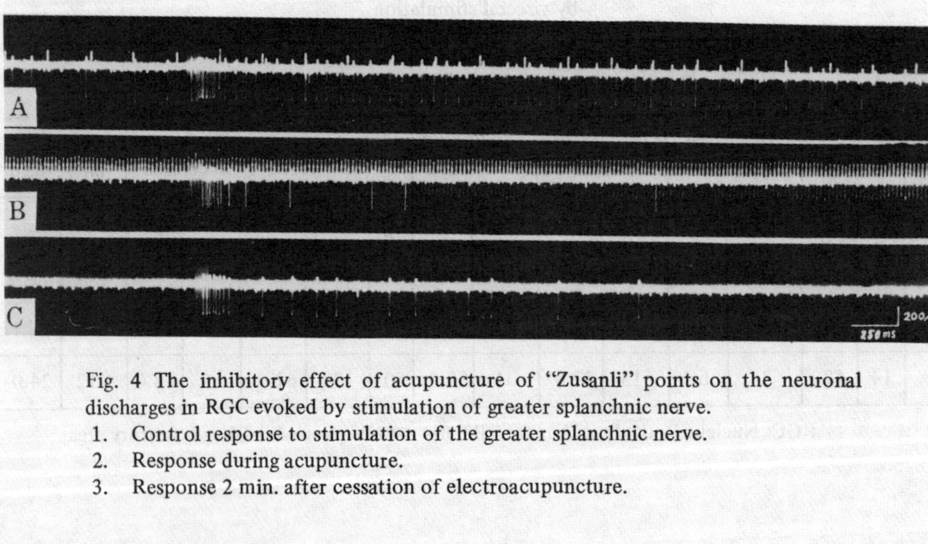

Fig. 4 The inhibitory effect of acupuncture of "Zusanli" points on the neuronal discharges in RGC evoked by stimulation of greater splanchnic nerve.

1. Control response to stimulation of the greater splanchnic nerve.
2. Response during acupuncture.
3. Response 2 min. after cessation of electroacupuncture.

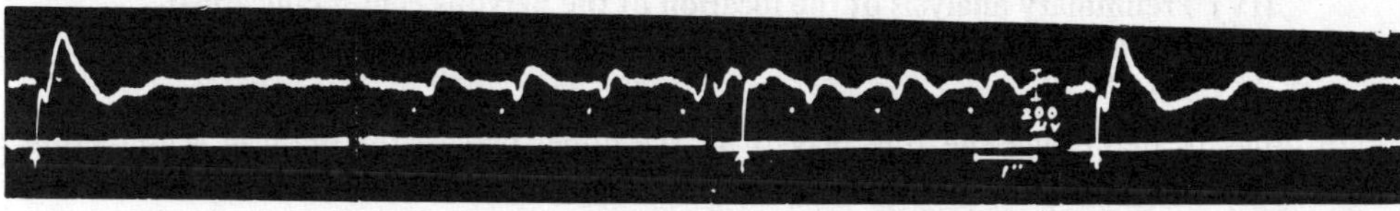

Fig. 5 The inhibitory effect of acupuncture on the evoked potential in RGC, showing the afferents from visceral organs and those from acupuncture points projected to the same region of bulbar reticular formation.

1. Evoked potential in RGC elicited by stimulation of splanchnic nerve.
2. Electro-acupuncture on "Zusanli" points only.
3. 1 repeated during acupuncture.
4. 1 repeated after acupuncture.

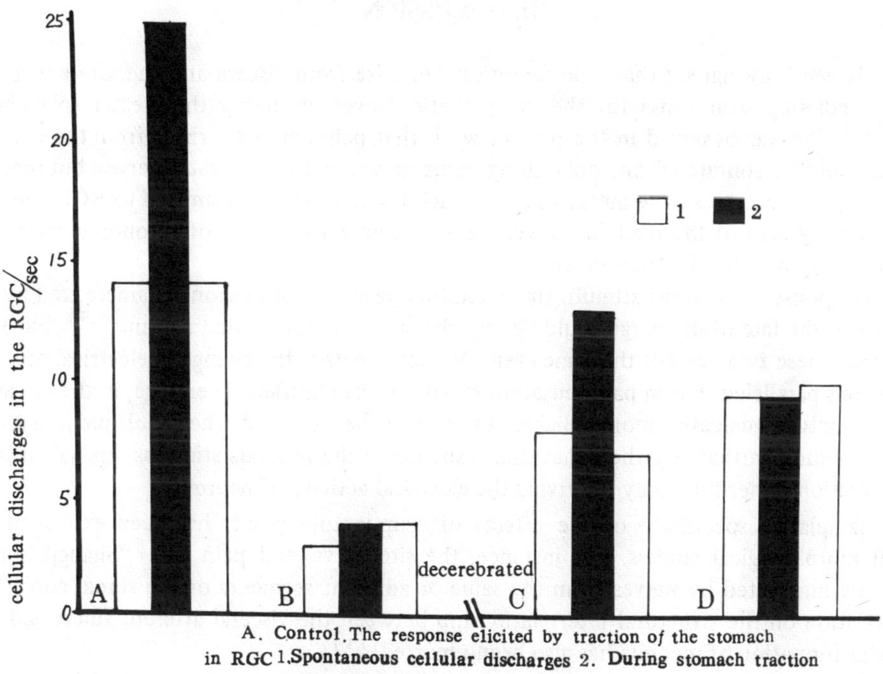

Fig. 6 The unit response of an RGC neuron elicited by stomach traction and its inhibition by acupuncture before and after decerebration.

1. Spontaneous discharges.
2. During stomach traction.
   A. Control response of an RGC neuron elicited by traction of the stomach.
   B. A repeated during acupuncture.
   C. D. A and B repeated after decerebration.

(IV) Preliminary analysis of the location of the nervous center concerned with the inhibitory effect of acupuncture on visceral pain

In order to determine the role played by the upper part of the brain in acupuncture analgesia, we transected the brain at various levels in 16 animals. When a transection was made at the upper margin of midbrain, the visceral painful responses and the inhibitory effect of acupuncture decreased, but the pattern of response was still maintained (Fig. 6).

It was not likely that the responses described above would be the result of fluctuations of blood pressure, because when the same pattern of pressor or depressor responses was evoked by traction of the stomach, different responses of RGC neurons could be elicited, viz., some of the neurons were excited, some were depressed, and others were not affected. Besides, the changes in blood pressure began much later than the unit responses of the neurons[5].

III. DISCUSSION

It is generally agreed that pain sensation can arise from viscera and the afferent nerve fibers mediating pain run with the sympathetic nerves, primarily the greater splanchnic nerve[6,7]. It was observed in the present work that pain impulses arising from the visceral organs could be conducted not only along vagus nerves and the somatic nerves, but mainly along splanchnic nerves. The messages of stomach traction were transmitted to RGC and the vagus sensory area of the medulla as well, and consequently a series of autonomic reactions accompanied by painful sensation were elicited.

In response to noxious stimuli, the excitatory response of neurons characterized by an increase of the rate of discharge could be regarded as a reaction related to pain[8,9], but it is clear that these two are not the same event. In fact, whether the change in electrical activity in neurons paralleled that in pain sensation remains to be clarified. Therefore, in the research of acupuncture analgesia, more reliable results may be obtained when multiple indices of pain, including particularly the behavioral response to the noxious stimulus, are taken into consideration rather than only observing the electrical activity of neurons.

The relative specificity of the effects of acupuncture points has been explained by recent morphological studies. For instance, the site of visceral pain and "Shangjizhong" point are innervated by nerves from the same or adjacent segments of the spinal cord. The investigation on the structural interrelationship between the visceral afferent fibers and the reticular formation of medulla has also been reported[11].

The results of our experiments indicated that the pain responses evoked by visceral stimuli were complicated and the inhibition produced by acupuncture was usually incomplete. These are consistent with the fact that the analgesic effect is not always satisfactory during gastrectomy under acupuncture anaesthesia.

Although the results of decerebrated animals indicated that a higher center in the brain was necessary for acupuncture analgesia, the reticular formation of medulla is actually also a place of convergence of impulses coming from the visceral organs and acupuncture points. It is well known that RGC is one of the major nuclei in bulbar reticular formation and most sensory ascending fibers send collaterals to this nucleus while passing by. Neurons in RGC can be activated by inputs originating from different regions of the body[12]. A large part of the afferent fibers carrying acupuncture signals ascend via the ventrolateral fasciculus of the spinal cord and reach the bulbar reticular formation including RGC. The signals carried by them may interact with the afferent activities elicited by the visceral nocuous stimuli at these levels. It seems from the results of the present investigation that the afferent activities from the points of acupuncture and from the visceral organs were often transmitted to the same area, even to the same cells in bulbar reticular formation. The inhibitory effect on the response evoked by visceral afferent may well be the results of interactions between these two kinds of afferent impulses. On the other hand, the impulses generated in RGC may be transmitted downward to the spinal cord and act on the pain-related cells in the dorsal horn to help to prevent further transmission of the pain messages from the primary station[13], and also they may go upward through the region of central tegmental fasciculus to Nucleus centrum medianum of thalamus, which constitutes a very important part of the central nervous system in controlling and modulating pain[9,14]. Therefore, the convergence and modulation of different sensory inputs in the bulbar reticular formation might play an important role in the mechanism of acupuncture analgesia[13,15].

IV. CONCLUSIONS

1. Experiments were performed on unanesthetized but immobilized cats and rabbits. The electrical stimulation of the central cut end of the splanchnic nerve and stomach traction were used as visceral nocuous stimuli, and the increase in the frequency of unit discharges in RGC was regarded as visceral painful responses. The peripheral afferent pathways of the visceral pain signals and their projection in the medulla were analyzed.

2. Electro-acupuncture at "Renzhong", "Shangjizhong" and "Zusanli" points could inhibit the visceral pain responses, but the effect was incomplete.

3. In decerebrated animals, the visceral pain responses in RGC and the analgesic effect of acupuncture were both reduced.

In conclusion, the bulbar reticular formation, in which the convergence and modulation of the impulses coming from the visceral organs and the acupuncture points take place, may play an important role in acupuncture analgesia.

REFERENCES

[1] 重庆医学院生理教研室针麻原理研究组：新医药学杂志，12：29，1975。

[2] 重庆医学院生理教研室针麻原理研究组：全国针刺麻醉研究资料选编，上海人民出版社，288 页，1975。

[3] 重庆医学院生理教研室针麻原理研究组：针刺麻醉(合订本)，81，1976。

[4] 重庆医学院生理教研室针麻原理研究组：新医药学杂志，5：43，1978。

[5] 黄仲荪等：科学通报，24：1140，1979。

[6] 杜焕基等：新医药学杂志，4：25，1975。

[7] Cannon B: *J. Physiol*, **105**:366, 1933.

[8] Casey KL: *Science*, **173**:77, 1971.

[9] 张香桐：中国科学，1：28，1973。

[10] Casey K K *et al*: *Advances in Neurology*, **4**:197, 1974.

[11] 中医研究院针灸经络研究所：针刺麻醉，3—4：25，1978。

[12] Amassian V B *et al.*: *J. Neurophysiol*, **6**:575, 1954.

[13] 沈 锷等：中华医学杂志，54：628，1974。

[14] Bowsher D *et al.*: *J. Neurophysiol*, **31**:288, 1968.

[15] 沈克飞等：科学通报，21：507，1976。

RESEARCH ON MECHANISM OF ACUPUNCTURE ANTI-VISCERALGIA

I. AN EXPERIMENTAL OBSERVATION ON INTEGRATION IN MEDULLA OBLONGATA

The lst Department of Physiology, Institute of Acupuncture and Moxibustion, Academy of Traditional Chinese Medicine

I. INTRODUCTION

As shown by a large amount of clinical practice, needling points over the body surface can relieve visceralgia. During surgical operations, acupuncture anesthesia brings about a certain effect in relieving the viscero-traction reaction (including visceralgia). According to ancient Chinese medical classics, acupuncture cures diseases by harmonizing the Yin with the Yang, invigorating the flow of "Chi" (vital energy) in Jing Luo, regulating the "Chi" and "Blood", and boosting positive factors and eliminating negative ones. The Jing Luo involves a part of structure and function of the nervous system, and is closely related to the brain. From the anatomical and physiological points of view, the nerve projections originating from the body surface and viscera to the central nervous system (CNS) always have some overlaps. It is the central nervous system which plays an important role in the connection of body surface and viscera, and it may be a main modulator in the regulating process of acupuncture analgesia. In order to study the possible afferent pathway of viscero-traction reaction (including visceralgia) and the integration of the afferent impulses of acupuncture stimulation and visceral traction at the medullary level, we have observed the changes in electro-activities of the neurons induced by stomach traction and the effect of acupuncture on them in the nucleus of the solitary tract and medial medullary reticular formation of the rat.

With the aim to determine the correlation between the changes in electro-activities of the neurons and pain, and its relation to acupuncture analgesia, a chronic microelectrode method was employed to study the interaction between the afferent impulses of acupuncture and viscera in the reticular gigantocellular nucleus (RGC), a relay station, to which splanchnic nerves and needling points are projected[1,2,3]. At the same time, the abdominal muscular discharge and behavioral responses of the animal were also observed.

II. MATERIAL AND METHODS

(I) Acute experiments

After anesthesia with urethane (1.2 gm/kg), male rats, weighing about 400 g, were placed in a stereotaxic apparatus to keep the 4th ventricle floor in a level position. Occipital craniotomy was performed, and the exposed obex was treated as the zero point. The recording sites of the solitary tract nucleus were 0.4–0.5 mm anterior to the obex, 0.4–0.5 mm lateral to the midline, and 0.3–0.8 mm in depth from the dorsal medullary surface. The recording sites of medial medullary reticular formation were 0.5–1.0 mm anterior to the obex, 0.5–1.0 mm lateral to the midline, and 1.7–2.5 mm in depth from the dorsal medullary surface.

Extracellular unit recordings were made with glass microelectrodes (tip diameter 1–2 μ, DC resistance 5–15 MΩ). The neuronal discharge was amplified and taped down. The data were analyzed by a medical computer or photographed in succession.

Viscero-traction stimulation was elaborately designed. The stomach body was fastened with a plastic cord which was drawn out from inferior abdomen. The mechanical traction was applied to the stomach by pulling out the cord 1.5–2.0 cm for ten seconds. There was a 5 minute interval between two successive tractions.

The Bei-Hang 57–6 model electro-acupuncture (EA) apparatus was used for stimulation, which had the following parameters: continuous biphasic electric pulses, frequency 100 c/s, intensity 2 mA. Points Zusanli on both sides or Renzhong — Juliao were stimulated with electro-acupuncture for ten minutes. The charges in the unit discharges induced by the stomach traction were recorded immediately and at 5, 10, 15, 20, and 30 minutes after cessation of acupuncture.

(II) Preparation of animal

Adult cats of both sex weighing 2 to 3 kg were selected on the basis of apparent good health and reasonable disposition. They were anesthetized with sodium pentobarbital (40 mg/kg i.p.). Then the cats were operated on under aseptic conditions. The left splanchnic nerve was separated behind the peritoneum and cut. Its central end was placed on a pair of platinum electrodes for stimulation and the electrodes were put in a small box made of plexiglass. Then wax (melting point 39.5°C) was poured into the box for insulation. The leading wire of the electrode was drawn out from the back of the animal for stimulation. A pair of recording electrodes of stainless steel were embedded in the abdominal muscle. The animal's head was fixed on a stereotaxic apparatus which was inclined 21° forward.

A craniotomy was made 6–7 mm anterior to the occipital protuberance and 1.0–1.5 mm lateral to the midline. The base of the microelectrode manipulator was fixed horizontally on the skull. On the 4th or 5th day after the operation, the first experiment was made. The cat was put into a shielded box 80×80×80 cm in dimensions. The animal was kept in a waking condition and was able to move freely in the box.

(III) Stimulation

Visceralgia was mimicked by electric stimulation applied to the splanchnic nerve. Trains of square waves (100–200 ms) were provided by a DISA stimulator (pulse duration 1 ms, frequency 100 c/s).

The intensity enough to induce the animal's behavioural responses, such as shrinking, avoidance and vocalization etc., might be used as the visceralgia stimulation. The intensity of the stimulation ranged from 10 to 20 volts.

Points Pishu of both sides were stimulated with electro-acupuncture for ten minutes. Continuous biphase electric pulses were provided by the electro-acupuncture apparatus at a frequency of 100 c/s, and the adequate intensity was selected for each animal.

The responses of the animal caused by visceralgia stimulation were determined immediately and at 5, 10, 15, 20 and 30 minutes after cessation of acupuncture.

Records:

The extracellular unit recordings were made with glass microelectrodes. The recording sites, which were in the rostrum of the gigantocellular nucleus, were 16.5–18.5 mm beneath the cerebellar surface.

The method of collection and analysis of the experimental data was similar to that mentioned above.

After the experiments, the recording site of the electrode was identified by the Prussian blue method.

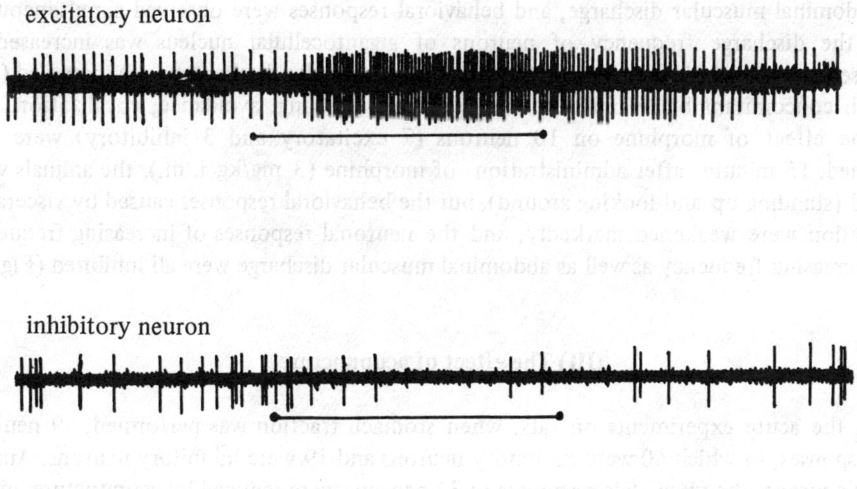

Fig. 1 Effect of stomach traction on neuronal discharge. The bar shows duration of stomach traction.

III. RESULTS

(I) Effects of stomach traction or electric stimulation of the splanchnic nerve on single unit activity in medulla oblongata

In the acute experiments of rats, we analyzed 59 neurons having responses to the stomach traction. Among these, 19 neurons were located in the solitary tract nucleus, and the others were in the medial medullary reticular formation. When the stomach was pulled, some neurons did not respond but the others showed changes in discharge manifested mainly in two patterns, viz., increase or decrease in discharge. We call those cells showing increase in discharge excitatory neurons and those showing decrease in discharge inhibitory neurons (Fig. 1).

In the chronic experiments on cats, the responses of 107 neurons of the reticular gigantocellular nucleus caused by the electrical stimulation of the splanchnic nerve were observed. The patterns of response were similar to those in the acute experiments. Among the 107 neurons, there were 58 neurons (54%) which gave the response of increasing frequency. 16 neurons (15%) showed the response of decreasing frequency. There were no significant changes in the remaining 33 neurons (31%).

(II) The relationship between the changes of neuronal discharge and pain

In the chronic experiments, the electro-activities of the reticular gigantocellular nucleus, the abdominal muscular discharge, and behavioral responses were observed simultaneously. When the discharge frequency of neurons of gigantocellular nucleus was increased or decreased by splanchnic stimulation, the abdominal muscular discharges were increased (Fig. 2) with concomitant behavioral responses such as shrinking, avoidance, vocalization, etc.

The effect of morphine on 10 neurons (7 excitatory and 3 inhibitory) were also examined. 15 minutes after administration of morphine (3 mg/kg i. m.), the animals were excited (standing up and looking around), but the behavioral responses caused by visceralgia stimulation were weakened markedly, and the neuronal responses of increasing frequency and decreasing frequency as well as abdominal muscular discharge were all inhibited (Figs. 3, 4).

(III) The effect of acupuncture

In the acute experiments on rats, when stomach traction was performed, 59 neurons had responses, in which 40 were excitatory neurons and 19 were inhibitory neurons. Among the 59 neurons, the visceralgia responses of 32 neurons were reduced by acupuncture, giving an effective rate of 54%.

The effect of acupuncture on the excitatory neurons was indicated by a suppressing effect on the increasing frequency response caused by the stomach traction, and the effective rate was 60%. The effect of acupuncture on the inhibitory neurons was indicated by the releasing effect on the decreasing frequency response caused by the stomach traction, and the effective rate was 42.1%.

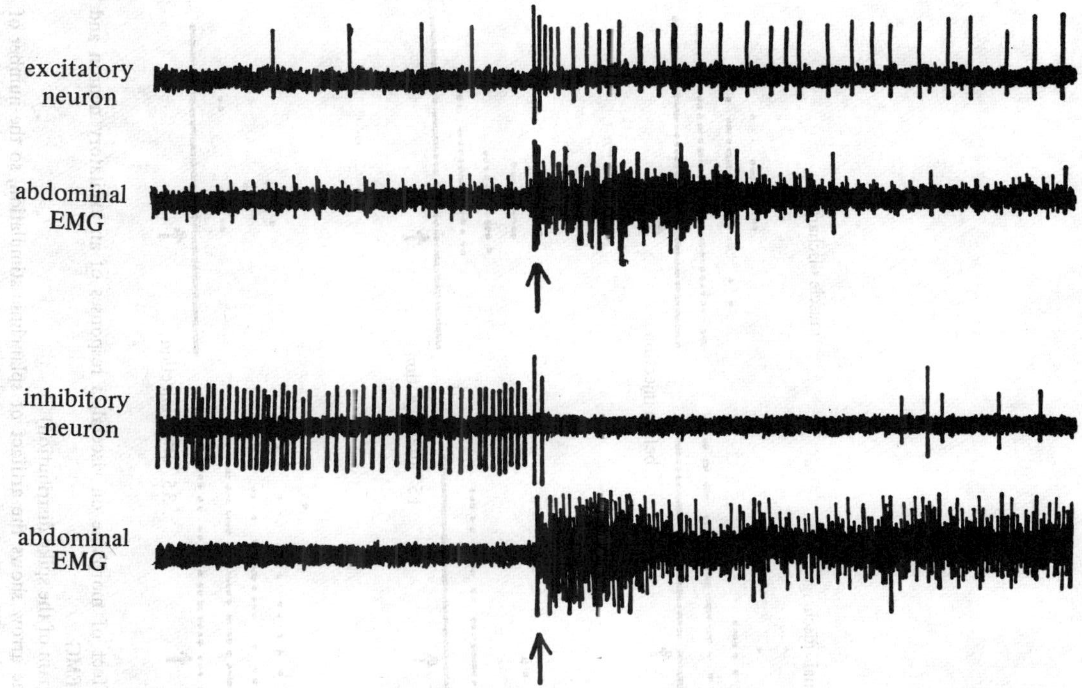

Fig. 2 The changes of RGC unit activity and muscular discharge caused by visceral noxious stimulation (The arrow shows splanchnic stimulation).

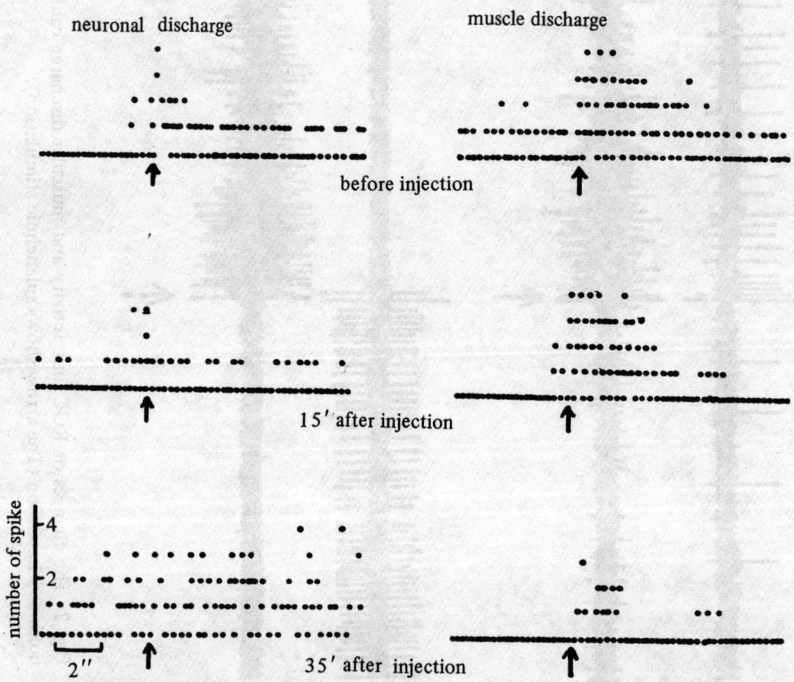

Fig. 3 Effect of morphine on visceralgia responses of an excitatory neuron and abdominal EMG
(The histogram of the spike distribution)
Note: The arrow shows the artifact of splanchnic stimulation, so the number of spike at this time includes the count of stimulus artifact.

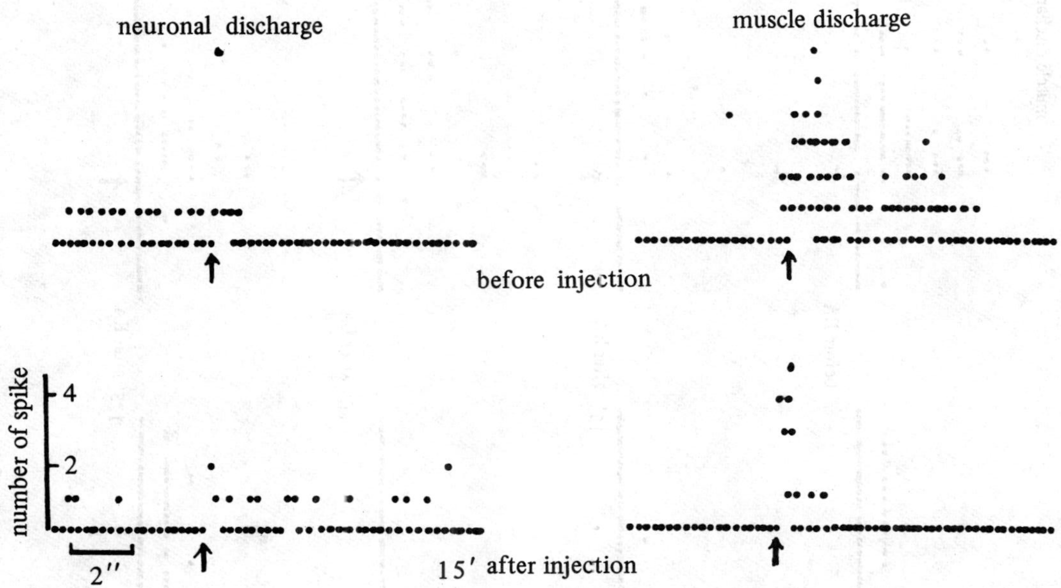

Fig. 4 Effect of morphine on visceralgia responses of an inhibitory neuron and abdominal EMG.
Note: The same as above.

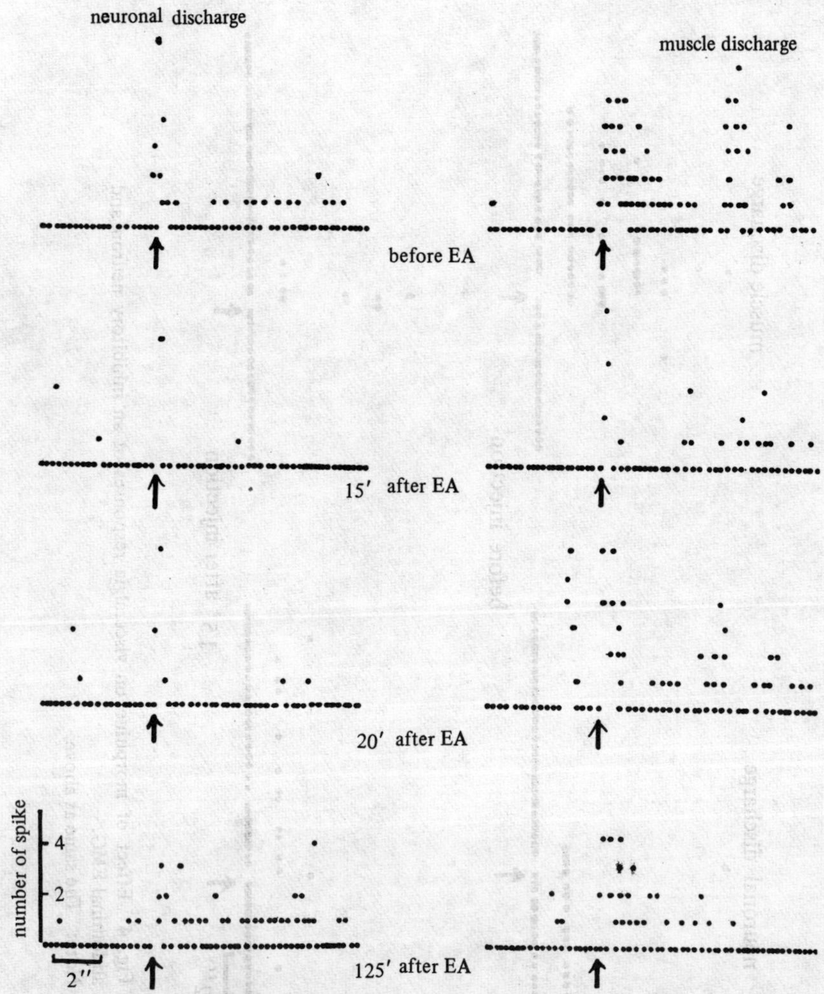

Fig. 5 Effect of EA on the visceralgia responses of an excitatory neuron and abdominal EMG.
Note: The same as above.

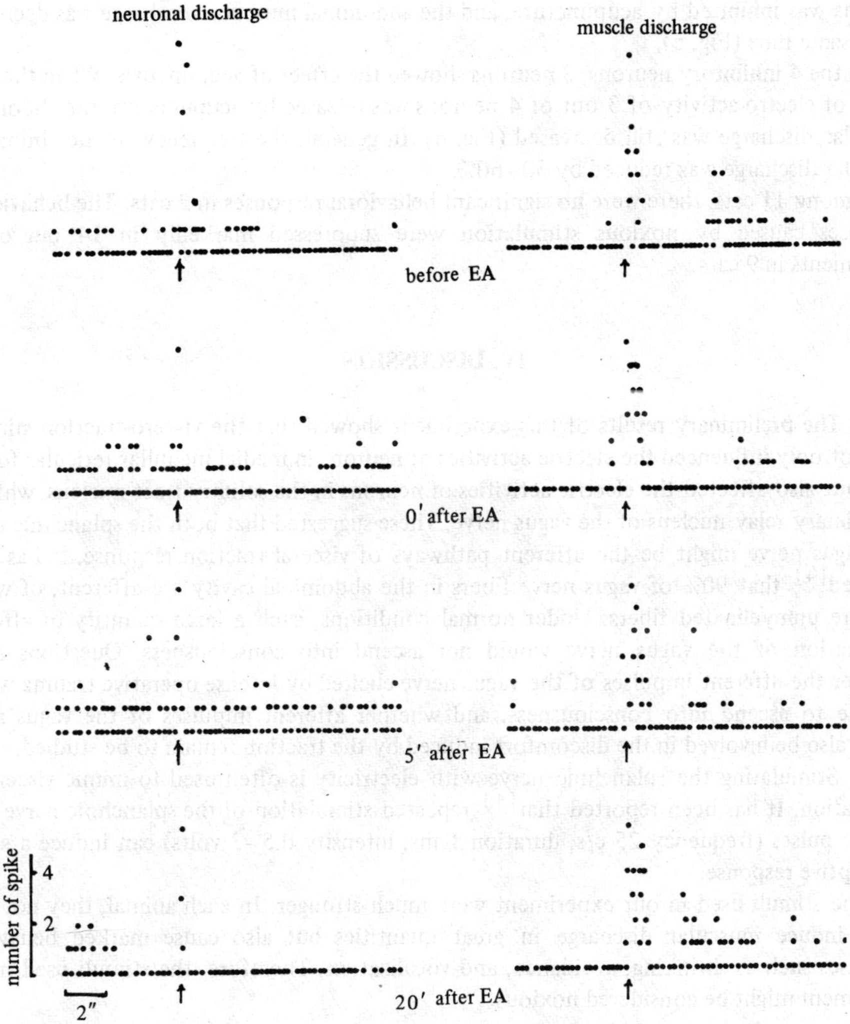

Fig. 6 Effect of EA on the visceralgia responses of inhibitory neuron and abdominal EMG.
Note: The same as above.

In the chronic experiments, the effect of acupuncture on 24 neurons (excitatory neurons 20, inhibitory neurons 4) was observed. The electro-activities of 12 out of the 24 neurons were influenced not only by the acupuncture but also by the visceralgia, which means that visceralgia and acupuncture can change the spontaneous discharge of the neurons separately. Both signals converged on the same neuron. In this neuron these two kinds of signals were interacting between each other. The result of this interaction was suppression of the responses caused by visceralgia. It means that the activities of the central nervous system might be effectively regulated by the electro-acupuncture. In the 20 excitatory neurons, 15 neurons showed the regulating effect of the acupuncture. The electro-activity of 9 out of 15 neurons was inhibited by acupuncture, and the abdominal muscular discharge was decreased at the same time (Fig. 5).

In the 4 inhibitory neurons, 3 neurons showed the effect of acupuncture. When the inhibition of electro-activity of 3 out of 4 neurons was released by acupuncture, the abdominal muscular discharge was still decreased (Fig. 6). In general, the frequency of the abdominal muscular discharge was reduced by 30–60%.

Among 11 cats, there were no significant behavioral responses in 2 cats. The behavioural responses caused by noxious stimulation were suppressed markedly in 14 out of 25 experiments in 9 cats.

IV. DISCUSSION

1. The preliminary results of this experiment showed that the viscero-traction stimulation not only influenced the electric activities of neurons in medial medullar reticular formation, but also affected the electric activities of neurons in the solitary tract nucleus, which is the primary relay nucleus of the vagus nerve. These suggested that both the splanchnic nerve and vagus nerve might be the afferent pathways of visceral traction response. It has been reported[4] that 90% of vagus nerve fibers in the abdominal cavity are afferent, of which 99% are unmyelinated fibers. Under normal conditions, such a large quantity of afferent information of the vagus nerve would not ascend into consciousness. Questions as to whether the afferent impulses of the vagus nerve elicited by intense operative trauma would be able to ascend into consciousness, and whether afferent impulses of the vagus nerve would also be involved in the discomfort induced by the traction remain to be studied.

2. Stimulating the splanchnic nerve with electricity is often used to mimic visceralgic stimulation. It has been reported that[5] repeated stimulation of the splanchnic nerve with electric pulses (frequency 25 c/s, duration 1 ms, intensity 0.5–3 volts) can induce a stable nociceptive response.

The stimuli used in our experiment were much stronger. In each animal, they not only could induce muscular discharge in great quantities but also cause marked behavioral responses such as shrinking, avoidance, and vocalization. Therefore, the stimuli used in the experiment might be considered noxious.

It has been reported[6] that the neurons of the gigantocellular nucleus show two different responses to noxious stimulation; one of them is the increasing frequency response and the other, decreasing. In our experiment the neurons of the gigantocellular nucleus showed the same twotypes of responses. When we stimulated the splanchnic nerve with intense electricity, in many cases these responses might last for 10 to 20 seconds, and without adaptability. In view of the fact that morphine has an effect on both of these responses, it could be assumed that the responses of the neurons are related to pain. The relationship between excitatory and inhibitory neurons should be studied further.

3. Gigantocellular nucleus of medulla oblongata is the convergent region of multiple sensations[7]. It is not merely related to nociperception[8,9,10], but is also involved in the regulation of analgesia. During the last few years, investigations showed that gigantocellular nucleus plays a certain role in acupuncture analgesia[11,12]. In our experiment, we have observed that both the visceralgia signal and acupuncture signal might arrive at this nucleus group and converge on the same neuron. Owing to the interaction between the two kinds of signals, in many cases, the response of neurons induced by a noxious stimulation would exhibit inhibitory properties. We suppose that the integration at the level of gigantocellular nucleus in medulla oblongata may be one form of action of acupuncture anti-visceralgia.

Takagi *et al.*[13] found that the nucleus reticularis gigantocellularis of the medulla oblongata of the rat is a highly sensitive area in the production of morphine analgesia. Other studies of electro-physiology have suggested that the nucleus reticularis gigantocellularis may descend to inhibit the neuronal activity of transmitting pain signals at the dorsal horn in the spinal cord[14,15], and ascend to inhibit the discharge of the pain-sensitive cells of the central lateral nucleus of the thalamus[16].

We also observed that stimulating the gigantocellular nucleus by electricity might have certain inhibitory effects on the visceralgia response. It is inferred that the gigantocellular nucleus might also mediate other actions of acupuncture analgesia besides the integrative action. Accordingly, we should pay more attention to the role of gigantocellular nucleus in acupuncture analgesia.

V. SUMMARY

1. When the stomach of the experimental animal was in traction or when electro-stimulation was applied to the splanchnic nerve, part of the neurons in medulla oblongata did not respond, but the others showed changes in discharge manifesting two main patterns, viz., the response of increasing frequency and that of decreasing frequency.

2. In waking cats, when the discharge frequency of neurons of gigantocellular nucleus was increased or decreased by splanchnic stimulation, the abdominal muscular discharge was all increased, with concomitant shrinking and/or avoidance, and/or vocalization of the animal.

3. All the above responses were inhibited in different degrees by electro-acupuncture.

4. The integration in the gigantocellular nucleus might be considered as one form of action of acupuncture antivisceralgia.

REFERENCES

[1] 上海生理研究所二室针麻组：«针刺麻醉临床和原理研究资料选编»上海人民出版社，155，1977。

[2] 重庆医学院生理教研室针麻原理研究组：针刺麻醉，81，1976。
[3] 刘 磊：针刺麻醉，105，1976。
[4] Abella, G.G. and Pease, H. L.: *Brain Res.,* **58**:465, 1973.
[5] 上海生理研究所针刺麻醉研究组：针刺麻醉理论研究资料选编，上海人民出版社，119，1973。
[6] Hector J. Leblanc & Glenn B. Gralipon: *Exp. Neurol.,* **42**:264, 1974.
[7] Casey, K. L. *et al.*: *Exp. Neurol.,* **25**:35, 1969.
[8] Casey, K. L. *et al.*: *Science,* **73**:77, 1971.
[9] Casey, K. L. & Keene, J. J.: *Advance in Neurology,* **4**:197, 1974.
[10] Guilbaud, G., Bessen, J. M. *et al.*: *Brain,* **63**:131, 1973.
[11] 张香桐：中国科学，4：465，1978。
[12] 上海生理研究所针刺麻醉研究组：针刺麻醉理论研究资料选编，上海人民出版社，154，1973。
[13] Takagi, H. *et al.*: *European J. Pharmacol.,* **45**:91, 1971.
[14] Takagi, H., Doi, T. and Kawasaki, K.: *Life Sci.,* **17**:67, 1975.
[15] Haber, L. H., Martin, R. F. *et al.*: *Brain Res.,* **153**:163, 1978.
[16] 沈克飞等：科学通报 21：507，1976。

RESEARCII ON MECHANISM OF ACUPUNCTURE ANTI-VISCERALGIA

II. EFFECT OF MORPHINE ANTAGONIST ON ELECTROACUPUNCTURE ANTI-VISCERALGIA

The lst Department of Physiology, Institute of Acupuncture and Moxibustion, Academy of Traditional Chinese Medicine

In our previous work, we have observed that the neuronal discharges of the bulb and the electromyograph of the abdominal muscle in response to traction of the visceral organs and electrical stimulation applied to the splanchnic nerve were found to be depressed by clectro acupuncture[1]. We supposed that acupuncture analgesia may be achieved through activating and strengthening the intrinsic pain and anti-pain regulating system. The discovery of opiate receptors in the brain[2] suggested the existence of an endogenous substance (or intrinsic ligand), for certainly they were not'designed' for narcotic drugs.

Since it was found that stimulating the periaqueductal gray (an established high morphinc cffcct area) could produce analgesia[3,4], similarities between morphine analgesia and stimulation-produced analgesia (SPA) have further been observed, such as both can activate the raphe magnus nucleus (NRM)[5] through dorsal lateral tract (DLT)[6] down to dorsal horn to block the transmission of nociceptive input[7,8], both have tolerance and show cross-tolerance to each other[9], and both analgesic effects can be antagonized by naloxone[10]. All these suggest that both SPA and morphine analgesia might activate the same intrinsic analgesic system.

In the course of finding out the intrinsic ligand for opiate receptor and exploring the intrinsic analgesic system, researchers have identified the endogenous morphine-like factors (MLF)[11]. Soon later a number of scientists reported that the distribution of MLF was quite similar to that of opiate receptor itself[12], that MLF showed its analgesic effect through stereospecific binding with opiate receptor[13], and that its analgesic effect could also be blocked by naloxone[14,15]. So it is supposed that the endogenous morphine-like factors may be included in the analgesic system and take part in analgesic effect.

If this is true, how does acupuncture work? Does the acupuncture also activate the analgesic system and elevate MLF level?

The aim of our experiment is to investigate the action of MLF in acupuncture anti-visceralgia in rats.

I. MATERIALS AND METHODS

Male rats weighing 350–450 gms were used. The left splanchnic nerve was separated post-peritoneally from the surrounding tissue and was ligated under ether and urethane (0.5gm/kg i.p.) anesthesia. A bipolar platinum electrode was implanted in the central end of the splanchnic nerve and several pieces of cotton soaked in paraffin were used for protecting the nerve. After the operation the rat woke up and crawled into a special holding, and then it was restrained.

The noxious splanchnic nerve stimulation which was a train made up of 10 pulses with 10 ms intervals (pulse duration 1 ms, unloading intensity 15–25V) was used as visceralgia stimulation. The abdominal EMG and ECG were recorded with concentric electrode and needle electrode respectively. The visceralgia stimulation could induce the abdominal muscle discharge and acceleration of heart rate. The muscle discharge was amplified by a preamplifier, transformed into direct current by a frequency integrater, and then written down in the X-Y recorder. The magnitude of the induced abdominal muscle discharge was expressed by the area of the integration curve of EMG (cm^2/min). The larger the area, the more the muscle discharge (Fig.1). The ECG was taped down and was fed to a medical computer to

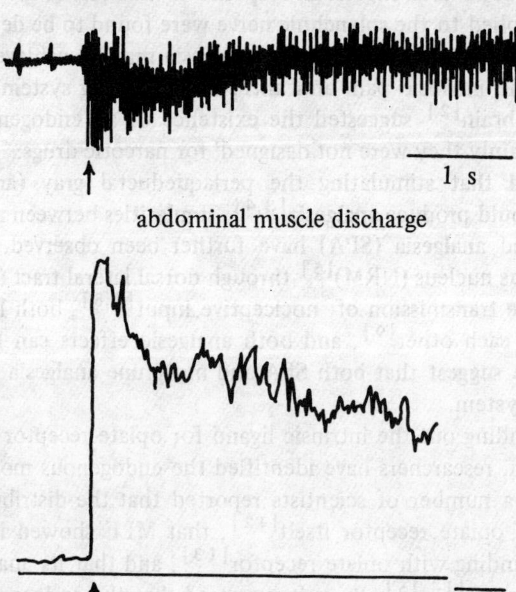

Fig. 1 Abdominal musele discharge induced by visceralgia stimulation.

make the R-R interval histogram (256 address, address time was 10 ms, vertical volume was 320 ms/ full scale). The higher the dot, the longer the R-R interval, and the slower the heart rate. The quantity of acceleration of heart rate was indicated by the difference between R-R intervals before and after splanchnic stimulation (Fig.2).

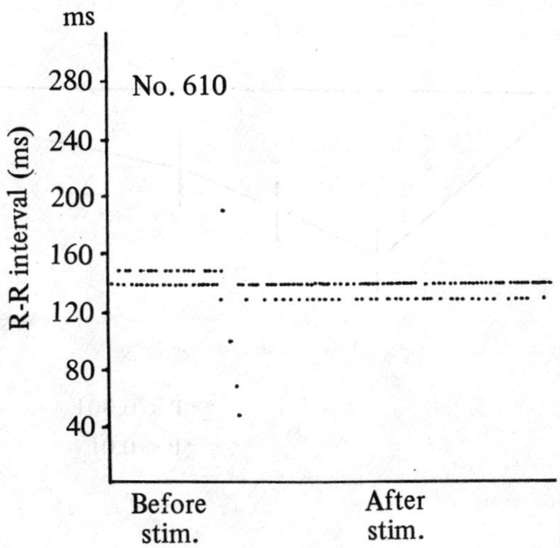

Fig. 2 R-R interval shortened by visceralgia stimulation (cardiac acceleration).

After these visceralgia responses had been repeatably stabilized, points "Xin Xue II" were stimulated bilaterally with type 57–6 acupuncture apparatus (spike wave, frequency 100 c/s and unloaded intensity 20V) for ten minutes.

Before acupuncture and immediately, 5, 10 and 20 minutes after cessation of acupuncture, the visceralgia responses were measured and the percentage of inhibition by electro-acupuncture (EA) was calculated.

The rats were divided into two groups: the control group and the experimental group. In the control group, saline was injected at the beginning of electro-acupuncture while in the experimental group, narcotic antagonist was injected, and the electro-acupuncture effects in both groups were observed comparatively. If comparative observation was made on the same rat, the interval between the two sessions of electro-acupuncture would be more than one and a half hours.

The drugs were made up with saline.

II. RESULTS

(I) Inhibition of visceralgia responses by electro-acupuncture

The abdominal muscle discharge induced by visceralgia stimulation was inhibited by electro-acupuncture. The percentage of inhibition in 15 rats at 0, 5, 10 and 20 minutes after cessation of electro-acupuncture was 37.0%, 25.5%, 17.2% and 9.1% respectively. The inhibitory effect of electro-acupuncture at 0 and 5 minutes was statistically significant ($p < 0.001$ and $p < 0.01$) (Fig.3).

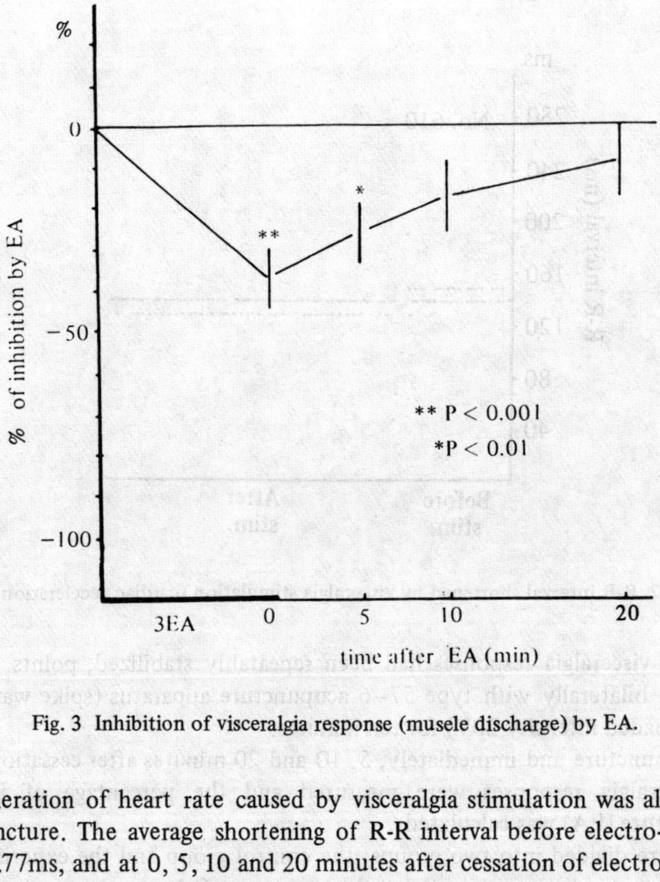

Fig. 3 Inhibition of visceralgia response (musele discharge) by EA.

The acceleration of heart rate caused by visceralgia stimulation was also inhibited by electro-acupuncture. The average shortening of R-R interval before electro-acupuncture in 18 rats was 5.77ms, and at 0, 5, 10 and 20 minutes after cessation of electro-acupuncture it was decreased to 2.10, 3.17, 4.47 and 5.29ms respectively. The inhibitory effect of electro-acupuncture at 0 and 5 minutes was also statistically significant ($P<0.001$, $P<0.01$) (Fig. 4).

So it is evident that visceralgia responses indicated by induced abdominal muscle discharge and cardiac acceleration were significantly inhibited by electro-acupuncture.

(II) The effect of morphine antagonist on electro-acupuncture anti-visceralgia

In our experiments, when the visceralgia response indicated by induced muscle discharge was nearly completely depressed by administration of morphine (5 mg/kg i.p.), naloxone in the dose 1 mg/Kg was injected peritoneally, then the visceralgia response was recovered even beyond the base line about 20 minutes later. It means that the inhibitory effect of morphine was reversed by naloxone. But how does the same dose of naloxone affect the acupuncture anti-visceralgia effect?

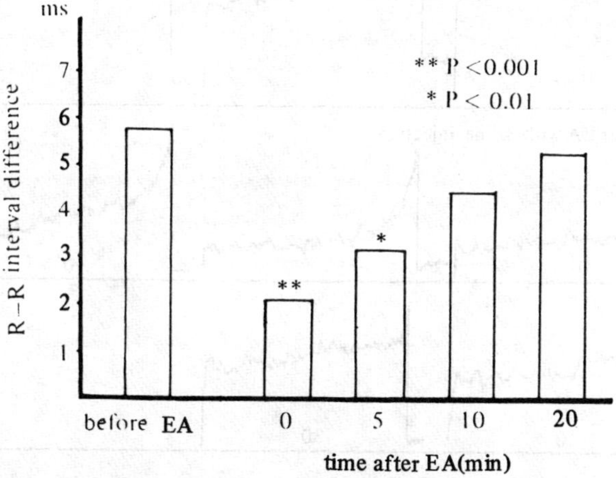

Fig. 4 Attenuation of visceralgia response by EA (cardiac acceleration).

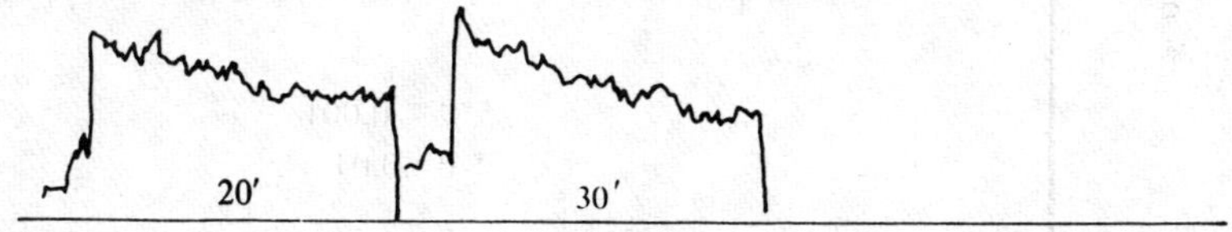

Fig. 5 Inhibition of visceralgia response by EA (musele discharge).

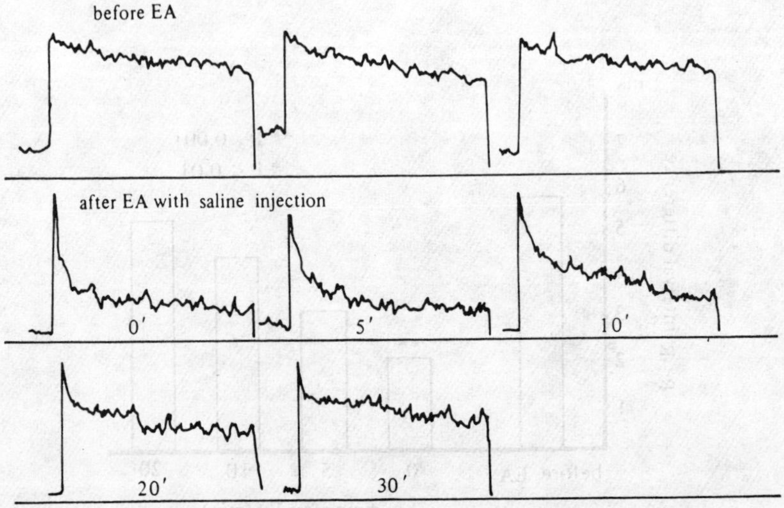

Fig. 6 Effect of acupuncture anti-visceralgia blocked by naloxone.

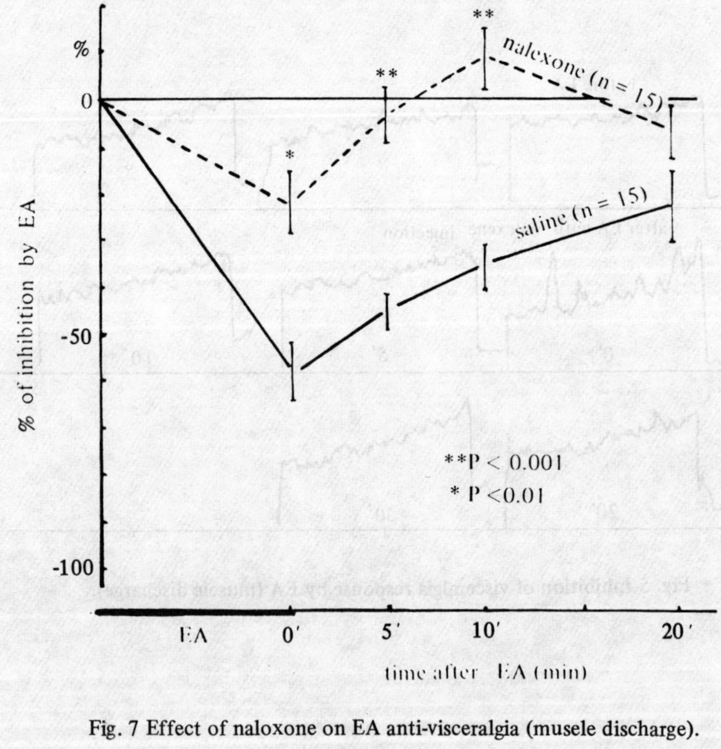

Fig. 7 Effect of naloxone on EA anti-visceralgia (musele discharge).

From Figs.5 and 6, we observed that the inhibitory effect of electro-acupuncture was blocked by naloxone in this case.

In the control group of 15 rats, at 0, 5 and 10 minutes after cessation of electroacupuncture the induced abdominal muscle discharge was reduced by 57.9%, 45.0% and 34.8% of the pre-acupuncture control value (as 100%), respectively, while in the naloxone group (n=15) it was reduced by 22.7%, 3.2% and +9.7% after electro-acupuncture, which means the visceralgia response was increased rather than decreased at 10 minutes, the percentage of facilitation being 9.7%.

This indicates that the acupuncture anti-visceralgia effect was partially blocked by naloxone. Immediately after cessation of acupuncture the percentage of blockage was 60.9% (P <0.01) and was nearly completely blocked 5 and 10 minutes after acupuncture its percentage of blockage being 92.4% and 100% (P<0.001), respectively. So it is evident that the acupuncture inhibitory effect is significantly but not completely blocked by naloxone (Fig. 7 and Table 1).

At the same time, the acupuncture inhibitory effect indicated by attenuation of cardiac acceleration was also blocked by naloxone. In the control group (n=9) before acupuncture the average shortening of R-R interval induced by visceralgia stimulation was 6.08 ms, and

Table 1. Effect of naloxone on EA anti-visceralgia (induced muscle discharge)

Time after EA (min.)	% of inhibition: Saline (S)	% of inhibition: Naloxone (N)	% of blockage*	t	P
0	57.9±5.77	22.7±6.73	60.79	3.689	<0.01
5	45.0±3.59	3.2±6.30	92.89	6.602	<0.001
10	34.8±5.55	0(+9.7)** ±8.20	100.00	5.055	<0.001

*% of blockage= $\frac{S-N}{S}\times 100\%$, ** % of facilitation.

Table 2. Effect of naloxone on EA anti-visceralgia (cardiac acceleration)

Time after EA (min.)	Decreased value of R-R interval difference (ms): Saline (S)	Decreased value of R-R interval difference (ms): Naloxone (N)	% of blockage*	t	P
0	4.75±0.50	1.88±1.19	60.42	4.948	<0.001
5	3.66±0.71	+1.54±1.32**	100.00	9.793	<0.001
10	4.23±0.81	+0.40±0.90**	100.00	9.666	<0.001
20	1.35±1.43	+0.82±1.28**	100.00	3.647	<0.01

* % of blockage = $\frac{S-N}{S}\times 100\%$, **increased values (ms)

at 0, 5, 10 and 20 minutes after cessation of acupuncture, it was decreased by 4.75, 3.66, 4.23 and 1.35ms, respectively. The percentage of inhibition was 78.1%, 60.4%, 69.5% and 22.7%, respectively. In the naloxone group (n=9), before acupuncture the average shortening of R-R interval induced by visceralgia was 4.02ms, and immediately after electro-acupuncture it was decreased by 1.88ms, the percentage of inhibition being 46.8%; but at 5, 10 and 20 minutes it was increased rather than decreased. It was increased by 1.54 ms, 0.40 ms and 0.82 ms, respectively. It shows that the acupuncture anti-visceralgia effect indicated by attenuation of cardiac acceleration is partially blocked by naloxone immediately after electro-acupuncture, the percentage of blockage being 60.4%, and is reversed at 5, 10 and 20 minutes after electro-acupuncture, the percentage of blockage being 100%. So the blocking effects of naloxone were significant (P<0.001) (Fig. 8 and Table 2).

In addition, the effect of another morphine antagonist, nalorphine, was also observed. Nalorphine exerts some inhibitory effect on visceralgia response (morphine-like effect) when the effect of acupuncture anti-visceralgia is not obvious (3 of 4 rats). If acupuncture exerts some inhibitory effect, then it would be partially blocked by administration of nalorphine at the beginning of needling, as shown in 3 of 4 rats (morphine antagonist effect). It shows that nalorphine has dual action on acupuncture anti-visceralgia, i.e., synergistic and antagonistic.

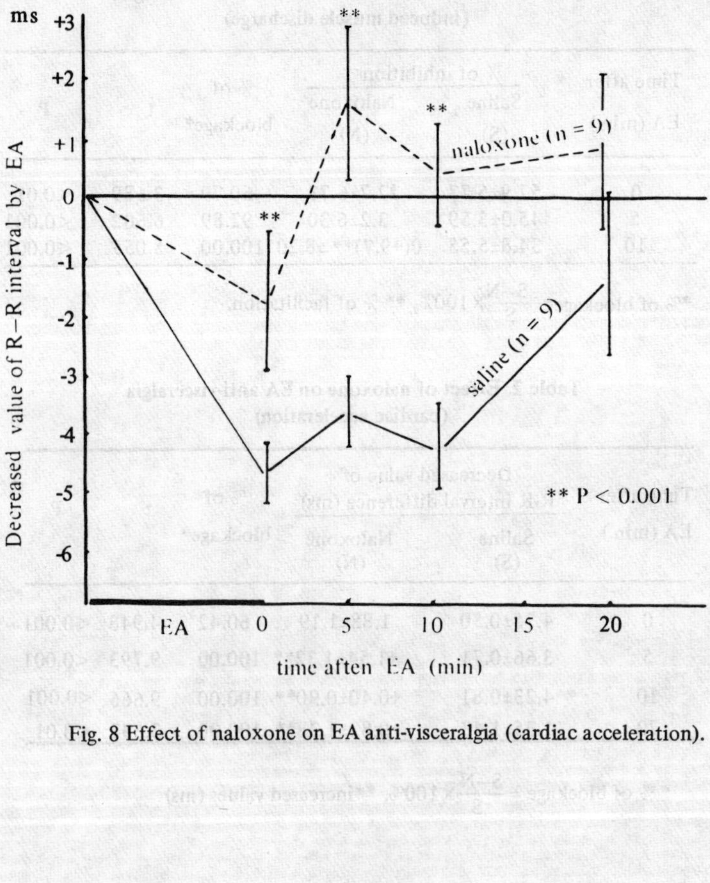

Fig. 8 Effect of naloxone on EA anti-visceralgia (cardiac acceleration).

III. DISCUSSION

1. From the above data it is inferred that the endogenous morphine-like substances may be involved in the intrinsic analgesic system and take part in acupuncture anti-visceralgia. It has been reported that the analgesic effect of acupuncture is partially blocked by administration of naloxone in man, cat, rabbit and mouse, and recently, in rat[16–23]. In the present study we also observed the same effect of naloxone on acupuncture anti-visceralgia in rats. Thus involvement of morphine-like substances might be considered as a common mechanism of acupuncture analgesia in various mammals to relieve somatic as well as visceral pain. The inconsistency of results obtained in rats may be due to difference in the models and indications. McClane[24] has taken notice of the difference in sensitivity of various indications used to examine the effect of morphine and morphine antagonist.

2. In view of the fact that acupuncture analgesia could be blocked by naloxone, we suppose that the mechanism of acupuncture analgesia may be similar to that of SPA and morphine analgesia. In that case, does acupuncture also indirectly activate the raphe magnus nucleus down to the spinal cord to prevent transmission of the nociceptive message? The preliminary result obtained in our experiments indicates that acupuncture may also activate the serotonergic system to produce the analgesic effect, because the acupuncture anti-visceralgia effect is depressed by a lesion of NRM. As for the relationship between the opiate system and the serotonergic system in acupuncture analgesia, it remains to be studied.

3. The same dose of naloxone as is enough to completely reverse the morphine inhibitory effect can only partially block the electro-acupuncture analgesic effect (especially immediately after cessation of acupuncture). It is assumed that the mechanism of acupuncture analgesia is more complicated than that of morphine. It might activate a non-opiate analgesic system directly besides the opiate analgesic system.

4. In our experiments, we could also see the facilitating action of naloxone in some cases (6 of 9 rats). About 20 minutes after administration of naloxone, the rat often showed restlessness and irregular respiration accompanied by an increase of the induced muscle discharge by nociceptive stimulation. This agrees with Bell & Martin's[25] report that naloxone may facilitate the C-fiber reflex, and Goldfarb's[26] report that naloxone may enhance the flexor reflex. They considered that it was due to the antagonization of natural occurring MLF by naloxone. From the viewpoint of the unity of opposites, we might speculate that when the operative trauma and the visceralgia stimulation induce the visceralgia responses, they may at the same time activate the analgesic system to elevate MLF to a tonic level, thus preventing the occurrence of excessive visceralgia responses, and naloxone blocks the action of MLF at tonic level to facilitate the visceralgia responses. But in some cases, naloxone had not any effect and even had a little inhibitory effect on visceralgia responses instead. Some factors of variation such as the tonic level of MLF, the amount of opiate receptors and the development of anti-pain ability, should be considered.

Buchsbaum[27] reported that in normal subjects the effect of naloxone on the pain threshold is varied. In some subjects the effect of naloxone on pain perception is varied. The pain-insensitive subjects found shocks significantly more painful after naloxone administration while the pain-sensitive subjects experienced them as less painful. These results suggest that individual difference in pain sensitivity may relate to differences in an endorphin system. It is inferred that the naloxone effect on pain response depends to a large extent on the levels of MLF. So one might consider that MLF also takes part in physiological regulation of pain and anti-pain. Acupuncture would strengthen the process of this regulation.

IV. SUMMARY

The studies were performed on the conscious but restrained rats. The splanchnic nociceptive stimulation was used as visceralgia stimulation, by which the abdominal muscle discharge and cardiac acceleration were induced. These visceralgia responses were significantly inhibited by needling "Xinxue II" points. The electro-acupuncture inhibitory effect on visceralgia responses was partially blocked (about 60%) by administration of naloxone (1mg/ Kg i.p.) immediately after termination of acupuncture and nearly completely at 5 and 10 minutes. This indicates the possible involvement of endogenous morphine-like substances in acupuncture anti-visceralgia. In addition, the possible physiological role of MLF in regulating pain and anti-pain was discussed.

REFERENCES

[1] The 1st Department of Physiology, Institute of Acupuncture and Moxibustion, Academy of Traditional Chinese Medicine.
[2] Pert, C. B. & Snyder, S. H. : *Science,* **179**:1011, 1973.
[3] Reynolds, D. V. : *Science,* **164**:444, 1969.
[4] Mayer, D. J.: *Science,* **174**:1351, 1971.
[5] Anderson, S. D. & Basbaum, A. I.: *Brain Res.,* **123**:363, 1977.
[6] Basbaum, A. I. *et al.*: *Pain,* **3**:43, 1977.
[7] Fields, H. L. & Basbaum, A. I.: *Brain Res.,* **126**:441, 1977.
[8] Fields, H. L. & Basbaum, A. I.: *Ann. Rev. Physiol.,* **40**:217, 1978.
[9] Mayer, D. J. & Hayes, R. L.: *Science,* **188**:941, 1975.
[10] Akil, H.: *Science,* **191**:961, 1976.
[11] Hughes, J. *et al.*: *Brain Res.,* **88**:295, 1975.
[12] Simantov, R. *et al.*: *Brain Res.,* **106**:189, 1976.
[13] Pert, A. *et al.*: *Brain Res.,* **136**:523, 1977.
[14] Hill, R.G *et al.*: *Nature,* **262**:604, 1976.
[15] Bradley, P. B. *et al.*: *Nature,* **261**:425, 1976.
[16] Mayer, D. J.: *Brain Res.,* **121**:368, 1977.
[17] Pomeranz, B.: *Life Science,* **19**:1757, 1976.
[18] Pomeranz, B.: *Exp. Neurol.,* **54**:172, 1977.
[19] 北医针麻组：中华外科杂志 15：192，1977。
[20] 上海市人体针刺镇痛协作组：医学情报交流 6：12，1977。
[21] Natt, J. G.: *Clin. Pharmacol. Ther.,* **15**:361, 1974.
[22] 岗 洁：日本生理学杂志 39：350，1977。
[23] 武重千冬：医学のあゆみ 105：595，1978。
[24] McClane, T. K. *et al.*: *Int. J. Pharmacol.,* **6**:29, 1967.
[25] Bell, J. A. & Martin, W. R.: *Europ. J. Pharmacol.,* **42**:147, 1977.
[26] Goldfarb, J. & Hu, L. W.: *Neuropharmacol.,* **15**:785, 1976.
[27] Buchsbaum, M. S. *et al.*: *Nature,* **270**:620, 1977.

RELATIONSHIP BETWEEN CEREBRAL CORTEX AND ACUPUNCTURE INHIBITION OF VISCERAL PAIN

Chen Peixi, Chen Zhuhua, Weng Jiwei,
Ren Huifang, Zhang Jinmei, Zhang Jinghang*,
Feng Jianqiang

(Research Laboratory of Acupuncture Anesthesia, Zhongshan Medical College)

The cerebral cortex is the highest portion of the central nervous system which is essential in sensory perception, especially in integration of sensation. Formation of visceral painful sensation and acupuncture sensation as well as their inter-action must take place here. So, in order to explore the mechanism of acupuncture anesthesia, it is necessary to study the relationship between the cerebral cortex and acupuncture inhibition of visceral pain. Recently a lot of clinical facts have demonstrated that the effect of acupuncture anesthesia depends mostly upon the physiological state of the subject. Some experimental data also showed that the cerebral cortex played a part in acupuncture anesthesia, while other data showed otherwise[1-4]. In view of such difference in opinion, this study is to observe the change in cortical evoked potential and unit discharge during stimulation of the splanchnic nerve initiating visceral pain, in order to explore the relationship between the cerebral cortex and visceral pain, and the acupuncture effect. This might contribute to the understanding of the mechanism of acupuncture anesthesia.

I. METHODS

Experiments were carried out on cats anesthetized with a single dose of chloralose and urethane at the beginning of surgical preparation, and then immobilized with Flaxedil and artificially ventilated. EEG and femoral arterial blood pressure were monitored throughout the experiment. Body temperature was maintained at 36.5–38.5°C. Recording of the responses was started 5hr after the initial anesthesia.

The splanchnic nerve was stimulated with electrical rectangular pulses of 0.1 msec in duration, and 20V in intensity every 1.3 sec. Stimulation parameters on "Neiguan" point or cortical "Neiguan" projecting area were 0.1–0.3msec, 4–6V, and 50 Hz.

The surface cortical evoked potentials were recorded with a silver ball electrode and averaged (n=100) through an addscope. Unit discharges were recorded in the contralateral

---

* Anhui Medical College.

cortical splanchnic projection area (post-sigmoid gyrus) with the glass microelectrode (resistance 5–20MΩ) which was connected to a microelectrode amplifier. The signals were amplified and the output from the amplifier was displayed on oscilloscopes. Extracellular spikes were counted by TQ-19 medical data processor, and the signals were also stored on a tape recorder for further analysis.

II. RESULTS

(I) Relationship Between Visceral Pain and Cortical Potential Evoked by Stimulating Splanchnic Nerve

In our 17 experiments, stimulating the proximal portion of the splanchnic nerve intensely (at such an intensity that could excite the C fiber) usually brought forth cortical evoked potential as well as elevation of blood pressure and vaso-constriction. The evoked potentials taken at 16 points of the contralateral cerebral cortical surface are shown in Fig. 1. The maximal evoked potential was at the middle part of post-sigmoid gyrus near crucial sulcus. Thus we called this part the splanchnic projecting area. These cortical evoked potentials consisted of two components, the early and the late components. The early component was of 10 to 14 msec latency and positive-negative-(positive) biphasic potential; the late component was of 150 to 350 msec latency and mono-or di-phasic (negative or positive) potential. When the intensity of stimulus was lower so that it could excite the A_β fiber only, the evoked potential grew faint or became a negative early response (component) and the late component disappeared. This showed that the late component was due to excitation of A_δ- and C-fiber. Since it was easily inhibited by intravenous injection of Demerol, the late component might be concerned in pain, or it might reflect abdominal visceral pain. Electroacupuncture on "Neiguan" point could inhibit this cortical splanchnic evoked potential, especially its late component.

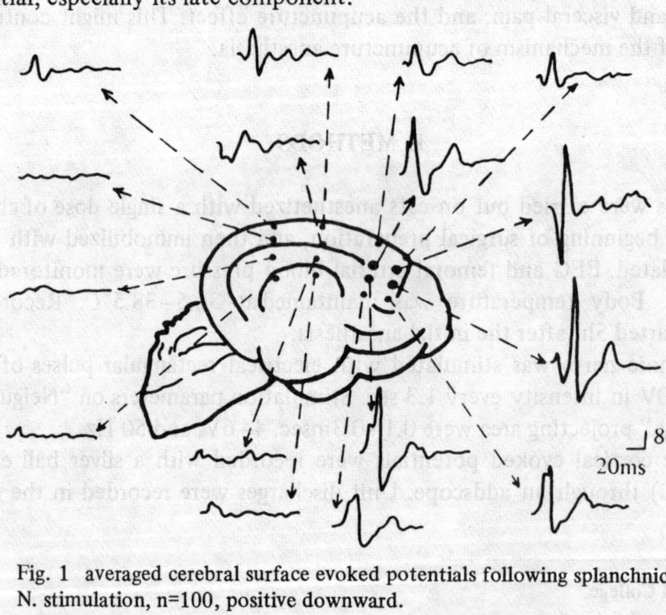

Fig. 1 averaged cerebral surface evoked potentials following splanchnic N. stimulation, n=100, positive downward.

(II) Relationship Between Visceral Pain and Cortical Unit Discharge by Stimulating Splanchnic Nerve and Effect of Electro-acupuncture

When a micro-electrode was inserted into the deep layer of the splanchnic projecting area, a number of spontaneous discharges were observed. Among 38 experimental trials when the proximal end of the splanchnic nerve was stimulated with a strong stimulus which could excite the C fiber, most of the spontaneous discharging units continued to give spikes, but the rate of discharge was unchanged; 86 units (we call excitatory units) showed an increase; 20 units (we call inhibitory units) showed a decrease; 3 units showed an increase at first and then a decrease; 2 units showed a decrease at first and an increase later. Fig. 2 showed the discharges of a cortical visceralgia excitatory unit. It showed that during stimulation of the splanchnic nerve, it took a long latent period for the discharge increase, then the discharging gradually increased and maintained a high level. After dismissing the stimulation the aftereffect lasted for a period before its gradual recovery. The middle part of Fig. 2 shows the change of discharging average frequency with an aftereffect of 120 sec.

Fig. 3 shows the discharges of a cortical visceralgia inhibitory unit. During stimulation of the splanchnic nerve, the unit discharges gradually decreased and then maintained a low level. After stopping the stimulus, recovery gradually took place.

According to the post-stimulus histogram, cortical unit discharges evoked by stimulating the splanchnic nerve might be classified into 2 classes (the early discharge and late discharge). The early discharges were of short latency (15 to 40 msec), 30 to 100 msec duration, and were coincident with the early component of the cortical evoked potential. The late discharges were of long latency (longer than 200 msec), long duration, and were coincident with the late component. There was a period of 100 to 200 msec between the early and late discharges, during which there was no (or lessened) discharge.

When the intensity of stimulus was weakened so that only the A_β fiber was activated, there was no effect on the unit discharge of the visceralgia excitatory unit. If the intensity was raised again to activate the A_δ fiber, its unit discharges increased once more (Fig. 4). This suggested that the increase in discharge was mostly due to excitation of both A_δ and C fibers. In addition, we also observed two units which received only A_β fiber afferent impulse have slightly increased discharge.

After intravenous injection of Demerol (5 to 10mg/Kg), 5 out of 6 animals showed inhibition of cortical unit discharge evoked by stimulating the splanchnic nerve (Fig. 5) with diminishing discharge, prolonged inhibitory period and lessening amplitude. Recovery took place gradually 30 min after injection. Thus it was suggested that the cortical splanchnic evoked discharge was also concerned in pain, and it might reflect upper abdominal visceral pain. Thus we call it cortical visceralgial discharge.

(III) Effect of Acupuncture on Cortical Visceralgial Discharges

Seven of our ten trials showed different degrees of acupuncture inhibition on cortical visceralgial discharges. Their discharges diminished, inhibitory period lengthened, latency prolonged, and recovery took place gradually after cessation of the acupuncture (Fig. 6). In

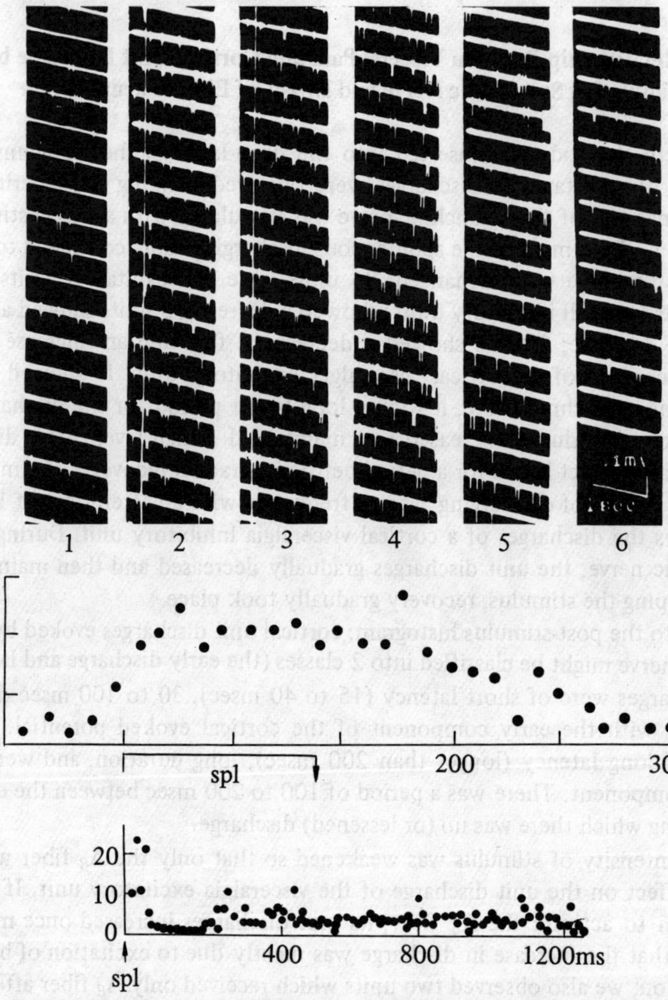

Fig. 2 Excitatory response of cortical neurons in postsigmoid gyrus to stimulation of splanchnic nerve (cortical visceralgia excitatory units).

Upper: the oscillograph of unit discharge, every horizontal line is the time sweep, from left to right (every 1.3 sec) and from up to down. The long longitudinal marks represent stimulation of spl. N.
1, before stimulation (spontaneous discharges).
2, 3 during stimulation of spl. N.
4, 5, 6 after cessation of stimulation

Middle: the average frequency histogram of spike ordinate=spikes per 10 sec. abscissa=time in sec., bin width 10 sec, spl indicates stimulation of spl. N.

Lower: the post-stimulus thme histogram, 20 repetitons, abscissae= time in msec., bin width 10 msec. Ordinate is calibrated in number of spikes/10 msec./20 rep. Arrow indicates stimulation of spl. N.

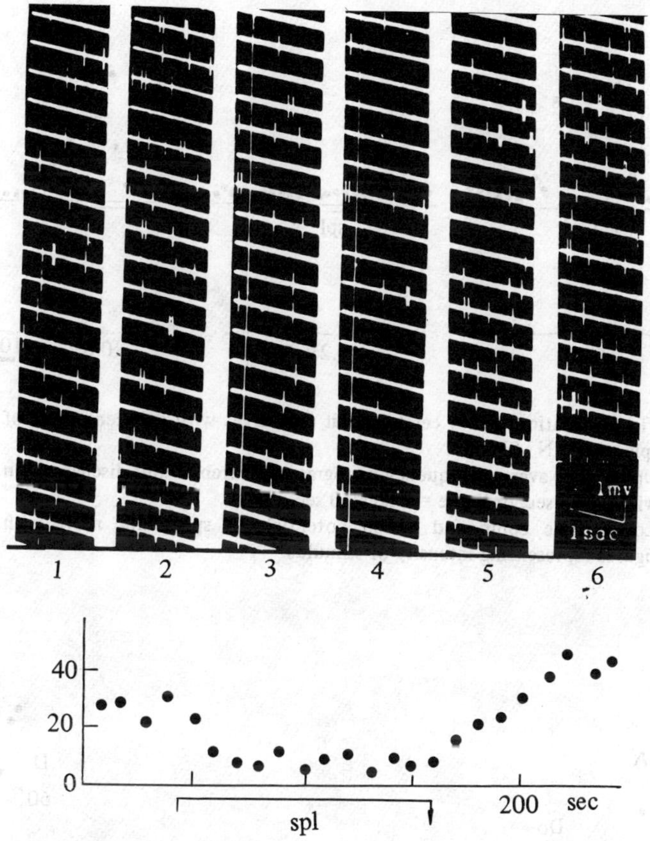

Fig. 3 Inhibitory response of cortical neurons to stimulation of splanchnic N. (cortical visceralgia inhibitory unit)
Upper: 1,2 before stimulation. 3, 4 during stimulation of spl. N. 5, 6 after cessation of stimulation.
Lower: average frequency histogram

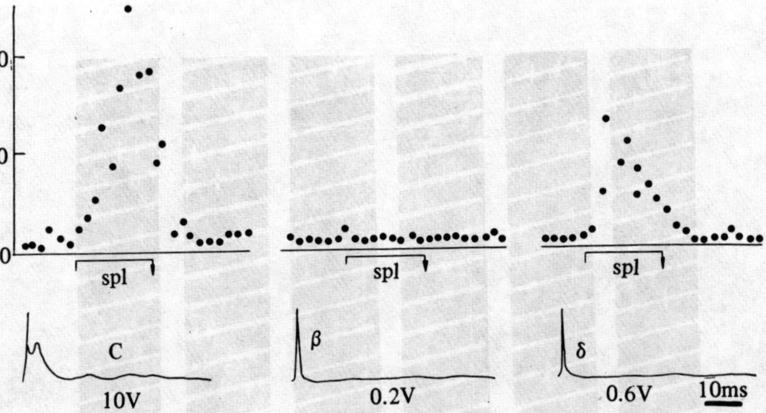

Fig. 4 Relationship of cerebral unit discharges with different kinds of splanchnic N fibers.
Upper: The average frequency histograms of cerebral unit discharge, bin width = 10 sec. ordinate = spikes/10 sec.
Lower: The compound action potentials of splanchnic nerve with figures representing intensity of stimulus.

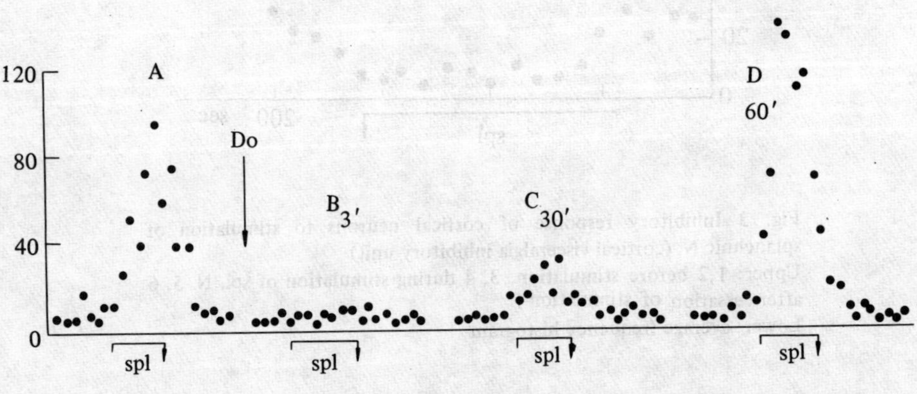

Fig. 5 Effect of Demerol on cortical splanchnic evoked discharge. A, before injection of Demerol. B, C, D 3 min, 30 min, and 60 min after injection respectively. D_0 indicates injection.

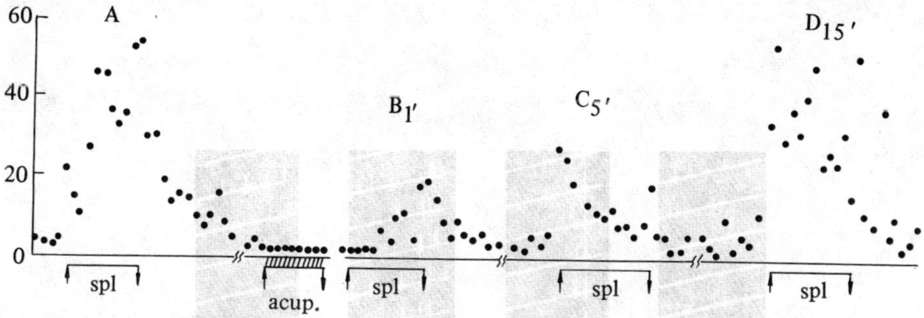

Fig. 6 Effect of electro-acupuncture of "Neiguan" point on cortical visceralgial discharge. A, before acupuncture, B, C, D, 1 min, 5 min and 15 min after cessation of the acupuncture respectively, ⊏⊐ indicates acupuncture.

one of the trials the visceralgial inhibitory units turned to show an excitatory effect (increase of discharge) during acupuncture.

(IV) The Cortical Evoked Potential and Unit Discharge During Stimulation of the "Neiguan" Point

Results of 4 experiments showed that stimulating the "Neiguan" point with an electric pulse of medium strength usually brought forth diphasic evoked potential at the surface of contralateral post-sigmoid gyrus. The potential of maximal amplitude could be recorded over a small area in front of the sulcus ansatus and behind the splanchnic projecting area. Thus we called it the "Neiguan" projecting area. If the microelectrode was inserted into a deeper layer of this area, the surface positive potential would change to a negative one. The highest negative "Neiguan" evoked potential could be recorded from the depth of 500 to 1000μ. This was the area of "Neiguan" excitatory units where stimulation of the "Neiguan" point would bring forth increased unit discharge, and recovery took place after stopping the stimulus. It was suggested that the "Neiguan" afferent signals might reach the cerebral cortex (SI). (Fig. 7)

(V) Effect of Stimulation of "Neiguan" Projecting Area on Cortical Visceralgial Unit Discharge

Our 4 experimental cases showed that the visceralgial discharge of cortical splanchnic projecting area was inhibited markedly by electro-stimulation of the "neiguan" projecting area, the rate of discharges lessened, the inhibitory period prolonged, and recovery took place gradually after its cessation (Fig. 8). In addition to the above results, facilitation took place at some units with an intensifying action on the visceralgial discharges. Thus it was suggested that the "Neiguan" projecting area might have some effect on the activities of the splanchnic projecting area. Thus the "Neiguan" projecting area might play some roles in the inhibitory effect of electro-acupuncture of the "Neiguan" point on cortical visceralgial discharges.

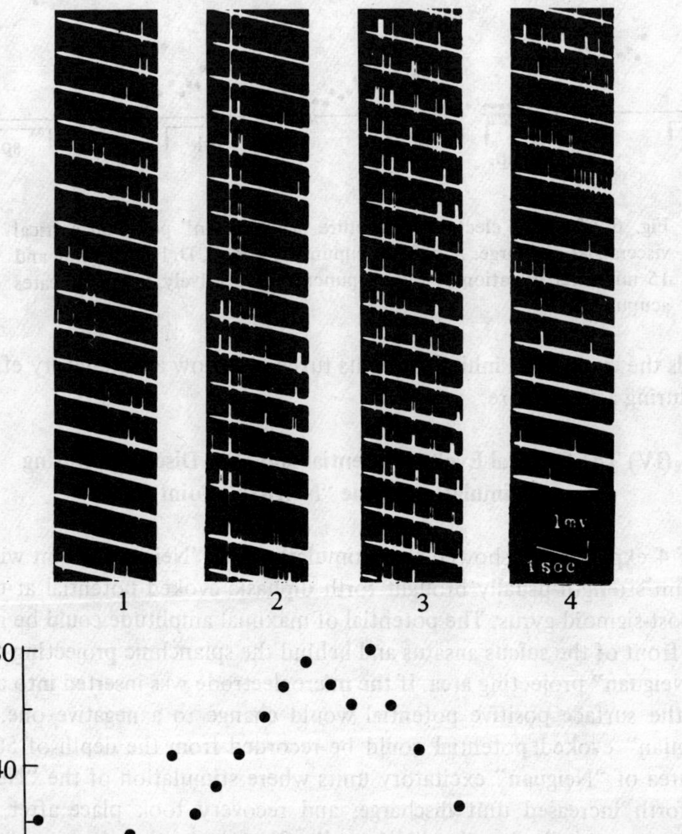

Fig. 7 Excitatory response of cortical neurons to stimulation of "neiguan" point (cerebral "Neiguan" excitatory unit).

Upper: 1, before stimulation, 2, 3, during stimulation of Neiguan point. 4, after cessation of stimulation.

Lower: average frequency histogram, Neiguan indicates stimulation of Neiguan point.

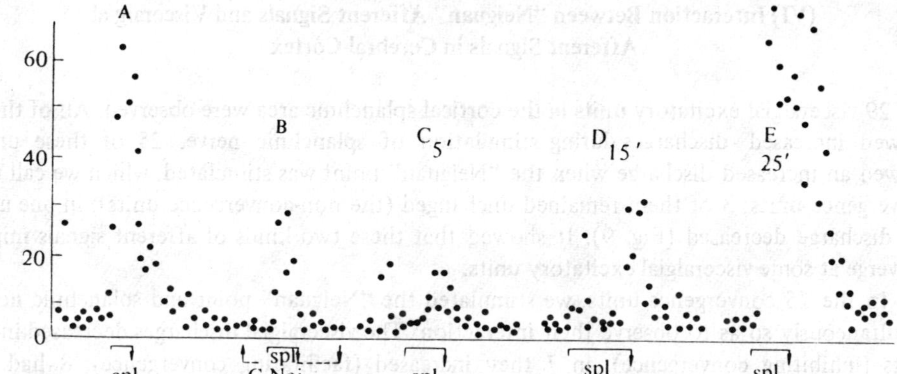

Fig. 8 Effect of stimulation of cortical "Neiguan" projection area on the cortical visceralgial discharge. A before stimulation of cortical "Neiguan" projection area, B, during stimulation, C, D, E 5 min, 15 min, and 25 min respectively after stimulation. CNei indicates stimulation of cortical "Neiguan" projection area.

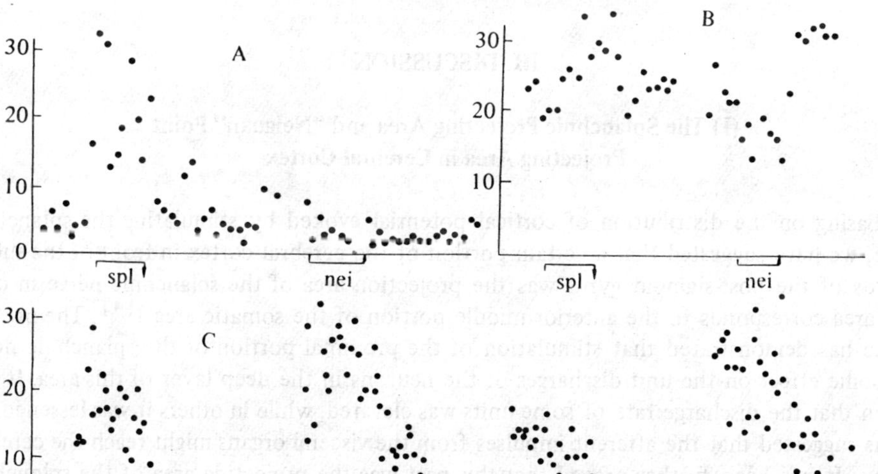

Fig. 9 Responses of 3 cortical visceralgial excitatory units to stimulation of "Neiguan" point. A, unchanged (non-convergence unit) B, decreased (Convergence unit), C, increased (convergence unit), inhibiting convergence. spl indicates stimulation of spl. N. "Nei" indicates stimulation of "Neiguan" point

(VI) Interaction Between "Neiguan" Afferent Signals and Visceralgial Afferent Signals in Cerebral Cortex

29 visceralgial excitatory units in the cortical splanchnic area were observed. All of them showed increased discharges during stimulation of splanchnic nerve. 25 of these units showed an increased discharge when the "Neiguan" point was stimulated, which we call the convergence units; 3 of them remained unchanged (the non-convergence units); in one unit the discharge decreased (Fig. 9). It showed that these two kinds of afferent signals might converge at some visceralgial excitatory units.

In the 25 convergence units, we stimulated the "Neiguan" point and splanchnic nerve simultaneously so as to observe their interaction. The visceralgial discharges decreased in 10 units (inhibiting convergence); in 7 they increased (facilitating convergence); 8 had no obvious change. This suggested that the interaction between them was rather complex. Its end result may be inhibitory or facilitatory, and the effect may be greater or smaller.

Finally we tried to get some idea of the relationship between acupuncture effect and convergence in 7 of our experimental cases. It seemed that acupuncture (of "Neiguan") inhibition of cortical visceralgial discharge was more powerful at the inhibiting convergence units than at the facilitating convergence units. These observations show that the effect of acupuncture is closely related to convergence.

III. DISCUSSION

(I) The Splanchnic Projecting Area and "Neiguan" Point Projecting Area in Cerebral Cortex

Basing on the distribution of cortical potential evoked by stimulating the splanchnic nerve, we have suggested that a certain portion of the cerebral cortex in front of the sulcus ansatus of the post-sigmoid gyrus was the projection area of the splanchnic nerve in cats. This area corresponds to the anterior middle portion of the somatic area I[4]. The present article has demonstrated that stimulation of the proximal portion of the splanchnic nerve had some effect on the unit discharges of the neurons in the deep layer of this area. It was shown that the discharge rate of some units was elevated, while in others it was lessened. So it was suggested that the afferent impulses from the visceral organs might reach the cerebral cortex. It has been further proved that this part was the projecting area of the splanchnic nerve (or the sensory area of the upper abdominal organs). As to the relationship between the cerebral cortex and visceral sensation there are different opinions[5–9]. We incline to consider that the cerebral cortex is concerned with the formation of visceral sensation.

As the "Neiguan" point was stimulated, cortical evoked potential could be recorded at the contralateral posterior sigmoid gyrus, with the maximal potential in front of the sulcus ansatus which was slightly posterior to the splanchnic projecting area. Thus we called it the "Neiguan" point projecting area. Stimulation of "Neiguan" point might also bring forth increased unit discharges at its deep layer. This further showed that the afferent impulse from "Neiguan" point might reach the cortical "Neiguan" projecting area which played some roles in the formation of acupuncture sensation. This process is not yet clear and needs further study. Nevertheless, it has been reported that the maximal potential evoked by stimulating the nerve of the forelimb of cat could also be recorded at the cortical "Neiguan" projecting area or in its vicinity[10].

(II) The Cortical Visceralgial Excitatory Unit and Inhibitory Unit

Stimulation of the splanchnic nerve usually brought forth excitation of both A_δ and C fibers, and consequently an increase in the unit discharges of the cortical splanchnic projecting area. But in case the intensity of stimulation was lowered so that only the A_β fiber was excited, the above increasing effect disappeared. It was suggested that this response in discharge was due to excitation of both A_δ and C fibers. Their characteristics were: prolonged latency, prolonged aftereffect and being easily inhibited by the analgesic dolantin. On account of these characteristics it might be concerned with pain sensation and might reflect the upper abdominal visceralgia. Thus we called these discharges the cortical visceralgial unit discharges, and these units, the cortical visceralgial excitatory units. On the other hand, stimulating the splanchnic nerve might also bring forth decrease in unit discharges. These we called the visceralgial inhibitory units.

At the projection area these two different kinds of units intermingled, but they responded differently to visceralgial stimulation, i.e., some were excited, and others were inhibited. They also responded contrarily to acupuncture. Interaction between these two different kinds of units might be concerned with integration of visceralgia.

(III) The Role of Cortical "Neiguan" Projection Area in Inhibition of Cortical Visceralgial Discharges by Electro-acupuncture.

When the "Neiguan" point was stimulated, the afferent impulses could reach the cortical "Neiguan" projecting area and elicit evoked potential and unit discharge. The cortical visceralgial unit discharge of the splanchnic projecting area could be inhibited by electro-stimulation of the cortical "Neiguan" projecting area. This experimental fact showed that the cortical "Neiguan" projecting area played an intermediate role in the inhibition of cortical visceralgial discharges by electro-acupuncture on "Neiguan" point. The question whether this action was due to spreading depression[11] from the cortical "Neiguan" projecting area to the splanchnic projecting area or whether it was through some other mechanisms should be further studied. In some experimental cases we saw that the discharges at the cortical splanchnic projecting area were enhanced during stimulation of the cortical "Neiguan" projecting area. It was obvious that the effect of the cortical "Neiguan" projecting area on the cortical splanchnic projecting area was rather complex; it might be exciting or inhibiting, and its action (inhibiting or exciting) might be determined by the frequency and intensity of the stimulus and the physiological state of these two projecting areas.

(IV) Interaction Between Visceralgial and "Neiguan" Point Afferent Signals in Cerebral Cortex

When the "Neiguan" point was stimulated, the rate of unit discharge increased in some cortical visceralgial excitatory units. It was shown that afferent signals from "Neiguan" point and visceral pain could converge at these cortical units. These two afferent signals interacted with each other resulting in inhibition or facilitation. In inhibitory convergency visceralgial discharges were diminished, and in facilitating convergency enhanced. Again the inhibitory effect of acupuncture on "Neiguan" point was obvious in the cortical units of inhibitory convergency, but it was rather dim in the facilitating units. This showed that inhibitory convergency might be the fundamental basis of electro-acupuncture inhibition on visceralgia. It was stated previously that the visceral and somatic afferent signals might converge in other parts (besides the cerebral cortex) of the central nervous system[12–14]. Thus the visceralgial integration might take place at several levels of CNS. But, which is the most important level is a question that has not yet been solved.

The above results are consistent with the opinion that "acupuncture anesthesia is the resulting effect of interaction between the pain signals and acupuncture signals in the central nervous system."[5]. They may interact in the cerebral cortex, which thus plays some roles in acupuncture inhibition on visceralgia.

IV. SUMMARY

1. There was found in the cat a cortical splanchnic projection area in the anterior middle portion of the post-sigmoid gyrus. Cortical visceralgial excitatory and inhibitory units were observed in this area. When the contralateral splanchnic nerve was stimulated, the maximal cortical evoked potential could be recorded in this area, and the rate of discharge in visceralgial excitatory units increased. These cortical visceralgial discharges could be inhibited by Demerol and by acupuncture. It was suggested that afferent signals of visceral pain could reach the cerebral cortex.

2. When the "Neiguan" point was stimulated, the maximal cortical evoked potential was recorded at the posterior middle portion of contralateral post-sigmoid gyrus. Stimulation of "Neiguan" point might also evoke increased unit discharges at its deep layer. Thus we called it the cortical "Neiguan" projection area. The visceralgial discharge of the cortical splanchnic projection area could be inhibited by stimulating this area. It showed that the afferent signal from "Neiguan" piont might reach the cerebral cortex, and the cortical "Neiguan" projection area might play an intermediate role in the inhibition of cortical visceralgial discharge by electro-acupuncture on "Neiguan" point.

3. The afferent signals of visceral pain and those from "Neiguan" point could converge to the visceralgial unit of the cortical splanchnic projection area. The results of interaction between these two afferent signals might be inhibiting or facilitating cortical visceralgial discharge.

From the above results, it is suggested that the cerebral cortex probably plays an important role in the mechanism of acupuncture inhibition on visceral pain.

REFERENCES

[1] 中山医学院生理教研组：新医学（5）：55，1974。

[2] 中医研究院针灸经络研究所生理组：新医药杂志（6）：28，1976。

[3] 北京市中医研究所：针刺麻醉（2）：28，1978。

[4] 中山医学院针麻原理研究室：针刺麻醉（2）：14，1978。

[5] 张香桐：中国科学（1）：28，1973。

[6] Amassian, V. E.: *J. Neurophysiol.,* **14**:433, 1951.
[7] Downmann, C.B.B.: *J. Physiol.,* **113**:434, 1951.
[8] Langhof, H. & Rubia, E.J.:*Pflüger. Arch. Ges. Physiol.,* **312**:18, 1969.
[9] Newman, P.P.: *J. Physiol.,* **160**:284, 1962.
[10] Osearsson, O.& Rosen, I.: *Experientia,* **19**:206, 1963.
[11] Krnjevic, K.: *Nature,* **201**:1294, 1964.
[12] Selzer, M. & Spencer, W.A.: *Brain Res.,* **14**:349, 1969.
[13] Hancork, M.B. *et al.*: *J. Neurophysiol.,* **83**:46, 1970.
[14] Macleod, J.G.: *J. Physiol.,* **140**:462, 1958.

PART I
RESEARCHE ON THE MECHANISMS OF ACUPUNCTURE, MOXIBUSTION AND ACUPUNCTURE ANESTHESIA
(2)

ROLE OF CENTRAL NEUROTRANSMITTERS IN ACUPUNCTURE ANALGESIA

Han Jisheng, Tang Jian, Ren Minfeng,*
Zhou Zhongfu, Fan Shaoguang,
Qiu Xuecai
(Research Group of Acupuncture Anesthesia, Beijing Medical College, Beijing)

I. INTRODUCTION

(I) The effect of acupuncture analgesia in human beings[1]

Our study of acupuncture analgesia (AA) began during the years of 1965 to 1966 in a general survey of the effect of acupuncture in healthy volunteers and also in some patients with neurological disorders. In a group of 66 individuals given acupuncture at "Hoku", there was a rise in pain threshold of the skin in about 2/3 of the cases which attained its maximal effect in about 30 minutes and declined thereafter exponentially with a half-life of about 15–17 minutes. Judging from the slow and regular changes in pain threshold induced by acupuncture, we imagined that there could have been certain chemical agents mobilized by the acupuncture stimulus within the body to bring about the analgesic effect. We also found that the effect could be blocked by local infiltration of procaine at the point of acupuncture, and was absent in case the acupuncture was applied to the afflicted extremities of those paraplegic or hemiplegic patients. Since the transmission of afferent impulses arising from the point of acupuncture into the CNS is a prerequisite for effective acupuncture analgesia, we inclined to look for the putative analgesic agents within the CNS.

(II) Cerebro-ventricular perfusion studies in rabbits[2]

Experiments were carried out in 1972, using the rabbit acupuncture model. Needling of the "Zusanli" point or finger pressing of the "Kunlun" point brought about a rise in pain threshold of the skin around the nostrils and the mouth, represented by the prolongation of the latency of the head-withdrawal reaction upon thermal irradiation. When a ventricular perfusate was drawn from the analgesic donor rabbit in the course of finger-acupuncture and injected into the ventricle of another normal recipient animal, the latter showed an elevation of pain threshold also. The perfusate drawn from a rabbit under the same conditions

*Present address: Gansu Institute of New Medicine and Pharmacology.

except for acupuncture was ineffective in this regard. This implied that some effective chemical substrate with analgesic effect might have been produced in the brain of the donor rabbit in the course of acupuncture analgesia.

(III) The role of central neurotransmitters in AA

Central neurotransmitters subserve the materialistic basis for the transmission of nerve impulses within the CNS. Since 1973, our interest has been focused mainly on the study of the role of central neurotransmitters in acupuncture analgesia. The scheme of our research involved two parallel and reciprocal lines of study: (1) Does acupuncture bring about any changes in the content and turnover rate of the central neurotransmitters? (2) Could the effect of acupuncture analgesia be modified by selective alteration of the functional status of these neurotransmitters? For each kind of neurotransmitters under study, the nature of its effect on AA was determined both qualitatively (being facilitatory or inhibitory) and quantitatively (with regard to the magnitude of its effect, dose-response time-response effects, etc.). Efforts were made also to localize its site of action in the CNS, and to as certain the interrelationships between various neurotransmitters.

Aside from the clinical and experimental studies in healthy individuals and patients, we have also established three different kinds of models of acupuncture analgesia in laboratory animals. They are: (1) The rabbit finger-acupuncture model described above[3]; (2) The vocalization model in rats, in which electroacupuncture was given to bilateral "Zusanli" and "Sanyinjiao" points and vocalization test with electrical stimulation of the tail by subcutaneous electrodes was used for assessment of pain[4]; (3) The rat tail-flick acupuncture analgesia model: Electro-acupuncture was given as above, and radiant-heat tail-flick test was adopted for assessment of pain[12].

The content of 5-hydroxytryptamine (5-HT), dopamine (DA) and norepinephrine (NE) in the brain was determined by spectrofluorophotometry, the opiate-like activity by radioreceptor assay and ACh by bioassay in leech dorsal longitudinal muscle preparations.

Seven years' study in our laboratory revealed that central 5-HT, endogenous opiate-like substances (OLS) and acetylcholine (ACh) have a facilitatory effect on acupuncture analgesia (AA), while catecholamines (CAs, including NE and DA) and endogenous anti-opiate substrates (AOS) have an antagonistic effect. The effects of these neurotransmitters on AA are introduced briefly as follows.

II. THE ROLE OF 5-HT

(I) Lowering of cerebral 5-HT content

Intraventricular injection of parachlorophenylalanine (PCPA), which lowered cerebral 5-HT content by inhibition of synthesis, attenuated the effect of AA significantly[5]. Similar results were obtained in rats given intraperitoneal injection of PCPA[9].

With regard to the sites of action of central 5-HT, many authors have demonstrated the role of descending fibers from the raphe nuclei in both morphine analgesia (MA) and AA. In order to evaluate the effect of ascending serotonergic pathways, 5,6-dihydroxytryptamine (5,6-DHT), the chemical denervator of serotonergic fibers, was injected into the medial forebrain bundle of rats[21]. A significant reduction in the effect of AA following the selective lowering of forebrain 5-HT content as a result of 5,6-DHT injection implied that ascending serotonergic fibers may play an important role in AA.

It is worthwhile to mention here that when the cerebral 5-HT content was seriously lowered by PCPA or 5,6-DHT, the effect of AA was significantly attenuated but not totally abolished. This implies that cerebral 5-HT is an important factor but not the sole determinant in AA.

(II) Increase in the functional activity of central 5-HT

The effect of AA is significantly augmented in rabbits given intravenous injection of pargyline to reduce the degradation of 5-HT[6], and also in rats given intraperitoneal injection of 5-hydroxytryptophan (5-HTP) to increase the synthesis of 5-HT[9]. That the amount of 5-HTP effective in augmenting AA upon intraventricular injection was only 1–2% of the effective dose for intraperitoneal injection evidenced a central site of action[21]. Clomipramine, which selectively blocked the reuptake of 5-HT at serotonergic nerve terminals and accentuated serotonergic functional activities was found to be effective clinically in potentiation of the effect of acupuncture anesthesia for the extraction of impacted last molar in a double-blind study[13].

(III) The effect of electroacupuncture on the activity of central serotonergic neurons

Cerebral 5-HT content rose significantly in the course of electroacupuncture analgesia[21]. Recent studies revealed that there was a positive correlation between the cerebral 5-HT increment and the effectiveness of AA with a coefficient of correlation of 0.59, which was statistically very significant ($P<0.001$)[28].

Turnover studies revealed that during AA, both synthesis and utilization of central 5-HT were facilitated; while the rate of synthesis exceeded its utilization, central 5-HT content increased[21]. The electrophysiological group of our laboratory have also found a significant increase in the rate of unit discharge of N. raphe dorsalis during and within 10 minutes after electroacupuncture. The results are quite in line with those obtained in neurochemical studies.

It can be concluded from above that central 5-HT is an important link mediating AA.

III. THE ROLE OF ENDOGENOUS OPIATE-LIKE SUBSTANCES

(I) The effect of blockade of central opiate receptors on AA

It has been demonstrated that opiate antagonists antagonized the effect of AA partially both in man (Mayer et al., 1977; Jiang et al., 1978) and in mice (Pomeranz et al., 1976). Observations were made in rabbits and rats in our laboratory also.

The effects of AA in rabbits were partially antagonized after intraventricular injection of naloxone (40μg/100μl)[10]. Localization studies in discrete brain areas revealed that bilateral slow infusion of naloxone (2μg in 5μl on each side within 20 minutes) through chronic *indwelled* cannulae was effective in antagonizing AA significantly at N. accumbens, amygdaloid nucleus, the habenulae and also periaqueductal grey (PAG)[29]. Same amount of naloxone given to the caudate nucleus, hippocampus, internal capsule, the thalamic tissue around the habenular nucleus, and the *tectal region in the midbrain* was totally ineffective. Nor was it effective when it was injected into the lateral ventricle or cerebral aqueduct.

We were puzzled indeed when we found that the results of experiments of intraventricular injection of naloxone in rats were quite different from those of rabbits. The dose of naloxone (20μg in 50μl infused within 16 minutes) was certainly strong enough in blocking the effect of 10mg/kg of morphine given subcutaneously, but it failed to block AA[34]. However, the fact that microinjections at bilateral N. accumbens[22] or habenulae[35] were also effective in blocking the effect of AA gives affirmative support to the importance of OLS as a substrate mediating AA in rats just like it is in rabbits. So there is an explanation for the failure of intraventricular injection of naloxone in the blocking of AA in rats.

(II) The effect of blockade of OLS degradation on AA

The released enkephalins were known to be rapidly destroyed by carboxypeptidase A or the enkephalinase. Should OLS play an important part in AA, measures which retard its enzymatic degradation would have raised the effectiveness of AA. We found recently that intraventricular injection of 200μg of D-phenylalanine, the peptidase inhibitor, enhanced the effect of AA in rabbits significantly and this augmenting effect could be completely reversed by narcotic antagonist naloxone[36]. This is another sample stressing the importance of OLS for mediation of AA in rabbits.

(III) Changes in cerebral OLS activity during AA

Rats were given electroacupuncture for 30 minutes and decapitated for determination of cerebral OLS activity in the whole brain. There was a significant rise after acupuncture which ran parallel with the effect of AA; the better the analgesic effect, the higher the OLS activity raised. A positive correlation was found between them ($r=0.61$, $P<0.01$)[15], and this was also verified in recent study[28].

As we proceeded further for localization studies, the brain was severed into 3 segments: the telencephalon, the diencephalon and the brainstem. The results indicated that the portion of the brain that was best correlated was found in the telencephalon. Some correlation was noticed in the brainstem also, and no correlation in the diencephalon including caudate-putamen[17]. Further analysis revealed that it was the septum-accumbens in the telencephalon and the midbrain portion in the brainstem that actually counted, and the OLS contents therein were intimately correlated with the effects of AA[33]. The results were in line with blockade of AA by microinjection of naloxone at N. accumbens and midbrain PAG mentioned above.

(IV) Changes in the blood OLS activity during AA[32]

The effect of AA in 21 healthy volunteers given single needle acupuncture at "Sanyanluo" was observed and correlated with changes in blood OLS activity in venous blood samples. In those with excellent analgesic effects, the OLS activity in the postacupunctural blood sample was significantly higher than the control level taken before acupuncture, while in those with poor results, OLS activity did not rise significantly. The effect of AA was found to be well correlated with the blood OLS activity ($r=0.645, P<0.01$) This implied that blood OLS activity was in some way related to the analgesic effect of acupuncture.

IV. THE INTERRELATIONSHIP BETWEEN 5-HT AND OLS

The above data shows the important roles of 5-HT and OLS in AA, and it would be a question of great interest and significance to observe whether these two neurochemical substrates were functionally interrelated with each other.

(I) The effect of blockage of opiate receptors on central 5-HT

Rats given intraventricular perfusion of naloxone (20μg within 16 minutes) were decapitated immediately at the end of infusion for determination of 5-HT and 5-HIAA content in the whole brain. There was an elevation of 5-HT over the control group by 14% ($P<0.01$) and 5-HIAA by 16% ($P<0.05$), indicating that blockade of the effect of OLS led to an increase in the turnover of central 5-HT.

(II) The effect of decrease in central 5-HT content on cerebral OLS activity[20]

3–5 days after the injection of different dosages of PCPA and 5,6-DHT in rats, there was a significant elevation in cerebral OLS activity in association with the reduction of central 5-HT content. The percentage change of OLS activity (y) was found to be negatively correlated with that of 5-HT content (x) in a linear regression equation: $y=164.8-0.64x$. The coefficient of correlation (r) was found to be -0.74 and was statistically very significant ($n=50, p<0.001$). The equation implies that with a reduction of the cerebral 5-HT content to 50% of its normal level, the cerebral OLS activity might be raised to 132.8% of its normal value (taken as 100%).

The fact that the functions of 5-HT and OLS were interrelated, i.e., the impairment of function in one aroused a compensatory increase in the other, might be helpful to the explanation of the following experimental phenomena: (1) in rats, the effect of AA was not reduced after intraventricular infusion of a large amount of naloxone[33]; (2) intraventricular injection of naloxone, which induced a partial blockade of the effect of AA in rabbits, was ineffective when central 5-HT was elevated by pargyline[10]; (3) some of the rats retained a fairly good effect of AA even though the cerebral 5-HT content was reduced to less than 20% of its normal level[20].

(III) Changes in the central 5-HT content and CLS activity during electroacupuncture in normal rats[25, 28]

Rats were given electroacupuncture for 30 minutes. After that, the brains were removed after decapitation and sectioned into 2 equal halves for the determination of central 5-HT content and OLS activity separately. Correlation of the neurochemical findings with the effect of AA in individual rats revealed that rats with higher levels of both central 5-HT content and OLS activity generally exhibited excellent analgesic effects, those with elevation of either 5-HT or OLS a moderate analgesic effect, while those without any elevation or even a reduction in both showed a poor effect. The correlation of central 5-HT content (x_1, expressed as % of the normal level) and OLS activity (%, x_2) with the effect of AA (y, the average % increase in pain threshold over the basal level) can be expressed in a regression equation: $y=0.64x_1+0.46x_2-75$ ($r=0.69$, $n=27$, $P<0.001$). The equation stresses the importance of 5-HT and OLS in AA, and also indicates that the reduction of any one of them would not seriously impair the effectiveness of AA if the other one would have been raised significantly.

(IV) Correlation of central 5-HT content and OLS activity with the effect of AA in PCPA-treated rats[20]

As mentioned above, the reduction of central 5-HT content after PCPA was accompanied by a spontaneous rise in cerebral OLS activity. The trend of elevation of OLS was even more marked when electroacupuncture stimulation was given to these animals. Correlative analysis of these 3 factors revealed that, inasmuch as the decrease in cerebral 5-HT had been compensated by a rise in OLS, the rats retained a fairly good effect of acupuncture analgesia. While in those rats, the cerebral OLS activity failed to make up for the loss in 5-HT, the effect of AA was almost completely abolished. The results of observation in a group of 51 rats may be expressed in a regression equation: $y=0.61x_1+0.48x_2-62$ ($r=0.60$, $P<0.01$) which was very similar to that obtained from normal rats (*cf. IV. (III)*). The consistency of the general equation under different experimental conditions might well indicate the existence of a substantial interrelationship between central 5-HT and OLS with regard to the effect of AA.

(V) The effect of simultaneous blockade of 5-HT and OLS on AA in rats[11, 33]

Intraperitoneal injection of a small dose of PCPA (200 mg/kg) reduced the cerebral 5-HT content by 52% ($P<0.01$); at the same time, the effect of AA was reduced by 19% only ($P>0.05$). Intraventricular perfusion of naloxone (20μg) had no apparent effect on AA also. But the effect of AA was reduced very significantly when these 2 measures were given in combination (–59%, $P<0.005$). The results implied that the antagonistic effect of naloxone could have been manifested in case there is a reduction in cerebral 5-HT. When naloxone was given in association with large doses of PCPA (320 mg/kg ip, plus 10 mg/kg ivt), so that both the effects of 5-HT and OLS were blocked, the effect of AA was totally abolished.

Summary: The effect of AA in rats seems to be intimately related with the content and the extent of mobilization of cerebral 5-HT and OLS, and these two neurochemical substrates were found to be closely interrelated and functionally compensatory to each other.

V. THE ROLE OF ACETYLCHOLINE

(I) The lowering of functional activity of central ACh

Blocking of synthesis of ACh by intraventricular injection of 10 or 20 μg of HC-3 reduced the effect of AA significantly in a dose-dependent manner[7, 18]. There is a likewise reduction in the effect of AA when the central *unscarinic* receptors were blocked by atropine given intraventricularly to rabbits[2] or intraperitoneally to rats and also by benztropine given intraventricularly to rats[37]. The results implied that central ACh may be one of the important substrates concerning the mechanism of AA.

(II) Increase in the functional activity of central ACh[37]

The blocking effect of HC-3 on AA could be partially reversed by choline chloride, the precursor of ACh, although choline did not affect AA in itself. Rats given eserine by the subcutaneous route also showed an increase in the effect of AA.

From the results stated above, it follows that central 5-HT, OLS and ACh seem to be the important factors mediating the analgesic effect of acupuncture. Here below we are going to discuss the action of some of the neurochemical factors that have an antagonistic effect.

VI. THE ROLE OF CATECHOLAMINES

(I) The effect of DA

Intraventricular injection of apomorphine, the DA receptor agonist, reduced the effect of AA, while spiroperidol, the DA receptor antagonist, strengthened it[19]. Droperidol, another DA antagonist, was also effective in augmenting AA[8]. Clinical application of this drug has been proved to be helpful in increasing the effectiveness of acupuncture anesthesia in thyroidectomy (The First Attached Hospital of Peking Medical College, 1976). Therefore, central DA might have an antagonistic action on the effect of AA.

(II) The effect of NE

DOPS, the immediate antecedent of NE, may be decarboxylated directly to NE in the body, thus by passing the stage of DA formation. Given by the intraventricular route to rats, DOPS (25–200μg) induced a dose-dependent increase in the content of central NE, and a concomitant decline in the effect of AA[16]. Selective destruction of ascending noradrenergic fibers by microinjection of 6-OHDA, the chemical denervator of noradrenergic fibers, into bilateral medial forebrain bundles in rats, reduced the cerebral NE content and accentuated the effect of AA significantly[19]. Intraperitoneal injection of NE, which raised the NE level in the blood but not in the brain due to the presence of blood brain barrier, did not impart any significant influence upon AA[19]. This implies that it is the cerebral NE which is antagonistic to the effect of AA.

(III) The effect of α-receptors

In the experiments with rabbits, intraventricular injection of α-agonist clonidine antagonized AA, while α-antagonist phentolamine augmented it[19]. Similar results were also obtained upon intraperitoneal injection of these two drugs in rats[19]. The antagonistic effect of DOPS which could be easily decarboxylated to NE in the brain, could be partially reversed by α-antagonist phentolamine, but not by β-antagonist propranolol[31]. Thus the effect of NE in antagonizing AA might be brought about through the activation of α-receptors.

(IV) The effect of β-receptors

Rabbits were given intraventricular injection of β-receptor agonist isoproterenol or β-receptor antagonist propranolol, and no apparent effect on AA was noticed[19]. However, propranol given intraperitoneally or intraventricularly to rats, attenuated the effect of AA significantly[31]. Clinical application of propranolol in surgical operations also revealed a detrimental effect on acupuncture anesthesia (The First Attached Hospital of Peking Medical College, 1976).

Summary: Central NE exerts an antagonistic effect via α-receptors and an augmentative effect via β-receptors on AA. While the overall effect of DOPS which might exert both of these opposing actions after its transformation to NE was to attenuate AA, the α-effect might be the one that predominated. The precise physiological effect of different receptors, however, should be analyzed according to the site of action.

(V) Localization studies of the effect of NE-α[36]

In rabbits with indwelled intracranial cannulae directed to the habenulae or PAG, microinjection of clonidine resulted in a definite antagonistic action on AA, and phentolamine an augmentatory effect. Microinjection of clonidine into N. accumbens had some antagonistic effect also, while injections given to the amygdaloid nucleus were ineffective. This implies that N. habenula and PAG might be the effective site of action of central NE in antagonizing the effect of AA.

(VI) Changes in central NE content and turnover during AA

The contents of central NE in the brain and spinal cord were significantly lowered in the course of electroacupuncture in rats. Turnover studies revealed that electroacupuncture stimulation accelerated the synthesis of central NE as well as its release for utilization. While the rate of release exceeded that of synthesis, the cerebral content of NE dropped consequently[24]. Tracer studies with ^{14}C-NE in rats denoted also that the metabolism of NE was accelerated during electroacupuncture[14].

As the general trend in the action of NE was antagonistic to AA as mentioned above, the accelerated metabolism of cerebral NE in the course of electroacupuncture as demonstrated in turnover studies makes us believe that the antagonistic action should have paralleled the facilitating one throughout the course of acupuncture, although in the majority of cases the facilitatory action may predominate. Similar situations are not rarely seen in the physiological regulation of the bodily functions such as those found in the innervation of the heart in which an increase in vagal tone often accompanies the strengthening of sympathetic activity although the latter may predominate.

So far our discussion has been limited to CAs within the brain. Recently in preliminary study in spinal animals (which ordinarily exhibited a minimal analgesic effect upon electroacupuncture), administration of clonidine exhibited an augmenting effect on AA which was in direct contrast to the antagonistic effect seen in intact animals. This adds further to the complexity of the problem with regard to the effect of central CAs in acupuncture analgesia counteraction of DA and α-receptor in one part and β-receptor in the other, cerebral α-effect on one hand and spinal α-effect on the other, etc.

VII. ACUPUNCTURE TOLERANCE AND ENDOGENOUS ANTI-OPIATE SUBSTRATES

(I) The phenomenon of acupuncture tolerance[26]

Recently it has been proved by numerous authors that endorphins, just like morphine, may develop tolerance upon repeated administrations. It is conceivable that the large amount of OLS liberated in the brain upon long term repeated electroacupuncture could have induced a similar tolerance state that would curtail the effect of AA.

In our experiments in rats given electroacupuncture continuously for more than one hour at 3 volts under sparse and dense waves, the effect of AA declined gradually. Significant reductions in the analgesic effect were also noticed in rats given electroacupuncture repeatedly at hourly intervals for 2–3 sessions with increasing strengths of 1–2–3 volts for 30 minutes in a single session. We take this phenomenon of gradual decline in the effect of AA following prolonged or repeated electroacupunctures as "acupuncture tolerance". It could not be accounted for by local tissue damage at the point of acupuncture, since it persists after the point of needling has been changed. Neither could it be explained by the depletion of cerebral OLS as a result of excessive release, because cerebral OLS activity in acupuncture-tolerant rats was still higher than normal.

(II) Cross-tolerance with morphine

In case the development of acupuncture tolerance came about as a result of prolonged action of OLS upon opiate receptors, a cross-tolerance to morphine might be expected. Results of experimentation in this regard include 3 different aspects as follows:

(1) Injection of morphine into acupuncture-tolerant rats gave rise to a weak analgesic effect only[26].

(2) While the effect of morphine (6 mg/kg sc) was significantly lowered upon repeated

administration every 2 hours for 5 times, the effect of electroacupuncture given thereafter was not attenuated, thus indicating a one-way cross-tolerance between AA and MA[26].

(3) In chronic morphine-tolerant rats given morphine injections (5–50mg/kg) thrice daily for 8 days, the effect of AA was significantly attenuated[27].

(III) Endogenous anti-opiate substrate (AOS)[27]

The discovery of endogenous opiate-receptor agonist ("endogenous morphine") in the brain leads to the question: is it possible to find an endogenous opiate antagonist ("endogenous naloxone") in the brain also? Ungar (1976) succeeded in the extraction of an anti-opiate fraction from the brain of morphine-tolerant rats. Following similar procedures, we have also found something with an anti-opiate activity in acupuncture-tolerant rats. It is characterized by:

(1) Competition with ^{3}H-morphine in binding with opiate receptors;

(2) Antagonism of the inhibitory effect of morphine upon the contraction of mouse vas deferens induced by electrical stimulation;

(3) Antagonism of MA upon intraventricular injection in normal rats;

(4) Antagonism of AA upon intraventricular injection in normal rats.

The last point was certainly of special interest to us, since naloxone injected intraventricularly to rats failed to antagonize the effect of AA, although it was effective in counteracting MA. In this sense, the physiological activity of endogenous AOS seemed to be stronger than that of naloxone.

VIII. THE EFFECT OF CYCLIC NUCLEOTIDES

It is well known that the effect of various neurotransmitters are interpolated by cyclic nucleotides. A close interrelation was also found between the mechanism of MA and cyclic nucleotides. For example, opiates may antagonize the effect of CA in activating adenylcyclase.

We have found that intraventricular injection of cAMP in rats antagonized both MA and AA in a dose-dependent manner within the range from 50 to 400 μg[23]. Recently we have also noticed that intraventricular injection of cGMP was effective in augmenting both MA and AA[38]. All these results seem to point to a common underlying mechanism between MA and AA concerning cyclic nucleotides.

IX. CONCLUSION

(I) Central neurotransmitters implicated in AA

When the signals of acupuncture enter the CNS, it excites numerous neurones into action and various neurotransmitters are released. Among them some have a facilitatory action on AA (e.g., 5-HT, OLS and ACh), while others may have an antagonistic effect (e.g., NE-d, DA, AOS, etc.) (Fig.1).

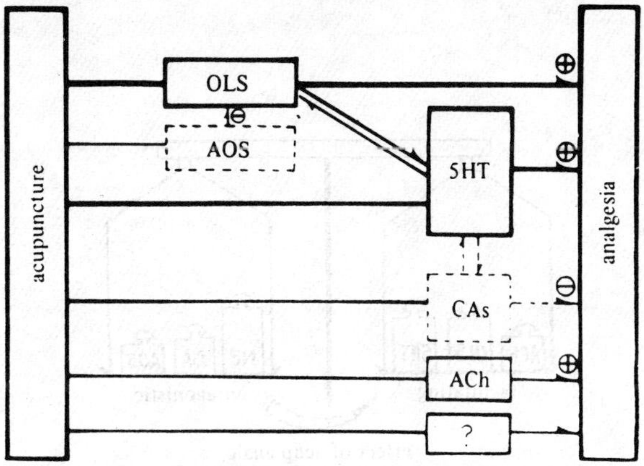

Fig. 1 Central neurotransmitters implicated in acupuncture analgesia.

Under ordinary conditions, there is some sort of equilibrium between the actions of these two groups of agents just like the balance of weights on the two sides of a scale, and the effect of AA is therefore kept at its ordinary level. Certainly, there could be a difference among different individuals and either of the two sides may predominate over the other. This might be one of the intrinsic mechanisms responsible for individual variations in the effectiveness of AA.

In the study of the roles of central neurotransmitters in AA, various pharmacological and physiological procedures have been taken to tilt the balance. When measures were taken to add some weight on the left side of the scale (e.g., increase of functional activity of 5-HT by 5-HTP, pargyline and clomipramine, or that of ACh by eserine, and that of OLS by bacitracin or D-phenylalanine) or to reduce the weight on the right side of the scale (e.g., blockade of α-receptors by phentolamine, destruction of ascending noradrenergic fibers by 6-OHDA, or blocking of DA receptors by spiroperidol or droperidol), the effect of AA could be augmented.

On the contrary, the effect of AA would be attenuated, when measures were taken to reduce the weight on the left side of the scale (e.g., decrease in the functional activity of 5-HT by PCPA or 5,6-DHT, blockade of opiate receptors by naloxone) or to add some weight on the right side (e.g., stimulation of DA or α-receptors by their agonists apomorphine and clonidine, increase in central NE after DOPS, or the production of endogenous AOS induced by repeated electroacupuncture).

It seems that the result of AA is effected by the conjoined actions and intricate interactions of various neurotransmitters in different brain areas; among them, 5-HT and OLS seem to be the key links.

(II) The neural pathways and the related neurotransmitters in AA

Now we would like to draw a sketch about the neural mechanism of AA, taking for reference the various works of other laboratories here and abroad, especially the excellent

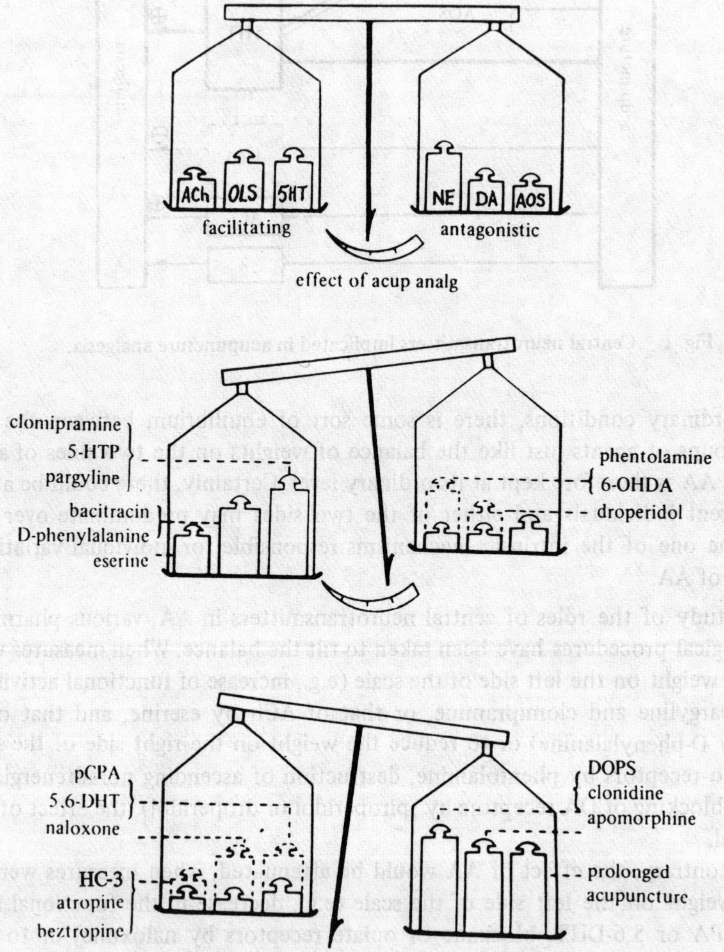

Fig. 2 The effect of altering the functional activity of central neurotransmitters on acupuncture analgesia.

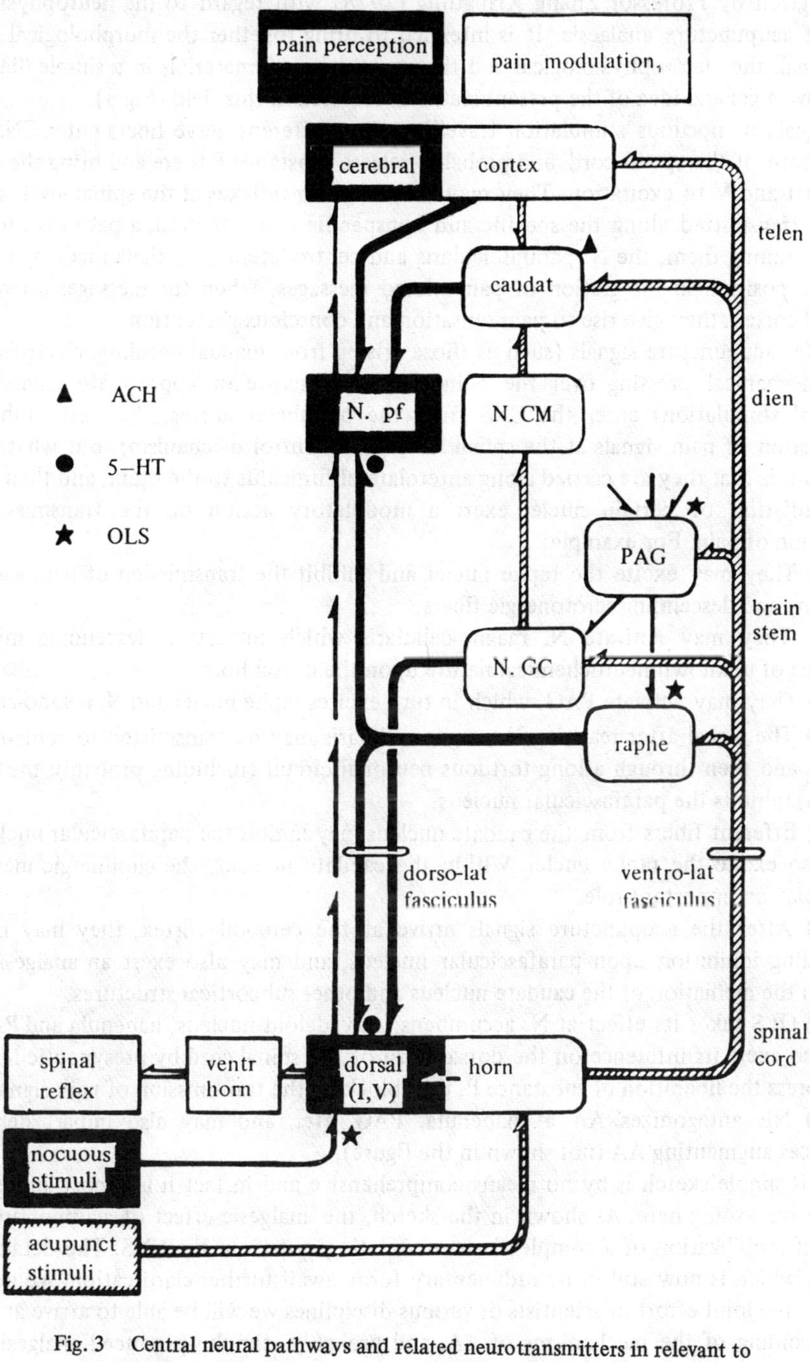

Fig. 3 Central neural pathways and related neurotransmitters in relevant to acupuncture analgesia.

review given by Professor Zhang Xiangtung (1978) with regard to the neurophysiological basis of acupuncture analgesia. It is intended to bring together the morphological and the functional, the electrophysiological and the neurochemical materials in a simple diagram so as to have a general idea of the present status of research in this field (Fig.3).

Signals of nocuous stimulation travelling along afferent nerve fibers enter CNS at the dorsal horn of the spinal cord, and probably release substance P there and bring the neurons of layer I and V to excitation. They may arouse motor reflexes at the spinal level, and may also be transmitted along the specific and nonspecific pain-conducting pathways to higher centers; among them, the N. parafascicularis and centro-lateralis of thalamus may occupy a strategic position in integration of pain-related messages. When the messages arrive at the cerebral cortex, they give rise to pain sensation and conscious perception.

After acupuncture signals (such as those arising from manual needling, electroacupuncture, mechanical pressing over the points of acupuncture or appropriate transcutaeous electrical stimulation) enter the CNS from the peripheral nerves, they may inhibit the transmission of pain signals at the spinal level (gate control mechanism). But what is more important is that they are carried along anterolateral funiculus to the brain, and then through the mediation of certain nuclei exert a modulatory action on the transmission and perception of pain. For example:

(1) They may excite the raphe nuclei and inhibit the transmission of pain signals via ascending and descending serotonergic fibers.

(2) They may activate N. magno-cellularis which imparts a descending inhibitory influence of unknown neurochemical nature upon the dorsal horn.

(3) They may activate PAG, which in turn excites raphe nuclei and N. magno-cellularis.

(4) The signal after reaching N. magno-cellularis may be transmitted to centro-median nucleus and then through a long tortuous neuronal circuit (including probably the caudate nucleus) inhibits the parafascicular nucleus.

(5) Efferent fibers from the caudate nucleus may inhibit the parafascicular nucleus and may also excite the raphe nuclei. Within the caudate nucleus, the cholinergic mechanism might play an important role.

(6) After the acupuncture signals arrive at the cerebral cortex, they may impart a descending inhibition upon parafascicular nucleus, and may also exert an analgesic effect through the mediation of the caudate nucleus and other subcortical structures.

(7) OLS takes its effect at N. accumbens, amygdaloid nucleus, habenula and PAG, and may also exert its influence on the dorsal horn of the spinal cord by presynaptic inhibition to suppress the liberation of substance P, thus blocking the transmission of pain signals.

(8) NE antagonizes AA at habenula, PAG, etc., and may also impart descending influences augmenting AA (not shown in the figure).

This simple sketch is by no means comprehensive and in fact it is almost impossible to include everything here. As shown in the sketch, the analgesic effect of acupuncture is the result of mobilization of a complex pain-modulating system in the CNS. The details of the system, which is now still in its rudimentary form, await further clarification. We hope that through the joint effort of scientists of various disciplines we will be able to arrive at a better understanding of the mechanisms of AA, and probably stimulus-produced analgesia (SPA) and MA as well.

---

*The work was accomplished with the joint efforts of the members attending at Classes on the Research of Acupuncture Anesthesia from 1974to 1978.

REFERENCES

[1] 北京医学院基础部针麻原理研究组：中华医学杂志（3）：151，1973。

[2] Research Group of Acupuncture Anesthesia, Peking Medical College: *Scientia Sinica,* **17**:112, 1974.

[3] 北京医学院基础部针麻原理研究组生理组：北京医学院学报（1）：18，1974。

[4] ——: *Ibid,* (3):170. 1974.

[5] ——: 科学通报 **20**：483，1975。

[6] ——: *Ibid,* **20**;532, 1975.

[7] ——: 北京医学院学报（4）：224，1975。

[8] ——: *Ibid,* (2):75.1976.

[9] ——: 新医药学杂志（3）：133，1976。

[10] ——: 中华外科杂志 **15**：192，1977。

[11] 韩济生等：生理学报 **30**：201，1978。

[12] 任民峰 韩济生：Ibid 30：204。1978。

[13] 赵福运等：北京医学院学报（2）：79，1978。

[14] 周仲福等：Ibid（3）：147。1978。

[15] 汤 健 韩济生：Ibid（3）：150，1978。

[16] 韩济生等：Ibid（4）：209。1978。

[17] 汤 健等：Ibid（4）：212，1978。

[18] 任民峰等：Ibid（4）：214。1978。

[19] 北京医学院基础部针麻原理研究组生理组：中华医学杂志（3）：129，1978。

[20] 韩济生等：Ibid（12）：721。1978。

[21] Han, C.S. *et al.*: *Scientia Sinica,* **22**:91, 1979.

[22] 范少光等：北京医学院学报（1）：1，1979。

[23] 邱学才等：Ibid（1）：4。1979。

[24] 韩济生等：生理学报 **31**：11，1979。

[25] 韩济生等：北京医学 **1**：31，1979。

[26] 汤 健等：Ibid **1**：34，1979。

[27] Han. J.S. *et al.*: *National Symposia of Acupuncture and Moxibustion and Acupuncture Anesthesia* Abstracts, p. 492. Beijing, 1979.

[28] Liang, X.N. *et al.*: *Ibib*,, ,p. 490.

[29] Zhou, Z.F., *et al.*: *Ibid.*, p. 487.

[30] Xu, S.L., *et al.*: *Ibid.*, p. 493.

[31] Ren, M.F., *et al.*: *Ibid*, p. 441.

[32] 苏树伊等：针刺麻醉（2）：53，1979。

[33] 张万琴等：Ibid（3）：1979。

[34] 范少光等：科学通报，待发表。

[35] 涂宗苹等：北京医学院学报，待发表。

[36] 韩济生等：动物学报，待发表。

[37] 周仲福等：待发表。

[38] 邱学才等：待发表。

ENDORPHIN AND ACUPUNCTURE ANALGESIA*

Zhang Anzhong, Pan Xiaopin, Xu Shaofen,
Cheng Jieshi, Mo Wanying
(Acupuncture Analgesia Research Cooperative Group, Shanghai First Medical College)

Endorphin belongs to a group of endogenous opiate peptides. Some prove themselves to be neurotransmitters or modulators; the others may be neurohormones[1]. There are various physiological functions of these opiate peptides, analgesia being one of them. The regional distribution of endorphins and opiate receptors in the brain is consistent with the pain pathway[2] and with the active position of analgesia in the brain produced by microinjection of morphine[3] and electro-stimulation[4] as well. This suggests that the endorphin is related to analgesia and may be one of the important components of the central analgesic system[5].

Since 1975, we have been studying the interrelationship between endorphin and acupuncture analgesia. There are several kinds of endorphins which differ in regional distributions and functions. It seems necessary to separate them and to study the roles of these peptides individually. The elevation of pain thresholds in humans[6,7] and rabbits[8] after electroacupuncture was reversed by naloxone; and the elevation of endorphin activity in the CSF[9] and some rabbits nucleus (central grey, caudate nucleus, nucleus accumbens, etc.) was found after acupuncture[8]. Injection of naloxone (2μg/2μl/3min), the opiate antagonist, into the lateral ventricle or central grey of the rabbits significantly decreased the effect of acupuncture analgesia. Intravenous injection of naloxone (0.4mg/kg) significantly antagonized the analgesic effect of moderate electroacupuncture, but superstrength electroacupuncture did not. The effects of acupuncture on responses both to somatic and visceral pain were also partially antagonized by naloxone. Our results showed that the endorphins took part in acupuncture analgesia from presynaptic to receptor site. However, the functions of endorphins are not limited to analgesia only, and the transmitters or modulators of the central analgesic system are not limited to endorphins either. So acupuncture analgesia is a comprehensive result of multifactors, and further studies are necessary for other neurotransmitters or moderators regarding the mechanism of acupuncture analgesia. This report summarizes our work in the past few years.

---

*A Summary of the Studies in this Acupuncture Analgesia Research Cooperative Group.

I. ANALGESIC EFFECT OF ENDORPHINS

From the acetone extract of human brain we found a fraction, called "fraction 29"[10], which showed opioid activities in the mouse vas deferens bioassay (Fig.1) and radioreceptor assay. Fraction 29 was eluted from a Sephadex G-10 column in the void column of 1.8–2.4, and the Rf values of thin layer chromatography on silica gel G were found to be 0.50 and 0.60. The chromatographic pattern of fraction 29 in polyamide layer sheet is, however, different from those of enkaphalins. No activity of fraction 29 was detected when it was incubated with chymotrypsin at 37°C. It showed that there was analgesic effect on rabbits during ventriculo-injections. This effect could be reversed by naloxone (Fig.2). The potassium iontophoretic dolorimetry was used to measure pain threshold in the rabbit experiments.

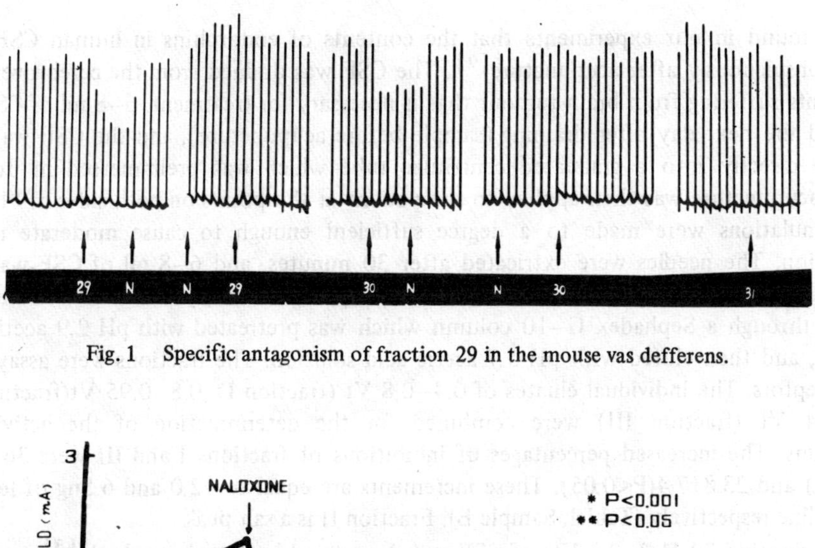

Fig. 1 Specific antagonism of fraction 29 in the mouse vas defferens.

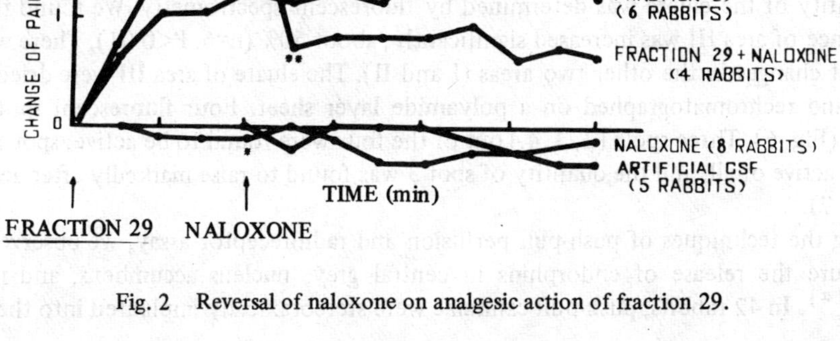

Fig. 2 Reversal of naloxone on analgesic action of fraction 29.

When the acetone extract of human brain stem was eluted from a column of Sephadex G-10 and the eluate was lyophilized and assayed by radioreceptors, seven active peaks were obtained, including fraction 29 (peak VI) (Fig. 3).

In normal cases, endorphins are bound to the opiate receptors partially in the brain[11, 12]. We assume that fraction 29 might also be bound to the opiate receptors. For the proof of this, we isolated the synaptic plasma membrances (SPM) from human brain stem and then extracted the morphine-like substances from the synaptic plasma membranes by 0.1 N HCl. The extract was neutralized, lyophilized and then eluted from a column of Sephadex G–10. The eluates were assayed by radioreceptors. The elution profile of the extract from synaptic plasma membranes on Sephadex G–10 column in terms of radioreceptor blocking activity (Fig. 4) corresponds with that of human brain stem, including fraction 29 (peak VI).

II. RELEASE OF ENDORPHINS BY ACUPUNCTURE

We found in our experiments that the contents of endorphins in human CSF were raised conspicuously after acupuncture[9]. The CSF was drained from the cerebroventricle of patients suffering from brain tumour that is necessary for treatment. 6–8 ml of CSF was collected the next day after draining (sample before acupuncture), and the CSF was drip-dropped directly into a graduated centrifuge tube which was preimmersed in dry ice. Electro-acupuncture was then applied to the patient at the points on both sides of "Hegu". The stimulations were made to a degree sufficient enough to cause moderate muscle contraction. The needles were extricated after 30 minutes, and 6–8 ml of CSF was then collected (sample after acupuncture). The CSF was purified first by ultrafiltration and then running through a Sephadex G–10 column which was pretreated with pH 2.9 acetic acid solution, and then eluted with pH 5.7 acetic acid solution. The fractions were assayed by radioreceptors. The individual eluates of 0.4–0.8 Vt (fraction I), 0.8–0.95 Vt(fraction II), 0.95–1.4 Vt (fraction III) were combined for the determination of the activity of endorphins. The increased percentages of inhibitions of fractions I and III were 36.6±8.6 ($P<0.05$) and 23.8±7.4($P<0.05$). These increments are equal to 12.0 and 6.5ng of leucine-enkephaline respectively (Tablel, Sample B). Fraction II is a salt peak.

The fraction 29 (1.8–2.4 Vt) of CSF was dansylated by Gray's method[13] and then chromatographed on a polyamide layer sheet (Fig. 5). We arbitrarily divided the fluorescent spots into three areas (I, II, III), and then eluted separately with methanol from the sheet. The quantity of the eluate was determined by fluorescent spectrometry. We found that the fluorescence of area III was increased significantly, about 50% ($n=6$, $P<0.01$). There were no significant changes in the other two areas (I and II). The eluate of area III were dried under vacuum and rechromatographed on a polyamide layer sheet. Four fluorescent spots were obtained (Fig. 6). Three spots (2, 3, 4,) out of the four were found to be active, spot 3 being the most active of all, and the quantity of spot 3 was found to raise markedly after acupuncture (Fig. 7).

Using the techniques of push-pull perfusion and radioreceptor assay, we observed after acupuncture the release of endorphins in central grey, nucleus accumbens, and nucleus caudate[14]. In 42 rabbits, push-pull cannulae were stereotaxically implanted into the above

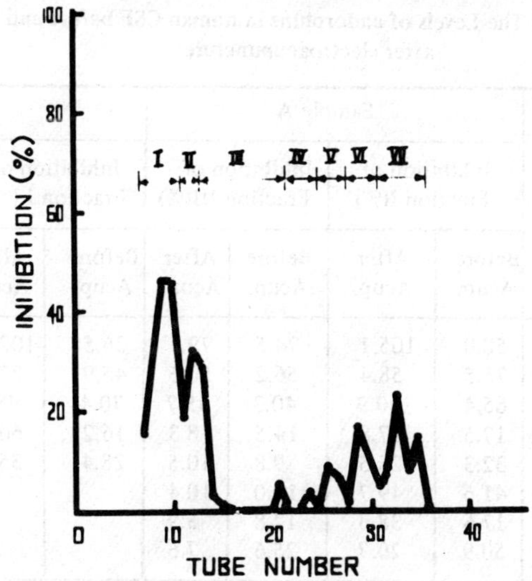

Fig. 3 Elution profile of the extracts of human brain stem on Sephadex G–10 in terms of radioreceptor blocking activity.

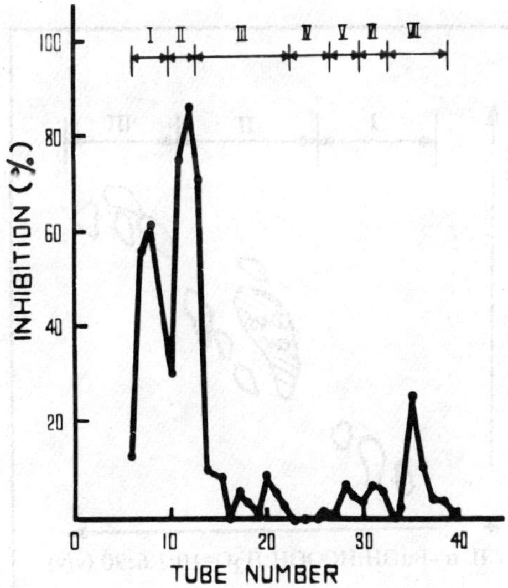

Fig. 4 Elution profile of the extracts of SPM in terms of radioreceptor blocking activity.

Table 1. The Levels of endorphins in human CSF before and after electroacupuncture

No.	Name	Sex	Age	Sample A				Sample B			
				Inhibition of Fraction I(%)		Inhibition of Fraction III(%)		Inhibition of Fraction I (%)		Inhibition of Fraction III (%)	
				Before Acup.	After Acup.	Before Acup.	After Acup.	Before Acup.	After Acup.	Before Acup.	After Acup.
1	Shen	M	24	58.0	105.1	74.5	79.7	36.5	102.4	30.9	62.3
2	Zhu	M	41	75.5	58.4	56.2	50.5	45.9	87.2	22.9	65.5
3	Wang	M	25	65.4	60.9	40.3	55.7	70.4	95.0	29.7	69.2
4	Mou	M	45	17.5	37.8	14.5	8.3	16.2	60.3	9.6	12.7
5	Koa	M	22	32.3	25.5	9.8	10.5	28.4	35.3	6.2	8.8
6	Fan	M	14	41.6	49.7	11.0	10.4				
7	Bie	F	33	17.6	38.3	12.8	5.9				
8	Shi	F	41	50.9	20.7	25.6	7.6				

Notes: M=male; F=female
Sample A=CSF was collected immediately after draining
Sample B=CSF was collected in the next day after draining

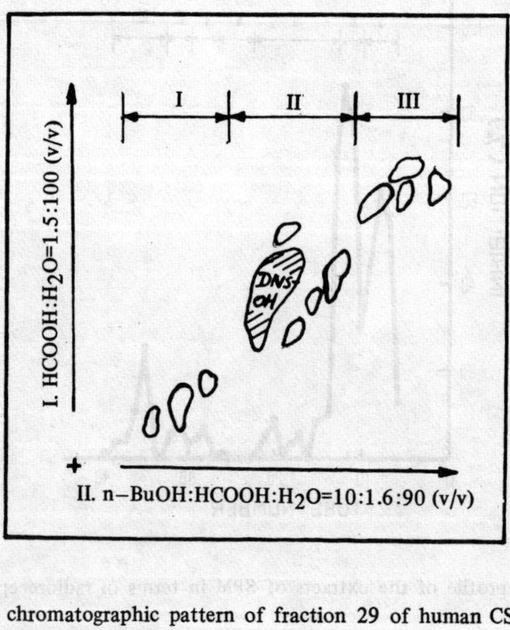

Fig. 5 The chromatographic pattern of fraction 29 of human CSF on polyamide layer sheet.

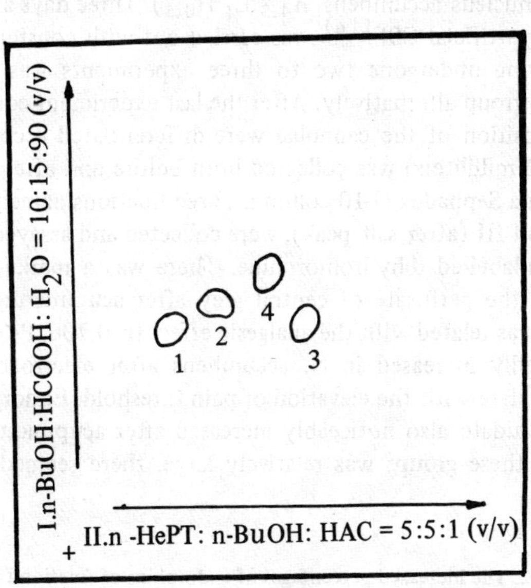

Fig. 6 The chromatagraphic pattern of fraction 29-III of human CSF.

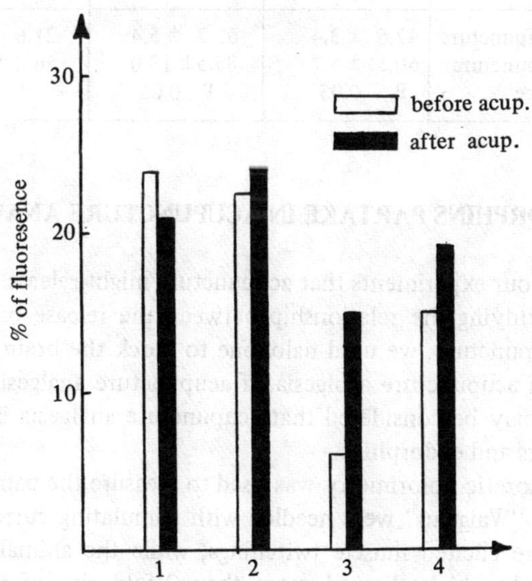

Fig. 7 The levels before and after acupuncture of fraction 29-III of human CSF.

mentioned nuclei according to Sawyer's atlas[15] (central grey, $P_{9.5}$ L_1 $H_{-1.5}$; nucleus caudate, A_2 L_3 $H_{3.5}$; nucleus accumbens, $A_{4.5}$ L_1 $H_{0.5}$). Three days after operation, push-pull perfusion by using artificial CSF[16] was carried out with constant rate and temperature. Each animal having undergone two to three experiments was treated as acupuncture group and control group alternatively. After the last experiment completed, the animals were killed and the position of the cannulae were differentiated according to histological procedure. Perfusate (2 milliliters) was collected both before and after electroacupuncture, and was eluted through a Sephadex G-10 column. Three fractions namely, I (prior to the salt peak), II (salt peak) and III (after salt peak), were collected and assayed for opiate receptor affinity against tritium-labelled dihydromorphine. There was a marked increase of endorphin on fraction I in the perfusate of central grey after acupuncture analgesia, and the increase of endorphin was related with the analgesic effect ($r=0.706$, $P<0.05$). The release of endorphins also markedly increased in N. accumbens after electroacupuncture, but the increment did not correlate with the elevation of pain threshold. Endorphins in fraction I in perfusate of nucleus caudate also noticeably increased after acupuncture. However, as the individual variation in these groups was relatively large, there seemed to be no statistical significance.

Table 2. The increased percentages of endorphins of fraction I in perfusate of central grey, nucleus caudate, and nucleus accumbens after acupuncture

Nucleus	Central grey	N. Caudate	N. Accumbens
Before acupuncture	47.6 ± 3.4	62.2 ± 5.4	21.6 ± 7.4
After acupuncture	60.5 ± 5.7	85.5± 13.0	56.3 ±10.3
Significance	P 0.05	P 0.05	P 0.01

III. ENDORPHINS PARTAKE IN ACUPUNCTURE ANALGESIA

We have found in our experiments that acupuncture might release brain endorphins[8]. For the purpose of studying the relationship between the release of endorphins and the analgesic effect of acupuncture, we used naloxone to block the brain opiate receptors and observed its effects on acupuncture analgesia. If acupuncture analgesia can be antagonized by naloxone, then it may be considered that acupuncture analgesia is related to the functions of opiate receptors and endorphins.

Potassium iontophoretic dolorimetry was used to measure the pain threshold in rabbits. Unilateral "Hegu" and "Waiguan" were needled with stimulating current 7.5–8.0 mA. The strength of acupuncture elicited muscle twitchings, while the animals were still kept in a quiet state. The animals which showed more than 2-fold rise of pain threshold during acupuncture at 20 minutes were selected to receive further experiments. These animals were divided into two groups, i.e., naloxone group and saline control group. Each animal of the naloxone group and saline group was given an intravenous injection of naloxone (0.4mg/kg) or normal saline (1 ml/kg) during acupuncture. After five minutes, the acupuncture analgesia of 75% of the animals was found to be reversed by naloxone, the average reversal of the naloxone group being 41%. It differed significantly from that of the saline group (P<0.005). After reversal, the pain threshold gradually increased and returned to its initial levels within 15 min[17] (Fig. 8).

Besides behavioral observation, we have used electrophysiological and biochemical methods to observe antagonized effect of naloxone on acupuncture analgesia. It was found that inhibitory action of electro-acupuncture upon cortical potentials evoked by tooth pulp stimulation on rabbits was antagonized by naloxone (P<0.01)[18].

We also used push-pull perfusion method and competitive protein binding assay to observe the changes of cAMP levels of the perfusate in the nucleus caudate before and after acupuncture. The level of cAMP was decreased by acupuncture significantly[19] (P<0.05). Both acupuncture analgesic effect and decreased levels of cAMP could be reversed by naloxone.

We further used the slow microinjection of naloxone (2 μg/ 2μl/ 3 min) into the central grey in rabbits. The dosage was only 1/10 of an intraventricular-effective dose and 1/400 of an intravenous-effective dose. It was found that the pain threshold was increased 206% at 20 min during acupuncture. The average reversal of pain threshold by naloxone was 33%, and

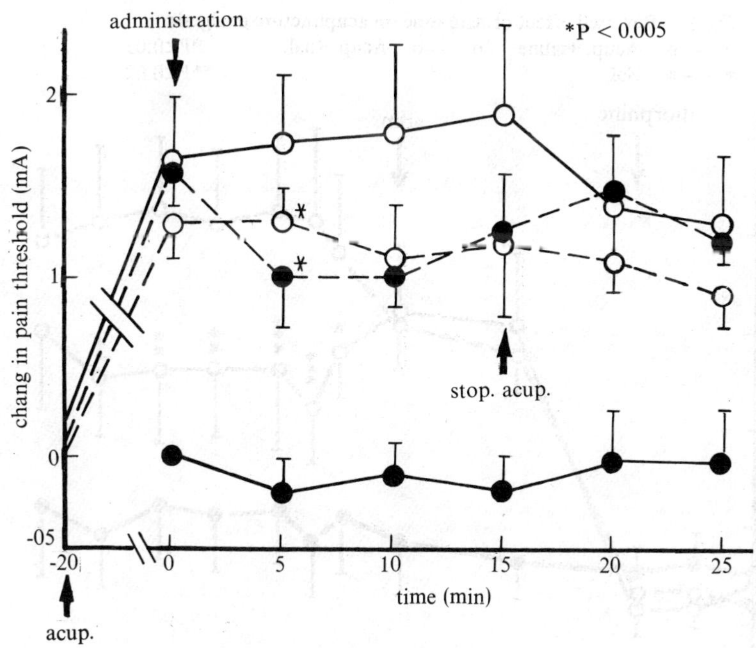

Fig. 8 The different effect of naloxone on acupuncture analgesia produced by different electro-stimulation.

o---o Super. stim. +Nal. o---o Mod. stim. +Saline

●---● Mod. stim. +Nal. ●——● Nal.

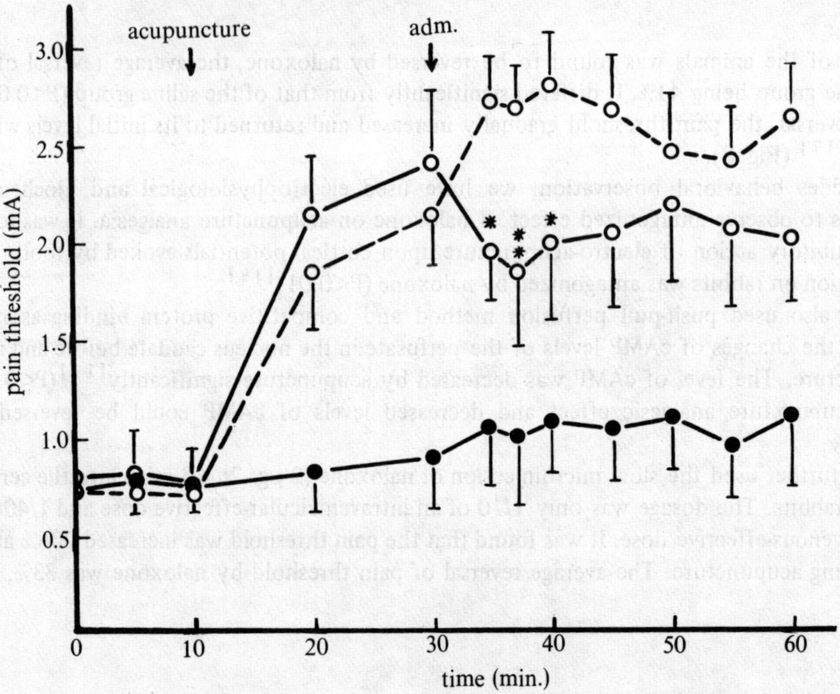

Fig. 9 Reversed effect of naloxone on acupuncture analgesia

o---o Acup. +saline   o——o Acup. +nal.   *P<0.01
●——● Nal.   **P<0.02

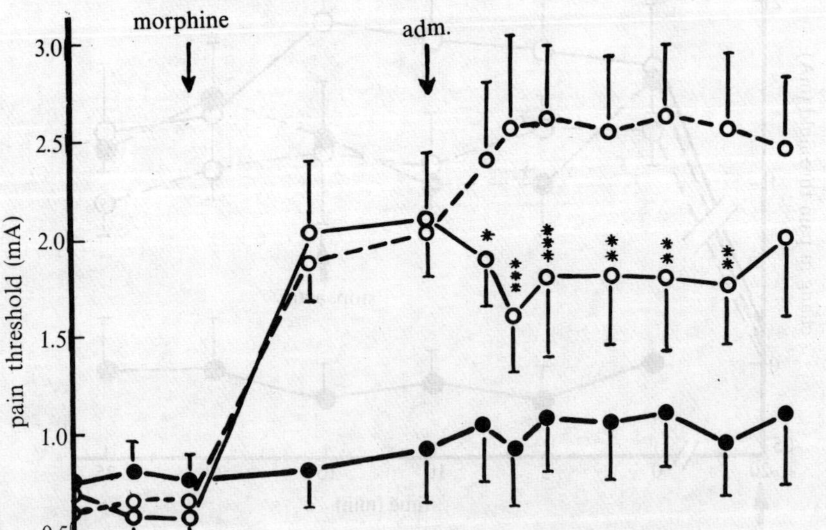

Fig. 10 Reversed effect of naloxone on morphine analgesia

o---o Morphine + saline   ●——● Nal.   *P<0.05   ****P<0.01
o——o Morphine+nal.   **P<0.02

the decrement was significantly different from that of the saline controls ($P<0.01$). While the electroacupuncture was continued, the reversed effect of naloxone could be maintained 10 min (Fig. 9). The analgesic effect of morphine (5 mg/kg iv) could be also antagonized by naloxone, and the basal pain threshold was not influenced by naloxone[20] (Fig. 10).

IV. DISCUSSION

Based on the properties observed from the eluting void column of Sephadex G–10 column, R_f values on thin layer chromatograhy, pattern of polyamide layer sheet chromatography, and ready inactivation by chymotrypsin, fraction 29 is obviously quite different from enkephalin and may be a new morphine-like substance[10].

From the results of radioreceptor assay of the eluting fraction of human CSF, there are seven active peaks (I-VII). Peak VI is fraction 29, and peak II is salt fraction. Fraction 29 not only exists in the human brain extract, but also exists in the human CSF[9].

The contents of endorphins of fractions I and III in human CSF are raised significantly after acupuncture[9]. However, in the perfusate of central grey, nucleus caudate, and nucleus accumbens, fraction I is increased markedly after acupuncture, but fraction III varies very much, and is of no significance. Because the quantity of endorphin of fraction III in 2 ml of the perfusate is very small, it is very difficult to determine the real values at the lower limit of the sensitivity of radioreceptor assay.

The analgesic effect of moderate-strength electroacupuncture (with stimulating current of 7.5–8.0 mA) can be reversed by naloxone (0.4 mg/kg iv) but the analgesic effect of superstrength electroacupuncture (with stimulating current of 12.5–15.0 mA which makes the rabbits struggle hard) cannot be reversed by naloxone. The analgesic potencies of these two kinds of acupunctures are rather alike, yet their responses to naloxone are markedly different, which suggests that the mechanism of analgesia produced by different strengths of electroacupuncture is also different. The analgesic effect of moderate strength acupuncture may partially be due to the activity of opiate receptors, while the superstrength electroacupuncture may be the stress analgesia. This result is similar to that of the levels of endorphins in human CSF collected the next day after being drained and the patients are in a quiet state. The endorphin is raised markedly after acupuncture. But the variations in the samples immediately collected after draining (before and after acupuncture) are extremely great and the statistical significance is not obtainable (table 1). It also may be due to the stress of operation.

As the naloxone (2 μg/2μl/3 min) is microinjected into the central grey of the rabbit, the analgesic effect of acupuncture is reversed 33% by naloxone. The analgesic effect of morphine (5 mg/kg iv) is reversed 35% by naloxone. This experiment indicates that the functions of central grey are very important in acupuncture analgesia as well as morphine analgesia in the central analgesic system.

Since central grey is an important relay of the central pain pathway, it receives convergent and somatotropically organizes somatosensory input, then inhibits the input of noxious stimuli in the dorsal horn of the spinal cord, via a descending inhibiting pathway. This negative feedback mechanism might be the main part of central analgesic mechanism. Acupunctural signals may get to central grey by way of the somatosensory input path, thus activating the central analgesic mechanism.

According to our investigations, it may be suggested that the endorphins partake in acupuncture analgesia from presynaptic level to receptor sites. The studies on endorphin release and antagonist microinjections indicate that the endorphins are closely related to acupuncture analgesia. The functions of endorphins play a far more important role than just analgesia, and the analgesic neuropeptides in the central system consist of more than endorphins, which should be further studied.

V. SUMMARY

The contents of endorphins of fractions I, III and 29 in human CSF are increased significantly after electroacupuncture. Using the techniques of push-pull perfusion, we have observed the release of endorphins after acupuncture in central grey, nucleus caudate and nucleus accumbens. It shows that endorphins are related to the acupuncture analgesia. Electroacupuncture may increase the pain thresholds of rabbits, inhibit the cortical potentials evoked by tooth pulp stimulation on rabbits, and decrease cAMP levels of the perfusates in the nucleus caudate. These effects can be reversed by naloxone. Our results show that the endorphins partake in acupuncture analgesia from presynatic levels to receptor sites.

REFERENCES

[1] Hughes, J. *et al.*: *Nature,* **258**:577, 1975.

[2] Nauta, W. J. H.: *Neurosci. Res. Prog. Bull.*, **13**:84, 1975.

[3] Tortella, E.C. *et al.*: *Fed. Proc.*, 37:237, 1978.

[4] Mayer, D. J. *et al.*: *Brain Res.*, 68:73, 1974.

[5] Li, C.H. *et al.*: *Nature,* **263**:239, 1976.

[6] Mayer, D. J. *et al.*: *Brain Res.,* **121**:368, 1977.

[7] 江振裕等：动物学报 **24**：1，1978。

[8] Zhang Anzhong, *et al.*: *National Symposia of Acupuncture and Moxibustion and Acupuncture Anesthesia,* p 481, Beijing, 1979.

[9] Pan Xiaoping, *et al.*: *National Symposia of Acupuncture and Moxibustion and Acupuncture Anesthesia.* p. 479, Beijing, 1979.

[10] 上海第一医学院针麻原理研究协作组：中华医学杂志 58：611，1978。

[11] Pert, C. B. *et al.*: *Science,* **179**:1011, 1973.

[12] Smith, T.W. *et al.*: "Enkephalins: Isolation, Distribution and Function," in *Opiate and Endogenous Opioid Peptides* (Ed Kosterlitz), p.57–62, Amsterdam, 1976.

[13] Gray, W.R., *Methods in Enzymology* vol. XI (Ed. Hirs C.H.W.), Academic Press Inc. N.Y. 1967, p. 139–155.

[14] Zhang Anzhong, *et al.*: *National Symposia of Acupuncture and Moxibustion and Acupuncture Anesthesia.* p. 480, Beijing, 1979.

[15] Sawyer, C.H. *et al.*: *J.Comp.Neurol.,* **101**:801, 1954.

[16] Pappenheimer, J.R. *et al.*: *Am. J.Physiol.,* **203**:763, 1962.

[17] Zhang Anzhong, *et al.*: *National Symposia of Acupuncture and Moxibustion and Acupuncture Anesthesia,* p. 484, Beijing, 1979.

[18] 程介士等：中华医学杂志 **59**：257，1979。

[19] 许绍芬等：科学通报 **24**：761，1979。

[20] 上海第一医学院基础医学部针麻研究组：上海第一医学院学报 **5**：186，1978。

ENKEPHALIN INVOLVEMENT IN ACUPUNCTURE ANALGESIA—RADIOIMMUNOASSAY

Zou Gang, Yi Qingcheng, Wu Shixiang,
Lu Yixin,* Wang Fansheng, Yu Yuegui,
Ji Xinquan, Zhang Zuxuan,** Zhao Dandan
(Shanghai Institute of Materia Medica, Academia Sinica)

In recent years the discovery of endogenous morphine-like peptides (endorphins)[1] has given a new impetus to the research of the intrinsic antinociceptive mechanism of the nervous system[2]. Attention has naturally been paid to the role of these substances in acupuncture analgesia. Indirect support for this postulate was provided by naloxone partial reversal of human acupuncture analgesia[3]. However, naloxone can reverse analgesia produced by many factors[4]; it is thus necessary to measure directly the alterations of endorphin contents in acupuncture. Sjölund et al.[5] reported that electric acupuncture of the lower limb could increase endorphin levels in cerebrospinal fluid (CSF) collected by lumbar puncture. Han *et al.*[6], using radioreceptor assay, also found an increase of total morphine-like substance in the whole brain of rats after electric acupuncture. Since there are varieties of endogenous morphine-like substances differing in distribution and probably also in function[2, 7], it seemed necessary to measure them separately in order to explain the theory of acupuncture analgesia. Therefore we have set up radioimmunoassays (RIA) for met- and leu-enkephalin, the main endorphins in the brain, and employed it in determining the changes of enkephalin contents in the brain and CSF during acupuncture.

I. METHODS

(I) Establishment of RIA for enkephalin

Met- and leu-enkephalin differ only in one amino acid in the carboxyl terminals. In preparing immunogens, therefore, polylysine was linked through succinic acid to their N-terminals according to Theres[8]. The rate of condensation was 90%. Every 2.3 lysine residues were condensed with one met-enkephalin, and every 3.2 lysine residues with one leu-enkephalin. Rabbits were innoculated intradermally in multiple sites. Antisera were

* Shanghai Research for Hypertension.

** Visiting investigator from the Department of Biology, Nanjing University.

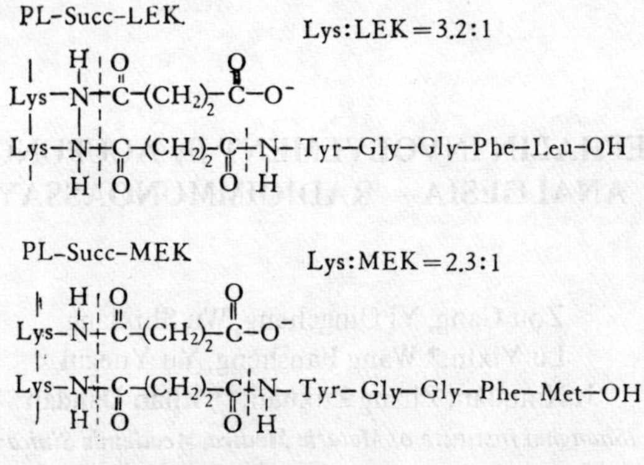

Fig. 1 Two enkephalin immunogens.
PL, Polylysine; succ, succinic acid; LEK, leu-enkephalin; MEK, met-enkephalin; lys-lysine.

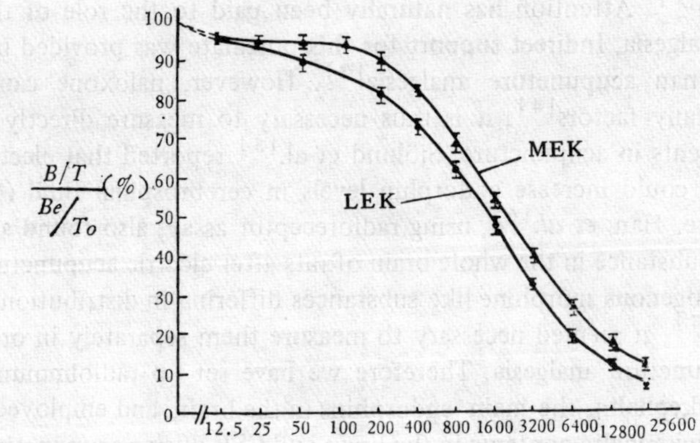

Fig. 2 RIA Competitive inhibition curves of two enkephalins.

obtained after 3–6 months and were used at a dilution of 1:5,000 in RIA, and the keff of the antisera was 10^9 litre/mole. ^{125}I-labelled enkephalins were prepared by Chloramine T method, and purified by DEAE-Sephadex A-25 column chromatography. During RIA, free and bound ^{125}I-enkephalins were separated with double antibody technique. The competitive inhibition curves (Fig. 2) showed that the smallest assayable amount of leu-enkephalin was 18 pg, and that of met-enkephalin was 130 pg. There were no conspicuous cross reactions between β-endorphin and these two antisera, as shown in Fig. 3. Eight peptides, i.e., vasopressin, oxytocin, angiotensin I & II, bradykinin, TSH, insulin, LRH and morphine and naloxone also showed no noticeable cross reactions when 10 ng of which were added into each assay tube. The cross reaction of met-enkephalin with the antiserum of leu-enkephalin was 3.3%, while that of leu-enkephalin with the antiserum of met-enkephalin was less than 1%. The detailed procedure of setting up the RIA for enkephalins will be published elsewhere[9].

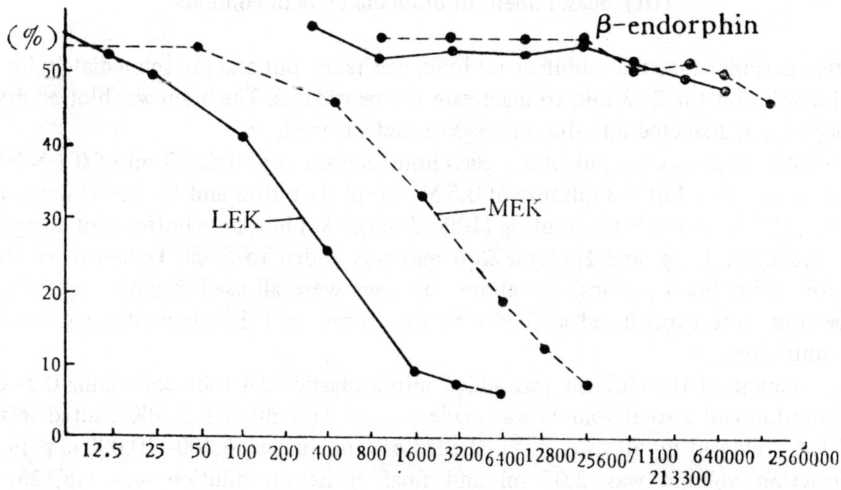

Fig. 3 Rate of cross reaction between β-endorphin and leu-and met-enkephalin antisera..

(II) Pain threshold evaluation and method of acupuncture

1. Rabbits. Rabbits weighing about 2 kg of both sexes were restrained in wooden boxes or hung up in cotton pocket for pain threshold evaluation with potassium iontophoresis. One electrode was fixed on each ear tip. Sudden struggle after closing the circuit was taken as the pain response, and the electric current in mA at this moment was recorded[10]. Pain threshold was measured once every 10 min for 3 times, and the average was taken as the basal pain threshold. Manual twirling of the acupuncture points Zusanli on both hind legs continued for 30 min. After withdrawal of the needles, pain threshold was again measured. The rabbit was decapitated immediately and brain dissected or 1 ml of CSF was taken by cisternal puncture under local anesthesia. Enkephalin contents were then determined by RIA.

2. Rats. Rats weighing 200–220 g of both sexes were restrained in lucite containers. Electrodes for pain stimulation were fixed on the tail and tail-flick response latencies were determined by a Beihung 57–9A skin pain stimulator[11]. In later stage, we used the radiant heat method. The latency was measured every 5 min for 3 times, and the average taken as the basal pain threshold. Electric acupuncture was carried out with two stainless steel needles through the acupuncture point Huantiao of both hind thighs with a G 6805 therapeutic stimulator for 30 min. The wave form was "dense and sparse";pain threshold was measured again 5 sec after the cessation of electric acupuncture. Rats were decapitated and brain dissected immediately. Enkephalin contents were measured by RIA.

(III) Measurement of brain enkephalin contents

After decapitation, the rabbit or rat brain was taken out and put immediately into boiling saline solution for 2–3 min to inactivate the peptidases. The brain was blotted dry with filter papers and dissected into discrete regions and weighed.

Rat brain regions were put into a glass homogenizer containing 3 ml of 0.1 N HCl and homogenized. One ml of 7:3 mixture of 0.5 M phosphate buffer and 1N NaOH was added to adjust to pH 7.8. Then PELH solution (100 ml of 0.1 M phosphate buffer containing EDTA 0.11g, lysozyme 1 mg, and Hibitane 200 mg) was added to 5 ml. Owing to the heavier weight of rabbit brain regions, the above solutions were all used in double quantity. The homogenates were centrifuged at 3,300 Xg for 30 min and the supernatants stored below –20°C until assay.

Supernatant of 0.5–0.7 ml was added into a plastic RIA tube containing 0.3–0.5 ml PELH solution and a total volume was made of 1 ml. One ml of 1:2, 500 diluted antiserum was added, followed by 50 μl of ^{125}I-labelled enkephalin (ca. 6,000–10,000 c. p. m.). The final reaction volume was 2.05 ml and final antiserum dilution was 1:5,125. After incubation at 4°C for 24 hr, 30 μl of 1:12 diluted normal rabbit serum and 60 μl or sheep anti-rabbit γ-globulin were added in sequence into each assay tube, which was incubated at 4° C for another 20 hr. After centrifugation at low temperature, the supernatant was discarded and the radioactivity in the precipitate was counted in a single channel gamma-spectrometer. The percentage value of B/T in each tube was calculated. The enkephalin content was read from the standard curve of the same experiment, and finally converted into pg per mg wet weight of brain tissue. Each assay tube had its duplicate.

II. RESULTS

(I) Alterations in regional enkephalin contents during acupuncture analgesia

1. Rabbits. Measurement of pain threshold in seven control rabbits every 10 min for 5 times showed no noticeable changes. Two enkephalin contents expressed in wet weight were highest in hypothalamus and striatum, next in brainstem and cortex, and lowest in hippocampus and thalamus. Six rabbits of the acupuncture group showed a change of 79.1± 8.0% rise in pain threshold after manual needling ($P<0.001$). The most prominent increases in regional enkephalin contents were in the hypothalamus (1.6–1.8 times, $P<0.005$) and the striatum (1.6–1.7 times, $P<0.01$) (Fig. 4). Alterations in other brain regions were of no statistical significance.

2. Rats. Pain threshold measurements in 6 control rats every 5 min for 4 times showed no noticeable changes. Enkephalin contents were measured in hypothalamus, striatum, nucleus accumbens, thalamus and brainstem. Contents in unit wet weight were found to be much higher in the rat brain than in rabbit, and the level in the rat thalamus was not so low as that in the rabbit. Pain threshold increased prominently in 6 rats of the electric acupuncture group, being 92±22% higher than the basal pain threshold ($P<0.01$). The

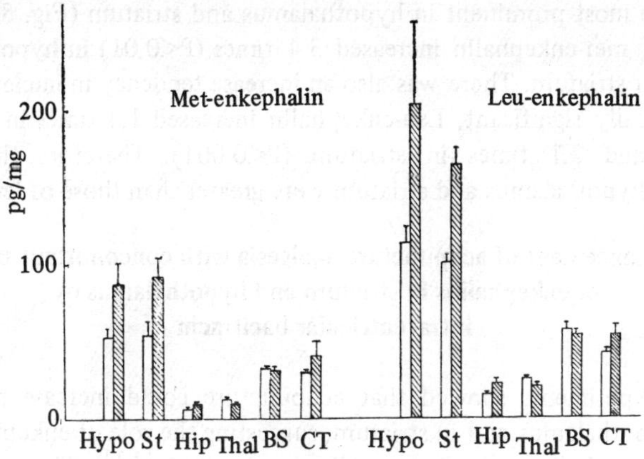

Fig. 4 Effect of acupuncture on rabbit brain regional contents of enkephalins.
White wolumn, control group;
Striated column, acupuncture group;
Hypo, hypothalamus;
St, striatum;
Hip, hippocampus;
Thal, thalamus;
BS, brainstem;
CT, cortex.

Met-Enkephalin Leu-Enkephalin Pg/mg Hypo St HiP Thal BS CT Hypo St HiP Thal BS Ct

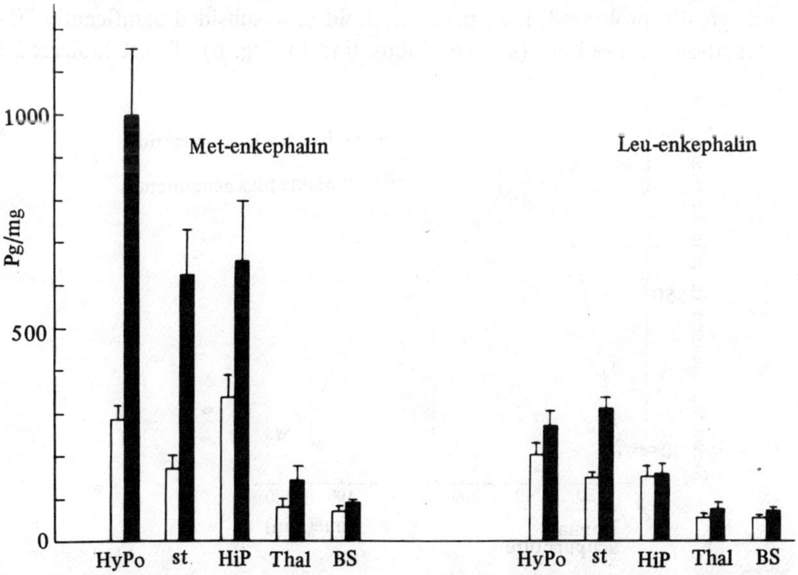

Fig. 5 Effect of acupuncture on rat brain regional contents of enkephalins.
White column Control group
Striated colum n Acupuncture group
See other abbreviations in Fig. 4.

increases were also most prominent in hypothalamus and striatum (Fig. 5). Compared with the control group, met-enkephalin increased 3.4 times ($P<0.01$) in hypothalamus and 3.6 times ($P<0.005$) in striatum. There was also an increase tendency in nucleus accumbens but it was not statistically significant. Leu-enkephalin increased 1.4 times in hypothalamus (P approach 0.05), and 2.1 times in striatum ($P<0.001$). Therefore the increments of met-enkephalin in hypothalamus and striatum were greater than those of leu-enkephalin.

(II) Enhancement of acupuncture analgesia with concomittant increase of enkephalins in striatum and hypothalamus by intraventricular bacitracin

The above experiments showed that acupuncture could increase prominently both enkephalins in hypothalamus and in striatum, suggesting the role of enkephalins in acupuncture analgesia. Enkephalins degraded rapidly in the brain[12]. The peptidase inhibitor bacitracin retarded their degradation *in vitro*[12–14] and potentiated their analgesic effect *in vivo*[15]. Therefore, intraventricular administration of bacitracin was used to observe whether there was an enhancement in acupuncture analgesia in order to search for the possible relation between alterations in enkephalin levels and analgesic effect.

1. Enhancement of acupuncture analgesia. Five control rabbits with intraventricular injection of 0.05 ml saline solution showed a prominent increase in pain threshold after manual acupuncture. The raised threshold gradually subsided and virtually returned to pre-acupuncture level 30 min after the cessation of needling (see dotted line in Fig. 6). Five rabbits in the bacitracin group showed no change in pain threshold 10 min after intraventricular injection of 50 ug/0.05 ml. Although the amplitude of increase in the bacitracin plus acupuncture group was similar to that in the saline plus acupuncture group, the duration of analgesia was greatly prolonged, i. e., pain threshold only subsided significantly 70–80 min after the cessation of needling (see continous line in Fig. 6). T test indicated that the

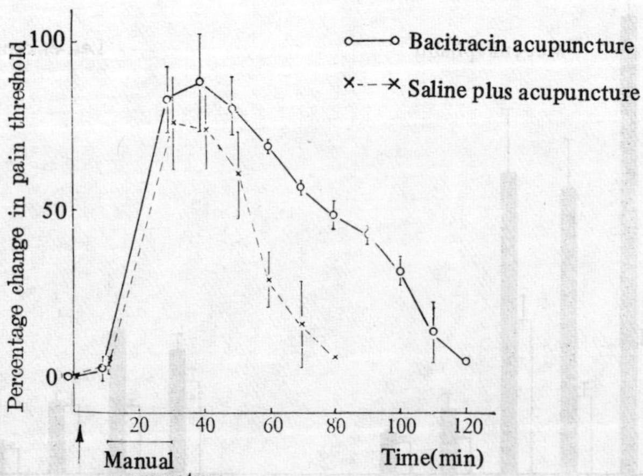

Fig. 6 Enhancement of acupuncture analgesia by intraventricular bacitracin
Arrow designates intraventricular injection of bacitracin

difference of analgesic areas between saline manual acupuncture group and bacitracin plus acupuncture group was obviously significant ($P<0.001$). This experiment indicated that the enhancement of acupuncture analgesia by intraventricular bacitracin was mainly in the prolongation of analgesia.

2. Effects on the alteration of enkephalin contents induced by acupuncture. Twelve rabbits with indwelling intraventricular cannulae were divided randomly into 3 groups: (1) bacitracin, (2) saline plus manual acupuncture, and (3) bacitracin plus manual acupuncture. Same dosage of bacitracin was used. Rabbits in groups 2 and 3 were decapitated 30 min after the cessation of needling, and those of group 1 were decapitated at the corresponding time. Measurement just before decapitation showed that pain threshold was still very highly elevated in group 3, but had already returned to preacupuncture level in the saline plus acupuncture group (group 2). The difference was obviously significant ($P<0.01$). The regional enkephalin contents are presented in Fig. 7. It could be seen that the most prominent increases were again in the hypothalamus and in the striatum. In the former region, the content in group 3 was 40% higher than the contents in groups 1 and 2. Met-enkephalin increased very markedly ($P<0.01$) and leu-enkephalin increased markedly ($P<0.05$). In the striatum, the contents of both enkephalins increased even more, being 2–3 times the content of the bacitracin group ($P<0.01$) and 50–100% higher than the content of saline plus acupuncture group ($P<0.05$ and <0.01). These results effectivelt substantiated the postulate that the bacitracin prolongation of acupuncture analgesia is due to retardation of the enzymatic breakdown of enkephalins.

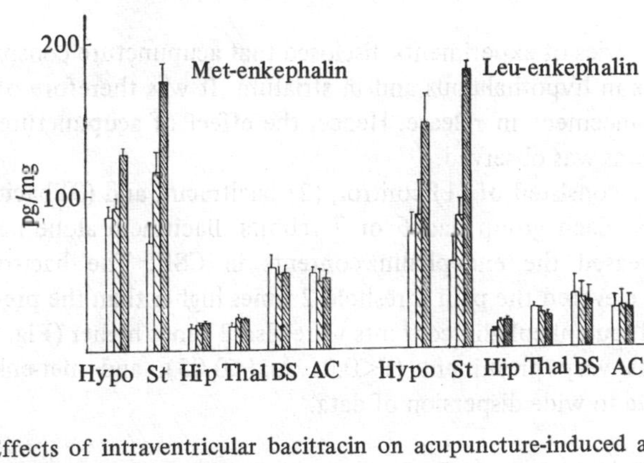

Fig. 7 Effects of intraventricular bacitracin on acupuncture-induced alteration of brain enkephalin contents.
White column, intraventricular bacitracin; striated column, intraventricular saline plus acupuncture; black column, intraventricular bacitracin plus acupuncture; decapitated and dissected at 30 min after the cessation of needling.
AC, nucleus accumbens; other abbreviations see Fig. 4.

3. Naloxone reversal of the bacitracin-prolonged acupuncture analgesia. Bacitracin inhibited many peptidases. In order to gain further support that bacitracin enhancement was actually mediated by endogenous morphine-like substances, naloxone reversal experiments were carried out. Five rabbits were injected with bacitracin and manually acupunctured as above. Naloxone 0.2 mg/kg was administered intravenously 30 min after the cessation of

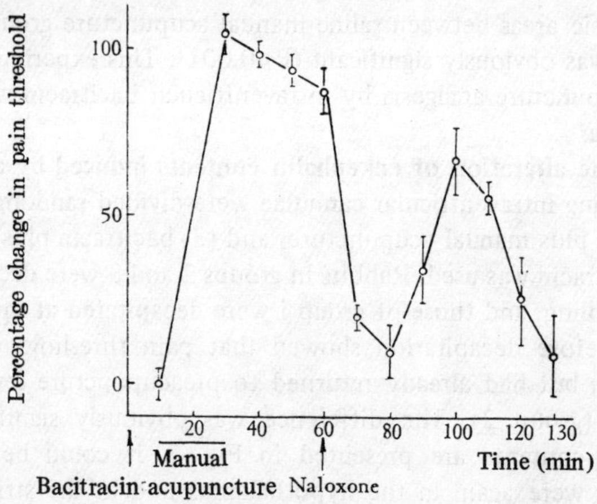

Fig. 8 Naloxone reversal of bacitracin prolonged-acupuncture analgesia.

needling, and prominent reversal of acupuncture analgesia was observed (Fig. 8) for about 30 min.

(III) Increased levels of enkephalins in the cisternal CSF of rabbits during acupuncture

The above two series of experiments disclosed that acupuncture conspicuously increased enkephalin contents in hypothalamus and in striatum. It was therefore of interest to see if there was also enhancement in release. Hence, the effect of acupuncture on cisternal CSF content of enkephalins was observed.

The experiment consisted of (1) control, (2) bacitracin, and (3) bacitracin plus manual acupuncture groups. Each group had 6 or 7 rabbits. Bacitracin alone neither elevated the threshold nor increased the enkephalin contents in CSF. The bacitracin plus manual acupuncture group elevated the pain threshold 2 times higher than the pre-acupuncture level ($P<0.01$). Met- and leu-enkephalin contents were also 2 times higher (Fig. 9), the increase of leu-enkephaline was very prominent ($P<0.01$ and <0.05), and met-enkephalins P value approached 0.05 due to wide dispersion of data.

(IV) Acceleration of enkephalin biosynthesis by acupuncture

Enkephalin contents in hypothalamus, striatum and CSF were increased by acupuncture. It has been reported that cycloheximide, the protein-synthesis inhibitor, might inhibit the incorporation of tritium-labelled tyrosine into enkephalins in vitro[16]. To study the mechanism of increase in enkephalin contents by acupuncture, we observed its *in vivo* effect with intraventricular injection[17] on acupuncture analgesia and met-enkephalin contents in hypothalamus and in striatum.

Thirty-eight rats were divided into 4 groups: (1) control, 10 rats, (2) electric acupuncture, 10 rats, (3) cycloheximide, 9 rats, and (4) cycloheximide plus electric acupuncture, 9

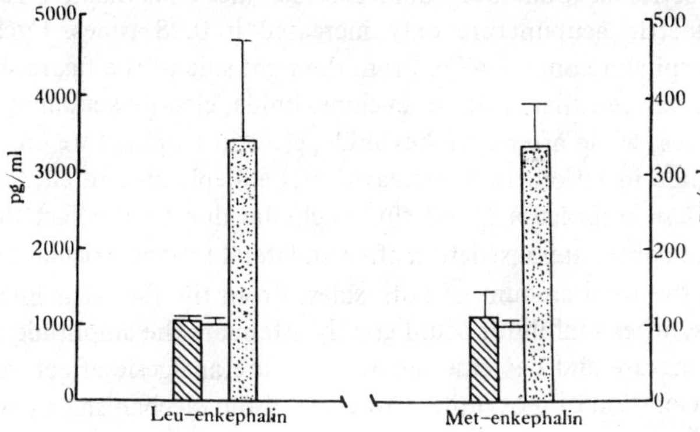

Fig. 9 **Increased enkephalin levels of cisternal cerebrospinal fluid of rabbits during acupuncture.**
Striated column, Control;
White column Intraventricular bacitracin
Dotted column Intraventricular bacitracin plus manual acupuncture

rats. The dosage of cycloheximide was 500μg/10μl. Experiments were performed 24 hr after cycloheximide injection.

The results of pain threshold measurement of acupuncture analgesia are as follows: As compared with the control group, pain threshold increased 206±32.8% in the electric acupuncture group with a very significant difference (P<0.001), while it increased only 43% in the cycloheximide plus acupuncture group. Cycloheximide injection alone did not prominently change the pain threshold, i.e., only about 11 % increase (P>0.05). Metenkephalin contents were determined in the hypothalamus and in the striatum—two regions with most prominent increase of enkephalins during acupuncture, as illustrated in Fig. 10. From the left side of the figure denoting hypothalamus, it can be seen that, without

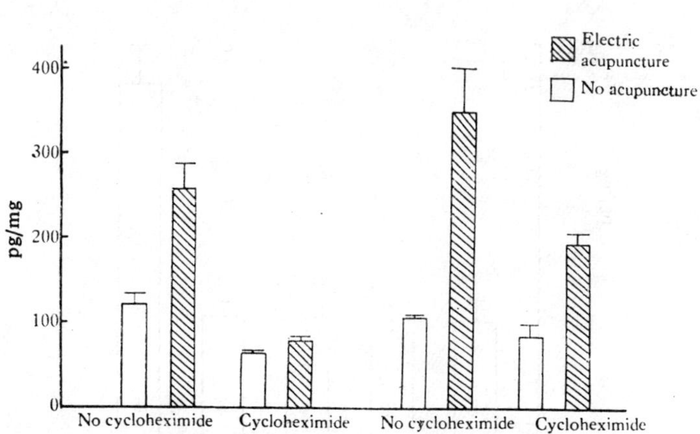

Fig. 10 **Effect of intraventricular cycloheximide on acupuncture-induced alteration of met-enkephalin contents in hypothalamus and striatum.**

cycloheximide, electric acupuncture could increase met-enkephalin 1.13 times, but after cycloheximide, electric acupuncture only increased it 0.28 times. Cycloheximide alone decreased met-enkephalin content 47%. From the right side of the figure showing the results in striatum, it can be seen that, without cycloheximide, electric acupuncture increased met-enkephalin 2.2 times, while after cycloheximide, electric acupuncture only increased it 1.23 times. Cycloheximide injection itself decreased met-enkephalin content 20%. The effect on the striatum was less conspicuous, and this might be due to the fact that cycloheximide could not reach the contralateral striatum after unilateral intraventricular injection, but what we measured was the total amount of both sides. From the fact that intraventricular injection of a protein-synthesis inhibitor could greatly attenuate the amplitude of met-enkephalin increase by acupuncture and decrease the acupuncture analgesic effect, a conclusion could be drawn that acceleration of biosynthesis was one of the mechanisms by which acupuncture increases enkephalin content.

(V) Effect of surgical isolation of hypothalamus on met-enkephalin therein and acupuncture analgesia

Acupuncture greatly elevated enkephalin contents in the hypothalamus and in the striatum. There have been many reports suggesting a role of caudate nucleus, a constituent part of the striatum, in acupuncture analgesia, but relatively few on hypothalamus. In addition to enkephalinergic neurones, β-endorphinergic nerve cell bodies reside exclusively in the basal hypothalamus[18,19]. Therefore we isolated the hypothalamus from the rest of the brain with Halasz knife, and observed its effect on met-enkephalin content therein and acupuncture analgesia in order to know the role of enkephalinergic and /or β-endorphinergic neurones in the hypothalamus.

Experiments were performed in five groups: (1) normal control, (2) hypothalamus isolation, (3) hypothalamus isolation plus electric acupuncture, (4) sham operation (mere insertion of the Halasz knife without circumsection), and (5) sham operation plus electric

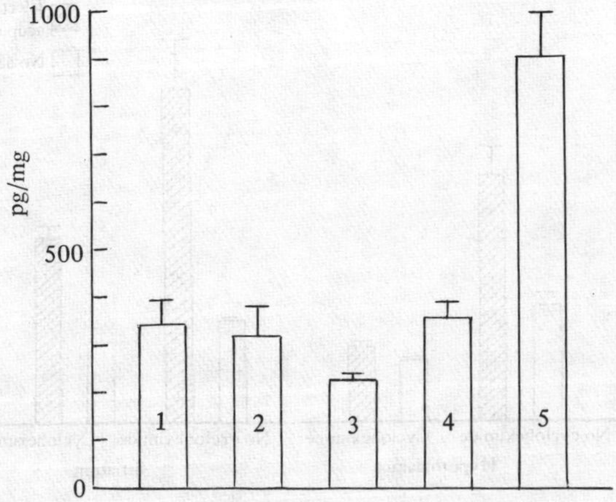

Fig. 11 Effect of hypothalamus isolation on met-enkephalin content there in.

acupuncture. No noticeable change in pain threshold was found in groups 1, 2 and 4 within 60 min. Group 5 showed a marked increase in pain threshold after acupuncture, and the difference between group 4 and group 5 was very significant ($P<0.005$). Pain threshold of group 3 could still be elevated but not to such an extent as that of group 5. There was a significant difference between them ($P<0.05$). These results indicated that hypothalamus isolation attenuated but did not eliminate acupuncture analgesic effect.

The weight of isolated hypothalamus was 12–14 mg. Met-enkephalin contents are shown in Fig. 11. Group 5 increased markedly, and a significant difference existed between group 5 and the other four groups ($P<0.001$). Group 3 decreased a little rather than increased, but the decrease was not significant from groups 1, 2 and 4. This experiment indicated a role of hypothalamus in acupuncture analgesia but it was not the sole mechanism.

III. DISCUSSION

This paper indicates that acupuncture could prominently increase brain enkephalin contents in specific regions, i. e., hypothalamus, striatum, and probably also nucleus accumbens. Furthermore, similar results were obtained on two animal species though acupunctured differently. All these speak in favor of the assumption that enkephalin plays a role in acupuncture analgesia. Further support came from the bacitracin experiments. Intraventricular injection of bacitracin itself had no analgesic effect, but could effectively prolong acupuncture analgesia. Corresponding enhanced increases of enkephalin contents were also observed. This prolonged analgesia could be reversed by the opiate antagonist naloxone. Injection of bacitracin alone did not elevate brain and CSF contents of enkephalines, but prominently enhanced the increase by acupuncture, indicating that the enkephalinergic neurones were in a low level of activity at resting state, but greatly activated during acupuncture.

In regard to the mechanism of the elevation of enkephalin level, according to the fact that acupuncture no longer increased met-enkephalin content in the hypothalamus after deafferentation, the incoming impulses were essential. Besides, after intraventricular injection of cycloheximide, the protein-synthesis inhibitor, the amplitude of met-enkephalin increase by acupuncture was greatly reduced, indicating that acupuncture accelerated enkephalin biosynthesis and consequently increased enkephalin contents. Other mechanisms remain to be studied.

Hypothalamus isolation attenuated electric acupuncture analgesia. Because β-endorphinergic nerve cell bodies resided exclusively in the basal hypothalamus, after isolation, the extrahypothalamic projections of β-endorphinergic fibres should degenerate. It was thus possible that the reduction of acupuncture analgesia after hypothalamus isolation could be attributed partly to the elimination of the functions of β-endorphinergic neurones.

According to microinjection studies[21, 22], the most affective sites of morphine action located in the periventricular are periaqueductal gray (PVG-PAG). Hypothalamus can be considered as an integral part of the PVG of the third ventricle. The striatum constituting the lateral walls of the two lateral ventricles may release enkephalins into the CSF during acupuncture and then act on the PVG-PAG to induce analgesia. But the brain regions we measured were still too big and homogenized, and the high density of enkephalins localized in a small area might be masked. Therefore, we cannot rule out other regions such as periaqueductal gray as sites where enkephalin content may also be increased by acupuncture. In this respect immunohistochemical studies may yield fruitful results.

IV. ABSTRACT

Since there are several endogenous morphine-like substances differing in distribution and probably also in function,[2, 7] it seemes necessary to study their roles in acupuncture analgesia separately. Therefore we set up a sensitive and specific radioimmunoassay (RIA) for met- and leu-enkephalin, and employed it in determing the changes of enkephalin contents of rabbits and rats in the brain regions and CSF during acupuncture. The main results are as follows: (1) two enkephalins increase markedly in hypothalamus and in striatum during acupuncture analgesia; (2) prior intraventricular bacitracin enhances the acupuncture analgesia with concomittant increased contents of enkephalins in the brain and CSF; (3) cycloheximide, the proteinsynthesis inhibitor, reduces the enkephalin-increasing effect of acupuncture, indicating that one of the mechanisms by which acupuncture elevates the enkephalin levels is the acceleration of biosynthesis; (4) after surgical isolation of rat hypothalamus, the effect of electric acupuncture is attenuated. This indicates that hypothalamus takes part in acupuncture analgesia.

REFERENCES

[1] Hughes, J.: *Brain Res.*, 88:295, 1975.

[2] 邹 冈 易庆成: 生理科学进展 **9**: 2, 1978。

[3] Mayer, D.J., *et al.*: *Brain Res.,* **121**:368, 1977.

[4] Hayes, R., *et al.*: *Science,* **196**:600, 1977.

[5] Sjölund, B., *et al.*: *Acta Physiol. Scan.*, **100**:382, 1977.

[6] 韩济生等: 生理学报 **30**: 201, 1978。

[7] Rossier, J., *et al.*: *Proc. Nat. Acad. Sci. USA*, 74:5162, 1977.

[8] Therese, E.H.: *J. Clin. Endocr.*, **29**:1349, 1969.

[9] 陆以信等: 脑啡肽的放射免疫测定,待发表。

[10] 易庆成等: 中国科学 **20**: 113, 1977。

[11] 易庆成等: 科学通报 **22**: 43, 1977。

[12] Meek, J.L., *et al.*: *Neuropharmacology,* **16**:154, 1977.

[13] Minneman, K.P. and Iversen, L.L.: *Nature,* **262**:313, 1976.

[14] Miller, R.J., *et al.*: *Biochem. Biophys. Res. Comm.*, **74**:1311, 1977.

[15] 邹 冈等: 甲一脑啡肽及其它数种神经肽脑室内注射镇痛效应的观察,待发表。

[16] Sosa, R.P. *et al.*: *FEBS Lett.*, **84**: 195, 1977.

[17] Hong, J.S., *et al.*: *Brain Res.*, **160**:192, 1979.

[18] Bloom, F.E., *et al.*: *Proc. Nat. Acad. Sci. USA*, 75:1591, 1978.

[19] Watson, S.J., *et al.*: *Nature,* **275**:226, 1978.

[20] Hala'sz, B. and Pupp, L.: *Endocrinology,* 77:553, 1965.

[21] Tsou, K. and Jang, C.S.: *Scientia Sinica,* 13:1099, 1964.

[22] Pert, A. and Yaksh, T.L.: *Brain Res.*, 80:135, 1974.

EFFECT OF INTRACEREBRAL MICROINJECTION OF NALOXONE ON ACUPUNCTURE AND MORPHINE-ANALGESIA IN THE RABBIT

Zhou Zhongfu, Du Mingyi, Wu Wenying,
Jiang Ying,* Han Jisheng
(Research Group of Acupuncture Anesthesia, Beijing Medical College)

The discovery of the uneven distribution of endogenous opiate-like substances (OLS) in brain substrates and their coexistence with opiate receptors have prompted an intensive survey of their possible participation in a series of physiological and pathological events. The study of the possible role of OLS in acupuncture analgesia (AA) has proceeded along two parallel and reciprocal lines. Blockade of opiate receptors with narcotic antagonist naloxone has been proved to decrease the effectiveness of AA in humans[1, 2], monkeys[3], cats[4], mice[5] and rabbits[6]. On the other hand it was found that acupuncture increased the OLS content in cerebrospinal fluid (CSF) in humans[7, 8]. In rats, electroacupuncture raised the content of OLS in the brain by 33% and the amplitude of increase in individual animals was found to be positively correlated with its analgesic effect[9]. All these data point to the conclusion that the central OLS is important for the mediation of AA.

After the importance of OLS in AA is ascertained, efforts are directed to the problem of its site of action. There are certain brain areas such as the nucleus accumbens, amygdala, habenula and periaqueductal grey (PAG) which are rich both in opiate receptors and endogenous OLS[10−12]. Some of them have been proved to play an active role in morphine analgesia (MA)[13, 14]. In the present study we attempted to evaluate the possible involvement of OLS in these brain areas for the mediation of AA by injectinga minute amount of narcotic antagonist naloxone into bilateral target nuclei and monitoring its effect on AA. For the sake of comparison, parallel experiments were also performed on the same animal to observe the effect of microinjection of naloxone on MA.

I. MATERIALS AND METHODS

1. Implantation of intracranial cannulae. Male rabbits weighing about 2.4kg each were used. The animal was anesthetized with sodium pentobarbital (30mg/kg) and mounted on a stereotaxic apparatus. Stainless steel cannulae with outer diameter of 0.9mm were implanted and fixed on the skull bilaterally. The coordinates selected according to Bureš[15] and

*Present address: Nanjing Pharmaceutical College.

Sawyer's[16] atlas were as follows: nucleus accumbens, A6.0, L1.2, H8.5; amygdala, P2.0, L6.0, H15.0; habenula, P5.0, L1.5, H7.5; periaqueductal grey, P9.5, L1.0, H10.0; inferior horn of lateral ventricle, P3.0, L8.5, H12.5; third ventricle, P5.0 Lo, H9.0. A stainless steel wire with a plastic cap was inserted into the cannula to keep it sealed. During the experiment, an injection tube with outer diameter of 0.4mm was introduced into the guide cannula and protruded out of it for 1.5mm to reach the injection site. The experiments were started one week after the surgical operation and completed in 5 weeks.

2. Algometry and acupuncture. The rabbits were hung up with their eyes covered. Radiant heat was applied to the skin around the nostrils and mouth and the latency of head withdrawal reaction was recorded as the "pain threshold". Assessments were carried out every 5 minutes for 3 times. The latencies of the first 3 measurements were averaged as the basal pain threshold. After that, the animal was given constant rate intracerebral injection which lasted for 20 minutes. Ten minutes after the beginning of intracerebral injection, the animal was given either an intravenous injection of morphine (4mg/kg) or a session of "finger acupuncture" which consists of rhythmic finger pressing (2/sec) of the Kunlun point for 10 minutes. Nociceptive tests were then made every 10 minutes for a total of 5 measurements. The values were compared with the basal pain threshold and expressed in percentage changes, taking +200% as the cut-off value so as to avoid burning of the skin. The method has been described in detail elsewhere[17, 18].

For the sake of comparison, some of the animals were given electroacupuncture with the needles inserted into point Zusanli and Kunlun and electrified with DZ-62 electronic stimulator which delivered a series of dense and sparse impulses, the amplitude of the main wave being 1.5V. Electroacupuncture lasted for 10 minutes which was followed by nociceptive tests as stated above[18].

3. Intracerebral and intraventricular injection. Constant rate intracerebral injections were given through two injection tubes introduced into bilateral guide cannulae simultaneously, the rate of injection being 0.25ul/min. The volume injected in each side was 5μl during a period of 20 minutes.

Injection into the third ventricle was made through a single cannula at a rate of 0.5μl/min. A total of 10μl was injected within a period of 20 minutes. The animal was injected with naloxone solution (0.4μg/ul) in the drug group and artificial CSF in controls.

4. Verification of the injection site. The animal was killed by overdose of sodium pentobarbital. 30ml of 10% formaline containing 1% potassium ferocyanide was injected into each side of the carotid arteries. An electrode of the same length as the injection tube, insulated except for the tip, was introduced into the guide cannula. The brain tissue at the tip of the electrode was stained blue by the anode current (1mA, 15sec) passing through the intracranial electrode with the reference electrode placed in the rectum. Serial sections of 1mm thickness were made for examination of the injection sites.

Those animals used only for intraventricular injection were killed and decapitated. The head was fixed in 10% formaline for at least one week. 1–2μl of methylene blue solution was then injected through the same injection tube used during the *in vivo* experiment and serial brain slabs of lmm thickness were made to examine whether the dye was injected into the ventricle.

II. RESULTS

1. The analgesic effect of finger-acupuncture (FA) and electroacupuncture (EA). The pain threshold change measured immediately after the cessation of FA in a group of 37 rabbits was 169±9.2% (mean±SE) higher than the basal level, while that of EA group (32 rabbits) was 136±13.8% (cf. Tab. 1, Fig. 1). The effect of FA seemed to be higher than that of EA, although the difference was not statistically significant. However, if we took the mean value of the 5 nociceptive tests, the mean acupuncture effect (MAE), as the index of AA, then the effect of FA (75±7.3%) would be significantly higher than that of EA (53±7.2%) ($P<0.05$). In order to obtain a higher rate of analgesic effect FA was used throughout the study.

2. The effect of microinjection of naloxone into bilateral accumbens on MA and AA in rabbits.

(1) Antagonism of MA by microinjection of naloxone into bilateral accumbens: Intravenous administration of 4mg/kg of morphine brought about an elevation of pain threshold on an average of 176±18.8% higher than the basal level 10 minutes after the injection and 192±6.5% half an hour after the injection in the normal control group (n=11). If morphine was injected superimposedly upon bilateral intra-accumbens naloxone infusion, the pain threshold elevation 30 minutes after morphine was found to be only 18±8.4% which was significantly lower than that of the control group ($P<0.001$)(cf. Fig. 3, Tab. 1). Injection of naloxone into the septal area seemed also to exert some antagonistic effect on

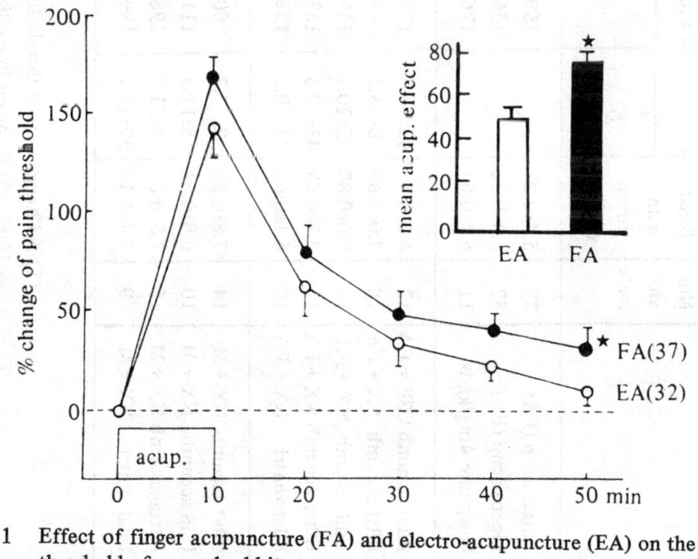

Fig. 1 Effect of finger acupuncture (FA) and electro-acupuncture (EA) on the pain threshold of normal rabbits.

Vertical bar shows the standard error, numerals in brackets denote the number of animals. The inset shows the change of mean acupuncture effect, i.e., the mean value of the pain threshold changes in five successive nococeptive tests taken after the acupuncture session. *denotes $P<0.05$.

Table 1. The effect of microinjection of naloxone into nucleus accumbens on AA and MA in rabbits

	No. animals	Basal pain thresh (sec)	% Change of Pain threshold after FA or morphine iv					
			0′	10′	20′	30′	40′	50′
Finger acup (FA)	37	5.4±0.27		169± 9.2	79±12.8	50±11.1	41± 8.5	32± 8.9
Electroacup (EA)	32	6.4±0.32		136±13.8	61±13.4	35±10.1	22± 7.1	9± 6.3
Morphine 4mg/kg iv	11	6.5±0.67		176±18.8	175±19.1	192± 6.5	185±15.6	176±19.3
Bilat accumb CSF + FA	12	5.2±0.45	42±17.5	173±17.8	98±23.1	75±21.6	39±10.5	48±17.2
Bilat accumb NX + FA	18	7.0±0.63	6± 5.5	49± 7.1	35± 7.6	11± 5.2	3± 6.4	0± 5.3
Unil accumb NX + FA	11	7.0±0.80	22±20.9	149±18.1	85±23.2	63±22.1	51±23.0	61±20.0
Extra-accumb NX + FA	13	7.7±0.69	33±17.6	183± 9.7	91±16.2	51±12.2	40±10.1	39±12.1
Bilat ventri NX + FA	10	6.1±0.61	21±10.1	178±15.8	99±21.8	36±10.1	52±20.0	25±15.2
Bilat accumb NX + M	14	7.8±0.89	2± 7.3	60±17.0	52±15.0	18± 8.4	11± 8.3	9± 6.0
Unil accumb NX + M	10	6.8±0.54	15±11.3	111±25.6	92±25.4	126±25.0	121±25.0	97±28.5
Extra-accumb NX + M	5	7.5±0.81	39±21.2	198± 2.1	156±49.0	123±54.7	153±49.3	99±49.8
Bilat ventri NX + M	9	7.4±1.10	39±14.1	189±11.1	189±11.1	178±14.3	169±21.7	147±20.3

(1) % Change of pain threshold was calculated taking basal pain threshold as 100%. (2) 0′ means immediately before FA or morphine injection, but 10 minutes after the begining of intracerebral infusion. (3) Numerals in the table are mean±SE.

MA, while injection into caudate-putamen or inferior horns of the lateral ventricle had no significant effect(Fig. 2, Tab. 1).

(2) Antagonism of AA by microinjection of naloxone into bilateral accumbens: In rabbits injected with artificial CSF into bilateral accumbens, finger acupuncture of Kuanlun point caused an elevation of pain threshold by 173±17.8% (n=12); while in animals injected

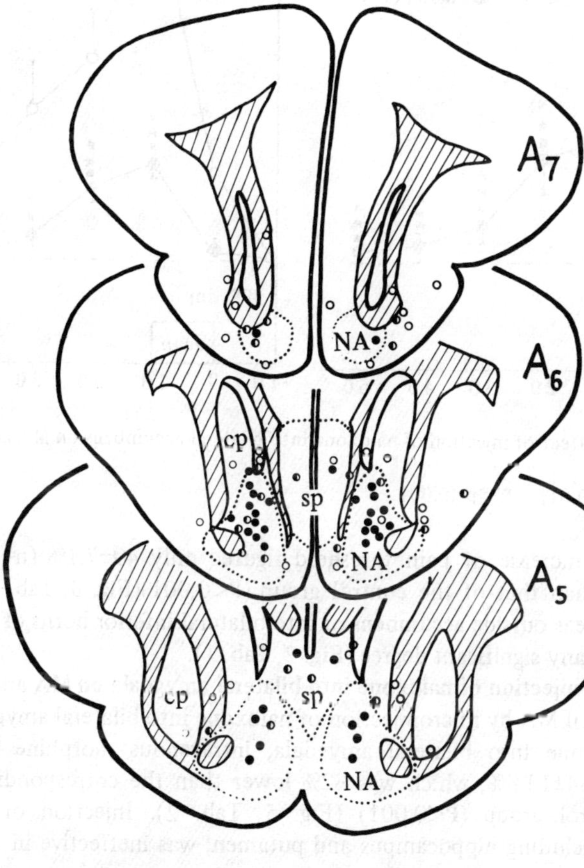

Fig. 2 The effect of injection of naloxone in nucleus accumbens on morphine analgesia (MA) and acupuncture analgesia (AA) in rabbits.

The site of injection and its effect on MA and AA are shown by different symbols in 3 coronary sections (A7, A6, A5) of the rabbit brain. NA: nucleus accumbens; Sp: septum; V: anterior horn of the lateral ventricle; CP: caudate-putamen. Black dot denotes the site where injection of naloxone blocks both MA and AA, i.e., the pain threshold change did not exceed 60% when it was taken 30 minutes after morphine injection or immediately after 10 minutes' finger acupuncture. Semiblack dot denotes the site where injection of naloxone causes partial block of MA and / or AA, i.e., the pain threshold elevation after morphine and/or acupuncture treatment are within the range of 60–120%. Circle denotes the site where injection of naloxone has no concern with MA and AA, the increase of pain threshold after morphine or acupuncture treatment being > 120%. The same symbols are used in Figs 4, 6 and 8.

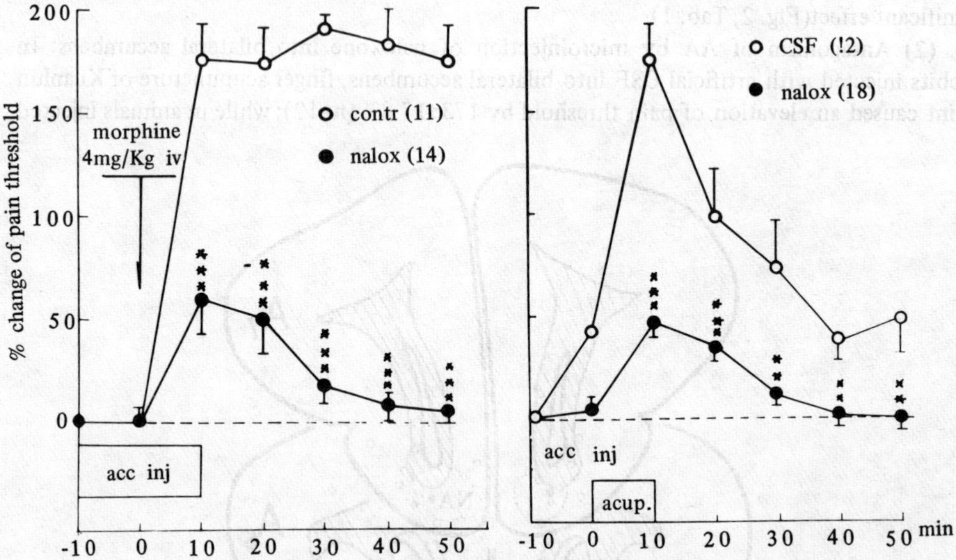

Fig. 3 The effect of injection of naloxone into bilateral accumbens on MA and AA.

**denotes p<0.01, ***p<0.001.

with naloxone, the increase of pain threshold figured only 49±7.1% (n=18), which was significantly lower than that of the control group (P<0.001)(Fig. 3, Tab. 1). Injection of naloxone to brain areas outside accumbens or into bilateral inferior horns of lateral ventricle did not affect AA in any significant degree (Fig. 2, Tab. 1).

3. The effect of injection of naloxone into bilateral amygdala on MA and AA in rabbits.

(1) Antagonism of MA by microinjection of naloxone into bilateral amygdala: In rabbits injected with naloxone into bilateral amygdala, intravenous morphine raised the pain threshold by only 34±13.8%, which was 82% lower than the corresponding value (192± 6.5%) in the control group (P<0.001) (Fig. 5, Tab. 2). Injection of naloxone into neighboring areas, including hippocampus and putamen, was ineffective in this regard (Fig. 4, Tab. 2).

(2) Antagonism of AA by microinjection of naloxone into bilateral amygdala: In a group of 17 rabbits in which naloxone was injected into bilateral amygdala, FA brought about an elevation of pain threshold by 58±14.0% which was only 32% that of the CSF control group (184±11.9%, n=7). The difference between these two groups was statistically very significant (P<0.001) (Fig. 5, Tab. 2). No significant attenuation of AA was observed when naloxone was injected to neighboring areas such as hippocampus and putamen (Fig. 4, Tab. 2).

4. The effects of injection of naloxone into bilateral habenula on MA and AA in rabbits.

(1) Antagonism of MA by microinjection of naloxone into bilateral habenula: In a group of 13 rabbits in which the injection cannulae hit bilateral habenula, injection of naloxone decreased the effectiveness of MA by 76% (P<0.001) (Fig. 7, Tab. 3). The same

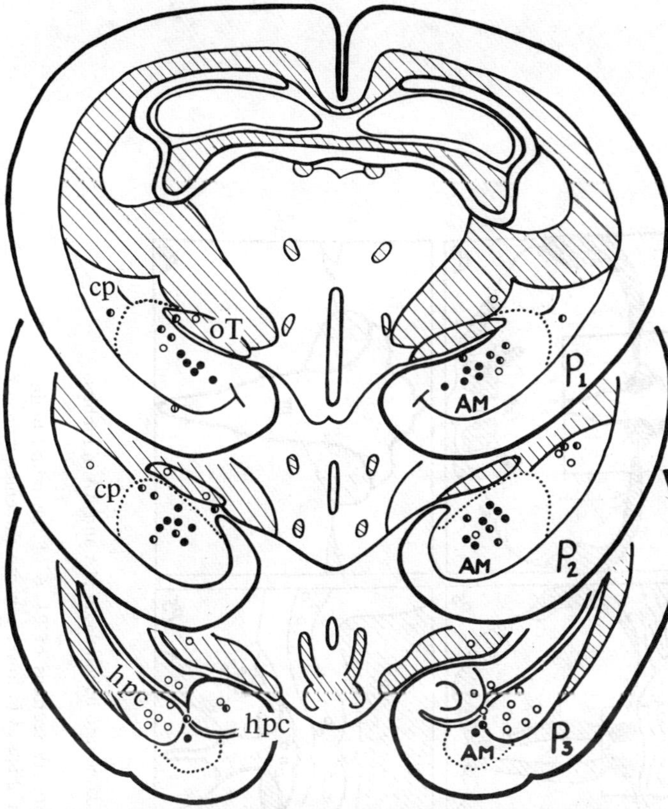

Fig. 4 The effect of injection of naloxone into amygdala on MA and AA in rabbits.

The three coronary brain sections are reconstructed from the atlas of Sawyer et al (16) and Bures et al 15. AM: amygdala, Hpc:hippocampus.

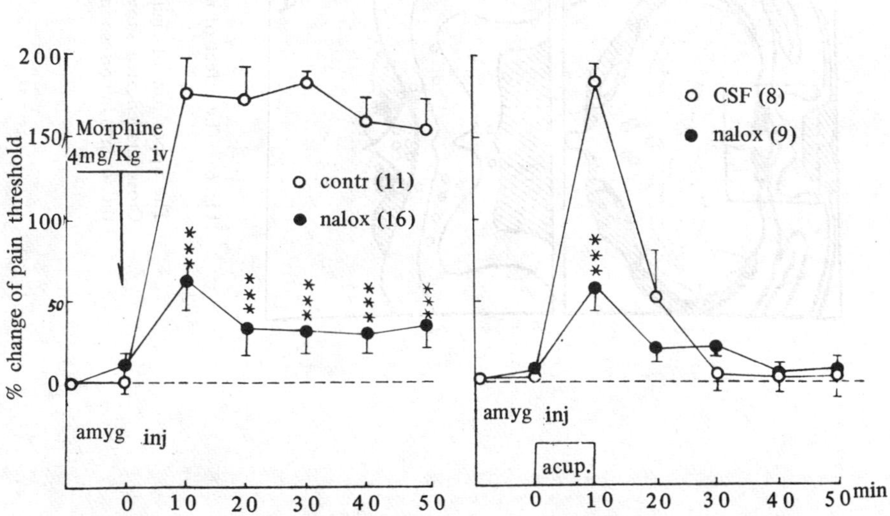

Fig. 5 The effect of injection of naloxone into bilateral maygdala on MA and AA in rabbits.

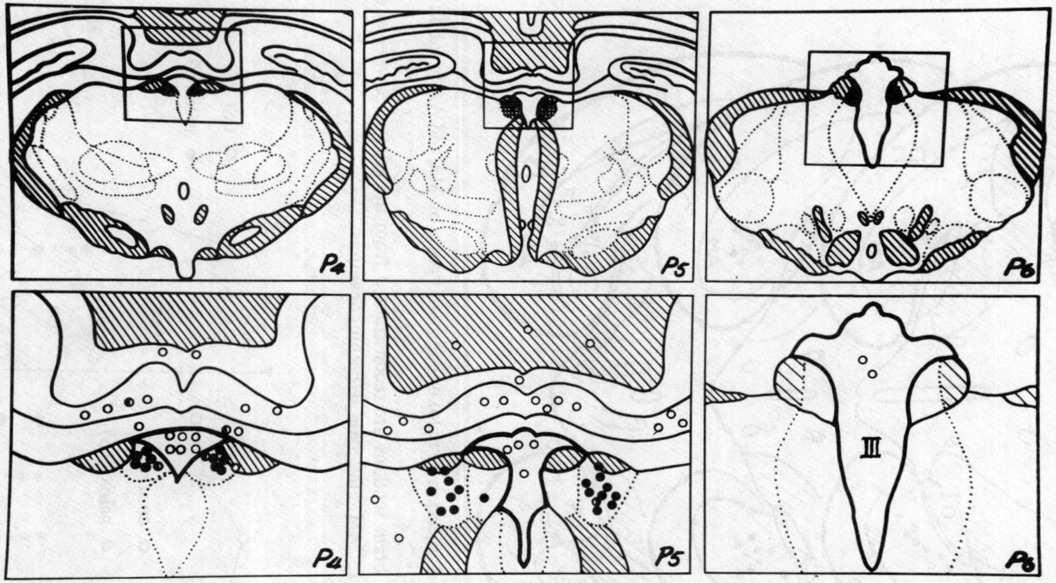

Fig. 6 The effect of injection of naloxone into habenula on MA and AA in rabbits.

The upper row of figures exhibits coronary sections of P4–6 of the rabbit brain. Cross shaded area shows the habenula. Figures in lower row are the enlargment of the squares in corresponding upper drawings.

Table 2. The effect of microinjection of naloxone into amygdala on AA and MA in rabbits

	No. animals	Basal pain threshold (sec)	% Change of pain threshold after FA or morphine					
			0′	10′	20′	30′	40′	50′
Bilat amygd CSF + FA	8	7.2±0.65	7± 7.4	184±12.0	51±29.3	4±11.8	5±10.8	3±12.7
Bilat amygd NX + FA	17	6.2±0.53	4± 6.2	58±14.0	20± 8.6	21± 5.5	5± 5.3	7±10.0
Unil amygd NX + FA	9	6.0±0.75	28± 19.5	109±26.0	98±28.1	42±21.8	25±12.0	48±19.0
Extra-amygd NX + FA	9	9.2±0.65	13±27.2	192±8.4	149±26.2	63±20.9	22±10.6	25±13.1
Bilat amygd NX + M	16	7.2±0.52	11± 7.2	65±18.4	38±13.8	34±13.8	31±13.1	36±13.6
Unil amygd NX + M	9	6.8±0.65	17±17.2	167±21.4	119±32.7	118±33.0	110±29.8	118±31.0
Extra-amygd NX + M	11	8.4±0.62	−1±11.0	200± 0.0	200± 0.0	194± 4.7	168±17.9	186±11.1

Table 3. The effect of microinjection of naloxone into habenula on AA and MA in rabbite

	No. animals	Basal pain threshold (sec)	% Change of pain threshold after FA or morphine					
			0′	10′	20′	30′	40′	50′
Bilat haben CSF + FA	14	6.9±0.44	0± 5.0	166±13.3	30±10.1	12±11.7	−1± 4.9	16±10.9
Bilat haben NX + FA	14	6.6±0.49	−6± 5.1	15± 8.2	14± 7.8	6± 4.2	5± 6.8	−2± 1.4
Unil haben NX + FA	4	5.9±0.91	6± 4.8	108±18.1	17± 7.4	51±16.9	29±14.0	28± 9.6
Extra-haben NX + FA	4	9.0±0.73	38±25.1	198± 2.0	48±16.2	9±17.3	−9±16.7	-14±13.1
III ventricle NX + FA	10	8.9±0.56	23±13.8	175± 9.8	83±16.2	36±11.4	27± 8.7	11±10.8
Bilat haben NX + M	13	6.0±0.41	−1± 5.7	66±19.4	62±18.0	47±19.7	63±19.7	28±17.5
Unil haben NX + M	4	5.7±0.72	28±12.5	105±44.2	105±40.2	86±42.2	65±46.5	52±49.8
Extra-haben NX + M	4	9.7±0.68	19±27.3	200± 0.0	198± 2.5	186± 8.3	148±48.5	149±48.0
III ventricle NX + M	9	10.7±0.73	14± 9.2	196± 3.8	178±18.8	175±21.2	160±20.3	162±23.2

Table 4. The effect of microinjection of naloxone into PAG on AA and MA in rabbits

	No. animals	Basal Pain threshold (sec)	% Change of pain threshold after FA or morphine					
			0′	10′	20′	30′	40′	50′
Bilat PAG CSF + FA	12	5.4±0.44	27±12.1	158±19.6	80±18.2	49±19.5	35±11.6	26±11.3
Bilat PAG NX + FA	17	6.9±0.53	−6± 6.5	39±15.4	16± 9.3	11± 8.9	−7± 4.5	−5± 7.0
Unil PAG NX + FA	5	5.4±0.93	20±22.2	143±22.0	27±17.1	13±15.1	12±16.5	18±17.5
Extra-PAG NX + FA	4	5.2±0.25	6±19.0	171±22.0	132±40.7	66±52.5	67±55.1	43±46.3
Bilat PAG NX + M	16	6.5±0.47	28 ± 7.4	106±20.2	55±16.4	48±18.4	16± 9.2	26±13.6
Unil PAG NX + M	5	6.7±0.85	24±16.5	119±33.3	74±33.8	59±37.7	54±38.6	56±51.3
Extra-PAG NX + M	4	6.6±0.96	33±42.1	191± 8.8	191± 8.8	171±29.5	173±16.3	191± 8.8

amount of naloxone when injected into corpus callosum, head of hippocampus or the third ventricle was of little effect on MA (Fig. 6, Tab. 3).

(2) Antagonism of AA by microinjection of naloxone into bilateral habenula: In a group of 14 rabbits injection of naloxone into bilateral habenula abolished almost completely the effect of AA. The pain threshold elevation in CSF control group was 166±13.3% while in the naloxone group only 15±8.2% ---a drop of 91% (P<0.001)(Fig. 7, Tab. 3). No significant attenuation of AA was noticed when naloxone was injected into the neighboring areas, such as corpus callosum, head of hippocampus or the third ventricle (Fig. 6, Tab. 3).

5. The effect of injection of naloxone into bilateral periaqueductal grey (PAG) on MA and AA in rabbits.

(1) Antagonism of MA by microinjection of naloxone into bilateral PAG: Intravenous injection of 4mg/kg of morphine raised the pain threshold by 48±18.4% in a group of 16 rabbits when naloxone was infused into bilateral PAG, a figure which was only one fourth that of the control group (P<0.001) (Fig. 9, Tab. 4). The same amount of naloxone when injected outside PAG or inside the aqueduct had no significant effect on MA (Fig. 8, Tab. 4).

(2) Antagonism of AA by microinjection of naloxone into bilateral PAG: In a group of 12 rabbits injected with artificial CSF into bilateral PAG as control, FA raised the pain threshold by 158±19.6%. When naloxone was injected instead of CSF, the effect of AA was found to be 39±15.4%, which was only one fourth that of the control group (P<0.001) (Fig. 9, Tab. 4). Injection of naloxone to the vicinity of PAG or into the aqueduct exhibited no blocking effect on AA (Fig. 8, Tabs.3, 4).

6. The effect of unilateral injection of naloxone into nucleus accumbens, amygdala, habenula or PAG on MA and AA. In some of the animals one of the cannulae hit the target nucleus with the other inserted to the neighboring area or the ventricle. The results of unilateral naloxone injection into the target nucleus on MA and AA are shown in Fig. 10.

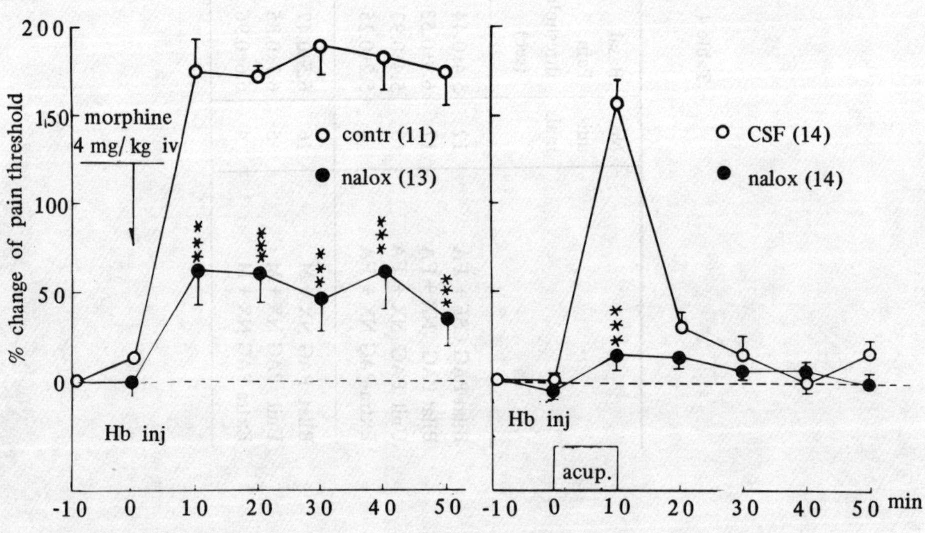

Fig. 7 The effect of injection of naloxone into bilateral habenula on MA and AA in rabbits.

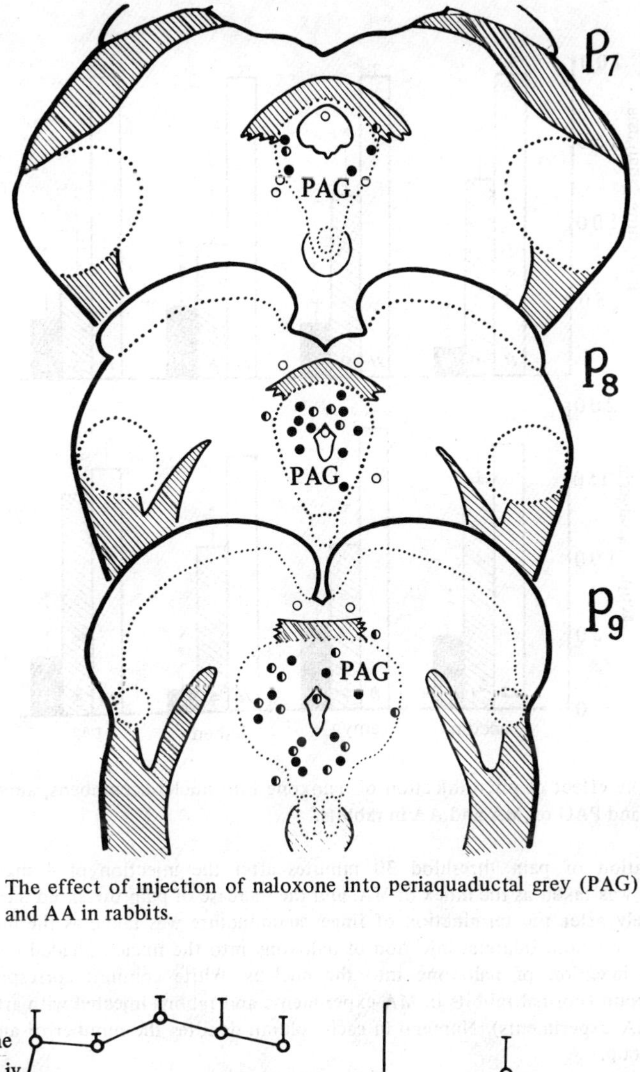

Fig. 8 The effect of injection of naloxone into periaquaductal grey (PAG) on MA and AA in rabbits.

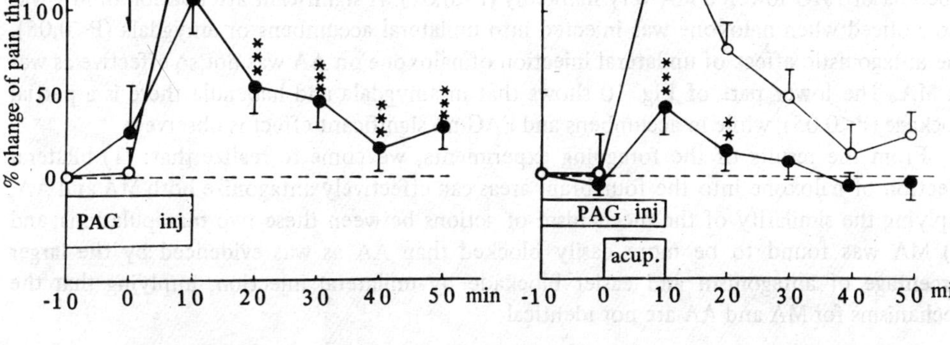

Fig. 9 The effect of injection of naloxone into bilateral PAG on MA and AA in rabbits.

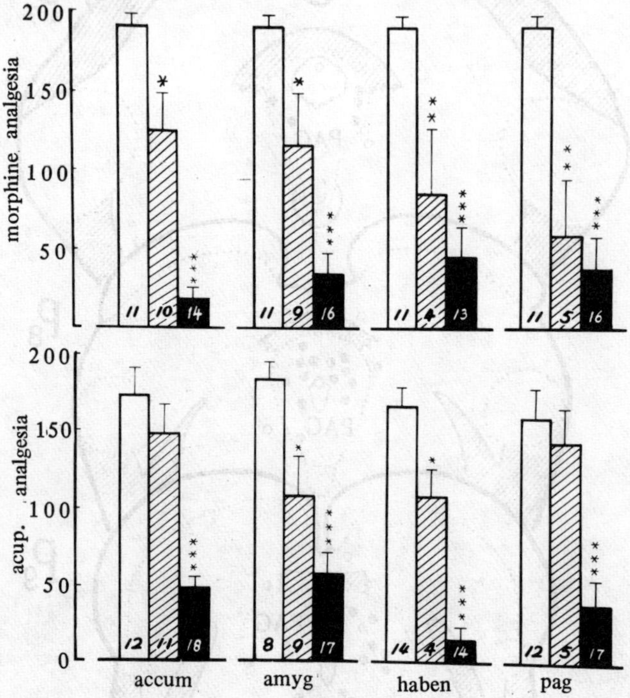

Fig. 10 The effect of microinjection of naloxone into nuclei accumbens, amygdala, habenula and PAG on MA and AA in rabbits.

The elevation of pain threshlod 30 minutes after the injection of 4 mg/kg of morphine was taken as the index of MA, and the increase of pain threshold measured immediately after the termination of finger acupuncture was taken as the indix of AA. Black column: bilateral injection of naloxone into the nuclei. Shaded column: unilateral injection of naloxone into the nucleus. White column: corresponding control group (normal rabbits in MA experiments and rabbits injected with artificial CSF in AA experiments). Numeral in each column denotes the number of amimals in each group.

The upper part of the figure shows the effect on MA. Unilateral injection of naloxone into habenula or PAG lowered MA very markedly ($P<0.01$). A significant attenuation of MA was also noticed when naloxone was injected into unilateral accumbens or amygdala ($P<0.05$). The antagonistic effect of unilateral injection of naloxone on AA was not so effective as was on MA. The lower part of Fig. 10 shows that in amygdala and habenula there is a partial blockage ($P<0.05$), while in accumbens and PAG no significant effect is observed.

From the results of the foregoing experiments, we come to realize that: (1) bilateral injection of naloxone into the four brain areas can effectively antagonize both MA and AA, implying the similarity of the mechanism of actions between these two manipulations; and (2) MA was found to be more easily blocked than AA as was evidenced by the larger percentage of antagonism and easier blockade by unilateral injection, implying that the mechanisms for MA and AA are not identical.

III. DISCUSSION

The nucleus accumbens of the mammalian brain has been reported to contain very high concentrations of OLS[10–12] and considerable amounts of enkephalinergic nerve endings[10]. Recently it was reported that electrolytic lesion of nuclei accumbens resulted in significant attenuation of AA in the rat[19]. In order to clarify whether the OLS contained in nucleus accumbens plays an active role in AA, we examined the changes of OLS activity in area"septumaccumbens" of the rat brain following 30 minutes' EA and found that there was a marked increase in OLS activity in this brain area. Regression analysis revealed that the amplitude of increase of OLS in individual animals was well correlated with the effectiveness of AA[20]. In line with this was our recent finding that microinjection of naloxone into bilateral accumbens brought about a marked decrease in the effect of AA in the rat[14].

Concerning morphine analgesia, Costa et al. reported that the antinociceptive effect induced by 15mg/kg of morphine could be blocked by microinjection of naltrexone, an opiate antagonist, into the nucleus accumbens of the rat[13]. Similar results were obtained in our laboratory using naloxone instead of naltrexone[14]. All these results pointed to the same conclusion that, as far as rats are concerned, the opiate receptors in the nucleus accumbens seemed to play an important part both in MA and in AA. In the present study we used rabbits as experimental animals and got very similar results, thus further strengthening the conclusion obtained from the rat.

Amygdala constitutes one of the main structures in the limbic system. The medial and central amygdala were reported to be rich in opiate receptors[21] and endogenous opioids[10–12], and were supposed to be related with the affective component of the pain experience. The results of the present study indicated that injection of opiate antagonist into bilateral amygdala blocked both MA and AA significantly, implying that either exogenous or endogenous opioids could act on the opiate receptors in the amygdala, thus exerting its analgesic effect.

The habenular complex recieves its main afferents from septum, accumbens and amygdala and sends its main efferents via habenulo-interpeduncular tract to interpeduncular nucleus which is in turn related to other structures in the lower brain stem[22]. The habenular complex may thus be regarded as a vital link which funnels informations from the forebrain to the midbrain structures[11, 23, 24]. Wang et al. reported that electric stimulation of habenula caused inhibition of unit discharges of nucleus raphe magnus[25], the importance of which in AA has repeatedly been proved[20, 21]. The results of the present study indicated that naloxone blockade of opiate receptors in habenula antagonized MA very significantly and AA almost completely. Taking this divergent evidence together we could postulate that exogenously administered morphine or endogenously released OLS during acupuncture may inhibit the activities of habenula neurons, thus releasing the raphe nuclei and the serotoninergic system from the descending inhibitory influence and turning it into a state of activation so as to exert its powerful antinociceptive effect. Further experimentation is necessary for the verification of this hypothesis.

There is strong evidence supporting PAG as one of the most important sites of action for MA[21, 27–31]. For AA, it has been reported that the OLS content in the perfusate from PAG of the rabbit increased significantly during the course of EA[32]. The results from this study indicated that naloxone blockade of opiate receptors in bilateral PAG blocked both MA and AA, implying that the opiate receptors in PAG were of ultimate importance for both MA and AA. It is worthy to mention that unilateral injection of naloxone blocked MA ($P<0.01$) but not AA ($P>0.05$). This discrepancy may indicate a qualitative difference in mechanisms of action between MA and AA, suggesting a more complicated mechanism for AA. Alternatively, it may suggest only a quantitative difference in that the amount of naloxone diffusing from the injection site to the opposite side is sufficient to antagonize the action of 4mg/kg of morphine but insufficient for blockade of AA.

From the aforementioned data emerges another problem. How could it be explained that the effect of MA or AA can be antagonized by injection of naloxone in only one brain area, since the intravenously administered morphine and endogenously released OLS must have activated opiate receptors in multiple brain areas? Fisher and Courey in their study of the physiology and pharmacology of drinking suggested a cholinergic circuit in the brain for the control of thirst-drinking behavior in the rat. They found that injection of muscarinic blocking agent at any point in the circuit would inactivate the function of the whole system and reduce the amount of drinking[33]. Similarly, one may postulate a pain modulating neural circuit in the brain which utilizes OLS as its neurotransmitter or neuromodulator and blockade of any point in the circuit would interrupt the whole function. This seems to be a problem deserving of further investigation.

IV. CONCLUSION

1. Finger acupuncture of Kuanlun point or electroacupuncture of Zusanli and Kuanlun points in the rabbit raised the pain threshold of the skin more than 100% higher than the basal level. The mean analgesic effect of finger acupuncture was significantly higher than that of electroacupuncture.

2. The analgesic effect induced by finger acupuncture of Kuanlun or intravenous injection of morphine was antagonized by 70–90% by bilateral injection of naloxone into one of the four brain areas, i.e., accumbens, amygdala, habenula and PAG, suggesting the functional importance of opiate receptors in these brain areas in mediating MA and AA and also the similarity of mechanisms of action between MA and AA.

3. By using the same dose of naloxone, MA was found to be more easily blocked than AA as was evidenced by the larger percentage of antagonism and easier blockage by unilateral injection, implying a more complicated mechanism for AA.

REFERENCES

[1] Mayer, D.J., *et al.*: *Brain Res.*, **121**:368, 1977.

[2] 江振裕等: 动物学报 24: 1, 1978。

[3] 黄 晔等: 中华医学杂志 58: 196, 1978。

[4] Pomeranz B. *et al.*: *Exp. Neurol.*, **54**:172, 1977.
[5] Pomeranz, B and Chiu D: *Life Sci* **19**:1757, 1976.
[6] 北京医学院基础部针麻原理研究组：中华外科杂志 **15**：129，1977。
[7] Sjolund. B., *et al.*: *Acta Physiol. Scand*, **100**:382, 1977.
[8] 上海第一医学院针麻原理研究协作组：上海第一医学院学报 **5**：13，1978。
[9] 汤 健，韩济生：北京医学院学报（3)：150，1978。
[10] Simantov, R. *et al.*: *Proc. Natl. Acad. Sci. USA*, **74**:2167, 1977.
[11] Hughes, J. *et al.*: *Nature* **258**:577, 1975.
[12] Snyder. S.H.: *Nature*, **257**:185, 1975.
[13] Costa, E. *et al.*: *Neuropharmacology*, **16**:323, 1977.
[14] 范少光等：北京医学院学报（1)：1，1979。
[15] Bures, J 等著，范世藩、江振裕译，«电生理学方法»，上海科技出版社，1963。
[16] Sawyer, C.H. *et al.*: *J. Comp. Neurol.*, **101**:801, 1954.
[17] Research Group of Acupuncture Anesthesia, Peking Medical College: *Scientia Sinica* , **17**:112, 1974.
[18] 北京医学院针麻原理研究组生理组：北京医学院学报（1)：18，1974。
[19] 张德星等：生理学报 **30**：95，1978。
[20] Zhang, W.Q. *et al.*: *Abstracts of National Symposia of Acupuncture and Moxibustion and Acupuncture Anesthesia*, Beijing, p.486, 1979.
[21] Yasuko, F. *et al.*: *Science*, **185**:105, 1974.
[22] Mountcastle, V.B. (ed): *Medical Physiology*, 13th ed, vol 1, p229, Mosby, 1974.
[23] Wang, R Y. and Aghajanian, G.K.: *Science*, **197**:89, 1977.
[24] Herkenkam, M. Nauta, W.J.H.: *J. Comp. Neurol.*, **173**:123, 1977.
[25] Wang, S. *et al.*: *Abstracts of National Symposia of Acupuncture and Moxibustion and Acupuncture Anesthesia*, Beijing, p.384, 1979.
[26] 陕西省中医研究所针麻原理研究室：陕西新医药（5)：59，1975。
[27] 江振裕等：中华医学杂志 **57**：611，1977。
[28] 屠曾宏等：生理学报 **30**：51，1978。
[29] Urca, G. *et al.*: *Science*, **182**:490, 1973.
[30] Yasuko, F, *et al.*: *Science*, **182**:490, 1973.
[31] Jaquet, Y.F.,and Marls, N.: *Science*, **194**:632, 1976.
[32] 上海第一医学院针麻研究组，同位素中心实验室：上海第一医学院学报 **5**：17，1978。
[33] Fisher, A.E. and Coury, J.N.: *Science*, **138**:691, 1962.

EFFECTS OF NALOXONE ON ANALGESIA PRODUCED BY DIFFERENT STRENGTHS OF ELECTROACUPUNCTURE

Zhang Anzhong, Zeng Dayun, Zhang Lingmei
(Laboratory of Neuropharmacology)

Cheng Jieshi, Ye Zhijun, Ou Shupei
(Laboratory of Neurophysiology)
(Research Departement of Acupuncture Analgesia, Shanghai First Medical College)

The discovery of opiate receptors and endorphins in the brain has given an important clue to the further investigation of the mechanism of acupuncture analgesia. The relationship between effects of acupuncture, especially its analgesic effect, and opiate receptors together with their transmitter system is now a subject of general interest. Mayer[1] and the Shanghai Cooperative Research Group of Acupuncture Analgesia[2] found that the morphineantagonist naloxone could reverse the acupuncture analgesic effect on the humanbody. But experiments on the animals led to different results. Pomeranz[3] reported that naloxone could markedly antagonize the effect of electroacupuncture analgesia on mice. The Shanghai Institute of Physiology[4] and our laboratory[5] also observed the reversal effect of naloxone on acupuncture analgesia in monkeys and rabbits respectively. However, Mclennan[6] could not demonstrate the same result on rabbits. Since 1976, the effect of morphineantagonists levallorphan and naloxone on electroacupuncture analgesia has been studied in rabbits in our laboratory. It was found that the effect of these two antagonists on acupuncture analgesia varied with the dosage, time of administration, the parameter of electroacupuncture and the functional state of animals. This discovery may give an explanation for the different results of the animal experiments mentioned above.

I. METHOD

The experiments were performed on rabbits of both sexes (body weight 2-2.8kg). They were divided into two groups.

1. One group of animals was kept in a quiet state during the experiment. The pain threshold of the ear skin was measured with a potassium ion electro-phoretic dolorimeter at intervals of 3 minutes. The somatic defensive reaction was taken as indication of pain. It was found that the pain threshold was quite stable under these conditions. The points corresponding to "Hegú" and "Waiguan" were electrically needled by the electroacupuncture apparatus model G 6805. The pulse frequency of the apparatus output was 2–3 c/s. The strength used was graded into two categories: (a) Moderate strength ranged between 7.5–8 mA, which caused only moderate muscle contraction of the animal forelegs but in general the animal kept quiet; (b) Superstrength, ranged from 12.5 mA to 15mA, which caused animal stress showing overall agitation and struggle.

Rabbits showing a more than two-fold rise in pain threshold at the 20th minute during electroacupuncture were considered as "acupuncture effective" and were chosen for further studies.

2. In another group of animals under intravenous chloralose/urethane anesthesia (respective mixtures of chloralose and urethane, 30–50mg/kg and 0.3–0.5g/kg). the cortical potential evoked by tooth pulp stimulation was recorded. An upper incisor tooth was cut off and concentric electrodes were inserted into the sectioned tooth cavity. The skull overlying the contralateral sensorimotor cortex was drilled open, and the exposed cerebral dura was covered with warm liquid paraffin. Recording was started, when the animal regained sensation. The tooth pulp was stimulated with single rectangular pulse (0.5 msec in duration, 30–90V of amplitude). Biggest evoked potentials could be evoked by this strength of stimulation. Evoked potentials (EP) were led by silver electrode placed on the exposed dura. Into the TQ 19A data processor via a preamplifier were fed the signals of EP, which were averaged (20 times, interval 3–5 sec) by the processor and then recorded on a X-Y plotter. Points "Hegu" and "Neiguan" were electrically needled with moderate strength or superstrength as before.

II. RESULTS

1. Experiments in pain thresholds. The acupuncture effective rates in the moderate strength acupuncture group (37 animals) and the superstrength acupuncture group (12 animals) were 70% and 66% respectively. The percentages of the rising pain threshold between these two groups were shown to be of no statistical difference.

At the 20th min during acupuncture, some animals of both groups were injected with naloxone 0.4 mg/kg intravenously, and the others were injected with normal saline as control. It was found that the analgesic effects of moderate strength acupuncture were markedly reversed by naloxone in 10 out of 14 animals. At the 5th minute after naloxone injection the average decrease rate in pain threshold of the whole group was 41%, which differed significantly from the control group ($P<0.005$). The reversed pain threshold then rose again gradually and nearly reached the preinjection level after 15 min following the naloxone injection. However, the analgesic effect of superstrength acupuncture was not reversed by naloxone. There was only 1 out of 10 animals showing a decreased pain threshold at the 5th minute after naloxone injection; the average pain threshold of the whole group at that time was not statistically different from that before naloxone injection.

Both the pain thresholds of the saline control group (12 animals) and the naloxone control group remained unchanged during the corresponding experiment (Tab. 1, Fig. 1).

2. Experiments in cortical evoked potential. Experiments were performed on 15 rabbits. While the tooth pulp was stimulated with single rectangular pulse on the rather stable background of spontaneous electric activities of the cerebro-cortex, a biphasic potential that

Table 1. Effective rate of analgesia produced by two different strengths of acupuncture and reversed by naloxone

Strength of acup.	Number of rabbits	Acup. effective rabbits (number and %)	Rise (%) of pain threshold	Reversal (%) of pain threshold by naloxone
Mod.	37	26 (70%)	187 %	40%
Super.	12	8 (66%)	200 %	–6 %

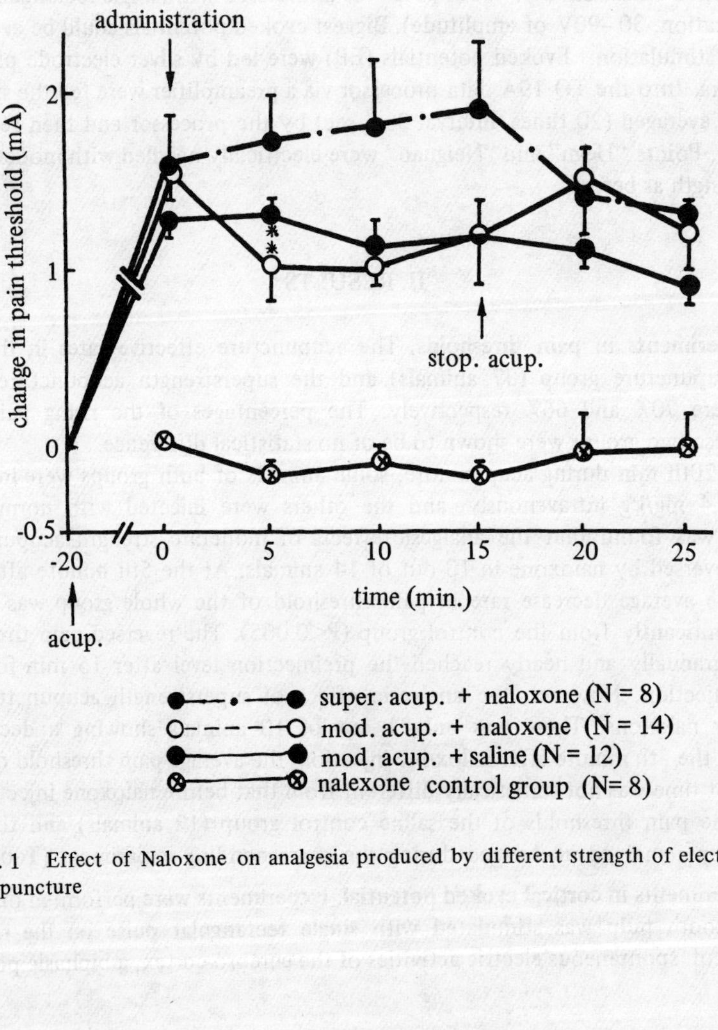

Fig. 1 Effect of Naloxone on analgesia produced by different strength of electro-acupuncture

showed a downward positive wave followed by a negative one was recorded from the cortical somatosensory area. The amplitude of the positive wave ranged from 100 μV to 500 μV while that of the negative wave was only about a few dozen μV. The positive wave was taken as index for statistical analysis, but in some experiments, the pike to pike amplitudes of positive-negative waves were simultaneously taken for statistical treatment.

When the amplitude of the evoked potentials remained stable, electrical needling of "Hegu" and "Neiguan" points with moderate strength markedly depressed these potentials (their amplitudes decreased by 50–80 μV on the average). The response recovered in a few minutes after cessation of acupuncture. In order to examine the effect of naloxone on the inhibitory action of needling, naloxone (0.4mg/kg) was injected intravenously to the rabbits two minutes before the electric needling. The inhibitory action of needling on the evoked potentials was reversed by naloxone in 13 out of 15 animals. The effect of naloxone was shown at the first minute of electroacupuncture (at the 3rd minute after naloxone injection) and lasted about 13–17 minutes. An hour later, the antagonistic effect of naloxone disappeared completely, and the inhibitory action of needling on the evoked potentials reached nearly to the pre-injection level. The inhibitory action of electroacupuncture upon evoked potentials of tooth pulp stimulation decreased on an average by 21 μV within the 3–17 minutes after naloxone injection, accounting for 36% of the total decrease by needling. It was seen that the inhibitory action of acupuncture on the evoked potentials between the above-mentioned two groups revealed a significant difference ($P<0.01$) (Fig. 2).

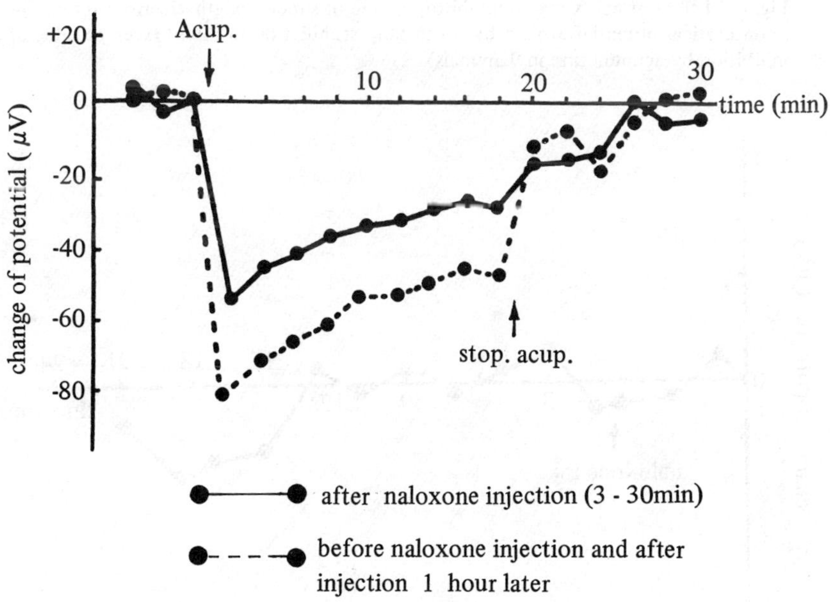

Fig. 2 Antagonistic effect of Naloxone on inhibitory action of moderate electro-acupuncture upon cortical pontential evoked by tooth pulp stimulation in rabbit (average value of inhibition by acupuncture in 15 animals)

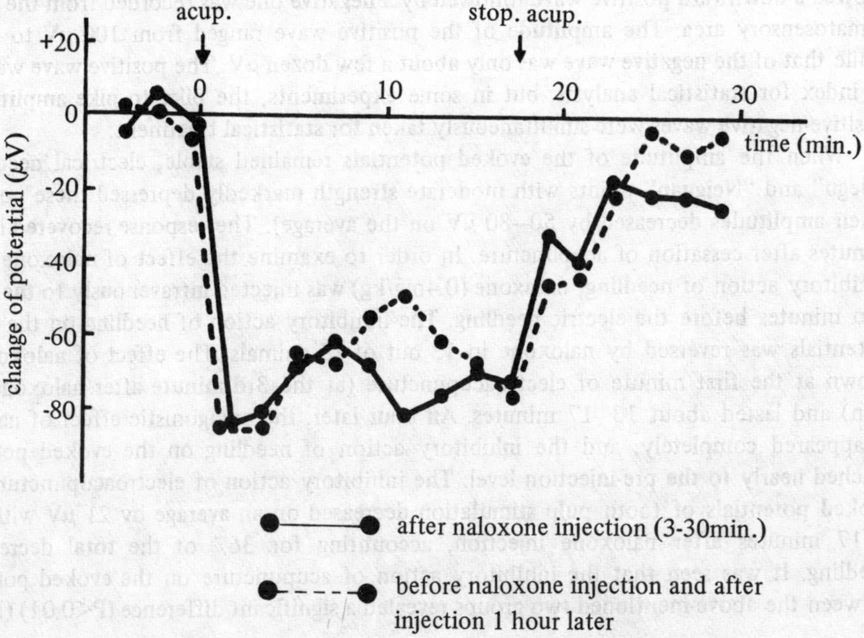

Fig.3 Effect of naloxone on inhibitory action of superstrength electroacupuncture upon cortical potential evoked by tooth pulp stimulation in rabbit (average value of inhibition by acupuncture in 9 animals)

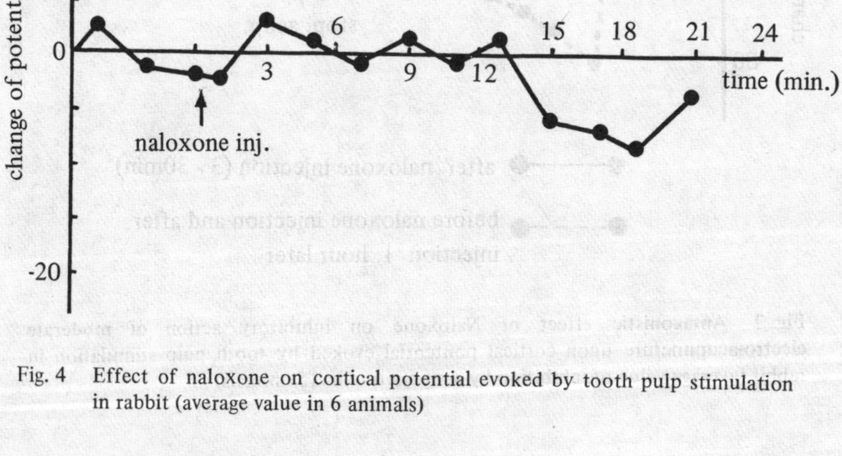

Fig. 4 Effect of naloxone on cortical potential evoked by tooth pulp stimulation in rabbit (average value in 6 animals)

The second part of this experimental group was performed on 9 rabbits treated with superstrength electroacupuncture. It was found that the superstrength electroacupuncture decreased the amplitude of the evoked potential by 60–80 μV on the average before and after naloxone injection. There is no obvious difference between these two. It shows that the inhibitory effect of superstrength electroacupuncture was not reversed by naloxone. (Fig. 3).

Control experiments were performed on 6 rabbits. It was observed that naloxone injection alone had no effect on the tooth pulp evoked potentials ($P<0.4$). (Fig. 4).

III. DISCUSSION

The results from both groups of our experiments indicate that the analgesic effect of moderate strength electroacupuncture is antagonized by naloxone, but the effect of superstrength electroacupuncture is not. This suggests that the analgesic effect of moderate strength acupuncture may result from the activity of opiate receptors and the analgesic effect of superstrength acupuncture may not. This may illuminate the different results reported by different authors.

In the present experiment, the analgesic potency of the superstrength acupuncture which gave rise to the wild struggle of the animals was not greater than that of the moderate strength acupuncture (Tab. 1). It has been reported that the superstrength acupuncture acted as a stress stimulus and caused a stress analgesia, which was not reversed by naloxone in a regular dose[7, 8], or might be partially antagonized by a large dose of naloxone (10 mg/kg)[9]. It indicated that endorphin was not a major factor in stress analgesia. During stress response the release of β-endorphin from the pituitary markedly increased. However, it was reported that intravenous injection of 8mg/kg β-endorphin to the rat did not cause any analgesic effect[10].

Some previous work in our laboratory[11, 12] showed that the sympathic tone decreased and the plasma cortisol level also tended to decrease during acupuncture in the human body. It obviously differed from stress response. Recently the plasma cortisol level of the two grades of electroacupuncture strength was compared in rabbits. It was found that the cortisol level during the moderate acupuncture strength tended to decrease, but not significantly. However, cortisol level was significantly increased ($P<0.05$) by superstrength acupuncture. Section of the postero-lateral columns of the spinal cord could remove the analgesia produced by morphine and acupuncture, but could not remove the stress analgesia[13]. It is likely that there should be different descending pathways of these two analgesic effects.

Our results suggest that the analgesia produced by different strengths of electroacupuncture may likely occur through different mechanisms. The analgesia of the moderate strength acupuncture may partially result from the activity of opiate receptors, and its mechanism differs at least in some aspects from that of "stress analgesia". On the other hand, the analgesia of superstrength acupuncture may be a kind of "stress analgesia".

REFERENCES

[1] Mayer, D.J. *et al.*: *Brain Res.*, **121**:368, 1977.

[2] 上海市人体针刺镇痛实验协作组：医学情况交流 **6**：12，1977。

[3] Pomeranz B, *et al.*: *Life Sci.*, **19**:1757, 1976.

[4] 黄晔等：中华医学杂志 **58**：196，1978。

[5] 程介士等：中华医学杂志 **59**：257，1978。

[6] Mclennan, H. *et al.*: *Pain*, **3**:229, 1977.

[7] Goldstein, A. *et al.*: *Life Sci.*, **18**:599, 1976.

[8] Hayes, R.L. *et al.*: *Neurosci. Abstr.*, **2**:939, 1976.

[9] Bodnar, R.L. *et al.*:*Fed Proc.*, **26**:1010, 1977.

[10] Rossier, J, *et al.*: *Nature*, **270**:618, 1977.

[11] 曹小定等：针刺镇痛效果与交感机能活动的关系，本论文集。

[12] 上海第一医学院针麻研究室神经药理组：两种电针强度对家兔血浆皮质醇的影响，待发表。

[13] Mayer, D.J. *et al.*: *Pain*, **2**:379, 1977.

EFFECT OF MORPHINE TOLERANCE ON ACUPUNCTURE ANALGESIA

Zhang Anzhong, Xu Shaofen, Zhang Lingmei,
Zeng Dayun
(Research Department of Acupuncture Analgesia, Shanghai First Medical College)

It has been reported that acupuncture analgesia could be antagonized by naloxone[1,2], indicating that the mechanism of acupuncture analgesia is related to the opiate receptor. Does this cross-tolerance occur between morphine and acupuncture analgesia? Our experimental results have revealed the nonentity of cross-tolerance between morphine and acupuncture analgesia, and that the analgesic effect of acupuncture occurring in the morphine tolerant rabbits could also be antagonized by the morphine antagonist levallorphan. Small doses of para-chloroamphetamine (PCA) had no prominent effect on the acupuncture analgesia of control rabbits, but it did completely abolish the acupuncture analgesia of tolerant rabbits.

I. MATERIALS AND METHODS

1. Drugs.

(1) Levallorphan hydrochloride synthesized by Shanghai Institute of Medicinal Industry was given intravenously as 3% solution in distilled water at a dose of 3 mg/kg.

(2) PCA synthesized by Shanghai Institute of Materia Medica, Academia Sinica, was freshly prepared before subcutaneous injection at a dose of 1 mg/kg, and treated with electroacupuncture 24 hr later.

(3) Morphine Hydrochloride produced by Qinghai Pharmaceutical Factory.

2. Animals. Healthy rabbits of both sexes weighing 2 kg were used.

3. Evaluation of pain threshold. The potassium iontophoretic dolorimeter was used to measure the analgesic effects of acupuncture and morphine. The defense reaction of the head and forelimbs was taken as the pain response, and the electric current in mA at that moment was recorded as the pain threshold. The basal pain threshold was obtained from the average value of 3–4 determinations before the acupuncture. Then, the electroacupuncture was carried out on one limb at the points corresponding to the "Hegu" and "Waiguan" of a man, using a G-6805 electroacupuncture apparatus with a frequency of 2 pulses/sec and a voltage about 7.5–8 mA which is sufficient to cause slight twitches of the forelimb. The pain threshold was measured at an interval of 10 minutes, and it was raised after the 10–20th minute of acupuncture and reached the maximum at the 40–60th minute. If the electroacupuncture was prolonged, the raised pain threshold gradually subsided down and got back to the pre-acupuncture level at the 120th minute when the tolerance of electroacupuncture was produced.

4. Tolerance to morphine. Two methods were used to establish the morphine tolerance:

(1) The method of using morphine intravenously infused within 8 hours[4]. Morphine hydrochloride 50mg/kg was dissolved in 5% glucose raline solution and intravenously infused into the conscious animals from a continuous infusion apparatus within 8 hours. The rate of infusion was 10–15 ml/hr and in control experiments the rabbits were infused with 5% glucose saline solution only. The pain threshold was measured in the whole course of infusion. It was found that an increase of analgesi a was observed, and the peak of analgesia was reached at about the 2nd hr of infusion, then the level of analgesia began to decline and returned gradually to the pre-infusion level at about the 8th hr of infusion. When this tolerance phenomenon was established, the experiments could be carried out on the next day.

(2) The method of morphine subcutaneous injection for a week—modified Herz's method. In rabbits, increasing doses of morphine up to 120 mg/kg per day were injected in the subcutaneous tissue at the back of neck. The dose schedule of the 1–7th day was as follows: 20, 40, 60, 80, 100, 120, and 120 mg/kg per day. The animals showed loss of appetite, constipation and decrease of body weight. Hence it was not so safe as in the method of intravenous infusion, since the decrease of body weight was not observed in the latter case. In the control group, the rabbits were only injected with normal saline.

Tolerance to morphine was verified by a nonresponse in pain threshold to a test intravenous injection of morphine 5 mg/kg. In individual rabbits the withdrawal syndrome was precipitated by an intravenous injection of naloxone 0.4 mg per rabbit. It is characterized by the rabbits' struggling, squeaking, mydriasis, etc. soon after the injection. After experiments, a dose of 20 mg/kg of morphine subcutaneously was injected twice daily to prolong the tolerance of morphine.

5. Statitics. Using t test and Wilcoxon examination.

II. RESULTS

1. Tolerance to morphine was established in 13 rabbits by the method of intravenous infusion or subcutaneous injection. It was verified by a nonresponse in pain threshold to a test injection of morphine (5 mg/kg), but when the same dose of morphine was given to control rabbits, the pain thresholds were markedly increased (Fig. 1).

The morphine tolerant rabbits and control rabbits were all under electroacupuncture; the pain threshold was markedly increased (Fig. 2), and the analgesic effect of acupuncture occurred both in the tolerant rabbits and in the control rabbits (Fig. 2). There was no statistically significant difference between the tolerant rabbits and the control rabbits at the end of 10 and 20 minutes ($P<0.05$). The two groups of rabbits were also under electroacupuncture; as the pain threshold rose markedly, levallorphan 3 mg/kg was given intravenously to both groups in 7 morphine tolerant rabbits and 5 control rabbits when the electroacupuncture was being continued. The acupuncture analgesia of all rabbits were reversed by levallorphan, except in one of the control rabbits, and the peak of reversal was at the 10th

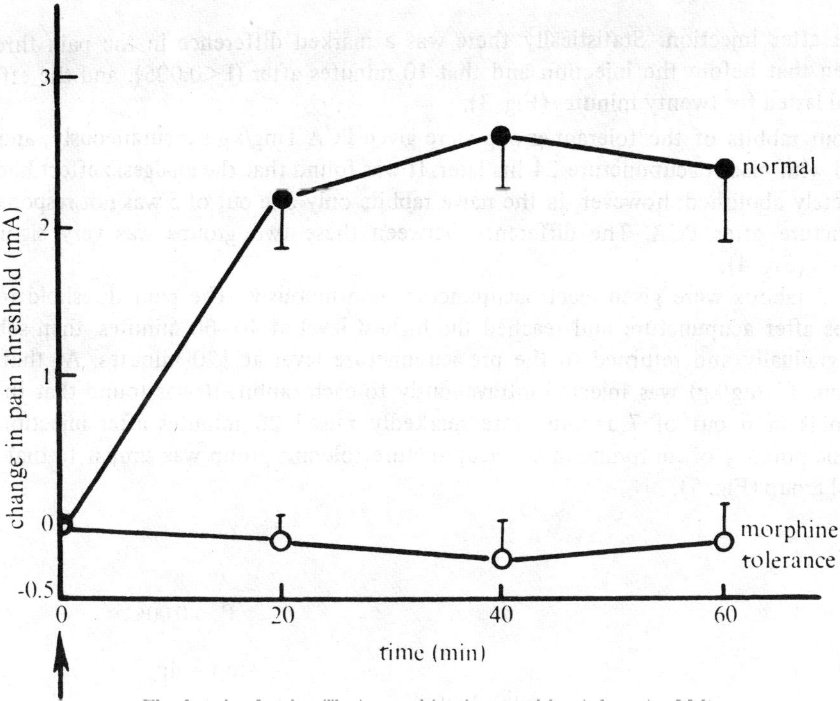

Fig. 1 Analgesic effect morphine in morphine tolerant rabbits.

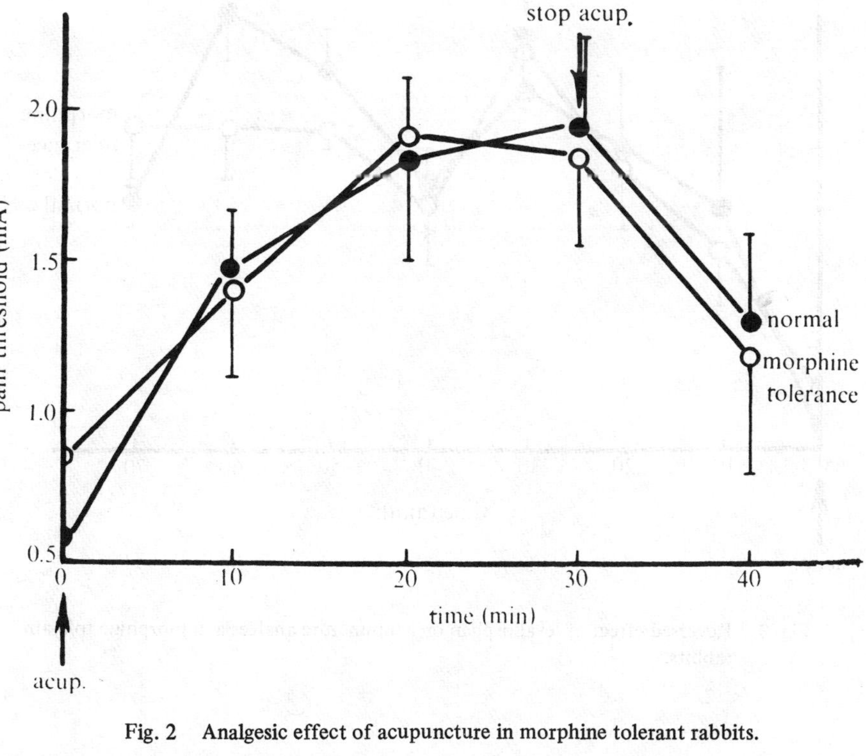

Fig. 2 Analgesic effect of acupuncture in morphine tolerant rabbits.

minute after injection. Statistically there was a marked difference in the pain threshold between that before the injection and that 10 minutes after ($P<0.005$), and the effect of reversal lasted for twenty minutes (Fig. 3).

Four rabbits of the tolerant group were given PCA 1mg/kg subcutaneously, and were treated with electroacupuncture 24 hrs later. It was found that the analgesic effect had been completely abolished; however, in the naive rabbits only one out of 5 was not responsive to acupuncture after PCA. The difference between these two groups was very significant ($P<0.01$) (Fig. 4).

2. 7 rabbits were given electroacupuncture continuously. The pain threshold rose 20 minutes after acupuncture and reached the highest level at 40–60 minutes, then subsided down gradually and returned to the pre-acupuncture level at 120 minutes. At that time, morphine (5 mg/kg) was injected intravenously to each rabbit. It was found that the pain thresholds in 6 out of 7 rabbits were markedly raised 20 minutes after injection. The analgesic potency of morphine in the acupuncture tolerant group was similar to that in the control group (Fig. 5).

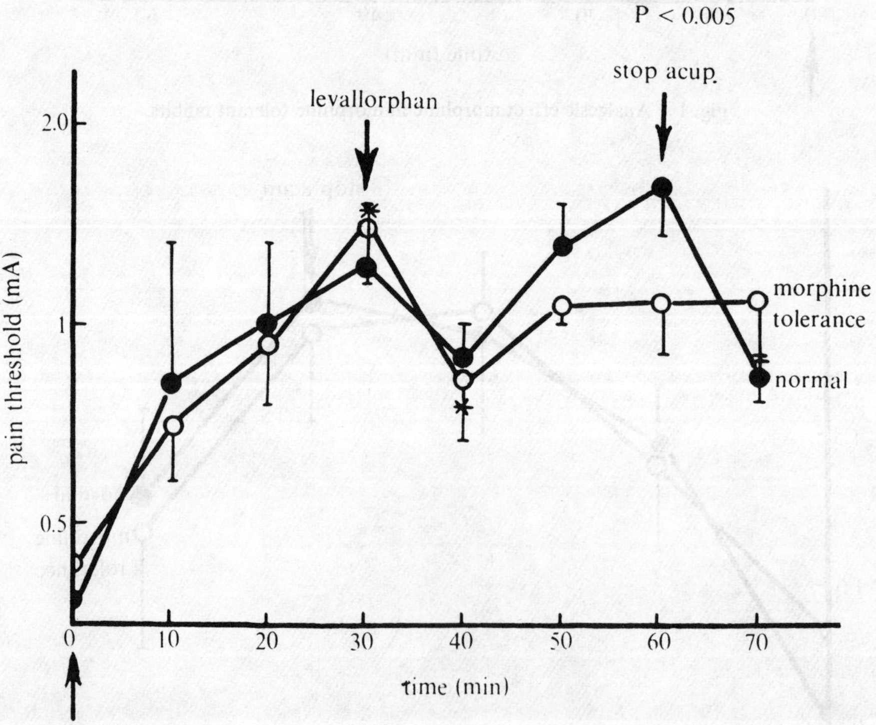

Fig. 3 Reversed effect of levallorphan on acupuncture analgesia in morphine tolerant rabbits.

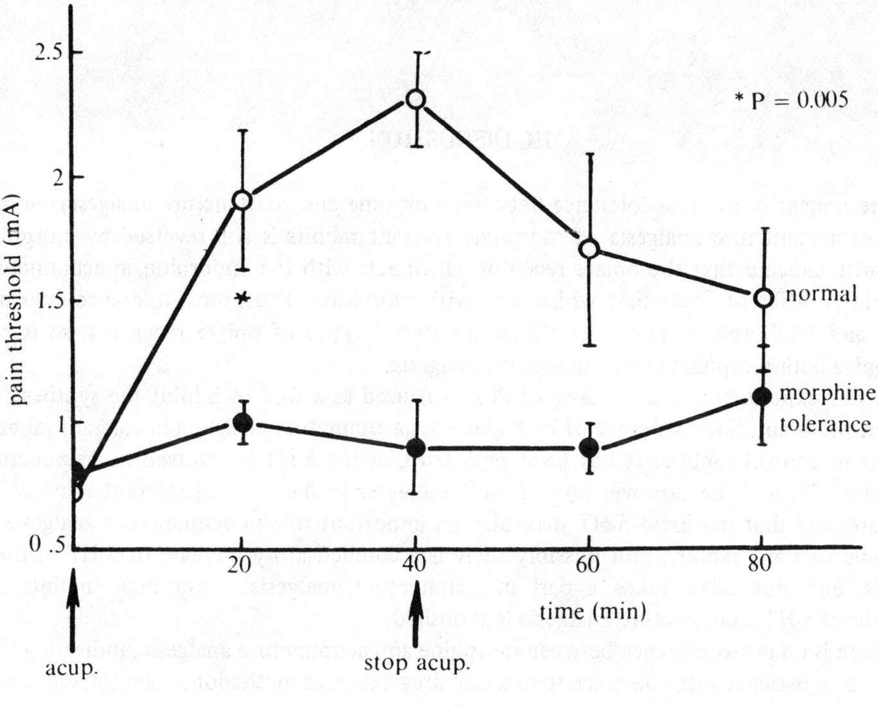

Fig. 4 Acupuncture analgesia after 24 hours of PCA.

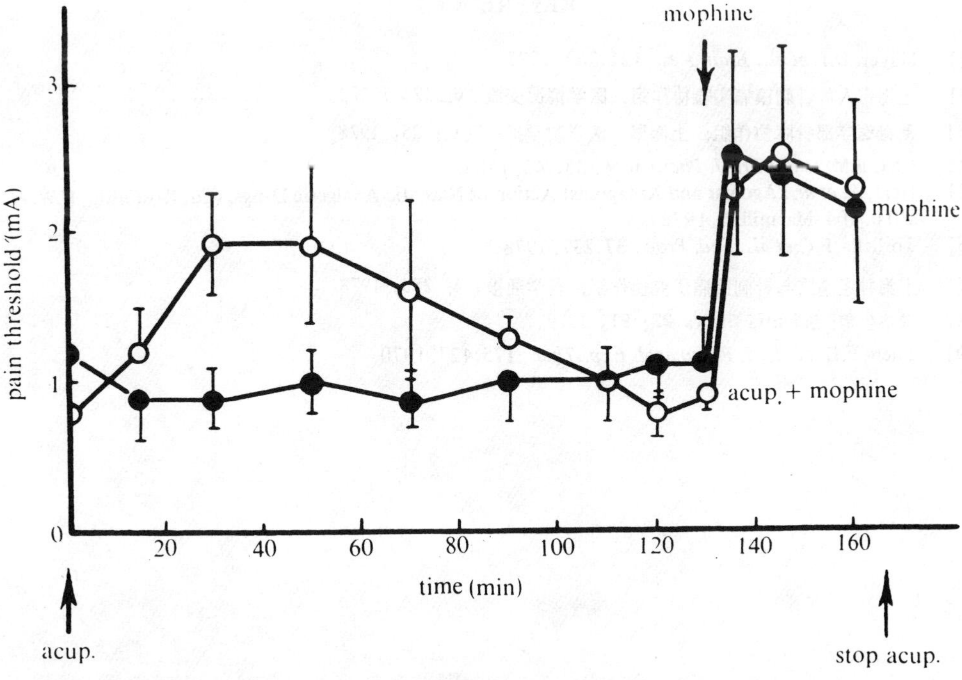

Fig. 5 Analgesic effect of morphine occurred in the acupuncture tolerant rabbits.

III. DISCUSSION

The nonentity of cross-tolerance between morphine and acupuncture analgesia and the effect of acupuncture analgesia of morphine tolerant rabbits is still reversed by morphine antagonist indicate that the opiate receptor which acts with the endorphin in acupuncture analgesia is different from that which acts with morphine. Thus, cross-tolerance does not occur, and levallorphan may have effects on several types of opiate receptors, so it can antagonize both morphine and acupuncture analgesia.

In our experiment, a small dose of PCA was used as a tool to inhibit the synthesis of 5-HT in the brain. Such a dosage of PCA abolishes acupuncture analgesia in tolerant rabbits, but not in control rabbits. It has been reported that the 5-HT is involved in acupuncture analgesia[7,8], and the turnover rate of 5-HT increases in the brain of tolerant animals[9]. It is supposed that the brain 5-HT may play an important role in acupuncture analgesia in morphine tolerant rabbits, and possibly there is a compensatory increase of 5-HT in these animals, and this 5-HT takes a part in acupuncture analgesia. After PCA inhibits the synthesis of 5-HT, acupuncture analgesia is abolished.

There is no cross-tolerance between morphine and acupuncture analgesia, indicating that chronic pain patients with tolerance to narcotic drugs, such as methadon, dolantin, etc. could also be treated with acupuncture as a pain-inhibiting measure.

REFERENCES

[1] Mayer, D.J. *et al.*: *Brain Res.,* **121**:368, 1977.

[2] 上海市人体针刺镇痛实验协作组：医学情况交流 **6**: 12，1977。

[3] 基础医学部针麻协作组：上海第一医学院学报 5(1): 25，1978。

[4] Cox, B.M. *et al.*: *Bri. J. Pharmacol.,* **33**:245, 1968.

[5] Herz, A. *et al.*: **Agonist and Antagonist Action of Narcotic Analgesic Drugs,** (Ed. Kosterlitg, H.W. *et al.*) p. 104, Macmillan, 1972.

[6] Torllella, F.C. *et al.*: *Fed. Proc.,* **37**:237, 1978.

[7] 上海神经递质与针刺镇痛研究协作组：科学通报，**4**: 253，1978。

[8] 韩济生等: Scientia Sinica **22**: 91，1979。

[9] Shen, F.H. *et al.*: *J. Pharmacol. Exp. Ther.,* **175**:427, 1970.

CENTRAL 5-HYDROXYTRYPTAMINE, OPIATE-LIKE SUBSTANCES AND ACUPUNCTURE ANALGESIA

Han Jisheng, Tang Jian, Fan Shaoguang,
Ren Minfeng*, Zhou Zhongfu, Zhang Wanqin,**
Liang Xinan***
(Research Group of Acupuncture Anesthesia Beijing Medical College, Beijing)

Acupuncture therapy is one of the classical methods for combatting painful ailments in the traditional Chinese medicine. The clinical applications of acupuncture anesthesia in recent years have further promoted the study of acupuncture analgesia (AA). Recent advances in the research regarding morphine analgesia (MA) and stimulation-produced analgesia (SPA), and the discovery of endogenous opiate-like substances in the brain have increased the study of pain and analgesia to new heights. It seems that although different procedures are adopted in AA, MA and SPA, they could activate one and the same pain modulating system in the CNS which imparts an inhibitory influence on the transmission and perception of nociceptive stimulus within the body. Numerous neurotransmitters have been implicated in this system; among them 5-hydroxytryptamine (5-HT) and endogenous opiatelike substances (OLS) might be the key links. In this paper, we shall discuss the interrelationships between 5-HT, OLS and the effect of AA.

I. THE INTERRELATIONSHIP BETWEEN 5-HT AND AA

1. Effect of lowering of cerebral 5-HT content on AA. Rats were given electroacupuncture (2-15 Hz) at bilateral "Zusanli" and "Sanyinjiao" points with gradually increasing strengths from 1 to 3 volts. There was a significant rise in pain threshold as measured by the radiant heat tail-flick test[1]. The lowering of cerebral 5-HT content following the intraperitoneal injection of parachlorophenylalanine (PCPA), the 5-HT synthesis inhibitor, or intracerebral injection of 5,6-dihydroxytryptamine (5,6-DHT), the serotonergic chemical denervator, was accompanied by a parallel decrease in the effect of AA. A significant positive correlation was found between the % change of central 5-HT (x) and the effect of AA (y, % change of pain threshold ever the basal level) (Fig. 1), expressed in an equation of

---

Present address: * Gansu Institute of New Medicine and Pharmacology,
**Zunyi Medical College.
***Guangxi Medical College.

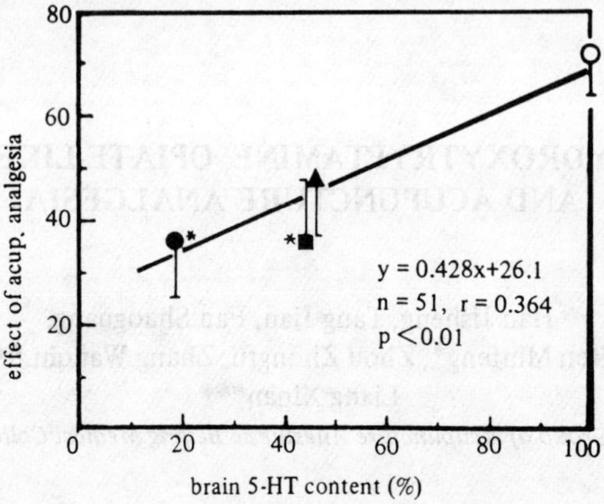

Fig. 1 The relationship between cerebral 5-HT and the effect of acupuncture analgesia.

Abscissa denotes % of 5-HT content of the whole brain, taking the average content in normal rats (655±19 ng/g) as 100%. Ordinate denotes the average pain threshold changes in 30 minutes of electroacupuncture. The solid regression line in the figure is based on the regression equation calculated from the data of 51 rats: 20 normal rats (○), 7 rats injected with 200 mg/kg of PCPA ip (▲), 12 rats injected with PCPA 320mg/kg ip plus 10mg/kg ivt(●) and 12 rats treated with 5,6-DHT, 75μg ivt plus 25μg injected into bilateral medial forebrain bundle (■). The average value of the four groups and their standard errors are also shown for reference. *denotes $p<0.05$ as compared with the normal control group.

linear regression: $y=0.428x+26.1$ ($r=0.364$, $n=51$, $P<0.01$)[2]. It can be seen from the equation that the effect of electroacupuncture in rats is closely related to the cerebral 5-HT content. In addition, the effect of AA would not be totally abolished, even though the content of central 5-HT falls to a very low level. This implies that central 5-HT is an important factor but not the sole determinant of AA.

2. Changes in the cerebral 5-HT content during AA. As reported previously, there was a significant rise in cerebral 5-HT content during AA in rats[3]. In a recent study, we have further proved that the % increase in amplitude of central 5-HT (y) was positively correlated with the effect of AA (% increase of pain threshold, x) in the regression equation: $y=0.30x-4.7$ ($n=27$, $r=0.59$, $P<0.001$)[4] (Fig 2). This gives further affirmative support to the important role of 5-HT in AA.

II. THE INTERRELATIONSHIP BETWEEN OLS AND AA

1. Effect of blockade of opiate receptors on AA. It has been proved separately by Mayer in human beings[5] and by Pomeranz in mice[6] and cats[7] that the effect of AA could be partially abolished by opiate receptor antagonists. We have obtained similar results in rabbits[8], implying that OLS is implicated in AA; but we failed in our experiments with the rat tail-flick acupuncture analgesia model. The dose of naloxone (20μg in 50μl infused

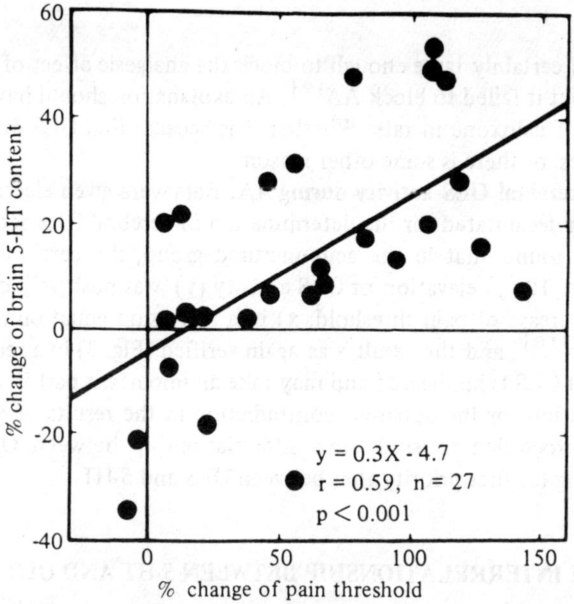

Fig. 2 Changes of cerebral 5-HT content during acupuncture analgesia in the rat. 27 rats were decapitated after 30 minutes of electroacupuncture, and their brains removed. Half of the brain was used for measurement of 5-HT spectroflourophotometrically. The ordinate denotes the % change as compared with the normal control value. The oblique line is the regression line from the equation shown in the figure.

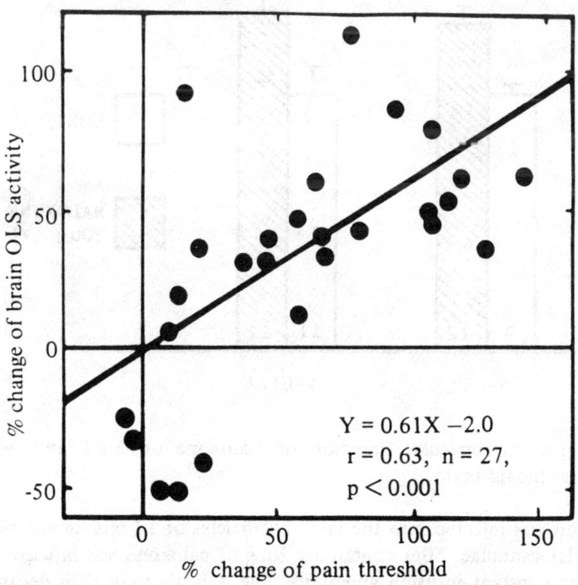

Fig. 3 Changes of cerebral OLS activity during acupuncture analgesia in the rat.

27 rats were decapitated after 30 minutes of electroacupuncture. Half of the brain was removed for determination of opioid activity by radioreceptor assay. The ordinate denotes the % change as compared with the normal control value. The oblique line is the regression line from the equation shown in the figure.

within 16 minutes) was certainly large enough to block the analgesic effect of morphine (10 mg/kg sc) completely, but it failed to block AA[9]. An explanation should have been sought for the ineffectiveness of naloxone in rats: Whether it is because that OLS does not take its part in AA in this species, or there is some other reason.

2. Changes in the cerebral OLS activity during AA. Rats were given electroacupuncture for 30 minutes and then decapitated for the determination of cerebral OLS activity by radioreceptor assay. It was found that in the acupunctured group, the cerebral OLS activity increased conspicuously. The % elevation of OLS activity (y) was positively correlated with the effect of AA (% increase of pain threshold, x) in a regression equation: $y=0.56x-7.1$ ($r=0.61$, $n=20$, $P<0.01$)[10], and the result was again verified (Fig. 3) in a recent study[4]. This implies that central OLS is implicated and may take an important part in AA in rats.

Aiming at a resolution for the apparent contradiction in the results of experiments in rats and rabbits, we proceeded to study the interrelationship between OLS and other neurotransmitters, taking for first priority that between OLS and 5-HT.

III. THE INTERRELATIONSHIP BETWEEN 5-HT AND OLS

1. Effect of blockade of opiate receptors on cerebral 5-HT. After the rats were given intraventricular infusion of naloxone (20μg within 16 minutes), they were decapitated immediately for the determination of 5-HT content, which increased by 14% on average over

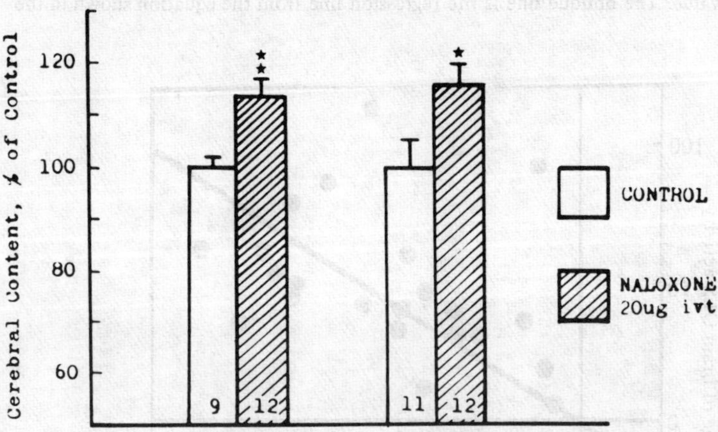

Fig. 4 Effect of intraventricular injection of Naloxone on 5-HT and 5-HIAA content of the rat brain.

Naloxone solution was injected into the lateral ventricles of 12 rats implanted with chronic ventricular cannulae. 50μl containing 20μg of naloxone was infused within 16 minutes using constant infusion apparatus. The animals were then decapitated and their brains removed for determination of 5-HT and 5-HIAA spectroflourophotometrically. The contents were expressed as % of the control value from 11 normal rats. *denotes $p<0.05$, **$p<0.01$ as compared with the normal control.

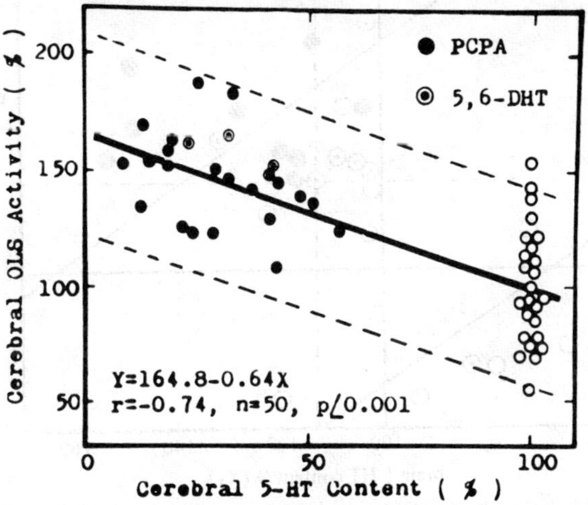

Fig. 5 The effect of lowering of cerebral 5-HT content on brain opioid activity in the rat.

rats were sacfificed 3 days after PCPA injection (•) or 5 days after 5,6-DHT treatment (O), and their brains removed for determination of 5-HT content and OLS activity. The corresponding values of the normal control rats (o) were taking as 100%. Full line in the figure represents the regression line from the data of 50 rats, and the dotted lines the 95% confidence limits.

the control group ($P<0.01$), and 5-HIAA by 16% ($P<0.05$). The results imply that the blockage of endogenous OLS activity brought about an acceleration in the metabolism of central 5-HT (Fig 4).

2. Effect of lowering of central 5-HT on cerebral OLS activity. The decrease in cerebral 5-HT content (x) following the administration of PCPA or 5,6-DHT was accompanied by a corresponding increase in central OLS activity (y), and a high negative correlation was found between their relative contents expressed as % of normal ($r=-0.74$, $n=50$, $P<0.001$). The regression equation ($y=164.8-0.64x$) implied that a decrease in the cerebral 5-HT content effected a spontaneous increase in central OLS activity (Fig 5).

The existence of an intimate functional interrelationship between central 5-HT and OLS, the impairment of function in either of them being compensated by an automatic elevation in the other, helps to explain the following experimental phenomena:

(1) The effect of AA was not totally abolished, even though the cerebral 5-HT content was reduced to less than 20% of its normal level (cf., section I, 1).

(2) Blockage of cerebral OLS activity did not attenuate the effect of AA significantly in rats (cf., section II, 1).

(3) Intraventricular injection of naloxone which induced a partial blockage of the effect of AA in normal rabbits was ineffective in those in which the cerebral 5-HT content had been elevated by the injection of pargyline[7].

IV. THE INTERRELATIONSHIPS BETWEEN 5-HT, OLS AND AA

1. Change in the cerebral 5-HT content and OLS activity during AA in normal rats[4].

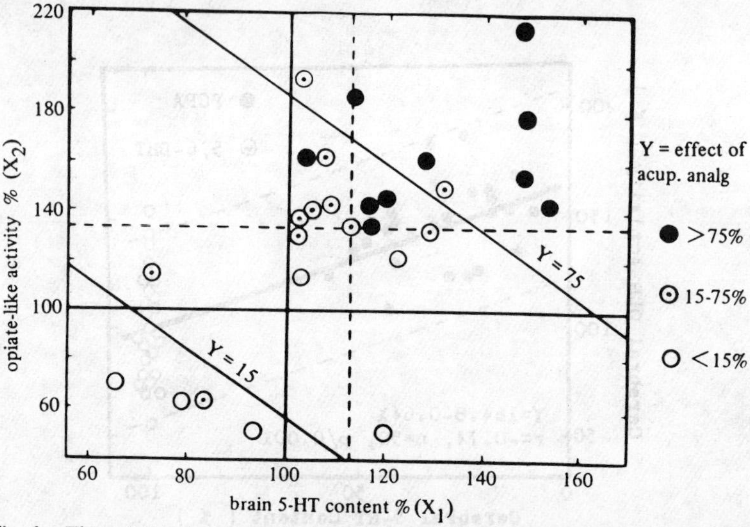

Fig. 6 The relation between the acupuncture analgesic effect and the changes of 5-HT content and opioid activity in the brain of the rat.

Rats were killed immediately after 30 minutes' electroacupuncture and their brains removed for determination of 5-HT content and opioid activity. The values were expressed as % of the normal control. The effect of acupuncture analgesia (% increase of pain threshold after electroacupuncture, Y) is positively related with the cerebral 5-HT content (X_1) and the OLS activity (X_2), as shown by the regression equation $Y=0.64X_1+0.46X_2-75$. The two oblique lines are the regression lines to predict the neurochemical changes when Y=15(minimal acupuncture effect) and Y=75 (excellent acupuncture effect).

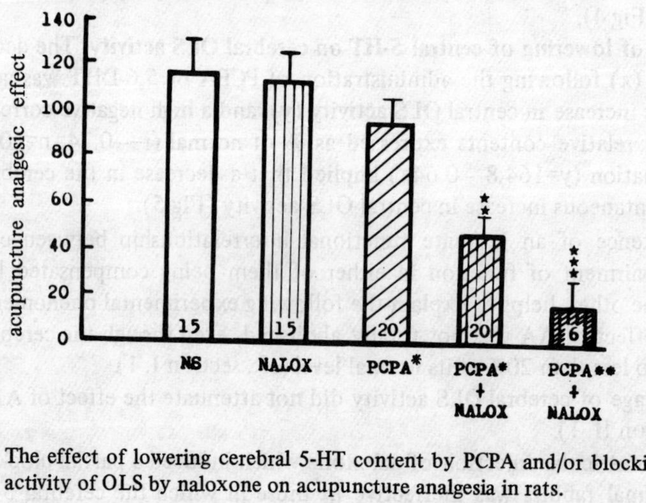

Fig. 7 The effect of lowering cerebral 5-HT content by PCPA and/or blocking the activity of OLS by naloxone on acupuncture analgesia in rats.

Ordinate denotes the % increase of pain threshold after 10 minutes of electro-acupuncture. Numerals in columes denote number of animals in each group. NS: intraventricular injection of 20µl of normal saline. NALOX: ivt infusion of 20µg/50µl of naloxone in 16 minutes. PCPA*: PCPA 200mg/kg ip. PCPA**:PCPA 320mg/kg ip plus 10 mg/kg ivt. **P<0.01, ***p<0.001 as compared with the NS group.

In a group of 27 rats given electroacupuncture for 30 min, the cerebral 5-HT content and OLS activity were determined simultaneously after decapitation at the end of electroacupuncture. It was found that rats with high levels of both central 5-HT content and OLS activity generally exhibit excellent analgesic effects, those with elevation of either 5-HT or OLS a moderate analgesic effect, while those with no elevation or even a reduction in both showed a poor effect (Fig. 6). The interrelationships between central 5-HT content (%, x_1), OLS activity (%, x_2)(Fig. 6) and the effect of AA (% increase in pain threshold, y) can be expressed by the regression equation: $y=0.64x_1+0.46x_2-75$ ($r=0.69$, $P<0.001$).

From the above equation we denote that central 5-HT and OLS are important factors determining the effect of AA, and the effect of AA is related to the joint action of these neurotransmitters. In order to ascertain the general significance of the equation, the experiment was repeated under conditions of reduced 5-HT.

2. The interrelationships between 5-HT, OLS and the effect of AA in PCPA-treated rats. As mentioned above, the reduction of central 5-HT content after PCPA was accompanied by a spontaneous rise in cerebral OLS activity. The trend of elevation of OLS was even more marked when electroacupuncture was given to these animals. Correlative analysis of central 5-HT content and OLS activity with the effect of AA in individual rats revealed that, inasmuch as the decrease in cerebral 5-HT had been compensated by a rise in OLS, the rats retained a fairly good effect of AA. While in those rats, where in the cerebral OLS activity failed to make up for the loss in 5-HT, the effect of AA was almost completely abolished. The results of observation in a group of 51 rats may be expressed in a regression equation: $y=0.61x_1+0.48x_2-62$ ($r=0.60$, $P<0.01$), which was very similar to that obtained in normal rats (cf. section IV,1). The consistency of the general equation under different experimental conditions may well indicate the existence of a substantial interrelationship between central 5-HT and OLS with regard to the effect of AA.

3. The effect of simultaneous blockade of 5-HT and OLS on AA in rats[8]. Intraperitoneal injection of a small dose of PCPA (200 mg/kg) reduced the cerebral 5-HTcontent by 52% ($P<0.001$); at the same time, the effect of AA was reduced by 19% only ($P>0.05$). Intraventricular infusion of naloxone (20 μg) had no apparent effect on AA also. But the effect of AA was reduced very significantly when these 2 measures were given in combination (−59%, $P<0.005$). The results implied that the antagonistic effect of naloxone could have been manifested in rats in cases where there was a reduction in the functional activity of central 5-HT. When naloxone was given in combination with large doses of PCPA (320 mg/kg ip plus 10 mg/kg ivt), both the effects of 5-HT and OLS were blocked, and the effect of AA was almost totally abolished (−82%, not significantly different from the basal pain threshold, see Fig. 7).

V. CONCLUSION

1. The effect of AA in rats seems to be intimately related to the cerebral 5-HT content and OLS activity, and the extent they were mobilized in the course of acupuncture.

2. There seems to be an intimate interrelationship and a functionally compensatory mechanism between 5-HT and OLS in the CNS.

REFERENCES

[1] Jen, M.F. and Han, C.S.: *Acta Physiol. Sinica,* **30**:204, 1978. (In Chinese)

[2] Han, C.S., *et al.*: *National Med. J. China,* **58**: 721, 1978. (In Chinese)

[3] Han, C.S., *et al.*: *Scientia Sinica,* **22**:91, 1979.

[4] Liang, X.N., *et al.*: *To be published.*

[5] Mayer, D.J. *et al.*: *Brain Res.,* **121**:368, 1977.

[6] Pomeranz, B and Chiu, D.: *Life Sci.,* **19**:1757, 1976.

[7] Pomeranz, B. *et al.*: *Exp. Neurol.,* **54**:172, 1977.

[8] Research Group of Acupuncture Anesthesia, Peking Medical College: *Chinese J. Surg.,* **15**:192, 1977. (In Chinese)

[9] Fan, S.G. *et al.*: *Kexue Tongbao,* **1979**, in press.

[10] Tang, J. and Han, C.S.: *J. Peking Med. College,* **(3)**:150, 1978. (In Chinese)

ROLE OF BRAIN SEROTONERGIC AND CATECHOLAMINERGIC SYSTEMS IN ACUPUNCTURE ANALGESIA

Jin Guozhang, Zhang Zhende, Yu Leiping,
Han Yifan, Xu Jian, Feng Jie,
Pan Jiancui*
(Shanghai Institute of Materia Medica, Academia Sinica)

Serotonine (5-HT) and catecholamines, as essential neurotrans mitters in the brain, have important physiological functions. In recent years, several transmitters, such as 5-HT, DA, NA, etc. have been demonstrated to be able to actively participate in pain perception and acupuncture analgesia[1-11]. Elucidating the relationship between neurotransmitters and acupuncture analgesia (AA) will be helpful for understanding the mode of action and the material basis of AA . We have systematically studied the relationship between central 5-hydroxytryptaminergic system and AA , and showed that the normal functioning of the 5-HT system was indispensable for AA [6-8]. Our viewpoint has been accepted. However, the effect of catecholamines in AA is still uncertain, because this is a complicated and contradictory problem. In the following, we would give a survey on our recent work about the role of the monoaminergic transmitters on AA .

I. METHODS

(I) Acupuncture Analgesia in Rats[7-8]

Rats weighing 190–220g were used. A pair of electrodes were fixed on the distal one-third part of the tail, the negative electrode being placed at the proximal end. A cutaneous electric nocuous stimulation was applied, and the strength of current was increased in parallel with the duration of stimulation. The animal usually responded firstly with a tail-flick and then with a squeak. The latencies (sec) of both responses were taken

---

Abbreviations: DA– dopamine; NA–noradrenaline; 5-HTP– 5-hydroxytryptophan; 5HT 5-hydroxytryptamine; 5-HIAA–5-hydroxy-indoleacetic acid; 5,6-DHT 5,6-dihydroxytryptaimine; PCA–p-Chloroamphetamine; HVA– Homovanillic acid; EAC– electric acupuncture; AA– acupuncture analgesia.

* Fudan University, Shanghai.

separately to represent the pain threshold. Two pairs of acupuncture needles were separately inserted into the bilateral points which corresponded to "Huantiao" and "Zusanli" points on human beings, the needles on the "Huantiao" pionts being used as the negative electrodes. In some cases only one pair of needles was inserted into the bilateral "Huantiao" pionts. The Shanghai G-6805 type transistor therapeutic apparatus was used for electric acupuncture (EAC), and the dense-sparse biphasic waves were adopted. The duration of acupuncture lasted 30 min.

At the beginning of the experiment, we kept the animals calm in the individual cages for 30 min. Then the pain thresholds were measured every 5 min for three times. The mean value was taken as the "basic pain threshold" (BPT). The animal was then given the drug to be tested; the pain thresholds (as "post-medication threshold") were again measured. And then, EAC was applied to the rat; after the cessation of EAC the pain thresholds were again measured every 5 min for three times which was designated as the "post-acupuncture threshold". The "Least Significant Difference" statistics method was used to assess the effect of drugs on AA . Usually, each experiment consisted of four groups: 1) Saline, 2) Drug, 3) Saline +Acupuncture, and 4) Drug + Acupuncture.

After AA test, most of the animals were decapitated and the heads were immediately immersed into the dry ice-acetone or liquid nitrogen. Each brain was homogenized with acidic butanol, and centrifuged. A definite amount of the supernatant was aspirated into the centrifuge tube with stock, and 0.1 N HCl and heptane were added. After shaking, the upper layer and lower layer were used separately to determine the amounts of 5-HT, DA, NA and 5-HIAA by spectrofluorometric analysis[12–14].

(II) Acupuncture Analgesia in Rabbits[15]

Rabbits weighing 1.7–2.0kg were used, and two platinum electrodes were placed on the skin of the two ears. The pain thresholds were measured by means of K^+ iontophoretic technique. The head turning response was taken as indication. Two rabbits showing the similar BPT were chosen for paired experiment. One of the paired rabbits was given EAC (continuous pulses with a frequency of 2–4 c/s) at the bilateral "Hegu" and "Waiguan" points for 15 min, and the other was used as control (without EAC).

After the EAC test, the animal was decapitated immediately. Brain tissue was homogenized with 0.4 N $HClO_4$, and centrifuged (15,000 × g, 30 min. 0°C). The supernatant was passed through the gel permeation chromatography[16, 17]. Brain NA, DA, HVA and 5-HIAA were sequentially separated by Sephadex G-10 and QAE-Sephadex A-25 and measured by the spectrofluorometric method (Fig. 1).

(III) Acupuncture Analgesia in Cats

The viscero-somatic reflex activities elicited by splanchnic nerve stimulation were recorded from the 11th intercostal nerve in Flaxedil immobilized cats, and that was used as the index of visceral pain reaction which could be inhibited by the stimulation of the common peroneal nerve (0.2 ms in duration, 100 c/s of frequency). The inhibitory effect

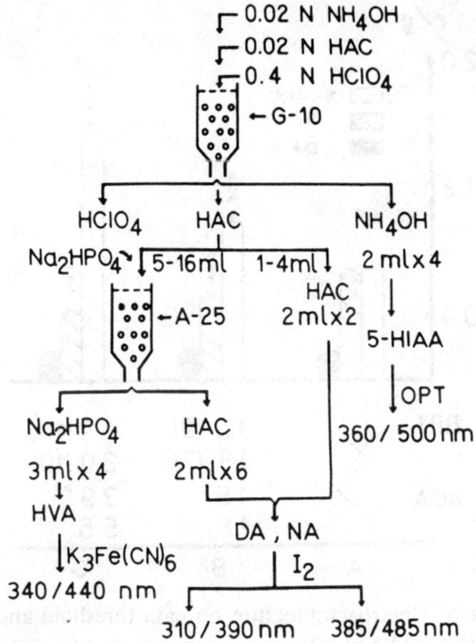

Fig. 1 Diagram on the method used for separation of NA, DA, HVA and 5-HIAA in rabbit brain.

G-10: Sephadex G-10. A-25: QAE-Sephadex A-25.

was used as an index of electric acupuncture analgesia (AA)[6]. This experiment was repeated after drug administration. Then the effects of the drug on AA were observed and the concentrations of brain 5-HT and 5-HIAA were determined.

(IV) Spectrofluorometric Analysis of 1-Tryptophan and 1-Tyrosine in Brain Tissues and Plasma[18]

The brain tissues of rat were homogenized with 0.4 N $HClO_4$, and the supernatant was passed through Dowex 50 X 2 (200–400 mesh) to separate brain tryptophan. The eluates were adjusted to pH 10 by 1 M K_2CO_3, and the natural fluorescence (280/360 nm) was measured. The concentrations of plasma 1-tryptophan were determined according to Denckla[19].

Brain tyrosine and plasma tyrosine contents were assayed spectrofluorometrically[20].

II. RESULTS

(I) Acupuncture Analgesia and Brain Levels of Monoamines

Rats were divided into 3 groups: (1) normal, (2) pain measurement, and (3) EAC and pain measurement. Figure 2 shows the effect of AA . And the brain levels of monoamines

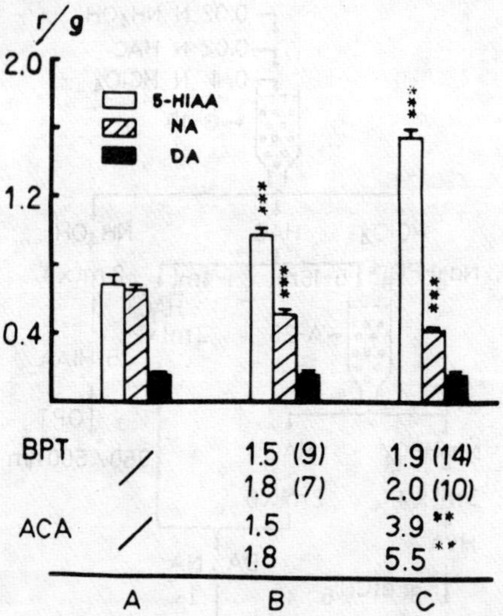

Fig. 2 The effects of electroacupuncture on pain threshold and brain contents of DA, NA, and 5-HIAA in rat.

A: contol group, B: pain measurement group, C: acupuncture group. BPT and ACA in sec. of squeak. Numerals in parenthesis represent the number of animals. **:P<0.01, ***: P<0.001.

were measured as follows. The rats which exhibited AA after EAC, had their brain contents of 5-HIAA markedly increased and NA significantly decreased. The amount of 5-HIAA increase was in the order of group 3, 2, and 1, but the brain contents of NA were in the reverse order. The brain contents of DA had no significant difference among these 3 groups (Fig. 2). Therefore, AA was accompanied by a decrease of brain NA contents and an elevation of brain 5-HIAA levels.

(II) Role of Brain Serotonergic System in Acupuncture Analgesia

1. Effect of electroacupuncture on the brain levels of 5-HT and 5-HIAA. In order to observe more accurately the relationship between AA and brain 5-HT neuronal activity, liquid nitrogen (–180°C) was used for quick freezing of the tested rats. Right after the final measurement of pain threshold, the animals (both acupuncture and nonacupuncture groups) were immediately immersed into the liquid nitrogen for a few minutes, then they were decapitated and transferred to a refrigerator for reelevation of temperature; after that the brain 5-HT and 5-HIAA contents were assayed.

The results showed that the BPT was 1.9 sec. After EAC, the pain threshold was raised to 7.0 sec (tail-flick) and 7.9 sec (squeak) respectively. At the same time, the brain 5-HT increased significantly in comparison with the nonacupuncture group, and the 5-HIAA content increased still more prominently. This indicated that there is an augmentation of 5-HT biosynthesis and oxidative deamination (Table 1). Brain 5-HIAA is a valid index for testing brain 5-HT neuronal activity.

2. Effect of electroacupuncture on the transportation of 1-tryptophan through blood-brain-barrier. It is well known that 1-tryptophan is the precursor of 5-HT. The brain content of tryptophan is derived from the transportation of tryptophan from plasma. During the transportation, there is a competitive inhibitory effect between the plasma tryptophan and tyrosine[21].

Table 1. The effects of electric acupuncture on pain threshold and the activity of Serotonergic neurons in rats

Group	BPT (squeak)	ACA (sec)	5-HT	5-HIAA
			(Mean±S.E. in ng/g brain)	
EAC	1.9 (16)	7.9***	1327 ± 50 (12)	539 ± 36 (12)
PM	1.7 (15)	1.9	1081 ± 58 (8)	370 ± 10 (8)
P value	>0.5	<0.001	<0.01	<0.001

PM: pain measurement.
***: ACA in comparison with BPT, P<0.001.
Numerals in parentheses represent the number of animals.

Table 2. The effects of electric acupuncture and Probenecid on the contents of 1-tryptophan and tyrosine in brain and plasma

Test		Non-EAC	EAC	NS	Probenecid
1-Tryptophan	Plasma	32.58±1.44 (18)	41.72± 1.82** (18)	18.76±0.93 (7)	9.12±1.70** (11)
	Brain	5.02±0.16 (15)	7.59±0.24** (15)	3.91±0.05 (7)	7.08±0.28** (11)
Tyrosine	Plasma	31.82±3.52 (8)	39.56±1.75* (16)		
	Brain	13.59±1.52	17.10±1.03		

Mean ± S.E. μg/g brain wt. or μg/ml plasma.
*: P<0.05, **: P<0.01, EAC in comparison with Non-EAC, or Probencid with NS.

After EAC, as soon as the rats exhibited AA , the brain levels of 1-tryptophan were determined and were found to be elevated significantly in comparison with the non-acupuncture rats, whilst the brain levels of tyrosine had no significant changes (Table 2). It indicated that the influence of amino-acids transportation via BBB by EAC is likely to be selective for tryptophan.

3. The augmentation of AA by an enhancement of 5-HT neuronal activity.

(1) Exogenous 1-tryptophan: Under the loading of 1-tryptophan (100 mg/kg, i.p.), the rats' BPT and pain threshold 60 min after the medication were quite similar to the saline control group. After EAC, the AA of the treated group was more potent than that of the control group (Table 3).

Table 3. The effects of serotonergic drugs on electric acupuncture analgesia

Drugs (mg/kg, ip.)	BPT	Post-Med. Threshold	A A	P value
NS + AC	1.7 (17)	–	4.9	<0.01
1-Try + AC (100)	1.7 (18)	–	6.8	<0.001
NS + AC	2.1 (10)	2.4	6.7	<0.01
Pro + AC (200)	1.7 (10)	3.6	9.1**	<0.01
NS + AC	1.6 (18)	1.3	3.7	<0.05
5HTP + AC (75)	1.3 (24)	1.5	9.1**	<0.001
NS + AC	1.6 (18)	1.4	4.6	<0.001
PCA + AC (5)	1.5 (20)	1.6	2.6**	<0.01
NS + AC	1.6 (12)	–	3.9	<0.01
Cin + AC (20)	1.7 (11)	–	1.9***	>0.5

1-Try: 1-tryptophan, pro: Probenecid, Cin: cinanserin,
*:P<0.05, **:P<0.01, ***: P<0.001, the group of NS+AC in comparison with the group of drug + AC.

In the other two groups of rats without EAC, the brain 5-HT and 5-HIAA contents of the loading group were higher than those in the control group (Table 4), indicating that the loading dosage of 1-tryptophan stimulated the activity of 5-HT neurons. It is thus suggested that the enhancement of 5-HT neuronal activity may potentiate the AA in consequence.

(2) Endogenous 1-tryptophan: Probenecid can convert plasma bound 1-tryptophan into free form, and subsequently elevate brain level of 1-tryptophan via BBB (Table 2).

60 and 90 min after administering this drug (200 mg/kg, i.p.) the post-medication threshold in rats was increased, but the amount of the increase was not significant in comparison with that of the control group. After the application of EAC, the pain threshold of the treated group was raised markedly with a potent aftereffect, which differed from the control group very significantly (Table 3).

(3) Exogenous 5-HTP: The BPT and post-medication threshold of the group treated with 5-HTP (75 mg/kg, i.p.) and the control group were quite similar. But after EAC was applied to these two groups, the pain threshold of the treated group elevated severalfold, and differed very significantly from the control (Table 3).

If rats were first loaded with 5-HTP then treated with EAC, the brain 5-HT and 5-HIAA contents of the treated group were much higher than those of the controls which were only loaded with 5-HTP without EAC (Table 4). It indicates that EAC enhances the 5-HTP decarboxylation and 5-HT oxidative deamination.

4. The attenuation of AA by a depression of 5-HT neuronal activity.

(1) 5,6-DHT: Following intra-ventricular injection of 5,6-DHT (500–1,000μg/0.12–0.2 ml) to cats, the inhibitory effect on viscero-somatic reflex resulting from the common peroneal nerve stimulation (IEA) was attenuated (Fig. 3)[6]. In 3–10 days after the 5,6-DHT injection the IEA diminished to a large extent and a significant decrease in 5-HT and 5-HIAA contents of diencephalon, midbrain-pons, medulla and spinal cord occurred (Fig. 4).

Table 4. Effects of drugs on the brain contents of 5-HT and 5-HIAA

Drugs	Rats (No.)	5-HT		5-HIAA	
NS	15	1.31 ± 0.02		0.45 ± 0.06	
1-Try	13	1.59 ± 0.06**		0.73 ± 0.08**	
NS	10	1.10 ± 0.02	*** (NS vs 5HTP)	0.34 ± 0.06	*** (NS vs 5HTP)
5HTP	9	1.62 ± 0.08	* (5HTP vs 5HTP + AC)	2.17 ± 0.10	*** (5HTP vs 5HTP + AC)
5HTP + AC	9	1.94 ± 0.10		3.59 ± 0.06	
NS	20	1.28 ± 0.05	*** (NS vs PCA)	0.51 ± 0.03	*** (NS vs PCA)
PCA	19	0.84 ± 0.06	* (PCA vs PCA + AC)	0.24 ± 0.03	*** (PCA vs PCA + AC)
PCA + AC	20	1.03 ± 0.05		0.42 ± 0.04	

Mean ± S.E. μg/g brain tissue, * P<0.05, ** P<0.01, *** P<0.001.

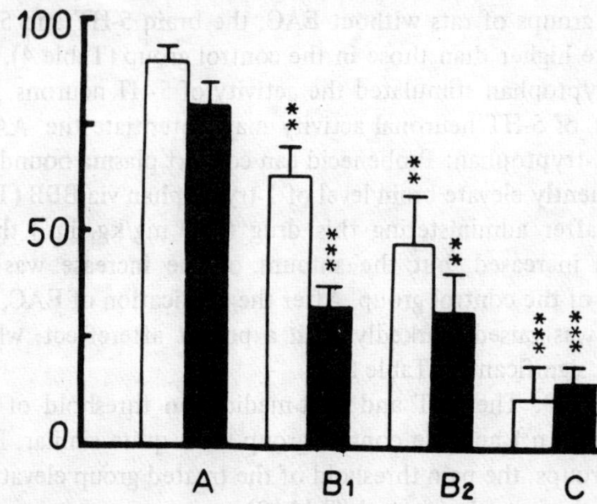

Fig. 3 The inhibitory effects of 5,6-DHT and PCA on the acupuncture analgesia in cats.

The longitudinal axis represent the % change of viscerosomatic reflex activities. A: group intraventricular injected with vesicle, B_1 : injected with 5,6-DHT 3–4 days later, B_2 : injected with 5,6-DHT 8-10 days later; C: group intraperotoneally or intravenously injected with PCA. Blank blocks represent the viscero-somatic reflex activities before or during EAC; black blocks represent the viscero-somatic reflex activities after EAC. **: $P<0.01$, ***: $P<0.001$.

A progressive degeneration of 5-HT descending nerve terminals and the acute functional destruction of nuclei raphe were observed.

(2) p-Chloroamphetamine (PCA): PCA is a selective inhibitor of brain tryptophan hydroxylase. In 4 cats, after the injection of PCA (5 mg/kg, i.p. or i.v.) a sharp decrease in IEA happened (Fig. 3).

Rats showed mild excitation after the injection of PCA (5 mg/kg), and the EAC was not applied until the next day when normal behavior had been restored. After the application of EAC, though the pain threshold of the treated group still increased, the degree of increase was much less obvious than that of the control group. These experiments showed that PCA markedly weakened the AA (Table 3). At this time, both the brain 5-HT and 5-HIAA contents of the PCA treated group were significantly reduced (Table 4). This may indicate that the 5-HT neurons are functionally inhibited.

However, the experiment showed that despite the inhibitory effect of PCA on the brain 5-HT synthesis, acupuncture process was still able to increase both brain 5-HT and 5-HIAA as we compared these results with of the control group receiving PCA alone. Thus, it is suggested that EAC may activate tryptophan hydroxylation.

(3) Cinanserin: This drug is known as a blocking agent on 5-HT receptors. If rats were given this drug (10 mg/kg, i.p.), immediately before EAC, the potency of depressive action of AA was found to be weaker than that of the control group; and the AA was completely abolished when the dose of cinanserin was increased to 20 mg/kg (Table 3).

These results indicate that the depression of 5-HT neuronal function may give rise to an attenuation of AA. Therefore, it is reasonable to suppose that the normal function of 5-HT neurons is indispensable for AA..

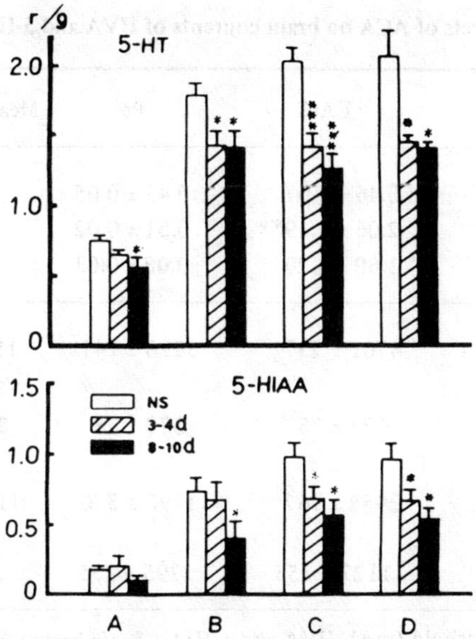

Fig. 4 The effects of 5,6-DHT on brain contents of 5-HT and 5-HIAA in cats.

A: spinal cord, B: medulla, C: pons-midbrain, D: diencephalon. The contents of 5-HT and 5-HIAA were determined on 3–4 days and 8–10 days after intraventricular injection of 5,6-DHT.

*:P<0.05, **: P<0.01, ***:P<0.001.

(III) Function of Brain Dopaminergic System and AA

Because in our previous study it was difficult to ascertain the relationship between the DA-neuronal function and EAC in rats[8], we used the rabbits as experimental models instead.

In the paired experiment, rabbits of the acupuncture group exhibited the AA, while the control group had no analgesia. In the acupuncture group, the contents of HVA and 5-HIAA in caudate and diencephalon-midbrain increased significantly in comparison with those in the control group (Table 5). Thus the EAC activated not only DA neurons, but also 5-HT neurons; the latter coincided with the above mentioned experiments of rats.

Apomorphine is an agonist of DA-receptor. The increase of the AA in rabbits given apomorphine (7 pairs) was significant by using statistical analysis of variance (F=13.6, P<0.001). Thus, DA neurons activated by the drug prompted the AA.

(IV) Role of Brain Noradrenergic System in AA

Based on the results from section (I), it was presumed that the more the brain level of NA lowered, the greater the AA manifested. In order to prove this presumption we utilized the drugs acting specifically on the NA-system to investigate the relationship between the

Table 5. The effects of ACA on brain contents of HVA and 5-HIAA in rabbits

	Test	EAC	PM	Mean of Difference	P value
	BPT	0.46 ± 0.07	0.43 ± 0.05	–	>0.5
	PT after EAC	2.06 ± 0.19**	0.51 ± 0.02	–	<0.01
	Elevated PT	1.60 ± 0.20	0.08 ± 0.03	–	<0.001
HVA	Caudatum	4761 ± 237	3228 ± 241	1533 ± 170	<0.001
	Diencephalon-mid brain	677 ± 76	378 ± 78	299 ± 51	<0.01
5HIAA	Diencephalon-mid brain	2988 ± 767	1798 ± 376	1190 ± 458	<0.05
	Medulla	1127 ± 155	795 ± 155	332 ± 66	<0.05

mean ± S.E. in pain theshold (mA), HVA and 5-HIAA (μg/g brain wt) of 8 pairs of rabbits.

NA-system and AA, such as α-mpt (tyrosine hydroxylase inhibitor), sodium diethyl dithiocarbamate (DDC, DA-β-H inhibitor), phenoxybenzamine (α-adreno-receptor antagonist) and clonidine (α-agonist). But the results were so variable that no definite conclusion could be drawn.

It is possible that the systemic injection of drugs may impose a complicated influence on the results. In order to overcome this complication, we used the method of micro-injection of drugs into certain brain regions.

The micro-injection techniques were described in another paper of this volume[22]. Following the micro-injection of NA (3μg/3μl) into the ventromedial hypothalamus, a striking potentiation of AA was observed 3 or 24 hr later. The AA was elevated 2–3 times in comparison with the degree of AA produced before injection (P<0.001). This potentiating effect was antagonized by naloxone (0.8 mg/kg, i.p.) which was injected just before acupuncture, while the original AA value (the degree of AA produced in the rats not injected with NA) remained the same. However, no matter whether the animal was given NA or not the AA effect was completely abolished by intraventricular injection of phenoxybenzamine (0.1 mg/kg/100μl) 5 hours before EAC. If EAC was applied 8 hours after the medication, the antagonistic effect of phenoxybenzamine was partially diminished (Fig. 5).

Obviously, the micro-injection of NA caused a striking potentiation of AA, which was mediated by α-adreno-receptors of ventral ascending NA bundle and in which the opiate receptors located in the ventromedial hypothalamus also took an active part.

III. DISCUSSION

Numerous neurophysiological experiments have shown that the AA resulted from the

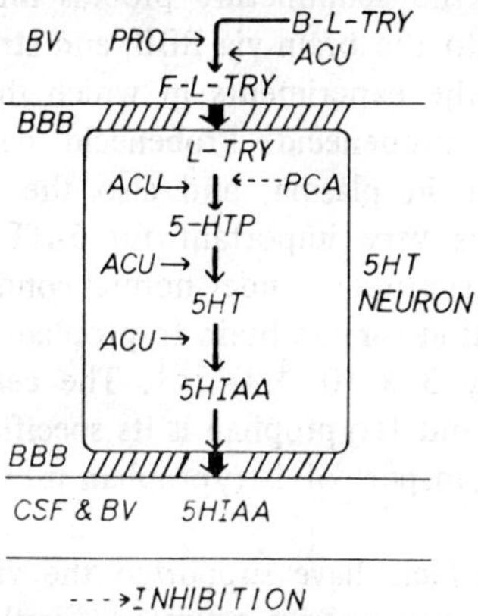

Fig. 5 **The effect of micro-injection of noradrenaline into ventro-medial hypothalamus on acupuncture analgesia.**

PBZ: phenoxybenzamine intraventricularly injected (0.1 mg/kg/100μl); naloxone intraperotoneally injected (0.8 mg/kg). 3° and 24° represent NA (3μg/3μl) injected after 3 and 24 hours respectively,

interaction between the acupunctural afferent impulses and nocuous stimuli; such interaction exists in all levels of the CNS including the cerebal cortex, the thalamus, the brainstem and the spinal cord[23–26]. As a result, the acupuncture effect inhibits the perception of pain. Monoaminergic neurons are involved in this complicate interaction. EAC may, on the one hand, activate several sorts of neurons which synergize the AA , and on the other hand, may inhibit other neuronal activities which diminish the antagonistic effect upon AA . The activity level of the neurons can be demonstrated by the amounts of the neurotransmitters biosynthesized or by the amounts of catabolic products of transmitters. For instance, the brain contents of 5-HIAA and HVA were used as the valid indices reflecting the activities of 5-HT and DA neurons respectively. In this report, drugs which act specifically on the activity of monoaminergic systems were chosen to investigate the relationship between these systems and AA . The results are discussed as follows:

1. The Normal Function of Brain Serotonergic System is Indispensable for Acupuncture Analgesia. We draw the conclusion that the normal function of brain 5-HT system is indispensable for AA from the following facts[6–8]: (1) It has been shown that 5,6-DHT can reduce the AA , and at the same time selectively destroy the central 5-HT neurons, and the brain contents of 5-HT and 5-HIAA markedly decreased concomitantly. (2) PCA was used to depress the tryptophan hydroxylation, and as a result, 5-HT neuronal activity was inhibited. Following the injection of PCA, brain 5-HT and 5–HIAA as well as ACA were reduced. (3) If the activity of 5-HT receptor was blocked by cinanserin, an attenuation or abolition of AA was observed. Our results are concurrent with those data reported elsewhere by other authors utilizing 5,6-DHT[27], PCPA[9, 28] as well as Cyproheptadine[28].

2. The Enhancement of Brain 5-HT Neuronal Activity During Acupuncture Process. Our work[18] showed that the acupuncture process might accelerate the transport of 1-tryptophan from plasma into the brain via BBB, and strengthen 5-HT neuronal activity. There results coincide with the experiments in which the animals were pretreated with exogenous 1-tryptophan or probenecid. Probenecid has the effect of elevating the endogenous free 1-tryptophan in plasma, and also the brain 1-tryptophan. The brain 1-tryptophan concentration is very important for 5-HT neuronal activity, because the concentration of the brain 1-tryptophan under normal conditions (about $4.5{-}2.5 \times 10^{-5}$M) is not an optimum concentration for the brain tryptophan hydroxylase activity (the Km of this enzyme is approximately 3×10^{-4}M)[29]. The central tryptophan hydroxylase is present only in 5-HT neuron and 1tryptophan is its specific substrate. Thus, it is suggested that the acceleration of the transport of 1-tryptophan into the brain is an important factor involved in AA.

Moreover, the following facts have supported the viewpoint (Table 4) that during the acupuncture process 5-HT neurons are activated. Firstly, EAC can partially restore the inhibition of the tryptophan hydroxylation induced by PCA; secondarily, EAC can enhance the decarboxylation of exogenous 5-HTP and convert the 5-HTP into 5-HT; thirdly, EAC can enhance oxidative deamination of the endogenous 5-HT, and greater amounts of 5-HIAA are produced. Based on these findings, it is suggested that EAC can activate the three steps of metabolism in 5-HT neurons, i.e., hydroxylation, decarboxylation, and deamination (Fig. 6).

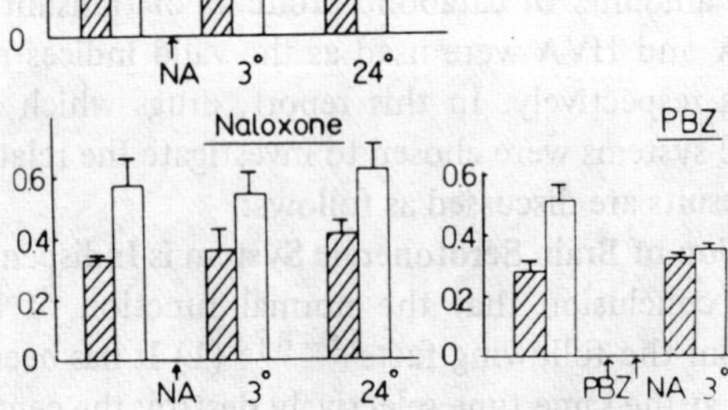

Fig. 6 Diagram showing the effect of the electroacupuncture on the 5-HT neuronal activities and transportation of 1-tryptophan.

ACU: electroacupuncture, Pro: probenecid, BV: blood vessel, BBB: blood-brain-barrier, CSF: cerebrospinal fluid, B-1-TRY: bound 1-tryptophan in plasma, F-1-TRY: free 1-tryptophan in plasma.

To sum up, EAC can elevate the brain contents of 1-tryptophan, 5-HT and 5-HIAA, and strengthen 5-HT neuronal activity which in turn enhances the AA .

3. What Roles do Catecholamines Play in AA ? The roles of CA in EAC are very complicated and results reported in the literature are contradictory[8, 10, 15, 30–34]. Several factors may influence the AA , for example: animal specics used for acupuncture, routes of medication, methods of microanalysis of neurotransmitter and its catabolic metabolites, etc. Owing to the various experimental conditions, different results were obtained. Our work revealed that if we used rats as experimental animals and used solvent to extract HVA, it was impossible to investigate the brain DA-neuronal activity[8]. When rabbits as experimental animals and gel permeation chromatography as the method to separate DA and HVA were used, it was found that the AA was accompanied by an activation of DA neurons[15]. Our results differ from the other reports[2, 10, 32] because the rabbits have less stress reaction and more contents of HVA, and Sephadex used for separation is more sensitive and accurate.

As to NA, many reports concluded that the mormal function of NA in the brain was antagonistic to AA [2, 4, 10, 30, 31], but we have a different opinion with regard to this problem[8]. The discrepency is due to the fact that systemic injection of adrenergic drugs may induce complicated and non-specific effects on the NA- system. If this factor is neglected, it is difficult to find out the exact role of NA on AA . We may doubt the reliability of the results obtained under such circumstance. Only by using the micro-injection of drugs into brain tissues can these defects be avoided. By using the micro-injectiong method, some authors[31] found that the AA was augmented by micro-injection of 6-OHDA into locus coerulus or NA-asceding dorsal bundle in rats. Thus, they considered that the normal function of dorsal ascending NA bundle was antagonistic to AA . However, in our work micro-injection of NA into the ventromedial hypothalamus, in which the ventral ascending NA bundle innervated, caused a striking potentiation of AA . Therefore, we suppose that the function of ventral ascending NA bundle differs from the dorsal NA bundle, it can potentiale the AA . Of course, further investigation is required. In fact, it is possible that the various nuclei, innervated separately by ventral or dorsal NA bundle, exert different effects on AA .

It has been shown that when neurotransmitters were injected into the ventromedial hypothalamus, only NA exhibited more specific effect than DA and 5-HT[22]. The potentiation of NA on AA was induced later, lasted longer, and was mediated by μ-adreno-receptors and opiate receptors. These features which may be related to the effects of endorphine, ACTH, etc. are very worthwhile to be clarified.

IV. CONCLUSIONS

(1) The experiments from rats rabbits and cats indicated that the normal function of brain serotonergic system is indispensable for the acupuncture analgesia. Acupuncture process activates the function of 5-HT neurons in brain of rats or rabbits; it also accelerates the 1tryptophan transportation from blood into brain. The brain concentration of 1-tryptophan is probably an important factor involved in acupuncture analgesia.

(2) Acupuncture analgesia was accompanied with an activation of rabbits' brain

DA-neuronal activity which might be also activated by apomorphine, and prompted the ACA in turn.

(3) In rats, acupuncture analgesia was accompanied by a lowering of brain contents of NA. Following the micro-injection of NA into ventromedial hypothalamus, a striking potentiation of acupuncture analgesia was found. The potentiation was induced later, lasted longer, and was mediated via μ-adreno-receptors and the opiate receptors were also involved in this effect.

REFERENCES

[1] 湖南医学院针麻原理研究组：中华医学杂志。**53**: 478，1973。

[2] Research Group of Acupuncture Analgesia, Beijing, Medical College: *Scientia Sinica*, **17**(1): 112, 1974.

[3] 中医研究院针灸经络研究所生化组：新医药学杂志，(2): 131，1976。

[4] 陕西中医研究所针麻原理研究室：陕西新医药，(2): 66，1976。

[5] Yi Chingcheng, *et al.*: *Scientia Sinica,* **20**: 113, 1977.

[6] Du Huanji, *et al.*: *Acta Zoologica Sinica,* **24**:11, 1978.

[7] Shanghai Coordinating Group for Research on Neurotransmitters and Acupuncture Analgesia: *Kexue Tongbao,* **23**: 253, 1978.

[8] Kin Kuochang, *et al.*: *Acta Physiol. Sinica,* **31**: 121, 1979.

[9] Han Chisheng, *et al.*: *Scientia Sinica,* **22**: 91, 1979.

[10] Biochemical Group, Institute of Acupuncture Academy of Traditional Chinese Medicine: in the abstract of *National Symposia of Acupuncture and Moxibustion and Acupuncture Anesthesia.* June 1–5, Beijing, pp. 427–428, 1979.

[11] Yu Guangdi, *et al.*: *Ibid.*, pp.433–434, 1979.

[12] Curzon, G. and Green, A.R.: *Brit. J. Pharmacol.,* **39**: 653, 1970.

[13] Chang, C.C: *Int. J. Neuropharmacol.,* **3**: 643, 1964.

[14] Shellenberg, M.K. and Gordon, J.H.: *Anal. Biochem.*, **39**: 356, 1971.

[15] Yang Fangzhong, *et al.*: *Acta Biochem. et Biophys.*, 1979, to be published.

[16] Karasawam, T., *et al.*: *Life Sci.*, **15**: 1465, 1974.

[17] Westerink, B.H.C. and Korf, J.: *J. Neurochem.*, **29**: 697, 1977.

[18] Zhang Zhende, *et al.*: *Acta Physiol. Sinica,* **31**: 163, 1979.

[19] Bloxam, D.L. and Warren, W.H.: *Anal. Biochem.*, **60**: 621, 1974.

[20] Udenfriend, S.: *Fluorescence Assay in Biology and Medicine.*, Academic Press, New York, pp.130–134, 1962.

[21] Gessa, G. L. and Tagliamonte, A.: *Adv. Biochem. Psychopharmacol.,* **11**: 119, 1974.

[22] Pan Jiancui and Zhang Shengmei: in the abstract of *National Symposia of Acupuncture and moxibustion and acupuncture anesthesia.*, June 1–5 1979, Beijing, p. 457.

[23] Chang, H. T.: *Scientia Sinica,* **16**: 25, 1973.

[24] Wu, C.P., *et al.*: Inhibitory effect of produced by simulation of afferent nerves on responses of cat dorsolateral fasciculus fibres to nocuous stimulus. *Scientia Sinica,* **17**: 688, 1974.

[25] Chiang Chenyu, *et al.*: *Scientic Sinica,* **18**: 651, 1975.

[26] Du Huanji and Chao Yanfang: *Scientia Sinica,* **19**: 137, 1976.

[27] Yih Chingcheng, *et al.*: *Kexue Tongbao,* **22**: 43, 1977.

[28] Mclennan, H., *et al.*: *Pain,* **3**: 229, 1977.

[29] Wurtman, R.T. and Fernstrom, J.D.: in *Perspectives in Neuropharmacol.*, (Snyder, S.H. ed.), Oxford University Press, New York, pp.143–197, 1972.

[30] Physiological Section of the Acupuncture Analgesia Mechanism Reseach Group, Department of Preclinical Basic Science, Beijing Medical college: *National Med. J. China,* **58**: 129, 1978.

[31] Zhang Dexing, *et al.*: *Kexue Tongbao*, **23**: 117, 1978.
[32] 中医研究院针灸经络研究所生化组：中医药研究参考，(7)：8，1977。
[33] Ye Weiling, *et al.*: *Kexue Tongbao.*, **22**: 367–368, 1977.
[34] Feng Ziaochen, *et al.*: *Kexue Tongbao.*, **23**: 314–315, 1978.

EFFECT OF MICROINJECTION OF NORADRENALINE INTO HYPOTHALAMUS ON ACUPUNCTURE ANALGESIA

Pan Jiancui , Zhang Shengmei
(Fudan University, Shanghai)

I. INTRODUCTION

Both 5-hydroxytryptamine (5-HT) and noradrenaline (NA) are the important neurotransmitters within the brain. Recently it has been generally accepted that 5-HT is necessary during the process of acupuncture analgesia (AA)[1–5], whereas the effect of NA on AA. is still unclear[3, 6–9]. It is possible that the NA fibers innervating various nuclei exert different actions on AA.

Recently the hypothalamus has been shown to be an important area contributing to the effect of AA [10–14]. But there are several kinds of neurotransmitters which are located in different nerve endings, among which the distribution of the NA ventral bundle fibers of hypothalamus is especially noticeable[15, 16].

In order to investigate the relationship between the NA ventral bundle and AA , we have microinjected NA through the base of the rat skull into the ventromedial area of the hypothalamus. We have also microinjected other transmitters or drugs into the same region in comparison with the effect of NA. The experimental results show that only NA has a significant effect on AA .

II. METHODS

Experiments were performed on 71 albino rats, weighing 200–250 g. During the experiment, the rat was put into the celluloid cage, and a pair of electrodes set at the one third of the distal of the tail for stimulation. When the gradient square waves were increased progressively to elicite a tailflick response, the current intensity was recorded as pain threshold (PT). The mean of PT determined every 5 minutes for three times was taken as the basic pain threshold (BPT). The electric acupuncture (EAC) inducement was given to the rats at bilateral "Huantiao" points by using G-6805 transistor therapeutic apparatus for 30 minutes. The PT was again measured at the begining of 15th, 20th, 25th and 30th minute in the duration of EAC. The average of PT after EAC minus BPT was used as AA .

Afterwards, the rat was anesthetized with ether and was put with abdomen turned upside on the operation table. A longitudinal incision was made on the cervical skin, and the skull bone was exposed, after dissection of the digastric muscle. The location of injection was at 4.0–4.5 mm in front of the 'T' suture between the basiocoipital and basisphenoid

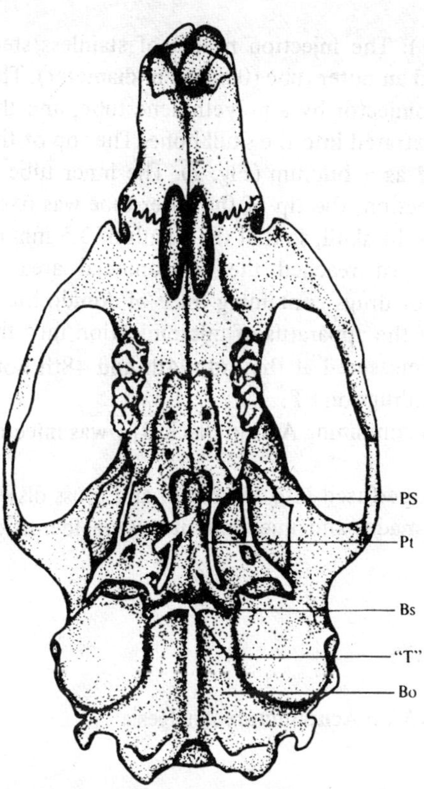

Fig. 1 The ventral view of the skull of rat.
B O: Basioccipital
B S: Basisphenoid
P S: Presphenoid
P t: Pterygoid
'T' : T Suture
Arrow indicates the localization of the injection.

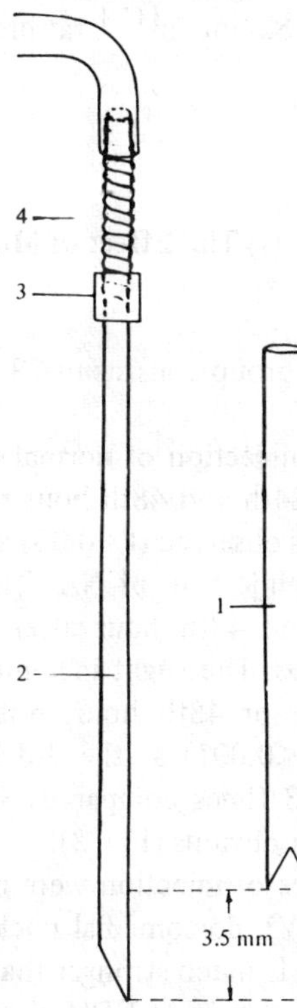

Fig. 2 The needle of microinjection
1. 0.8 mm in diameter of outer layer.
2. 0.4 mm in diameter of inner layer.
The inner layer is 3.5 mm longer than the outer layer.
3. movable celluloid tube.
4. fixed wire.

bones, 0.5 mm lateral to the middle line (Fig. 1). The injection needle of stainless steel consists of an inner tube (0.4 mm in diameter) and an outer tube (0.8 mm in diameter). The top of the inner tube was connected to the microinjector by a polyethylene tube, and the oblique section of the outer tube was directly penetrated into the skull bone. The top of the outer tube has a symmetric oblique section used as a fulcrum (Fig. 2). The inner tube is 3.5mm longer than the outer one. During the injection, the tip of the outer tube was fixed to the skull, and the inner tube penetrated through the skull, so that the length of 3.5 mm of inner tube was implanted into the brain and just reached the ventromedial area of hypothalamus. Then the solution of transmitters or drugs containing trace of Amido Black B_{10} (as a visual indicator) was injected slowly by the apparatus of microinjection into the ventromedial area of hypothalamus. The PT was measured at the 3rd, 24th and 48th hour after injection respectively to observe the effect of drugs on PT.

In the control experiment, normal saline (NS) containing Amido Black B_{10} was injected in the same manner.

At the end of experiment, 10% formalin was perfused into the brain, and gross dissections of histological sections of the brain were made, and injection sites were identified according to Skinner's[17] rat brain atlas.

III. RESULTS

(I) The Effect of Microinjection of NA on Acupuncture Analgesia

The NA group consists of 23 rats and the control group 12 rats.

1. Microinjection of normal saline. The BPT, measured before or after injection of NS(3 μl) at 3rd, 24th and 48th hour respectively, were the same. After the application of EAC, the AA was observed ($P<0.05$) at 3rd and 24th hour, but it was faint ($P>0.05$) (Fig. 3).

2. Microinjection of NA. The effects of drugs on PT were determined respectively at 3rd, 24th and 48th hour after injection of NA (3μg/3μl) into the ventromedial area of hypothalamus. The slight increment of PT caused by injection of NA 3 hours later, but not at the 24th or 48th hour, was observed. Following the EAC the AA was markedly increased ($P<0.001$) at the 3rd hour, and lasted a long time until the 24th hour. The PT elevated 2–3 times compared with pre-acupuncutre. At 48th hour, the effect of NA on EAC was not obvious (Fig. 3).

The sites of injection were mostly at the ventromedial nucleus (HVM), periventricular nucleus (HPV), dorsomedial nucleus (HDM) and arcuate nucleus (ARC). The effect of EAC in the HVM is much stronger than those in HPV, HDM and ARC. When the NA was injected into the dorsal part of HDM or massa intermedia, the effect on AA was slight (Figs. 4,5). It is worthwhile to mention here that the effect of NA on AA has presented before us three characteristics: (1) the effect of NA appeared only by induction of EAC with much stronger potentiating effect; (2) this potentiating effect persisted even to the 24th hour; (3) the effect showed a site-specificity.

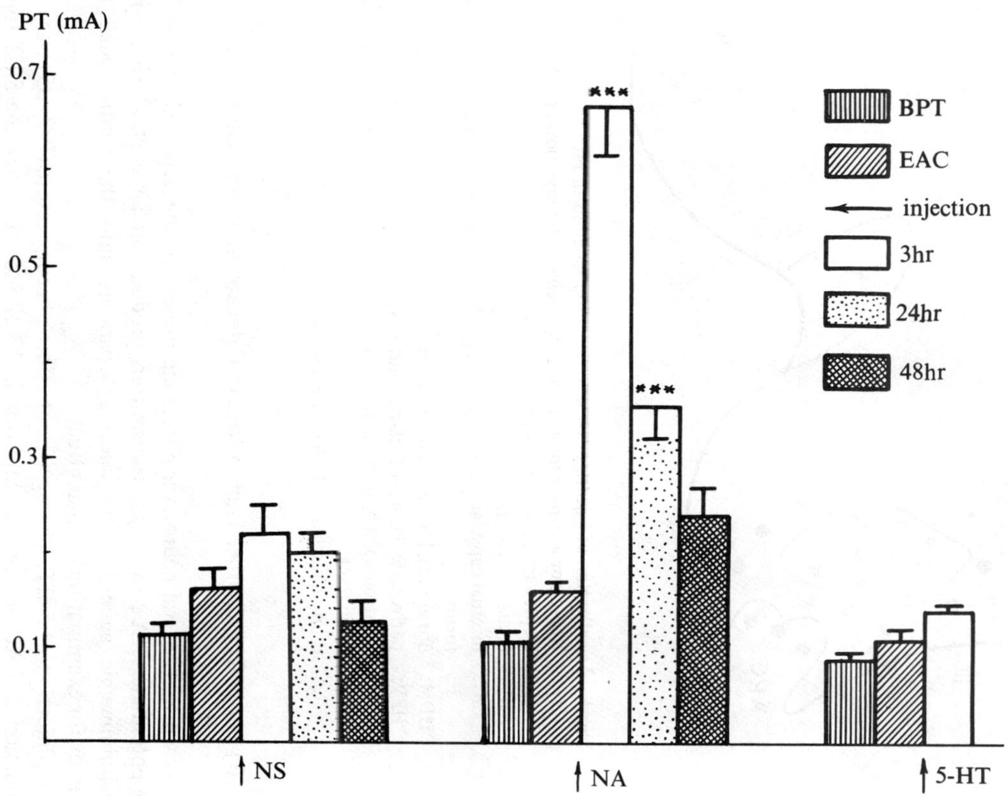

Fig. 3 Effects of microinjection of the neurotransmitters on acupuncture analgesia.
P T: Pain threshold (mA, Mean ± s_x))
***: P<0.001

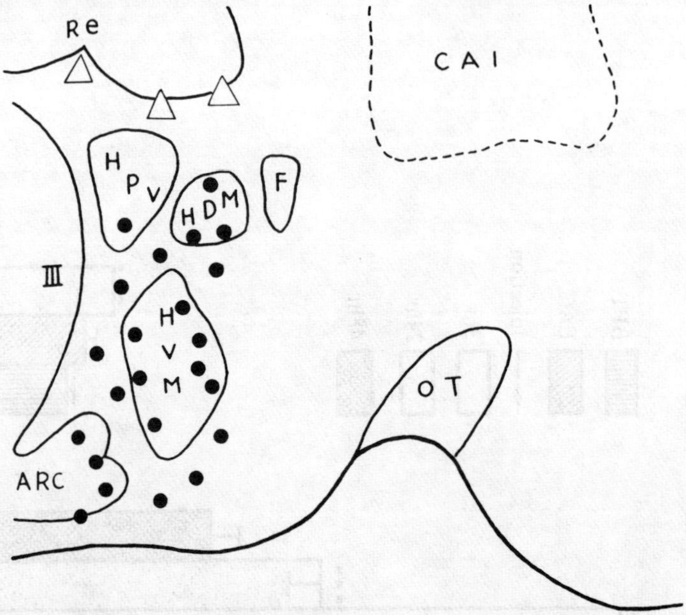

Fig. 4 Localization of injecting NA into the hypothalamus of rat.
● : Represent a significant acupuncture analgesia by injection of NA.
Δ : Represent no significant effect.
ARC: arcuate nucleus.
CAI: internal capsulae,
F: fornix,
HDM: dorsomedial hypothalamus nucleus,
HPV: periventricular hypothalamus nucleus,
HVM: ventromedial hypothalamus nucleus,
O T: optic tract,
Re: reunion nucleus, III; the third ventricle.

(II) The Effect of Other Transmitters or Catecholamine Agonists on AA

It is known that several neurotransmitters are present in the hypothalamus. As NA can markedly potentiate AA , can other transmitters produce similar effects? Thus 5-HT, DA and catecholminergic agonists were injected separately into the ventromedial area of hypothalamus for examination of their effect.

1. Microinjection of 5-HT. The significant effect of acupuncture ($P<0.05$) was observed by an induction of EAC before drug injection in 13 albino rats. Then the 5-HT ($6\mu g/ 3\mu l$) was injected into the ventromedial area of hypothalamus. The BPT was not significantly different at the 3rd hour after injection. The effect of AA was still retained, but the increment of AA was not significant in comparison with that before and after injection of drug. There was the same effect in a few rats observed at the 1st, 24th and 48th hour. It was found that 5-HT could not obviously potentiate AA . Therefore, we suggested that 5-HT in the hypothalamus was not possible to participate in the effect of AA .

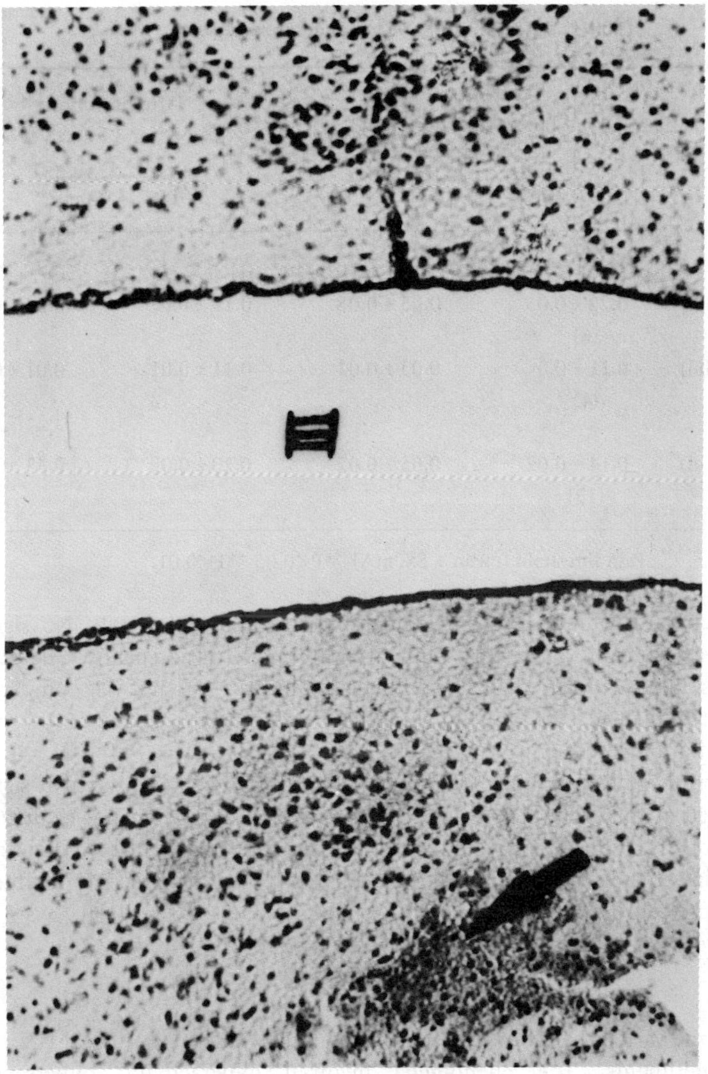

Fig. 5 Transverse section of the rat's hypothalamus after injection of NA. An arrow showing the localization of the injection of NA (containing trace of Amido Black B_{10}).

2. Microinjection of dopamine. This group consists of 13 albino rats. A slight increase in BPT (P<0.05) was observed at the 3rd hour after injection of DA (3μg/3μl). The value of induction of EAC was about 1.5 times that of BPT, in comparison with the EAC (P<0.01). It was proved that the effect of DA was slight potentiation, and it lasted shorter in comparison with NA (Table 1).

Table 1. Effect of drugs on acupuncture analgesia

Drugs	Before injection		After injection for 3 hours	
	BPT	Acup	BPT	Acup
Ad (3μg/3μl)	0.22 ± 0.05 (6)	0.05 ± 0.08	0.19 ± 0.03	** 0.35 ± 0.01
1-PA (2.5μg/5μl)	0.11 ± 0.0 (4)	0.03 ± 0.04	0.11 ± 0.01	0.01 ± 0.01
DA (3μg/3μl)	0.14 ± 0.02 (13)	0.05 ± 0.02	* 0.20 ± 0.02	** 0.33 ±0.07

Pain threshold (mean ± S$\bar{x}$, mA) *P<0.05 **P<0.01.

3. Microinjection of adrenline. This group consists of 6 albino rats. No significant change in BPT was observed at the 3rd hour after injection of adrenaline (3μg/3μl). The value of EAC was about 2 times of BPT after injection of drug, when it was compared with EAC (P<0.01). It explained that the α-angoinst had potentiation similar to NA, but the duration of potentiation was short.

4. Microinjection of isoprenaline. This group consists of 4 albino rats. No significant effect was observed at the 3rd and 24th hour after injection of isoprenaline (2.5μg/5μl) on PT and AA (Table 1). It might be stated that the β-angonist had no effect. Therefore, the NA could potentiate the AA which might be mediated by α-adreno-receptor, without any relationship with β-receptor.

(III) Behavior Reactions

We observed the various behavior reactions of the rats by microinjection of NA, 5-HT or DA in the experiments. The phenomena involved hyperactivity, hypersensitivity, hyperphagia and hyperuresis by microinjection of NA in the rats. Besides, there were dullness, quiet and hypersomia (sleepyhead) by microinjection of 5-HT in the animals. Some rats died for hypophagia after microinjection of DA. These phenomena showed that the transmitter microinjected into the ventromedial area of hypothalamus thereby aroused the vegetative functions and emotion of the animals.

(IV) DISCUSSION

The first point we would like to stress here is the advantage of our microinjection technique in exploration of the functions of the hypothalamus directly through the base of the skull where the brain is in immediate contact. It is much better than approaching the hypothalamus even stereotaxically to inject or stimulate through the dorsal surface of the skull. By the latter way, much more brain tissues and structures would be spared of the physiological symptoms, and thus the nuclear specificity was diffcult to obtain.

Besides, the dye Amido Black B_{10} was used to accompany any solution injected in order to mark the specific site in the hypothalamus for microscopic examination[18]. So far, we have not met with any interference with the physiological effects.

As to the effect of NA on AA, some authors assigned NA to produce an antagonistic effect on AA mediated by α-adrenoreceptor[7]. When a lesion was made electrically on the locus coerulus of brain stem, or the ascending dorsal bundle of NA neurons was selectively destroyed by means of microinjection of 6-hydroxydopamine, the NA function was much weakened, and the AA in these cases was much strengthened[6–8]. Therefore these authors also suggested that the function of NA was to antagonize AA. However, our experiments were contradicting to their results and revealed a significant potentiating effect of AA after microinjection of NA into the ventromedial area of hypothalamus innervated by the NA ventral bundle. This contradiction might be due to the fact that the NA ascending dorsal bundles innervated the other nuclei, which had other specific physiological functions than the NA ventral bundle. Consequently the contrary effect on the AA had inevitably resulted. Here comes to the fore the problem of specificity of the brain nucleus or nuclei group in addition to the chemically specific transmitter such as NA, a problem worthy to be clarified. We observed the strong potentiating effect on AA by microinjection of NA into HVM at the 3rd hour, which retained evidently after the 24th hour. This fact leads us to infer that first of all the effect must be referred to the function of the α-receptor in the HVM, and then in succession the other hypothalamus substances including endorphine, ACTH, etc.[19–20]. Besides, within the hypothalamus there concentrate a number of cell bodies of the endophine neurons[25, 26], whose fiber conections are widely related to the preoptic area, the medial eminence of the hypothalamus, the central gray and the locus coerules of the brain stem, etc. Apparently all of these areas take part integratively in the pain process.

Further research is considered to look for the specialities of NA on the ventral and dorsal bundle, particularly the mechanism of NA taken by HVM on AA..

IV. SUMMARY

After microinjecting of NA, 5-HT, DA, adrenaline or isoprenaline into the VM of hypothalamus and on AA, the results were as follows:

1. The microinjection of NA into the ventromedial area of hypothalamus had a much stronger potentiating effect on AA which lasted for 24 hours. It was mediated by α-

adrenoreceptor, and not by β-receptor. This potentiating effect is more specific in the ventromedial area of hypothalamus than in other neighboring nuclei.

2. When the DA was microinjected into the ventromedial area of hypothalamus, the potentiating effect was slight and lasted shorter in comparison with the NA. The 5-HT had no potentiating effect, so we suggested that the 5-HT injected in the ventromedial area of hypothalamus did not participate in acupuncture analgesia.

We'd like to express our acknowledgement to Professor Jin Guozhang (Shanghai Institute of Materia Medica, Academia Sinica) for his helpful suggestions.

REFERENCES

[1] 陕西中医研究所针麻原理研究室：陕西新医学，5：29，1975。
[2] 北京医学院基础部针麻原理研究室生理组：新医学杂志，3：37，1976。
[3] 清水隆雄等：日本薬理雜志，**70** (4)：167，1974。
[4] 陕西省中医研究所针麻原理研究组：陕西新医学、5：53，1975。
[5] 上海神经递质与针刺镇痛研究协作小组：科学通报，**4**：253，1978。
[6] 陕西省中医研究所针麻原理研究室：陕西新医学，1：66，1976。
[7] 北京医学院基础部针麻原理研究组：中华医学杂志，**58** (3)：129，1978。
[8] 张德星等：科学通报，**23** (2)：17，1978。
[9] 金国章等：生理学报，**31** (2)：121，1979。
[10] 唐仲良等：复旦学报(自然科学报)，1：13，1978。
[11] 陈宜张等：全国针灸针麻学术讨论会，论文摘要(二)，会议学术处编，23，1979。
[12] 林葆城等：全国针灸针麻学术讨论会，论文摘要(二)，会议学术处编：22，1979。
[13] 中山大学生物系针麻原理研究组：中山大学学报(自然科学版)，1：40，1977。
[14] 邹 冈等：全国针灸针麻学术讨论会，论文摘要(二)，会议学术处编：134，1979 。
[15] Lindvall, O. *et al.*: *Actaphysiologica Scand. Suppl.*, **412**, 1974.
[16] Davision, A.N.: *Biochemical Correlates of Brain Structure and Function.* p.137, Academic Press. Lond and N.Y. 1977.
[17] Skinner, J.E.: *Neuroscience Laboratory Manual.* p.197, Philadelphia. 1971.
[18] 莽克强等：聚丙烯酰胺凝胶电泳，科学出版社，54，1975。
[19] 北医基础部针麻原理研究组：中枢神经介质概论，第1版，科学出版社，1977。
[20] Prunty, F. T. G *et al.*: *Modern Trends in Endocrinology-4.* p.13, Lond. 1973.
[21] Li, C. H. *et al.*: *Proc. Nat. Acad. Sci.*, **73**: 1821, 1976.
[22] Goldstain, A.: *Science*, **193** (4258): 1081, 1976.
[23] Woodbary, D. M.: *Pharmacol. Rev.*, **10** (2): 275, 1958.
[24] Jolla, L.: *Science*, **197**: 1367, 1977.
[25] Bloom, F.: *Proc. Nat. Acad. Sci.*, **75**(3): 1591, 1978.
[26] Weston, S. T.: *Science*, **200**(4344): 964, 1978.

ROLE OF CHOLINERGIC NERVES IN ELECTROACUPUNCTURE ANALGESIA

—INFLUENCE OF ACETYLCHOLINE, ESERINE, NEOSTIGMINE AND HEMICHOLINUM ON ELECTROACUPUNCTURE ANALGESIA

Guan Xinmin, Yu Bi, Wang Caiyuan,
Liu Xiaochun

(Department of Acupuncture Anesthesia Research, Wuhan Medical College)

It was found in our previous experiments that an increase of central acetylcholine (ACh) content in certain regions of the brain and a tendency of increased cholinesterase (ChE) activity in some nerve tissues (both central and peripheral) were associated with an elevation of pain threshold during the operation of electroacupuncture analgesia[1–8]. For the purpose of furthei investigation of the role of cholinergic nerves in electroacupuncture analgesia the present study was designed according to the metabolic pathway of the cholinergic neurotransmitter by using pharmacological tools to raise or to reduce the effective concentration of ACh, and its influence on electroacupuncture analgesia was observed.

I. MATERIALS AND METHODS

Animals. 791 rats (body weight 180–250g) were divided randomly into 4 main groups, each given a different drug and the main group was again subdivided according to the different dosages into several smaller groups. In each smaller group, a portion of the animals received injection of drug (or drugs) only while the others received drug followed by electroacupuncture.

Drugs. Eserine: Injection physostigmini salicylatis produced by People's Drug Manufacturers of Tianjin.

Neostigmine: Injection neostigmine methylsulfurici produced by Drug Manufacturers of Shanghai.

Acetylcholing Chloride (ACh): made by Shirgia Drug Factory of Shanghai.

Hemicholinum (HC-3): Aldrich (95%).

Conditions of electroacupuncture. Type G-6805 electroacupuncture apparatus was used. The needles were punctured into the points coresponding to "Zusanli" and electroacupuncture was given for 20 minutes. The current intensity for acupuncture accorded with the limit of endurance of animals without giving vocal response and the frequency used was 500 Hz per minute.

Measurement of threshold. The rats were held in special canvas bags, and the pain threshold was determined by the apparatus made by ourselves. 2 electrodes were inserted under the skin on both sides of the middle portion of rat tail. The pain thresholds were represented as milliamperes required for initiating vocalization response in the rat. Three measurements of steady pain thresholds should be obtained before the beginning of the experiment.

Determinations of ACh and ChE. At the end of 20 minutes of electroacupuncture, the brain was removed following decapitation and different regions of the brain were dissected on a cold glass stage according to the atlas in Craige's Neuroanatomy of rat[9]. The ACh concentration in different regions was estimated on toad's rectus abdomins muscle[10], and the ChE activity was determined by Herstrin's colormetric method[11].

Route for administration. ACh and eserine were given subcutaneously, HC-3 intraventricularly, and neostigmine subcutaneously or intraventricularly.

The intraventricular injection was performed according to Noble's technique[12].

II. RESULTS

(I) Influence of the exogenous ACh on Electroacupuncture Analgesia

1) The analgesic effects of ACh. The results were as follows. There was no analgesic effect after injection of ACh subcutaneously (0.5mg/kg). However, the analgesic effect could appear if eserine was given immediately before injection of ACh. In eserine plus ACh (0.25mg/kg each) group the pain threshold was raised 0.221 mA higher than that of simple eserine group ($P<0.05$). The results are shown in Table 1.

Table 1. Analgesic effect of ACh

Treatment	Dosage (mg/kg)	No. of animals	Pain threshold Mean ± SE
Saline		51	0.044 ± 0.003
ACh	0.5	20	0.050 ± 0.001
Eserine	−0.25	25	0.149 ± 0.024
Eserine plus ACh	aa 0.25	43	0.370 ± 0.010

2) The influence of ACh on electroacupuncture analgesia. It was found that the analgesic effect in ACh (0.5 mg/kg) electroacupuncture group was equivalent to that in the saline-electroacupuncture group. In other words, no influence was found on the effect of electroacupuncture analgesia after a simple injection of ACh. But it could be elevated by ACh (0.5 mg/kg) plus eserine (0.25 mg/kg) as shown in Fig. 1.

These results indicate that the elevation of pain threshold by electroacupuncture might be related to the increase of the effective concentration of ACh.

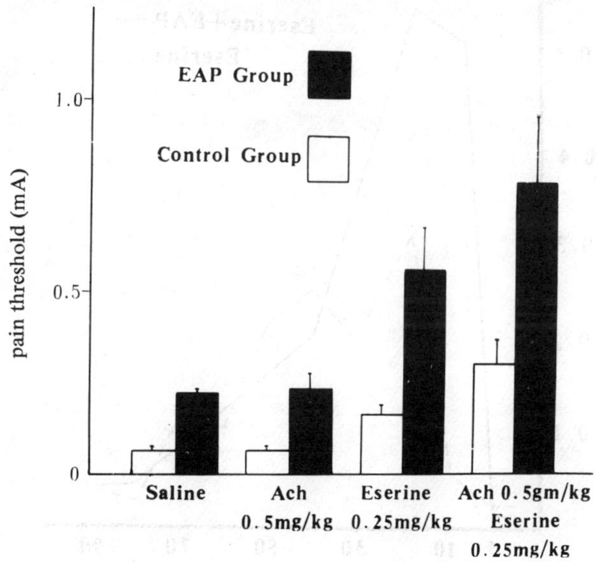

Fig. 1 Influence of ACh on Electroacupuncture Analgesia.

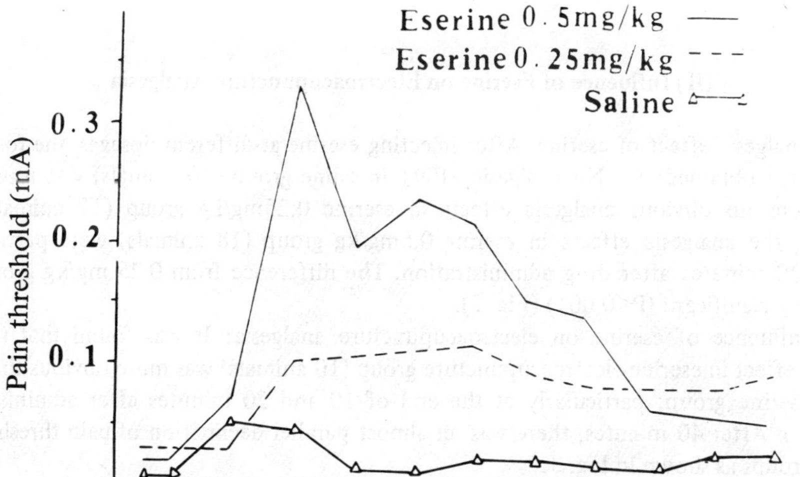

Fig. 2 Influence of various dosages of eserine on analgesia in rats.

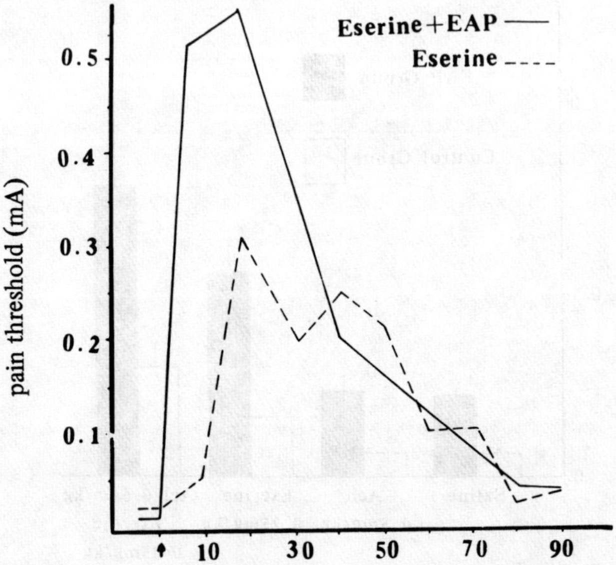

Fig. 3 Influence of eserine (0.5mg/kg) on electroacupuncture analgesia of rat.

(II) Influence of Eserine on Electroacupuncture Analgesia

1) Analgesic effect of eserine. After injecting eserine at different dosages, the following results were obtained: (a) No analgesic effect in saline group (10 animals) was found. (b) There were no obvious analgesic effects in eserine 0.25mg/kg group (17 animals). (c) However, the analgesic effects in eserine 0.5mg/kg group (18 animals) were particularly obvious 20 minutes after drug administration. The difference from 0.25 mg/kg group was statistically significant ($P<0.001$) (Fig. 2).

2) Influence of eserine on electroacupuncture analgesia: It was found that (a) The analgesic effect in eserine-electroacupuncture group (10 animals) was more obvious than that of the eserine group, particularly at the end of 10 and 20 minutes after administration ($P<0.001$). After 40 minutes, there was an almost parallel declination of pain thresholds in these 2 groups as shown in Fig. 3.

(b) Similar changes could also be observed between the eserine (0.25mg/kg) electroacupuncture group and simple eserine group, and their peak effects also presented at 20 minutes.

3) Influence of various dosages of eserine on electroacupuncture analgesia: Because the peak effects of eserine-electroacupuncture and eserine group all occurred at 20 minutes, the changes of pain threshold at this moment were observed with emphasis. The results were shown in Table 2.

Table 2. Influence of eserine on electroacupuncture analgesia in rat

Groups		Drug giving group			Drug electroacupuncture group		
		Group No.	No. of animals	Pain threshold(mA) Mean ± SE	Group No.	No. of animals	Pain threshold(mA) Mean ± SE
Saline		1	51	0.044 ± 0.003	2	29	0.200 ± 0.007
Eserine (mg/kg)	0.125	3	9	0.124 ± 0.038	4	15	0.193 ± 0.063
	0.25	5	25	0.149 ± 0.024	6	39	0.513 ± 0.157
	0.5	7	42	1.260 ± 0.204	8	42	2.071 ± 0.246

The results of statistical analyses were as follows: (a) The pain threshold in eserine group of different dosages was obviously higher than that of the saline control group (1:3, P<0.05; 1:5 or 1:7, P<0.001), and the analgesic effect became more prominent following the increment of eserine dosages, (3:5, P<0.05; 5:7 and 7:9, P<0.001). (b) The pain thresholds of both normal and eserine-treated rats could be augmented by electroacupuncture (1:2 and 5:6, P<0.001; 7:8, P<0.02). (c) The pain thresholds of eserine-electroacupuncture group were much higher than that of electroacupuncture group (2:6, P<0.05; 2:8, P<0.001). (d) The electroacupuncture analgesic effect also became more prominent following the increment of eserine dosages (6:8, P< 0.001).

The results denote that the analgesic effect of electroacupuncture can be augmented by eserine and there was obvious dose effect relationship in the analgesic effect of eserine.

(III) Influence of Eserine and Electroacupuncture on ACh Concentration in Rat Brain

56 rats were divided into 4 groups: control, electroacupuncture, eserine (0.5mg/kg) and eserine-electroacupuncture group. The results were shown in Tables 3 and 4.

From analysis of variance, P<0.05. Q test showed that there was significant difference in ACh content in thalamus as compared with that of the other three groups.

Table 3. Influences of eserine and electroacupuncture on ACh content in thalamus

Group	Control	EAP*	Eserine	Eserine-EAP*
ACh content ($\bar{X}$ r/g)	1.572	1.927	2.019	2.099

* EAP: Electroacupuncture

Table 4. Influences of eserine and electroacupuncture on ACh content in caudate nucleus

Group	Control	EAP*	Eserine	Eserine-EAP*
ACh content ($\overline{X}$ r/g)	2.022	2.455	3.437	3.571

*EAP: Electroacupuncture.

The estimation of ACh in caudate nucleus also showed very significant difference (P<0.01). Q test showed significant differences in eserine group, or eserine-electroacupuncture group as compared with the control. If T test was used it also showed a statistically significant difference between control and electroacupuncture group (P<0.05).

The results indicated that the analgesic effect of eserine was accompanied by a marked increase in cerebral ACh content. Not only in simple electroacupuncture group but also in eserine-electroacupuncture group, the increase of pain thresholds was coincident with the increase of ACh content of rat brain.

(IV) Influence of Eserine and Electroacupuncture on ChE Activity in Rat Brain

Table 5.

Groups	Cortex Mean ± SE	Caudate nucleus Mean ± SE	Thalamus Mean ± SE
Saline	24.848 ± 1.61 (27)	50.264 ± 0.74 (38)	25.344 ± 1.13 (38)
Eserine	16.475 ± 1.72** (22)	45.638 ± 1.79* (34)	17.960 ± 0.63** (33)
Eserine -EAP	20.376 ± 1.30 (21)	48.239 ± 1.24 (41)	18.095 ± 0.83 (40)

The asterisk shows statistically significant difference with saline group.
** P<0.001 * P<0.05 (Figures in brackets indicate the number of animals.)

The results showed: (a) 20 minutes after giving eserine (0.5 mg/kg) ChE activity in rat brain decreased obviously; (b) ChE activities inhibited by eserine in different regions of brain might vary; (c) ChE activity could be raised further by electroacupuncture even in the condition that ChE had been inhibited by eserine, and the increasing degree of ChE was not the same in different regions of the brain.

(V) Influnce of Neostigmine on Electroacupuncture Analgesia of Rat

1) Neostigmine administered intraventricularly:

The variance analysis indicated a statistically very significant difference (F<0.01). The analgesic effect of neostigmine upon intraventricular administration was related to its dosage (significant difference exists among drug groups). The electroacupuncture analgesic effect could be augmented by neostigmine injection. Comparing the 2.5 μg-electroacupuncture group with 2.5 μg drug group or 1μg-electroacupuncture group, the differenc was statistically significant.

2) Neostigmine injected subcutaneously:

Table 6. Analgesic effect of neostigmine given intraventricularly and its influence on electroacupuncture analgesia

The dosage of Neostigmine	Drug group		Drug EAP group	
	Animals	Pain threshold Mean (mA)	Animals	Pain threshold Mean (mA)
1.0 μg	8	0.24	7	0.80
2.5 μg	6	1.26	6	2.23
5.0 μg	4	2.65		
10.0 μg	4	3.50		

The variance analysis showed that there was significant difference (F<0.01). No analgesic effect was found after subcutaneous injection of small dosage of neostigmine, but the pain threshold was apparently elevated by administrating larger dosage (0.5 mg/kg). (There were significant differences between 0.5 mg/kg group and the other groups.) The electroacupuncture analgesic effect, however, could be augmented by injecting neostigmine 0.125 mg/kg subcutaneously. There was significant difference between 0.125 mg/kg-electroacupuncture group and 0.125 mg/kg drug group or 0.05 mg/kg-electroacupuncture group.

(VI) The Influence of HC-3 on Analgesic Effect of Eserine and Electroacupuncture

After injecting HC-3 40μg each intraventricularly the animals were divided into eserine (0.5 mg/kg) group (16 rats) and eserine (0.5 mg/kg)-electroacupuncture group (17 rats). The experiments began in 4–6 hours, day 2 and day 3 respectively following the injection of HC-3. The influence of HC-3 on the analgesic effect of eserine and eserine-electroacupuncture were observed. It was discovered that in 4–6 hours after injection of HC-3 the analgesic effect of eserine and eserine-electroacupuncture vanished entirely. However on the second

Table 7. Analgesic effect of neostigmine given subcutaneously and its influence on electroacupuncture analgesia

The dosage of neostigmine (mg/kg)	Durg group		Drug EAP group	
	Animals	pain threshold Mean (mA)	Animals	Pain threshold Mean (mA)
0.05	17	0.037	18	0.154
0.125	16	0.038	15	0.790
0.5	5	1.760		
Saline	51	0.044	29	0.200

day the inhibiting effect was subsided somewhat and the analgesic effect began to appear. In the third day the analgesic effect increased further (Fig. 4). In 4–6 hours after giving HC-3 intraventricularly the inhibitting effect was outstandingly obvious. In the meantime, if the HC-3 treated animals received an additional injection of ACh (0.5 mg/kg) following administration of eserine as eserine-ACh group (14 rats) and another group given eserine-ACh-electroacupuncture (19 rats), it was found that inhibitting effect of HC-3 was inverted in certain degree due to the direct supply of ACh, and the effect of electroacupuncture analgesia appeared again ($P<0.001$).

The preceding results apparently indicated that the analgesic effects of eserine and electroacupuncture were inhibited by reducing the ACh content in rat brain and this inhibiting effect could be abolished by giving ACh. Hence our data may consititute sufficient evidence to suggest that the brain ACh level plays an important role in electroacupuncture analgesia. To summarize the results mentioned above, the pain thresholds and acupuncture analgesia of rats can be augmented by injecting exogeneous ACh or ChE inhibitor (eserine or neostigmine) to raise the ACh level directly or indirectly; The analgesic effect may be inhibited by reducing ACh level (as with HC-3). Further more this inhibiting effect can be inverted by an additional injection of ACh resulting in a reappearance of the analgesic effect of electroacupuncture.

III. DISCUSSION

(I) The Role of Cholinergic Nerves in Analgesia

Since eserine and neostigmine are all ChE inhibitors, the hydrolysis of ACh released from the synapse or administered extrinsically can be prevented and the concentration of ACh at nerve endings can be raised to such a degree as to show its cholinergic effect or to augment the effect of ACh[13, 14]. Therefore, the analgesic effect of eserine and neostigmine is related to the increase of ACh concentration in nerve endings. It is also found that the analgesic effect of eserine was accompanied by an elevation of brain ACh level.

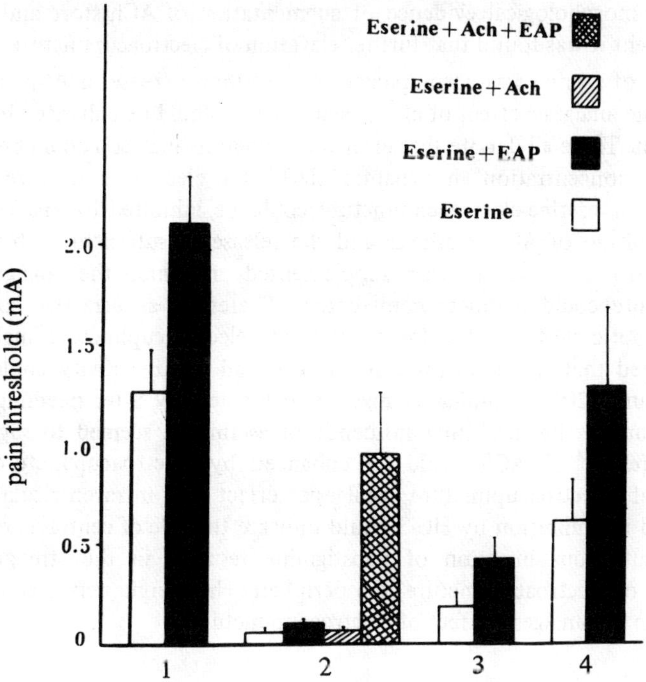

Fig. 4 Influence of HC-3 on eserine, ACh and electroacupuncture (EAP) analgesia.
1. HC-3 not injected of HC-3 2. 4-6H after injection of HC-3
3. 2nd day after injection 4. 3rd day after injection of HC-3

These facts as mentioned above prove that ACh is one of the important neurotransmitters implicated in analgesia.

Because eserine can pass through the blood-brain barrier, the analgesic effect of eserine injected subcutaneously may indicate the effect of cholinergic nerves in both central and peripheral nervous systems. However the effect of cholinergic nerves in analgsia has been proved by the analgesic effect of neostigmine which was injected intraventricularly and can not pass the blood-brain barrier and by the inhibiting effect of HC-3 on the analgesia yielded by eserine. The present results agree with the reports of Jacob (1972) and Spercr (1972)[15]. But the analgesic effect of subcutaneous injection of neostigmine should denote a peripheral effect of cholinergic nerves. Hence the foregoing evidence discloses that the analgesic effect of cholinergic nerves may be related not only to the central nervous system but also to the peripheral one.

(II) The Role of Cholinergic Nerves In Electroacupuncture Analgesia

It has been found in our laboratory that after electroacupuncture, the pain threshold as well as the ACh content was elevated. The analgesic effect was also accompanied by an increase of both the amount of clear synaptic vesicles and the width of synaptic cleft under electron microscope[16-18]. These ultrastructural changes following electroacupuncture seem to be the morphological evidence of augmentation of ACh store and release. In the present experiment it was found that further elevation of electroacupuncture analgesia effect by the injection of eserine was accompanied by a further increase of ACh concentration in the rat brain. The analgesic effect of electroacupuncture could be enhanced by an additional injection of ACh. These all denote that electroacupuncture analgesia could be augmented by increasing ACh concentration in synaptic cleft. But electroacupuncture analgesia and analgesic effect of eserine-electroacupuncture could be inhibited by HC-3[19]. This was due to the inhibition of ACh synthesis and the release of sufficient ACh at the synapse. However, meanwhile, if ACh was supplemented in time, the analgesic effect of electroacupuncture could reappear immediately. Therefore, an effective concentration of ACh at the synaptic cleft may be closely related to electroacupuncture analgesia effect. It has been reported that the concentration of ACh and AChE activity could be raised by electroacupuncture [20]. A similar change of AChE activity after needling could also be observed even under the inhibiting influence of eserine. It seemed to suggest that both synthesis and release of ACh could be enhanced by electroacupuncture. Besides, the enhancement of electroacupuncture analgesia effect by intraventricular injection of neostigmine and its inhibition by HC-3 could indicate the role of central cholinergic nerves. Since the subcutaneous injection of neostigmine resulted in the strengthening of the analgesic effect of electroacupuncture, the peripheral cholinergic nerves could also take an important role in the analgesic effect of electroacupuncture.

IV. SUMMARY

The results of 6 experiments (in a total of 791 rats) are reported including the effect of ACh, eserine, neostigmine and hemicholinum on electroacupuncture analgesia and the changes of ACh content, as well as ChE activity in the brain after needling. Besides, the role of cholinergic nerves in electroacupuncture analgesia was preliminarily discussed.

REFERENCES

[1] 武汉医学院针麻研究室：武汉医学院学报(增刊) (2)：98，1976。

[2] 武汉医学院针麻研究室：针刺麻醉 1：68，1978。

[3] 武汉医学院针麻研究室：新医学杂志 (1)：24，1975。

[4] 武汉医学院针麻理论研究小组：针刺麻醉原理的探讨，人民卫生出版社，402 页，1974。

[5] 武汉医学院针麻理论研究小组：针刺麻醉原理的探讨，人民卫生出版社，405 页，1974。

[6] 熊希凯等：全国针灸针麻学术讨论会论文摘要(二)，109 页，1979。

[7] 武汉医学院针麻研究室附二院针麻组：武汉医学院学报(增刊) (2)：61，1976。

[8] 武汉医学院针麻研究室等：武汉医学院学报(增刊) (2)：57，1976。

[9] *Craige's Neuroanatomy of the Rat.* (Revised and expanded by W. Zeman). Academic press, New York, 1963.

[10] Chang, H.C. and Gadum.J.H: *J. Physiol.*, **79**:225. 1933.

[11] Hestrin, B.S.: *J.Biol. Chem.*, **180**:249, 1949.

[12] Noble, E.P. *et al.*: *Life Sciences*, **6**:281, 1967.

[13] 上海第一医学院等：医用药理学：人民卫生出版社，373 页，1977。
[14] 上海第一医学院等：医用生物化学：人民卫生出版社，713 页，750 页。1979。
[15] 北京医学院基础部针麻原理研究组：中枢神经介质概论，科学出版社，61 页，258 页，1977。
[16] 武汉医学院针麻研究室，电子显微镜室：全国针麻研究资料选编；上海人民出版社，571 页，1977。
[17] 武汉医学院针麻研究室，电子显微镜室：针刺麻醉 (2—3) 期：96 页，1977。
[18] 武汉医学院人体解剖教研室，电子显微镜室：全国针刺麻醉研究资料选编，上海人民出版社，564 页，1977。
[19] 艾民康等：全国针灸针麻学术讨论会论文摘要(二)，111 页，1979。
[20] 杨静霞等：全国针灸针麻学术讨论会论文摘要(二)，105 页，1979。

ACTION OF SYMPATHETIC NERVE AND ITS MEDIATOR IN MECHANISM OF ACUPUNCTURE ANESTHESIA

Yan Huijin, Xu Chengtao, Chen Mengqin
Liu Bochun, Chen Houlan
(Department of Physiology, Institute of Basic Medical Sciences, Chinese Academy of Medical Sciences)

Cai Liangwan, Xu Caimin
(Department of Biochemistry, Institute of Basic Medical Sciences, Chinese Academy of Medical Sciences)

Li Huizhen,Wei Yue, Fu Guanying
(Department of Cellular Biology, Institute of Basic Medical Sciences, Chinese Academy of Medical Sciences)

During application of acupuncture anesthesia for either major or minor operations, an induction period of 20–30 minutes, which begins just after the insertion of the needle and feel of some sensation, is absolutely necessary before performance of incision or other operative procedures. It is assumed that a series of functional regulations might take place in the body within this period and some chemical substances might be produced against the pain resulting from the operation. This paper is limited to observing the possibility of whether the sympathetic nerve and its mediator are involved in the functional regulation or not.

I. METHODS

The investigating subjects are patients of gastro-duodenal ulcer and affections of thyroid gland who had received operations under acupuncture anesthesia. Acupuncture points used were "Renzong" (Du 26) and "Chengjiang" (Ren 24). Upon part of the patients, supplementary points were added . The frequency of the electric stimulation applied upon most of the cases was 60,000 times/minute, and part of them 6,000 and a few 600. The effect of acupuncture anesthesia was graded according to the national unified atandard. The relationship between the efficacy of acupuncture anesthesia and the change of sympathetic activity was observed depending upon the following indices before and after induction and during the progression of the operation on a majority of the same patients;

1. Galvanic skin reflex: Two 2X3 cm size square electrodes were placed on the dorsum and palm of the hand respectively, and a piece of gauze, which had been soaked with saline, was put between the skin and the electrode. The Galvanic skin reflex was recorded on a polygraph, and the time constant was 2 seconds. The amplitude of the Galvanic skin reflex was indicated by millivolts.

2. Digital skin temperature: A transistorized thermometer was used for the measurement of the digital skin temperature; the detector of the instrument was fixed at the dorsum of the distal phalange of the middle finger near the nail bed. The room temperature was kept within the range of 1°C.

3. Heart rate and digital plethysmogram. The change of pulse wave of the distal phalange of the index finger was recorded with a photoactive resistance plethysmographic transducer. The speed of running of the record paper was 1.25 mm or 2.5 mm per second, and the time constant was 0.3 second. The amplitude and frequency were measured with the units of millimeter and number of pulsation of one minute. It revealed that the frequency of the pulse wave was identical to the heart rate.

II. RESULTS

(I) Relationship between the change of the sympathetic function and the effectiveness of acupuncture anesthesia

1. Change of Galvanic skin reflex. Galvanic skin reflex became active transitorily upon potential amplitude at the beginning of perception of needle sensation upon 99 case (Fig. 1), and then it was going to be inhibited in the process of induction. After induction for 20 minutes, 47 patients had an anesthetic efficacy of grade I and the mean decrease of the amplitude of the Galvanic skin reflex was 0.57 ± 0.20 mV (Table 1). The difference is predominant comparing Grade III ($P<0.05$). This indicates acupuncture induction could suppress Galvanic skin reflex and is correlated with effectiveness of acupuncture anesthesia. It is worthy to be noted that Galvanic skin reflex upon patients of Grade III was very active at the begining of perception of needle sensation and the increase of the amplitude was more marked than that of the patients of Grade I ($P<0.05$), but the inhibitory action after 20 min induction was just the contrary.

Table 1. The change of Galvanic skin reflex after 20 min acupuncture induction upon 99 patients

Grades	No. of cases	The value of change (mv) (mean value ± stand error)	P
I	47	−0.57 ±0.20	<0.01
II	41	−0.91 ± 0.60	>0.10
III	11	−0.45 ± 0.26	>0.10

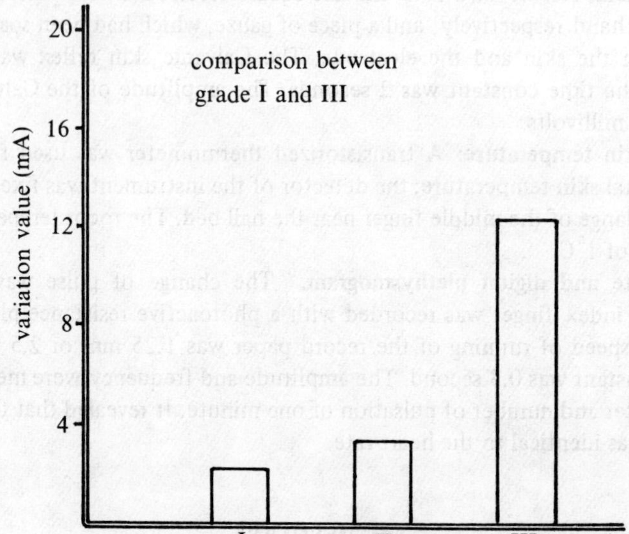

Fig. 1 The variation of the galvanic skin reflex during acupuncture.

2. Change of digital skin temperature. On 82 cases, the digital skin temperature was slightly decreased for a little while at the beginning of occurrence of acupuncture sense, then it undulated or increased gradually. After 20 minutes induction the mean value of the digital skin temperature of most patients was increased (Table 2). Comparison of pre-and postacupuncture upon patients of Grade I and II shows the difference is very significant statistically, but none upon Grade III.

Table 2. Changes of digital skin temperature after 20 min acupuncture induction upon 82 patients

Grades	No. of cases	The value of change of skin temperature (°C) (mean value ± standard error)	P
I	40	0.93 ± 0.20	<0.01
II	33	0.78 ± 0.33	<0.05
III	9	0.75 ± 1.09	>0.05

3. Changes of heart rate. Generally there was no apparent change of heart rate at the early stage of presence of acupuncture sensation. But during induction, it gradually decreased and this decrease became more marked at the time of 20 minutes. This change of heart rate was more or less similar among 101 cases including Grade I, II and III, but there is no statistical significance upon Grade III (Table 3).

Table 3. Changes of heart rate after 20 min acupuncture induction upon 101 patients

Grades	No. of cases	The value of change (beat/min.) (mean value ± standard error)	P
I	48	−1.81 ± 0.65	<0.01
II	42	−2.59 ± 0.62	<0.01
III	11	−1.32 ± 1.54	>0.30

4. Changes of digital plethysmogram. The amplitude of plethysmogram in 99 cases showed a sharp reduction at the beginning of development of acupuncture sensation. It gradually regained near or over its original height after 10 minutes induction in the majority of the patients and it increased greatly at the time of 20 minutes, but it has no statistical significance.

Based on the facts mentioned above, it might be concluded that the enhanced Galvanic skin reflex, reduced amplitude of plethysmogram and the slight decline of digital temperature at the beginning of acupuncture and their gradual change into the opposite directions in the period of induction are due to development of inhibitions which depress the activity of the sympathetic nervous system. These changes are more evident after induction for 20 minutes and they are related to the efficacy of acupuncture anesthesia to a certain degree. Therefore, the better the anesthesia, the more evident is the depth of inhibition of the activity of the sympathetic nervous system (Fig. 2).

(1) Determination of plasma dopamine-β-hydroxylase (DβH): Dopamine-β-hydroxylaseenters into blood in company with NA during its release. The amount of release of both substances is proportional. Since DβH is not reabsorbed, its activity can be used to reflect NA level. Plasma DβH activity was determined by the method of Nagatsu and Underfriend[1]. Copper ion was used to replace N-ethylmaleidamine. Blood samples were taken before and after induction from 106 patients who had been subjected to subtotal gastrectomy, thyroidectomy and so on (Table 4).

Table 4. Change before and after induction of DβH activity upon 106 cases

Efficacy of acupuncture anesthesia	No. of cases	Changes of DβH activities (from before to after induction)			P
		increased	decreased	no change	
I	29	8	21	0	<0.05
II	63	19	39	5	<0.005
III	14	10	2	2	>0.5

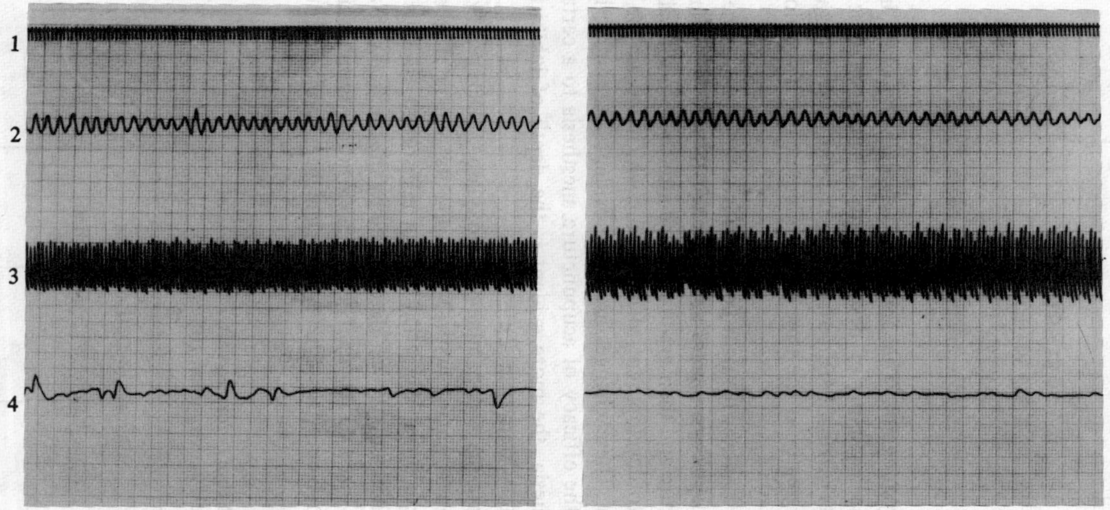

Fig. 2 The changes of galvanic skin reflex and amplitude of digital plethysmogram before and after acupuncture induction.

1. Time interval (sec)
2. Respiratory movement
3. Digital plethysmogram
4. Galvanic skin reflex

Table 4 shows that the DβH activity decreased from before to after induction upon most cases of grade I (excellent) and grade II (good) (72% and 62% respectively), but increased in most of the cases of grade III (seemed to be fair 71%). The general tendency of DβH activity of grade I and grade II is below 0;the former is –0.85μm/min /litre and the latter is –1.03 μm/min/litre. It is statistically significent ($P<0.05$). The general tendency of DβH activity of grade III is increased and the mean value of grade III is ±0.374μm/min/litre.

During the performance of operation 31 cases out of the 106 were investigated upon DβH activity and most cases showed a regain of the activity but it did not reach the level prior to induction, and a few decreased continuously instead of rising. Comparing the level during operation with the level before induction, the mean value of decrease is –1.01μm/min/litre which is statistically significant ($P<0.025$).

The results seemed to support the hypothesis that acupuncture anesthesia may modulate the autonomic nervous system by decreasing the release of transmitters from sympathetic nerve endings.

(2) The observation of histofluorescence of NA of the wall of the stomach and omentum major and minor.

By using the techniques of histofluorescence, the number of adrenergic nerves and the amount of its neurotransmitter NA may be determined[2], and this is a benefit for the investigation of the activity of the sympathetic nervous system during acupuncture anesthesia (Figs. 3, 4).

Based on the number of nerves and their varicosities and the intensity of histofluorescence as semi-quantitative analysis, symbol"+" was used for denoting the content of NA. The results were favorable. The content of NA of omentum major of 21 cases of Grade I was from "++" to "+++" (42.8%), and 0 mentum minor of 20 cases and stomach of 16 cases were 50% and 25%, respectively. Upon grade II, the omentum major of 29 cases was 41.4%, minor of 25 cases 52%, and stomach of 26 cases 30.8%. Upon 11 patients of Grade III the Na content of both omentum major and minor was below "++", (Fig. 2) and only "+" in the wall of stomach. Comparing the decrease of plasma DβH of patients of Grade I and II, it is obvious that the release of Na decreased.

III. DISCUSSION

In the process of acupuncture anesthesia after 20–30 min induction, the sympathetic activity is in a relatively inhibitory state which is evidenced by a decrease of skin galvanic reflex, increase of digital skin temperature and plethysmographic amplitude and the decrease of heart rate[3, 4]. Simultaneously, in the blood, DβH is decreased, while in the tissue (stomach and omentum) NA seems to be increased. All these changes are more predominant upon successful patients of acupuncture anesthesia as Grade I. Furthermore, on the same patient blood samples were taken before and after induction for bioassay of cathecholamine (CA). It was found that the blood CA of Grade I patients showed decrease after induction, being statistically significant. It was confirmed by means of analysis of α and β blocking agents (phentolamine and propranolol) that the mean component of blood CA in blood was NA[5].

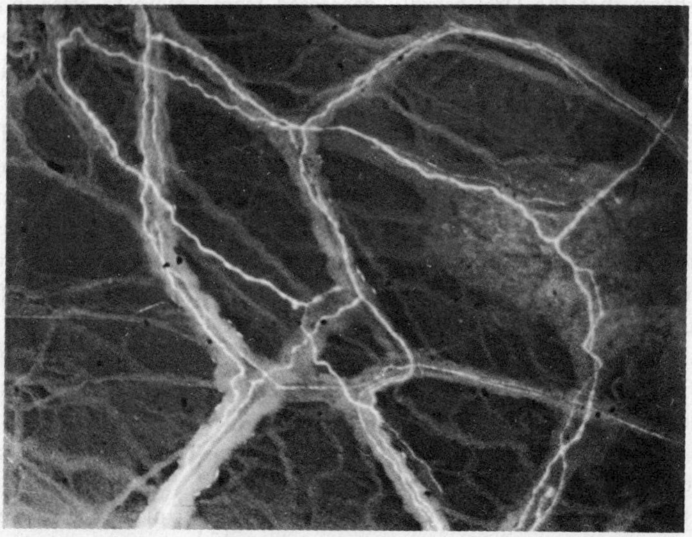

Fig. 3 Histofluorescence of adrenergic nerves in omentum majus stretch preparation, NA content "ttt" magnification : 150×.

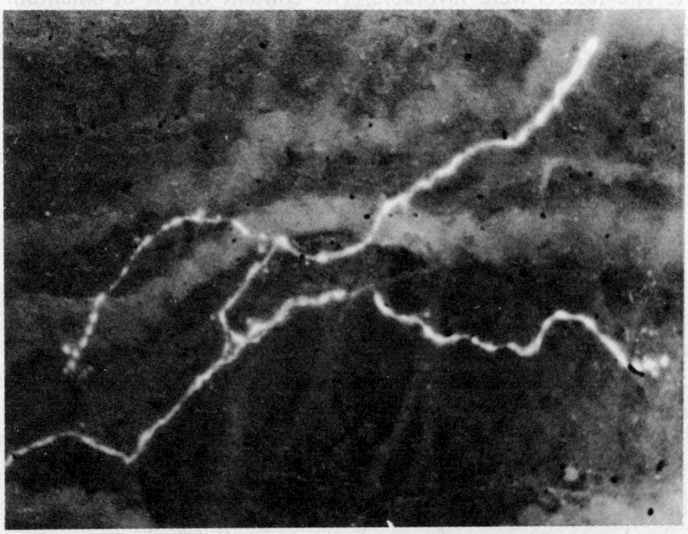

Fig. 4 Histofluorescence of adrenergic nerves in omentum majus stretch preparation, NA content "t" magnification : 150×.

When the sympathetic activity is inhibited by acupuncture the tension of the patient is diminished; the disorder of the physiological activity is decreased; and the pain response from operation may be alleviated. These changes agree with the theory of Chinese traditional medicine that needle puncture has the action of quieting the heart and smoothing the nerve.

Furthermore, with the decrease of the constrictor substance NA, relaxation of the blood vessel naturally follows, thus allowing opening of the path to regulate "Qi" and blood. Hence it fits with one dictum of Chinese medicine that "when it is open, there is no pain". Therefore it may be deduced that during acupuncture anesthesia, the depression of the sympathetic activity and the diminution of sympathetic mediator may be of great significance to explain in one way the mechanism of acupuncture anesthesia.

Whether the central sympathetic center and its mediator may also be concerned in the mechanism of acupuncture anesthesia is a problem under study. The role of the parasympathetic nerve and its mediator in the mechanism of acupuncture anesthesia is also being investigated.

IV. CONCLUSION

103 cases of subtotal gastrectomy done under acupuncture anesthesia are observed. Evidence is presented to show that the sympthetic nervous activity of the Grade I patient shows relative depression after 20–30 min induction. It is suggested that this inhibition of sympathetic activities and the diminution of the sympthetic mediator NA may be one mechanism of acupuncture anesthesia.

REFERENCES

[1] Nagatus, T. and Underfriend, S.: *Clin. Chem.*, **18**(9):980, 1972.
[2] Jonsson, G.: *Prog. in Histochem. and Cytochem.*, **2**:315, 1971.
[3] Wang, G.H.: *Am. J. Physic. Med.*, **36**:295, 1957;37; 35, 1958.
[4] Grenfield, A.D.M.,In "Hand Book of Physiology", Sec. 2, circulation, vol. II. Am. Physiol. Society, Washington, D. C. pp.1325–1351, 1963.
[5] To be published.

STUDY OF ROLE OF HUMORAL FACTORS IN CENTRAL ACTION OF ACUPUNCTURE ANALGESIA

Chen Mengqin, Zheng Yongfang, Xue Zuohong*, Wen Yunyi, Nie Zaimin*, Zhang Baozhen

(Department of Physiology, Institute of Basic Medical Science, Chinese Academy of Medical Sciences)

Acupuncture analgesia is a rather complicated process in which multiple factors are involved. Besides the action of the central nervous system, how do the humoral factors work in this process? Is there any relationship between the variations of humoral factors in the peripheral blood and the central action of acupuncture analgesia? These are very important questions that have to be answered in the study of the principle of acupuncture anesthesia. In 1971 and 1972, we demonstrated preliminarily that electroacupuncture in one of the cross-circulated cats induced the release of some humoral factors which were carried through the blood stream into its counterpart to play a role in the central action of acupuncture analgesia. These humoral factors seemed to be related to adrenocortical hormone and monoamines.

I. METHOD

Two adult cats of the same sex weighing each about 2–3kg were used in each experiment. The animals were anesthetized with chloralose (80 mg/kg body weight) intraperitoneally, tracheae cannulated, the common carotid arteries isolated on one side, and the major splanchnic nerves dissected postperitoneally from the back on the other side. The central ends of the nerves of both cats were stimulated with a Disa stimulator (square wave, intensity 5–15 V, duration 0.1–0.5 msec, single or repetitive at frequency of 1 cps) simultaneously as the pain stimulus. The cerebral cortical potentials of both cats evoked by the stimulation of the major splanchnic nerves were recorded oscilloscopically with a small silver electrode on the medial portion of the sulcus ansatus. Heparin (10 mg/kg body weight) was given intravenously. The isolated common carotid arteries of the two cats were cross-connected with polythene tubes, i.e., the cephalic end of the artery of one cat was connected with the cardic end of the artery of its counterpart, and vice versa. About 200 ml of 5% glucose saline solution was given by intravenous drip to each cat throughout the experiment.

*Present address: Department of Acupuncture Anesthesia Research in this institute.

Electroacupuncture was applied with a Model 6–26 transistor electro-stimulator made by ourselves to one of the animals at the needling points corresponding to "Weishu", "Neiguan", "Zusanli" or "Shangqiu" points in man. Two pairs of acupuncture points were stimulated in each experiment. The frequency and the intensity of the electro-needling were 45 Hz. and 5–45 V, respectively. The inhibitory effect of electroacupuncture on the cortical splanchnic evoked potential (CSEP) of both acupunctured donor and unacupunctured recipient cats were observed as an indicator of the pain response. The criterion of the inhibitory effect was mentioned in our previous work[1] The electroacupuncture on the donor stopped until the inhibition on the CSEP of the recipient appeared. Generally, if the inhibition did not appear, the electro-needling would be discontinued at the 60th minute. There was only one experiment in which the electro-needling was prolonged to 65 minutes. The experimental arrangement is shown in Fig. 1.

The relationship between the inhibition on CSEP of the recipient and the plasma corticosterone content had been investigated. In the second series of experiments, plasma corticosterone was estimated for the blood samples taken by means of a T tube from the carotid artery of the donor before electro-needling, 1 minute before the cessation of needling and 30 and/or 60 minutes after the cessation of needling respectively. The modified fluorescence method as described by Silber et al.[2] and Steenburg et al.[3] was employed to estimate the plasma corticosterone content. The recovery rate was 88.46%. In part of the experiment, when the inhibition of CSEP of the recipient produced by the action of electro-needling on the donor had recovered, the median eminence of hypothalamus of the donor was burnt with DC current (10 mA, 30–90 Sec.) by means of Horsley-Clarke stereotaxic instrument and Jasper's Atlas. The same electro-needling trials and estimation of corticosterone content were repeated after destruction. The animal's head was fixed by perfusing with 10% Formalin solution after experiment, and histological examination was then taken to locate the burnt area in the brain.

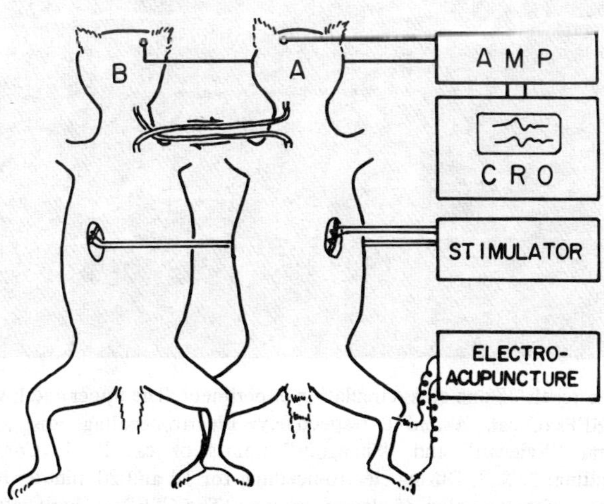

Fig. 1 The schematic diagram of the cross-circulation experiment in cats. Detail see text.

In the third series of experiments for studying whether the inhibitory effect of the recipient by electro-needling on the donor had anything to do with monoamines, reserpine (0.5–0.8 mg/kg body weight) was given intraperitoneally to the animals 24–48 hours prior to experiment. The animals were divided into 3 groups. In the first group, both the donors and the recipients were reserpinized; in the second group only the donors were reserpinized; and in the third group only the recipients were reserpinized. Then, the inhibitory effect on the CSEPs of the recipients and the estimation of plasma corticosterone were observed and made again.

II. RESULTS

(I) The Effect of Electro-needling the Donor on the Cortical Evoked Potential of the Recipient

In the cross-circulation experiment, generally the CSEP of the acupunctured cat itself would be inhibited after 5–15 minutes of electroacupuncture. When the intensity and stimulating time of electroacupuncture on the donor were increased to a certain degree, the partial or complete inhibition on the CSEP of the recipient took place in most cases (Fig. 2). The inhibition was indicated mainly in that the CSEP minimized to approach the baseline or to overlap with it, or decrease in the amplitude of CSEP and/or the prolongation of the

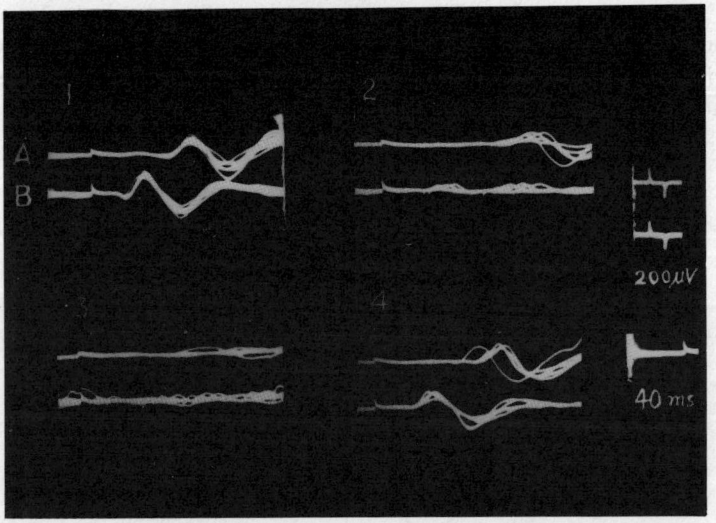

Fig. 2 The result of one cross-circulation experiment. The upper and lower tracings are the CSEPs of cats A and B respectively. Electro-needling was applied on the bilateral "Neiguan" and "Shangqiu" points of cat B. 1. Control before electro-needling; 2. & 3. During electro-needling for 10 and 20 minutes respectively; 4. 10 minutes after cessation of electro-needling, The CSEPs of both cats recovered. Note the CSEP of cat A showing some inhibition during electro-needling at 10th minute, and being completely inhibited at 20th minute.

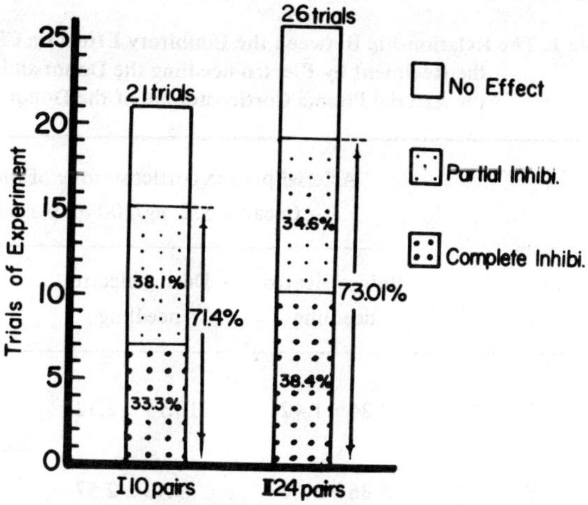

Fig. 3 Inhibitory effect on the CSEP of the recipient by electro-needling the donor in the cross-circulation experiments on cats. The results of the first and second series are shown. There were 21 trials in the series 1 with 10 pairs of animals, and 26 trials in the series 2 with 24 pairs of animals.

latent period. The shortest time of the appearance of inhibition of the CSEP in the unacupunctured redcipient by electro-needling on the donor was 10 minutes, with the majority of them between 35–55 minutes. There was only one case of 65 minutes. The CSEPs of both cats recovered after acupuncture, with the unacupunctured cat regaining it first. The time for complete recovery was generally 5–15 minutes. In a few experiments, electro-needling on the donor only inhibited the CSEP of itself, but could not do so with the CSEP of the recipient, or even occasionally potentiated the latter. Two series of experiments were performed by the same method.

In the first series of the experiments with 10 pairs of animals, complete and partial inhibition of the CSEPs in the unacupunctured cats occurred 7 (33.3%) and 8 (38.19%) times, respectively, in a total of 21 trials of electro-needling. The total inhibition rate was 71.4%. There was no inhibition in 3 trials and increased potentiation in another 3 trials.

In the second series of experiments with 24 pairs of animals, only two pairs of the cross-circulated cats were electroacupunctured one by one. In the other 22 pairs only one animal was electroacupunctured for the determination of plasma corticosterone in the donors. Complete inhibition and partial inhibition of CSEPs of the recipients occurred 10 (38.46%) and 9 (34.61%) times respectively in 26 trials of electro-needling on the donors. The total inhibition rate was 73.07%. No inhibition was seen in 4 trials, and in another 3 trials potentiation was observed. The results of these two series of experiments were similar (Fig. 3).

(II) The Relationship Between the Inhibition on CSEP of the Recipient and the Plasma Corticosterone Content of the Donor

In the second series of experiments with 24 pairs of animals in which the estimation of corticosterone content was carried out, the complete inhibition and partial inhibition of

Table 1. The Relationship Between the Inhibitory Effect on CSEP of the Recipient by Electro-needling the Donor and the Arterial Plasma Corticosterone of the Donor

Inhibitory Effect on the Recipient	cases	Arterial plasma corticosterone of the donor (mean ± S.E. μg/100 ml plasma)		
		Before electro needling	During electro needling	After electro needling
Complete Inhibition	9	7.24 ± 1.42	10.19 ± 2.32*	12.20 ± 3.30*
Partial Inhibition	8	3.86 ± 1.06	9.43 ± 2.57	5.36 ± 1.61
No Effect	7	8.78 ± 1.87	11.42 ± 2.64	13.81 ± 0.33

*P<0.05 compared to "Before electro-needling."

CSEPs of the recipients occurred 9 and 8 times respectively in a total of 24 trials of electro-needling on the donors; no effect and augmentation of the CSEPs of recipients were seen in the remaining 7 trials.

The plasma corticosterone content was estimated in blood samples taken from the crossed-carotid arteries of the donor cats before acupuncture, 1 min before, and 30 to 60 mins after the cessation of needling respectively.

The results are shown in Table 1.

The results showed that in the cases of complete inhibition, the corticosterone content was significantly increased during and after acupuncture, but in both the partial inhibition and no inhibition trials, such differences showed no statistical significance. It seems that the inhibition effect of acupuncture may be connected with the plasma corticosterone level. The relationship between the inhibitory effect on the CSEP of the recipient by electro-needling the donor and the plasma corticosterone content of donor cat is shown in Figs. 4 and 5.

In 7 cases of these cross-circulation experiments, when the CSEP of the recipient cat had been inhibited by the action of electro-needling on the donor cat and had recovered, the median eminence of the hypothalamus and part of the pituitary stem in the donor cat were burnt with D.C. current. After destruction, the trials of electro-needling and the estimation of corticosterone were repeated as before. Consequently, in 4 cases of them, the effects of electro-needling the donor on both the elevation of plasma corticosterone and the inhibition of CSEP of the recipient cat were completely undone by this process, and the histological examination after the experiment revealed the complete destruction of the median eminence (Fig. 6). In the other 3 cases the burnt sites were found in the hypothalamus rather than the median eminence; complete inhibition and partial inhibition of the CSEP of the recipients occurred in 2 and 1 of them, respectively. From these results, we suggest that the release

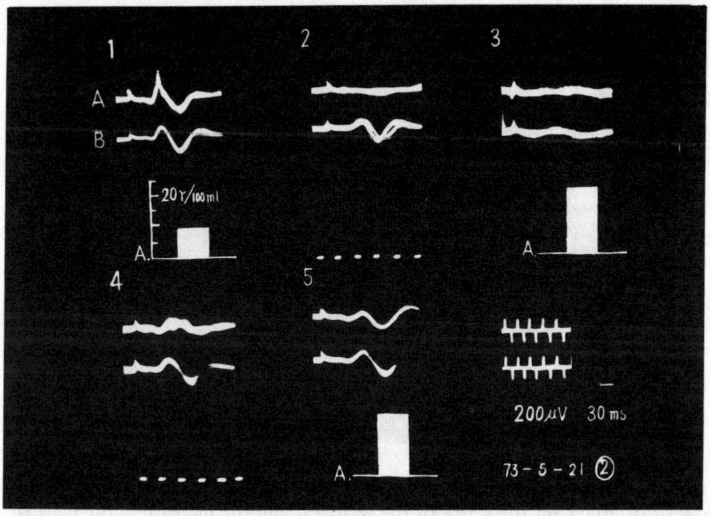

Fig. 4 The result of one cross-circulation experiment. The upper and lower tracings are the CSEPs of cats A and B respectively, while the columls represent the corticosterone levels of arterial plasma of cat A in corresponding time. The needling points "Weishu" and "Neiguan" on cat A were stimulated. 1. Control before electro-needling; 2. During electro-needling for 10 minutes; 3. During electro-needling for 45 minutes, note the inhibition of the CSEP on cat B and the elevation of the corticosterone level of cat A; 4. At the 5th minute after cessation of needling; 5. At the 30th minute after cessation of needling, the CSEPs of both cats reappeared.

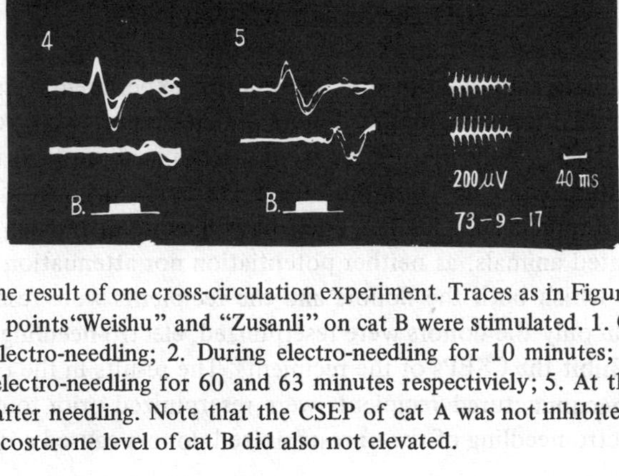

Fig. 5 The result of one cross-circulation experiment. Traces as in Figure 4. The needling points "Weishu" and "Zusanli" on cat B were stimulated. 1. Control before electro-needling; 2. During electro-needling for 10 minutes; 3. & 4. During electro-needling for 60 and 63 minutes respectiviely; 5. At the 50th minute after needling. Note that the CSEP of cat A was not inhibited while the corticosterone level of cat B did also not elevated.

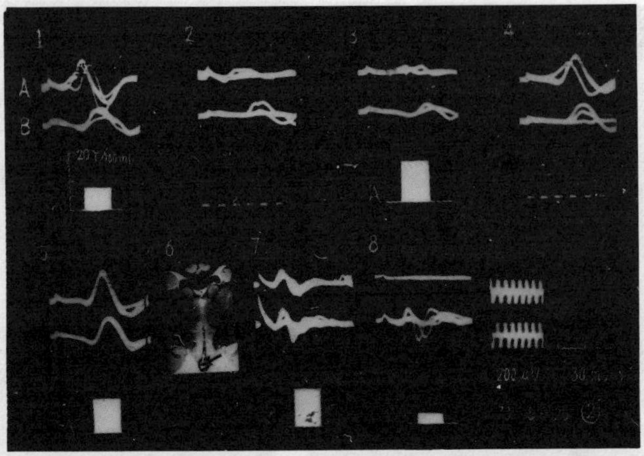

Fig. 6 Influence of destruction of the median eminence of the donor on the inhibitory effect on the CSEP of the recipient and the increase in the plasma corticosterone of the donor produced by the electro-needling on the donor. Traces as in Figure 4. The needling points "Weishu" and "Zusanli" of cat A were stimulated. 1. Control before electro-needling; 2. During electro-needling for 15 minutes; 3. During electro-needling for 48 minutes; the CSEP of cat B was partially inhibited, while the plasma corticsterone of cat A was markedly increased; 4.5 minutes after cessation of needling; 5. 50 minutes after cessation of needling, the CSEPs of both cats reappeared; 6. A photograph of histological section showing the destruction of the median eminence of cat A; 7. 15 minutes after destruction of the median eminence, no electro-needling was applied. 8. At 40th minute of electro-needling after destruction of the median eminence, the CSEP of cat B could not be inhibited again, and the level of plasma coticosterone of cat A could not elevated also.

of the adreno-cortical hormone prompted by electro-needling is effected via the pituitary, and also that the inhibitory effect on the CSEP of the recipient may be connected with this hormone.

(III) The Action of Reserpine

21 pairs of cats were employed in the 3rd series of experiments. Animals were divided into 3 groups: (1) in 10 pairs, both the donors and recipients were reserpinized prior to experiment; (2) in 6 pairs, only the donors were reserpinized; and (3) in 5 pairs, only the recipients were reserpinized. After reserpinization the inhibitory effect of electro-needling on the CSEP of the donor itself remained unchanged, i.e., no difference was found between them and the untreated animals, as neither potentiation nor attenuation were observed. But in the first group in which both the donors and the recipients were reserpinized and in the second group wherein only the donors were reserpinized, electro-needling on the reserpinized donors could not inhibit the CSEPs of the recipients. The results in the other 3 pairs of cats, in which only the unacupunctured recipients were reserpinized prior to experiment, showed in contrast, that electro-needling of the unreserpinized donors caused complete inhibition of

the CSEP of the recipient in one case and partial inhibition of the CSEP of the recipient in 4 cases. It suggest that in a pair of cross-circulated animals, whenever the donor is reserpinized, electro-needling on the donor cannot inhibit the CSEP of the recipient, no matter whether the recipient is reserpinized or not.

The plasma corticosterone contents of the donors in these three groups mentioned above were estimated. The results are shown in Table 2. It can be seen that in the first group of 10 pairs of animals, both the donors and the recipients treated with reserpine, the mean value of of the plasma corticosterone content in these 10 reserpinized donors before electro-needling is 4.816 ± 0.86μg/100 ml plasma. The mean value of the plasma corticosterone content of 24 normal cats before needling is 6.56 ± 0.92μg/100 ml plasma; there is a highly significant difference between them ($P<0.01$). It is believed that the significant decrease in plasma corticosterone is due to the action of reserpine. In the group in which only the donors were reserpinized, the donors' plasma corticosterone content estimated did not represent the real value, because the donors' blood had mixed with that of their unreserpinized counterparts. Therefore, this mean value was higher than that of the animals which were all reserpinized, both donors and recipients. The changes in plasma corticosterone content before and after electro-needling in the first and second groups showed no significant difference. But in the 3rd group in which only the recipients were reserpinized, not only the inhibition on the CSEP of the recipients was induced by electro-needling of the donors, but also the mean value of corticosterone of the donors' arterial plasma was higher than that of the donors in the former two groups. It seems that the inhibitory effect of acupuncture may be related with the corticosterone content. Statistical analysis was not done because the number of cases studied were too few. A record of one experiment in which both the donor and the recipient were reserpinized is shown in Fig. 7.

Table 2. The Relationship Between the Inhibitory Effect on CSEP of the Recipient by Electro-needling the Donor and the Arterial Plasma Corticosterone of the Donor After Reserpinization

Reserpinization Prior to Experiment	Inhibitory Effect on the Recipient	Cases	Arterial Plasma Corticosterone of the Donor (mean ± S.E. μg/100ml plasma) Before Electro-needling	During Electro-needling	After Electro-needling
Both Donor and Recipient	No Effect	10	4.81 ± 0.86	6.40 ± 0.94*	5.32 ± 0.56*
Donor Only	No Effect	6	6.72 ± 0.56	7.86 ± 0.44*	8.67 ± 0.67*
Recipient Only	Complete Inhibition	1	9.38 ± 1.59	10.34 ± 0.97	12.82 ± 2.63
	Partial Inhibition	4			

* $P>0.05$ Compared to "Before electro-needling".

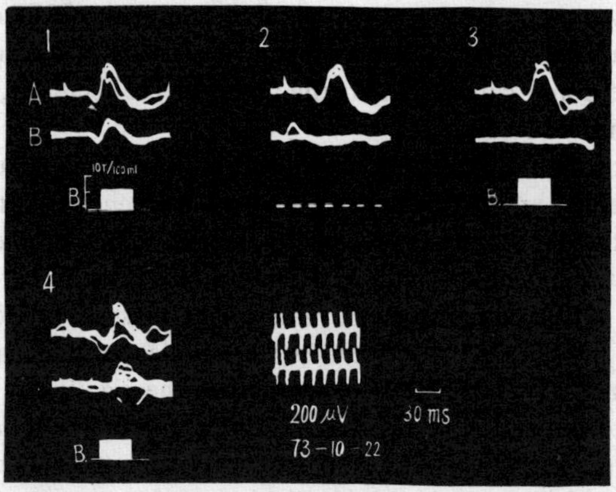

Fig. 7 A result of one experiment in which both the donor and recipient were reserpinized prior to experiment. Traces as in Figure 4. The needling points "Weshu" and "Zusanli" of cat B were stimulated. 1. Control before electroneedling; 2. & 3 During electro-needling for 50 and 59 minutes respectively; 4. 5 minutes afterc̶s cessation of electro-needling. No inhibition on the CSEP of cat A and no elevation of corticosterone content in cat B appeared.

III. DISCUSSION

By means of cross-circulation–a classical method to study the action of humoral factors in vivo- it is found experimentally that electro-acupuncture of one of two cross-circulated animals may induce the release of certain humoral factors which are carried by the blood stream into the other one to play a role in the central action of analgesia.

Purpura mentioned that the EEG arousal could be observed in one of the animals when the bulbar reticular formation of its counterpart was stimulated for 30–80 seconds in the cross-perfusion experiment[4]. It indicates that the stimulating of a certain part of the central nervous system of one of a pair of animals may induce the release of some humoral factors which are carried by the cross-circulated blood stream into the other one to affect the electrical activity of its cortex. Since acupuncture may play an important role in modulating the central and peripheral functions, it may induce the release of some humoral factors in one animal to affect the central nervous system of another via the cross-circulated blood stream.

What are the humoral factors that are liberated to affect the central nervous system by the action of acupuncture? We believe it is the adrenocortical hormone, for, in the first place, acupuncture may induce the release of this hormone[4]. We had studied the changes in plasma corticosterone content in the vena cava of the chloralosed cats before and after acupuncture, and found that the plasma content of this hormone increased after electroneedling. Further, adrenocortical hormone was shown to cross the blood-brain barrier rapidly into the brain[6, 7, 8]. The results of our experiments described above also show that while the CSEP of the recipient cat is inhibited by electro-needling of the donor cat, the level of corticosterone of the arterial plasma in the donor is increased significantly during acupuncture. In 7 cases of the experiment on destruction of the median eminence of the donor cat, the CSEPs of all 7 recipients were inhibited by electro-needling of the donors before the destruction was made. In 4 cases of them, the median eminence of the donors was completely destroyed, which was confirmed by histological examination after the experiment, but the CSEP of the recipients could not be inhibited again by electro-needling of the donors after the destruction. In contrast, in 3 other cases of them, the median eminence was still intact after the destruction process due to technical error; the CSEP of the recipient was completely inhibited in 2 cases and partially inhibited in one case by electro-needling of the donors. This suggests that not only the effect of the acupuncture on the release of adrenocortical hormone is possibly effected via the hypothalamus-pituitary pathway, but also that there may be a relationship between the inhibition of the CSEP of the unacupunctured recipient and the plasma corticosterone level of the acupunctured donor. It is well known that the exogenous corticosterone is taken up predominantly by the hippocampus, the septum and some other limbic structures in the brain and localized over the cell nuclear region in the neuron[9], and affects the neuronal activity[10, 11]. Dafny et al. suggested that the central effect of adrenocortical hormone may be realized via the monoamine transmitters in the brain[12], and it is possible that this is the way and manner in which the adrenocortical hormone modulates the functional state of the brain, and therefore, participates in the central action of acupuncture analgesia.

The result of the cross-circulation experiment in reserpinized animals shows evidently that in 16 cases in which the donor cats were reserpinized prior to cross-circulation, the CSEPs of the recipients cannot be inhibited by electro-needling of the donors; but in 5 other cases, electro-needling of the unreserpinized donors could inhibit the CSEP of their unacupunctured counterparts which were reserpinized prior to the experiment. This suggests that failure to inhibit the CSEP of the recipient by electro-needling of the reserpinized donor may be related with the changes in some humoral factors caused by reserpinization of the donor. Our experiment also shows that the level of plasma corticosterone of the reserpinized animals is significantly lower than that of the controlsdue to the exhaustion of ACTH by reserpine since it is reported that reserpine may induce the release of ACTH from the pituitary via the action of monoamine transmitters[13, 14]. However, we assume that the exhaustion of monoamine substances in the donor by reserpine may be more important in annulling the inhibitory effect of acupuncture. The actions of brain monoamines in the mechanism of acupuncture analgesia have been studied in many laboratories in this country[15, 16]. It is worthwhile to note whether the monoamines in the circulating blood really cross the blood-brain barrier into the brain to modulate the central nervous activity, since exogenous serotonin and other monoamines may act on certain regions of the brain in which the blood-brain barriers are believed to be incomplete[17, 18, 19]. For further studies on these problems, the following experiments are being performed in our laboratory.

At first, the changes of bio-active substances in the plasma of the cat during acupuncture are studied by means of blood bath organ technique. The result revealed that electro-acupuncture may induce the release of monoamines into the peripheral blood of the cat, mostly the catecholamines from the adrenal gland. In part of the experiment, the release of serotonin associated with the release of catecholamine was also observed[20].

Second, intracarotid injection of noradrenaline, adrenaline or serotonin may inhibit the

CSEP of the cat, and potentiate the inhibitory effect of electroacupuncture on the CSEP[21]. These studies support the result obtained from the cross-circulation experiments described above, and suggest that electroacupuncture on the needling points may induce the release of peripheral monoamine substances which may enter the brain to play a role in the inhibition of CSEP.

IV. SUMMARY

1. Electro-needling of the donor of two crosscirculated cats may inhibit the CSEP of its unacupunctured counterpart. The total inhibition rate is 71–73%. The results of two series of 47 trials of acupuncture in 34 pairs of cats are similar.

2. Estimation of the plasma corticosterone content of the blood taken from the acupunctured donor's carotid artery shows that there is a relationship between the content of plasma corticosterone of the donor and the inhibitory effect on the CSEP of the unacupunctured recipient, i.e., while the electro-needling of the donor may inhibit the CSEP of the recipient completely, the content of the donor's plasma corticosterone increases significantly after acupuncture.

3. Electroacupuncture of the reserpinized donor cat cannot cause the inhibition of the CSEP of the recipient cat. However, if the donor cat is not reserpinized, the inhibitory effect on the CSEP will be obtained, although the recipient has been reserpinized prior to the experiment. This result suggests that the humoral factors released by the effect of acupuncture on the donor animal to affect the central nervous system of the recipient animal may be one or more of the monoamine substances. The further studies with the blood-bath organ technique and the experiment of intracarotid injection of monoamine substances have confirmed this result.

REFERENCES

[1] 郑永芳等：针刺麻醉，1979。4 (3): 59—64。
[2] Silber, R. H. *et al.*: *Clin. Chem.*, **4**:278,1958.
[3] Steenburg, R.W. *et al.*: *J. Clin. Endocr.*, **24**:875, 1964.
[4] Purpura, D. P.: *Am. J. Physiol.*, **186**:250, 1956.
[5] 陕西省中医研究所：针灸原理研究参考资料，74 页，陕西省中医研究所，1972。
[6] Abelson, D. *et al.*: *J. Endocr.*, **12**:87, 1955.
[7] Christy, N. P. *et al.*: *J. Clin. Invest.*, **40**:1997, 1961.
[8] Butte, J. C. *et al.*: *Endocrinology*, **92**:1775, 1973.
[9] McEwen, B. S. *et al.*: In "The Structure and Function of Nervous Tissue, Vol. V, Structure and Physiology III", Edited by Bourne, G. H., p. 205, Academic Press, 1972.
[10] Pfaff, D. W. *et al.*: *Science*, **17**:394, 1971.
[11] Michal, E. K.: *Brain Res.*, **65**:180, 1974.
[12] Danfy, N. *et al.*: *Brain Res.*, **59**:257, 1973.
[13] Montanari, R. *et al.*: *Brit. J. Pharmacol* **18**:337, 1962.
[14] Westermann, E. P. *et al.*: *J. Pharmacol. Exper. Therap.*, **138**:208, 1962.
[15] 北京医学院基础部针麻原理研究组：中国科学，(1): 98，1974。
[16] 金国章等：生理学报 31 (2): 121，1979。
[17] Koella, W. P. *et al.*: *Am. J. Physiol.*, **211**:926, 1966.

[18] Leimdorfer, A. *et al.*: *Am. J. Physiol.*, **157**:116, 1949.
[19] Weil-Malherbe, H. *et al.*: *J. Neurochem.*, 8:55, 1961.
[20] 文允镒等：针刺麻醉，1979，**4** (4)：49—54。
[21] 郑永芳等：针刺研究　1980，**5** (1)：48—53。

COMMON BASIS OF ELECTROACUPUNCTURE ANALGESIA AND MORPHINE ANALGESIA

Zhang Zuxuan, Zhang Yuanzhen, Yu Qixiang,
Li Chunbao
(Department of Biology, Nanjing University)

Chen Rongsan
(Coordination Chemistry Institute, Nanjing University)

The correlation of twelve metal ions with electroacupuncture analgesia in mice was studied. At first, it was found that a decrease of calcium ion (Ca^{2+}) content in the brain enhanced the analgesic effect of electroacupuncture, while an increase of Ca^{2+} content lowered or abolished its effect. Other cations, such as potassium, sodium, lithum, copper, strontium, barium, zinc, cobalt, ferrum, magnesium and aluminum, had no effect on electroacupuncture analgesia[1]. During the electroacupuncture analgesia, the decrease of Ca^{2+} content in the brain was always simultaneously accompanied by an increase of magnesium ion (Mg^{2+}) content. The analgesic effect was definitely related with the ratio of Mg^{2+}/Ca^{2+}. An appropriate increase of Mg^{2+}, and thereby an alteration of the ratio of Mg^{2+}/Ca^{2+}, prolonged the analgesic effect. When the ratio was about 8, the electroacupuncture analgesia was maximal. When this ratio was exceeded, the analgesic effect declined as the ratio increased, till over 15, it was entirely lost[2].

In order to determine the significance of Ca^{2+} in the physiologic function of the central nervous system with reference to electroacupuncture analgesia, the above findings were further attested by using chelating agents which combined with Ca^{2+} and Mg^{2+} of different instabilities. At the same time, the correlations of Ca^{2+} and Mg^{2+} with electroacupuncture analgesia, morphine analgesia and nonnarcotic analgesia were studied and compared.

I. METHODS

Experimental animals used were mice weighing 22–28 g each. They were picked at random (both sexes). The animals were treated on the basis of the electroacupunctue analgesia model made in our own laboratory[3]. The animals were killed by immersion in liquid nitrogen. The thalamus were separated and the ionic contents in the supernatant of the brain were determined by microcomplexometric titration[4].

The chelating agents used in the present work were analytical reagents. The aconitine used is a white crystal (E. Merck Co.). The chelating agents and analgesics were injected intraventricularly[5] or intracisternally[6], and Ca^{2+} was injected intraperitoneally. Animals of the corresponding control group received double distilled water of equal volume by the same route.

II. RESULTS

(I) Comparison of analgesic effect of chelating agents

As mentioned above, the electroacupuncture analgesia was closely related with the change in Ca^{2+} and Mg^{2+} content in the brain of mice. For the purpose of further observing the significance of the value of Mg^{2+}/Ca^{2+} in electroacupuncture analgesia, five chelating agents which combined with Ca^{2+} and Mg^{2+} with different instabilities were attested and they were EGTA (2,2'-Ethylenedioxybis-ethyliminodiacetic acid), EDTA (Ethylenediamine tetraacetic acid), CDTA (Cyclohexane diamine tetraacetic acid), NTA (Nitrilotriacetic acid) and HEDTA (N-(2-Hydroxyethyl ethylene diamine triacetic acid)). Each of them was injected twice (4μmol/kg each time) into the lateral ventricle. In Table 1, instability constants of the five chelating agents for comparison and analysis were shown.

The above five chelating agents of the same dose (8μmol/kg) not only had some analgesic effect of their own, but also possessed a synergetic effect with electroacupuncture analgesia, i.e., enhancement of the pain threshold was always accompanied by an increase of the value of $\lg\frac{KMg}{KCa}$. Among the five chelating agents, the synergetic effect of EGTA was the highest, CDTA the next, and NTA the least. These results were in good agreement with published data on the brain[2].

(II) Effect of analgesia of drugs and electroacupuncture on contents of Ca^{2+} and Mg^{2+} in the brain

In order to demonstrate the relationship between electroacupuncture analgesia and morphine analgesia, and the effect of aconitine which had almost certain analgesic effect[7], and that of La^{3+}, the changes in the content of Ca^{2+} and Mg^{2+} in the brain were also observed.

Table 2 shows that double distilled water itself had no effect on the pain threshold of the animals. After administration of drugs or electroacupuncture, the pain threshold was raised remarkably with the Mg^{2+} content in the brain increased and the Ca^{2+} content decreased. This increased the ratio of Mg^{2+}/Ca^{2+} and showed that the analgesic effect of the above three drugs was similar to electroacupuncture analgesia.

(III) Effect of Ca^{2+} i.p. on analgesia of electroacupuncture and the drugs i.c. and on the changes in the contents of Mg^{2+} and Ca^{2+} in the brain

In the present series of experiments, animals which showed analgesic effect of drugs and electroacupuncture were selected. Each of them was injected intraperitoneally with Ca^{2+}

Table 1. Comparison of analgesic effect of chelating agents

Agents		Pain Threshold (sec)			Instability Constant		$\lg \frac{K\text{Mg}}{K\text{Ca}}$
		Before injection	First injection	Second injection	$\lg K_{Ca}$	$\lg K_{Mg}$	
Double Distillate	20μl(19)	3.7 ± 0.10	3.4 ± 0.20*	3.5 ± 0.20*			
NTA	8μmol/kg(20)	3.2 ± 0.10	4.3 ± 0.20*	5.1 ± 0.40*	−6.46	−5.46	1.00
HEDTA	8μmol/kg(20)	3.5 ± 0.11	9.2 ± 2.24*	12.6 ± 2.31*	−8.51	−7.00	1.51
CDTA	8μmol/kg(20)	3.4 ± 0.14	11.9 ± 2.30*	12.9 ± 2.20*	−12.50	−10.32	2.18
EDTA	8μmol/kg(20)	4.1 ± 0.24	11.8 ± 2.33	17.9 ± 2.30	−11.00	−8.69	2.31
EGTA	8μmol/kg(20)	3.5 ± 0.17	19.5 ± 2.12	23.7 ± 2.27	−10.97	−5.20	5.77

The K values of EDTA made use of values in 0.1M KNO_3 solution at 20°C. Each value represents the mean ± S.E. for 19–20 animals. Number of animals in parenthesis.
*P>0.05.

Table 2. Changes in contents of Ca^{2+} and Mg^{2+} in the brain when analgesic effects of drugs and electroacupuncture were positive

Groups		Pain Threshold (sec)		Content of Ions mg/100g Fresh Brain		Mg^{2+}/Ca^{2+}
		Before treatment	After treatment	Mg^{2+}	Ca^{2+}	
Double Distillate	20μl(20)	3.8 ± 0.10	3.7 ± 0.13*	6.76 ± 0.42	5.25 ± 0.24*	1.3
Aconitine	0.002mg/Kg(18)	3.2 ± 0.08	22.1 ± 22.0	13.52 ± 1.12	1.45 ± 0.01	9.3
Morphine	60μg/20μl(19)	4.1 ± 0.15	24.0 ± 2.10	16.79 ± 2.21	2.16 ± 0.20	7.7
La^{3+}	0.002mol/Kg(20)	3.2 ± 0.13	18.0 ± 3.03	11.42 ± 1.32	1.22 ± 0.12	9.4
Electro-acupuncture (effective)	(20)	3.8 ± 0.08	21.8 ± 2.15	21.41 ± 2.04	2.99 ± 0.20	7.2

Each value represents the mean ± S. E. for 18–20 animals. Number of animals in parentheses.
*P>0.05.

Table 3. Effect of Ca^{2+} i.p. on electroacupuncture analgesia and drugs i.c. and on the changes in Mg^{2+} and Ca^{2+} contents in the brain

Groups	Pain threshold (sec)			Ion Content mg/100g fresh Brain		Mg^{2+}/Ca^{2+}
	Before Treatment	After Treatment	Added Ca^{2+}	Mg^{2+}	Ca^{2+}	
Aconitine (20)	3.4 ± 0.11	30	3.8 ± 0.14	4.12 ± 0.14	12.10 ± 2.11	0.34
Morphine (20)	3.8 ± 0.14	30	4.4 ± 0.17	3.18 ± 0.09	10.27 ± 1.87	0.30
La^{3+} (20)	4.1 ± 0.17	30	3.9 ± 0.21	5.74 ± 0.81*	13.34 ± 2.14	0.40
Electroacupuncture (effective) (18)	3.6 ± 0.13	30	4.1 ± 0.74	3.17 ± 0.49	11.34 ± 1.87	0.30

Each value represents the mean ± S.E. for 18–20 animals. The control and dose are the same as in Table 2. Numerals in parentheses indicate the numbers of animals.
i.p. – intraperitoneally; i. c. – intracisternally.
* $P>0.05$.

(3.75 mmol/kg). When the pain threshold returned to the normal level, the animals were immersed in liquid nitrogen, and the contents of Mg^{2+} and Ca^{2+} in the brain were determined. The control group was subjected to the same treatments for observing the course of restoration of the pain threshold. The results are shown in Table 3 and Figure 1.

With the background of increased pain threshold caused by drugs or electroacupuncture, administration of Ca^{2+} by interperitoneal route led to marked decrease of the pain threshold. At the same time, besides the group treated with La^{3+}, the content of Mg^{2+} in the brain of the other groups decreased markedly, meaning a decrease of the ratio of Mg^{2+}/Ca^{2+}. The course of pain threshold restoration indicated that the pain threshold values of the four groups returned approximately to the normal levels, and the analgesic effects in all cases were reduced or inhibited by Ca^{2+} (see Fig. 1).

(IV) Effect of dl-allyldromoran on analgesia of electro-acupunctue and morphine

The results of the foregoing experiments showed that Ca^{2+} resisted persistently the analgesic effects of drugs and electroacupuncture. In the present group, dl-allyldromoran was used to further demonstrate the similarity between the analgesic effect of drugs and that of electroacupuncture.

As shown in Fig. 2, analgesic effect of electroacupuncture and morphine could be relieved by dl-allyldromoran but not that of aconitine and La^{3+}.

III. DISCUSSION

The above results show that the five chelating agents not only have some analgesic effect of their own, but also possess a synergetic effect with electro-acupuncture analgesia. Among

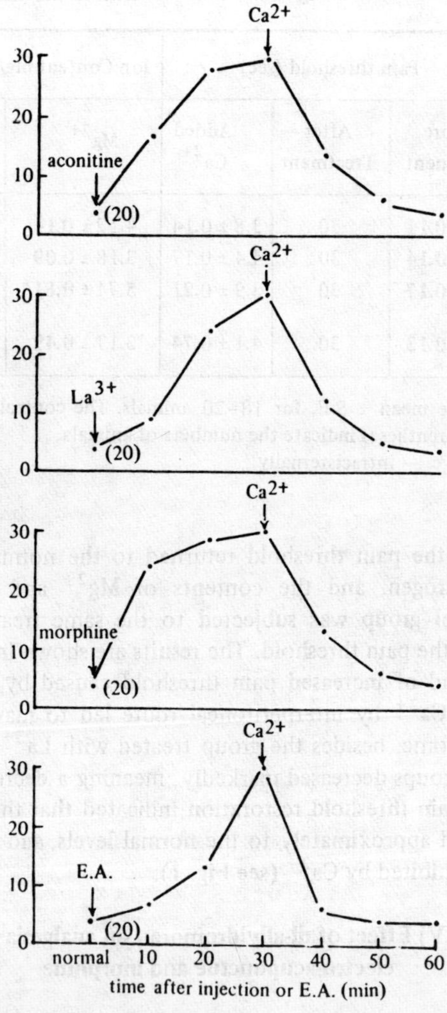

Fig. 1 Effect of Ca^{2+} (i.p.) on analgesia of electro-acupuncture and morphine, aconitine and La^{3+} (i.c.)

The first point represents the mean of 60 times response, the rest point represent respectively that of 20 times response. Site of arrow is the time of injection or E.A. the dose of drugs was same as Table 2.

Number of animals in parenthesis.

E.A.=Electro-acupuncture

i.p.=intraperioneally

i.c.=intracisternally

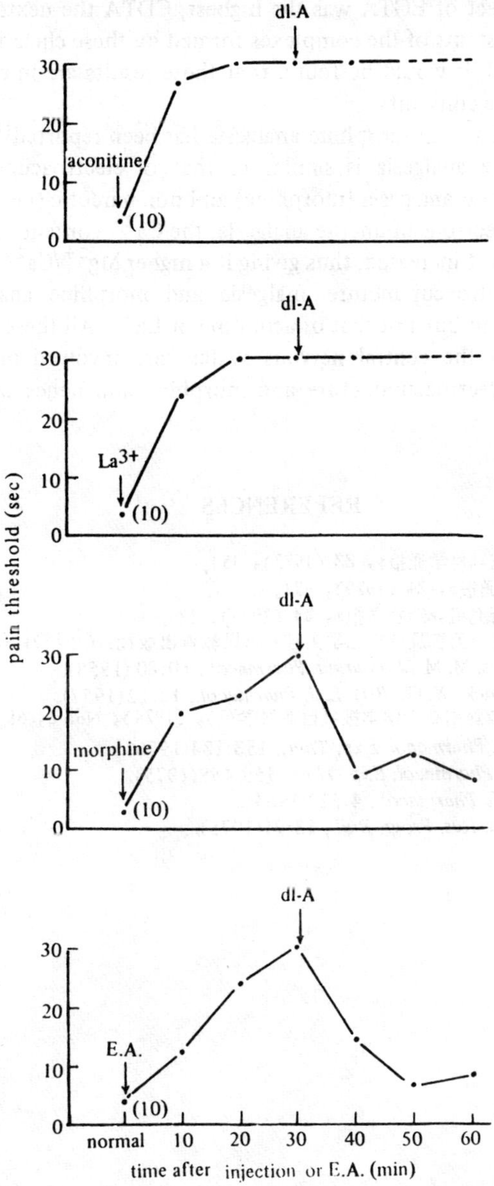

Fig. 2 Effect of dl-allydromoran on anagesia of electro-acupuncture and drugs
The first point represents the mean of 30 times response,, the rest points represent respectively that of 10 times response. Site of arrow is the time of injection or E.A. Except dl-allytromoran 50 g/kg, the dose of the rest drugs are same as Table 2.

Number of animals in parenthesis
E.A.=Electro-acupuncture
dl–A=dl-allydromoran

them, the synergetic effect of EGTA was the highest, CDTA the next, and NTA the least. When the instability constants of the complexes formed by these chelating agents with Ca^{2+} and Mg^{2+} are considered, it would be found that these results are in coincidence with the values calculated from the constants.

The significance of Ca^{2+} in morphine analgesia has been reported[8-10]. There is also suggestion that morphine analgesia is similar to that of electroacupuncture[11]. It was found that in both narcotic analgesia (morphine) and non-narcotic (i.e., aconitine or $LaCl_3$) analgesia, as well as in electro-acupunctue analgesia, the Ca^{2+} content in the brain decreased and the Mg^{2+} content in it increased, thus giving it a higher Mg^{2+}/Ca^{2+} ratio. It was further observed that both electroacupuncture analgesia and morphine analgesia were resisted locally by dl-allyldromoran but not that of aconitine or La^{3+}. All these observation indicate that Ca^{2+} and Mg^{2+} in the central nervous system are involved in the mechanism of analgesia produced by electroacupuncture and morphine and hence both have a common ionic basis.

REFERENCES

[1] 张祖暄,陈荣三,胡卫东,«科学通报», **22** (1977), 454.

[2] 张祖暄,陈荣三,«科学通报», **24** (1979), 471.

[3] 南京大学生物系针麻研究组,«动物学报», **24** (1978), 136.

[4] 陈荣三,黄孟健,钱可萍,«无机及分析化学实验»,人民教育出版社, (1978), 122.

[5] Lockett, M. F. & Davis, M. M., *J. Pharma. Pharmacol.*, **10**:80 (1958).

[6] Haley, T.J. & Mccormick, W. G., *Brit. L. J. Pharmacol.*, **12**:12(1957).

[7] 肖信生,余启祥,张祖暄,«南京大学学报»(自然科学版), (1974), No. 2, 68.

[8] Kakunaga, T. *et al.*: *J. Pharmacol. Exp. Ther.*, **153**:134(1976).

[9] Harris, R. H. et al., *J. Pharmacol. Exp. Ther.*, **159**:488(1975).

[10] Hano, K. *et al.*: *Jap. J. Pharmacol.*, **4**:227(1964).

[11] Mayer, D. J., *Neurosci. Res. Progr. Bull.*, **13**:94(1975).

Acknowledgments-Thanks are due to Prof. Dai Anbang for invaluable guidance, Prof. Zou Gang for advice and helpful comments on the manuscript.

ROLE OF HISTAMINE IN ACUPUNCTURE ANALGESIA

Lu Zusun, Cheng Jun
(Department of Biochemistry, Beijing Tuberculosis Research Institute)

Histamine is widely distributed in all the tissues and organs of the body. The content of histamine is highest in the skin, lung, and peripheral nervous tissue[1], but less in the brain which contains a certain amount of it[2]. Histamine has various physiological functions, one of which is related with pain sensation[3]. The nociceptive chemoreceptor may be stimulated by a number of chemical substances, i.e., histamine, 5-HT, and kinnins released by trauma and inflammation. The afferent impulses produced and transmitted centralpitally evoke pain. Therefore, histamine in the peripheral tissue is generally considered as a pain producing substance. Histamine in the brain may be a neurotransmitter, and some works show that it takes part in the pharmacological action of morphine[2, 4, 5, 6]. In order to find out whether histamine is involved in the mechanism of acupuncture analgesia or not, the present work has been carried out on rabbits, rats, and human beings.

I. THE CHANGED BLOOD CONTENT OF HISTAMINE IN PATIENT UNDERGOING PULMONARY RESECTION WITH ACUPUNCTURE ANESTHESIA

Pain may be initiated by an increase of the blood content of histamine resulting from the release of histamine during surgical trauma. In this work we have tried to study the rolo blood histamine played in acupuncture anesthesia by observing the changes in the blood histamine level in patients undergoing pulmonary resection with acupuncture anesthesia and correlating it with the efficacy of acupuncture anesthesia.

(I) Method

45 cases of lung resection for pulmonary tuberculosis were studied in 1975. The Sanyanlou acupuncture point was used as the main point. Venous blood was collected for histamine determination (Zacharie's method[7]) before electroacupuncture, after 20 minutes of acupunctural induction, at 1 hr after incision of skin and 4 hrs after the end of the operation. After the blood histamine was extracted, fluorescence was produced by condensation with 0-pH thalaldehyde alkaline solution.

(II) Result

In 28 cases, the average content of blood histamine was 103.3 ± 7.35 ng/ml before

Table 1. **Blood content of histamine of patients 1 hr after incision of skin (ng/ml)**

Grade	No. of Cases	Preinduction	1 hr after incision	Change in %	
I & II	36	118.1 ± 5.95	128.0 ± 8.40	+8.4%	P≐0.05
III & IV	9	128.1 ± 18.97	162.2 ± 26.87	+26.6%	

acupuncture and 102.6 ± 6.03 ng/ml after induction for 20 minutes, so it remained basically unchanged (P>0.05).

One hour after incision of skin, the blood level of histamine was elevated due to the release of histamine by surgical trauma (Table 1). The degree of elevation was related with the efficacy of acupuncture anesthesia. That is, it only increased slightly in patients of the good efficacy group (8.4%+), but more prominently in patients of Grades III and IV groups (26.6%+). The difference between the percentages of elevation of histamine in Grades I and II groups and Grades III and IV groups is just statistically significant (P≐0.05).

Examination of the change in each case separately found that in 25 out of 36 cases of the Grades I & II group, the content remained unchanged (vary within ±20 ng/ml), while in 6 out of 9 cases of the Grade III & IV group it was increased. The difference is also statistically significant (X^2=6.64, P=0.01).

The blood amount of histamine decreased 4 hrs after the ending of the operation. The average of 20 cases studied decreased from the preoperative level of 90.7 ± 5.66 ng/ml to 61.7 ± 6.13 ng/ml (P<0.01). This decrease had no connection with the efficacy of acupuncture anesthesia.

II. EFFECT OF PARENTERAL ADMINISTRATION OF HISTAMINE AND GLYCOGEN ON ACUPUNCTURE ANALGESIA IN RABBITS

In this experiment, blood histamine content was changed by injection of drugs and their effects on acupuncture analgesia were observed.

(I) Method

Rabbits weighing 2.5–3 kg irrespective of sex were used for determination of pain threshold by radiant heat focused on nosetip at room temperature of 20 ± 1°C[8]. Electro-acupuncture was carried out at the bilateral Sanyanlou point with a 71–1 Model stimulator with positive rectangular and negative spike waves (5 c/s). The stimulation intensity was just enought to cause contraction of forelimb muscles.

Electrostimulation was started 10 min after intraperitoneal injection of histamine phosphate (1 mg/kg) or 20 min after intravenous injection of glycogen (20 mg/kg). Blood content of histamine was measured according to the method mentioned above.

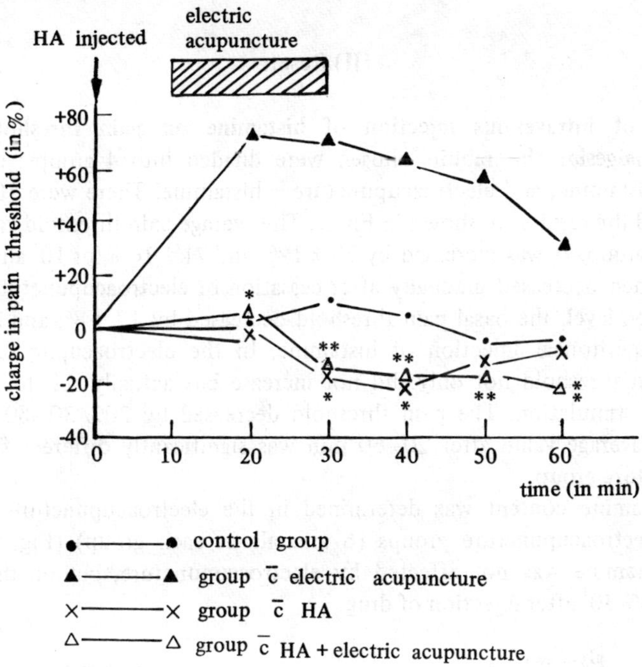

Fig. 1 Influence of intraperitoneal injection of HA on the analgesic effect of electric acupuncture in rabbits.

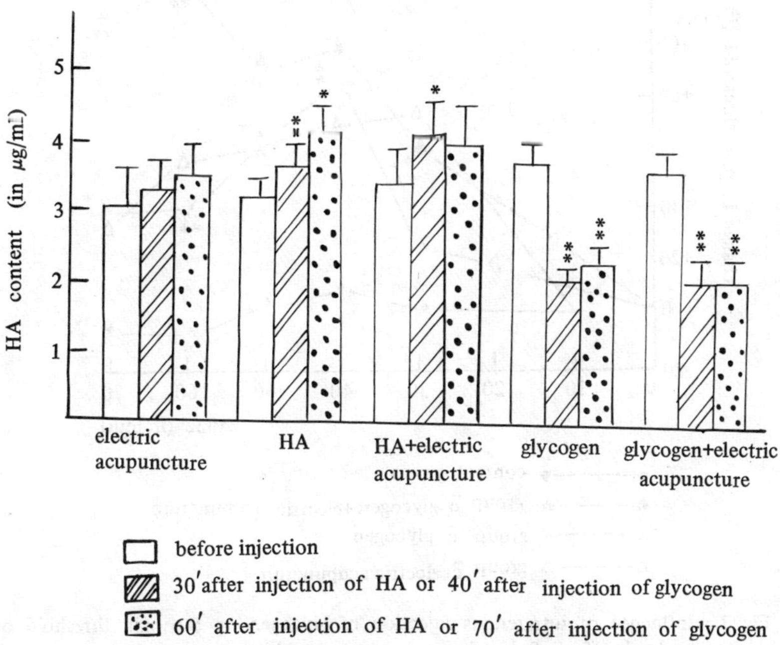

Fig. 2 Blood HA level in rabbits after injection of drugs.

(II) Result

1. Effect of intravenous injection of histamine on pain threshold and electro-acupuncture analgesia. The rabbits chosen were divided into 4 groups: control, electro-acupuncture, histamine, and electroacupuncture + histamine. There were 10–12 animals in each group, and the results are shown in Fig. 1. The average pain threshold varies within 10% in the control group. It was increased by 73 ± 19% and 71 ± 16% for 10′ and 20′ of electro-acupuncture, then decreased gradually after cessation of electroacupuncture. As compared with preinjection level, the basal pain threshold decreased by 17 ± 8% and 22 ± 8% 30′ and 40′ after intraperitoneal injection of histamine. In the electroacupuncture + histamine group, the pain threshold not only did not increase but actually fell to subnormal level during electric stimulation. The pain threshold decreased by 20% 30–60 min after drug injection. The average value after 20–60 min was significantly different from that of the electroacupuncture group.

Blood histamine content was determined in the electroacupuncture, histamine, and histamine + electroacupuncture groups (6 animals in each group) (Fig. 2). The blood content of histamine was not affected by electroacupuncture, but on the contrary was increased by 20% 30′ after injection of drug.

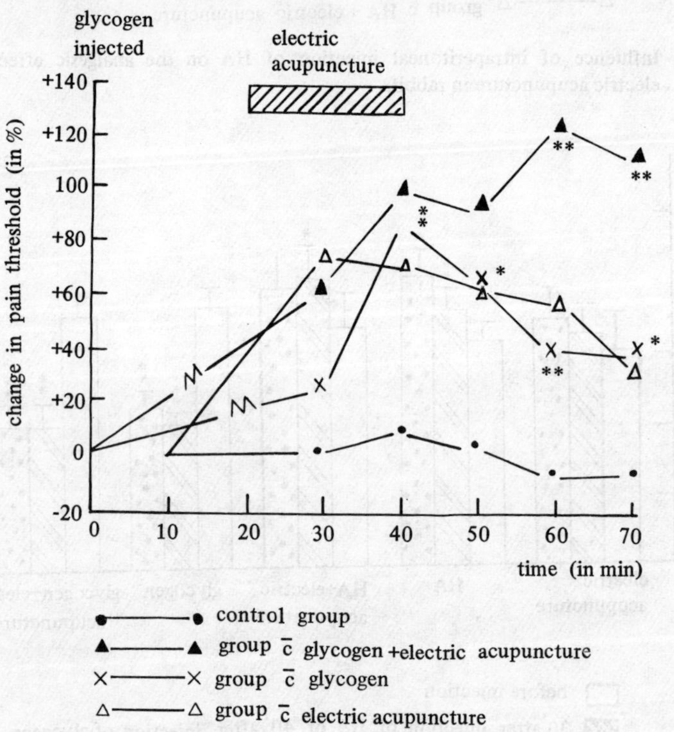

Fig. 3 Influence of intrarenous injection of glycogen on the pain threshold of analgesic effect of electric acupuncture in rabbits.

The result indicated that when blood histamine content was increased by injection of histamine and the animals became hyperalgesic, the analgesic effect of electroacupuncture was resisted or inhibited.

2. Effect of intravenous injection of glycogen on pain threshold and electroacupuncture analgesia. As shown in Fig. 3, 40–70 min after intravenous injection of glycogen, the pain threshold was elevated markedly as compared with that of the control. Since the pain threshold both during and after electrostimulation in the electroacupuncture + drug group was higher than that in the electroacupuncture group, the electroacupuncture analgesia was reenforced by injection of glycogen. The aftereffect also manifested more prominently in the group of drug injection. The average pain threshold 20 and 30 min after cessation of stimulation was increased by 126 ± 15% and 113 ± 15% in the drug injection group instead of 51 ± 12% and 32 ± 12% in the electroacupuncture group.

The blood content of histamine was decreased by 40% 40–70 min after glycogen injection.

From the results, it seems that when blood histamine content is decreased by intravenous injection of glycogen, the animal would become hypoalgesic and the analgesic effect of electroacupuncture would be reenforced.

III. EFFECT OF INCREASING BRAIN CONTENT OF HISTAMINE ON ELECTROACUPUNCTURE ANALGESIC EFFECT

In this experiment we tried to study the effect on electroacupuncture analgesia by increasing the brain content of histamine with intraperitoneal injection of histidine or intraventricular injection of histamine.

(I) Method

Demale rats weighing 150–240 g (in the histidine group) and 250 330 g (in the histamine group) were used. Pain thresholds were determined by radiant heat focused on the tails of the rats at room temperature of 20 ± 1°C[9]. Acupuncture was performed at the bilateral Zusanli point and the parameters of stimuli were as follows: biphasic irregular wave pulse, 130 c/min, 15–20 volts.

Electroacupuncture started 3 hrs after intraperitoneal injection of DL-histidine (1g/kg) and continued for 30 minutes. The pain threshold was evaluated before electroacupuncture, and once every 10 min during electroacupuncture. Histamine diluted with artificial C.S.F. to 10 μl was injected into the lateral ventricle of the rat according to Noble's method[10] with a specially made needle. The histamine content of the rat's whole brain was determined according to Anton's method[11] with some modification and the blood content of histamine was analyzed as before.

(II) Result

1. Effect of intraperitoneal injection of histidine. The average pain threshold of 28 animals injected with histidine 3 hrs before was 4.78 ± 0.20 sec, while it was 4.38 ± 0.12

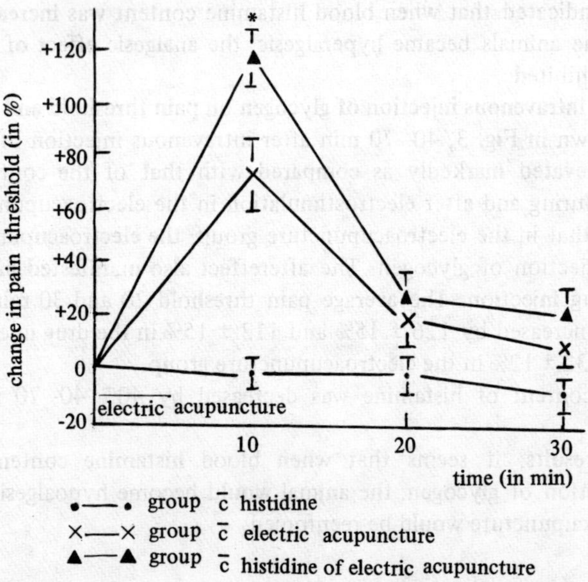

Fig. 4 Influence of intraperitoneal injection of histidine on the analgesic effect of electric-acupuncture in rats.

sec in 34 control animals injected with normal saline. The difference between the histidine groups and the control group was non-significant. Pain threshold measured at the 30 minutes interval 3 hrs after injection of histidine varied within 0.8%. Thus the basal pain threshold was not affected by histidine injection. The average percentage of elevation of pain threshold by electroacupuncture for 10 min was 117 ± 11% in the drug + electroacupuncture group (25 rats). As compared with 73 ± 13% in N.S. + electroacupuncture (26 rats), the difference between them is statistically significant ($P<0.05$) (Fig. 4). Therefore, the analgesic effect of electroacupuncture is enhanced by histidine injection.

The brain content of histamine determination showed 89 ± 3.9 ng/g brain tissue in the normal saline group and 166 ± 9.8 ng/g brain tissue in the histidine group, so that it is increased by 86% due to histidine injection. The blood content of histamine was 105 ± 7.6 ng/ml in the normal saline group and 105 ± 6.3 ng/ml in the histidine group.

2. Effect of intraventricular injection of histamine. On basal pain threshold: The animals used were divided into 4 groups: control[14], histamine 10 μg[8], histamine 30μg[17] and histamine 100 μg[14] group. Pain thresholds evaluated 30 min after intraventricular injection of histamine in these 4 groups were: 6.3 ± 0.47 sec, 6.7 ± 0.37 sec 10.6 ± 9.6 sec, 11.0 ± 12.4 sec, respectively. As compared with the control group, the basal pain threshold was not influenced by 10μg histamine injection, but greatly increased by 30 and 100 μg histamine injections.

On analgesic effect of electro-acupuncture: The pain threshold obtained 50 minutes and 4 hrs after intraventricular injection of 30 or 100 μg histamine, were 5.3 ± 0.41 sec and 5.8 ± 0.31 sec, respectively. It was 5.0 ± 0.35 sec. in the normal saline group. There were no significant differences among them (by variance analysis $F=1.036$, $P<0.05$).

It seems that the histamine, being catabolized after injection 1–4 hrs, does not affect pain threshold any more. Just at this moment electroacupuncture was applied for 10 min., and then pain threshold was determined at the end of stimulation. The amount of elevation of pain threshold was 58 ± 15% in the normal saline group and 97 ± 12% in the histamine + electroacupuncture group. The difference between them was statistically significant ($P<0.05$).

From the results, it looks likely that when histamine content of rat brain is increased to a certain degree, the pain threshold may be elevated and analgesic effect of electroacupuncture is enhanced.

IV. DISCUSSION

1. Many works[1, 3, 12, 13, 14] demonstrate that histamine is one of the chemical agents for initiation of cutaneous pain sensation. Even in the dilution of 10^{-18}, it can still induce burning or pain sensation. Histamine can be released by trauma, electric stimulation, burning of the skin and other tissues. Kinnin synthesis, which is under control of histamine, is also activated by these stimuli. The pain threshold may be greatly elevated by depletion of skin histamine content with agents releasing histamine such as compound 48/80. In the present work, it has been shown that a small amount of histamine injected intraperitoneally causes hyperalgesia, and decreasing histamine content by glycogen injection induces hypoalgesia. Thus it suggests that histamine in the peripheral tissue may serve as a pain-producing substance. However, some authors[15] consider that the histamine concentration required for producing pain is rather high, so it is more likely to cause itching rather than physiological pain.

2. The regulatory effect of acupuncture. The clinical data suggest that the underlying mechanism of acupuncture anesthesia lies in the activation of anti-nociceptive, and in the capability of anti-physiological disturbance of the body, such as the nervous, endocrinal, and immunological systems that take part in it. The effect of acupuncture on pain producing substances in the peripheral must not be overlooked. The role of kinnin and potassium ions has been reported[16]. By our observation in 1975, it was found that at 1 hr after incision of skin, while the operative trauma is most extensive, the blood content of histamine was increased in patients with poor efficacy of acupuncture, but it remained unchanged in patients with good efficacy. Observations were also made on 31 patients of similar conditions in 1977[17]. The results obtained were alike, that is, the blood level of histamine was elevated in patients with poor efficacy of acupuncture but remained unchanged in patients with good efficacy of acupuncture 1 hr after incision of skin. The increase was even more prominent in blood collected from incision wound. Recently an experimentation on 21 normal subjects was carried out by us[18]. The results showed that blood histamine level was not affected by hand acupuncture at Sanyanlou point, but the elevation of histamine induced by nociceptive stimuli could be inhibited. To summarize the results obtained we consider that acupuncture itself, unlike nociceptive stimuli, does not trigger off any change in the blood content of histamine, but by its regulatory effect it can inhibit the elevation of histamine caused by pain stimuli or traumatic injury. As to the regulatory effect of acupuncture, further investigation is needed.

3. Histamine in the brain[2, 4, 5]. Along with methodological improvement, a great advance has been achieved in this area. Currently, histamine is considered as a speculative neurotransmitter. Being synthesized by a specific histidine decarboxylase, histamine is stored in the synaptosome and released subsequently during depolarization. In the brain there are histamine receptors, but their exact physiological function is not well understood. We are interested in the fact that histamine has the pharmacologic action of morphine[6]. Our preliminary work indicates that histamine also has something to do with acupuncture analgesia.

4. About the drugs used. Due to the presence of blood-brain barrier, blood histamine is separated from brain histamine[19, 20]. Therefore, the histamine content either in the blood or in the brain may be altered intentionally by different drugs or the routes of medication. It has been demonstrated that systemic injection of histamine cannot penetrate through blood-brain barrier; it may lead only to increase of the blood level of histamine but without any affect on the brain content of it. Thus either blood or brain content of histamine can be increased respectively by intraperitoneal or intraventricular administration. Furthermore, after intravenous injection of glycogen to the rabbit, while the brain histamine is not affected, the blood level of histamine rises up within the first 1–2 min due to histamine release, but quickly drops down to a low level due to its retention in the lung[21]. According to our results, 40–70 min after intravenous injection of glycogen, the blood content of histamine decreased by 40%. It may be used as a tool for reduce blood histamine content. However, it is less specific, because blood 5-HT is also decreased by glycogen. Schwartz and his colleagues[22] showed that after intraperitoneal injection of L-histidine 500 mg/kg, the brain histamine content may be increased by 50%, and the highest level is reached within 3 hrs and remains for several hrs, but no effect is produced by D-histidine. Moreover, according to Abou et al.[19], histamine content of different brain areas may be increased by intravenous injection of L-histidine 500 mg/kg without any changes in blood histamine. Our results show that 3 hrs after DL-histidine injections (1 g/kg), the brain histamine content is increased by 86% in coincidence with the above mentioned works.

V. SUMMARY

1. The blood content of histamine of 45 cases of lung resection under electroacupuncture was measured with fluoro-spectrophotometric method. As compared with preacupuncture, the level of histamine did not change after 20 minutes of induction. Histamine content 1 hr after incision of the skin varies with efficacy of acupuncture analgesia. It changes slightly in the good efficacy group, but increased markedly in the poor efficacy group. Four hrs after the end of operation, histamine content decreased significantly.

2. When the blood histamine is increased by 20% with intraperitoneal injection of histamine (1 mg/kg), the pain threshold of rabbits decreased and analgesic effect of electroacupuncture is resisted. When histamine is decreased by 40% with intravenous injection of glycogen (20 mg/kg), the pain threshold is increased and analgesic effect of electroacupuncture is reenforced. Electric acupuncture of the bilateral Sanyanlou point does not affect the histamine level of normal human beings.

3. Pain threshold is elevated markedly in rat by intraventricular injection of histamine. Analgesic effect of electroacupuncture can be reenforced either by intraventricular injection of histamine or by intraperitoneal injection of histidine (1 g/kg) which causes the brain histamine content to increase by 86% 3 hrs later.

4. From account of our preliminary results, it sccms to indicate that histamine which serves as a pain producing agent in the periphery may resist the analgesic effect of acupuncture.

REFERENCES

[1] Успенский,В.И.:Гистамин,Медгиз,1963.

[2] Green, J.P.: In *Handbook of Neurochemistry,* vol. 4 Lajtha (Ed.) p.221, 1970.

[3] Rosenthal, S.R.: *Fed. Proc.,* **23**: 1108, 1964.

[4] Snyder, S.H. *et al.*: In *Perspectives in Neuropharmacology,* Solomon, H. Snyder (Ed.), P.43, 1972.

[5] Schwartz, J.C.: *Life Sci.,* **17**:503, 1975.

[6] Domino, E.F. *et al.*: *J. Pharmacol. Exp. Ther.* **184**: 18, 1973.

[7] Zachariae, H.: *Scand J. Clin. Lab. Invest.,* **15**:173, 1963.

[8] 北京市结核病研究所生化研究室等：针麻资料汇编，北京市结核病研究所情报资料室编，第99页，1976。

[9] 北京医学院基础部针麻原理研究组生理组：新医药学杂志，3：133，1976。

[10] Noble, C.P. *et al.*: *Life Sci.,* **6**: 281, 1967.

[11] Anton, A.H. *et al.*: *J. Pharmacol. Exp. Ther.,* **166**: 285, 1969.

[12] Edery, H. *et al.*: *J. Physiol.,* **169**: 568, 1963.

[13] НесТерепко,

[14] Lim, R.K.S.: *Ann. Rev. Physiol.,* **32**: 269, 1970.

[15] Keele, C.A. *et al.*: *Substances Producing Pain and Itch,* E.Arnold, London, 1964.

[16] 针刺调整作用专题座谈会：针刺调整作用研究进展概况(内部资料)，1975。

[17] 北京市结核病研究所等：结核病与肺部肿瘤，1：14，1979。

[18] Xu Shulian, *et al.*. *National Symposia of Acupuncture and Moxibustion and Acupuncture Anesthesia,* p.493, 1979.

[19] Abou, Y.Z. *et al.*: *Br. J. Pharmacol.,* **48**: 577, 1973.

[20] Snyder, S.H. *et al.*: *J. Pharmacol. Exp. Ther.,* **144**: 373, 1964.

[21] Waalkes, T. *et al.*: *Proc. Soc. Exp. Biol. Med.,* **101**: 122, 1959.

[22] Schwartz, J.C. *et al.*: *J. Neurochemistry,* **19**: 801, 1972.

SUBSTANCE P: ITS ANALGESIC EFFECT AND INFLUENCE ON CAUDATE NEURONAL ACTIVITY IN CONSCIOUS RABBITS

Zhang Chongli*, Sun Gongduo**, Yan Huijin***, Yang Kongshun****
Ye Liangqin*, Li Xuming**, Xie Yikuan***, Cheng Shaojie****,
Wang Hong*, Zhao Bingshun*, Jiang Yanjia**, He Guoliang+

I. INTRODUCTION

Substance P (SP) is a peptide consisting of eleven amino acids[1], which is universally present in the nervous tissue of all vertebrates[2], and has long been known to play an important role in the central nervous system[3–5] and to participate also in pain sensation[6–12]. There are some experiments indicating that SP may affect the pain sensation in two different ways: one being the analgesic effect in the brain[6–9], and the other, acting as a pain transmitter in the spinal cord[10–12]. In addition, it has been demonstrated that SP has analgesic effect if injected into the raphe nucleus of the midbrain, and the effect is blocked by naloxone pretreatment[7]. There are some reports demonstrating that the raphe nucleus play an important role in morphine analgesia and acupuncture analgesia[13–17]. On the other hand, there is evidence showing that the caudate nucleus may play an important role in acupuncture analgesia[21–22]. Owing to the close relationship between the raphe nuclei and caudate nucleus both in electrophysiological and morphological connections[22], a chronic experimental study was designed to investigate the role of SP in analgesia as well as its influence on the spontaneous neuronal firing of the caudate nucleus.

II. METHODS

1. **Analgesic experiments.** Twenty-two adult rabbits of both sexes weighing 2–2.4 kg were used. The analgesic effect was measured by the animal's response to potassium ion stimulation on the tail. The contraction of the tail and light struggle responses were taken as the criteria for pain tolerance threshold (MA). A cannula with an outer diameter of 0.9 mm

* Department of Endocrinology, Institute of Zoology, Academia Sinica.

** Department of Physiology, Guiyang Medical College.

*** Department of Physiology, Institute of Basic Medical Science, Chinese Academy of Medical Sciences.

**** Department of Physiology, Guiyang Traditional Chinese Medical College.

\+ Visiting research fellow from Jiangxi Medical College. The authors are indebted to Prof. C. Y. Chang for his valuable suggestions and reading of the manuscript.

was stereotaxically implanted under anesthesia with sodium pentobarbital for the injection of drugs. The coordinates of the raphe nuclei of the midbrain for implantation are $P_{9.5}$, R_{0-1}, $H_{-(5-6)}$ according to Sawyer's atlas of rabbit brain[24]. Experiments were started one day after the operation. First saline (5μl) and then SP (Beckman Co. 10 μg/5 μl saline) were injected into raphe nuclei. In a part of the animals, saline and SP were injected in the reverse order on the next day in order to rule out any interference produced by saline injection.

2. Electrophysiological Study. Twenty-one adult rabbits of both sexes weighing 2–2.5 kg were used. The cannula was stereotaxically implanted as above and the base of micro-manipulator was simultaneously fixed on the skull in the mirror position of the head of caudate nucleus[25–26]. The coordinates of caudate nucleus implantation are about A_{2-4}, L_{2-4}. Experiments were begun about 1–2 days after operation. Glass microelectrodes filled with 3 M KCl were used for recording the single unit activity in conscious animals under a restrained condition. The electrode resistance range from 5–25 megaohms was chosen. Electrical discharge of neurons picked up from the microelectrode, after being fed to a negative capacity-compensated cathode follower, was displayed on a double-beam oscilloscope (Model SBR–1) and recorded simultaneously with a type recorder.

The experimental sequence was as follows:

Recording of spontaneous neuronal firing (without any treatment)→injection of saline (5 μl) or SP (1.0 μg/5 μl saline)→recording of spontaneous neuronal firing→injection of SP or

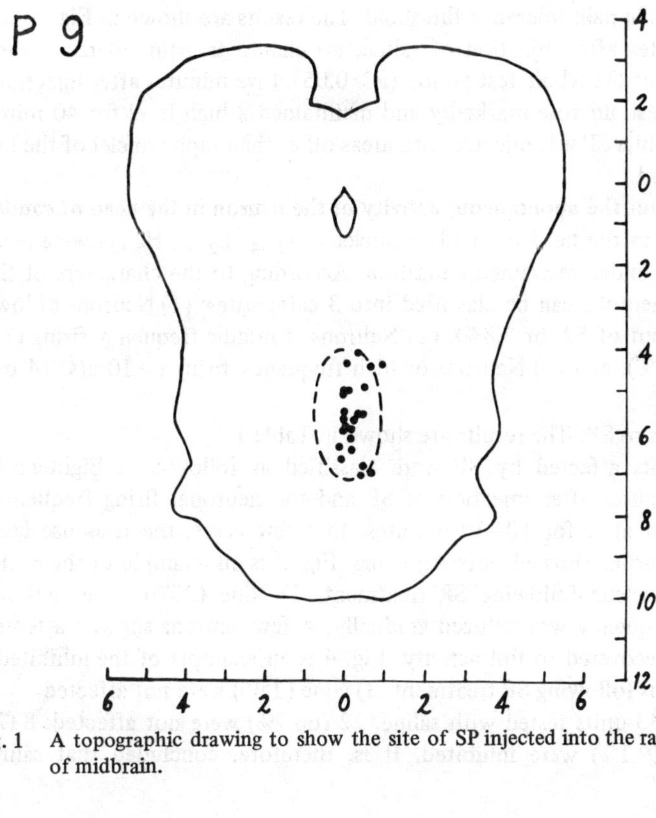

Fig. 1 A topographic drawing to show the site of SP injected into the raphe nuclei of midbrain.

saline→recording of spontaneous neuronal firing. The total sequence lasted about 40 min.

3. Identification of the site of cannula and microelectrode. After the completion of the experiments, a stainless steel needle electrode was inserted into the cannula and the recorded corresponding position of the glass microelectrode. The sites of the injection and the electrode were identified by passing an anodal current 100 μA for 30 sec and then the brain was fixed in 1% potassium ferrocyanide and 10% formalin. Frozen sections were made and the localization of the exact sites of injection and the electrode tip was checked microscopically. A topographic drawing to show the sites of SP injection is presented in Fig. 1.

4. Analysis of electrophysiological data.

(1) Unit discharges were fed into a computer (Type TQ–19) to draw sequence total pulse number histograms.

(2) Unit discharges were fed into a digital frequency meter and the pulse counts were statistically analyzed.

(3) Unit discharges were translated by a stimulator into square waves which were fed into the cathode of an oscilloscope and displayed as bright points, with each representing a spike. The tracings were photographed finally.

III. RESULTS

1. The changes in pain tolerance threshold. The results are shown in Fig. 2.

Twenty minutes after injection of saline, no change in pain tolerance threshold was observed throughout the whole test period ($P>0.05$). Five minutes after injection of SP, the pain tolerance threshold rose markedly and maintained a high level for 40 min ($P<0.01$). Moreover, in 7 rabbits SP was injected into areas other than raphe nuclei of the midbrain; no change was observed.

2. The effect on the apontaneous activity of the neuron in the head of caudate nucleus. Fifty-two neurons in the head of caudate nucleus (A_{2-4}, L_{2-4}, H_{6-3}) were recorded in 21 conscious animals under restrained condition. According to the characters of the neuronal firing frequency, neurons can be classified into 3 categorites: (1) Neurons of low frequency firing (<1 c/s, 2 out of 52, or 3.8%), (2) Neurons of middle frequency firing (1–10 c/s, 36 out of 52, or 69.2%), and (3) Neurons of high frequency firing (>10 c/s, 14 out of 52, or 27%).

(1). Responses to SP: The results are shown in Table 1.

Thirty-six units affected by SP were classified as follows: 1) Eighteen (50%) were activated 1–3 minutes after injection of SP and the neuronal firing frequency promptly increased and kept at it for 10–30 minutes. In a few cases, the response lasted over 40 minutes. Some neurons showed bursting firing. Fig. 3 is an example of the excited neurons of the caudate nucleus following SP treatment. 2) Nine (25%) were inhibited and the neuronal firing frequency was reduced gradually. A few neurons showed a temporary state of rest and then recovered to full activity. Fig. 4 is an example of the inhibited neurons of the caudate nucleus following SP treatment. 3) Nine (25%) were not affected.

However, in 33 units tested with saline, 22 (66.7%) were not affected; 8 (24.2%) were activated and 3 (9.1%) were inhibited. It is, therefore, concluded that saline does not

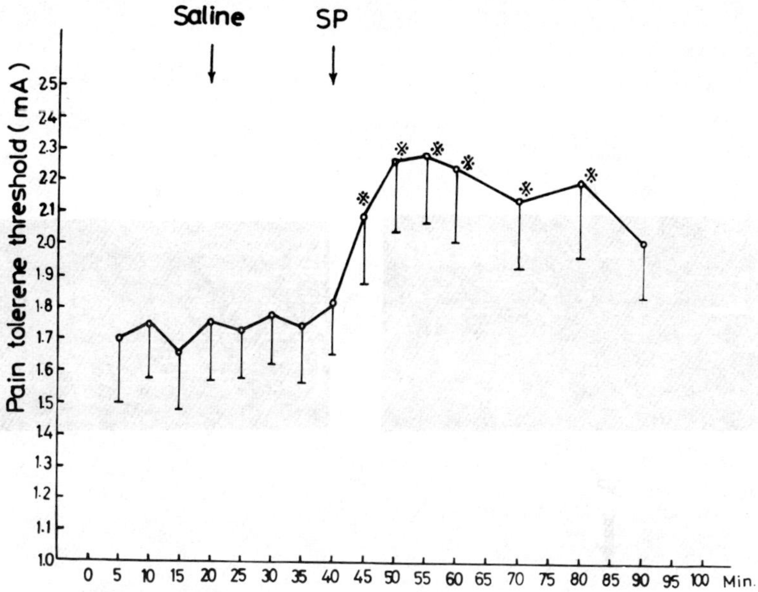

Fig. 2 The effect of SP microinjected into the midbrain raphe nuclei on pain tolerance threshold.
Number of rabbit: 1.5
* P<0.01 ° S.E.

Table 1. The Effect of SP microinjected into the raphe nuclei on caudate neurons

Drug of injection	Neurons of Caudate Nucleus			
	Total number of units	Number of units activated (% of total)	Number of units inhibited (% of total)	Number of units notaffected (% of total)
Substance P	36	18 (50)	9 (25)	9 (25)
Saline	33	8 (24.2)	3 (9.1)	22 (66.7)

significantly affect the spontaneous activity of the neurons of the caudate nucleus.

Statistical analysis (X^2 test) of the results from SP and saline shows a significant difference ($P<0.01$), the effect of SP being specific.

A particularly interesting phenomenon observed was that some of the resting neurons of caudate nucleus started a bursting firing after injection of SP into raphe nuclei of the midbrain, and some of such neurons lasted for a long time.

(2) Space distribution of neurons mo dulated by SP: In the present study, almost all of the neurons of middle frequency firing were activated caudate nuclei (17 out of 18, or 94.4%) following SP injection and most of them were found to be located in the superficial

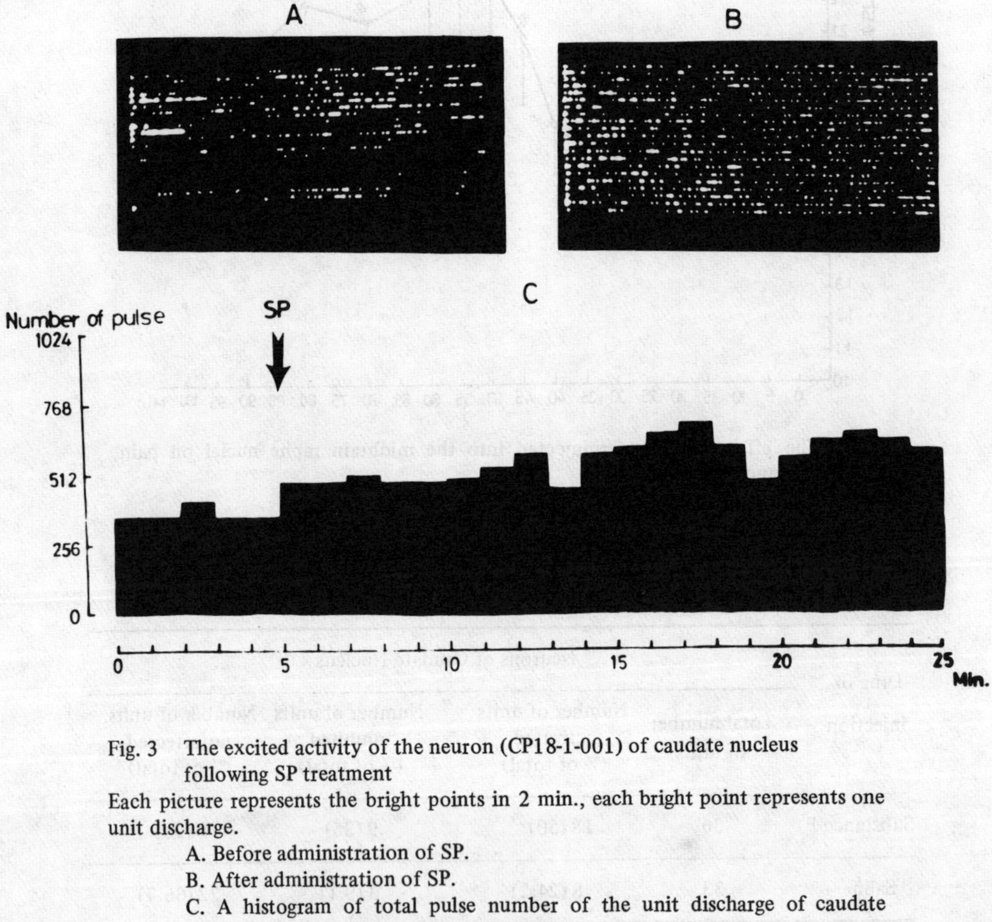

Fig. 3 The excited activity of the neuron (CP18-1-001) of caudate nucleus following SP treatment

Each picture represents the bright points in 2 min., each bright point represents one unit discharge.

A. Before administration of SP.

B. After administration of SP.

C. A histogram of total pulse number of the unit discharge of caudate nucleus before and after SP administration.

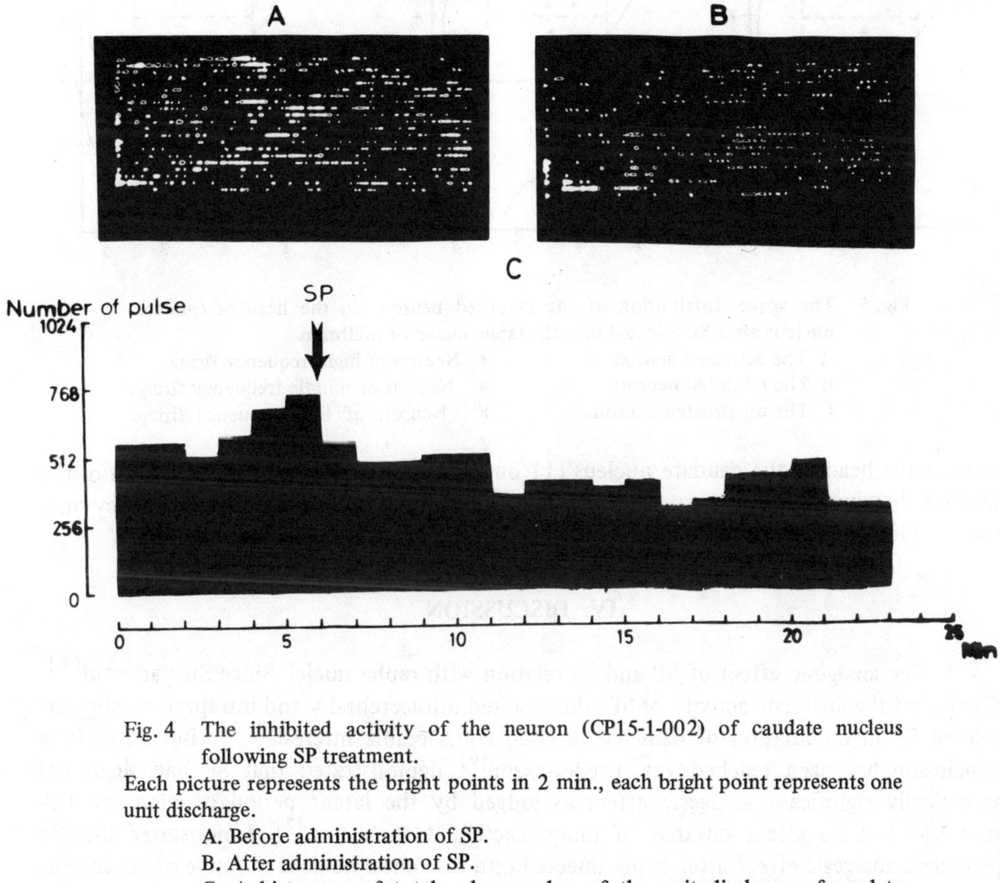

Fig. 4 The inhibited activity of the neuron (CP15-1-002) of caudate nucleus following SP treatment.

Each picture represents the bright points in 2 min., each bright point represents one unit discharge.

A. Before administration of SP.

B. After administration of SP.

C. A histogram of total pulse number of the unit discharge of caudate nucleus before and after sp administration.

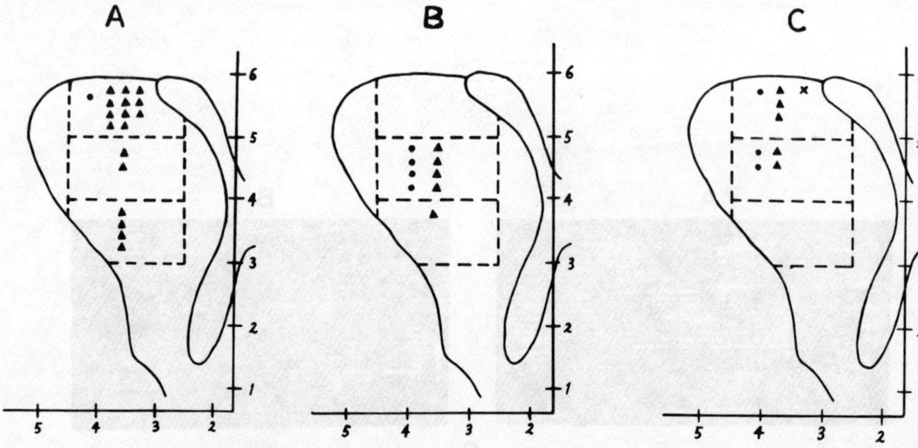

Fig. 5 The space distribution of the recorded neurons in the head of caudate. nucleus after SP injected into the raphe nuclei of midbrain

A The activated neuron. ● Neuron of high frequency firing.

B The inhibited neuron. ▲ Neuron of middle frequency firing.

C The un-affected neuron. × Neuron of low frequence firing.

layer of the head of the caudate nucleus (11 out of 18, or 61.1%, see Fig. 5A). Most of the neurons showing inhibitory response to SP injection were of middle and high frequency ones and were located in the middle layer of the head of the caudate nuclei (see Fig. 5B).

IV. DISCUSSION

1. The analgesic effect of SP and its relation with raphe nuclei. Since Stewart *et al*[6] discovered the analgesic activity of SP administered intracerebrally and intraperitoneally, the role of SP in modulation of pain has aroused considerable interest[8–9]. But no definite conclusion has been reached yet. Frederickson[9] demonstrated that SP had slight but statistically significant analgesic effect as judged by the latent period of hind-paw lick response, but no effect on that of jump reaction. Malick *et al*[7] demonstated that SP produced analgesic effect after being injected into the dorsal nucleus of raphe of rat and the effect was found to be blocked by naloxone pretreatment. The present experimental results show that a notable analgesic effect was promptly produced following injection of SP into the raphe nuclei of rabbit midbrain. If SP was injected into areas other than raphe nuclei, no analgesic effect was found. Unpublished results from this laboratory, however, could not confirm the above results if analgesia was tested by measuring the mice's tail-flick response to radiant heat as the criterion for pain and if SP was injected intracerebrally or intraperitoneally. The notion that the raphe nucleus is essential in the regulation of analgesic action is further verified in our experiments.

2. The modulation of SP on the spontaneous activity of neurons of the caudate nucleus after intra-raphe nuclei injection as well as its relation with analgesia. The relationship between caudate nucleus and analgesia has recently received considerable attention.

Experimental evidence demonstrated that the restricted stimulation of the superficial cells of the caudate nucleus suppresses the activity of the extralemniscal thalamic units but not that of the lemniscal system[28–30]. Preliminary studies indicate that stimulation of the head of caudate nucleus increases pain threshold[18–20]; and the destruction of this structure attenuates the analgesic effect produced by acupuncture[18, 19]. The intractable pain in terminal cancer patients can be temporarily relieved by self-controlled electrical stimulation of the caudate nucleus[20]. In addition, it has also been demonstrated that the afferent signals of electroacupuncture could be transmitted to the caudate nucleus[18, 26, 31]. Chang[21, 22] has suggested that the caudate nucleus may coordinate with the thalamus in the regulation of acupuncture analgesia. The present experiments show that the intra-raphe injection of SP could modulate the neurons of caudate nucleus (50% activated; 25% inhibited)- and the excited neurons showed response promptly and lasted for a relatively longer time. Almost all of the neurons in the superficial layer of the caudate nucleus were activated. It is, therefore, suggested that the analgesic effect of SP and its exciting effect on the neurons of the head of caudate nucleus via the raphe nuclei of the midbrain might be one of the analgesic mechanisms in the CNS.

V. SUMMARY

In the present study, a chronic experimental method was adopted. SP was injected into the rabbit raphe nuclei of the midbrain. The results are summarized as follows:

1. The change in pain tolerance threshold. Analgesic effect was measured by the animal's response to K^+ stimulus on the tail. Five minutes after the injection of SP (10 μg/5 μl saline), the pain tolerance threshold rose markedly and maintained a high level throughout the test period for 40 min ($P<0.01$). In the saline control group, on the other hand, no change was observed ($P>0.05$).

2. The effect on spontaneous activity of the neurons in the head of the caudate nucleus. By using chronic microelectrodes, 52 neurons in the head of the caudate nucleus were recorded in 21 conscious animals under restrained condition. Out of a total 33 units tested with saline, 22 (66.7%) were not affected, 8 (24.2%) activated and 3 (9.1%) inhibited. The result suggests that the spontaneous neuronal firing is not affected significantly by saline. However, in 36 units tested with SP, 27 (75%) were modulated, 18 (50%) activated, and 9 (25%) inhibited. The characteristics of modulation were prompt onset and long post-effect. In addition, neurons activated by SP were mainly of middle frequency and located in the superficial layer of the head of caudate nucleus.

From the results of the present experiment, it is concluded that the analgesic effect of SP is possibly mediated by the raphe nuclei. Since the caudate nucleus is implicated in analgesia as well as in acupuncture analgesia, it is, therefore, suggested that SP modulating the activity of neurons in the head of the caudate nucleus by way of the raphe nuclei of the midbrain may be one of the analgesic factors in the CNS.

REFERENCES

[1] Chang, M.M. *et al.*: *Nature New Biol.*, **232**:86, 1971.
[2] Lembeck, F. *et al.*: *Int. Rev. Neurobiol.*, **4**:159, Academic Press, New York and London, 1962.
[3] Leeman, S. E. *Life Sci.*, **15**:2033, 1974.
[4] Pernow, B.: *Acta Physiol. Scand.*, (Suppl. 105) **29**:1, 1953.
[5] Bury, R. W.: *Aust. J. Exp. Biol. Med. Sci.*, **55**(pt. 6):671, 1977.
[6] Stewart, J. M. *et al.*: *Nature*, **262**(5571):784, 1976.
[7] Malick, J. B. *et al.*: *Fed. Proc.*, **36**(3):994, 1977.
[8] Starr M. S. *et al.*: *Europ. J. Pharmacol.*, **48**:203, 1978.
[9] Frederickson, R. C. A. *et al.*: *Science*, **199**:1359, 1978.
[10] Henry, J. L. *Substance P, Nobel Symposium 37* (U.S. von Euler and B. Pernow, Eds.) Reven Press, N.Y., p.231, 1977.
[11] Randic, M. *et al.*: *Brain Res.*, **128**:164, 1977.
[12] Jessell, T. M. *et al.*: *Nature*, **268**:549, 1977.
[13] 江振裕等：中华医学杂志，55（10）：611，1977。
[14] 广西医学院针麻研究小组：动物学报，24（1）：29，1978。
[15] 韩济生等：中国科学，5：579，1978。
[16] Proudfit, H. K. *et al.*: *Brain Res.*, **98**(1):612, 1975.
[17] Way, E. L. *Fed. Proc.*, **31**:113, 1972.
[18] 上海第一医学院生理教研组：中华医学杂志，**55**（5）：336，1975。
[19] 上海生理研究所第二研究室针麻组：中华医学杂志，**55**（5）：340，1975。
[20] 上海第一医学院华山医院针麻研究协作组：中华医学杂志，55（6）：427，1975。
[21] 张香桐：中国科学，1：28，1973。
[22] 张香桐：中国科学，4：465，1978。
[23] Usunoff, K. G.: *Brain Res.*, **74**(1):143 1974.
[24] Sawyer, C. H. *et al.*: *J. Comp. Neurol.*, **101**:801, 1954.
[25] 孙公铎等：中华医学杂志，3：139，1978。
[26] 孙公铎等：科学通报，23（7）：447，1978。
[27] Schmidek H. H.: *J. Neurosurg.*, **35**:715, 1971.
[28] Feliz, P. *et al.*: *J. Neurophysiol.*, **30**:55, 1967.
[29] Rogers, D. K. *et al.*: *Brain Res.*, **56**:345, 1973.
[30] Lineverry, C. C. *et al.*: *Brain Res.*, **98**:110, 1975.
[31] 上海第一医学院基础医学部 生理学教研组针麻研究组：中华医学杂志，58（3）：135，1978。

POSSIBLE ROLE OF HYPOTHALAMUS-PITUITARY-ADRENAL SYSTEM IN ACUPUNCTURE ANALGESIA

Liu Xuegao, Yang Zijiang , Li Qinzhang
(Department of Biology, Jinan University, Guangzhou, China)

Huang Yiming, Xu Hao , Xiao Changqi
(Department of Biology, Zhongshan University, Guangzhou, China)

Liang Zhixi
(Physiological Division, Guangzhou Medical College, Guangzhou, China)

Acupuncture and moxibustion have been widely used in China as traditional, simple, and effective therapeutic methods for the relief of pain. Under acupuncture stimulation, it has been observed that there are very complicated physiological changes in the body. Early in the 1950s, Chinese research workers discovered that acupuncture stimulation could induce significant functional and morphological changes in the adrenal cortex. Early medical workers postulated that the pituitary-adrenal system might play some role in the coordina-ation of physiological disorders and the relief of pains following acupuncture. It has been reported that adrenocorticotrophin and cortical steroids possess certain analgesic effect[1, 2], and these substances are closely related to the spinal cord reflex, central nervous conduction, synaptic transmission and central excitability [1]. Quite recently numerous scientific investigations have indicated that the hypothalamus and pituitary gland can secrete certain endogenous opiate-like substances related to ACTH and β-lipotropin. Accordingly, a study was undertaken to explore the possible role of this system on acupuncture analgesia.

I. EFFECT OF INTRACEREBRAL STEROID IMPLANTATION ON THE PITUITARY-ADRENAL SYSTEM AND ACUPUNCTURE ANALGESIC EFFICACY IN RATS

Hydrocortisone pellets were introduced into the ventro-medial nucleus of the hypothalamus in rats (Fig. 2) by intracerebral implantation technique[3] (Fig. 1) according to Bernardis and Skelton's Atlas of rat hypothalamus[4]. The sham operated controls were implanted with the same amount of sucrose crystals in the same localization. The results revealed that unilateral steroid implant was effective in lowering significantly both adrenal weight and its ascorbic acid content. Through histological examination of the adrenal cortex,

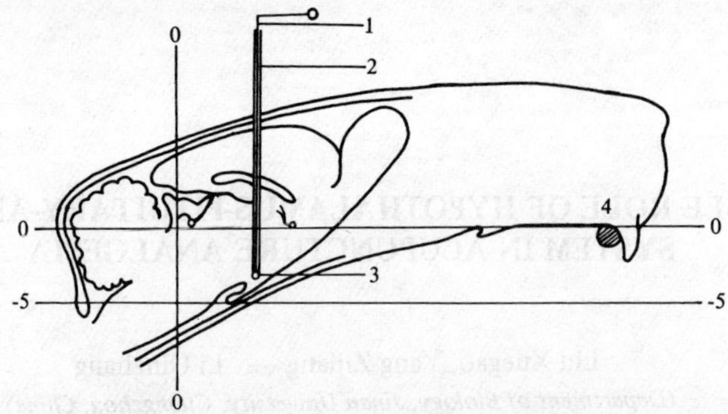

Fig. 1 Technique for intracerebral steroid implantation in rat.
1. Push bar; 2. Cannula; 3. Steroid pellet.
4. Fixation Plane for the upper jaw.

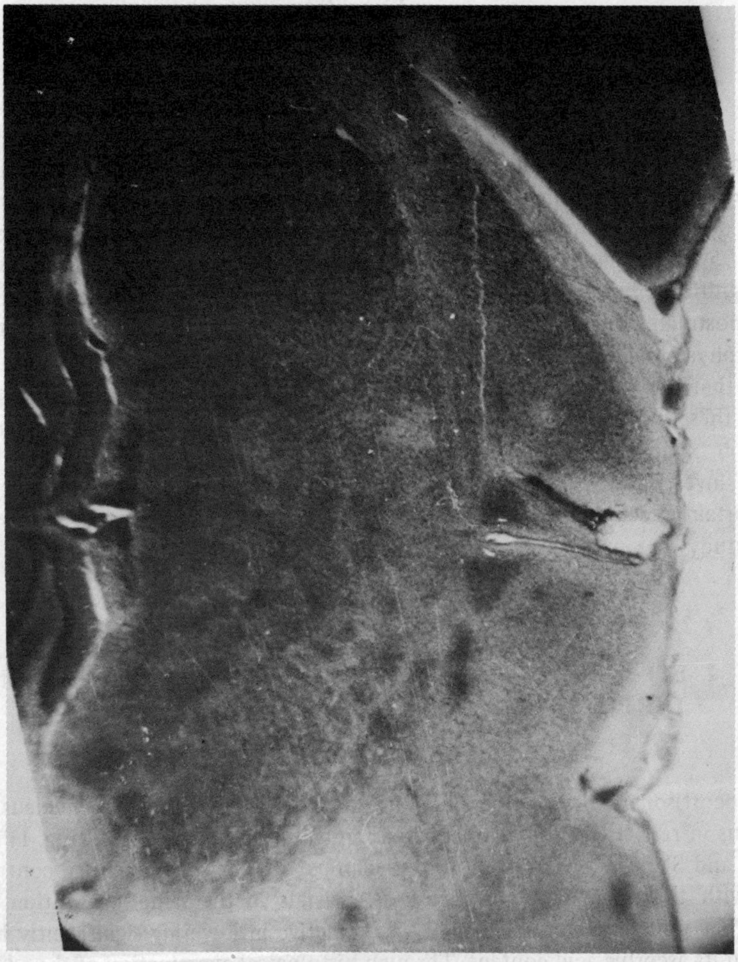

Fig. 2 Coronal section of experimental rat: hydrocortison implantation in ventromedial nucleus of hypothalamus.

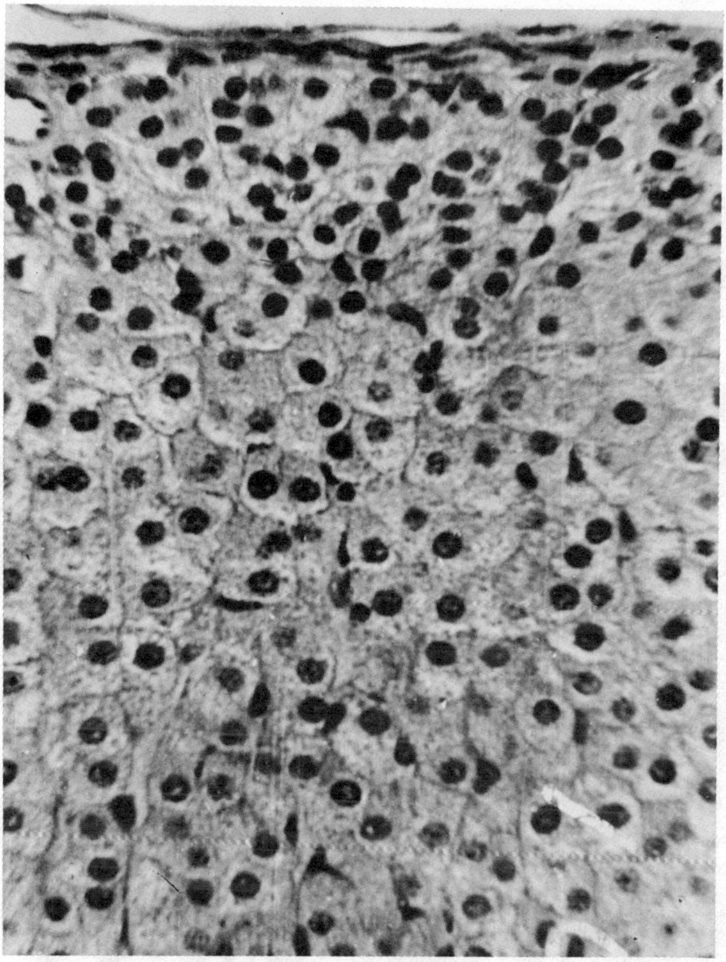

Fig. 3A Microscopic observation of the adrenal cortex of control rat: normal histological appearances.

different degrees of atrophic degeneration were also observed in the experimental animals. These implied that ventro-medial nucleus implantation of steroid hormone in rats might selectively block the pituitary-adrenal system through feedback mechanism (Fig. 3).

In the effectively steroid blocked animals, the pain threshold and acupuncture analgesic efficacy decreased significantly. Before steroid implantation, the acupuncture efficacy averaged 40.4%; two weeks after the implantation, it decreased to –7.8%. The amplitude of decrement was 48.2%. In sucrose implantation controls, it averaged 41.3% before the sham operation, and dropped to 14.9% after surgery, with an amplitude of about 26.4%; it was only about half the value of the experimental group (Fig. 4).

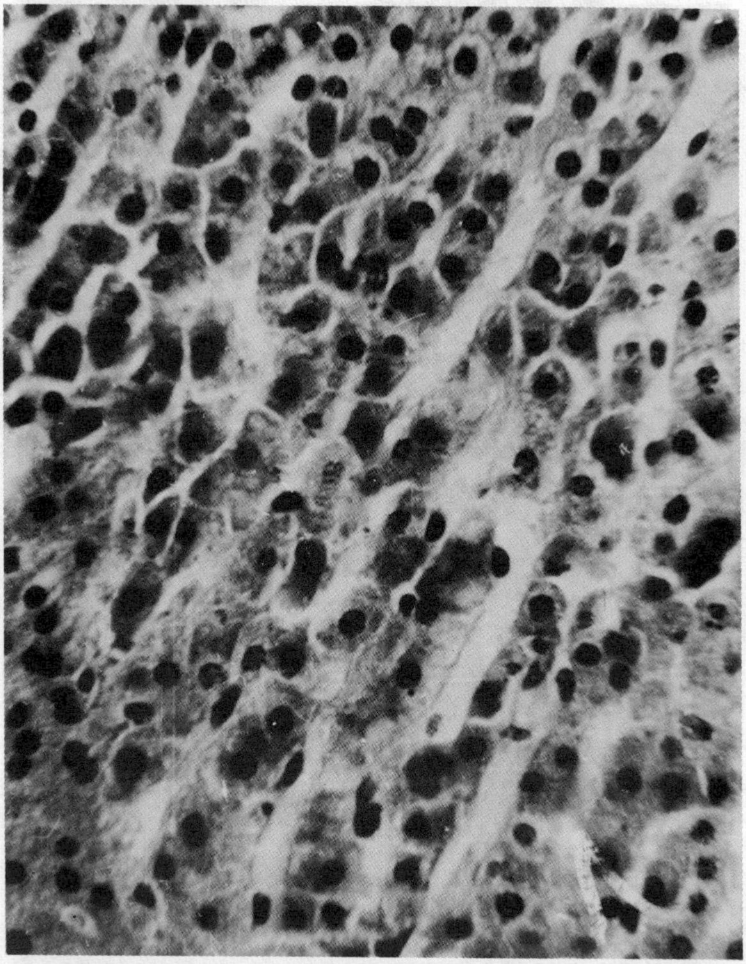

Fig. 3B Microscopic observation of the adrenal cortex of experimental rat: karyopykonosis abnormal histological appearances.

The adrenal weight and its ascorbic acid content were finally examined in the two groups of animals. The difference was quite significant. The adrenal weight of the control animals averaged 38.7mg or 0.27mg/g B.W.; ascorbic acid content averaged 161.3mg or 1.15mg/g B.W.; while in those effectively blocked experimental animals, the adrenal weight averaged 21.6mg or 0.16mg/g B.W.; ascorbic acid content averaged 89.4 or 0.66mg/g B.W. (Fig. 5).

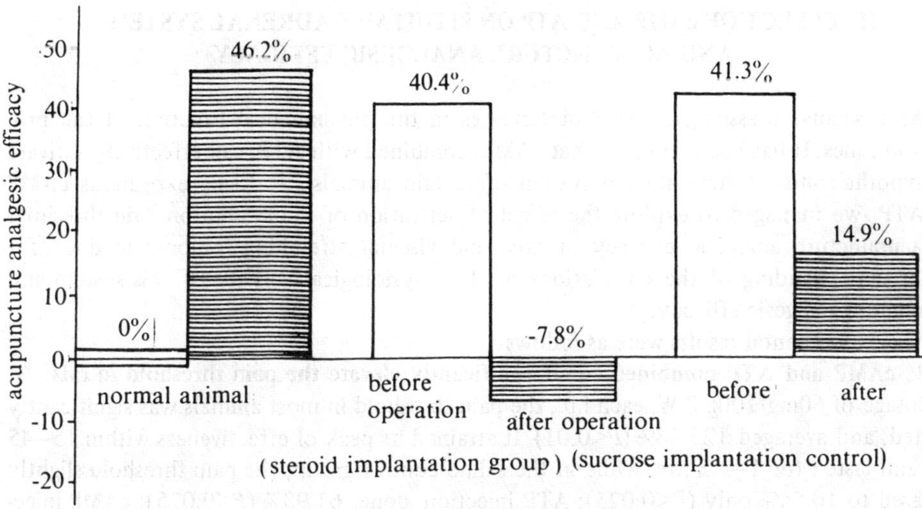

Fig. 4 Effect of intrahypothalamic steroid implantation on the acupuncture analgesic efficacy of rat.

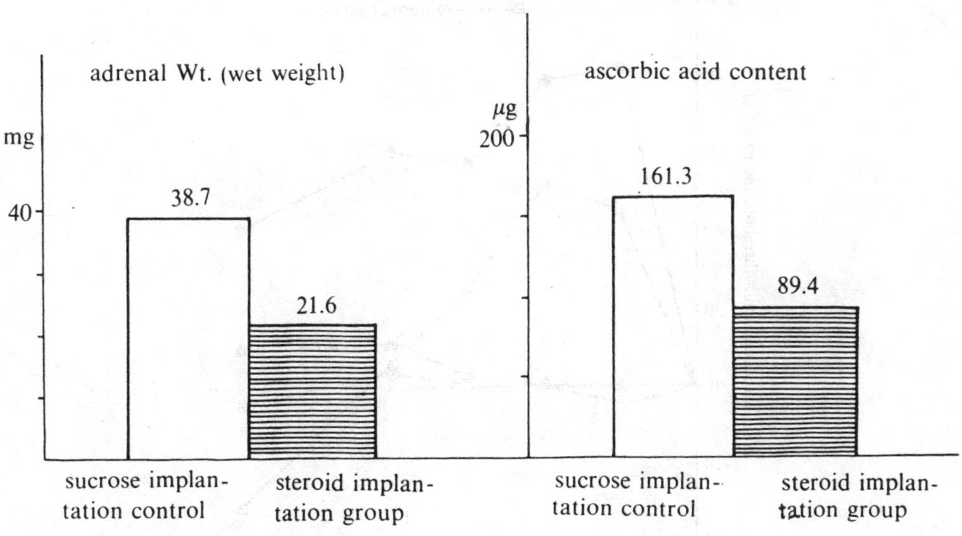

Fig. 5 Effect of hypothalamic steroid implantation on the pituitary-adrenal system of rat.

II. EFFECT OF cAMP AND ATP ON PITUITARY-ADRENAL SYSTEM AND ACUPUNCTURE ANALGESIC EFFICACY

As a second messenger, cAMP participates in the physiological function of the protein hormones. It has been reported that cAMP, combined with ATP, can effectively activate the hypothalamus-pituitary-adrenal system of certain animals[4]. Using exogenous cAMP and ATP, we managed to explore the effect of activation of the system on pain threshold and acupuncture analgesic efficacy in rats, and visceral stretching response in dogs, for further understanding of the correlations of the physiological activity of this system and acupuncture analgesic efficacy.

The experimental results were as follows:

1. cAMP and ATP combined could significantly elevate the pain threshold in rats: At the dosage of 60mg/100g B.W. each i.p., the pain threshold in most animals was significantly elevated, and averaged 125.18% (*P*<0.01). It attained its peak of effectiveness within 15–45 min, and lasted for 1–1.5 hrs; while in the saline control group, the pain threshold slightly increased to 10.54% only (*P*<0.025); ATP injection alone, 61.93% (*P*<0.025); cAMP injection alone, 15.20% (*P*<0.005). The difference in pain threshold elevations between cAMP

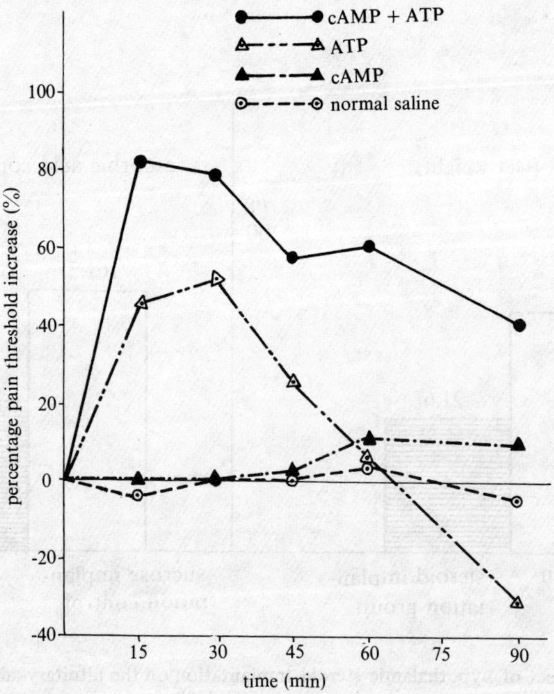

Fig. 6 Effect of i.p. cAMP. ATP injection on the pain threshold of rat.

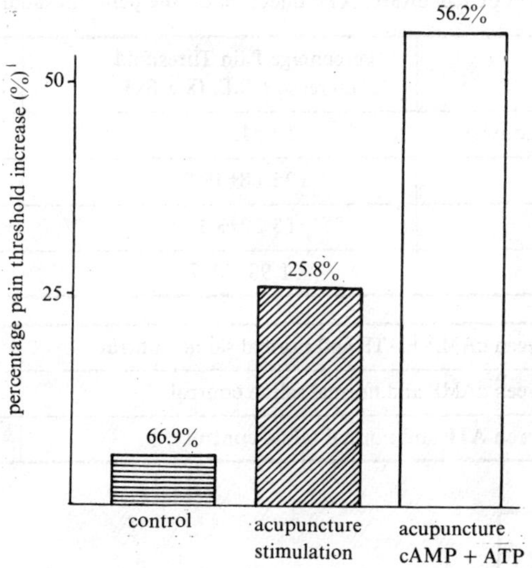

Fig. 7 Effect of acupuncture stimnlation and cAMP+ATP injection on the pain threshold.

+ ATP and the saline control group was statistically significant ($P<0.05$) (Fig. 6 and Table 1).

2. cAMP + ATP could significantly elevate the acupuncture analgesic efficacy in rats: When acupuncture stimulation was applied immediately aftor i.p. injection of cAMP + ATP 15mg/100g B.W. each, the pain threshold increased by 56.91% ($P<0.005$); while in the saline control, the elevation of the pain threshold averaged 25.8% only ($P<0.05$). In the 3rd no drug no acupuncture group, the pain threshold remained practically constant, and averaged 6.66% ($P<0.05$). The difference between the experimental and control groups was statistically very significant ($P<0.005$) (Fig. 7).

3. cAMP + ATP could also significantly inhibit the visceral stretching response in dogs: On the basis of the establishment of the dog visceral stretching response model[5], we tested the effect of cAMP + ATP on this response. Intravenous injection of cAMP + ATP, 25mg each in saline, was followed by 25mg in 30cc saline for i.v. infusion. 15, 30, 60, 90 and 120 min after the infusion, visceral stretching response was determined by using the abdominal pressure change as an index. The abdominal pressure elevation averaged 153.4mm H_2O before drug administration, 134.8mm H_2O 15min after infusion, and became more pronounced 30 min later, averaging 53.6mm H_2O, only 1/3 of the preinfusion level. It maintained at a low level for 120 min; the abdominal pressure response to visceral stretching stimulation at the end of the experiment averaged 79.6mm H_2O, only 1/2 of the pre-infusion level (Fig. 8).

Table 1. Effect of 1.p. cAMP, ATP injection on the pain threshold of rat

Group	Percentage Pain Threshold Increase ± S.E. ($\bar{x} \pm S\bar{x}$)	Significance Test (P Value)
Normal Saline Control	10.54±3.3	<0.025
cAMP + ATP	125.18±39.9	<0.01
cAMP	15.20±3.1	<0.005
ATP	61.93±21.7	<0.025
Difference between cAMP + ATP and normal saline control		<0.05
Difference between cAMP and normal saline control		>0.2
Difference between ATP and normal saline control		<0.05

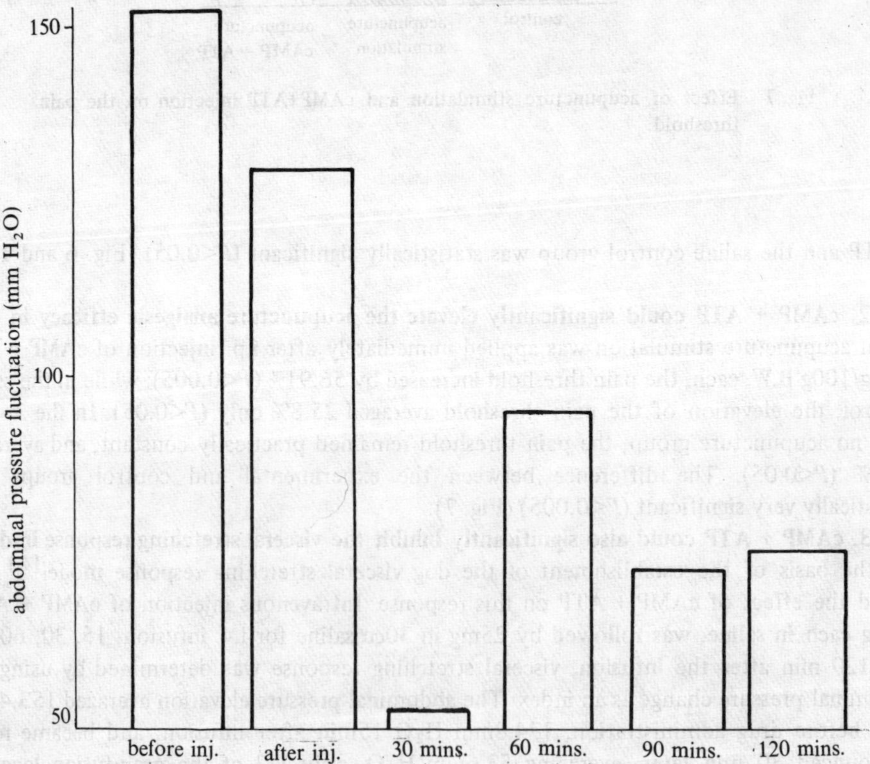

Fig. 8 Comparison of stomach stretching induced abdominal pressure fluctuation before and after CAMP+ATP injection.

III. A STUDY OF THE ACUPUNCTURE ANALGESIC EFFICACY AND ACIDOPHIL VARIATION OF DIFFERENT PEPTIC ULCER PATIENTS DURING GASTRECTOMY OPERATIONS

Based on the results of these previous animal experimentations, we have made some clinical observations on the relationship between acupuncture analgesic efficacy and the

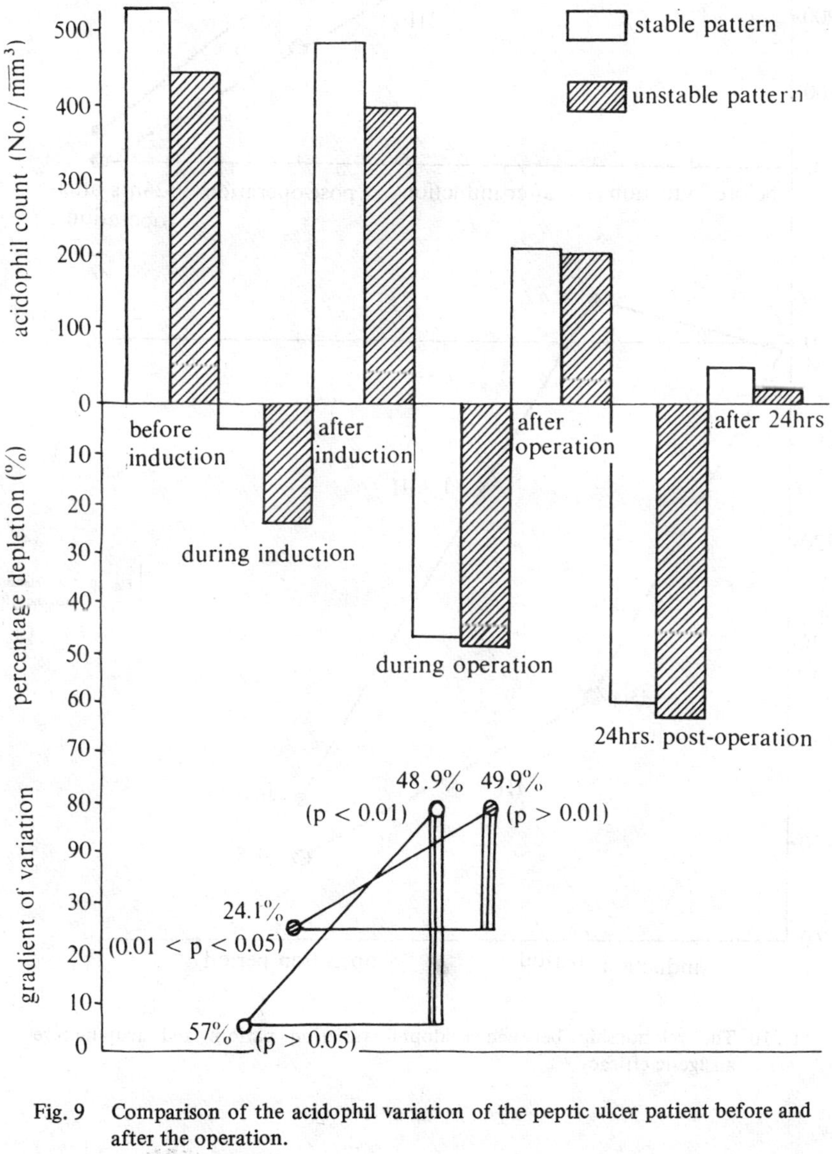

Fig. 9 Comparison of the acidophil variation of the peptic ulcer patient before and after the operation.

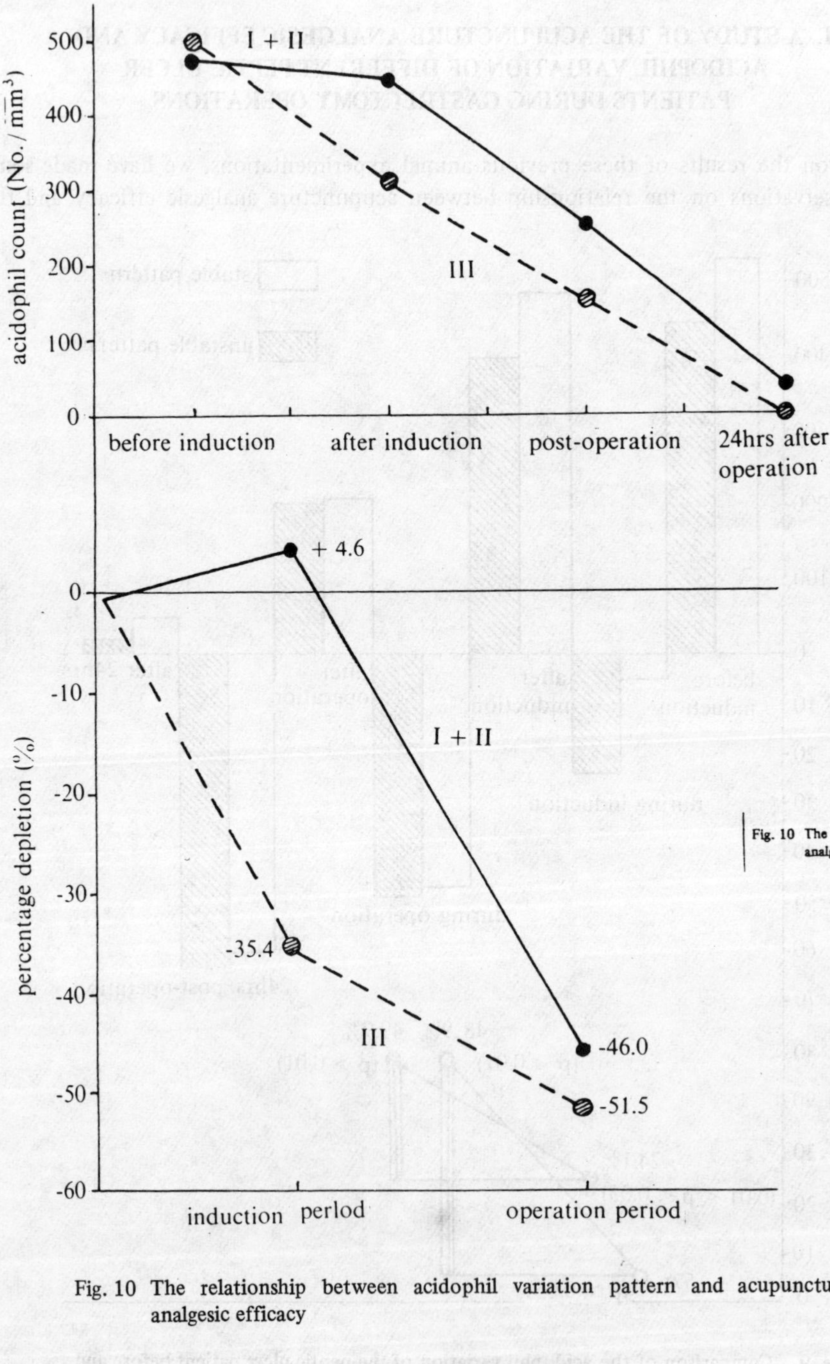

Fig. 10 The relationship between acidophil variation pattern and acupuncture analgesic efficacy

Fig. 10 The relatior analgesic effi

acidophil variation pattern of different peptic ulcer patients during operation.

According to traditional Chinese medicine, the basis of their physiological conditions and pathological symptoms, the patients with peptic ulceration can be classified into two groups:the weak-cold spleen-stomach type (pi wei xu han xing) and the stomach affected-by-liver-disorder type (gan qi fan wei xing). Using the acidophil depletion as a parameter, we found a significant difference between the activities of the hypothalamus-pituitary-adrenal system in these two different groups. One was designated as "stable excitation responding type" and the other as "unstable excitation-responding type". During the induction period of acupuncture anesthesia, the percentage of acidophil depletion of the first group was not significant, while the second group showed a significant drop. Consequently, the gradient of the percentage of acidophil depletion between the induction and the operation periods in the first group appeared to be greater than that of the second one (Fig. 9).

It was very interesting to note that the proportion of good acupuncture analgesic efficacy (Grades I and II) was higher in the first group than in the second group. Besides, most of the patients belonging to the good acupuncture efficacy categories (Grades I and II in the first and second group) showed the same acidophil variation pattern as that of the "adaptational stable type" (first group) (Fig. 10). The present data imply that the physiological activities of the hypothalamus-pituitary-adrenal system have some correlation with acupuncture analgesic efficacy.

In conclusion, the results of present investigation show that the hypothalamus-pituitary-adrenal system might play some role in acupuncture analgesia and personal variation in the efficacy of acupuncture analgesia.

REFERENCES

[1] Woodbury, D.M.: *Rev*. **10(2)**: 275, 1958.
[2] 浙江医科大学等; 中医药通讯,第 62 页，1973。
[3] Corbin, A., *et al.*: *Endocrinology* **76**(5): 811, 1965.
[4] Cook, D.B., *et al.*: *J. Endocrinol.* **(60)**: 65, 1974.
[5] 广州医学院　针麻原理研究组等: 广医通讯 (1): 34，1976。

RELATIONSHIP OF LIP-ACUPUNCTURE ANALGESIA WITH PITUITARY-ADRENOCORTICAL SYSTEM

Miao Ming*, Liu Huici, Gao Aili, Huang Weiqiu, Xu Bin, Yin Qizhang
(Research Group of Acupuncture Anesthesia, Suzhou Medical College)

In recent years there have been some reports concerning the relationship of acupuncture analgesia with the pituitary-adrenocortical system. After intracerebral implantation of corticosteroid, the adrenal cortex of the experimental rats became atrophied, and at the same time the analgesic effect of acupuncture was reduced significantly[1]. Hypophysectomy had the same effect, [but so were not the ACTH-maintained hypophysectomized rats[2].] A detailed study upon animal experiments as well as clinical observation was done by the Institute of Zoology, Academia Sinica. The results demonstrated that glucocorticoids did not play any role in acupuncture analgesia[3].

In view of the dissimilarity in experimental data and the importance of the pituitary-adrenocortical system in the regulation of function of an organism, it would be valuable to make a further investigation upon the role of this system in acupuncture analgesia. As one portion of the study of the mechanism of lip-acupuncture analgesia, this paper would report the influence of hypophysectomy on lip-acupuncture analgesia and plasma corticosterone level in rats.

I. METHODS

1. Model of acupuncture analgesia. Male adult rats, weighing 150–230 g, were used for study. The points of needling were those corresponding to Renzhong and Chengjiang of man on the upper and lower lips. Model G6805 stimulator was employed to give 14 trains/min alternately dense and sparse pulses, being 40 V. The pain threshold was measured by electrical stimulation of the tail of the rat with 57–9D type algesimeter, which provided a train of step-up square pulses of 0.1 msec duration with a frequency of 4610 cps. A step height of 0.1mA and a step width of 0.82 sec were selected. The lowest current intensity (mA), which is just necessary to provoke vocalization of the animals, was taken as an index of pain threshold.

2. Technique of hypophysectomy. Under ether anesthesia hypophysectomy was performed with a special aspirating needle according to Koyama's transauricular method[4]. The aspirates were verified histologically. 40,000 units of penicillin were given for 3 days

---

* Present address: Department of Biology, Fudan University.

after operation. 5% glucose saline was provided every day, and the room temperature was maintained at about 25°C. At the end of experiment both adrenals were extirpated and examined with histological technique. The surgical area of hypophysectomy was checked by visual inspection to examine whether there existed any pituitary residue. Some animals with sham operation of hypophysectomy were used as controls.

3. Plasma corticosterone determination. 0.3–0.4 ml blood was collected from the veins of the tail of the rat and plasma corticosterone was determined with the method of competitive protein binding analysis; the sensitivity of this method was 0.1ng[5].

4. Hormone administration. Corticosterone solution of 500μg/ml was prepared according to the method described by the Institute of Zoology[3], and was given intraperitoneally with a dose of 300μg per 100 grams of body weight. ACTH was diluted with distilled water to a concentration of 5 units/ml. A dose of 15 units/kg body weight was given intraperitoneally.

5. Experimental procedures. All the rats were placed in a warm experimental room which was temperature controlled (20±1°C) for 2 days prior to the experiment to avoid the environmental stress. It is well known that there exist diurnal rhythmical variations upon plasma corticosteroid level, therefore, the experiments were conducted at 8:00–11:00 A.M. regularly.

During the performance of the experiments the animals were restrained on the lip-acupuncture table. After the animals had become quiet, the basal pain threshold was first determined for 3 times, then blood sample was collected. Hereafter, electro-needling was given for 30 minutes. At the end of needling, pain threshold was determined for 3 times and the blood sample was collected again. The mean values of all pre-and post-needling data were compared. 1–2 weeks after the operation, the pre-and post-needling pain threshold and plasma corticosterone level were determined upon hypophysectomized, sham operated and normal control groups, respectively. After 2–3 days rest, ACTH or corticosterone intraperitoneally were given to the hypophysectomized rats. 10 minutes after administration of the drug, pain threshold and plasma corticosterone level were determined again before and after needling.

II. RESULTS

1. General changes after hypophysectomy. The body weight of hypophysectomized rats decreased progressively, but it was increased in the control and sham operated groups. A week later after hypophysectomy no plasma corticosterone could be detected by the method mentioned above (Table 2). Autopsy showed atrophy of adrenal cortex bilaterally and upon all the hypophysectomized rats no pituitary residue was found by the naked eye. All of this indicates that the removal of the pituitary gland by transauricular method was complete.

2. Effects of experimental condition on pain threshold and plasma corticosterone level (Table 1). Some normal rats were restrained on the lip-acupuncture table without electro-needling. The pain threshold and plasma corticosterone were determined at the same time interval as in the real application of electric needle of the experiment (30 minutes restraint corresponds to pre-electroneedling time, and 60 minutes restraint corresponds to

Table 1 Effects of experimental conditions on pain threshold and plasma corticosterone

	Pain threshold (mA)	Plasma corticosterone (μg/100ml)
Before restraint	0.76±0.11*(10)	9.63±0.25 (9)
30 min restraint	0.68±0.08(10)	14.45±0.89*** (6)
60 min restraint	0.79±0.11(10)	14.78±0.58*** (5)

postelectro-needling). The result indicated that the basal pain threshold remained stable; the plasma corticosterone level after 30 minutes restraint was 50% higher than that before restraint. The difference is very significant (P<0.001); but there was no significant difference statistically (P>0.05) between the values of restraint for 30 minutes and 60 minutes. Thus, it showed that the basal pain threshold and plasma corticosterone level had no significant variations within an hour restraint. Hypophysectomized and sham operated groups were treated with the same procedure and so were the results.

3. Effects of hypophysectomy on acupuncture analgesia and plasma corticosterone level (Table 2). After hypophysectomy the basal pain threshold elevated slightly but with no statistical significance. However, the analgesic effect of acupuncture decreased markedly. The pain threshold after electro-needling elevated only 13. 7±7.15% higher than that before electro-needling. At the same time, electro-needling promoted the pain threshold about 2 times upon both the control and the sham operated groups; the analgesic effect of

Table 2 Effects of lip-acupuncture on pain threshold and plasma corticosterone

	No of ani-mals	Pain threshold (mA)		Plasma corticosterone (μg/100ml)	
		Pre-acup	Post-acup	Pre-acup	Post-acup
Normal control	13	0.71±0.07	1.31±0.12*** (91.21±13.24%)	25.73±1.98	33.64±33** (28.78±6.90%)
Sham operation	15	0.63±0.04	1.33±0.16 (109.95±21.59%)	24.30±1.52	28.40±2.04** (26.73±6.71%)
Hypophysectomy	23	0.82±0.07	0.92±0.10 (13.87±7.15%)	0	0
Hypophysectomy +ACTH	12	0.55±0.03	0.90±0.10*** (65.92±16.10%)	0	2.04±0.50
Hypophysectomy +corticosterone	12	0.91±0.09	0.99±0.10 (10.27±6.60%)	0	23.06±2.08

Numerals in parentheses represent % of increase after acupuncture.

** P<0.01, *** P<0.001 as compared with pre-acupuncture. 0 represents that no presence of plasma corticosterone detected with the method of competitive prote in biuding analysis.

Values in tables 1 and 2 represent mean±S.E.M. Numerals in parentheses represent the number of anemals.

* The pain threshold was determined at the time when animals were just retrained.

*** P<0.001 as compared with the value before restraint.

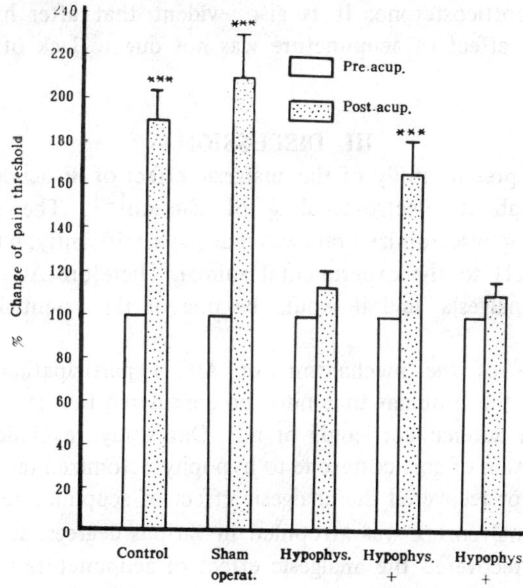

Fig. 1 Comparison of analgesic effect of lip-acupuncture of different groups.

Values of pre-acupuncture pain threshold are taken as 100%.

acupuncture was very predominant (P<0.001). Comparing the analgesic effect of acupuncture of hypophysectomized group with the other two groups, the difference was significant (P<0.05) (Fig.1). It is evident that upon hypophysectomized rats the analgesic effect of lip-acupuncture was diminished.

The results of corticosterone determination indicated that the plasma corticosterone of the hypophysectomized group could not be got both before and after electro-needling, but it increased about 30% after electro-needling (P<0.01) upon the other two groups. This shows that lip-acupuncture, which was used as a method to elicite the stress reaction, might prompt the release of corticosterone.

4. Effects of hormone administration on acupuncture analgesia upon hypophysectomized rats (Table 2). When ACTH was given, the basal pain threshold of hypophysectomized rats reduced obviously (P<0.001) and the analgesic effect of acupuncture was recovered. Electro-needling elevated pain threshold by 65.92±16.10%; the difference was very significant (P<0.001). On the contrary, injection of corticosterone made no apparent effect on basal pain threshold and no regain of the acupunctural analgesic effect (Fig. 1).

Determination of corticosteroid indicated that after administration of ACTH to the hypophysectomized rats the level of the plasma corticosterone was very low (2.04±0.50μg/100 ml), although the analgesic effect of acupuncture had been recovered. However, after corticosterone administration the plasma corticosterone elevated to a high level (23.06±2.08μg/100 ml), but the analgesic effect of acupuncture did not recover. This fact shows that there was no parallel relationship between the lip-acupuncture analgesia and the level of plasma corticosterone. It is also evident that after hypophysectomy the reduction of analgesic effect of acupuncture was not due to lack of corticosterone, but deficiency of ACTH.

III. DISCUSSION

The results of the present study of the analgesic effect of lip-acupuncture confirm our previous conclusion about electro-needling of Zusanli[2]. The analgesic effect of acupuncture upon hypophysectomized rats was reduced significantly, but it reappeared after administration of ACTH to the experimental animal. Therefore ACTH might play some role in acupuncture analgesia, and it would be one of the essential factors of such an analgesic process.

During the study of the mechanisms of ACTH participating in the process of acupuncture analgesia, the problem that must be considered first is whether the action of ACTH takes place via adrenal corticoids or not. Our study excludes such a possibility because: 1) administration of corticosterone to hypophysectomized rats neither affected the basal pain threshold, nor recovered the analgesic effect of acupuncture; 2) 1–2 weeks after hypophysectomy adrenal cortex was atrophied in various degrees, and at this time ACTH administration which recovered the analgesic effect of acupuncture resulted in only slight release of corticosterone; and 3) there was no parallel relationship between plasma corticosterone level and the analgesic effect of acupuncture. Thus, results of the present study support the conclusion reported by the Institute of Zoology, that glucocorticoids do not participate in acupuncture analgesia[3].

The alternative possibility was that ACTH participation in acupuncture analgesia was mediated by its central action. More recently, there were reports that ACTH has been detected in extensive areas of the brain[6–8], where it may function as a neuromodulator[9]. Furthermore, there was evidence that pituitary ACTH may reach the brain via the pituitary portal system[10, 11]. Therefore, it is quite possible that pituitary ACTH transported to the brain can modify or influence brain functions. The problem that has not been solved is how the brain ACTH participates in acupuncture analgesia. Recently, it has been pointed out by a number of authors that ACTH may bind to opiate receptors[12–14]. In this context, the analgesic effect of acupuncture may be reversed by opiate antagonist naloxone. Therefore, it is possible that the action of ACTH in acupuncture analgesia may be brought about by opiate receptors. Alternatively, there was some evidence that ACTH may increase the turnover rate of the cerebral serotonin (5-HT)[15], and a lot of experimental data have demonstrated that there exists a close relation between acupuncture analgesia and the serotoninergic neuronal system. Thus, the mode of action of ACTH in acupuncture analgesia is also probably mediated by this serotoninergic neuronal system.

Pomeranz attributed the loss of analgesic effect of acupuncture in hypophysectomized animals to deficiency of pituitary endorphins[16]. However, in our present work it was the injection of ACTH, not of endorphins, that restored the analgesic effect of acupuncture of the hypophysectomized rats. It implies that, although pituitary endorphins may play a certain role in acupuncture analgesia, it is not the soleone, some actions of pituitary ACTH must also be taken into consideration.

Moreover, our study indicates that lip-acupuncture, as a way to elicit the stress reaction of the animal, can excite the pituitary-adrenocortical system which, in turn, elevates the plasma corticosterone level. Although there is no parallel relationship between plasma corticosterone level and analgesic effect of acupuncture, the ACTH secreted by the pituitary during stress may be, presumably, involved in acupuncture analgesia.

It is found in the present work that ACTH can reduce the basal pain threshold. This indicates that ACTH may be involved in pain perception. This presumption is supported indirectly by the clinical observation that hypophysectomy may relieve intractable pain of late cancer[17]. In conclusion, it seems to us that the central action of ACTH is more complex, and it is worthwhile to further investigate its role in pain and analgesia.

IV. SUMMARY

1. With the experimental model of lip-acupuncture analgesia in rats, the effects of hypophysectomy on acupuncture analgesia and plasma corticosterone level were observed.

2. 1–2 weeks after hypophysectomy the analgesic effect of lip-acupuncture decreased, which could be reversed by injections of ACTH, but not of corticosterone.

3. Lip-acupuncture may produce a stress reaction and elevate the plasma corticosterone level, but there is no parallel relationship between the plasma corticosterone level and the lip-acupuncture analgesia.

4. According to the experimental data in the literature, the causes of reduction of the analgesic effect of acupuncture after hypophysectomy were discussed, and the lack of central actions of ACTH was presumed.

Our special thanks are expressed to the Department of Endocrinology, Institute of Zoology, Academia Sinica, for the supply of standard corticosterone, and to Mr. Yan Jianqun for typing the manuscript.

REFERENCES

[1] 中山大学生物系针麻原理研究组：中山大学学报(自然科学版)，(1)：40，1977。

[2] 苏州医学院生理学教研组：江苏医药(中医分册)，(2)：15，1976。

[3] 中国科学院动物研究所内分泌室针麻原理研究组：动物学报，24：71，1978。

[4] 小山良修：动物实验手技，48页。协同医书出版社，东京，1955。

[5] 缪 明等：动物学杂志 (2)：41，1980。

[6] Krieger, D. T. *et al.* : *Proc. Natl. Acad. Sci. USA,* **74**: 648, 1977.

[7] Krieger, D. T. *et al.* : *Brain Res.,* **128**: 575, 1977.

[8] Moldow, R. and Yalow, R.S.: *Proc. Natl. Acad. Sci. USA,* **75**: 994, 1978.

[9] Wood, P. L. *et al.* : *Life Sci.,* **22**:673, 1978.

[10] Bergland, R.M. and Page, R.B.: *Endocrinology,* **102**:1325, 1978.

[11] Bergland, R.M. and Page, R.B.: *Science,* **204**:18, 1979.

[12] Terenius, L.: *Europ. J. Pharmacol.,* **38**:211, 1976.

[13] Yasukawa, N. *et al.*: *Life Sci.,* **22**:1381, 1978.

[14] Czlonkowski, A. *et al.* : *Life Sci.,* **22**:953, 1978.

[15] File, S.E. and Vellucci, S.V.: *J. Pharm. Pharmacol.,* **30**: 105, 1978.

[16] Pomeranz, B. *et al.*: *Exp. Neurol.,* **54**:172, 1977.

[17] Moricca, G.: *Advances in Neurology,* **4**:707, 1974.

STUDY OF EFFECTS OF ACUPUNCTURE ON EXPERIMENTAL DEEP AND REFERRED PAINS

Zhou Shaoci, Weng Enqi

(Research Laboratory of Brain Function, Department of Biology, East China Normal University)

Ye Qiang, Wang Hua, Kang Yanping

(Shu Guang Hospital, Shanghai College of Traditional Chinese Medicine)

There have been several reports on the question of whether acupuncture points really produce any analgesic effects on a person receiving acupuncture therapy. Mayer[3], Chiang Chenyu[4] and some others gave proof of the actual analgesic effects of acupuncture by experimenting on the human body, applying the signal detection theory and observing the effect of a morphine antagonist, naloxone, on the analgesic effects of acupuncture. But such research was mostly limited to observations on dermalgia. Clinical observations led us to believe that the source of pains, including those due to surgical operations, is mainly located in the viscera and the deep-lying tissues. In other words, as a means of analgesia an acupuncture point must take into consideration its effect on deep and referred pains. The authors, therefore, felt that it was of immediate significance to study the effects of acupuncture on the experimental deep and referred pains in the human body.

I. METHOD

Altogether 116 persons in normal health were chosen as subjects for the experiment. A total number of 370 experiments were made. Of the 116 persons, 55 were men and 61 women, their age ranging from 20 to 44 years. They all had had an education above the average level, and were able to give a clear description of their sensations and such other changes taking place in them when needled. All the subjects were made to undergo two preliminary experiments in order to observe whether the nature and extent of the deep and the referred pains were steady, to see whether the formation of the pain sensation and the process of its disappearance were mutually related and in step with each other, and to see the subject's pain endurance and his degree of cooperation with the experimenter. After the preliminary experiments 44 persons were formally selected as the subjects for further experiments. The method adopted was that put forward by Kellgren with certain modification. An injection of 0.5 ml of 6% NaCl solution was given to the subject on his right interspinal ligament, between the $T_{10}-T_{11}$ segments and 0.5 cm to the midline of the vertebral column. This produced a region of deep and referred pain at the level from T_{11}–L_5. A detailed report about the nature of the deep and referred pains and the method of their determination and recording is given in a separate article[6].

During the entire process of experimentation the changes in the galvanic skin reflex and the vascular plethysmogram of the finger of the subject were recorded simultaneously. Then a piece of square filter paper of 2 cm^2 covered with plastic membrane was hermetically sealed and fixed to the back of the subject to measure the quantity of perspiration. The filter paper was taken off every three minutes and the weight of the quantity of perspiration therein quickly determined on a beam balance.

The acupuncture points were divided into two groups: the "distant segment group," such as Zusanli, Yanglingquan or Hegu, Zhigou and the "close segment group," such as the bilateral Zhangmen or Pishu, Weishu. To begin with, the manipulation of the acupuncture needle (such as the insertion or the pushing in of the needle and then the twirling or the twisting of the needle) was done by a specially appointed doctor or by one specialized in this line. As soon as the desired effects (such as the feelings of distention, sourness, etc.) were obtained, the needles were connected to the electric pulse stimulator (Type G6805) or to the mechanical manipulator (Type YQ23) for 20 minutes' induction, the strength of the stimulation being dependent on the subject's power of endurance. On 8 subjects who showed marked analgesic effects of acupuncture, a series of controlled placebo acupuncture experiments were carried out; that is, the needles were withdrawn immediately after their insertion into the needling points, and then the mechanical manipulator was employed so as not to let the subjects perceive that they were not actually receiving any acupuncture needling.

II. RESULTS

1. The Effects of Acupuncture Points on Deep Pain. The largest mean area of the deep and the referred pains formed by giving an injection of 6% NaCl solution to the 42 subjects was 54.7±14.4 square centimeters, and the length of time was 349±92 seconds. Control experiments proved that 20 minutes' sitting before acupuncture cannot produce any visible effect on the deep and the referred pains. A total number of 66 experiments were made on all the 42 subjects to see the effect of cupuncture points on deep pain, taking the close segment points for 31 experiments and the distant segment points for the other 35 experiments. The result was that nearly 70% of the subjects showed significant changes in their deep and referred pains as follows:

(1) The pain sensation was either reduced or completely lost, accompanied by a change in the nature of the deep sensation, for example, the change of the feeling of distention to that of tingling or aching.

(2) After an injection of NaCl solution, there was a slowdown of the tempo of intensification of the pain sensation or a delay of the appearance in time.

(3) Reduction in the extension of the referred pain zone.

(4) The shortening of the course of the disappearance of the deep pain ahead of time.

The changes mentioned above are the main basis on which we assess the analgesic effects of acupuncture. We can see from Table 1 given below that of the 31 experiments made with the acupuncture points in the close segment, 21 turned out to be effective, and of the 35 experiments with acupuncture points in the distant segment 24 were effective. The effective rates for the close and the distant segments were 67.7% and 68.6%, respectively, being very close to each other. Besides, experiments were made on 16 subjects to compare and contrast the analgesic effects of acupuncture points of distant segment needling with the needling of those of the close segment. But no statistical difference was found.

2. The Effects of Acupuncture on the Nature of Deep Sensation. Control experiments in the same individual were carried out on 20 subjects as follows.

Table 1 Rate of effectiveness of acupuncture points on deep and referred pains in both clese and distant segments.

Site of acupuncture	Number of cases	Effective cases	Effective rate (%)
Close segment	31	21	67.70
Distant segment	35	24	68.60
Total	66	45	67.65

On every individual subject two control experiments were performed. After giving an injection of 6% NaCl solution to the subject, a record of his feelings and sensations was made as reported by him. After this two more experiments were made to observe separately the effects of acupuncture points on the deep sensation both in the near and distant segments. The experimental results summed up are given in Table 2, which shows that the analgesic effects of acupuncture points in both the near and distant segments are very nearly

Table 2. The effects acupuncture points on various sensations of deep pain
(The results of control experiments on the same individual in 20 cases).

Experimental Cord / Cases No. / Feeling	Inj. NaCl (Control)	NalCl + Needling (Distant segment) Variation of the deep feeling: Disap-pearance	Redu-ction	Effec-tiveless	Variation rate (%)	NaCl + Needling (Close segment) Variation of the deep feeling: Disap-pearance	Reduc-tion	Effect-tiveless	Variation rate (%)
Pain	7	2	2	3	57.14	4	2	1	85.71
Distension	14	3	10	1	92.86	2	9	3	78.57
Sourness	9	2	6	1	88.89	2	9	3	77.78
Heaviness	3	3	0	0	100.00	1	0	2	33.33

the same. But the rate of disappearance of the pain sensation is comparatively much higher in the case of acupuncture points in close segments.

3. The Effects of Acupuncture on the Deep Pain Area and on the Changes of Its Duration. When a 6% NaCl solution was injected into the interspinal ligament, the feeling of pain appeared with a latency of 10 to 30 seconds, followed by an intensification of the feeling of pain, an enlargement of its area and the process of the formation of the referred pain area till a peak was attained. The results of the control experiments on the 14 subjects showed that the peak was reached within 1–2.5 minutes. After that there was a gradual weakening of the pain sensation until at about 5 minutes and a half it would disappear completely (see Figure 1). The graph in the figure shows that with the weakening of deep pain and the gradual reduction in the area of referred pain, there was a marked fall of the peak. In the experiments made on the same 14 subjects the area of referred pain was only 76.5–91.2% of the control. The difference between the two was distinctly of statistical significance ($P<0.05$). During this period the change in area was fairly steady, with practically no climaxing (attainment of the highest point). The average time for the disappearance of pain was 4 minutes 24 seconds.

4. Certain Effects of Acupuncture Points on the Changes in the Physiological Indices During the Formation of Deep Pain.

(1) The Heart Rate.

The increase in heartbeats accompanying the formation of deep pain is one of the distinct physiological changes. The result of the tests on 25 cases was that from the control

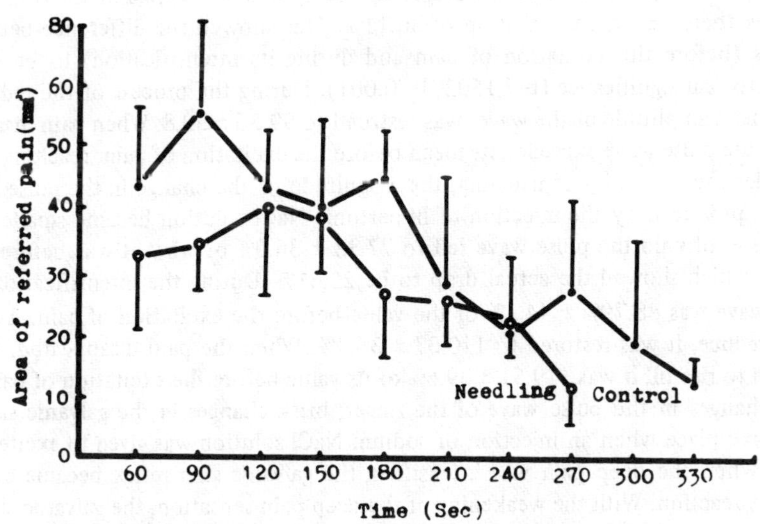

Fig. 1 Curves showing the effects of acupuncture points on the extent of deep and referred pains and on their duration. The upper curve shows results of control experiments, and the lower curve, under the conditions of electro-acupuncture. The ordinate indicates the area of deep and referred pain, while the abscissa, time of it's disappearance. (See text for details.)

average of 80.4±5.78 beats per minute, it increased to 87.24±6.44 beats per minute. The difference between the two was of marked significance ($t=6.345$, $P<0.0001$). There was practically no change in the mean of the heart rate during the process of intensification of the deep and referred pains. With the gradual reduction of pain, the heart rate started going down till it gradually returned to its original level. Under definite acupunctural points, control tests in the same individual were carried out on 25 cases (subjects). The average heart rate before needling was 80.4±5.78 beats per minute. During the period of induction one test was made every 5 minutes. The average rate after two tests was 78.86±5.4 beats per minute, slightly below the level before needling. The average heart rate determined during the pain sensation caused by the injection of solution was 79.44±3.06 beats per minute. The rate during the intensification of pain was 80.28±2.74 beats per minute. The contrast between such changes and the control tests constituted the most distinct statistical difference ($P<0.001$). Afterwards, when the pain sensation gradually decreased till complete disappearance and when the subject returned to normal, his heart rate remained steady between 76.8 and 78.72 beats per minute.

(2) The Changes in the Vascular Plethysmography of the Finger and in the Galvanic Skin Reflex after Injection of NaCl and the Effects on These Changes.

The results of experiments on 20 subjects indicated that during the formation of deep pain sensation, the amplitude of vascular plethysmogram of the finger became smaller. During the ten seconds before the excitation of pain, the mean of the wave magnitude was 100% and ten seconds after the excitation of pain, the mean of the wave magnitude dropped to 76.10 ± 31.82%. During the intensification of the deep and referred pains, there was a further drop in the pulse wave of the finger tip, being 69.89 ± 34.7% of the original value. That means there was an actual drop of 30.11%. This showed the difference between the two means (before the excitation of pain and during its intensification) to be of highly marked statistical significance ($t=7.1502$, $P<0.001$). During the process of the reduction of pain, the mean amplitude of the waves was restored to 99.36 ± 30.8. When pain disappeared, the rise in the pulse wave exceeded its mean before the excitation of pain, reaching 114.16% ± 7.9. Under the condition of needling, the magnitude of the change in the pulse wave due to the pain produced by the injection of hypertonic NaCl solution became smaller. During the excitation of pain the pulse wave fell to 77.38 ± 36.9% of what it was before the pain excitation, which showed the actual drop to be 22.61%. During the intensification of pain the pulse wave was 88.79% ± 44.1% of the value before the excitation of pain. As the pain began to reduce, it was restored to 110.07 ± 36.4%. When the pain disappeared, the pulse wave began to rise till it was 119.51 ± 39.6% of its value before the excitation of pain. Along with the changes in the pulse wave of the finger, brisk changes in the galvanic skin reflex began to take place when an injection of sodium NaCl solution was given to excite the pain sensation. When the deep pain was intensified, the galvanic skin reflex became even more active in its reaction. With the weakening of the deep pain sensation, the galvanic skin reflex showed a corresponding reduction till its complete disappearance. The waves in Figure 2a are the graphic representations of the reactions of the pulse wave and the galvanic skin reflex when a pain sensation was excited in the subject by giving him an injection of NaCl solution. Figure 2b constitutes the graphic representation of the records obtained 20 minutes after the needling of the bilateral Changmen of the selfsame subject. Under specified conditions of acupuncture, the changes in the pulse wave and the galvanic skin reflex during the pain

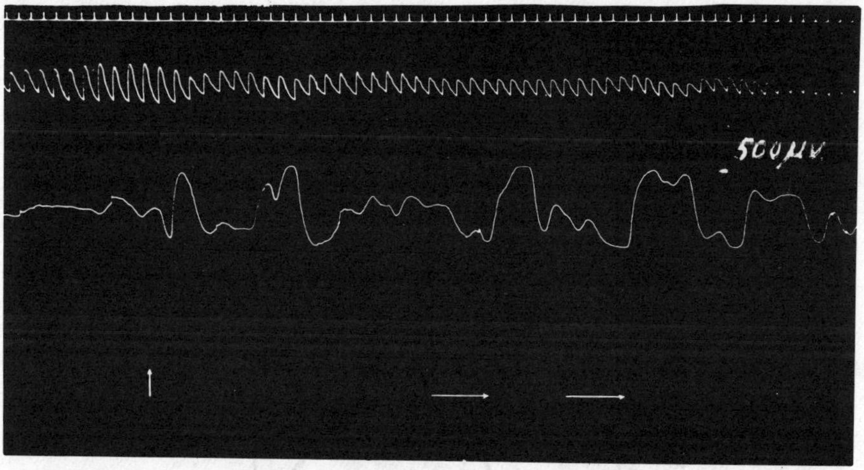

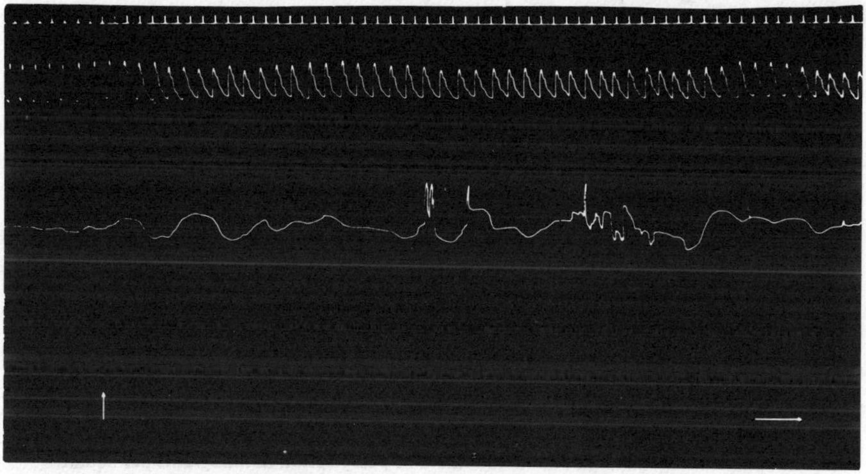

Fig. 2 Records showing the effect of acupuncture on the changes in plethysmogram and Galvanic skin reflex, elicited by NaCl injection.

Figure a shows the record of a subject made during an injection of NaCl solution.

Figure b shows a record from the same subject under the condition of electro-acupuncture of bilateral "Zhangmen".

The upper horizontal line shows the marks of time in second. The upper wave is the vascular plethysmogram of the finger and the lower wave the record of galvanic skin reflex. The vertical arrows indicate the injection of NaCl solution. The horizontal arrows indicate the complaint of the subject: "Intensification of the Feeling of Pain".

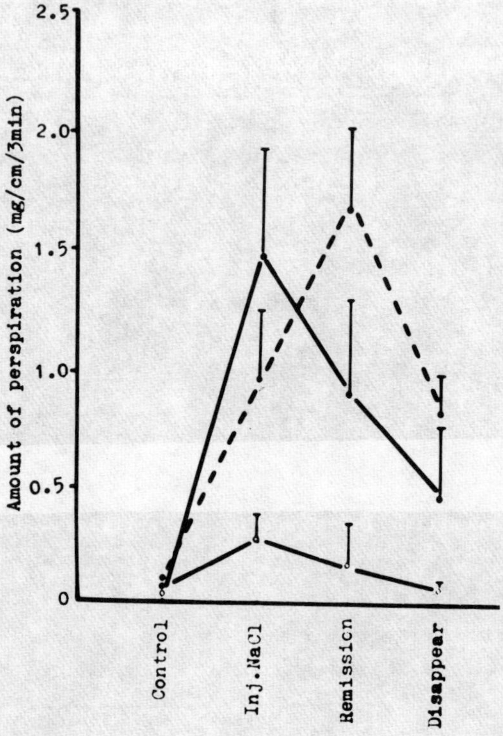

Fig. 3 Curves showing the effect of electroacupuncture on the changes in the quantities of perspiration during the formation of deep pain.

The curves with black dots represent the perspiration changes of control experiments. The curve below with small circles represents the changes of perspiration on the individuals that showed the effectiveness of acupuncture. The dotted curve shows the experimental results of individuals, on which the electroacupuncture did not have effected.

The ordinate indicates the quantities of perspiration in milligrams per square centimeter in every 3 minutes. The abscissa indicates the different stages of the formation of deep pain.

sensation produced by injecting NaCl solution were all much smaller than the controlled records of the reactions as represented in Figure 1a. There was no distinct change in the reactions of galvanic skin reflex either, during the stage when the pain sensation was intensified. The interference of the galvanic skin reflex was an illusory image created by the taking of the perspiration sample.

(3) Changes in the Quantities of Perspiration.

Samples of perspiration were collected from the backs of all the 34 subjects for quantitative determination. There was a marked increase in the perspiration induced by the excitation of pain sensation. The average value of the increase within 3 minutes was 2.04 mg/cm^2. With the diminishing of the pain sensation the quantity of perspiration gradually fell. In ten minutes after the disappearance of the pain sensation, perspiration nearly returned its level before the experiment. Under acupunctural conditions there was a marked decrease in perspiration during the pain sensation caused by the injection of NaCl solution. Figure 3 shows the graph indicating the results of the control experiments made on the same 13 subjects. In the control experiment, the quantity of perspiration, after the excitation of pain sensation, went up to 1.48 mg/cm^2, whereas in the 8 effective individual cases of acupuncture the increase in perspiration was only 0.4 mg/cm^2. It fell to 0.16 mg/cm^2 after the reduction of deep pain. In the 5 cases of non-effective acupuncture, the quantity of perspiration increased to 0.94 mg/cm^2 after the excitation of pain sensation. It continued to increase till it was 1.66 mg/cm^2 even after the reduction of pain, surpassing the quantity of perspiration induced during the pain sensation caused in the control experiments. After the disappearance of pain the perspiration level remained at 0.82 mg/cm^2.

5. The Effects of Acupuncture Points on Deep Pain Produced by NaCl Solution of Threshold Concentration. For this experiment 11 subjects were selected at random, and sodium chloride solution of threshold concentration (1.86–2.17% NaCl) was used to excite

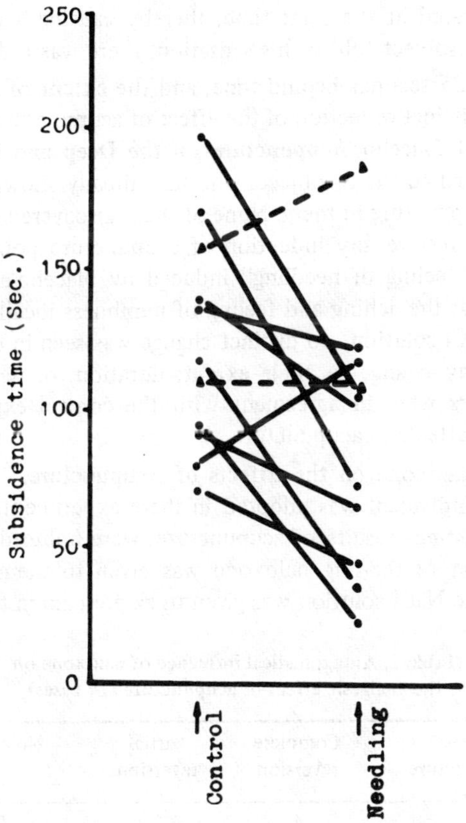

Fig. 4 Figure shows the effects of acupuncture on the subsidence time of deep pain prouced by the excitation of NaCl solution in threshold concentration.
The ordinate indicates the time in seconds. (See text for details.)

the sensation of pain, making a close observation of the effects of acupuncture points on the deep and referred pains excited by the injection of NaCl solution in threshold concentration. Among the 11 subjects chosen for this experiment, 4 were those who originally showed good acupunctural results, 4 were those showing no results, and the remaining 3 were those whose cases were difficult to decide. The results of the experiments were as follows:

Of the 11 subjects, 9 showed distinct acupunctural results, especially manifested in the disappearance or the reduction of the deep pain sensation and the abatement of the deep pain ahead of time. The remaining 2 subjects were purposely needled against the requirements of acupuncture, and shallow insertion of the needle produced no result. The changes in time for the disappearance of deep pain sensation under the specified controlled and acupuncture ctural conditions are shown in Figure 4. It can be seen in the figure that in the case of the two subjects who had shallow insertion of needles (shown by dotted lines in the figure), there was no indication of analgesic effects. But in the rest of the subjects there was a clear indication of the general tendency to shorten the course of time for the deep pain under the specified conditions of acupuncture. There was, however, one subject among them who was not interrogated at the right time, thereby causing a delay of 55 seconds. But according to what the subject told of his sensation, there was a distinct abatement of pain, the deep pain started 35 seconds behind time, and the extent of pain was rather indefinite. All these indicated a distinct reflection of the effect of acupuncture.

6. The Effects of Placebo Acupuncture on the Deep and Referred Pains. Placebo-acupuncture was applied to the 8 subjects who had already shown a clear indication of the analgesic effect of acupuncture in them. None of them discovered (or rather, perceived) that they did not actually receive any induction of acupuncture points. But 5 of the subjects reported about their "feeling of needling" induced by placebo-acupuncture. The other 3 subjects reported about the aching and feeling of numbness locally. When all the 8 subjects were injected with NaCl solution, no distinct change was seen in the formation of deep and referred pains, nor any change in their extent, duration, or nature. The changes in the physiological indicators were in agreement with the control experiment, there being no reflection of analgesic effects of acupuncture.

7. Influence of Naloxone on the Effects of Acupuncture. The method of making a control of the same individual was adopted in these experiments. Fourteen subjects, who had already shown distinct results of acupuncture, were induced for 12 minutes. Then an intramuscular injection of 0.8 mg naloxone was given to them, and 8 minutes later an injection of hypertonic NaCl solution was given to excite pain in them. It could be observed

Table 3. Antagonistical influence of naloxone on the analgesic effect of acupuncture (14 cases)

Site of acupuncture	Complete reversion	Partial reversion	No effect
Close Segment	4	2	0
Distant segment	3	1	4

that, due to the action of naloxone, of the 14 subjects (cases) there were 7 cases of complete reversion of the acupuncture analgesic effects. In the case of 3 subjects there was only partial reversion, and in the case of the remaining 4 subjects there was no clear indication of any changes in the analgesic effect of acupuncture (see Table 3).

Notable differences in the analgesic effects of acupuncture on different individuals can be brought about by naloxone. Reports on such actions of naloxone have already appeared in articles published before[4, 5, 8]. Considering the short duration of the reversing effect of naloxone and the method of intramuscular injection adopted for the present experiment, the question now is whether the non-reversion of the analgesic effects of acupuncture in the case of 4 subjects mentioned above is due to the non-uniformity of the rate of absorption of naloxone and the change in the time for the expected results (that caused a difference in analgesic effects on different individuals), both brought about by intramuscular injection. Therefore, under the conditions of acupuncture along with intramuscular injection of naloxone, two of the subjects were each given an injection of NaCl solution of threshold concentration into the deep part of musculi radialis every 5 minutes to excite a pain sensation so as to observe the time taken for the reversion of the analgesic effects of acupuncture by naloxone. The experimental results indicated that the time taken for the reversion of analgesic effects in the cases of the two subjects was between 15 and 20 minutes.

III. DISCUSSION

1. Before Kellgren's model of "Experimental Deep and Referred Pains" can be applied in the study of the analgesic effects of acupuncture, it must first of all be decided whether the model is positively steady. For the past several years, however, this model of Kellgren's has been considered as being steady, i.e., a model that can be repeated[7]. Experiments made by some authors in the year 1978[6] showed that the difference of deep and referred pains, excited by hypertonic NaCl solution, in individual cases was quite great. But so far as the same individual case was concerned, the nature of the pain sensation, its extent and its segmental distribution were all fairly steady. With such a wide selection of specimens as 116 subjects, a certain number of them chosen for the experimentation will definitely make such reproducibility of deep pain still more steady and reliable.

As necessitated by control experiments on the same individual, it is generally necessary for a subject to receive 4 to 6 injections of hypertonic NaCl solution to excite pain. This raises the question of whether there is any possibility of the formation of conditioned reflexive deep and referred pains. In order to answer this question, two of the subjects were each given four injections of 6% NaCl solution at different intervals. They were then injected with an equivalent dose (0.5ml) of sterilized physiological saline at the interspinal ligament. Experiments proved that the injection of physiological saline produced no extensive feeling of deep and referred pains except the locally formed sensation of pain due to the insertion of the needle. Therefore, it ruled out the possibility of the formation of deep pain sensation through conditioned reflex under the conditions arranged by us. In order to know whether re-injection of hypertonic NaCl solution has any possibility of creating an adaptibility of the subject to such deep sensation, two of the subjects were asked to volunteer for the experiment, though the authors had already made 8 to 20 repeated experiments on themselves. The experimental results showed no distinct change in the nature, extent, duration and distribution of the deep pain sensation. Hence, there is every reason to believe that the model put forward by Kellgren can be applied in the studies of analgesic effects of acupuncture.

2. The most distinct effect of acupuncture on the experimental deep pain was reflected in the changes in pain sensation (see Table 2). This was in complete agreement with the phenomenon observed earlier on the epidermis[4, 8]. It must be taken into consideration that the sensation of deep and referred pains produced by the injection of hypertonic NaCl solution is an intense feeling of discomfort, accompanied by violent changes in moods. Under acupunctural conditions, with the lessening and disappearance of the pain sensation, the changes in moods began to subside. These results confirmed once again that the clinical observations of the analgesic effects of acupuncture, and especially the analgesic effects on deep pain, can be further verified by experimental studies. Besides, under acupunctural conditions, the weakening of the chief complaint of deep aching, distention and the feeling of heaviness can be noticed, however, with the disappearance of the feeling of pain, the sensation of ache, distention, etc. is experienced in the affected region. Considering the fact that, during operations conducted under clinical acupuncture anesthesia, sensation of pain is very often converted into other milder feelings, such as aching, feeling of heaviness, etc., there is the possibility of looking upon the changes in the deep sensation as a different aspect of the indication of the effects of acupuncture.

3. Since there are different views on the actual analgesic effects of acupuncture up to now[1, 2, 9, 10], it has consequently become an important task in the experimental studies of acupuncture to avoid giving undue considerations to the subjective factors of the person experimented on, while attaching importance to his (the subject's) main complaints. One of the advantages of the model of "experimental deep pain" is that the changes in the deep sensation are not limited simply to the disappearance or the weakening of the pain sensation. It (the model) can enable the research workers to possibly carry on an overall examination of acupunctural effects within the range of the formation of deep and referred pain sensations, their disappearance and the other changes taking place in the subjects. The reduction of the extent of referred pain, delayed attainment of the peak, and the disappearance of deep pain ahead of time in the case of the 14 subjects (as represented in Fig. 1) under specified conditions of acupuncture — all these, in different aspects, put forward the objectiveness of the analgesic effects of acupuncture. Moreover, the determination of the physiological indices such as heart rate, vascular plethysmograph of the finger, galvanic skin reflex and perspiration on the back have similarly provided the basis in different ways to decide about the effects of acupuncture on the deep and referred pains. The experimental results showed that there existed a difference of acupunctural effects on the deep and referred pains in different individuals. In the experiment using 6% NaCl solution to excite pain, about 31.4 to 32.3% of the subjects showed no acupunctural effects. But this did not mean that acupuncture points did not have the least effect on the subjects. When a main sensation was excited in the "non-effective" individuals by using NaCl solution of threshold concentration, acupuncture points effected a change in the intensity of the deep and referred pains in all the individuals, the disappearance of pain sensation was ahead of time, and the acupunctural effect showed itself distinctly. This fact seems to hint that the

manifestation of analgesic effects of acupuncture is correlated with the intensity of pain excitation. When the intensity of the excitation of pain goes beyond a certain limit, the effect of acupuncture will most probably be overridden. That is to say, it will not be able to manifest itself. If this view is correct, then the examination of the analgesic effects of acupuncture should not simply be the study of acupunctural effects on the strong sensation of pain. It must also take note of the effects that can be produced by acupuncture on the weaker sensations in the same individual. This should especially be so when an experimental study is to be made with a limited selection of specimen subjects. With this view there can be, to a certain extent, a better understanding of the results of the experiments and the clinical observations made by Li (1975) and Modell (1976), and also of the reason for the difference in the results of the other experimental studies. Of course, the fundamental reason for the difference in the analgesic effects of acupuncture in individual cases is most probably the faintness (indistinctness) of the analgesic effects of acupuncture in a part of the individuals.

According to the experiments conducted by the authors, such feeble effects in a part of the individuals is almost similar to that produced (or induced) by 0.05 mg of fentanyl.

4. Mayer (1975, 1977), Sjölund (1976), Chiang Chenyu et al. (1978), Huang Yer and others (1978) proved that the analgesic effects of acupuncture could be reversed by naloxone, an antagonist of morphine receptors. And Sjölund (1977) also showed that the content of endorphin in cerebrospinal fluid increased. Thus the analgesic effects of acupuncture and the producing of the endogenous morphine-like substances can be linked together. The results obtained in the experiments (as mentioned in the present article) prove that the effects of acupuncture on the deep and the referred pains can similarly be counteracted, wholly or partly, by the injection of naloxone. This showed that the effect of acupuncture on deep pain was probably partly due to the formation of the endogenous morphine-like substances in the cerebrum. This is, therefore, an objective and realistically physiological effect. Besides, under the conditions of placebo-acupuncture, no change in the deep pain was observed; and this, too, explained the same thing as mentioned above (about the action of naloxone and the formation of morphine-like substances, etc.). However, even if it is so, we find it rather difficult to believe that it is possible to bring some influence to bear upon the experiments by avoiding the psychological factors wholly and absolutely. But the experiments made by Goldstein and some others (1975) confirmed that on account of the analgesic effect of hypnosis, there can be no reversion of the analgesic effects of acupuncture by naloxone. This fact seems to explain in a different way that the rising of the pain threshold is due to hypnosis and the analgesic effects of acupuncture do not proceed from the same mechanism. Therefore, the view which wholly attributes the analgesic effects of acupuncture to the results of hypnosis or psychological activity is probably one-sided and quite doubtable.

IV. SUMMARY

1. The deep and the referred pain produced by the injection of 6% NaCl solution into the interspinal ligament did undergo distinct changes under acupunctural conditions. The deep sensations disappeared in a part of the subjects. In the majority of the subjects the pain

and other deep sensations began to decrease. The duration of pain was shortened and the extent of referred pain diminished. The effective rate in this case was about 67.6%.

2. Acupuncture can convert the feelings of pain, bad ache and other discomforts produced by the injection of hypertonic NaCl solution into milder sensations such as dull ache, heaviness, etc. This is perhaps a different way of manifestation of the effects of acupuncture.

3. In the case of those individuals in whom acupuncture was effective, the change in heart rate was smaller than that in the control group when they were injected with NaCl solution to produce deep pain in them. The difference between the two was of highly distinct statistical significance ($P<0.001$). Besides, the changes in galvanic skin reflex, vascular plethysmogram of the finger and perspiration were far more steady and smooth compared with those of the control experiment group.

4. The effects of acupuncture on nearly 31.4% of the individuals were quite feeble. When a pain sensation was produced by injecting a solution of NaCl of threshold concentration, the effects of acupuncture began to be distinctly manifested in varying degrees as the deep pain sensation was comparatively milder.

5. The changes in the deep and referred pains caused by hypertonic sodium chloride solution could not be observed in the experimentation of placebo-acupuncture on 8 subjects.

6. Naloxone can, either wholly or partially, bring about the reversion of the analgesic effect of acupuncture on the experimental deep and referred pains. The reason for the absence of change in the analgesic effects in a part of the subjects was probably connected with the time taken for the manifestation of the effects of naloxone injected intramuscularly.

7. The results of the studies on the effects of acupuncture on the experimental deep and referred pains concerned have proved that the effects of acupuncture are an objective and realistically physiological reflection.

REFERENCES

[1] Kroger, W. S.: *Amer. J. Psychiat.*, **130**:855, 1973.

[2] Wall, P.: *HEW Scient.*, **64**: 31, 1974.

[3] Mayer, D. J. *et al.*: *Brain Res.*, **121**:368, 1977.

[4] 江振裕等：动物学报，24：1，1978。

[5] 北京医学针麻原理研究组：中华医学杂志，53：151，1973。

[6] 翁恩琪等：上海师范大学学报(自然科学)(4)：101，1980。

[7] Hockaday, J. M. *et al.*: *Brain*, **90**:481, 1967.

[8] 江振裕等：中国科学，16 (2)：157，1973。

[9] Modell, J. H. *et al.*: *Anesthesia* **and** *Analgesia.*, **55**:508, 1976.

[10] China, J. N. *et al.*: *Pain, 2:285, 1976.*

[11] Mayer, D. J.: *Neurosci. Res. Progr. Bull.*, **13**:94, 1975.

[12] Sjölund, B. and Eriksson, M.: *Lancet*, **13**:1085, 1976.

[13] 黄 晔等：中华医学杂志，58：193，1978。

[14] Sjölund, B. *et al*: *Acta Physiol. Scand.*, **100**:382, 1977.

[15] Goldstein, A. and Hilgard, E. R.: *Proc. Nat. Acad. Sci. U.S.A.*, **72**:2041, 1975.

PART I
RESEARCHE ON THE MECHANISMS OF ACUPUNCTURE, MOXIBUSTION AND ACUPUNCTURE ANESTHESIA (3)

STUDY OF RECEPTORS OF NEEDLING SENSATION AT SOMATIC ACUPUNCTURE POINTS

Hou Zonglian (C.L.Hou)
(Acupuncture Anaesthesia Mechanism Research Laboratory Xi'an Medical College, Xi'an)

I. INTRODUCTION

An acupuncture point is a point of needling sensation, i.e. a sensory one. In 1882, Blix discovered warm and cold points on the skin of the human body and there by laid the foundation for somatosensory physiology. However, as early as a few centuries B.C., acupuncture sensory points had already been discovered by our ancestors, and this discovery remains an important contribution to modern physiology.

As pointed out in traditional Chinese medicine, "the effects of moxibustion or acupuncture are determined by the effectiveness of acupuncture points" (Lingshu). Modern medical practice likewise shows that the stronger the needling sensation, the better the results of acupuncture therapy. Acupuncture treatment, acupuncture analgesia, and the study of the nature and properties of meridians all start from the needling sensation of acupuncture points. Therefore, elucidating the histologic foundation of needling sensation, i.e. the receptors of needling sensation, is of great significance both to the interpretation of the mechanism of acupuncture, moxibustion, and acupuncture analgesia, and to exploration of the essence of meridians.

In 1966, we located a point of soreness in deep muscular layers while pinching the acupuncture point "Hegu", but found none while pinching the skin or subcutaneous area. This happened also at other acupuncture points. We deduced therefore that the receptors of needling sensation at acupuncture points were deep receptors. In 1972, on the basis of this deduction, we made a series of studies[1,2,3] and then postulated as follows[4]:

(1) Needling sensations at the somatic acupuncture points occur in deep tissues, presumably due to the function of deep receptors.

(2) A constant regular relationship exists between the environment of an acupuncture point and the distribution of deep receptors receiving the needling sensation.

(3) When considering the different environments, it seens that each acupuncture point has its own deep predominant receptors.

(4) Receptors of needling sensation at "Hegu" and at other acupuncture points in thick muscles, especially on the extremities, are predominantly muscle spindles.

(5) Type I and II fibres, which are associated with the responses to stretching, have been considered by Gelfan et al.[5] to be unable to reach the sphere of consciousness. In order to solve this problem, we put forward the hypothesis of dual structure. By "dual structure"

we mean that muscle action potentials of acupuncture points are initiated by intrafusal muscles, while the afferent impulses of the needling sensation are transmitted by type IV (at that time, we thought that it was the same fibre which transmitted both needling sensation and analgesia). In muscle spindles, type IV fibres are distributed inside intrafusal muscles, and together the make up the receptors of needling sensation.

Since 1973, we have made a series of investigations based on the above postulates, which will be dealt with separately. The following is only a description of our study of needling sensation receptors at somatic acupuncture points.

(I) Needling sensation at somatic acupuncture points lies predominantly in deep tissues

1. The depth of "Hegu" point[1] . As the thickness of one's hand varies from individual to individual, it is impracticable to measure it in terms of its absolute depth. So we divided the hand from dorsum to ventrom into five equal parts to observe in which part the needling sensation exists. We found that the needling sensations from three acupuncture points were all in the 2/5–4/5 parts of the hand (measured from the dorsum). In order to find out their exact location, we made a cross-section of a corpse's hand at a level corresponding to "Hegu" point (Fig.1), and found that these parts were in thick muscular layers (the first musculi interossei dorsales and musclus adductor hallucis). Thus, it was established that needling sensation from "Hegu" point existed in the muscular layer, so its receptor must be in the deep receptor of the muscles.

2. Is there any needling sensation on or under the skin?[6] When the needling sensation is felt and muscular action potentials occur in the deep area of the acupuncture point, we observed 15 point-times (Hegu, Zusanli, etc). In all of them, no needling sensation was found either on or under the skin. This indicates that needling sensation occurs in deep tissues only.

3. The depth of the needling sensation[7] . In view of the limited number of cases in the above two experiments, we made further observation of five acupuncture points(Hegu,

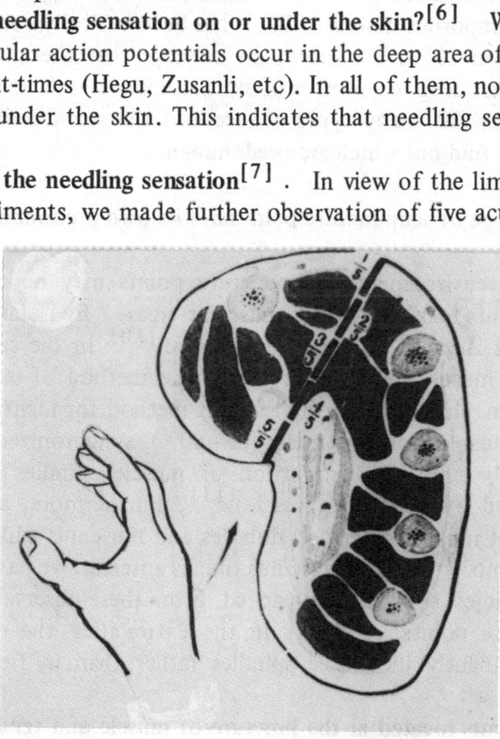

Fig 1 Depth of human needing sensation in Hegu area.

Zusanli, Chengshan, (Jiache and Zhongwan) in a series of 131 point-times to ascertain the location of the needling sensation. It was shown that at 2 point-times the depth of the needling sensation was below 5mm; at 22 point-times, below 5–10mm; and at 107 point-times, over 10mm. Postolating 10mm as the line of demarcation (probably too deep), the cases of needling sensation in superficial layers accounted for less than 19%.

From the above three experiments, it can be concluded that the needling sensation is certainly related to deep receptors, but not necessarily to superficial ones. It follows that the needling sensation receptors at somatic acupuncture points are predominantly deep receptors which constitute the material basis for needling sensation.

(II) Environment of acupuncture points and distribution of deep receptors

There are 5. main kinds of deep receptors: muscle spindles, tendon organs, Pacinian corpuscles, joint receptors and free nerve ending.

There is a rule governing the distribution of receptors in certain environments. Using this rule, if the environments in which certain acupuncture points exist are the spots where certain deep receptors are distributed, these receptors are the ones which receive the needling sensation. In other words, the environments link acupuncture points with their receptors. With knowledge of the environments of different acupuncture points, it is possible to estimate more precisely which receptors are distributed at each type of acupuncture point. We already noticed this important link in 1972. It has been basically confirmed by a series of investigations besinning in 1973. Therefore, the concept that the environments link acupuncture points with their deep receptors is of extraordinary significance. However, it is still necessary for us to study the many types of receptors that are distributed in certain acupuncture points, so as to find out which are predominant.

(III) Does each type of acupuncture point have its own predominant receptors?

According to their environments, acupuncture points may be classified as 5 types.

1. Acupuncture points located in thick muscular areas. By isolating nerve strands, we observed that, at points Zusanli[8], Hegu[9], Neiguan[10] in the cat, about 70–80% of the receptors are from muscle spindles (Table 1). The method of isolating nerve strands is considered by modern physiology to be the best method for identifying somatic receptors. The rate of muscular action potentials (65–80%), synchronized with the needling sensation, varies roughly with the proportion of muscle spindles (as muscular action potentials are discharged by intrafusal muscle)[11]. Furthermore, at Hegu and 2 other points [2,3], in the first musculi interrosei dorsales and musculus adductor hallucis and at Zusanli and 6 other points[12] in the musculus tibialis anterior, we have observed ally more microscopic muscle spindles, some closely packed. From these observations, we believe that at muscular acupuncture points, especially in the extremities, the receptors of needling sensation exist predominantly in muscle spindles rather than in free nerve endings and Pacinian corpuscles.

2. Acupuncture points located at the juncture of muscle and tendon. Previously, we postulated that tendon organs might be predominant in acupuncture points located at the

Table 1. The percentage of Muscle Spindles in certain Acupuncture points

Receptor / point	muscle spindles(%)	Tendon organs(%)	Pressor receptors(%)
Hegu	81.8	2.6	15.6
Neiguan	75.4	11.5	13.6
Zusanli	68.5	5.5	26
Chengshan	76.5	17.7	5.8

junctures of muscles and tendons. Nevertheless, after isolating nerve strands at Chengshan in the cat[13], we found that muscle spindles still accounted for 76.5% and tendon organs only 17.7% (Table 1), though figures for the latter were larger than those found at Hegu, Neiguan or Zusanli. Moreover, upon the application of histologic techniques and the method for isolating nerve strands (Fig. 2), we saw that,approximately in the center of Chengshan,there are more tendon organs, with muscle spindles at their periphery. This may be the characteristic of this type of acupuncture point.

3. Acupuncture points located near tendons. With the application of histologic techniques, we found Pacinian corpuscles densely distributed at the Kulun point[14]. In one case as many as 7 Pacinian corpuscles were packed together. Pacinian corpuscles have also been observed at the Quze point[15] by Anhui Medical College, at the toothache point[16] by the Institute of Zoology, Academia Sinica and at the tachong point by the Department of Histology and Embryology of our college. All these acupuncture points are located near tendons.

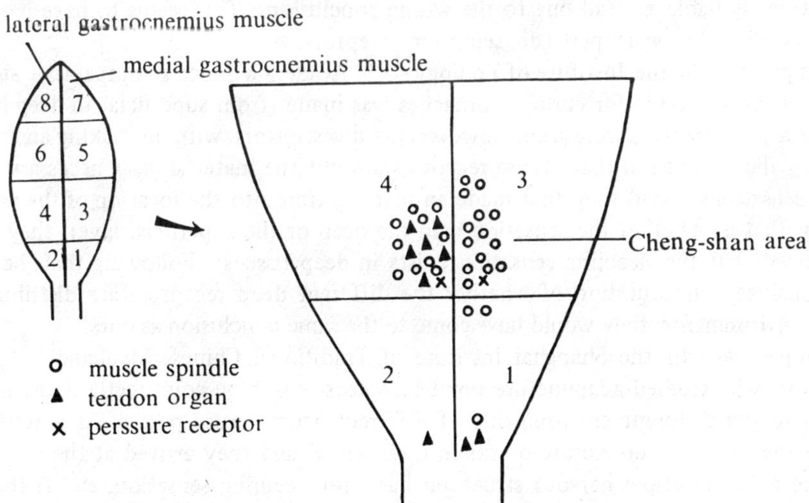

Fig 2 Distribution of receptors in Cheng-Shan area of the cat.

4. Acupuncture points on the scalp and elsewhere. We have observed 9 acupuncture points in areas ranging from Yintan to Baihui and from Zanzhu to Sizhukong. Since no receptors with capsules were found upon the application of histologic techniques[17], these must be free nerve endings.

5. Acupuncture points near joint capsules. Our study in this field is now in progress. According to previous studies by others, there are 3 kinds of receptors here, i.e. Ruffini-like bodies, Pacinian-like corpuscles and free nerve endings. Among them, Ruffini-like bodies might be the predominant ones; however, such a hypothesis remains to be substantiated.

II. DISCUSSION

1. The principle of integrating function with morphology. The work of exploring needling sensation receptors (the materiai basis of needling sensation) should be conducted in close cooperation with the study of the needling sensation. It is essential to locate the needling sensation first, and then to explore the area of its receptors (the material basis of needling sensation). Since 1958, quite a few morphologists have made observations deep under the skin and found no specific receptors there. On the other hand, some functionalists have observed that needling effects are produced in deep tissues, but they did not go on to look for the material basis of the needling sensation, i.e. receptors. As a consequence, despite the fact that both these groups of scientists have done a lot of work, they did not get the desired results. The reason is that they failed to combine the study of the needling sensation (or the study of acupuncture points where acupuncture effects are produced) with the exploration of its material basis; in other words, they failed to integrate functional with morphological study.

2. The principle of integrating analysis with synthesis. Without analysis, there would be no synthesis. For a scientist, one important tasks is to analyze the things he is studying. To synthesize anything without first analyzing it, or to explore it without first making a classification, is liable to lead one to the wrong conclusions. This seems to have happened in the work of exploring acupuncture sensation receptors.

Example one. In the Institute of Zoology[16], Academia Sinica a comparative study of three acupuncture points for curing toothaches was made (from superficial to deep layers), and quite a few receptors were seen. However, the investigators, without making an analysis, jumped to the conclusion that "these receptors are not the material basis necessary for all needling sensations". Had they first made an investigation into the location of the needling sensation, that is, whether the sensation is in the deep or the superficial layer, they would have realized that the needling sensation exists in deep tissues: Following that, had they further analyzed the question of whether the different deep receptors are distributed in different environments, they would have come to the same conclusion as ours.

Example two. In the Shanghai Institute of Traditional Chinese Medicine[18], those investigators who studied acupuncture point receptors with blue point method, did not pay attention to the different environments of different acupuncture points. As a result ther confused the various acupuncture points in their study, and they arrived at the conclusion that there exists multiple nervous structural basis for needling sensation, etc. If they had made an analytical study of acupuncture points with reference to their different environments, their conclusion would have been otherwise.

Example three. Not long ago, one of the morphologists working in our laboratory held that the receptors of the needling sensation at Hegu point include various types of receptors other than muscle spindles, and that nerve strands or trunks of different sizes had also been invelved in receiving stimulations[19]. The most important thing, as we see it is to determine which type of receptor plays the major role. Our conclusion that muscle spindles play the predominant role is derived from our experiments in isolating nerve strands. As shown in Table 1, with the isolation of nerve strands, it is possible in most cases to discover which nerve fibres come from pressure receptors and so forth. Since the majority of nerve fibres have been found to originate from muscle spindles (70–80%), it naturally follows that muscle spindles are the predominant receptors. More importantly, because the proportion of muscle spindles corresponds to the rate (65–80%) of coexistence of the needling sensation with muscular action potentials, and since the latter are known to be discharged from muscle spindles, our viewpoint that muscle spindles are predominant is reinforced. It seems improper to stick to the phenomena, and not to analyze in this manner. Departure from the analysis of things means a deparfore science, since one of the most important links of scientific work is the leap from the perceptual stage of knowledge to the rational stage, that is, from the perception of phenomena to the recognition of the essence of things. We are of the opinion that the correct scientific method is to collect ample material for our study, to analyze the different aspects of its development and to explore their relationship.

3. Inevitable and accidental connections. As stated above, in analyzing material, it is essential to discern which receptors or even which nerve bundles and trunks are materials necessary for the production of the needling sensation and which are unnecessary. For instance, deep receptors are indispensable for the formation of needling sensation while superficial receptors are dispensable. The former instance, therefore, is an inevitable connection. On the other hand, among those acupuncture points located in thick muscles, Neiguan is found to have been cut through by Nervi Medianus, but other points such as Hegu, Zusanli and so on have no nerve bundles in them. Hence, it can be said that the passing of nerve trunks through acupuncture points is an instance of accidental connection, that is, not the indispensable material basis for the needling sensation. However, some people put too much stress on the accidental connection, there by neglecting the main aspect.

4. Practice is the sole criterion of truth. Here I would like to say a few words about Gunn's classification of acupuncture points (Type I–IV).

(1) He pointed out that the Type I acupuncture point corresponds to a motor point. He added that the Type I acupuncture point had been proved to have something to do with the motor point itself[20]. However, as we know, an acupuncture point is a sensation point, which is a different thing from a motor point: they cannot be confused with one another. Gunn further stated that, as he had observed, the minimal electrical stimulation given to a motor point could relieve pain. However, as we see it, the contraction of extrafusal muscle is the result of stimulation of α fibres, whereas the relief of pain is the outcome of the stimulation of afferent fibres: Therefore it is wrong to confuse one with the other and to say that the exciting of the motor point could lead to pain relief. It is likewise wrong to regard a motor point as an acupuncture point, for the latter is a sensory point. Of course, these two may exist in the same environment, just as several symbiotic animals do; even so, we can only say that these animals are symbiotic, and not that they are of the same species. Using the same logic, although both the motor point and the acupuncture sensation point may

co-exist in the same environment, the former cannot be interpreted as the latter while the function of the former can also not neither be interpreted as that of the latter.

(2) Even in Gunn's work as in his classification of Type I acupuncture points, an acupuncture sensation point (i. e. acupuncture points) does not fully correspond with a motor point. He stated: "an example is that at the Hegu point in the first dorsal interosseus space of the hand, there exist the motor points of the first dorsal interossueus and the adductor pollicis brevis muscle", that is to say, these are two motor points. Actually, according to our observation, there are three acupuncture points (Hegu, Hubian and Posterior-Hegu) in the Hegu area[1], thus showing that even in Gunn's Type I acupuncture points, the motor point and the acupuncture sensation point (i. e. acupuncture point) do not coincide. Moreover, we have also observed that[3] muscle spindles near to Hegu and Posteror-Hegu point exist not only in the first musculi interossei dorsales, but also in the musculus aductor hallucis. Hence, it cannot be said that a certain motor point in these two muscles corrsponds to a certain point in two acupuncture points. This tends further to prove that a motor point cannot be taken as an acupuncture sensation point (i. e. acupuncture point).

(3) It is also inappropriate to take a low resistance point for an acupuncture sensation point (acupuncture point), for we have proved experimentally that these two never occur at the same point[1].

(4) Gunn seems to have connected the Type I acupuncture points with muscle spindles. Of Type I acupuncture points, some (such as Hegu, Waiguan, Qushi, Zusanli, and others) surely are predominantly muscle spindles, but it is worthy to note that no muscle spindles are found in facial expression muscles, whereas needling sensation receptors at some facial acupuncture points such as Taiyang and Jiache are found to be muscle spindles.

(5) As Gunn put it, if the Gate Control Theory of Melzack et al. for the perception of pain is to be invoked for a partial explanation of acupuncture analgesia, then it is interesting to note the fact that the afferent fibres with the largest diameter originate from the Type I_a fibres at the motor points[21]. However, Type I_a fibres do not originate from the motor points, but from muscle spindles. Also it has not yet been confirmed that they take part in the process of analgesia, although they are involved in the mono-synaptic reflex.

(6) Type II acupuncture points correspond to the focal meeting of superficial nerves in the sagittal plane, but whether or not it is a superficial nerve is uncertain. Our experiment [17] has indicated that on acupuncturing Yintang which belongs to the Type II points, a sensation of distension was elicited only when the needling approached the tunica adventitia of the bone, while the needling sensation from Zhongwan point was always found in deep layers (as deep as 5–10mm in 5 out of 16 cases and more than 10mm in 9)[7]. So it seems to us that the Type II acupuncture point does not belong to superficial nerves.

(7) A study of 3 points indicates that Type III acupuncture points do not belong to superficial nerves, either. The Neiguan point has been shown (by our laboratory[10], Shandong Medical College[22] and Anhui Medical College[15]) to have deep receptores with muscle spindles on acupunctureing Huantiao point, only deep stimulation could yield curative results. It has been estimated therefore that the receptor of Huantiao point belongs to muscle spindles. As to Chengshan point, Gunn himself has revised his original viewpoint and considered it to be a Type IV acupuncture point.

(8) As Type IV acupuncture points correspond to the junction of muscle and tendon, Gunn estimated that their receptors should be tendon organs. We have made the same sup-

position before. However, as mentioned above, we have revised our postulution since it was found experimentally that Chengshan point has many tendon organs in its centre and also muscle spindles at its periphery.

It seems to us that Gunn's viewpoints might have arisen from his deduction based only on the measurement of the low resistance point, without experimenting to find what type of receptors exist in each kind of acupuncture point.

5. Individuality, speciality and universality. Only through a comparative study of a large number of phenomena and processes which have been studied individually can we recognize universality. Our recognition process usually goes from individuality and speciality to finally arrive at universality. This principle should not be neglected in our research work. Nevertheless, investigators in some laboratories, while engaged in studying receptors of acupuncture points, have relied solely on investigation of the Zusanli point and they have tried to use the results of these investigations to expound on all other acupuncture point receptors. Naturally this is impracticable, because the correct conclusion can be arrived at only after more acupuncture points have been investigated. In this sense, our work is still far from adequate and further study has to be done before we can arrive at more precise conclusions. However, our preliminary conclusions are be summarized in the following section.

III. SUMMARY

1. Our research work has proven that the receptors of the needling sensation of an acupuncture point are mainly deep receptors.

2. The environment links an acupuncture point with its receptor. Basically there is a rule governing the existence of certain particularly deep receptors in given environments.

3. We have classified acupuncture points into 5 types according to their different environents. Our preliminary observations have shown that each type of acupuncture point has its own predominant receptors: a. Receptors of needling sensations located in thick muscles (especially on the extremities) are predominantly muscle spindles. b. For acupuncture points located at the junction of muscles and tendons, most tendon organs are found in their center and muscle spindles at their periphery. c. Pacinian corpusles seem to be predominate at the acupuncture point near the tendon. d. Receptors of the needling sensation from acupuncture points on the scalp are most likely nerve endings. e. Our study for the acupuncture points around joint capsules is just getting under way, but, based on the work done by others, Ruffini-like bodies seem to predominate in these locations.

REFERENCES

[1] 西安医学院针麻基础理论研究组：陕西新医药 1—2：17 1973。

[2] 西安医学院针麻基础理论研究组：陕西新医药 3：36 1973。

[3] 西安医学院针麻基础理论研究组：陕西新医药 4：28 1973。

[4] 西安医学院针麻基础理论研究组：陕西新医药 5：43 1973。

[5] Gelfan *et al.*: *Exptl. Neurol.*, 18:467, 1967.
[6] 李孝光等：未发表。
[7] 西安医学院针麻原理研究室：西安医学院学报 4：1 1976。
[8] 魏仁榆等：科学通报 4：184 1974。
[9] 西安医学院针麻基础理论研究组：西安医学院学报 1：56 1975。
[10] 西安医学院、山东医学院针麻原理协作组：西安医学院学报 4：18 1976。
[11] 西安医学院针麻原理研究室：西安医学院学报 4：34 1976。
[12] 西安医学院针麻基础理论研究组：西安医学院学报 1：45 1975。
[13] 西安医学院针麻原理研究室：西安医学院学报 4：81 1976。
[14] 关莲瑛等：陕西医药资料 4：43 1978。
[15] 安徽医学院针麻经络研究室：内部资料。
[16] 中国科学院动物研究所：1972 年全国针麻学习班资料选编之二 47 页 1974。
[17] 西安医学院针麻基础理论研究组：西安医学院学报 1：84 1975。
[18] 林文注等：全国针灸针麻学术讨论会论文摘要(二)：84 页 1979。
[19] 西安医学院针麻原理研究室形态组：西安医学院学报 4：50 1976。
[20] Gunn C_{c_1} *et al.*: *Am. J. Chin. Med.* 4:183, 1976.
[21] Gunn *Cc.*: *Am. J. Acupuncture* 5:51, 1977.
[22] 山东医学院解剖教研组 内部资料。

EFFECT OF ELECTROACUPUNCTURE AT POINT "ZUSANLI" ON ACTIVITY OF MUSCLE MECHANORECEPTORS AND AFFERENT FIBRES IN CATS

Tan Depei, Zhang Shujie, Mao Jianping

(Shanghai Institute of Physiology, Academia Sinica)

It has been pointed out[1] that most of the acupuncture points described in traditional Chinese medicine are located at the terminations of nerve branches where there is often on abundance of deep tissue. A previous study from this department[2] also indicated that selective blocking of the cutaneous nerve innervating the Hegu area did not markedly affect the analgesic effect of acupuncture, whereas infiltration of the deep tissues around the Hegu point with procaine entirely eliminated the analgesic effect. It is thus evident that the afferent signals from deep tissues are essential for producing acupuncture analgesia. In recent years, we[3,4] have studied the effect of acupuncture stimulation on the activity of various muscle mechanoreceptors including the stretch and pressure receptors by recording the unit activity of muscle afferents from isolated nerve filaments of a cat's anterior tibial nerve. It was found that the various kinds of muscle mechanoreceptors could be activated by manual acupuncture. A further analysis of the activity of the pressure receptors on the anterior tibial nerve showed that their receptive fields gathered around the point Zusanli, which was located in the region of the anterior tibial muscle, and that a large number of afferents belonged to group II fibers. Some receptors responsive to heavy pressure, possibly supplied by C fibres, responded with persistent discharges to manual manipulation of the needle inserted in the receptive fields. Sometimes a prolonged after-discharge lasting for minutes or even hours could be seen after the withdrawal of the needle. Since the electrical acupuncture is used more frequently than manual acupuncture for analgesia in China, this article is devoted to the study of the effect of electroacupuncture on the activity of the various kinds of mechanoreceptors and to the study of the related afferent fibres of the anterior tibial muscle.

I. METHODS AND RESULTS

Unit discharges of the fine filaments isolated from the anterior tibial nerve of a cat were recorded in the same way as previously reported[3,4]. The electroacupuncture was applied through an acupuncture needle inserted into the anterior tibial muscle at an area corresponding to the Zusanli point (see Jiang Kaicai et al[5]) by means of a metalic clip placed on the nearby tissue as an indifferent electrode. The stimulus intensity was adjusted so that a moderate muscle twitch was produced. The anterior tibial muscle was kept at the "maximal physiological length". The duration of the electroacupuncture was two minutes and the frequency was 5 or 50 Hz. Among the fifty four units investigated, eighteen were identified as heavy pressure receptors with unmyelinated nerve fibres, eleven as pressure receptors with myelinated nerve fibres, fifteen as muscle spindles and ten as tendon organs.

(I) Pressure receptors supplied by C fibres

Eighteen afferent units with conduction velocities of 0.2–1.68m/sec were investigated, and the receptive fields of nine of them were located within 1 cm around the point "Zusanli". All units tested responded to manual manipulation of the needle in their

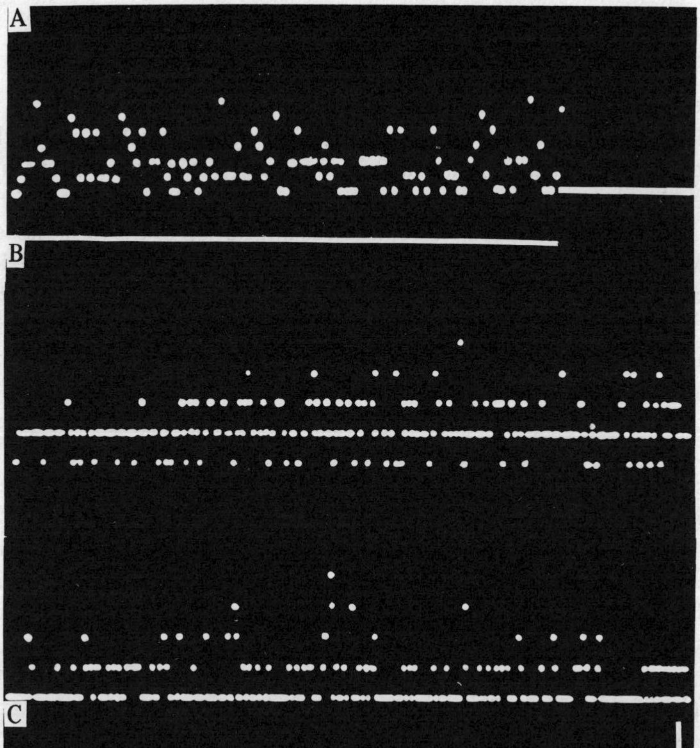

Fig 1 Discharges of a pressure receptor with myelinated nerve fibre in reponse to repetitive electrical stimulation of point "Zu-san-li".

All records are the sequential spike density histogram of unit discharges processed by a JSY-I type computer. The vertical position of the dots represents the number of spikes in each 200 msec. Vertical calibration: 4 spikes. A shows the discharges induced by pressing of receptive field. "–" represents the period of pressing. B and C show the discharges during the continuous electrical stimulation of 5 or 50 Hz respectively. Time mark: 8 sec. in A and 16 sec. in B and C.

receptive fields. Most units had no spontaneous activity although some gave persistent discharges after repeated heavy pressing at the receptive fields. A single electric stimulus delivered to the point "Zusanli" activated only one out of 18 units, the receptive field of which was very close to the point "Zusanli". The intensity of electric stimulus in this case was 1.6 mA. The other three units with receptive fields farther away gave no response to a single electrical stimulus to the "Zusanli" point, but would be excited by electrical stimulation of their receptive fields with stimulus intensities of 8, 4.2 and 3.4mA respectively. Each of these four units discharged 0.6–2.6 impulses/sec when electrical stimulation at the frequency of 5 or 50 Hz was delivered to the "Zusanli" point or to their receptive fields. For the remaining fourteen units, tetanic electrical stimulation of the point " Zusanli" for two minutes would neither evoke discharges nor have any detectable influence on the frequency of spontaneous discharges.

(II) Pressure receptors supplied by myelinated nerve fibres

Of the eleven units investigated, the receptive fields of six of them were found to be located within 1 cm of the "Zusanli" point. No spontaneous discharges were observed. All units tested belonged to group II afferent fibres and the conduction velocity of another unit

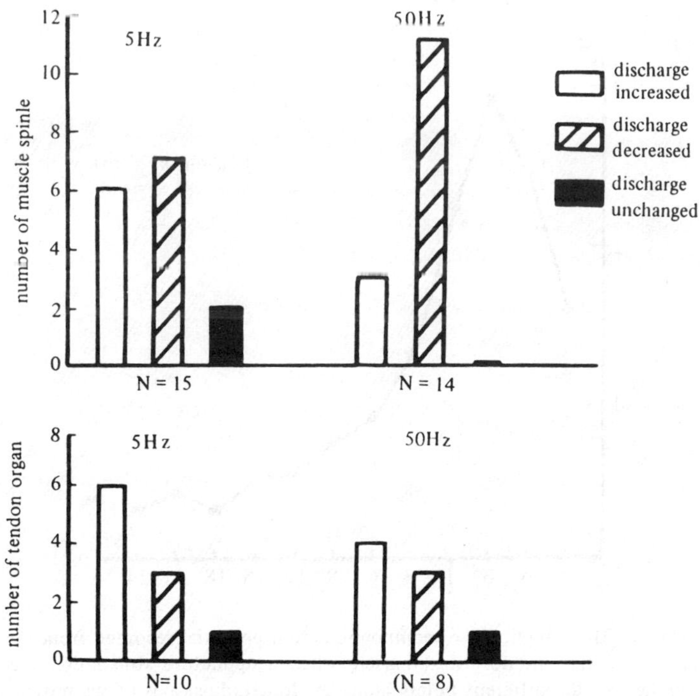

Fig. 2. Change in the discharge frequencies of muscle spindles (A) and tendon organs (B) of the anterior tibial muscle of a cat during the electrical stimulation of point "Zu-san-li" with 5 Hz or 50 Hz.

was not determined. Pressure exerted on the receptive fields produced afferent discharges with frequencies of 11.3–33 impulses/sec. All units except one delivered one or several spikes when single muscle twitches were evoked by single electric shocks applied to the nerve or to the point "Zusanli". During the tetanic contraction caused by the repetitive electrical stimulation of "Zusanli" point, they discharged with a frequencies ranging from 0.3 to 5.8 impulses/sec on 5 Hz and 0.08 to 5.1 impulses/sec on 50 Hz stimulation (Fig. 1). The difference of discharge frequencies caused by the stimulation of 5 Hz or 50 Hz was not significant statistically.

1. Muscle spindles. Of the fifteen muscle spindle units studied, two were supplied by group I afferent fibres while the other thirteen were from group II. When muscles were relaxed, some units had spontaneous discharges, while the others discharged only when the muscles were kept at the "maximal physiological length". Electrical stimulation of the point "Zusanli" with 5 Hz or 50 Hz frequency had diverse effects on different units. The discharge frequency of some units increased, that of others–lowered, and that of a very few units remained unchanged. (Fig. 2)

2. Tendon organs. In ten tendon organ units investigated, two were supplied by group I and eight by group II afferent fibres. One unit had spontaneous discharges when the muscle was relaxed, while the others began to discharge only when the muscle was kept at the "maximal physiological length". When a repetitive electrical stimulation of 5 Hz or 50 Hz was applied to the "Zusanli" point, the tendon organ units were also affected differently.

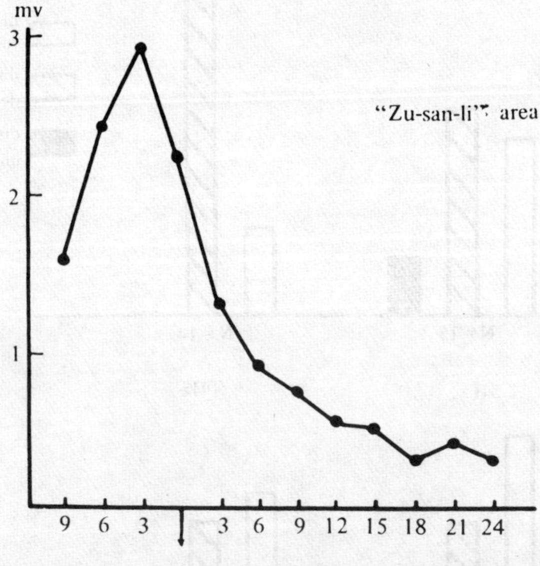

Fig. 3. The Amplitude of compound action potential recorded from the nerve of the anterior tibial muscle when acupuncture stimulation was applied to the different points along the longitudinal axis of the muscle. Distance between each point was 3 mm. Ordinate: The amplitude of action potentials recorded from the nerve of anterior tibial muscle (mv). Abscissa: distance of different stimulating points from the point "Zu-san-li" (mm). Points in the inset show the positions of stimulation.

The discharge frequency was found to be increased or decreased in different units and in only one unit, was the discharge frequency not markedly affected (Fig. 2).

The amplitude of the compound action potential recorded from the nerve to the anterior tibial muscle was investigated by applying the electro-acupuncture stimulus to different points along the longitudinal axis of the muscle. It was found that, when the stimulating needle was inserted into the area of the "Zusanli" point, a weak stimulus of 0.5 mA was sufficient to produce a small compound action potential. The amplitude of action potential increased with the increase in stimulus intensity and the largest amplitude recorded amounted to 1/2 or 1/3 of that produced by a supramaximal stimulus applied to the nerve. As a matter of fact, the largest action potential was recorded when the stimulating needle was close to the point at which the nerve entered the muscle and very close to where the point "Zusanli" was located. When the stimulating needle moved away from this point, the amplitude of the action potential decreased gradually (Fig. 3).

II. DISCUSSION

Bessou & Laporte (1960)[6] and Houk & Henneman (1967)[7] in their study on the activity of muscle spindles and tendon organs have pointed out that during a tetanic contraction of the muscle, some units discharged in a higher frequency while the others in a lower one. A similar phenomenon was observed in our experiments. It can be assumed that the acupuncture needle used for electrical stimulation might vary considerably in approximation to the active elements. From the result of the present study it seems evident that electro-acupuncture of "Zusanli" point could indirectly affect not only the activity of stretch and pressure receptors by causing muscle contraction, but also could directly excite the muscle nerve, since the entrance of the nerve into the muscle is very close to the point "Zusanli". Undoubtedly, the electrical stimulation could excite the large myelinated nerve fibes. One may wonder whether the stimulus in our case would also excite unmyelinated nerve fibres. This possibility, however, is considered unlikely. As described above, only one out of eighteen unmyelinated units could be activated by electrical acupuncture at the "Zusanli" point. This sole exception was probably due to the fact that the receptive field of this unit was very close to the point. We cannot rule out the possibility that a few unmyelinated units might be excited by the electrical stimulation of their receptive fields, but this would only happen when the intensity of the stimulus is so strong as to exceed the limit of human tolerance. On the other hand, manual needling of pressure receptive fields of unmyelinated nerve fibres often elicited afferent discharges.

III. SUMMARY

Electro-acupuncture of "Zusanli" point directly excited a part of the large nerve fibres of anterior tibial nerve; on the other hand, it affected the activity of various kinds of intramuscular mechanoreceptors by causing the contraction of the muscle. Most of the pressure receptors with myelinated nerve fibres were inactive when the muscle was relaxed, but could be activated by electro-acupuncture. Muscle spindles and tendon organs produced sustained discharges when the muscle was kept at the "maximal physiological length". Electro-acupuncture increased the discharges of some stretch receptors and decreased that of others. Pressure receptors innervated by C fibres responded to manual needling in the receptive fields, but could rarely be excited by electro-acupuncture. Tetanic contraction of the muscle produced by electro-acupuncture could not activate the heavy pressure receptors. or could it change the pattern of spontaneous discharges of the related C fibres.

REFERENCES

[1] 沈阳医学院针麻组：针刺麻醉原理的探讨，人民卫生出版社，68 页，1974 年。

[2] Chiang Chenyu et al.: *Scientia Sinica,* **14**: 210,1973.

[3] Wei Renyu : *Kexue Tongbao,* **18**: 184,1973.

[4] Wei Renyu : *Acta Zoologica Sinica,* **24**: 21,1978.

[5] 姜凯采等：上海中医学院学报，1：57，1960。

[6] Bessou P. and Laporte Y. : Symposium on Mussle Receptors, P.105, Hong kong University Press, 1962.

[7] Houk J. and Henneman E. : *J. Neurophysiol.,* **30**: 466,1967.

SOME OBSERVATIONS ON RECEPTIVE STRUCTURES IN CERTAIN ACUPUNCTURE POINTS AND THEIR AFFERENT PATHWAYS CONDUCTING "NEEDLING SENSATIONS" IN HUMAN BEINGS

Lin Wenzhu, Xu Minghai, Wang Zhiyu,
Dai Jingdian, Chen Guomei, Shen Jingyan
(Shanghai Institute of Traditional Chinese Medicine)

The so-called "needling sensations" usually referred to the patients' feelings of "soreness", "distension", "heaviness" and "numbness" elicited by acupuncture. Many clinical observations and experiments on the human body have shown that "needling sensations" are a prerequisite to the analgetic and therapeutic effects of acupuncture[1-3]. The present work is devoted to making observation of the correlation of the "needling sensations" with various receptive structures in certain acupuncture points and their afferent pathways.

I. THE TISSUE STRUCTURES OF "NEEDLING SENSATIONS" SPOTS OF ACUPOINTS

(I) Materials and methods

(1) Amputated human limbs were used as materials. Before anaesthesia for operation, points were selected on the extremity to be amputated and a syringe needle was used instead of an acupuncture needle. The needle was inserted slowly without other manipulations till some kind of "needling sensation" was reported. Then 1–2 μl of 1% methylene blue was injected in order to blue the spot near the tip of the needle. After the operation, the tissue piece with the blue spot was taken out and parts of the piece that had not been stained were removed. 1/4 skein of o-gauge operation thread was used to thread through the center of the blue spot. Continuous sections with thickness of 10–12 μm were prepared using the Cajal-Faworsky's silver impregnation method. An observation of the tissue structures' was made under a microscope around the center of the blue spot with a radius of 1.5mm. The spots at a certain depth which produced no sensation when stimulated by needling were treated as above.

(2) During an orthopedic operation under acupuncture anaesthesia those patients who were able to describe clearly how they felt were chosen. The exposed tissues such as blood vessel, nerve branch, muscle, muscle tendon and periosteum, that had been separated from their surrounding tissues, were stimulated by a needle or an eye forcep, and the patients'

feelings thus elicited were noted. Usually this kind of study was made when no tourniquet was used and when needling had stopped.

(II) Results

(1) General distribution of "needling sensation" spots

66 blue spots, among which 50 were "needling sensations" and the others non-"needling sensation", in 29 acupuncture points, including "Zusanli", "Sanyinjiao", "Neiguan", "Pianli", etc., from 42 adults were investigated. By stimulating these spots the nature of the sensations of the majority was "soreness" and "distension", and that of the minority was "heaviness", "numbness" and "with an electro-sensation". These sensations were distributed in the muscles, muscle tendons and surrounding tissues, nerve branches, blood vessels, joint capsules and subcutaneous connective tissues. Most frequently, they were found in deep tissues (Table 1).

(2) The microstructure of the "needling sensations" spots:

In the "needling sensations" spots which were about 1.5mm in radius away from the

Table 1. Distribution of "Needling Sensations" spots in various structures of acu-points

Structures	Soreness	Distension	Heaviness	Numbness	Electric-Sensation	Total
Muscle	6	9	1			16
Muscle tendon	10	5				15
Nerve branch	1	1		3		5
Blood vessel	1					1
Joint capsule		1			1	2
Periosteum	1	2				3
Subcutis	2	3	1	2		8
Total	21	21	2	5	1	50

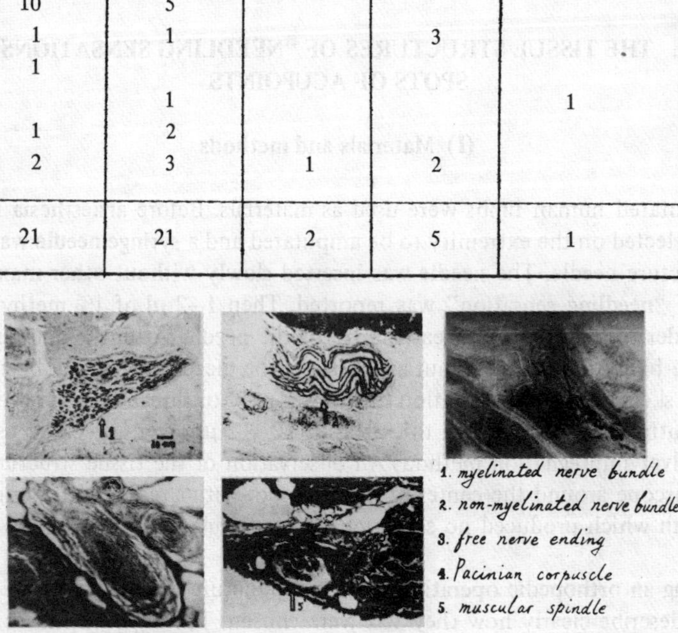

Fig. 1 Nerves and sensation receptors in the needling sensation point.

centre of the blue spot, various small nerve bundles composed of myelinated and non-myelinated fibers, free nerve endings, Pacinian corpuscles, muscular spindles (Fig. 1) and small blood vessels were found scparated from muscle fibers and connective tissues. No special structures could be identified. In "needling sensation" spots and non-"needling sensation" spots, the incidences of nerve structures were 82% and 23.08% respectively, with a significant difference ($P<0.01$), while those of blood vessels were 68% and 69.28%, with out significant difference ($P>0.05$). In each "needling sensation" spot, one or more kind of nerve structures was found. Nevertheless, the incidences of the small nerve bundles and free nerve endings were the highest. Their distribution is shown in Fig. 2.

The size of the myelinated nerve bundles and the number of their constituent nerve fibers in "needling sensation" spots were different from each other. The smallest nerve bundle was composed of several fibers whereas the biggest one had several hundreds of

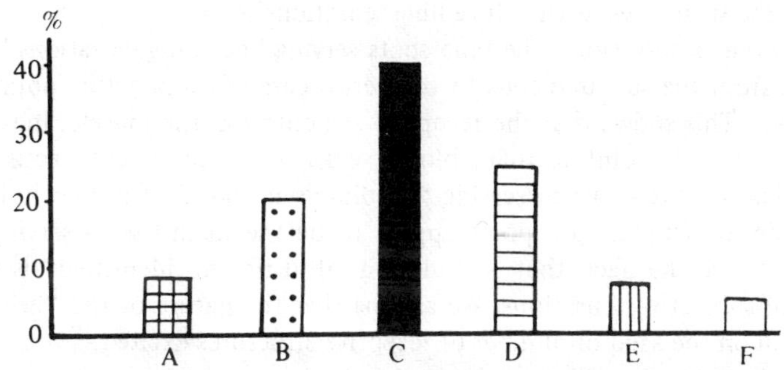

Fig. 2. Frequencies of nerves & receptors in "needing sensations" spots
A. Nerve Branch B. Non-myelinated Nerve Bundle C. Myelinated Nerve Bundle
D. Free Nerve Endings E. Pacinian Corpuscle F. Muscular Spindle

Table 2. Nature of sensations Elicited by stimulation of various structures in deep tissues of acu-points

Tissues stimulated	Soreness	Numbness	Distension	Heaviness	Warmth	Pain	Total
	6	30	13	2	1	4	56 cases
Nerve branch	10.71	53.57	23.21	3.57	1.79	7.15	100%
	3	4	1			12	20 cases
Blood Vessel	15.00	20.00	5.00			60.00	100%
	5	1	6			3	15 cases
Muscle	33.33	6.67	40.00			20.00	100%
	8	3	3			6	20 cases
Muscle tendon	40.00	15.00	15.00			30.00	100%
	10	1	2			4	17 cases
Periosteum	58.82	5.88	11.77			23.53	100%

fibers. The diameter of fibers varied from 1–10μm, but most of them were below 6μm.

(3) The patients' feelings elicited by stimulating blood vessels, nerves, muscles, muscle tendons or periostea.

In 56 cases, 128 stimulations of various tissues had been carried out. The results are shown in Table 2.

One can see from Table 2 that stimulation of the blood vessel, nerve, muscle, muscle tendon or periosteum may evoke various kinds of "needling sensations". It should be noted, however, that the incidences of the different "needling sensations" elicited varied the with different structures stimulated. The stimulation of nerve branches evoked "numbness" sensation predominantly; that of blood vessel, pain; that of muscle, tendon and periosteum, "soreness" and "distention".

(III) Discussion

(1) What are the structures serving "needling sensations"?

According to our observations, the blue spots serving "needling sensations" are located in various tissues from the subcutaneous to the periosteum of acupuncture points and most are in deep tissues. This shows that the receptive structures in the muscle, muscle tendon, periosteum, nerve branch, joint capsule, blood vessel wall and subcutaneous connective tissue have very likely, taken part in serving "needling sensations". On the whole, however, the deep tissues in an acupuncture point appear to be the main tissues serving "needling sensations". Based on the fact that stimulation of different identified tissues evoked different kinds of subjective sensations, We assume that the nature of the "needling sensations" may depend on the kind or number of receptive structures excited.

(2) Relations between "needling sensations" and nervous tissues

In histological study, certain nervous structures were found in most of "needling sensation" spots, whereas no nervous structures could be seen in the majority of non-"needling sensation" spots. The direct stimulation of a nerve branch could evoke several kinds of "needling sensations", which indicated the close relationship between them. The nerve structures, such as small nerve bundles and free nerve endings, were most frequently found in "needling sensation" spots and existed in almost all the points observed. However, nerve branches, pacinian corpuscles and muscular spindles could only be found in a few points. It showed that small nerve bundles and free nerve endings were likely to be the predominant receptive structures serving "needling sensations" in most of the points. No specific receptors serving the "needling sensations" of "soreness", "distention", "heaviness" and "numbness" respectively was found during the observation. However, it was shown that the nerve structures in the "needling sensation" spots serving mainly "soreness", "distension" and "heaviness" were small nerve bundles composed of small fibers, while those in the spots serving mainly "numbness" were mostly nerve branches containing large fibers. This suggests that the type or number of fibers excited to evoke "numbness" is different from that which elicits "soreness", "distension" and "heaviness".

(3) Relations between "needling sensations" and blood vessels

Blood vessels were seen in the tissue slices of "needling sensation" spots. Direct stimulation of the blood vessel could also evoke "needling sensations" though pain was felt frequently during stimulation. It was noted that there are rich nerve endings or nerve bundles at the blood vessel wall or perivascular connective tissues in "needling sensation" spots. Gross[4] claimed that pain is served also by afferents of autonomic nerves. In addition to somatic nerves, therefore, autonomic nerves on the blood vessel wall might have played a part in "needling sensations".

II. AFFERENT FIBERS AND PATHWAYS SERVING "ELECTRO ACUPUNCTURE SENSATIONS" AND "NEEDLING SENSATIONS (MANUAL MANIPULATION)"

(I) Types of afferent fibers identified by recording their electrical responses with a summation method

Experiments were made on 25 adults, among whom 6 were patients of cervical paraplegia. During the experiment, a subject of the experiment was lying in a supine position with his right arm relaxed as much as possible. A No. 32 needle was inserted slowly without twirling into the point "Neiguan" on the right side. After the "needling sensations" were elicited, the needle remained there and served as a stimulating electrode. An indifferent electrode was attached to the skin over the point "Weiguan" and its nearby region. An electric pulse of square wave, 0.1–1 (usually 0.5) msec in duration and 20–50 V in strength, delivered at a frequency of 1/sec, was used for stimulation. The recording electrodes took the form of two needles inserted into the point "Quze" and at the place 1 cm above it respectively. The electrical responses evoked were amplified and summated 50–500 times by a computer. Frequently, the sensations elicited by needling stimulation of "Neiguan" were soreness and distension, but the majority changed to numbness, numbness-distension or numbness-soreness as soon as the electric stimulation took place. The electrical response evoked by electric stimulation of "Neiguan" and recorded from "Quze" was a triphasic (positive-negative-positive) or diphasic (negative-positive) waveform of 2.22–60μV in amplitue and 1–2msec in duration. Its latent period was about 3msec. So the conduction speed was 55–78 m/sec (Fig. 3-1). In 7 cases, a second waveform of 1–2msec in duration and 1.2–11.98μV in amplitude, conducted at a velocity of 42–52 m/sec, could be recorded (Fig. 3–2). In one case, diring the falling phase of the first waveform, the second and third waveform were clearly seen. In addition, there was a fourth waveform of 3msec in duration and 4.6 μV in amplitude, with a conduction speed of 37 m/sec (Fig. 3-3).

Collins et al.[5] had stimulated the sensory nerves exposed during surgery in conscious patients. The compound action potentials of the nerves were recorded to correlate with the subjective sensations thus elicited. They found that the electrical activities of A_s fibers with a conduction speed of 25–30 m/sec could be recorded when the electric stimulation was 2–3 times as strong as that to activate A_r fibers. In the meantime, a distinct pricking pain was felt. On human bodies, Bland et al.[6] applied an electric pulse of 40–80 mA to the median nerve which was blocked by procaine at its proximal portion and they recorded the electric potentials of C fibers by means of a summating computer. In clinical practice, the strength of electro-acupuncture used is within a certain range so that the sensations elicited can be tolerated by the patient. Usually, the stimulating currents used in this observation

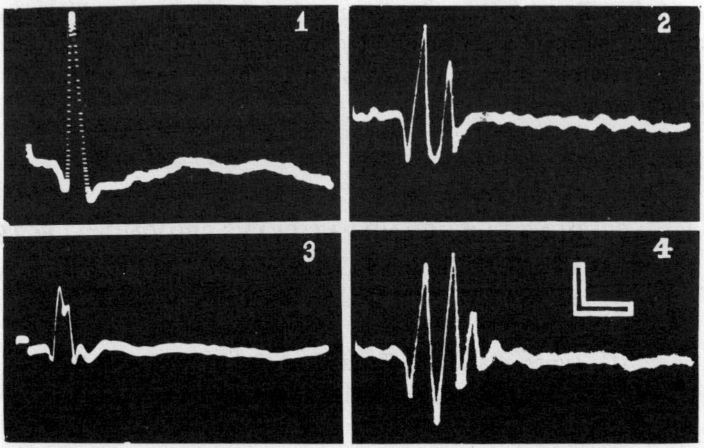

Fig. 3 Type of afferent fibres subserving electro-acupuncture sensation
(1) 240 responses averaged
(2), (4) 200 responses averaged
(3) 80 responses averaged
voltage: lmV; Time: 4msec

could only induce a response of 55–78 m/sec in conduction velocity. With a stronger stimulation, another response of 42–52 m/sec in conduction velocity could also be recorded. In the latter instance, the sensations elicited were so sharp that further increase in stimulus strength was refused. In patients suffering from cervical paraplegia whose upper limbs were anaesthetic, a much stronger stimulation could be tolerated, so the electrical activities of the smaller fibers, e.g. group III, could be recorded (Fig. 3-4). It is therefore assumed that the electro-acupuncture techniques curreatly used excite chiefly the larger fibers of group I and II.

(II) Investigation of the types of afferent fibers subserving needling and electro-acupuncture sensations by performing circulation blocking experiments

Experiments were carried out on 16 normal adults. A needle was placed in the point "Neiguan". After the feelings of soreness, distension or heaviness had arisen, a square wave of electric current of 0.1–0.5 msec in width was applied to it 1–10 times per sec. The strength of the pulse was adjusted to induce a sensation, predominantly of numbness. Then the blood flow to the forearm was blocked by a tourniquet with a pressure of 40 mmHg above the systolic pressure of the subject. Ten minutes later, the sensations of touch, pressure and pain on the skin over "Neiguan"and the "electro-acupuncture sensations" were examined every two minutes. The amount time in which each kind of sensations disappeared was recorded. After "electro-acupuncture sensations " disappeared completely, "Neiguan" was stimulated by raising, inserting and twirling the needle. In some subjects, the compound action potentials of nerve fibers, described before, were observed simultaneonsly. When touch and pressure sensations disappeared, the nerve impulses conducted at a velocity of

40–70 m/sec subsided too. The time by which each kind of sensations disappeared after blocking is as follows:

touch:	22.9 $\pm$4.01 min
pressure:	26.36 $\pm$4.16 min
pricking pain:	35.71 $\pm$4.81 min
"electro-acupucture sensations":	24.70 $\pm$4.55 min
"needling sensations":	37.30 $\pm$6.73 min

From these results it may be said that after the blood flow was blocked the "electro-acupuncture sensations" frequently disappeared with the touch-pressure sensations (served by group II fibers), and the "needling sensations" often disappeared with the pain sensations, the pricking pain sensations in particular. (served by group III fibers)

(III) Surveys of afferent pathways subserving "needling sensations" in patients suffering from nervous disorders

62 patients with documented nervous diseases were asked to report the feelings elicited by needling the points in affected parts in comparison with those elicited in normal parts. Similar reports were heard in the 5 or more needling treatments required in each case. The results were as follows:

(1) Diseases of peripheral nerves (8 cases)

In patients of polyneuritis and injured brachial plexus, no "needling sensations" could be induced in the affected parts where the sensations of pain and temperature had been lost. In the affected parts where the tactile sensation was severely impaired, the needling sensations could be elicited though weaker than normal.

(2) Spinal disorders (34 cases)

In transverse lesion of the cord below the affected level, all sensations were lost, and needling stimulation of the points in these parts could elicit no sensations at all.

In Brown-sequard syndrome caused by neoplasm, the "needling sensations" elicited were normal at the side of lesion where the motor function and deep sensibility were affected, but were impaired as much as the sensations of pain and temperature at the opposite side.

In tabes dorsalis, the deep sensibility was almost lost while the cutaneous sensation was impaired only slightly. The "needling sensations" elicited in the affected parts of the body were not greatly different from normal.

In syringomyelia, the "needling sensations" could not be aroused in the affected parts where the pain and temperature sensations were lost completely. However, if there was still a very slight sensation of pain left, a weak "needling sensation" could be elicited.

In hereditary ataxia, the pyramidal tracts, posterior fasciculi and anterior and posterior spino-cerebellar tracts on both sides were involved, while in the sequelae of polio, primarily the cells of ventral horn were involved. Nevertheless, needling sensations could be elicited in the affected parts of the body without obvious abnormal findings.

(3) Brain disorders (12 cases)

In cerebral hemorrhage, lesions of the knee and the hind limb of internal capsule and of other deeper structures of the hemisphere had has resulted in cases of hemiplegia and hemihypesthesia. Though "needling sensations" could be induced on the affected side, yet localization was inaccurate and the sensations were often referred to an area with an obscure border away from the point being stimulated. If the posterior third of the internal capsule was not involved and no sensory deficiency occurred, the "needling sensations" elicited on the side of hemiplegia were essentially normal.

Lesions of lenticula, globus pallidus and substantia nigra had no effect on "needling sensations".

(4) Miscellaneous (8 cases)

In anhidrosis, progressive muscular dystrophy, etc., and in one case of hysteria with unilateral paresis and anaesthesia, no abnormality in the "needling sensations" elicited was found.

From the observations mentioned above, the authors consider that the sensations elicited by needling the points are not directly related to the motor function of the nervous system.

They are closely related to the neural pathways for pain and temperature sensibilities.

(IV) Investigation of sensations elicited by stimulating the tooth pulp in comparison with "needling sensations."

An electric pulse of 1 msec in duration and 0.1–2 mA in strength delivered once per sec from a constant current stimulator was used to stimulate the tooth pulp which is known to be predominantly innervated by group III fibers in the human body. The stimulating electrode was a stainless steel rod of 1mm in diameter placed on the enamel surface. The "indifferent electrode" was a silvered copper plate of 7×3.5 cm^2 in size, placed on the skin of the forearm. 375 teeth in 50 subjects were investigated. The modalities of sensations thus evoked included soreness, distension, heaviness, numbness, cold, warmth, pain and

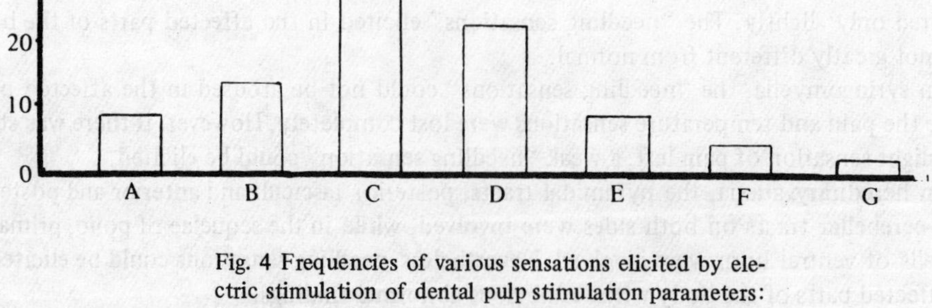

Fig. 4 Frequencies of various sensations elicited by electric stimulation of dental pulp stimulation parameters: 1 msec, 0.1–2mA, once per second. A. cold B. Pain C. Soreness D. Numbness E. Distension F. Warmth G. Heaviness

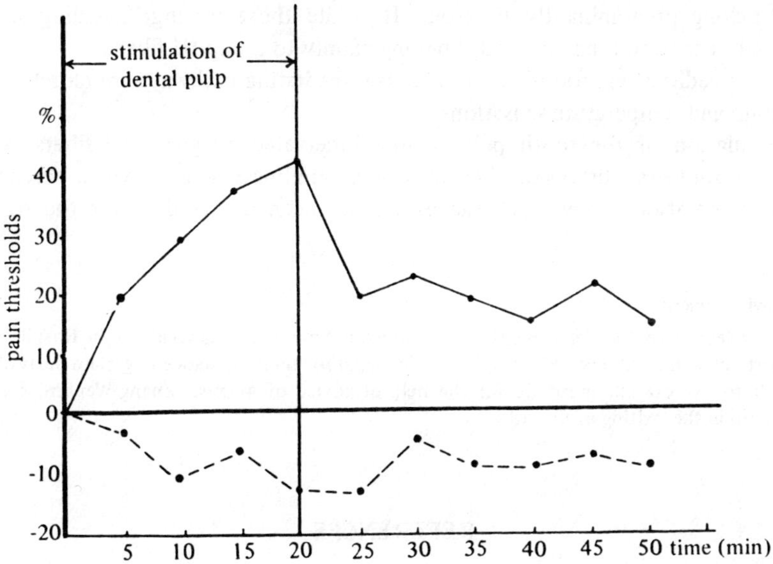

Fig. 5 Effert of electric stimulation of dental pulp on the pain thresholds of the skin.

electric sensations. The sensation reported most frequently was soreness (Fig. 4). In 35 teeth of 9 subjects, when the currents were increased to 5–10 mA, the nature of sensations induced was changed – mostly to a painful sensation. For a control, 11 denervated teeth in 5 subjects were stimulated with 1–20mA currents and no sensation arose.

In 20 subjects, pain thresholds measured by K^+ iontophoresis on the skin overlying the point "Yanqi" were determined before and during the stimulation of tooth pulp[2]. Fig. 5 illustrates the finding that pain thresholds increased steadily to about 140% during the 20 minutes stimulation of the tooth pulp.

III. SUMMARY

1. "Needling sensation" spots may be located in the different tissues of acupuncture points from subcutaneous tissue to periosteum, and were found mostly in deep tissues.

2. Stimulation of various tissues could evoke sensations of "soreness", "distention", "heaviness" and "numbness". However, the incidences of the sensory modalities evoked in different tissues are dissimilar. The stimulation of a nerve branch predominantly evokes a "numbness" sensation, that of tendon or periosteum "soreness", that of a muscle, "distention" or "soreness", and that of a blood vessel, pain.

3. The nervous tissues which respond to acupuncture and evokes "needling sensations" includes many structures. They are: small nerve bundles, free nerve endings, nerve branches and some encapsulated receptors. Among these, the small nerve bundles and free nerve endings are the most important receptive structures serving "needling sensations".

4. The afferent fibers serving "electro-acupuncture sensations" which is usually numbness belong predominantly to group II, while those serving "needling sensations" (soreness and distension predominantly) belong mainly to group III fibers.

5. The "needling sensations" of the central mediating pathways are closely related to those for pain and temperature sensations.

6. Stimulation of the tooth pulp mainly innervated by group III fibers can induce sensations of soreness, distension, heaviness and numbness, among which soreness is the predominant sensation. Some analgesic effect has been observed during the stimulation.

Acknowledgement

We are indebted to the departments of orthopedic surgery in Shanghai Ruijin Hospital, Shanghai Longhua Hospital, and Sixth People's Hospital of Shanghai for their assistance in certain parts of this work. We also wish to express our gratitude for the helpful advice of Messrs. Zhang Wenbin, Zeng Zhaolin and Qiao Yimin in the writing of this article.

REFERENCES

[1] 上海市针刺麻醉协作组：红旗杂志，(9)：59，1971。
[2] 北京医学院基础部针麻原理研究组：中华医学杂志，(3)：151，1973。
[3] 江振裕等：中国科学 (2)：157，1973。
[4] Gross D：医学参考资料 (6)：273，1975。
[5] Collins W. F. et al.: Arch Neurol (3): 381, 1960.
[6] Bland C. S. et al.: *Annual report from the institute of neurophysiology of the university of copenhagen,* September 1, 1970 to August 31, 1971, P. 31.

COMPOSITION OF AFFERENT FIBERS AT POINT "ZUSANLI" IN RELATION TO ACUPUNCTURE ANALGESIA—A FUNCTIONAL MORPHOLOGICAL INVESTIGATION

Lu Guowei, Xie Jingqiang, Yang Jin, Wang Yongning, Wang Qilin

(Laboratory of Acupuncture Anesthesia and Encephalology, Beijing Second Medical College)

The acupoint, being a specified stimulation point for acupuncture and moxibustion treatment, has already been used in traditional Chinese medicine for thousands of years. Its physiological properties and structural basis have long been subjects of interest, but are still little understood. In our previous endeavors, we found that the $A_{\beta\gamma}$ afferent fibers closely correlated to the transmission of analgesic impulses arising from the acupoints[1]. This seems to imply that there may be a certain characteristic pattern in regard to the composition and action of afferent fibers in local acupoints. Hence, in the present studies the point "Zusanli" was selected as a "target" (in view of the fact that the relative specificity of its analgesic effect had already been confirmed) and the characteristics of its innervation were explored.

I. METHODS

The experiments were carried out on rabbits and, to a lesser extent, on cats. The animals weighed each 2-3kg, and no discrimination was made in regard to species or sex. In order to determine the location or coordinates of an acupoint in animals, an analgesic experiment was performed as described previously[1]. By means of this experiment, several stipulations were made in methodology in this study. An acupoint of "Zusanli", the needling of which produced a marked analgesic effect, was defined as a "high-effective focus", and regarded as an acupoint in its original sense; and an acupoint of "Zusanli" without any analgesic effect was defined as a "non-effective focus", and regarded as the equivalent of a "non-meridian focus" anatomically. The latter was located 0.5 cm laterally from "Zusanli" and 1 cm in depth. In the present study, the "high-effective foci", regarded as experimental foci, were the main subjects of our study and both the "non-effective" and "non-channel" foci served as control foci.

The following four divisions were included in this study.

Establishment of the relative specificity of the location of point "Zusanli": To this end, points of "Quchi", "Zusanli" and "non-channel focus" were taken in turn according to an orthogonal design in one and the same individual, and their analgesic efficiency compared.

Determination of the velocity spectrum of afferent fibers: This was done on rabbits that had been needled for analgesia with a needle insulated except for its tip. After the typical effects of analgesia (conspicuous or absent) had been obtained, another needle was inserted into the "non-channel focus" according to the prescribed location. With these two needles remaining in situ, the spinal cord L_5-S_1 were exposed, and an oil bank filled with liquid paraffin kept at about 37°C was prepared above them. Gallamine triethiodine (2 mg/kg of body weight) or scoline (5 mg/kg of body weight) was injected intravenously to paralyze musculature, the animal being given artificial respiration. Then the filaments of the dorsal roots of the spinal nerves at $L_{6,7}$-S_1 were separated in accordance with the relevant methods[2-6]. Each filament was then twined round a platinum wire of 100μm in diameter and a monopolar lead applied to input the evoked discharges of afferent fibers to a Type TQ–19 medical data processor via a cathode follower and an amplifier. By using the bare-tipped needles in point "Zusanli" and "non-channel focus" as an effective electrode, repeated rectangular pulses of 0.03 msec duration at 20V strength and 4Hz frequency were transmitted via an isolator to a "high-" or "non-effective" focus and a "non-meridian focus" to stimulate afferent unit discharge, at the same time triggering into action a processor and a monitor oscilloscope. The latency and number of the evoked unit discharges were determined after the discharges of each filament had accumulated to 256 times at a unit interval of 20msec. When all the filaments of the related dorsal roots had been separated and recorded, the conduction distance between the effective electrode and recording electrode was measured with a thread, and the conduction velocity of each discharge unit and the spectrum of unit discharges were calculated accordingly.

Measurement of diameter spectrum of the afferent fibers: The animals to be used in this observation were first ventrorootomized to degenerate the efferent fibers. 30–50 days later, after all the efferent fibers in the area "Zusanli" had completely degenerated, analgesic experiments were made with a bare-tipped insulated needle to determine whether the point was a "high-effective focus" or not. Direct current of 10 mA intensity was then delivered through the needle and 1 percent pot. ferrocyanide in 10 percent formaline was perfused intracardially to mark the location of the stimulated foci with a "blue dot". The muscle tissue blocks containing the blue dots, each about 5 × 5 × 10 mm in size, were removed and stained with 0.5 percent osmic acid to demonstrate myelinated fibers. Transverse serial sections of 10μm in thickness were then excised and one section taken from every 10 for examination. Photomicrographs were taken of intramuscular fasciculi in a circular area with a 1.5 mm radius around the "blue dot", and the diameter and number of myelinated fibers measured on the photograph (enlarged 900 ×) according to the method described by Fernand and Young[7]. The measuring and counting were done by one person and checked by another.

Investigation of the ratio of myelinated and nonmyelinated fibers: This experiment was done on cats in which the ventral roots of the $L_{6,7}$ spinal nerves were also sectioned as above. The maneuvers and procedures were the same as used in the above studies, except that the silver nitrate staining method was used for demonstrating nonmyelinated fibers[8].

In order to assure the validity of the experiments in the present studies, the analgesic experiment and the subsequent analytic procedures were performed separately by different groups of persons according to the "blind method" principle. When the analgesic experiment had been accomplished by one special group of persons, the animal was transferred to another group for further physiological and morphological study without informing the latter group of the results of analgesia.

II. RESULTS

(I) The analgesic effects of needling "Zusanli", "Quchi" and "Non-channel" points

The acupuncture analgesic experiments were done on 23 animals, using the same maneuvers and procedures, and the pain-relieving effects were compared. It was found that a marked analgesic effect was obtained at "Zusanli" which happened to be at the same segmental innervation of the pain source, the "effective" ratio and "excellent and good" rate being in the order of 95.6 percent and 78.2 percent, respectively (Fig. 1, Table 1).

On the other hand, no apparent analgesic effect could be seen when the point "Quchi" (situated at a distance from the pain source) or "non-channel focus" (situated in the same segment as point "Zusanli", but not an acupoint) was acupunctured (Fig. 1, Table 1).

The difference in analgesic effect between point "Zusanli" and the two other points was very significant statistically (after the sign test, $P<0.001$).

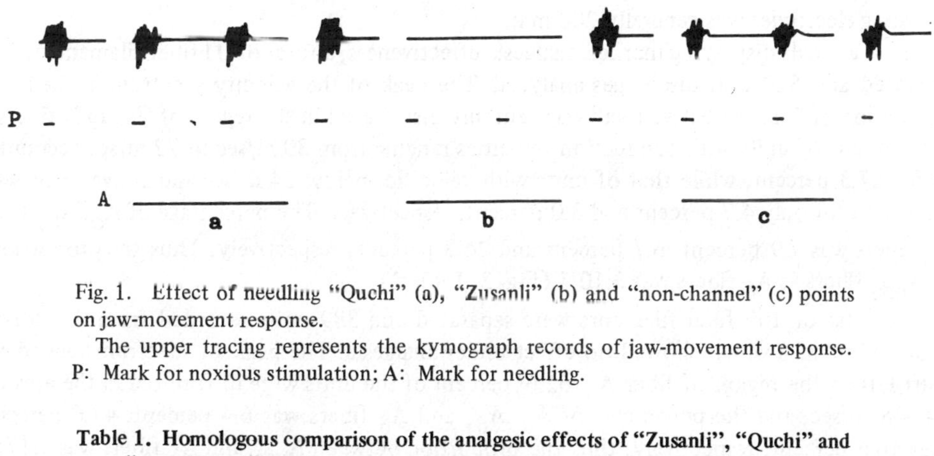

Fig. 1. Effect of needling "Quchi" (a), "Zusanli" (b) and "non-channel" (c) points on jaw-movement response.

The upper tracing represents the kymograph records of jaw-movement response. P: Mark for noxious stimulation; A: Mark for needling.

Table 1. Homologous comparison of the analgesic effects of "Zusanli", "Quchi" and "non-channel" points (numerals in parenthesis are the percentage of total)

	Total number of animals	Excellent	Fine	Moderate	Poor	Effectiveness	Excellent and fine
"Zusanli" point	23 (100)	6 (26.1)	12 (52.1)	4 (17.4)	1 (4.4)	22 (95.6)	18 (78.2)
"Quchi" point	23 (100)	0 (0)	0 (0)	1 (4.4)	22 (95.6)	1 (4.4)	0 0
"Non-meridian" point	23 (100)	0 (0)	1 (4.4)	1 (4.4)	21 (91.2)	2 (8.8)	1 (4.4)

The above experiments indicate that the analgesic effect produced by "Zusanli" is not only marked, but also possesses a certain relative specificity where nerve segments and point location are concerned. Particularly when compared with the effects produced by "non-channel points", the specificity of point "Zusanli" in the location or coordinate provided a useful precondition for further comparing the velocity and diameter spectra of channel and non-channel points. In light of the findings described above, analgesic experiments were no longer conducted in the following groups of experiments for the purpose of judging the location of "non-channel" points; however, in order to determine whether the location of "Zusanli" was a "high-" or "non-effective focus", analgesic experiments proceeded as usual.

(II) The velocity spectrum of afferent fiber of point "Zusanli" in relation to acupuncture analgesia.

A total of 210 fiber filaments were separated and 1481 unit discharges recorded in a total of 8 animals in which typical results had been produced by acupuncture analgesia and all their dorsal roots analyzed.

It was found that the effective positions for the needle tips were generally in the m. extensor digitorum common, and the distance between "high-" or "non-effective focus" and "non-channel focus" was usually 0.8 cm. The conduction distance between the effective and recording electrodes was generally 200 mm.

In 4 animals displaying marked analgesic effectiveness, a total of 111 fiber filaments were separated and 529 unit discharges analyzed. The peak of the velocity spectrum evoked by stimulation of "high-effective foci" was centrally distributed in the region of Group II fibers. The amount of units with conduction velocities ranging from 30 m/sec to 72 m/sec accounted for 87.3 percent, while that of units with velocities below 24 m/sec and above 78 m/sec accounted for only 4.7 percent and 8.0 percent, respectively. The percentage of A_{α}, $A_{\beta\gamma}$ and A_{δ} fibers was 7.9 percent, 6.7 percent and 24.3 percent, respectively. Thus the proportion of $A_{\alpha\beta\gamma}$ fibers vs A_{δ} fibers was 3.10:1 (Fig. 2, Table 2).

A total of 100 fiber filaments were separated and 389 units recorded from the dorsal roots of animals which showed no effect under analgesia. The peak of spectrum tended to shift left to the region of fiber A_{δ}. 62.6 percent of the units were distributed in the area of 24–48 m/sec, and the percentage of A_{α}, $A_{\beta\gamma}$ and A_{δ} fibers was 6.4 percent, 47.6 percent and 46.6 percent, respectively; thus the proportion between $A_{\alpha\beta\gamma}$ and A_{δ} fibers was 1.17:1 (Fig. 2, Table 2). On 192 of the dorsal roots of all the 4 animals displaying a significant effect under analgesia, as well as of 3 animals showing no effect, a total of 563 units evoked by stimulation of "non-channel foci" was also recorded. Similar to the "non-effective foci", their highest peak lay in the region of A_{δ} fibers; the number of A_{α}, $A_{\beta\gamma}$ and A_{δ} fibers made up 6.2 percent, 55.5 percent and 38.3 percent of the total, respectively; and the ratio of fibers $A_{\alpha\beta\gamma}$ to A_{δ} was 1.61:1 (Table 2). The difference in the ratio between "high-effective" and control foci was significant statistically (after White rank test, P<0.01) (Table 2).

These results suggest that the large fibers, especially $A_{\beta\gamma}$ fibers, are largely activated when "high-effective foci" for analgesia are being stimulated as compared with control ones, which seems to imply that the "high-effective foci", as acupoints, possess distinctive features in their afferent fiber composition.

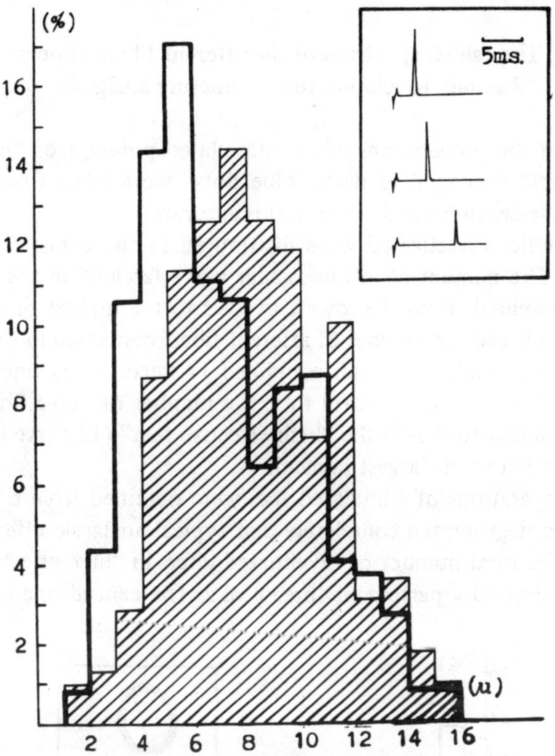

Fig. 2 Velocity spectrum of afferent fibers in "high-effective foci" (shaded area) and "non-effective foci" (open area).

Ordinate: Percentage of discharge units. Abscissa: Conduction velocity of discharge units expressed in terms of diameter with velocity diameter rate 6. The inset demonstrates afferent unit discharges plotted from the filaments No. 4 and 10 of a dorsal root in No. 8117 of a rabbit. Temperature in oil bank: 37°C; conduction distance: 207 mm.

Table 2. Proportion of discharge units of a fibers in "high-effective foci" and control foci (including both "non-effective" and "non-channel" foci)

	No. of foci recorded	No. of units recorded	Percentage of units A_α	$A_{\beta\gamma}$	A_δ	$A_{\alpha\beta\gamma} : A_\delta$ *
High-effective foci	4	529	7.9	67.8	24.3	3.10
Non-effective foci	4	389	6.4	47.6	46.0	1.17
Non-meridian foci	7	563	6.2	55.5	38.0	1.61

* The difference between "high-effective" and control foci is significant ($P<0.01$).

(III) The caliber spectrum of the afferent fibers of point "Zusanli" in relation to acupuncture analgesia

A great number of the preparations of the stimulated points, i. e., "high-", "non-effective" and "non-channel" foci marked with "blue dots" were taken from m. extensor digitorum common and a lesser number from m. tibilis anterior.

All the nerve bundles investigated were distributed in the connective tissue between muscle fiber bundles. The number of intramuscular nerve fasciculi in the stimulated points varied from animal to animal, from the lowest of 1–2 to the highest of 4–5 or more. The size of the nerve fasciculi and the number of afferent fibers contained in them also varied. In "high-effective foci", the smallest fasciculi contained 14 nerve fibers, and the largest might contain 173 afferent fibers. In the control foci, the number of nerve fibers present in the smallest fasciculi was similar to that in the "high-effective foci" (12 nerve fibers), but 66 was the highest number present in the largest fasciculi.

In this study, preparations of stimulated foci were obtained from 6 animals, in which the efferent fibers had degenerated completely and typical analgesic effects were achieved. In 5 of the animals, the total number of myelinated fibers in "high-effective foci" was 970. The caliber spectrum showed a pattern of three peaks. The central one lay in the region of

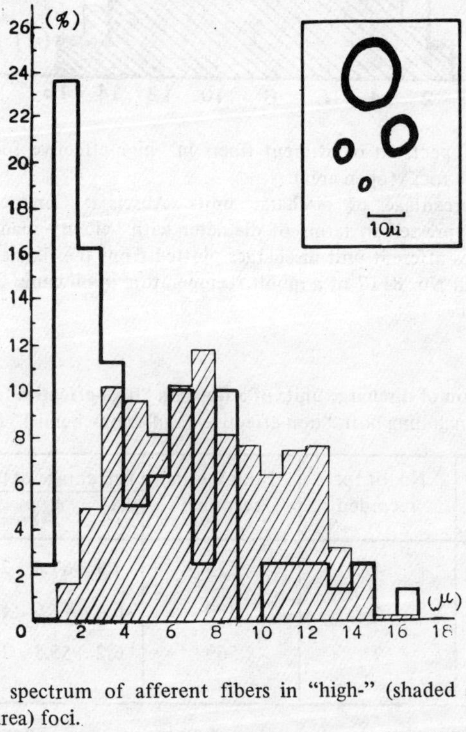

Fig. 3 Diameter spectrum of afferent fibers in "high-" (shaded area) and "non-effective" (open area) foci.

The inset displays the appearance under a microscope of myelinated fibers stained with osmic acid. Plotted from photograph No. 48, in rabbit No. 4.

Table 3. The percentages of different groups of myelinated afferent fibers in "high-effective" and control foci (including both "non-effective" and "non-meridian foci")

	No. of foci taken	No. of fibers examined	Percentage of fiber types I	II	III	(I + II) : III*
High-effective foci	5	970	22	52	26	2.8
Non-effective foci	1	66	10	31	59	0.7
Non-channel foci	2	192	15	36	49	1.0

* The difference between "high-effective" and control foci is significant ($P<0.05$).

Group II fibers. The percentages of Groups I, II and III fibers were 22 percent, 52 percent and 26 percent, respectively; the ratio of Groups I and II fibers to Group III fibers was 2.8:1 (Fig. 3, Table 3).

The peak of diameter spectrum of the intramuscular nerve fasciculi in one animal unresponsive to analgesia tended to shift to the left and was situated in the region of Group III fibers; the proportions of Groups I, II and III fibers were 10 percent, 31 percent and 59 percent, respectively; and Groups I and II/Group III ratio was about 1:1. The distribution of the afferent fibers of "non-meridian foci" in 5 animals with marked analgesic effects was similar to the "non-effective foci"; the percentages of various fiber groups were 15 percent, 36 percent and 49 percent, respectively; Groups I and II fibers/Group III fibers ratio was also about 1:1 (Fig. 3, Table 3)

The mean values of Group (I + II) to Group III fibers of the "high-effective" as compared to the two control foci showed a significant difference in statistics (after White rank test, $P<0.05$) (Table 3).

The above results suggest that the "high-effective foci", as an acupoint in its original sense, have more large fibers and more large Group II fibers in their afferent fiber composition in comparison with the two other controls.

(IV) The numerical ratio of myelinated fibers to nonmyelinated fibers at point "Zusanli" in relation to acupuncture analgesia.

In the present study, the preparations were examined in 9 animals in which the efferent fibers had degenerated completely and which showed typical reactions to acupuncture analgesia. The marked location of the stimulated points, the number of intramuscular nerve fasciculi in them and the number of nerve fibers contained in these fasciculi all resembled those seen in the studies of caliber spectra of afferent fibers described above. Under higher magnification, the myelinated and nonmyelinated fibers in the fasciculi could easily be distinguished. The axons of the myelinated fibers were usually thicker and stained brown or dark brown and a colorless "halo" could be seen around them. Those of the nonmyelinated ones were thinner and stained black. Most of the non-myelinated fibers were bunched in small bundles and situated in the interstices between the myelinated fibers, though some of them were dispersed. The cross sections of nonmyelinated fibers appeared as small black dots, and there was no "halo" around them (Fig. 4).

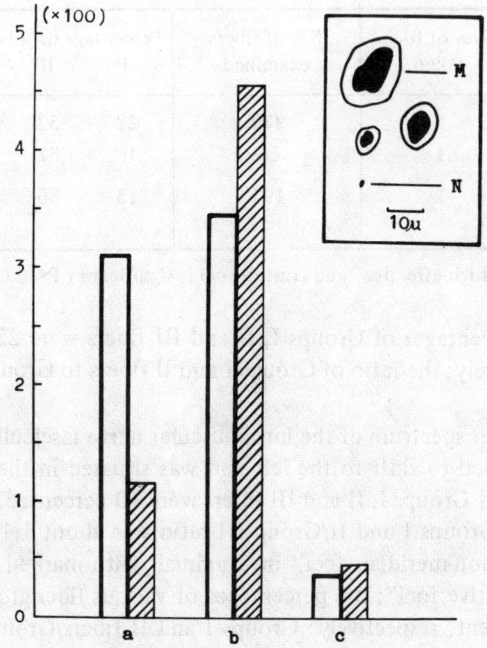

Fig. 4 Myelinated and non-myelinated fiber ratio in "high-effective" (a), "non-effective" (b) and "non-channel" (c) foci.

Ordinate: Mean values of myelinated (open bar) and nonmyelinated (shaded bar) fibers in each focus. The inset represents the appearance under a microscope of myelinated (M) and nonmyelinated (N) fibers stained with silver nitrate. Plotted from photograph No. 58 of cat No. 7.

Table 4. Numerical ratio of myelinated afferent fibers to nonmyelinated fibers in "high-effective" and control foci (including both "non-effective" and "non-channel" foci)

	No. of foci removed	No. of fibers examined	% of myelinated fibers	% of non-myelinated fibers	myelinated* / nonmeylinated
High-effective foci	5	2,127	73	27	2.7
Non-effective foci	2	1,599	44	56	0.8
Non-meridian foci	7	1,771	45	55	0.8

* The difference between "high-effective" and control foci is significant (P <0.01).

The total number of myelinated afferent fibers in the "high-effective foci" of 5 animals was 1550, and that of nonmeylinated ones was 577; thus the ratio of myelinated to nonmyelinated fibers was 2.7:1 (Fig. 4, Table 4). In two "non-effective foci", the total number of myelinated fibers was 690, and that of nonmyelinated fibers 909; thus the ratio of the two was 0.8:1. In 5 "non-effective foci" of the effective animals for analgesia, the total number of myelinated fibers was 640, and that of nonmyelinated ones 860; hence the ratio of the two was 0.7:1. In two "non-channel foci" of ineffective animals, the relevant values were 125, 146 and 0.8:1, respectively (Fig. 4, Table 4). The mean values of the ratio of myelinated to nonmyelinated fibers in "high-effective" as opposed to control foci showed a significant difference statistically (after White rank test, $P<0.01$) (Table 4).

Obviously the "high-effective foci", as meridian points, contain much moere myelinated fibers than nonmyelinated ones as compared with the control foci, i.e., "non-effective" and "non-channel" foci.

III. Discussion

The different analgesic effects produced by "Zusanli" and "Quchi" in regard to pain response induced by peroneal nerve stimulation may obviously be explained in terms of variations in segmental innervation, while the different effects shown by "Zusanli" and its neighbor point "non-channel focus" may perhaps be ascribed to the difference in location between them, for both of them belong to the same segment. We thus deemed it advisable to determine the properties of their constituents and compare the activity of their innervation.

It can be readily seen from the results that more large fibers and more Group II fibers are activated only when the "high-effective foci" are being stimulated. The velocity spectrum of afferent fibers induced by "high-effective focus" stimulation was manifestly different from that of the controls in the various respects: the distribution pattern, peak position and afferent fiber number. Most of the afferent fibers activated by "high-effective focus" stimulation are concentrated in the Group II fiber area; the number of Groups I and II fibers is 3.1 times that of Group III fibers, and over two thirds of the total number of myelinated afferent fibers are Group II fibers. In contrast, the velocity spectrum induced by stimulation of "non-effective" and "non-channel" foci is roughly the same in all aspects. Most of the fibers are situated around the Group III fiber area; the ratio of Groups I and II to Group III drops to 1.16 and 1.61, respectively, and the number of Group II and Group III fibers is almost equal. If the velocity spectrum data obtained from the individual points on relevant muscles, regardless of whether these points are "high-effective", "non-effective" or "non-channel" foci, are compared with those obtained from the muscle nerve trunks of a cat's soleus muscle and medial gastrocnemius muscle and with the diameter spectra of the proximal branch of m. tibialis anterior[9–14], it may be seen that the positions of the first peak of the two control foci are closely similar to those of the muscle nerve (4–6μm), except that the second peak shifts slightly to the left (10–12μm). On the other hand, the velocity spectrum of "high-effective foci" is obviously different from that of the muscle nerve; all the two peaks are situated within the area of Group II fibers (7–8μm and 11–12μm).

Similar to the findings of velocity spectrum, the distribution pattern, numerical relation and mean diameter of the afferent fibers in "high-effective foci" also manifestly differ from those in the two control foci. In "high-effective foci", the number of Groups I and II fibers is almost three times that of Group III fibers; and the number of Group II fibers makes up more than half of the total number of myelinated fibers. On the other hand, the diameter spectrum from "non-effective" and "non-channel" foci is alike in many respects: the number of Groups I and II fibers is almost the same as that of Group III fibers, and the proportion of Group II fibers is only about one third of the total. If diameter spectrum data from these three individual points within m. extensor digitorum common is compared with those of the relevant muscle (including m. extensor digitorum common mentioned above) nerve trunk, it will also be seen that the distribution pattern of the spectrum from both "non-effective" and "non-channel" foci is essentially similar to that from the muscle nerve trunk, in that it also shows a three-peak distribution pattern with a somewhat higher first peak; while that from "high-effective foci" shows its highest peak in the middle and the percentage of Group II fibers is larger, though three peaks also appear.

It is obvious that the findings of the diameter spectrum of these three foci are roughly similar to those of their velocity spectrum in all the principal respects. This seems to indicate that the distribution pattern of the velocity spectrum of afferent fibers is closely related to their natural local composition. As for the presence of some differences between the two kinds of spectra, these may be explained by the fact that caliber spectrum data is obtained solely from the intramuscular nerve fasciculi at the relevant points, whereas velocity spectrum data may not only be limited to the action of intramuscular nerve fasciculi, but may also include, in addition, the activities of the nerve branches, the nerve endings and the

Table 5. Comparison of the myelinated to nonmyelinated fiber ratios* in the whole trunk of muscle nerve and the intramuscular nerve fasciculi of some points within relevant muscles.

Authors	Microscope	Region studied			Findings
Ranson & Davenport (1931)	light	Nerve trunks of vastus medialis of m. quadriceps femoris			1:1
Landon & Preston (1963)	electron	Nerve trunks of vastus medialis of gastrocnemius			1:1
Stacey (1969)	electron	Nerve trunks of m. tibialis posterior			0.5:1
Lu et al. (1979)	light	Within m. extensor digitorum comon (or m. tibialis anterior)	Non-meridian foci	Intramuscular nerve fasciculi	0.8:1
			Non-effective foci		0.8:1
			High-effective foci		2.7:1

* Note: Since no sympathectomy was done in the present work, postganglionic sympathectic fibers may be included in the non-myelinated fibers listed here, but their quantity in the "high-effective", "non-effective" and "non-channel" foci can be regarded as an equal constant and ignored.

various sensory apparatus located in the vicinity of the effective electrode.

Fairly consistent results were also obtained in the study of myelinated/nonmyelinated ratio. Similar to the two kinds of spectra, the ratio in "high-effective foci" is also considerably different from that in both "non-effective" and "non-channel" foci, the number of myelinated fibers being 2.7 times that of nonmyelinated ones. There is no difference, however, in the ratio between the two control foci, both being below 1:1, which means that the number of nonmyelinated fibers is actually slightly higher than the myelinated ones. If the figures of the myelinated to nonmyelinated fiber ratio in these three points are also compared with those pertaining to the muscle nerve trunks[14–17], some interesting features will be noted (Table 5). It may be seen from Table 5 that the ratio value in the two control foci seen under an ordinary light microscope is somewhat lower than that in the muscle nerve (1:1), but somewhat higher than that in the muscle nerve seen under an electron microscope (0.5:1). On the contrary, the findings in the "high-effective foci" differ considerably from those in the muscle nerve, the myelinated/ nonmyelinated ratio in them (2.7:1) being much higher than that in the muscle nerve trunks whether at light or electron microscopelevel. The inevitable conclusion to be drawn from this is that one of the prominent features of the "high-effective focus", as a meridian point, is the predominance of myelinated fibers within it.

It has been shown above that the "non-effective" and the "non-channel" foci are closely similar in several respects. The former, therefore, may be considered as identical to the latter. This may be due to deficiency in precision in regard to the position and direction of needling or the explanation may lie in anatomical variations of point "Zusanli" in different animals. It can be assumed that the composition of afferent fibers is not the same in different parts of a whole muscle, for it has long been known that as the nerve proceeds to its distant end, it not only branches repeatedly but also becomes generally thinner[10, 14], and its composition changes as well[18]. Thus it is not surprising that the innervation of the meridian point, formed in the course of evolution, should be characterized by more myelinated, more large-sized and more Group II fibers.

Proceeding from the above analyses, it can be assumed that, since there are so many similarities between the "non-effective" and "non-channel" foci and the muscle nerve trunks which represent the total innervation of a whole muscle, these two categories of individual points within the muscle are able to represent the general properties of the muscle, so their numbers must be proportionately high. On the other hand, the tremendous difference between the "high-effective foci" and the muscle nerve trunks can only be considered as a specific property. In other words, the "high-effective foci" regarded as actual acupoints are only individual points within the relevant muscle. This situation corresponds with the numerical relationship between the non-channel and channel points in the body, i.e., more of the former and less of the latter.

The findings and analysis described above naturally raise a question of methodology in acupoint research. As stated above, the existence of such outstanding differencies between the three points in both the activity and composition of their afferent fibers would make it difficult to obtain stable and reliable results in acupoint research, if the acupoint is merely localized according to its surface position. The present study would seem to denote that efficiency for acupuncture analgesia may serve as a useful reference criterion for determining the coordinate of acupoints in animals, provided the animal's general condition is basically normal. In this sense, the "high-effective focus" in the present study may be regarded as a meridian point in its original sense. This, certainly, does not mean that the selection of other indicators, such as impedance and skin temperature, can be excluded. On the contrary, they are quite useful for the localization and study of acupoints.

IV. SUMMARY

1. "Zusanli" is the only point which has an inhibitory effect on pain response elicited by peroneal nerve stimulation, and no effect can be achieved by needling "Quchi" and "non-channel" points when these three points are being acupunctured in one and the same animal.

2. A "high-effective focus" or a "non-effective focus" and a "non-channel focus" can be distinguished in the area of "Zusanli" and its vicinity by means of analgesic experiments based on anatomical marks.

3. More large fibers and more Group II fibers can largely be activated by electrical stimulation of the "high-effective foci" of "Zusanli", whereas under the same conditions, similar results cannot be achieved by needling the other two foci.

4. More large-sized and more Group II fibers can be distinctly found in the "high-effective foci" in relation to their local afferent fiber composition, while the other two foci do not possess such characteristics.

5. Much more myelinated than nonmyelinated fibers exist in "high-effective foci"; in the other two foci, however, there are slightly less myelinated than nonmyelinated fibers.

6. The main distribution of myelinated, large-sized and Group II fibers in local acupoints and the methodological problem related to the localization of acupoint coordinates are discussed in the text.

REFERENCES

[1] 吕国蔚,梁荣照等: "足三里"针刺镇痛效应的外周传入神经纤维分析。中国科学, 1979, 5: 495—503。1979,5: 495–503.

[2] 吕国蔚,王齐林等: Proc. 5th Annual Symposium on Computer Applications in Medical care, p. 1089, 1981.

[3] Iggo, A.: The electrophysiological identification of single nerve fibers with particular reference to the slower conducting vagal afferent fibers in the cat, *J. Physiol.*, 1958, 142:110–126.

[4] Paintal, A.S.: Intramuscular propagation of sensory impulses, *J. Physiol.*, 1959, **148**: 240–251.

[5] Esplin, D.W.: Independence of conduction velocity among myeliated fibers in cat nerve, *J. Neurophysiol.*, 1962: **25**:805.

[6] Gasby, J.U. et al.: An analogue cross-correlator to study naturally induced activity in intact nerve trunks, *J. Neurophysiol.*, 1963, **26**:432–448.

[7] Fernand, V.S.V. & Young, J.Z.: The size of the nerve fibers of muscle nerves, *Proc. Roy. Soc. Biol.*, 1951, **139**;38–58.

[8] Naoumenko, J. & Feigin, I.: Stable silver solution for axonal staining in paraffin sections, *J. Neuropath. Exp. Neurol.*, 1967, 26: 669–673.

[9] Lloyd, D.P.C.: Neuron patterns controlling transmissions of ipsilateral hind limb reflex in cat, *J. Neurophysiol.*, 1943, **6**: 293–315.

[10] Lloyd, D.P.C. & Chang, H.T.: Afferent fibers in muscle nerves, *J. Neurophysiol.*, 1948, **198–208.**

[11] Rexed, B. & Therman, P.O.: Calibre spectra of motor sensory nerve fibers to flexor and extensor muscles, *J. Neurophysiol.*, 1948, **11**: 133–140.

[12] Hunt, C.C. & McIntyre, A.K.: An analysis of fiber diameter and receptor characteristics of myelinated

cutaneous afferent fibers in cat, *J. Physiol.*, **1960**, **153**: 99–112.
[13] Hagbarth, K.E. & Wohlfart, G.: The number of muscle-spindles in certain muscles in cat in relation to the composition of the muscles nerves, *Acta Anat.* (Basal), 1952, **15**: 85–104.
[14] Barker, D. et al.: *Muscle receptors,* Ed. by Hunt,C,C. 1974, P.173.
[15] Ranson, S.W. & Davenport, H.K.: Sensory unmyelinated fibers in the spinal nerves, *Amer. J. Anat.*, 1931, **48:331.**
[16] Landon, D.N. (ed.): *The peripheral nerve,* Chapman Hall, 1976, p.106.
[17] Stacey, M.J.: Free nerve endings in skeletal muscle of the cat, *J. Anat.*, 1969, **105**: 231.
[18] Sunderland, S.: *Nerves and nerve injuries,* 1968, p.6.

ANALYSIS OF AFFERENT FIBERS TRANSMITTING NEEDLING SIGNALS OF ACUPOINT

Lu Guowei, Zhao Guoshun, Liang Rongzhao,
Wang Yongning, Xing Weichang, Shi Guang
(Laboratory of Acupuncture Anesthesia and Encephalology, Beijing Second Medical College, Beijing)
(Acupuncture Anesthesia Group, Beijing Jishuitan Hospital, Beijing)

The previous work showed that the component of afferent fibers at an acupoint and the conduction of acupuncture analgesic signals are correlated mainly with large fibers, especially with Group II or $A_{\beta\gamma}$ fibers[1−2]. The effect of acupuncture analgesia is closely correlated with needling sensation in clinical practice. In order to acquaint ourselves with the peripheral process of needling sensation in normal persons and clinical cases, we compared the time relationship between the change of needling sensation at acupoints and the changes of tactual, positional, pain, and thermal sensations and of nervous electric reaction, etc. By obstructing the activities of the fine fibers at an acupoint with dilute novocaine, we observed the influence on needling sensation and acupuncture anesthesia effectiveness so as to find out the main afferent fibers which conduct the acupoint sensory impulses.

I. METHODS

The following three investigations were carried out in the present work:

(I) Comparing the relationship between the changes of needling sensation and the changes of deep and superficial sensations

(1) Arm tourniquet compression affecting large fibers preferentially. The left arm of the subject was compressed by a tourniquet whose pressure was higher than the systolic pressure by 40 mm Hg, in order to elicit a sensory variation as soon as the large fibers were affected. The time and order of the disappearance of the needling sensation were compared with those of other related sensations mentioned above.

25 cases of normal persons of about 25 years of age took part in the experiment. They were divided into two groups, the electric needling group and the manual needling one. There were 15 cases in the former and 10 cases in the latter. After tourniquet compression, the sensations mentioned above were examined separately at intervals of 10, 20, and 30 min in the manual needling group and of 10 min in the other group. The pre- and postcontrol observations were carried out before compression and after decompression, respectively.

The following methods were used in the examination of the various sensations:

a. The needling sensation in an acupoint: An acupuncture needle was inserted into point "Hegu" and appropriate needling sensation was elicited by manual manipulation or by electro-stimulation. Bei Hang 57–6 model electrostimulator was used for electro-stimulation with a frequency of 90 c/min and the voltage applied was recorded as the threshold of needling sensation.

b. The deep pain sensation: Its threshold in point "Hegu" was measured by a Type 626 pain threshold testor with an acupuncture needle inserted there as the stimutating electrode and a saline gauze over area "Waiguan" as a reference one.

c. The superficial pain: Its presence and disappearance were tested by a slight prick on the skin over area "Hegu".

d. The cold sensation: This was measured by a glass tube containing ice water at 0°C.

e. The tactual sensation: The skin over point "Hegu" was gently touched by a piece of cotton wool to check the presence of this sensation.

f. The position sensation: The fourth finger of the left hand of the subject was moved about for making out whether his evaluation of the direction of the movement is correct or not.

(2) Epidural and spinal anesthesia affecting small fibers preferentially: We compared the time and order of the variation of the needling sensation in acupoints (including "Guaumen", "Piguan" or "Zusanli") with those sensations related with the above.

29 cases of patients under epidural or spinal anesthesia took part in the experiment. They were also divided into two groups: the electric needling group and the manual needling group. After a catheter was inserted into the epidural space, the indices related to sensations were first examined, and the local anesthetic, Lidocaine, was injected immediately; relevant sensations were then tested at intervals of 5 min according to the methods mentioned above.

(II) Comparing the needle feeling level in acupoints with the electric response of the related nerve.

The subjects selected for the experiment were 13 cases of normal adults of about 23–25 years old. The experiment was done in room temperature of 18°C and the arm skin temperature was kept at 32°C.

In the course of the experiment, the subjects were in a sitting posture. Before the experiment, the skin of the left forearm was cleansed by a 75% alcohol solution. The subject's elbow was stimulated by a single square pulse, through a pair of silver electrode (ϕ 1cm), to find out the motor point of the median nerve and the electrodes were placed there for recording. The needle inserted into point "Neiguan" in the same side was taken as the effective stimulating electrode, and a copper plate (6×4 cm^2) applied on the back of the forearm was used as the reference electrode (Fig. 1).

In experimentation, (1) first, the "Neiguan" point was stimulated by square pulse of 0.03 msec duration at 4 Hz, making the subject feel only a slight needling sensation with relative low strength; (2) the relatively strong "adequate needling sensation" was then evoked by increasing the intensity of the stimulation; (3) finally, a stronger stimulation was delivered for eliciting a strong needling sensation accompanied with pain sensation.

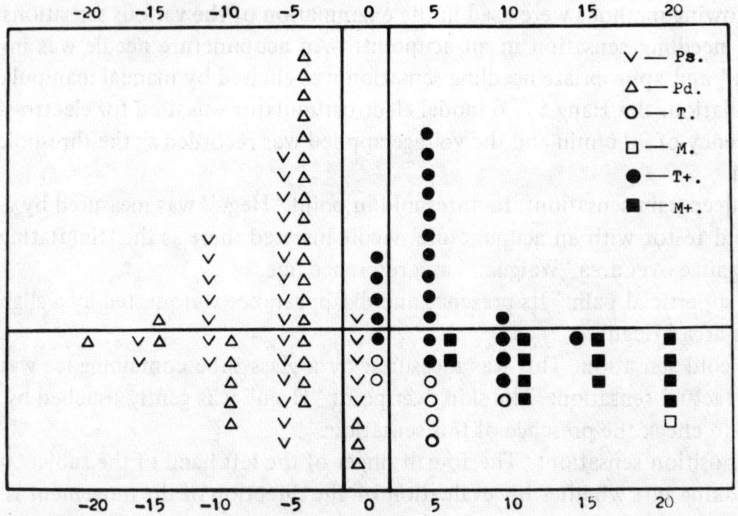

Fig. 1 Relative time of the disappearance of needing sensation and other related sevsations in the course of epidural anaesthesia (Taking the time of the vanishing of needling sensation as zero).

The upper position of the figure is the electric needling group (15) cases ; and the lower position is the manual needling group (14 cases).

V --- Ps. Superficial pain; Δ---Pd. deep pain; □---M. position sensation; ○---T. tactile; ●---T+. unvanishing tactile; ■---M. unvanishing position sensation abscissa represent time of vanishing.

The nature, degree, location and conduction direction of the needling feeling in each level were recorded separately at the same time. The electric reaction of the median nerve was induced and fed into an amplifier, and averaged by a TQ-19 model medical data processor for 256 times at 20 and 200μsec, and its wave form, amplitude, duration and latency were recorded. According to the latency and conduction distance from the effective electrode to the distant recording electrode, the conduction velocity of compound action potential was counted. In order to display the slow action potential, the signal was averaged usually to 512 times, even to 1024 times at 200μsec unit time.

(III) Comparing the change of needling feeling with the change of pain threshold following the blocking of local anesthetic in an acupoint

The work was carried out on normal persons and on surgical patients under acupuncture anesthesia. The observations were as follows:

(1) Observation of needling feeling: The change of needling sensation was observed before and after the injection of 0.1% novocaine into acupoints. The subjects in the experiment were 22 cases of students (the point examined was "Hegu") and 40 cases of patients of tubal ligation ("Sanyinjiao" point was used). The nature and degree of needling feeling and tolerance to electric current were recorded separately before and after injection of local anesthetics.

(2) Observation of analgesic effect: 22 cases of students mentioned above taken as subjects were divided into experimental and control groups. The influence of drug injection on pain threshold of the skin over "Hegu" point was compared according to the methods of cross design and "three blind".

(3) Observation of acupuncture anesthetic efficacy: The subjects in the experiment were patients operated on for abdominal tubal ligation, caesarean section, cystotomia urinae, herniaplasty and nephrectomy. No choice in the patients, surgeons and anesthetists was made. The patients were divided at random into test (120 cases) and control (74 cases) groups. Their clinical effectiveness was compared under identical conditions.

The practical procedure of local anesthetic blocking was as follows: After the acupoint was punctured by needle (gauge 5) and needling feeling appeared, 1 ml (into "Hegu") or 3–5 ml (into "Sanyinjiao") of 0.1% novocaine and 0.1% dicaine were injected there. An electric acupuncture current was then turned on and the acupoint was stimulated. In normal persons, the stimulation freguency was 196 c/min and the intensity was 17 mV. In patients, the frequency was 1200–1800 c/min and the intensity of stimulus was gauged by the patients' tolerability.

Needling sensation was described by the subjects' verbal report. Pain threshold was measured by a self-made 626 model pain threshold testor. In experimentation, the effective electrode (ϕ1cm) was placed on the skin over point "Neiguan," and the referance electrode (5×5 cm^2) was put on the skin over "Waiguan" point in the same side of the forearm. The current value by which stabbing pain could just be induced was determined as the pain threshold. The efficacy of acupuncture anesthesia was evaluated in accordance with the national unified criteria.

II. RESULTS

(I) The variation of needling feeling of "Hegu" point and other related sensations in the course of arm tourniquet compression

In 15 cases of the electro-needling group, after the arm was compressed by the tourniquet, the average time of the disappearance of deep pain, superficial pain and cold

Table 1. The average threshold of needling feeling and pain sensation in 15 cases of electro-needling group

	Pre-control		After tourniquet compression				Postcontrol	
Time (min)	0	10	0	10	20	30	0	10
Needling sensation threshold (V)	2.4	2.4	2.5	2.8	4.1*	10.4*	4.2	3.1
Pain threshold (mA)	0.96	0.93	0.96	0.82	0.95	0.84	1.26	0.69

*$P < 0.05$ in comparison with pre-control, after sign test.

sensation in area "Hegu" was 32, 29.5 and 26.5 min, respectively, and that of position sensation in the fourth finger and cutaneous tactile sensation in "Hegu" area was separately 25 and 24.5 min. The average time of the disappearance of electro-needling feeling of "Hegu" point was 23.5 min. No obvious alteration of deep pain threshold could be seen in the course of compression for 30 min, while the threshold of electro-needling feeling rose markedly at the 20th min and 30th min and was conspicuously different from that before compression ($P < 0.05$) (Table 1).

The variation in manual needling sensation was similar to that of electro-needling feeling, though the time of the disappearance of manual needling feeling was somewhat scattered. Except that the time of the vanishing of deep pain was significantly longer than that of other sensations ($P < 0.01$), there was no difference between them.

(II) The variation of the needling sensation and other related sensations in the course of epidural anesthesia

During the course of epidural anesthesia, both deep and superficial pain disappeared first in all cases. The time of the vanishing of tactual and position sensations were later than that of deep and superficial pain in all 29 cases. The time of the vanishing of position sensation was markedly later than that of the tactile in 8 out of 14 cases, and in the other 6 cases the position sensation did not disappear together with tactile sensation during the course of observation. Most of the needling sensation dropped off or disappeared after the pain sensation vanished, but it did not vanish in some persons during observation. Taking the time of the vanishing of electro-needling feeling as the standard, the time of the vanishing of other sensations was compared with that of the needling one (Fig. 1, upper part). In 29 cases, excepting 5 and 3 cases whose needling feeling disappeared simultaneously with superficial and deep pain, respectively, the time of the vanishing of the needling sensation in 24 and 26 cases was, respectively, obviously later than that of superficial and deep pain. On the other hand, needling feeling disappeared earlier than that of tactile and position sensation in most of the 29 cases, excepting a few cases whose needling feeling vanished together with superficial and deep sensations. As stated above, the time of the disappearance of the electro-needling sensation was usually later than deep and superficial pain and earlier than touch and position sensation. The difference among them was significant ($P < 0.01$).

Taking the time of the vanishing of manual needling feeling as criterion in comparison (Fig. 1, lower part), the time of the disappearance of manual needling sensation was scattered, but it was also generally later than deep and superficial pain, earlier or close to that of the touch and position sensation.

(III) The variation of the needling sensation and other related sensations in the course of spinal anesthesia

In 40 cases under spinal anesthesia, the superficial and deep pain, manual needling sensation, slight tactile and position sensations also disappeared in the same order as in epidural anesthesia, their average values being 3.4, 3.8, 8.1, 10.9 and 25.9 min, respectively (Table 2).

Table 2. The time of the disappearance of needling sensation and related sensations during spinal anesthesia

	Superficial pain	Deep pain	Needling feeling	Tactile sensation	Position sensation
mean + S.E.	3.4 ± 0.5	3.8 ± 0.7	8.1 ± 1.6	10.9 ± 2.2	25.9 ± 5.8
P		>0.05	<0.01	>0.05	<0.01

Except superficial pain, a few of the other four sensations did not vanish in the course of observation (one case each of deep pain and manual needling sensation; slight tactile, 2 cases; and position sensation, 11 cases.). It is easy to see that the needling feeling disappears between superficial and deep pain and tactual and position sensation, and it is even near to the latter. The difference between them was significant in statistics ($P < 0.05$).

(IV) The accompanying change of electric activity in median nerves during the variation of needling feelings in "Neiguan"

When electric needling of the "Neiguan" point caused a slight needling feeling (including slight numbness, distension or heaviness and heat in the local portion of the acupoint, as well as a slight "scurry" sense directed to the thumb, middle or index finger), a compound action potential with lower amplitude and a conduction velocity of 76.4 m/sec could be recorded in half of the subjects. Its wave presented a positive-negative biphasic form; sometimes there also appeared a positive-negative-positive (triphasic) or monophasic one. No visible slow action potentials were recorded in all subjects with "slight needling feeling" (Table 3).

When electric needling of the "Neiguan" point induced an adequate needling sensation (a stronger feeling of numbness, distension or heaviness and heat conducting towards fingertips without any pain or unbearable sensations), the electric reaction with an average conduction velocity of 73.7 m/sec could be recorded by the electrodes placed on the cutaneous surface of the median nerve at the elbow in all subjects. The form of the action potential was biphasic, triphasic or monophasic (Fig. 2, Table 3). No slow action potential was recorded in these subjects. In one-third of the examinees, action potential with conduction velocity of 45.3 m/sec could also be recorded.

Table 3. The average value of compound potential in the median nerve during slight and adequate needling sensation

	Latency (msec)	Amplitude (μV)	Duration (msec)	Conduction velocity (m/sec)
Slight needling feeling	3.05	28.4	1.61	76.4
Adequate needling feeling	3.13	53.8	1.82	73.7

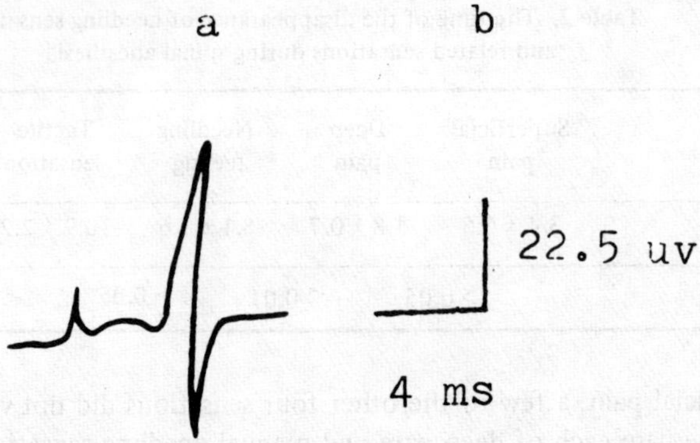

Fig. 2 Compound action potential in median nerve at the level of appropriate needling feeling.

With the increment of the strength of electric needling, a strong "needling sensation" of unbearable pain was produced, and a slow action potential with conduction velocity less than 36 m/sec could be recorded occasionally. In 5 out of 12 cases the action potentials of lower amplitude were recorded for 6 times, their conduction velocity being 36.8, 14.5, 10.7, 7.8, 4.6 and 1.8 m/sec, in monophasic or biphasic form.

(V) The variation of needling sensation, pain threshold and acupunctural analgesic effect following the blocking of acupoints with dilute local anesthetic

(1) The effect of acupoint blocks on needling sensations:

Before blocking, the complaints of needling sensation were generally a feeling of soreness, numbness, distension and heaviness. When an acupoint was injected with dilute novocaine, the degree of the needling sensation diminished and its nature became gentle under identical stimulation parameters as that without blocking. With the increase of the stimulation intensity, a rather strong needling sensation could occur but was not accompanied by unbearable pain. The strength of stimulation which could be tolerated was 0.5–1.0 time greater than that before injection and this strength was unbearable for the control group whose acupoint was injected with normal saline.

(2) The effect of acupoint blocks on the pain threshold of the skin:

As shown in Fig. 3, in the test group whose acupoint was infiltrated with 0.1% novocaine in advance, the pain threshold on the skin of ipsilateral arm tended to rise instantly after the needle was inserted and the current through the needle was turned on. After turning on the current for 30 and 40 min, the threshold was significantly increased as compared with the value before needling ($P < 0.05$). On the contrary, in a control group blocked by saline, the threshold rose insignificantly for a short duration of about 20–30 min after needling, then dropped gradually and returned to the same level as that before acupuncture about 50 min after needling (Fig. 3). It may be seen that the increment of pain threshold in the test group was not only faster and more notable, but also more lasting.

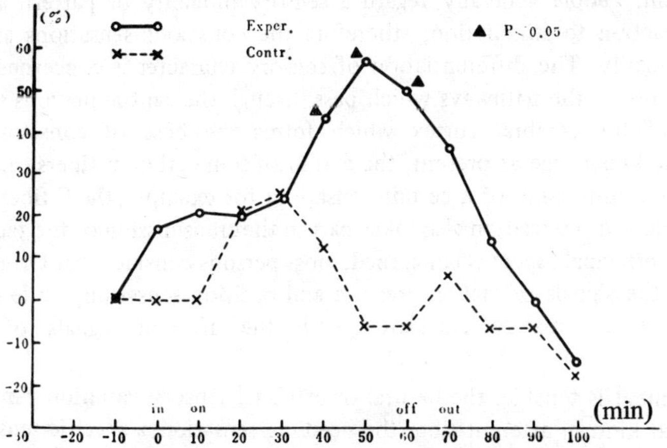

Fig. 3 Effect of local anesthetic block in point "Hegu" on pain threshold of the skin of ipsilateral forearm.

Ordinate: Percentage of change of pain threshold, Abscissa: Relative time scale, taking the inserting time as zero; "in", "on", "of" and "out" indicate respectively the instant time of inserting of the needle, turning on and turning out the electric current through the needle, and drawing the needle out.
o — o: Experimental group; X---X: Coutrol group.
△: P<0.05 in comparison with pre-control value.

(3) The influence of acupoint blocks on acupunctural analgesic efficiency:

In clinical practice, the rate of success of acupuncture anesthesia of the group blocked by novocaine and the control group was, respectively, 95.3% and 94.4%, and there was no marked difference between them; But the rate of excellence of these two groups was very different: it was 80.8% in the former and 50% in the latter; the rate was raised by 30.9% as compared with that of the control ($P < 0.01$) (Table 4).

Table 4. The influence of the blocking of an acupoint on acupuncture anesthesia efficiency

	Total cases	Average operation duration(min)	Excellent	Good	Fair	Failure	Excellent & good rate (%)
Control group	74	46	8	29	33	4	50.0
Experimental group	120	46	12	85	18	5	80.9

III. DISCUSSION

(I) The relationship between sensory modality and sensory afferent fibers

The study of needling sensation belongs to the category of that of sensory physiology.

In sensory physiology, the relationship of sensory modality with sensory afferent fibers is a complex problem. People generally regard a sensory modality or pattern as a subjective characteristic reaction to stimulation; therefore the conscious sensations are different in character or modality. The differentiation of sensory character is concerned with sensory organs, afferent fibers, the pathways which pass through the central nervous system and the final neurons of the cerebral cortex which forms the base of conscious experience. According to the knowledge at present, the action of some afferent fibers cannot be simply identified by the transmission of a certain sensation; for example, the C fiber which mainly transmits pain and warm sensation also takes part in the transmission of the tactile signal[3]. But so far as the principal aspect is concerned, most persons consider that Group II fibers are correlated with the signals of tactile, pressure and position sensation, while Group III and Group IV fibers are mainly correlated with the afferent signals of pain-thermal sensations[4].

If this argument is tenable, the natural or artificial sensory variation can be utilized to find out by what kind of afferent fiber the needling sensation, a specific sensory pattern, is transmitted.

(II) The variation of sensory pattern and the afferent fiber of needling sensation

The experimental results of the present work show that the sensory variation elicited by arm tourniquet compression is contrary to that elicited by epidural or spinal anesthesia in the order of the appearance of sensory variation, but the variation of electro-needling sensation appeared between the appearance of pain-thermal sensation (or tactile-position sensation) variation and tactile-position sensation (or pain-thermal sensation) variation. It is nearer to that of tactile and position sensation. This indicates that the diameter of the afferent fibers transmitting electro-needling sensation belongs chiefly to Group II and Group III fibers, the number of the former being much more than the latter. A change of the manual needling sensation also appears between that of pain-thermal sensation and tactile-position sensation, but its distribution is more dispersive. This may be correlated with the strength of manual acupuncture. When the strength of manual acupuncture is weak, Group II fibers are excited mainly, but when the strength is strong, besides Group II fibers, Group III fibers are also excited.

(III) The component of needling sensation and the sensory afferent fibers

As each kind of sensation generally has its own conductive fibers, this argument may probably be right, so we used the method by Collins, et al.[5] to compare directly the relationship of subjective complaints with the evoked nervous action potential in our study.

The needling sensation is generally described as the feeling of soreness, numbness, distension, and heaviness. We consider that, as the studies and their results about needling sensation in the present study are quite different, so we take the stronger sensation, which does not accompany pain but elicits soreness, numbness, distension, heaviness, etc., as an adequate or actual needling sensation.

During an experiment, when the examinee experiences an adequate and suitable needling sensation, nervous action potentials of 73.7m/sec velocity can be recorded. Seeing that the threshold of the electric stimulation of the afferent fiber is lower than that of the efferent fiber[6,7], the component of high conductive velocity recorded in our study may be an antidromic action potential of the efferent fiber. But the action of the afferent fiber caused by real needling sensation may appear after that potential. It is the portion of slower conduction velocity, which corresponds to the portion of Group II fibers. And as the slower potential had not been recorded in the level of "slight" and "adequate" needling sensation, it can be said that the component of needling sensation of soreness, distension, heaviness and numbness is transmitted mainly by Group II fibers.

When the needling sensation exceeded the general level, and became unbearable and accompanied with pain, the recorded slower potential which wasn't recorded in "slight" and "adequate" needling sensation, appeared similar to the electric reaction potential of Group III and even Group IV fibers.

This result conforms to the opinion that one would feel no pain if only the large fibers are stimulated[5], and that the pain is transmitted by small fibers[8]——which is the result obtained by direct recording of electric reaction potential from human nerves. The result shows that, when the needling sensation is unbearable and accompanies pain, the small fibers take part in the action, and the small fibers are not so important as the large fibers in the effect for conduction of the needling sensation of general soreness, distension, heaviness and numbness, etc.

(IV) The needling sensation at the acupoint blocked by local anesthetic

Result (V) shows that, after the acupoint was blocked by a local anesthetic of lower concentration, the needling sensation elicited by identical stimulating strength became rather gentle in its character, and often drops off by degrees. This may be correlated with the blockage of another component (Group III fibers) which transmits needling sensation. As the strength of stimulation is increased further, the needling sensation may recover and even surpass the original level but it may not elicit pain and other uncomfortable sensations which may occur before the blocking. This result indicates further that the rather gentle and adequate needling sensation is in close relationship with the action of Group II fibers; but the action of Group III fibers is correlated with the painful and unbearable components of needling sensations.

(V) The needling sensation of an acupoint and the effect of acupuncture

Clinical practice shows that good needling sensation generally is conditional to good efficacy in acupuncture analgesia and therapeutic treatment. The fact that the pain threshold and analgesic effect can be elevated by blocking an acupoint, may correlate with the maintaining or even enhancing of the needling sensation by strong stimulation. This coincides with the observation that the effect of acupuncture anesthesia may be improved by blocking the acupoint in an animal experiment, and the analgesic effect enhanced by strong stimulation after blocking the nerve trunk with local anesthetic[1]. This result indicates that the signal of needling sensation and that of acupuncture analgesia are virtually of the same kind; both of them are transmitted by Groups II and III fibers, most of them being Group II fibers.

This opinion is in keeping with the report that small fibers are inhibited by large fibers [8,9] as well as with the report of the mechanism of acupuncture anesthesia by inference reported at home and abroad[11,12].

It should be noted here that in our present experiment we blocked the acupoints with a local anesthetic far away from the operative area or the area for testing the pain threshold in order to simplify the theoretical analysis. But in actual application, the blocking can be applied at the point near the operative area, so that, not only the conduction of the small fibers in the operative area can be blocked to attain local anesthesia partially, but also the action of the large afferent fibers can be augmented and the effect of acupuncture analgesia therefore will be much better. We have made some trial observations, the results demonstrating that it really has a better effect.

IV. SUMMARY

This article analyzes and discusses the time relationship of the afferent fibers between the variation of the needling sensation at an acupoint and the variation of deep and superficial sensation and of accompanying nervous action potentials.

The results show that:

(1) The volleys of electro- and manual-needling sensations are carried mainly by Group II fibers and partially by Group III fibers.

(2) The subjective complaints of appropriate needling sensation are correlated with the electric activity of the large fibers.

(3) Increasing the activity of the large fibers and/or decreasing the action of the small ones contribute to higher efficiency of acupuncture analgesia.

REFERENCES

[1] Lu Guowei et al.: Role of peripheral afferent nerve fibers in acupuncture analgesia elicited by needling point Zusanli, *Scientia Sinica*, 1979, 6: 680–692.

[2] Lu Guowei et al.: The composition of afferent fibers at point "Zusanli" in relation to acupuncture analgesia, In this issue.

[3] Douglas, W.W. et al.: Non-medullated fibers in the saphenous nerve which signal touch, *J. Physiol.*, **139**: 383–399, 1957.

[4] Brobeck, J.R.: Physiological basis of medical practice ed. 19, p. 74, Williams and Wilkins, Baltimore, 1973.

[5] Collins, Jr.W.F. et al.: Relation of peripheral nerve fiber size and sensation in man, *Archs. Neural.* (Chicago), 3: 381–385, 1960.

[6] Kugelberg, E.: Accommodation in human nerves, *Acta Physiol. Scand.*, 8(24) Suppl., 46–51,1944.

[7] Sunderland, S.S.: Nervous and nerve injuries, p. 191, Livingstone, Edinburgh, 1972.

[8] Schmidt, R.F.: Fundamentals of neurophysiology, ed. 3, p. 62, Springer, Berlin, 1975.

[9] 中島英亲等: 针麻醉效果のメカニズムに対する推論。麻醉 **23**: 448—54, 1974。
23: 448–54, 1974.

[10] Holmgern, E.: Increase of pain threshold as a function of conditioning electrical stimulation, Am. J. Chin. Med., 3: 133–42, 1975.

[11] Li C.L.: Neurological basis of pain and its possible relationship to acupuncture analgesia, *Am. J. Chin. Med.,* 1:61–72, 1973.
[12] 久场襄：ハリ麻醉，克诚堂出版株式会社，东京，1974。

AN ANALYTICAL STUDY OF THE AFFERENT FIBRES FOR IMPULSES OF ACUPUNCTURE ANALGESIA

Chen Longshun, Tang Jingshi, Fan Li
Wang Kemo, Yan Jianqun
(Acupuncture Anesthesia Mechanism Research Laboratory (Director: Professer C. L. Hou), Xian Medical College, Xian)

Acupuncture has been experimentally shown to be able to excite various types of fibres[1,2]. However, opinions differ as to which type of fibre is responsible for the conveyance of analgesic impulses. While some consider that large-sized fibres are connected with analgesia[3,4], more insist that with the participation of type III fibres, the analgesic effects will be better[5,6]. As far as the role of type IV fibres in the action of analgesia is concerned, some authors take a negative attitude, but their findings are found to be inadequate[3,7].

In this study, pain stimulations were exerted on the somatic nerves to elicit reflex movements of the lower jaw and the reactions of the vascular movement; they were taken as objective indices of the two different kinds of pain responses. The stimulation strength was increased progressively so as to be able to excite different types of fibres in turn; in the meantime, the anode-blocking method was used to block all types of fibres in a successive way, and analgesic effects in them were evaluated from type to type. It was our purpose to find out which types of afferent fibres play the main role in acupuncture analgesia.

I. METHODS

Rabbits, with an average body weight of 2.5 kg or so, both female and male, were used for experiments when awake. One of the animals was placed with its head fixed, but its lower jaw allowed to make free movements, the waves of which, through the transducer, were imported into an oscillograph and displayed. The peroneal nerve in the hind-limb was exposed, with its neighboring nerves cut off. An oil trough was set up. On the peroneal nerve (from its distal to proximal ends) were placed an electrode of electric needling, an Ag-AgCl electrode, a recording electrode and an electrode of pain stimulation. Electrodes of electric needling and pain stimulation were connected separately with the stimulators through the isolators, while the recording electrode was attached to an oscillograph to display action potentials through a pre-amplifier. During the operation, the subcutaneous and muscular layers were soaked with a bit of 1% novocaine. The experiment usually started one to two hours after the operation when the animal was rather steady.

The pain stimulations used were of single square-wave, 0.3 msec pulse duration; their intensity was just strong enough to excite A_δ wave or C wave and to elicit the steady movement of the lower jaw. Pain stimulations proceeded at the interval of 2'30". Electric pulses from the electrodes of electric needling with the speed of 5 times per second and the pulse duration of 0.2 msec were applied successively to stimulate those peroneal nerves innervating "Zusanli" point. Analgesic effects occurring in the various types of fibres were observed after different intensities of stimulation were given for 15 minutes to fibres of types I, II, types I, II, III and types I, II, III, IV, respectively, simulating the stimulation of electric needling. While the anode-direct current passed through the Ag-AgCl electrode, the current intensity was scrupulously regulated to block the action of types I and II fibres, or types I, II, III fibres and the analgesic effects produced by exciting the fibres of type III or type IV and types III, IV were then observed. All the changing patterns of action potentials were displayed on an oscillograph for taking photographic recordings, and were put into one TQ-19 medical computer to monitor their changes. Each experiment consisted of 3 phases: (i) control, (ii) needling, and (iii) withdrawal of the needle; but the number of experiments differed from animal to animal.

II. RESULTS

(I) Characteristics of the reflex movement of the lower jaw[8]

After pain stimulation was applied to the rabbits which were awake, there invariably appeared the reflex movements of the lower jaw with regularity, which presented a compound, multi-directional form of waves. Their latency period averaged 200 msec, the duration ranged from 400 to 600 msec, and the mean amplitude was 40mV. At the same time, repeated stimulations were applied to check whether there was any effect of adaptation and the effect of morphine and so on, thereby to verify the pain responses. The results have shown that in the course of 1–2 hours, no adaptation phenomenon was seen with regard to the movements of the lower jaw. However, after injecting morphine with the dosage of 4 mg/kg, the reflex responses were inhibited, which persisted for 100 minutes or even longer, and subsequently the preinjection level of responses was gradually restored.

(II) Analgesic effects of acupuncture on the reflex movements of the lower jaw[8]

Among 23 animals in a series of 90 experiments, needling was shown to have analgesic effects of different degrees on the reflex movements of the lower jaw (Fig. 1).

Analgesic effects on the reflex movements of the lower jaw were classified into four grades, according to the percentage of wave-amplitude changes. Grade I (complete inhibition) —— the movements of the lower jaw completely disappeared, or their average wave-amplitude fell by 80% or more. Grade II (apparent inhibition) —— a large proportion of the movements of the lower jaw could not be seen, or their average wave-amplitude fell by 80–50%. Grade III (slight inhibition) —— the movements of the lower jaw decreased

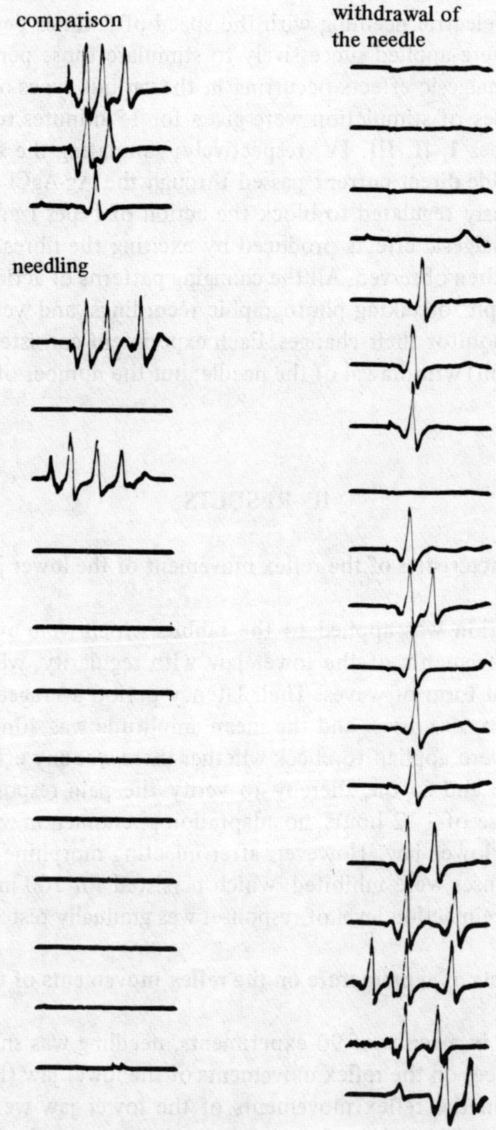

Fig. 1 Inhibitory effects of needling "Zusanli" point in rabbits on movements of the lower jaw Exp. R22

slightly, or their average wave-amplitude dropped by about 50–20%. Grade IV (no inhibition action) —— the movements of the lower jaw basically showed no changes, or their average wave-amplitude fell below 20%. According to the above gradation, in a series of 90 experiments, 81(90%) produced analgesic effects (inclusive of Grades I, II, III), 51 of which exhibited complete or apparent inhibition, amounting to 56.7% in all. The results also showed that the duration of acupunctural aftereffects was related with its inhibitory extent; that is to say, the stronger the inhibition, the longer the aftereffects.

As is known, the analgesic action caused by needling "Zusanli" points is transmitted to the center through the peroneal nerve. Electric pulses simulating electric needling were therefore successively applied to stimulate directly those peroneal nerves in order to show the effects of analgesia on pain response. Their effective rates were then compared with those of electro-needling of "Zusanli" points. By means of X^2 statistical method, it was found to be $P > 0.05$, i.e., with no significant difference in their effective rates; however, aftereffects were different. Needling the acupuncture point was shown to have longer aftereffects than stimulating the nerve-trunk, the longest up to about 3 hours. This characteristic has placed us in an advantageous position, for it enabled us to study the types of afferent fibres for impulses of acupuncture analgesia by simulating electro-needling of the nerve trunk.

(III) Analysis of analgesic effects produced by exciting different types of fibres[9]

The above results have shown that, by simulating electro-needling of the peroneal nerves, the analgesic effects caused by needling "Zusanli" points with electro-acupuncture could be reflected. By employing electric stimulation to excite the peroneal nerves and increasing the stimulation strength progressively to elicit the excitation of small fibres and then the smaller ones in turn, the roles played by the various type of fibres in the process of analgesia might also be revealed.

The results of our experiments have proved that upon exciting the various types of fibres of the peroneal nerve (Table 1), analgesic effects on pain response did occur.

It was shown in Table 1 that the excitation of types I, II fibres actually brought about a certain extent of analgesic effects, while exciting types I, II, III fibres could obviously strengthen them. However, if the strength of the stimulation was further increased to make type IV fibres excited too, then there was no significant difference between the analgesic effects of them. In terms of the rate of excellence, the percentage of the various types of fibres was in the order of 36.5% < 63% < 86%. It implied therefore that if the excitation of types I, II fibres was superimposed by that of types III fibres, analgesic effects would be considerably enhanced; if type IV fibre was further excited, the analgesic effects would be even more apparent (Fig. 2).

It is worth mentioning that, in some animals which had no response to the excitation of types I and II fibres, by exciting their type III or types III and IV fibres with augmented stimulation we could still induce apparent analgesic effects in their bodies. In 8 out of 9 cases, exciting type III fibres was effective; in 7 other cases, exciting types III and IV fibres brought about complete inhibition in all cases. In no case was there found any analgesic effect after exciting types I and II fibres; when types III or III, IV fibres were further excited, analgesic effects tended to decrease or even disappear altogether. This fully proved that types III and IV fibres have stronger inhibitory effects upon pain response than types I and

Table 1. Analgesic effects of exciting different types of fibres

Inhibitory gradation / Type of fibres	Cases (percentage in brackets)				Effective	Excellent
	Grade I	Grade II	Grade III	Grade IV	rate	rate
Types I, II	1(4.5)	7(32)	4(18)	10(45.5)	54.5	36.5
Types I, II, III	3(19)	7(44)	5(31)	1(6)	94.0	63.0
Types I, II, III, IV	3(21.5)	9(64.5)	1(7)	1(7)	93.0	86.0

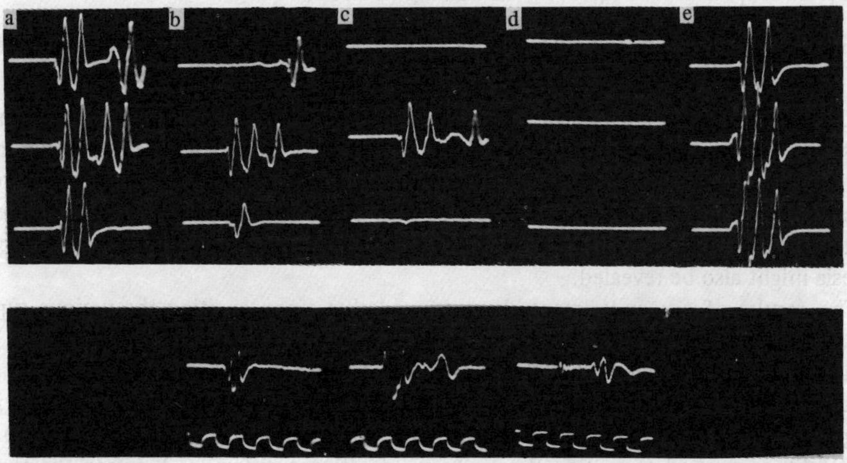

Fig. 2 Analgesic effects of exciting various groups of fibres
Above: changes of the lower jaw movement
Below: action potentials of the peroneal nerve
a. comparison, b. analgesic effects after exciting type I, II fibres. with intensity 1.5V, c. analgsic effects after exciting type I, II, III fibres. with intensity 3V, d. analgsic effects after exciting type I, II, III, IV fibres. with intensity 22V, e. withdrawing the needle.
Calibration: b.c. 2ms, 100μV, d. 20ms, 50μV. Exp. R72–2.

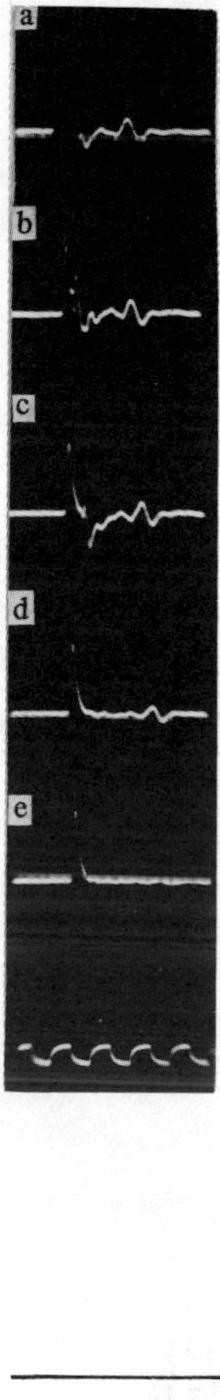

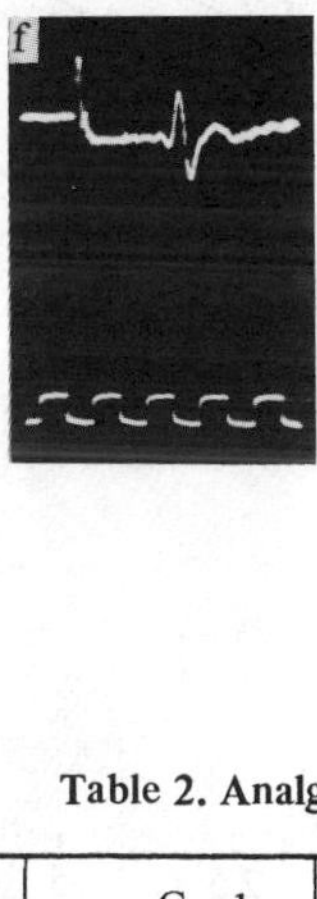

Fig. 3 Influence of the polarizing current on action potentials of the peroneal nerve
a. $A_{\epsilon\beta\gamma\delta}$ waves of the peroneal nerves
b. Using the current 60μA
c. On using the current 70μA, A_{α} a wave disappeared and $A_{\beta\gamma}$ wave decreased ;
d. On using the current 80μA, $A_{\alpha\beta\gamma}$ waves disappeared, but δ wave remained ;
e. $A_{\alpha\beta\gamma\delta}$ waves disappeared altogether by increasing the current 90μA,
f. $A_{\alpha\beta\gamma\delta}$ waves diappeared, but C wave remained when the current was 90μA.;
Calibration: a-e. 2ms, 200μA, f. 20ms, 100μV.

Table 2. Analgesic effects of exciting various groups of fibres

Inhibitory gradation / Type of fibres	Grade I	Grade II	Grade III	Grade IV	Number of experiment series	Effective rate	Excellent rate
Types I, II	1	4	7	11	23	52.0	21.7
Type III	2	6	5	4	17	76.5	47.1
Type IV	7	7	2	2	18	89.0	77.8
Types III, IV	4	1	0	0	5	100.0	100.0

II fibres.

(IV) Influence of D.C. anode-blocking of large-sized fibres on analgesic effects[10]

Considering that in the above experiment the excitation of the various types of fibres might bring about some compound reaction to the stimulation, and, moreover, it remained not quite certain whether the smaller the, fibres, the stronger the analgesic effects would be, we used the D.C. anode-blocking method to block the actions of the various types of fibres, from large to small ones in a successive way, so as to ascertain the role of small fibres in acupuncture analgesia.

First, we observed the effects of D.C. anode-blocking on the various waves of action potentials in the peroneal nerve (Fig. 3).

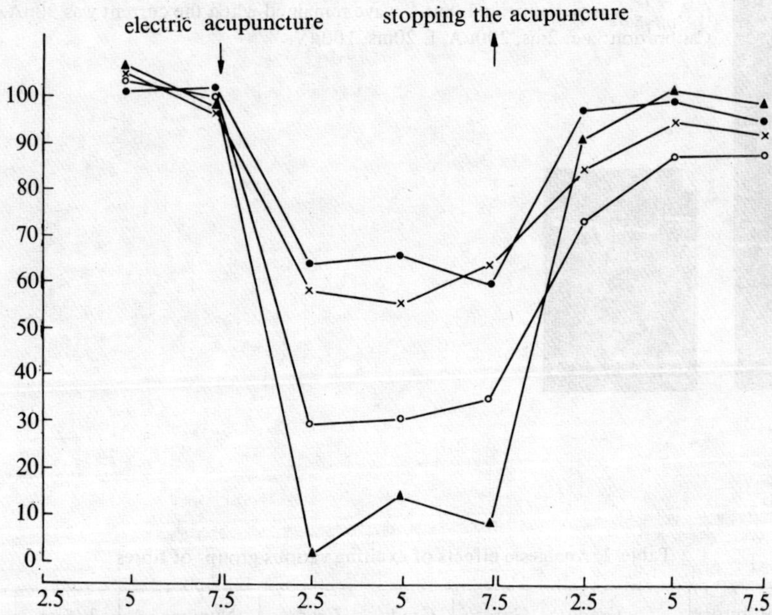

Fig. 4 Comparison of analgesic actions in various types of fibres

(1) These curves denote the changes of the wave-amplitude of the lower jaw movements (in percentage)

(2) Vertical axis denotes the changes of the wave-amplitude (in percentage); horizontal axis, the processes of acupuncture analgesia in needling (before needling; during needling; after withdrawing the needle)

" . " shows analgesic effects after exciting type I, II fibres

"X" shows analgsic effects after exciting type III fibres (with type I, II fibres being blocked)

"o" shows analgsic effects after exciting type IV fibres (with type I, II, III fibres being blocked)

"▲" shows analgesic effects after exciting type III, IV fibres (with type I, II fibres being blocked)

The arrow pointing downward indicates electric acupuncture; the arrow pointing upward indicates stopping the acupuncture.

After the current intensity was further increased, C wave began to fall and then disappeared completely. Properly managed, different strengths could be employed to block the various waves in the following order: $A_{\alpha} \rightarrow A_{\beta\gamma} \rightarrow A_{\delta} \rightarrow$ C wave. On the contrary, by successively decreasing the current intensity, the waves would be restored in the reverse order. This clearly showed that the current of a certain intensity could be first utilized to block the large-sized afferent fibres and when the intensity was increased, it would then be able to block smaller and smaller fibres[15,16]. In this way, the strength of $\beta\gamma$,δ and C waves reflected in analgesic effects on pain response could be evaluated.

In each series, analgesic effects of types I and II fibres were first observed; and then, after D.C. anode-blocking, the analgesic effects of the fibres of type III, type IV and types III, IV were investigated respectively.

Our findings have shown that after types I and II fibres had been blocked, by exciting fibres of type III, type IV and types III, IV analgesic effects could still be produced, as shown in Table 2. In terms of the rate of effectiveness, there was no significant difference between type III and type IV, and between type IV and types III, IV fibres; however, significant difference existed between type III and types III, IV. If the rate of excellence was to be considered, the outcome was: type III < type IV < types III, IV. It indicated that the analgesic effects of type IV fibres were larger than those of type III, and that if the excitation of type III fibres was followed by the excitation of type IV fibres, the analgesic effects were shown to be markedly larger than those by only exciting one of them. The results of this experiment can be seen in Fig. 4.

There was some similarity in the analgesic effects between type I and type II fibres on the one hand and type III on the other. This might be due to the fact that type III fibres were also somewhat affected during the anode-blocking. There was significant difference between the analgesic effects of type I, II and type IV fibres, and highly significant difference between those of types I, II and types III, IV fibres. Therefore, the analgesic effects in various types of fibres are I, II < III < IV < III, IV.

(V) Analysis of types of afferent fibres for the analgesic effects of needling on the pain reaction of the vascular movement[11,12]

In this study, the reaction of the vascular movement, which reflects the function of the autonomic nerve, was used as an index of pain. The same method as above-mentioned was employed with the purpose of using another model of analgesia to find out which types of afferent fibres are concerned in acupuncture analgesia.

Rabbits, immobilized and awake, were used. Pain stimulation was of long serial square-wave; frequency, 3 times per second, lasting for 5 sec; pulse duration 0.3 msec. Stimulation strength was great enough to excite A_{δ} and C waves so that the reactions of steady vascular movement might be induced and transmitted through the transducer into a four-channel physiogram to be recorded. When pain stimulation was applied, waves in diphasic form and with regularity would appear. At this time, the changes in blood pressure were recorded, and evaluated with reference to the characteristics of pain reaction. Analgesic effects of needling on the reaction of the vascular movements were expressed in Grades I, II, III, IV, in terms of the temporal rate of wave-amplitude.

The results were that, upon needling "Zusanli" points of 11 animals, the rate of effec-

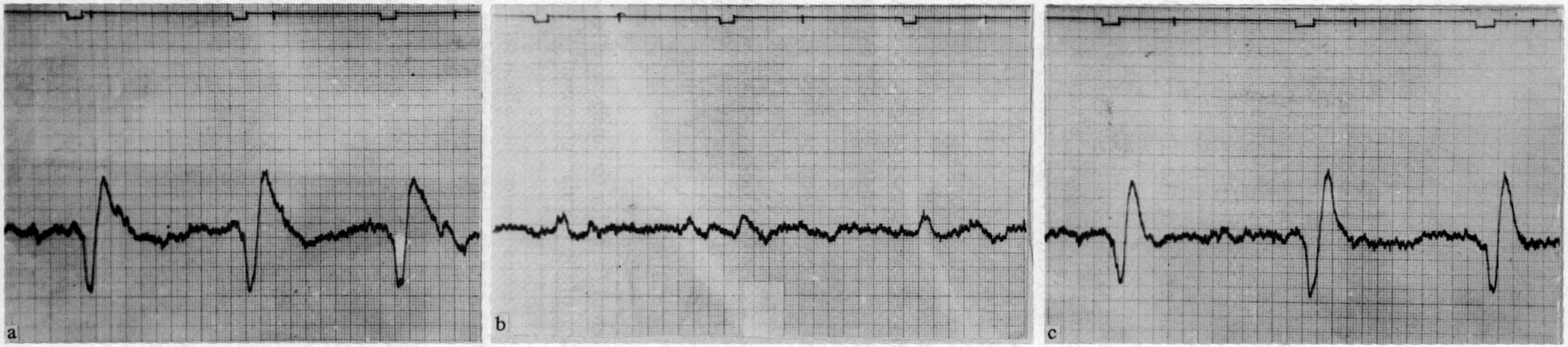

Fig. 5 Influence of needling on the vascular movement to pain responses
a, Before needling, b. After 20 min. needling (electro-needling "Zusanli" point, 10cps, 18V) c. 35 min. after needling withdrawal
Upper line: sign of pain stimulation. Parameters of stimulation: 3 cps, pulse width 0.3ms, intensity 25V
Lower line: the vascular movement to pain response

tiveness in a series of 17 experiments was 88% and the rate of excellence 47% (Fig. 5). As for analgesic effects appearing in the various types of fibres, it was found in a series of 45 experiments on 20 animals that the rate of effectiveness accounted for 36.8% upon exciting types I and II fibres; 77.8% upon exciting types I, II, III fibres; and 76.4% upon exciting types I, II, III, IV fibres. However, the rate of effectiveness rose to 88.8% during the excitation of fibres of type III and of types III, IV when types I and II fibres were blocked. Similarly, it was shown that small-sized fibres obviously had stronger analgesic effects than large-sized ones.

III. DISCUSSION

From the present study, it was evident that the smaller the excited fibres, the stronger their analgesic effects will become; in other words, the afferent fibres for acupuncture analgesia are predominantly small-sized fibres. Nevertheless, some researchers in other laboratories held that the action of large-sized fibres in the central nervous system may inhibit those of small fibres, and consequently they postulated that the afferent fibres for acupuncture analgesia are predominantly large-sized fibres whereas small-sized fibres play no apparent role in the course of analgesic effects.

According to our study, it is certain that large-sized fibres exerted their analgesic effects, but the rate of effectiveness was low. If, however, on the basis of the excitation of large-sized fibres there was added the excitation of type III fibres, this might markedly strengthen their inhibitory effects on pain response. Our observation was quite similar to that made in the Shanghai Research Institute of Physiology and so on [5,6,13]. Nevertheless, some doubts still existed as to whether the better result obtained by elevated stimulation strength was not due to the excitation of type III fibres, but due more to the excitation of type I, II fibres. Since the difference between the thresholds of large-sized and small-sized fibres were as large as 2–5 times, it is unimaginable that after types I and II fibres have been excited, more of them could be excited by further increasing the stimulation. This has been further borne out by the fact that in some animals which had no response to the excitation of types I and II fibres, exciting their type III or types III and IV fibres with augmented stimulation could still induce very apparent analgesic effects. After blocking type I and II fibres with the D.C. anode, the excitation of small-sized fibres produced stronger analgesic effects than largesized ones. A comparison was made between large-sized and small-sized fibres by the statistical X^2 method, showing that the difference was highly significant[10]. These facts indicated that the existence or non-existence of the action of large-sized fibres has no obvious relationship with analgesic effects; thus, large-sized fibres are not the main afferent fibres for acupuncture analgesia.

The opinion as to whether type C fibres might interfere with analgesic actions remains a controversial question. In our experiments, it was seen that when we, on the basis of the excitation of types I, II, III fibres, increased the stimulation strength to make type IV fibres further excited, then the rate of excellence rose from 63% to 86%; when we used the D.C. to block types I, II, III fibres and merely excited type IV fibres, the rate of analgesic effectiveness was 89%; if the current was further increased to block all the fibres of types I, II, III, IV then analgesic effects immediately disappeared. It was also observed in some research units which applied the method of isolating nervous strands that the unit-discharge caused by needling "Kunlun" point was elicited mainly through small-sized fibres, particularly type C fibres[14]. It is not difficult to understand that type C fibres not only do not interfere with analgesic action, but, conversely, play their definite role in analgesia. Then, could a stronger stimulation lead to a facilitation of excitement, a lowered threshold or an increased discharge of pain-sensitive neurons? Our attention was attracted by the following phenomenon: when we applied a current which was just strong enough to approach the threshold to stimulate type IV fibres, the animal trembled a bit but soon recovered. A measurement of its reaction showed that the animal obviously still kept its inhibitory action on pain response.

Therefore, it follows that the analgesic effects in the various types of fibres are in the following order: Types I, II < III < IV; that is, the smaller the fibres, the stronger their analgesic action. At this point, our views are also at variance with the gate control theory which propounds the idea of the inhibition of small-sized fibres by large-sized ones as one of its evidences[17-20].

It has been accepted by most people that small-sized fibres (inclusive of A_δ and C waves) are related closely with the transmitting of impulses of pain sensation as well as pain stimulation. The result of this study tends to show that small-sized fibres exert analgesic action and may inhibit pain responses. Then, how to explain it? Recent studies have shown that although needling may excite various fibres of types I, II, III, IV, it would not induce pain if those fibres connected with pain sensation are not touched. It follows that even though both pain and needling sensation are transmitted through types III and IV fibres, they are not necessarily the same fibres. It may be considered that the small-sized fibre taking part in analgesic action and the small-sized fibre conveying the impulses of pain sensation are possibly not the same fibres. Of course, the mechanism of acupuncture analgesia is connected not only with the function of peripheral nerves, but also, even more important, is through the action of afferent fibres, which trigger the anti-pain function in the centres and release nervous mediators from some of them, thus accomplishing the purpose of analgesia to convert the sensation of pain.

Are the afferent fibres for needling sensation and those for analgesia one and the same thing? According to traditional Chinese medicine, "the essence of acupuncture lies in the access of strength and its effectiveness" (Lingshu). Likewise, modern medicine postulates that the stronger the needling sensation, the better the results of acupuncture. They all denote that the intensity of needling sensation has a close relation with the effects of acupuncture therapy. In recent years, our work has shown that impulses of needling sensation are mainly transmitted by small-sized fibres[21]. Now, the present study has further proved that small-sized fibres are better able to inhibit the effects of pain response. Therefore, our deduction is that the afferent fibres for impulses of needling sensation and those for impulses of analgesia seem to be the same fibres.

IV. SUMMARY

1. In rabbits which were awake, pain stimulations were applied to the somatic nerves to elicit the reflex movements of the lower jaw and the reaction of vascular movement, both of which were taken as objective indices of pain responses.

2. By steadily increasing the stimulation strength to successively excite the various types of fibres in the peroneal nerve innervating "Zusanli" point, it was shown that the exciting of the different types of fibres could produce different degrees of analgesic effects, yet when the excitation of fibres of types I, II was superimposed by exciting the fibres of types III or IV, analgesic effects could be markedly raised.

3. By means of the anode-blocking of various types of fibres (beginning from large-sized fibres and then down to small-sized ones), it was found that small-sized fibres play the main role in the mechanism of acupuncture analgesia.

4. Our findings have shown that the smaller the fibres, the stronger the analgesic actions, that is, type IV > type III > types I, II, in terms of their analgesic effects.

REFERENCES

[1] 西安医学院针麻基础理论研究组：西安医学院学报（1）：56，1975。
[2] 西安医学院针麻原理研究室：西安医学院学报（4）：56，1976。
[3]
[4] 江苏省江苏医院针麻研究组：中华医学杂志（6）：360，1974。
[5] 沈　锷等：中华医学杂志　54（10）：628，1977。
[6] 上海第一人民医院针麻研究室：同神经电针对人体痛的感觉和情绪成分的影响。内部资料，1977。
[7] 张香桐：中国科学　（4）：465，1978。
[8] 陈隆顺、唐敬师：陕西医学资料（4）：1，1978。
[9] 陈隆顺、唐敬师等：陕西医学资料（4）：8，1978。
[10] 唐敬师等：陕西医学资料（4）：15，1978。
[11] 陈隆顺、奕力：陕西医学资料（4）：23，1978。
[12] 陈隆顺、奕力等：针刺对血管运动痛反应的抑制效应的传入纤维分析。内部资料，1978。
[13] 吴建屏等：中国科学　（5）：526，1974。
[14] 上海生理研究所：针刺麻醉（2）—3:9，1977。
[15] Mendell, L.M. and Wall, P.D.: *J. Physiol.,* **172**:274, 1964.
[16] Sassen, M. and Zimmermann, M.: *Pfluger Arch.,* **341**: 179, 1973.
[17] Anderson, S.A. and Aolmgren, E.: *Amer. J. Chin. Med.,* **4**:331, 1975.
[18] Zimmermann, M.: *Science,* **160**:896, 1968.
[19] Frang, D.N. & Iggo, A.: *Science,* **162**:1140, 1968.
[20] Carregal, E.J.A.: Pain Research and Treatment, p.7–33, Academic Press, New York, San Francisco, London, 1975.
[21] Hou Zonglian: *Chin. med. J.,* **4**:223, 1979.

THE AREA (SENSITIVE AREA) OF THE PRODUCTION OF TRACTION PAIT OF STOMACH, ITS AREA OF ORIGIN AND AFFERENT PATHWAY

Yu Pin, Li Zhennian, Zhang Kun, Li Guizhen,
Lu Yongli, Jiang Shuxue
(Research Group of Acupuncture Anesthesia, Zhongguo Medical College)

Among the tractive reactions of the stomach, tractive pain is the key problem of the "three problems" to be solved in an operation of the stomach. Information on the theoretical study of tractive pain are scarce; only a few reports of clinical or physiological study dwelling on the subject of its pathway to the centers have been published[1,2,3,4], but they are still in controversy. Yet no information on the study of the area (sensitive area) of the production of gastric tractive pain and its pathway has so far been reported. This article deals with the investigation carried out in subtotal gastrectomy under acupuncture anesthesia in order to establish, by experimental morphology, the area (sensitive area) of the production of gastric tractive pain and also make an observation of the quantity, property and origin of the nervous constituents and the afferent pathway in an attempt to elucidate the mechanism of the production of visceral tractive pain and the theory of inhibiting visceral tractive pain by acupuncture so as to make acupunctural anesthesia more acceptable and improve, on the basis of morphology, the forms of gastrectomy.

I. STUDY OF THE PERIPHERAL NERVOUS PLEXUSES OF THE GASTRIC ARTERIES

During gastrectomy, intense pain occurs as traction, ligation and severance of the vessels in the mesogastrium are performed. At the same time the pulse rate, the blood pressure and the amount of perspiration have apparently risen, but the digital blood-volume lowered[5]. To make clear of the situation of the production of tractive pain during gastrectomy, the tunica adventitia of gastric arteries, stained with silver impregnation method was seen dispersing with only a small quantity of fibrous reticulum of sensory nerves, while in the mesogastrium of cats and guinea pigs, stained with methylene blue *in vivo,* only a few sensory nerves were found. Neither of the two can explain how the intense tractive pain is produced. But we find that the perivascular nervous plexuses running with the gastric arteries greatly outnumber the nervous constituents in the above two kinds of structures. Therefore, thorough observations of the quantity and the property of the perivascular plexuses in the region operated upon have been made.

(I) The Quantity of the Peripheral Nervous Plexuses of the Gastric Vessels

The cross-sectional areas of the peripheral nervous plexuses of the gastric vessels of 6 human stomachs were measured. The part measured was just where the traction and severance of vessels were performed in an operation, i.e., the peripheral nervous plexuses around the left gastric artery in gastropancreatic plica, the peripheral nervous plexuses around the second-terminal branch of the left gastric artery, the peripheral nervous plexuses around the right gastric artery, the peripheral nervous plexuses of the right gastroepiploic artery and the peripheral nervous plexuses around the second-terminal branch of the left gastroepiploic artery. Results of the measurement are shown in Table 1.

The sizes of the cross-sectional areas of the perivascular nervous plexuses are: the peripheral plexus of the left gastric artery (in gastropancreatic plica) (Fig. 1) > the peripheral plexus of the second-terminal branch of the left gastric artery > the peripheral plexus of the right gastroepiploic artery > the peripheral plexus of the right gastric artery > the peripheral plexus of the second-terminal branch of the left gastroepiploic artery (Fig. 2). Their ratio is 34:13:7.5:2.6:1.

(II) The Quantity of Myelinated Sensory Nerve Fibres in the Peripheral Plexuses Around the Gastric Blood Vessels

The acid osmium impregnation method is used in the experiment. On the sections thus made from the perivascular plexuses of four human stomachs, the numbers of myelinated sensory nerve fibres of the peripheral plexuses are counted and their calibres measured (Table 2).

Table 1. The area of transverse section and branch-number of peripheral nervous plexuses around gastric vessels

	Lt. Gas. A. (in plica)		Br. 2 of Lt. Gas. A.		Rt. Gas-epip. A.		Rt. Gas. A.		Br. 2 of Lt. Gas-epip. A.	
	Area (mm^2)	Br.-No.	Area (mm^2)	Br.-No.	Area (mm^2)	Br.-No.	Area (mm^2)	Br.-No.	Area (mm^2)	Br.-No.
Newborn	0.051	14	0.023	16	0.017	9.3	0.018	9.3	0.0039	5.3
3 yr. ♂			0.082	15	0.035	14	0.024	10	0.003	4
19 yr. ♀	1.16	26.6	0.432	18	0.213	10	0.065	15	0.015	5
46 yr. ♀	0.67	33	0.250	26	0.143	10	0.0779	15	0.041	11
50 yr. ♀			0.290	20	0.176	10	0.029	17	0.0115	4
53 yr. ♂	0.42	37	0.296	26	0.117	10	0.061	13	0.021	5
Average	0.75	32.2	0.317	22.5	0.162	10	0.058	15	0.022	6.25

The average numbers are from the last 4 adults.

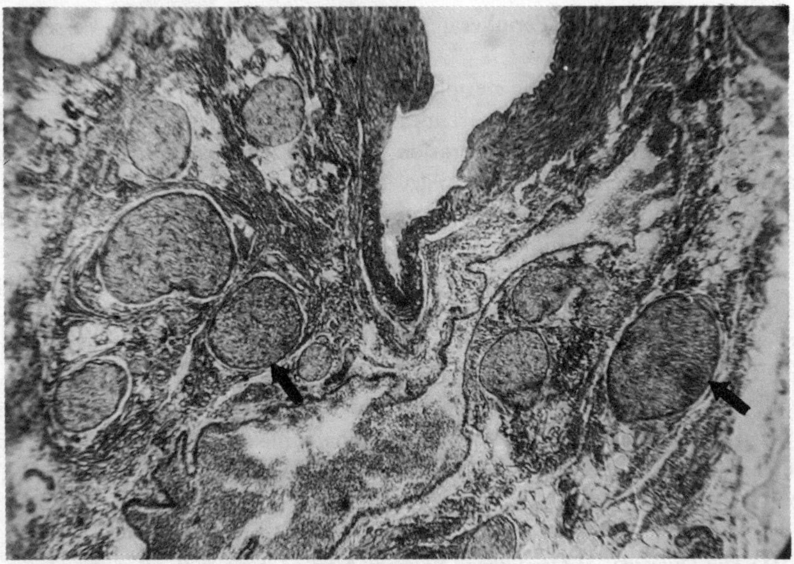

Fig. 1 The peripheral plexus(↑) of the left gastric artery. H.E. method 100X.

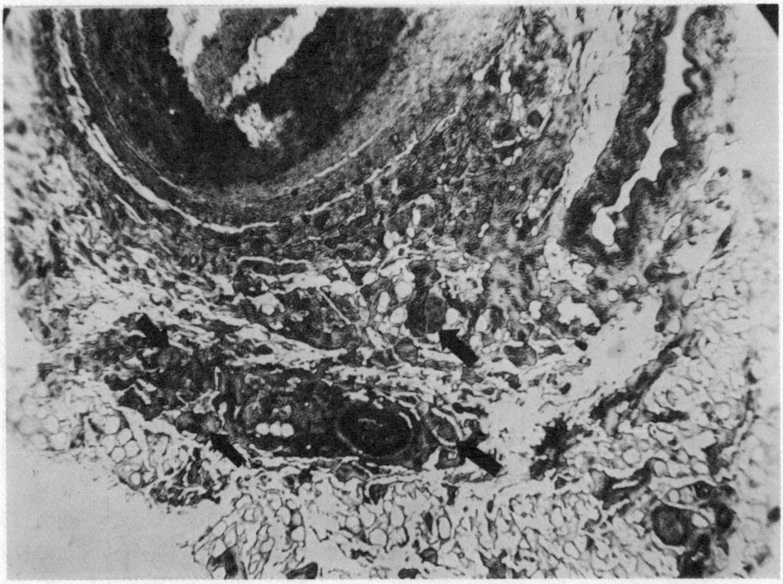

Fig. 2 The peripheral plexus(↑) of the right gastric artery. H.E. method 100X.

Table 2. Numbers of myelinated fibers of the peripheral plexus around the different blood vessels of the human stomach

	Gas. Br. of Lt. Gas. A.		Rt. Gas-epip. A.		Rt. Gas. A		Br. 2 of Lt. Gas-epip. A.		Total
	No. of N.f.	Br.	No. of N.f.	Br.	No. of N.f.	Br.	No. of N.f.	Br.	
Newborn	149	21	77	6	20	7	13	7	259
7 yr. ♀	341	22	113	12	56	11	6	4	516
9 yr. ♂	279	13	139	9	34	13	17	8	469
Adult ♂	376	26	167	22	65	9	8	4	616

As shown in Table 2, the myelinated nervous fibres are very few in number, amounting to only 469 — 616 (not including the numbers of a newborn child), but the numbers of non-myelinated nervous fibres are much more. In such plexus, there are fewer myelinated nervous fibres with long and moderate diameters (2–7μ) than those with short diameter (1–2μ). As there are no skeletal muscles in the stomach, a great part of the fibres here are sensory nervous ones. From the above, it may be thought that the visceral nerves controlling the stomach are quite different from the somatic nerves controlling the trunk. The

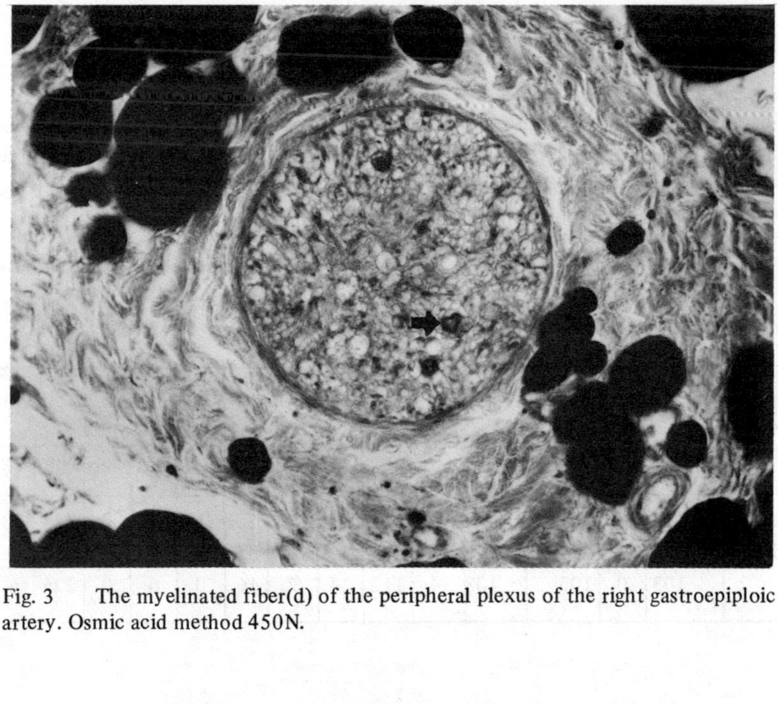

Fig. 3 The myelinated fiber(d) of the peripheral plexus of the right gastroepiploic artery. Osmic acid method 450N.

difference lies in the fact that in the stomach the myelinated nerve fibres are fewer in number than the non-myelinated ones, especially the C fibres. This coincides with the observations made by Hora[6] on the stomachs of dogs. The comparison of the numbers of the myelinated nerve fibres in gastric perivascular plexus is: fibres in the peripheral plexuses of the left gastric artery > fibres in the peripheral plexuses of the right gastroepiploic artery (Fig. 3) > fibres in the peripheral plexuses of the right gastric artery > fibres in the peripheral plexuses of the second-terminal branch of the left gastroepiploic artery.

(III) The Origin of Myelinated Sensory Nerve Fibres in the Peripheral Plexuses of Gastric Vessels

The left greater splanchnic nerve under the diaphragm or the left vagus nerve in the neck was severed separately. After five days, the gastric perivascular plexuses were taken out, stained using the acid osmium impregnation method and isolated under a cubic anatomic magnifier, and the total number of their myelinated nerve fibres and the number of those degenerated were then counted. The results are shown in Table 3.

It is shown that the proportion of the degenerated nerve fibres in the perivascular plexuses is very large when the left greater splanchnic nerve is severed (Fig. 4); but the proportion is very small when the left vagus nerve is severed, and the degenerated fibres may also be looked upon as parasympathetic preganglionic fibres (Fig. 5). So a great part of the myelinated sensory fibres of the peripheral plexuses around the above-said four gastric vessels originate from the greater splanchnic nerve and only a few originate from the vagus nerve.

(IV) The Origin of Non-myelinated Sensory Nerve Fibres of the Peripheral Plexuses Around Gastric Vessels

In order to elucidate the origin and the proportion of the non-myelinated sensory nerve fibres of the gastric perivascular plexuses, the left greater splanchnic nerve or the left vagus nerve were severed separately in dogs. Five days later the peripheral plexuses were taken out and observed under light and electron microscopes.

Table 3. The degeneration of the myelinated fibers of the peripheral plexus around the four gastric blood vessels of the dog

Part of severance	Lt. Gas. A.			Rt. Gas-epip. A.			Rt. Gas. A.			Br. 2 of Lt. Gas-epip. A.			Total		
	Nor.	Deg.	Tot.	Nor.	Deg.	Tot.	Nor.	Deg.	Tot.	Nor.	Deg.	Tot.	Nor.	Deg.	Tot.
N. spl. maj.	128	33	161	82	30	112	12	3	15	1	7	8	223	73	296
N. vag. sin. 1	231	1	232	20	0	20	34	1	35	30	1	31	315	3	318
N. vag. sin. 2	103	0	103	108	4	112	14	2	16	0	0	0	225	6	231

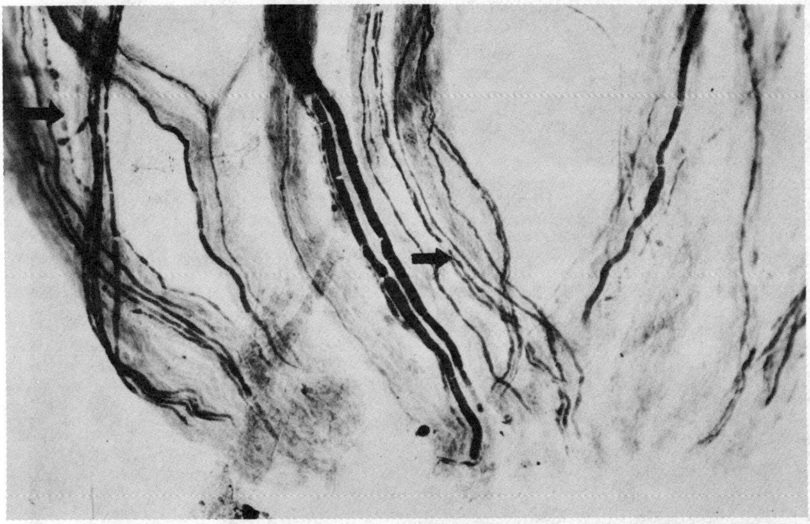

Fig. 4 A number of the myelinated fibers(↑) degenerated in the peripheral plexus of the left gastric artery. 5 days after the left greater splanchnic nerve had been cut in the dog. Osmic acid method isolated specimen. 100×.

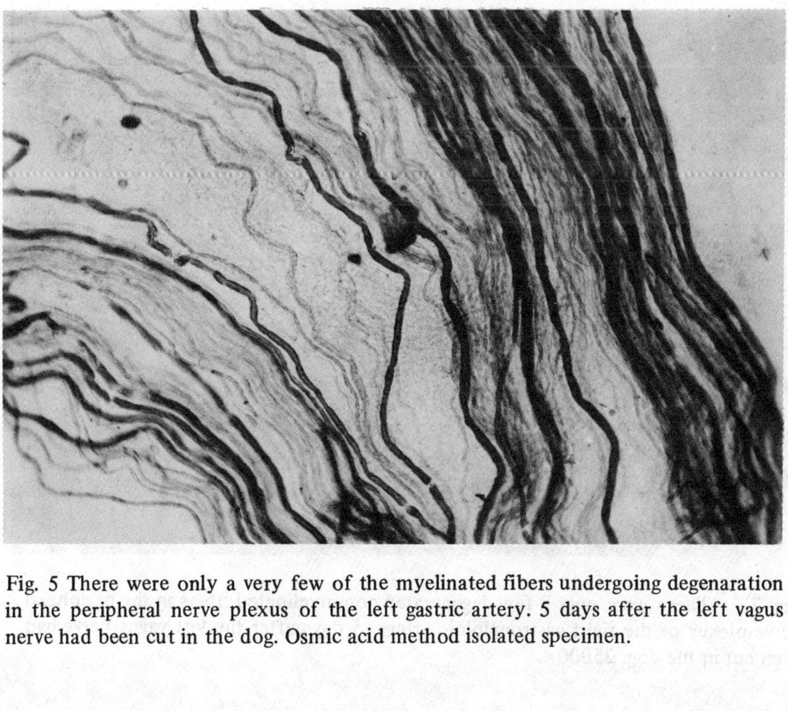

Fig. 5 There were only a very few of the myelinated fibers undergoing degenaration in the peripheral nerve plexus of the left gastric artery. 5 days after the left vagus nerve had been cut in the dog. Osmic acid method isolated specimen.

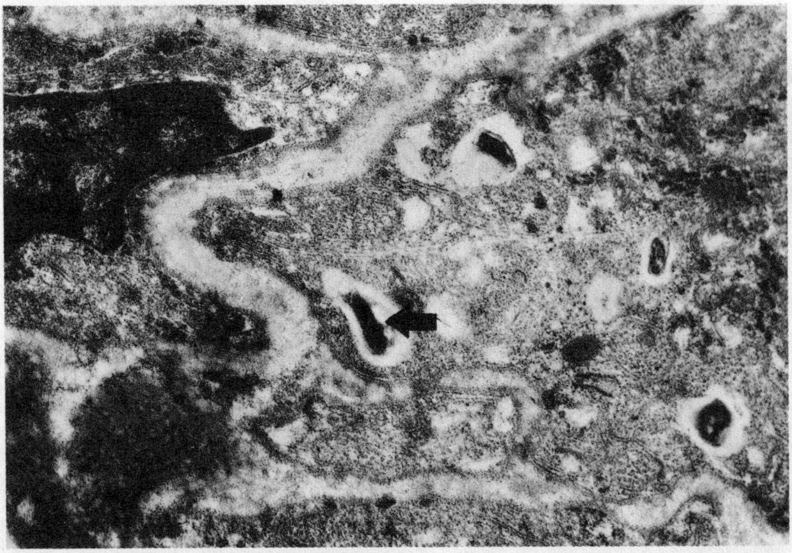

Fig. 6 There were a considerable number of the degenerated non-myelinated fibers(↑) in the peripheral nerve plexus of the right gastro-epiploic artery. 5 day after the left greater splanchnic nerve had been cut in the dog. 25000×.

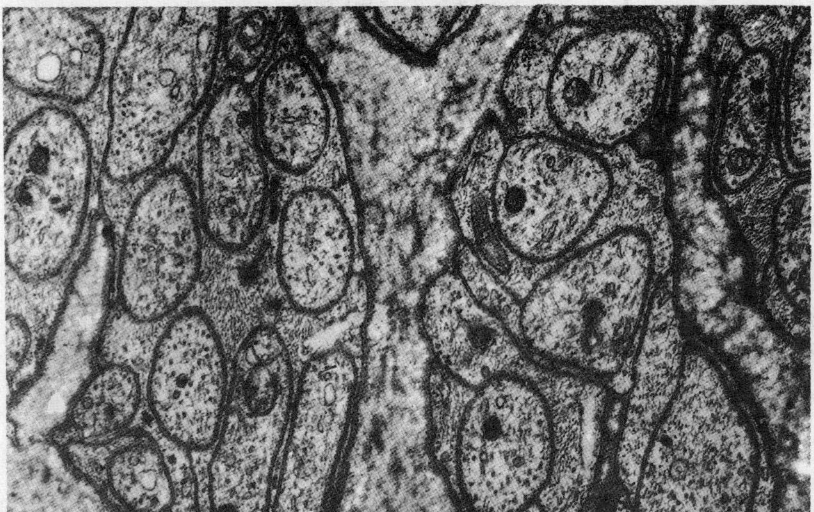

Fig. 7 There were only a few degenerated non-myelinated fibers in the peripheral nerve plexus of the right gastroepiploic artery. 5 days after the left vagus nerve had been cut in the dog. 25000×.

In the cases when the left splanchnic nerve was severed, a greater number of non-myelinated sensory nerves in the perivascular plexuses and gastric walls were seen degenerating on the specimens when stained with the silver impregnation method, and a greater number of non-myelinated sensory nerve fibres were seen degenerating on the specimens for electron microscopy (Fig. 6). In the cases when the left vagus nerve was severed, the numbers of the degenerate non-myelinated sensory nerve fibres were much less both on the light-microscopic specimens stained with the silver impregnation method and on the electron-microscopic specimens (Fig. 7). Therefore, it can be seen that non-myelinated sensory nerve fibres (C fibres) in the gastric perivascular plexus are numerous in number and that a great part of them originate from the greater splanchnic nerve.

(V) Centric Sites Where the Sensory Nerve Fibres of the Peripheral Nervous Plexuses Around the Gastric Vessels or the Greater Splanchnic Nerve Project

To make clear the centric sites where the sensory nerve fibres of the gastric peripheral nervous plexuses of the vessels or of the greater splanchnic nerve project, two methods were used in our research work. First, four dogs and five rabbits were used. The greater splanchnic nerves on one side of these animals were cut. The spinal ganglions were taken out from the dogs after five days and from the rabbits after twelve days, and serial sections made from them were investigated after staining with crystalline violet. The second was the horseradish peroxidase method. Three cats and five rabbits were used. Their gastric perivascular plexuses were injured and horseradish peroxidase was used to smear on the injured parts. After two days the material was taken out and then made into slides for observation. With the first method, the cells of the spinal ganglions from the upper thoracic segment to the terminal thoracic segment, particularly a large number of the smaller cells of them, were seen to

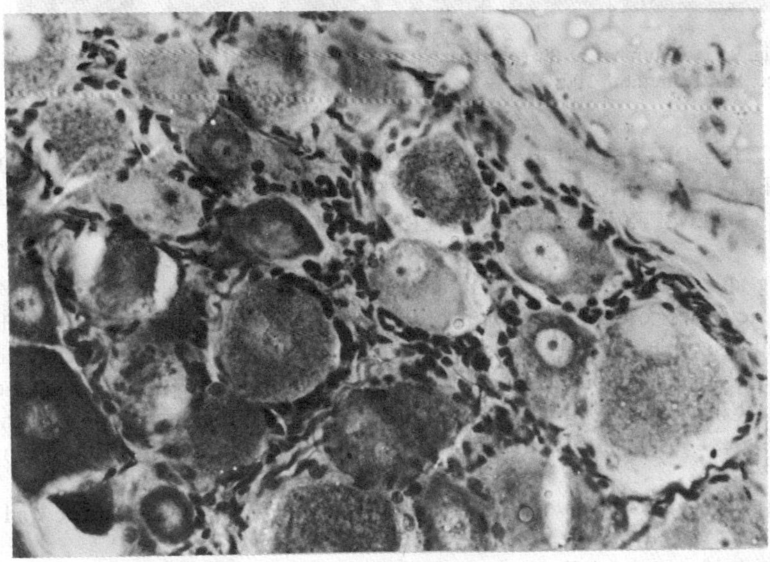

Fig. 8 The small neurons of the spinal ganglion (T. 5) showed chromatolysis. 5 days after left greater splanchnic nerve had been cut in the dog. Nissl method. 400×.

undergo conspicuous retrograde degeneration (Fig. 8). With the second method, the cells of the spinal ganglions were seen labelled with horseradish peroxidase everywhere on the spinal ganglions from the upper thoracic segment to the terminal segment; the cells of the spinal ganglions in the lower thoracic segment were found to be very numerous in number (Fig. 9). However in the nodular ganglions of the left and right vagus nerves there were seen only a small quantity of nerve cells containing horseradish peroxidase.

It may be seen from the above observations that the area where the nervous fibres of painful sensation in the perivascular plexuses of the gastric vessels project to the centers is, in the main, the spinal cord, especially that of the lower thoracic segments.

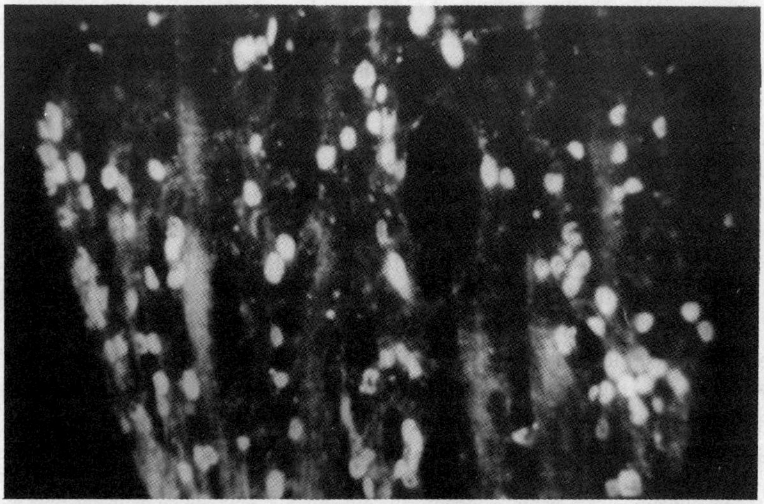

Fig. 9 A number of the spinal ganglion cells were labelled by horseradish peroxidase. H.R.P. method. 100×.

II. STUDY OF THE TYPE AND DISTRIBUTIVE DENSITY OF THE SENSORY NERVE–ENDINGS (NERVOUS RECEPTORS) AND THE DISTRIBUTIVE DENSITY OF SENSORY NERVE FIBRES IN GASTRIC WALL

During an operation, the exploring and the drawing of the stomach not only interfere with the activities of the peripheral nervous plexuses of the gastric vessels in the mesogastrium but also affect and stimulate the gastric wall itself on a large scale. The patient, with his stomach being explored and drawn, may feel to a certain degree the tractive pain and have nausea or vomiting. It is then necessary to make an investigation of the various sensory nervous constituents in the gastric wall and their proportions in distribution.

(I) The Types of Nervous Receptors in Different Layers of the Gastric Wall

Due probably to the difficulty of the silver impregnation method, only two articles on the investigation in this respect are referred to at present, the Yshigawa study[7] on human stomachs and the Триторьва study[8] on stomachs of animals.

In demonstrating the nervous constituents in the human gastric wall with the silver-impregnation technique, we observed: (1) that around the gland alveolus in the gastric mucosa there were small nervous receptors with a few branches, some of which had one branch attached to the gland alveolus and another to the smooth muscles (polyceptor), and it was for this reason that these receptors were classified as mechanical receptors and chemoreceptors in some literature[9,10]; (2) that some fine terminal branches of sensory fibres were on the wall of the small vessels, forming tiny branchy receptors, which, as described in Lim's report[11], could cause visceral pain when bradykinin was injected into the animal arteries; (3) that there were branchy receptors of various sizes in intermuscular nervous plexuses; and (4) that large numbers of branchy receptors of various sizes were in the muscular coat (Fig. 10). The appearances of the receptors, as we know, are multiple; some are composed of a thick myelinated sensory nerve fiber (the trunk) which branches and rebranches as a tree does. Some have a trunk which continuously branches out into small branches in its course, becoming slenderer and slenderer in the end; some have a trunk with large joints close to one another just like bamboo-joints and between the joints the trunk grows thinner, with small branches stretching out at the joints. The ends of all the above receptors are very slender and eventually are attached to the smooth muscles. Receptors in the muscular coat vary in size, some of them being considerably large, spreading extensively. According to the sizes of their trunks we classify them into three types: the large-sized (diameter of the trunk-fibre exceeding 2μ), the medium-sized (diameter between $1-2\mu$) and the small-sized (diameter under 1μ).

The function of the receptors in the muscular coat may be mechanical because these receptors are in the muscular coat and their slender ends are attached to the muscle fasciculus so that any variation of the muscular tone of the stomach may stimulate them. The degeneration of the receptors in the gastric muscular coat, observed after the severance of

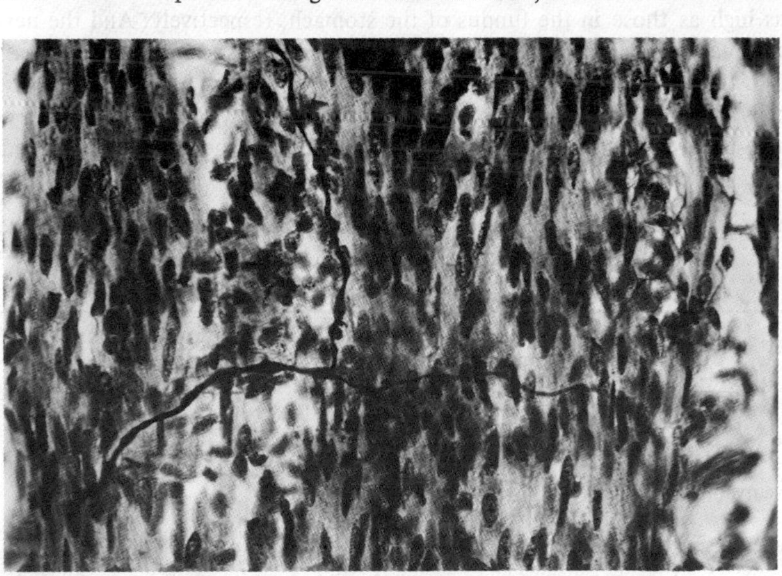

Fig. 10 The large sized mechanical receptor of the muscular coat of the human stomach. Bielschowsky's method. 200×.

the greater splanchnic nerve or vagus nerve of one side in dogs, proves that some of the impulses of the receptors are transmitted to the centers through the greater splanchnic nerve while others are transmitted through the vagus nerve. This can also justify the presumptions of other scientists in the past that the sensory nerve fibres of the sympathetic or vagus nerves can form receptors in the gastric muscular coat, that an increase in the tone of gastric muscular coat may result in pain in the depths of the stomach, that an expansion of the gastric muscular coat may result in vomiting, and that the former travelled to the centre through the sympathetic nerve and the latter through the vagus nerve. Thus, the mechanical receptors, under strong stimulation, may be associated with pain in the depths of the stomach, and with vomiting and nausea.

(II) The Distributive Density of the Nervous Receptors in the Muscular Coat of the Different Portions of the Stomach

The method used in the present study is as follows. Horizontal sections were made of the muscular coat of the different portions of the stomach. One section out of every six was prepared using the silver impregnation method. The number of large and medium-sized receptors and that of the nerve fibres with big and medium calibres in each prepared section were determined with the aid of a microscope. The area of every section was measured and the density of the above-mentioned nerves in the muscular coat of the different portions of the stomach calculated. The results obtained are given in Table 4.

As shown in Table 4, the large- and medium-sized receptors and the nerve fibres with big and medium calibres are the most numerous in the pylorus and the lesser curvature; they are less in number in the greater curvature and still less in the fundus of the stomach. The large- and medium-sized receptors in the pylorus and the lesser curvature are 14 and 6 times, 4 and 2 times, as high as those in the fundus of the stomach, respectively. And the nerve fibres with big and medium calibres are likewise 15 and 6 times, 5 and 7 times, as high as those in the fundus of the stomach, respectively.

Clinically, when extensive traction or exploration of the pylorus and the lesser curvature is done, the tractive pain and reactions are marked, but when the same procedures are

Table 4. The ratio of the distributive density of the receptor and nerve fiber in the muscular coat of the different portions of human stomach

Portions	Receptor		Nerve fiber	
	Large-sized	Median-sized	Thick calibre	Median calibre
Pyloric	14.92	23.41	50.64	351.32
Lesser curvature	5.65	11.82	28.97	393.69
Greater curvature	2.05	8.88	12.15	102.12
Fundus	0.94	5.35	3.45	68.99

carried out in the greater curvature and the fundus of the stomach, they are slight. This corresponds to the density of the mechanical receptors in the muscular coat of the stomach and it is accordingly believed that these mechanical receptors are one of the sites where the tractive pain and reactions are produced and that the sensitivity of the gastric wall to traction is greater in the pylorus and the lesser curvature than in the greater curvature and the fundus of the stomach. Also, the density of the sensory nerves is consistent with that of the motor nerves of the muscular coat in the different regions of the stomach[12].

III. DISCUSSION

(1) The perivascular nervous plexus of the stomach is the main site where tractive pain is produced (the sensitive area). One of the reasons for this is that the structural feature of the perivascular nerves is similar to that clinically seen in the tractive pain of the stomach, that is, myelinated nerve fibres in these nervous plexuses are much too few while non-myelinated sensory nerve fibres (C fibres) are numerous. The latter serve as afferent pathways of dull pains, and their location is indefinite, and when they are in action, there appear marked symptoms of the vegetative nervous system (increased blood pressure, increased pulse rate, increased perspiration and reduced volume of the digital blood vessels). The tractive pain, which is quite different from the pain felt at the time when the abdomen is opened and closed, coincides with the symptoms of the vegetative nervous system as complained, by the patient. Another reason is that the number of the perivascular nerves of the stomach (the left gastric artery > the right gastroepiploic artery > the right gastric artery > the second terminal branch of the left gastroepiploic artery) is coincident with the tractive pain felt by the patient and the objective physiological-index showing the degree of the pain when the above vessels are being handled during the operation. When the left gastric artery is being handled, intensive traction occurs in the perivascular nervous plexuses of this artery. As the plexus has the most numerous fibres, it receives the greatest stimulation and consequently the patient complains of the most intense tractive pain, and a peak in the objective index showing the degree of pain appears. When the right gastroepiploic artery is being manipulated, the patient complains of great, even greater, pain because there exist a great number of nerve fibres in this plexus. As the right gastroepiploic artery and the right gastric artery are handled consecutively in a short time, another peak in the objective index reflecting pain appears as a result of the indices overlapping each other. The perivascular nerves of the second terminal branch of the left gastroepiploic artery are the smallest in number and, in consequence, most patients had no reaction at all and there was only a slight change in the index of pain sensation while it was being manipulated.

We are of the opinion that according to the number of the perivascular nerves in the different portions of the stomach, the degree of sensitivity to traction, ligation and severance is in the following order: the left gastric artery > the right gastroepiploic artery > the right gastric artery > the second terminal branch of the left gastroepiploic artery.

(2) We believe that the mechanical receptors in the muscles of the stomach are one of the sites where tractive reactions of the stomach, including tractive pain, are produced when traction or exploration of the gastric wall is done. We also believe that the sensitivity of the

gastric wall to traction and exploration is the greatest in the pylorus and the lesser curvature; it is less in the greater curvature and still less in the fundus of the stomach, depending upon the density of the mechanical receptors (the pylorus > the lesser curvature > the greater curvature > the fundus). This is consistent with the patient's pain and reactions to traction, that is, the reaction is most intense when the pylorus is being pulled or explored, and it is less intense when traction or exploration is done in the greater curvature and still less in the fundus of the stomach.

(3) There is at present a controversy in opinions over the afferent pathways of the tractive pain in the stomach. Some people maintain that it is by way of the greater splanchnic nerve. Others believe that it is via the greater splanchnic nerve and the vagus nerve. But there has been no morphological evidence to support these beliefs. Judging from the above-mentioned experimental materials, we maintain that the tractive pain in the stomach is conveyed mainly by the greater splanchnic nerve. The reasons are: (1) in the first of the two groups in which the greater splanchnic nerve or the vagus nerve of one side was severed, degeneration occurred in most of the myelinated and non-myelinated nerve fibres of the perivascular nervous plexuses of the stomach as seen under a light microscope or an electron microscope, whereas very few showed degeneration in the second group; (2) in the group in which the greater splanchnic nerve of one side was severed, retrograde degeneration was found in most of the spinal nerve cells, especially those small ones, from the upper to the lower thoracic segments; (3) in the group in which horseradish peroxidase was used, the sensory nerve fibres of the perivascular nervous plexuses of the stomach were found to carry horseradish peroxidase to the spinal ganglion cells from Th.3—Th.13 segment, whereas only a small number of the cells of the nodular ganglions of the vagus nerve contained this enzyme. This shows that a large part of the sensory nerve fibres of the perivascular nervous plexuses of the stomach originate from the cells of the spinal-ganglions, especially the small cells which give off C fibres and are the afferent pathways for dull pains[13–15] and which are distributed to the peripheral nervous plexuses of the stomach via the greater splanchnic nerve[16–18].

The spinal cord receives sensations through its many segments and at the same time provides plenty of C fibres to receive them. This is distinct from the sensation of a particular part of the trunk or limbs which enters into only a few segments of the spinal cord. The incomplete anesthesia induced by acupuncture for gastric operations may be related to the multiple segmental innervation of the stomach. This is a point to be considered in the selection of points for acupuncture anesthesia for gastric operations.

(4) During a gastric operation under acupuncture anesthesia, it is advisable to reduce as much as possible tractive or other intense stimulation to the above described sensitive area so as to mitigate tractive pain in the stomach. When the blood vessels of the stomach are being handled, it is desirable to clamp first the blood vessels distal to the stomach and then those proximal to the stomach so that the patient suffers only once the tractive pain in the viscera caused by the clamping of the perivascular nervous plexuses.

IV. SUMMARY

(1) The perivascular nervous plexus of the stomach is the main site where tractive pain in the stomach is produced (the sensitive area). The degree of sensitivity is in the following

order: the left gastric artery > the right gastroepiploic artery > the right gastric artery > the second terminal branch of the left gastroepiploic artery.

(2) The mechanical receptors in the muscular coat of the gastric wall are one of the morpho-structural bases for the production of the tractive reactions of the stomach when traction is done on the gastric wall. The degree of sensitivity of the different portions of the gastric wall is as follows: the pylorus > the lesser curvature > the greater curvature > the fundus.

(3) The tractive pain in the stomach is conveyed to a number of segments of the spinal cord mainly by way of the greater splanchnic nerve, especially the lower thoracic segment. Only a little pain passes through the vagus nerve.

(4) Based on the above-mentioned results of the study, a suggestion is put forward for improving the selection of points and operative techniques in order that the effect of acupuncture anesthsia may be enhanced.

REFERENCES

[1] Herrin, C. and Meek, W.J. : *Amer. J. Physiol.,* 144 : 720, 1945

[2] Sheehau, D.: *J. Anot. Lond.,* 67 : 233, 1933

[3] Liaoning Cooperative Group of Acupuncture Anesthesia: *National Symposia of Acupuncture and Moxibustion and Acupuncture Anesthesia,* 171, Beijing, 1979.

[4] Cheng Daozhi, et al.: *National Symposia of Acupuncture and Moxibustion and Acupuncture Anesthesia,* 171, Beijing, 1979.

[5] Research Group of Acupuncture Anesthesia, Zhongshan Medical College: *National Symposia of Acupuncture and Moxibustion and Acupuncture Anesthesia,* 171, Beijing, 1979.

[6] 原正美：福岛医志，**7**，531，1957。

[7] 石川久三郎：東醫會誌，**146**，616，1972。

[8] Гилинский,Е.Я.:Изд. АН.СССР.М-Л,1958.

[9] Колосов,Н.Г.:Иннервочия Внутренных Органов и Сердечно Сосудистой Системы.М-Л,1954.

[10] Davenport, H.W.: *Physiology of the Digestive Tract,* 1971.

[11] Lim R.K.S. : *J. Comp. Neurol.,* 118: 269, 1962.

[12] Melmen ,Е.Р.:Архив Анатомий Гистологии и Эмбрнолотий 8:62, 1962.

[13] Schofield, G.C.: *Am Physiol. Society,* 1968.

[14] Strong, O.S. and Elwyn, A. : *Human Neurology,* 1957.

[15] Ranson, S.W. : *The Anatomy of the Nervous System,* 1962.

[16] Amassian, V.E. : *J. Neurophysiol.,* 14, 445–460, 1951.

[17] Meleod, J.G. : *J. Physol.,* 140, 462–478, 1958.

[18] Ray, B.S. and Meill, C.L. : *Ann. Surg.,* 126, 709-724, 1947.

ELECTRON MICROSCOPIC AND FLUOROHISTOCHEMICAL OBSERVATIONS OF NERVES IN HUMAN STOMACH WALL REMOVED DURING OPERATIONS UNDER ACUPUNCTURE ANESTHESIA

Yü Yi, Pang Junyun, Guo Yanru

(Department of Acupuncture Anesthesia, Institute of Basic Medisciences, Chinese Academy of Medical Sciences)

It has been shown in clinical practice that a close relationship exists between the effectiveness of acupuncture anesthesia and the functional state of the vegetative nervous system[1]. The purpose of this investigation is to study morphologically the changes in the transmitters of vegetative nerves brought about by a difference in the effectiveness of acupuncture anesthesia admininistered. We have investigated the changes in the ultrastructure of these nerves of the stomach wall with an electron microscope, the changes in the sympathetic transmitters in the stomach wall by fluorescent-histochemical methods, and the changes in monoamine oxidase activity associated with the metabolism of sympathetic transmitters.

I. MATERIALS AND METHODS

(I) Selection of Cases and Gradation of the Effectiveness of Acupuncture Anesthesia

Patients suffering from gastroduodenal ulcer and subject to subtotal gastrectomy were selected. Six points, Renzhong, Chengjiang, Zusanli, Pishu, Neiguan and Xinshu, were used[2]. Operations were performed after 30 minutes induction. Specimens of major omentum and stomach were taken during operations, and sections for electron microscope and histochemistry were prepared immediately. Based on the clinical manifestations (pain, traction response and muscle contraction, etc.) and physiological changes (heart rate, blood pressure and pulse quality, etc.) of patients during operations, the results of acupuncture anesthesia were classified into 3 grades: Grades I (excellent), II (good) and III (poor).

(II) Preparation of Sections for Electron Microscopic Studies and Examination Method

Specimens of 44 cases were all excised from about the middle part of the greater curvature of the stomach, about 5×5 mm^2 of the whole layer. Mucosa, submucosa and muscularis were dissected separately. Each layer was cut into small blocks, about 1 mm^3 in size and was fixed in glutaraldehyde solution (4°C) for 1 hr. After being washed with phosphate buffer, the tissue blocks were dipped in 1% osmic acid, dehydrated by acetone, and embedded in Epon 618. The ultrathin sections were stained with uranyl acetate and lead citrate for contrast. About 20 continuous sections on 2 copper meshes were examined for every one specimen. If any type of varicosities or nerve terminals was encountered, the number of vesicles in every type of them was counted. The number of vesicles contained in varicosities or nerve terminals of individual nerve fibres was classified into 3 gradients; the first gradient was "less than nine", the second one ranged from 10–19, and the third one was "more than 20". The results were then treated statistically and compared with the effectiveness of acupuncture anesthesia.

(III) Preparation of Specimens for Fluorescent-histochemical Examinations

Surgically removed samples of major omentum were obtained from 194 patients subjected to subtotal gastrectomy under acupuncture anestheisa. Parts of definite sites on major omentum were stretched on clean slides rapidly and dried. Noradrenaline was demonstrated by using Flack's[3] formaldehyde-induction method. Blocks (about 2 × 1.5 cm^2) of 61 cases, cut from parts of the greater curvature of the stomach adjacent to the cardiac orifice, were rapidly frozen in pentane or isopentane pre-cooled in dry ice. Cryostat sections, 25μ thick, were prepared with microtome at –20 —— –18°C, and were treated with a mixture of sucrose-phosphoric acid-glyoxylic acid (SPG Method)[4]. Fluorescent examination was carried out immediately with a microscope and photographs were taken. The fluorescence intensity depends upon the noradrenaline content in nerve fibres. According to the number of fluorescent nerve fibres per unit area and to the fluorescence intensity, the results were recorded as "weak" (±), "mediate" (+) and "intense" (++) and then compared with the effectiveness of acupuncture anaesthesia.

(IV) Preparation of Specimens and Estimation Method for Monoamine Oxidase (MAO)

Cryostat sections, 10μ thick, obtained from the stomachs of 43 cases with microtome were stained by Glenners' method[5]. The positive enzyme reactions were shown by violet-blue granules distributed in nerve cells and the nerve fibres. Depending on the size, quantity and density of violet-blue granules, the relative enzyme activity was determined as weak (±), mediate (+) or strong (++). Finally, the results were compared with the effectiveness of acupuncture anesthesia.

II. RESULTS

(I) Electron Microscopic Observations

We divided the nerve terminals observed with the electron microscope into 3 types according to the different vesicles contained in them. (Fig. 1). The agranular vesicles, contained primarily in the 1st type of nerve terminals, were 300–500 Å in diameter, enveloped by a thin layer of membrane, transparent and without dense core. It is usually recognized that acetylcholine is stored in these agranular vesicles and the nerve terminals containing such vesicles belong to cholinergic nerves. The small granular vesicles, abundantly contained in the 2nd type of nerve terminals, were 400–600 Å in diameter, with a mem-

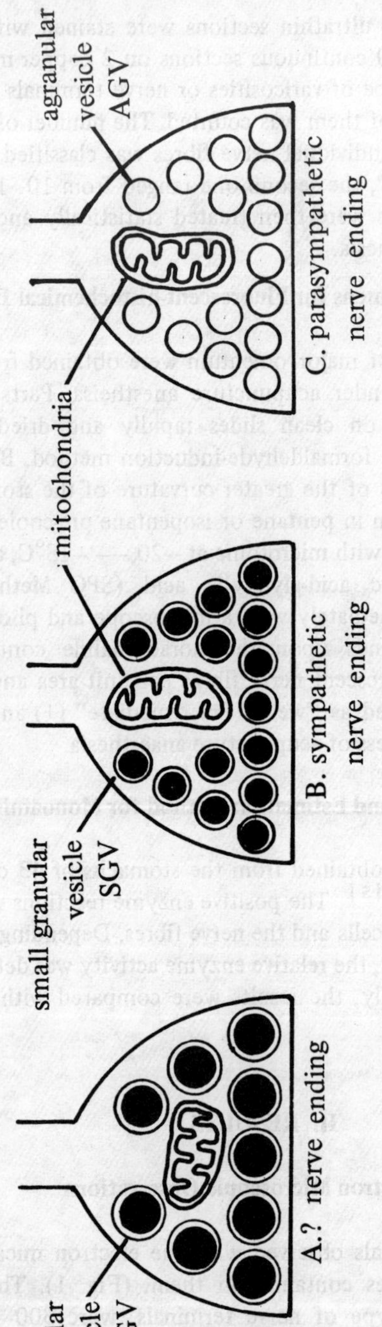

Fig. 1 Three types of nerve ending in the stomach wall

brane and an electron dense core, and with a halo between the dense core and the membrane. It is usually considered that noradrenaline is stored in these small vesicles and the nerve terminals containing such vesicles belong to adrenergic nerves. The 3rd type of nerve terminals contained many large granular vesicles, which were similar to small granular vesicles in structure, but larger in size (1000–1700 Å in diameter) and lower in electron density. It is still unknown what kinds of transmitters might be stored in these large vesicles and what the character of nerve terminals containing such large granular vesicles might be.

During observations, we could not find any apparent change in the number of agranular vesicles contained in cholinergic fibres and also of the small granular vesicles contained in adrenergic nerves. But an important fact was that the nerve terminals containing large granular vesicles were found easily and a bigger quantity of large granular vesicles were contained in individual nerve terminals in more cases (50%) of Grade I; such nerve terminals were not easily found and only a few large granular vesicles were contained in individual nerve terminals in most cases (67%) of Grade III (Table 1, Figs. 2–5). Because the character of the large granular vesicles in nerve fibres of the stomach wall remains unclear so far, we have tried to carry out some qualitative examinations using 3 methods as follows.

Specimens of the stomach wall were fixed with potassium dichromate, potassium permanganate or glutaraldehyde solutions or the mixture of the three, any of the above which would react with noradrenaline and produce electron-opaque precipitates. As a result, the dense cores in either large or small granular vesicles were well preserved. This indicated that the large granular vesicles also contained catecholamines.

Secondly, we found that the large granular vesicles in the nerves of the stomach wall were very similar in many ways, e.g., size (1000–2000Å), ultrastructure and chemical features (chromaffinic), to the chromaffin granucles of chromaffin cells in adrenal medulla. This supported the belief that noradrenaline or adrenaline was contained in the large granular vesicles.

Finally, specimens of the stomach wall from 20 cases were simultaneously examined electron-microscopically and fluorescent-histochemically. It was found that the number of the large granular vesicles was parallel with the fluorescence intensity in 14 cases.

Generally speaking, we have found that the nerve terminals of the 3rd type contained a bigger quantity of large granular vesicles in cases of more effective acupuncture anesthesia than in cases of less effective acupuncture anesthesia, and that the transmitter contained in

Table 1. Correlation between the number of large granular vesicles in a single nerve ending and effectiveness of acupuncture anesthesia

Grade	Total Number of Cases	Number of LGV		
		20– Number of Cases (%)	10–19 Number of Cases (%)	0–9 Number of Cases (%)
I	20	11 (55)	4 (20)	5 (25)
II	18	5 (28)	4 (22)	9 (50)
III	6	1 (16.5)	1 (16.5)	4 (67)

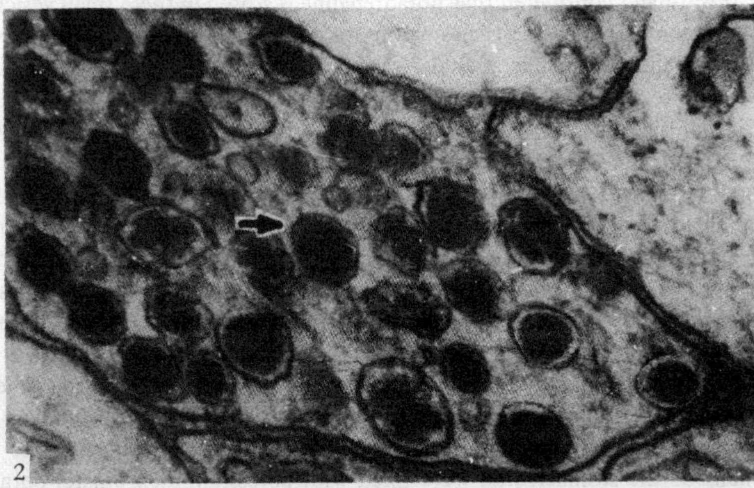

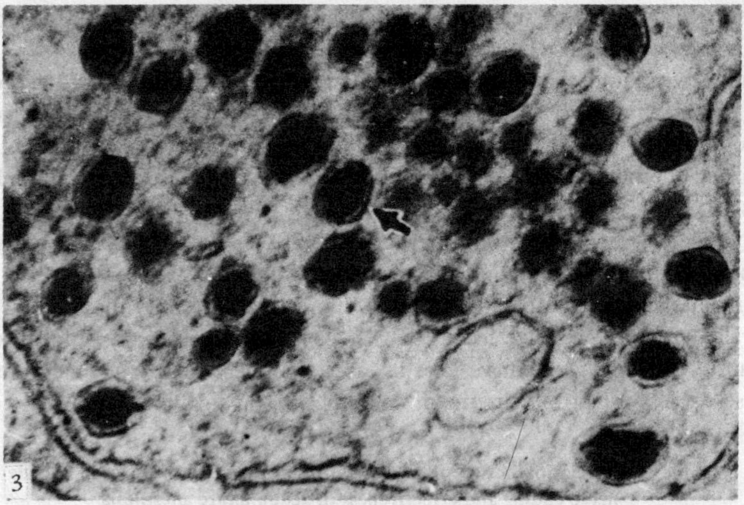

Figs. 2 & 3 show numerous large granular vesicles in individual nerve terminals. Operations performed under acupuncture anaesthesia of grade I 40,000×

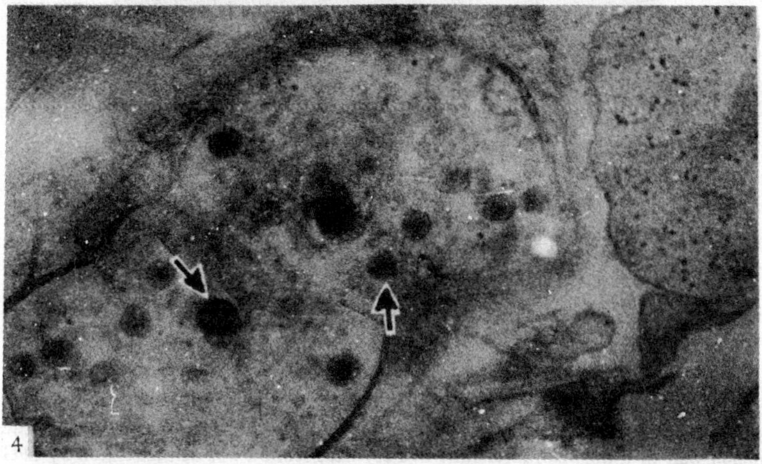

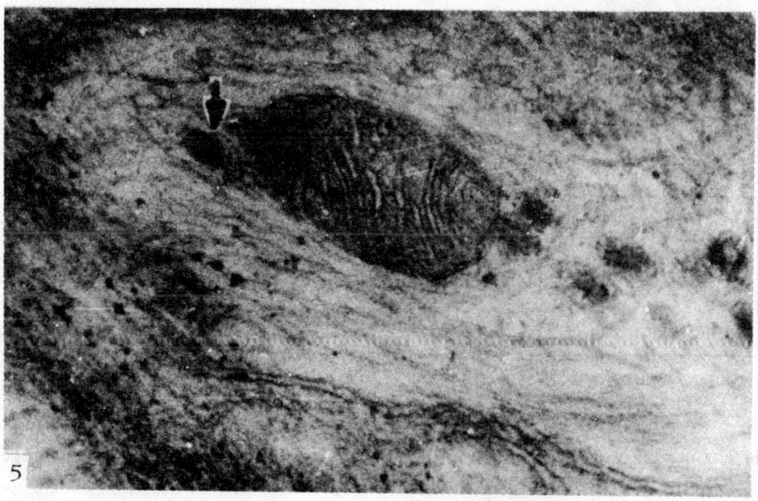

Fig. 4 & 5 Fluorescent micrographs of adrenergic nerves in the stomach wall and major omentum surgically removed from patients subjected to subtotal gastrectomy under acupuncture anaesthesia. Noradrenaline in adrenergic nerves was demonstrated by using formaldehyde-induced fluorescence or SPG methods.

Illustration of Plates (I)

Electron micrographs of individual nerve terminals of type III in muscularis of the stomach wall surgically removed from a patient subjected to subtotal gastrectomy under acupuncture anaesthesia.

↑ shows large granular vesicle

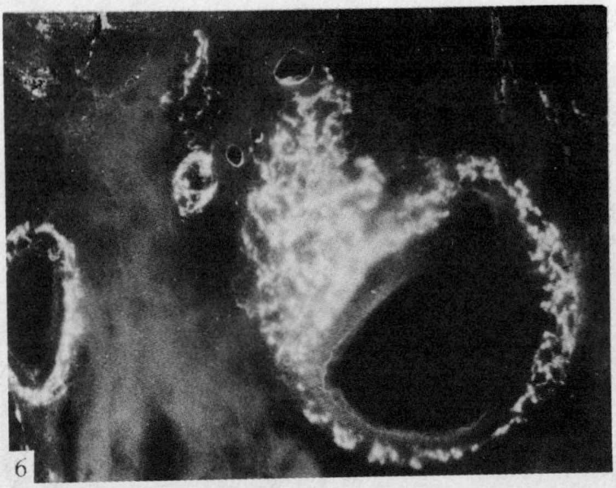

Fig. 6 shows intensive fluorescence in adrenergic nerves about blood vessels in the stomach wall of a dog. Noradrenaline in a cryostat section was demonstrated by SPG method 197×

Table 2. The correlation between the fluorohistochemical changes of transmitter of adrenergic nerve fiber of omentum major and effectiveness of acupuncture anesthesia

Grade	Total Number of Cases	Fluorescence Intensity		
		Weak Number of Cases	Moderate Number of Cases	Intense Number of Cases
I	124	22 (17.7)	38 (30.6)	64 (51.6)
II	54	22 (40.7)	18 (33.3)	14 (25.9)
III	16	9 (56.2)	1 (6.3)	6 (37.5)

Table 3. Correlation between the fluorohistochemical changes of transmitter of adrenergic nerve fibre of stomach wall and effectiveness of acupuncture anaesthesia

Grade	Total Number of Cases	Fluorescence Intensity		
		Weak Number of Cases %	**Moderate** Number of Cases %	**Intense** Number of Cases %
I	31		2 (38.7)	19 (61.3)
II	20	7 (35.0)	7 (35.0)	6 (30.0)
III	10	5 (50.0)	4 (40.0)	1 (10.0)

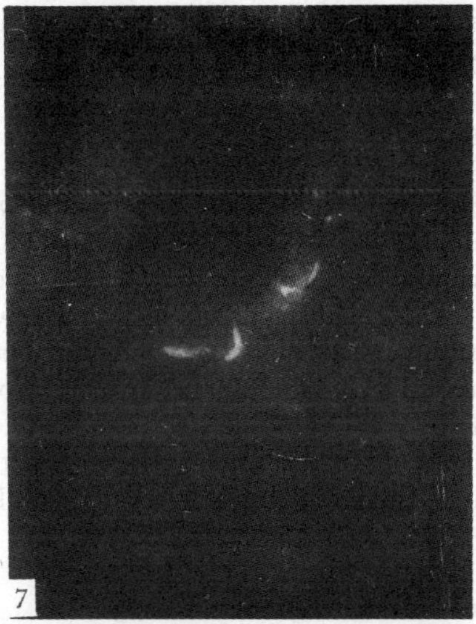

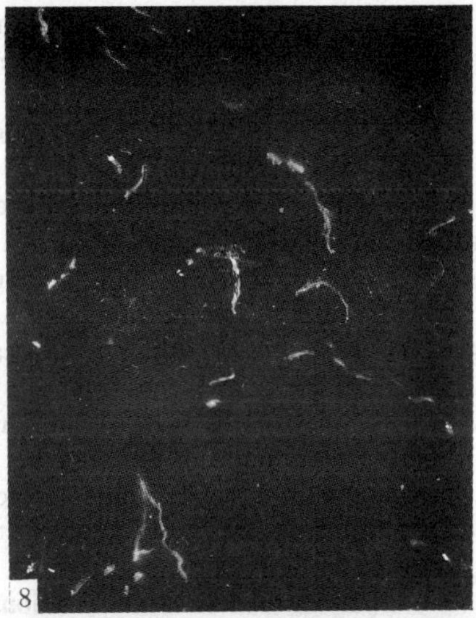

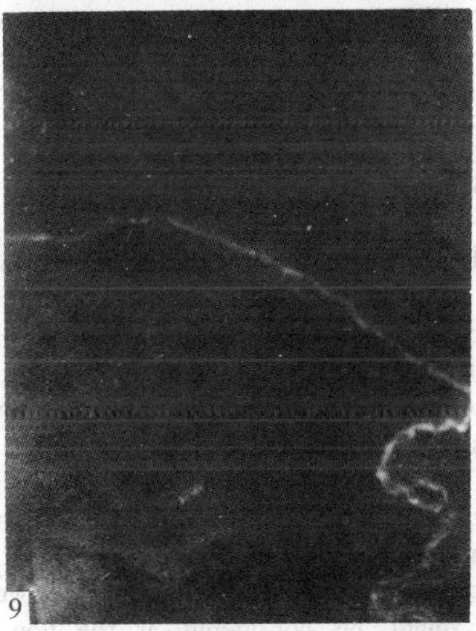

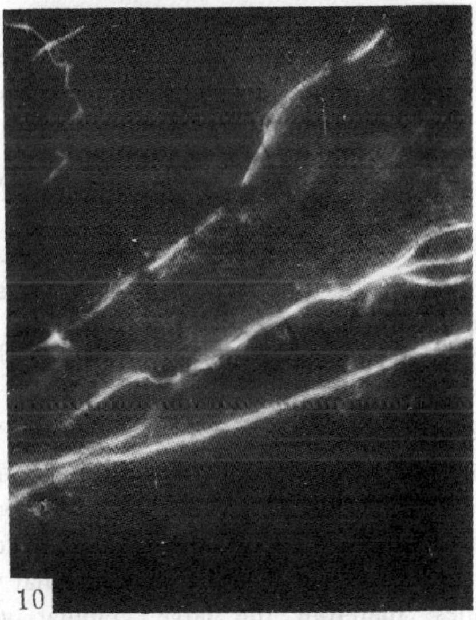

Fig. 7 shows less intensive fluorescence in adrenergic nerves in the stomach wall of a patient subjected to subtotal gastrectomy under acupuncture anaesthesia of grade III. Noradrenaline in cryostat section was demonstrated by SPG method 640 ×

Fig. 8 shows intensive fluorescence in adrenergic nerves in the stomach wall of a patient subjected to subtotal gastrectomy under acupuncture anaesthesia of grade I. Noradrenaline in cryostat section was demonstrated by SPG method 640 ×

Fig. 9 shows less intensive fluorescence in adrenergic nerves in the major omentum of a patient subjected to subtotal gastrectomy under acupuncture anaesthesia of grade III. Noradrenaline in stretch preparation was demonstrated by formaldehyde-induced fluorescence method 750 ×

Fig. 10 shows intensive fluorescence in adrenergic nerves in major omentum of a patient subjected to subtotal gastrectomy under acupuncture anaesthesia was demonstrated by formaldegyde-induced fluorescence method 750 ×.

the large granular vesicles in most likely noradrenaline; therefore the terminals containing the large granular vesicles might be considered as sympathetic.

(II) Fluorescent-histochemical Observations

In major omentum, fluorescent adrenergic nerve fibres were usually accompanied with or surrounded by blood vessels. And in tissues of the stomach wall, a certain amount of fluorescent adrenergic nerves could be found in many areas, e.g., plexus muscularis, intercellular space of muscles, submucosa, basal parts of mucosa epithelium, and blood vessel wall (Fig. 6). The results showed that, in most cases of Grade I, the amount of fluorescent adrenergic fibres and the fluorescence intensity were marked in a range from "+" to "++", especially in the tissues of the stomach wall; none of the cases of Grade I was less than "+".

From Tables 2 and 3, it was seen that the content of noradrenaline in adrenergic nerves was increased with the effectiveness of acupuncture anesthesia in a sequence: Grade I > Grade II > Grade III.

(III) Histochemical Observations on the Monoamine Oxidase Activity

Specimens of 43 cases have been examined. The results showed that the enzyme activity in the nerves of the stomach wall in cases of more effective acupuncture anesthesia was higher than that in cases of less effective acupuncture anesthesia.

III. DISCUSSION

Opinions still differ about the character of the large granular vesicles. In 1968, Silva[6] pointed out that the large granular vesicles could be identified with a positive cholinesterase reaction which fact tended to indicate that the large granular vesicles were closely concerned with cholinergic innervation. Burnstock[7] reported that the stimulating of the sympathetic nerves had resulted in changes in structure, morphology and the number of the large granular vesicles. Tranzer[8] and Jaim-Etcheverry's[9] study showed that sympathetic nerve terminals of cat vas deferens and iris contained many large granular vesicles, in which noradrenaline was stored. It was also reported that the large granular vesicles contained a great amount of chromogranins and dopamine-β-hydroxylase and a little amount of noradrenaline, and that the large granular vesicles become small after liberation of biogenic amines; therefore the large granular vesicles might be considered as the younger vesicles[10–12]. We did not examine the chemical features and functions of the large granular vesicles directly, but we observed similarities between the large granular vesicles and the chromaffins in morphology, ultrastructure and size. At the same time, we discovered that, in most cases, the fluorescence intensity of noradrenaline was positively related to the number of the large granular vesicles in the stomach wall. These findings tended to indicate that the large granular vesicles were the places where noradrenaline was stored and the terminals containing larger granular vesicles were sympathetic in nature. We might also consider that many large granular vesicles and intensive fluorescence in cases of more effective acupuncture anesthesia probably were associated with the accumulation of sympathetic transmitter noradrenaline. Some other authors[13–15] reported, however, that

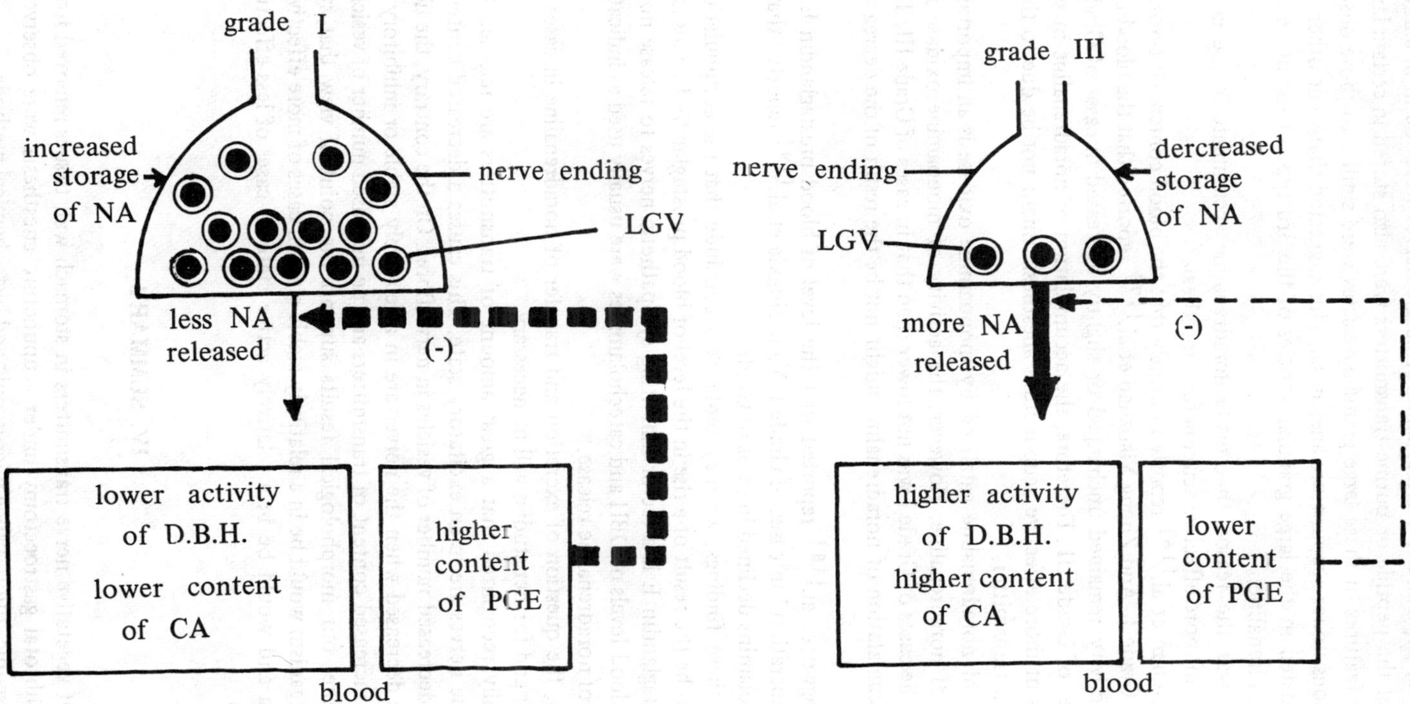

Fig. 11 Diagram of the release of sympathetic nerve transmitters under acupuncture anaesthesia

peptide neurons, peptide nerve fibres and purinergic nerves were found in animal digestive tracts, and that the peptide or purine transmitters were also stored in certain large granular vesicles. Some features of these large granular vesicles were similar to those observed by us during operations under acupuncture anesthesia. This suggested that some other transmitters might have existed in the large granular vesicles of the 3rd type of the nerve terminals in addition to noradrenaline.

But what was the reason that made noradrenaline accumulate in the large granular vesicles in cases of more effective acupuncture anesthesia?

Liang Zhihquan et al.[16] reported recently that the blood content of tyrosine decreased in cases of Grade I. And Zheng Xiaozhao et al.[17] reported that the blood dopamine-β-hydroxylase activity remained unchanged or slightly decreased in cases of Grade I and increased in cases of Grade III. Therefore, the accumulation of noradrenaline in sympathetic nerves in cases of more effective acupuncture anesthesia might not be due to the excessive synthesis of this transmitter.

Oxidation of noradrenaline catalized by monoamine oxidase is an important degradation pathway of noradrenaline. However, the activity of monoamine oxidase in stomach wall nerves in the cases of Grade I was not lower than that in cases of Grade III. This indicated that the accumalation of noradrenaline might not be the result of the decreased degradation of NA.

Zhou Lungwu et al.[18] reported that the level of blood prostaglandin E apparently rose "during operation" in cases of Grade I. Yang Jingxia et al.[19] reported that the blood level of catecholamins declined in cases of Grade I.

Based on these findings, we may tentatively conclude that the accumulation of noradrenaline might be the result of a rise in the level of blood prostaglandin E. This is due to the fact that prostaglandin E is a factor inhibiting sympathetic nerves to release noradrenaline and that the blood levels of DBH and catecholamines were usually used as indicators reflecting the degree of noradrenaline release.

Of course, the question of excretion and transfer of noradrenaline in cases of Grade I are still unclear and further studies will be necessary.

It is usually recognized that a great amount of transmitters are released from nerve fibres when the nerves are in an excitatory state. This causes a decreased content of transmitters and a decreased number of vesicles in nerve fibres. On the contrary, the liberation of transmitters is decreased when the nerves are in a relatively stable or inhibitory state. And this causes an increased content of transmitters and an increased number of vesicles in nerve fibres. Therefore, our morphological results support the point of view that sympathetic nerves of an organism would be in a relatively stable state in cases of more effective acupuncture anesthesia and would be in a relatively active state in cases of less effective acupuncture anesthesia.

IV. SUMMARY

Changes of vegetative nerve transmitters in stomach wall tissues removed from patients subjected to subtotal gastroectomy under acupuncture anesthesia were observed by using electron microscopic, fluorescence microscopic and histochemical methods.

Results, observed in most cases of more effective acupuncture anesthesia, are as follows: increases in the amount of terminals and varicosities of sympathetic nerve fibres containing large granular vesicles and in the number of the large granular vesicles containing transmitters in individual terminals or varicosities.

Preliminary studies about the character of the large granular vesicles showed that these vesicles with similarities to chromaffin granules in animal adrenal medulla might be a possible site for the storage of noradrenaline.

Intense fluorescence observed in adrenergic fibres of the stomach wall and major omentum indicated that more noradrenaline might exist in sympathetic nerves. A parallel relationship between the number of the large granular vesicles and the intensity of fluorescence was observed by combination of two examinations in individual specimens. Higher activity of monoamine oxidase was present in sympathetic nerves of the stomach wall.

The results obtained in most cases of less effective acupuncture anesthesia were for the most part contrary to that mentioned above.

Our results tend to support the viewpoint that sympathetic nerves were in a relatively stable or inhibitory state in cases of more effective acupuncture anesthesia.

REFERENCES

[1] 周 舒：针刺麻醉资料汇编，中国医学科学院 P.33 1979。
[2] 钟守先等：同上 P.7 1979。
[3] Falck, B. et al. : *J.Histochem. Cytochem.*, 10 : 348, 1962.
[4] J. C. de la Torre and Surgeon, J.W. : *Histochem.*, 49 : 81, 1976.
[5] Glenner, G. et al.: *J.Histochem. Cytochem.*, 5:591, 1957.
[6] Silva, D. G. et al. : *Anat. Rec.*, 162:157, 1968.
[7] Burnstock, G.: *Pharmacol. Rev.*, 24:509, 1972.
[8] Tranzer, J.P. and Thoenen, H.: *Experientia*, 24:484, 1968.
[9] Jaim-Etcheverry, G. et al.: Ad*vance Cytopharmacol.*, 1:343, 1971.
[10] H"o"kfelt, J.: *In "Frontiers in Catecholamine Res."*, p.439, 1973.
[11] Geffen, L.B. and Livett, B.G.: Physiol. Rev., 51:98, 1971.
[12] Bloom, F.E.: *J.Histochem. Cytochem.*, 4:21, 1973.
[13] Bishop, A.C. et al.: *Gut*, 18:962, 1977.
[14] Bryant, M.G. et al.: *Lancet*, 1:991, 1976.
[15] Larsson, L.I. et al.: *Histochemistry*, 54:173, 1977.
[16] 梁植权等：针刺麻醉资料汇编，中国医学科学院 P.217，1979。
[17] 郑肖剑等：同上 P.104 1979。
[18] 周隆武等：同上 P.154 1979。
[19] 杨静霞等：同上 P.91 1979。

SOMATOTOPIC PROJECTION OF THE RAPHE NUCLEI TO SPINAL DORSAL HORN IN THE CAT —A HORSERADISH PEROXIDASE STUDY

Ju Gong, Shu Siyun
(The Fourth Medical College of the PLA)

It has been well established that raphe nuclei project to the spinal cord. By using modified Gudden's method as early as 1960, Brodal et al.[1] discovered that the medullary raphe nuclei in the cat, including the nucleus raphe magnus, nucleus raphe pallidus, and nucleus raphe obscurus, project to the spinal cord. A sparse projection from the nucleus raphe pontis was also found. Dahlström and Fuxe[2] and Fuxe[3], using fluoresence histochemistry, found that, in the rat, the medullary raphe nuclei project to the anterior, lateral, and dorsal horns of the spinal cord. Recently, in the different species of animals, the raphe-spinal projection relation has been confirmed with the horseradish peroxidase and autoradiographic techniques[4-11]. But in all these morphological studies, the problem of somatotopic localization in this projection system had not been taken seriously. Crutcher et al.[10] were the only people who mentioned that this projection might be loosely organized in opossum. Whether the raphe-spinal projection is somatotopically localized has much to do with the understanding of its function.

Electrical stimulation of the nucleus raphe magnus tends to inhibit the response of the spinal cord to nociceptive stimuli. The activities of the dorsal root fibers, interneurons of the dorsal horn and the spinothalamic tract neurons may also be influenced[8,11-16]. Du et al.[17] have proved that electrical stimulation of the brain stem raphe nuclei of the cat may inhibit the viscerosomatic reflex provoked by stimulating the greater splanchnic nerve. Among the medullary raphe nuclei, the nucleus raphe magnus is the most potent, with the nucleus raphe pallidus second and the nucleus raphe obscurus the least in effectiveness. Du and Zhao[18] further showed that the destruction of the nucleus raphe magnus and its adjacent area markedly reduced the inhibitory action of acupuncture on the viscerosomatic reflex. Du et al.[17] concluded that the ventral part of the nucleus raphe magnus (including probably a part of the nucleus raphe pallidus) and its adjacent reticular formation might be the center of a strong pain modulating mechanism of the brain stem, and it might be, at the same time, the most important and final station through which is mediated the modulation and control on the transmission of pain signals and on pain reflexes in the spinal cord by the higher centers of the central nervous system. They inferred that this mechanism might be activated during acupuncture analgesia. It is generally accepted that by acupuncturing a specific point, a definite area of analgesia might result[19,20]. It is thus evident that the problem of somatotopic localization is significant in the analysis of the role of the raphe-spinal projection in acupuncture analgesia.

I. MATERIAL AND METHOD

Horseradish peroxidase (HRP) was injected into the dorsal horn of the cervical or lumbar intumescence (C_7 or $L_{4,5}$) in 11 cats, of which 7 were cervical and 4 lumbar injections. Of the 11 cases, 3 cervical and 3 lumbar ones gave satisfactory results, on which the following analysis was based. The results of the remaining cases were in full accord with those 6 cases.

Operations were performed under nembutal anesthesia. The lamina of the 6th cervical or 4th lumbar vertebra was removed and the cat was mounted on a spinal column stabilizing device. The dorsal medium sulcus of the spinal cord was identified as the site for locating the point of injection. The dura at the determined injection point was picked by a small hook and a minute hole cut with a pair of scissors. A micropipette containing a 30% HRP aqueous solution (Dong Feng, RZ 2.5 or 3.1) was connected to a microsyringe with a plastic tube, which was then inserted to the desired depth (centering at lamina V of Rexed). All the injections were on the right side of the spinal cord. Two points were injected in each case, and 0.1–0.2μl was injected at each point with an interval of several millimeters. The micropipette was left for 20 minutes after injection. The animals were allowed to survive for 2.5–4.5 days and then a solution of cold 3% paraformaldehyde - 1% glutaldehyde in 0.1*M* phosphate buffer (pH 7.4) was perfused through their aorta. Immediately afterwards, the brain and the spinal cord were removed and the injected spinal segment and the brain stem immersed in the same fixative for 24 hrs at 0–4°C. The injections and survival periods are shown in Table 1.

We have compared Graham and Karnovsky's diaminobenzidine method[21] with Mesulam's benzidine method[22] and found that when examined under a light microscope, Mesulam's benzidine technique is much more sensitive than the diaminobenzidine technique [23]. Mesulam's technique was thus adopted in this study, but the concentration of nitrofer-

Table 1. Injections and survival periods

Cat No.	Body Weight (kg)	Spinal Segment	30% HRP			Survival Period (days)
			RZ	Speed of injection (min./0.1μl)	Volume (μl) per injection	
$C_{11\text{-}11}$	2.5	C_7	2.5	50	0.1	3
$C_{11\text{-}27}$	2.25	C_7	3.1	20	0.2	3
$C_{11\text{-}28}$	2.25	C_7	3.1	20	0.2	2.5
$C_{11\text{-}21}$	2.5	L_4	3.1	45	0.15	3.5
$C_{11\text{-}25}$	3.0	L_5	3.1	18	0.2	4
$C_{11\text{-}26}$	3.15	L_4	3.1	18	0.2	4.5

ricyanide in the stabilizing solution was modified to 1.5% or 2%. Serial frozen sections in 40μm were cut. After coloration the sections were mounted. Every other section was counterstained with neutral red. The sections were examined under darkfield illumination.

II. RESULTS

The injected areas of each case are shown in Fig. 1. The extents of two injections in each case are largely the same. Fig. 1 shows the slightly larger injection points. Around the needle track is a dark blue area, sometimes intermingled with brown reaction product. Around this central area is a lighter peripheral zone. The central areas of all the cases are largely located in the dorsal horns. In some cases they extend in varying degrees ventrally.

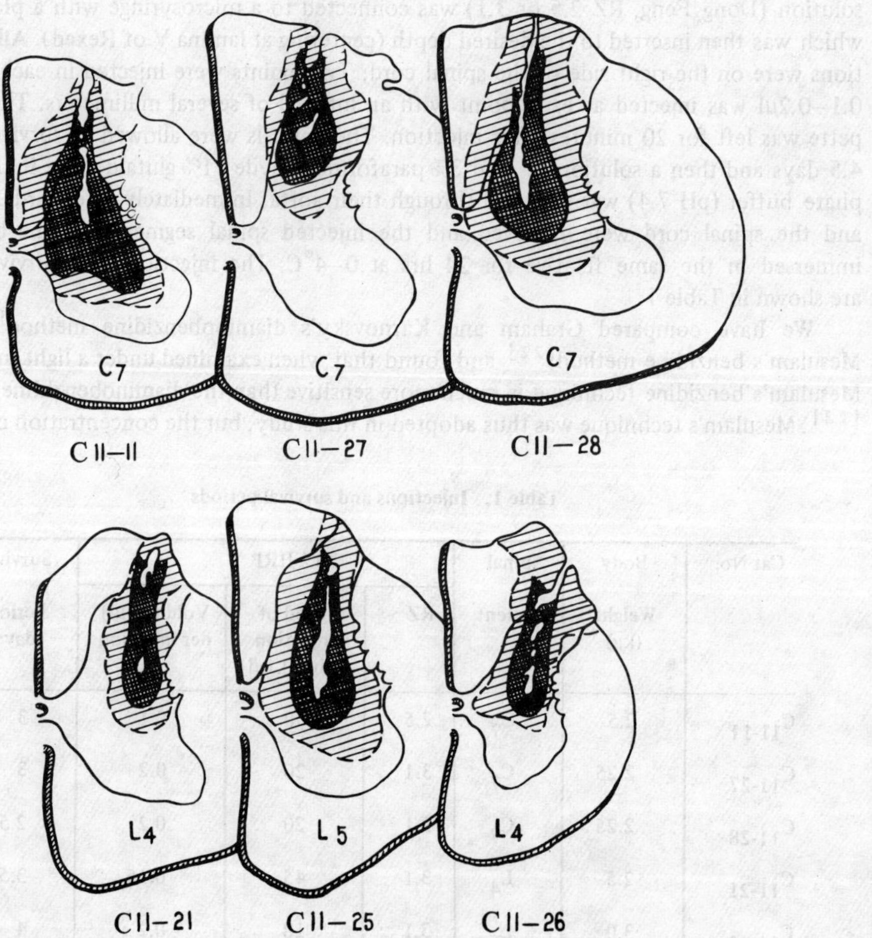

Fig. 1 Extent of injection. Crossed area:center of injection. Hatched area:peripheral zone.

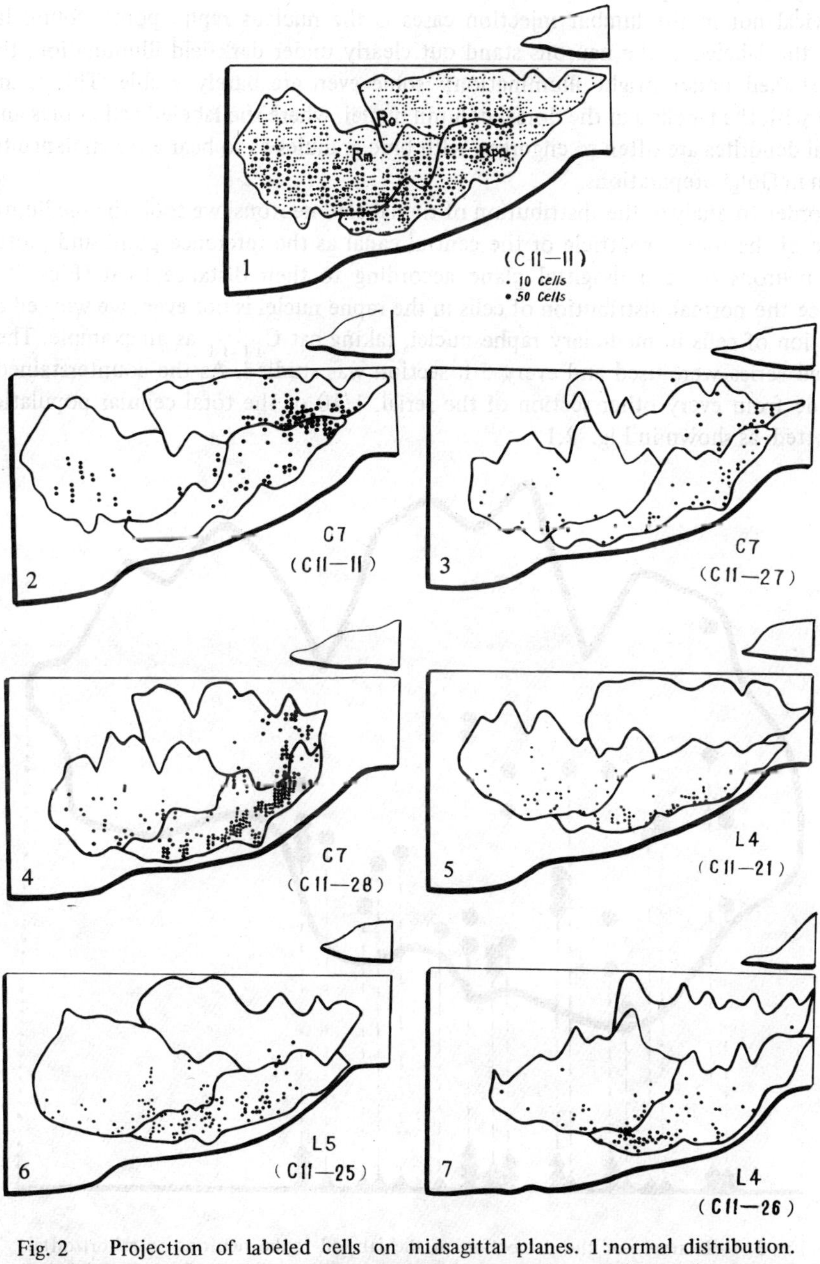

Fig. 2 Projection of labeled cells on midsagittal planes. 1:normal distribution. 2–4:cervical injection cases. 5–7:lumbar injection cases. Rm: nucleus raphe magnus. Ro:nucleus raphe obscurus. Rpa:nucleus raphe pallidus.

In C_7 injection cases, many labeled cells are found in the nucleus raphe magnus, nucleus raphe pallidus, and nucleus raphe obscurus (Figs. 8–10). In L_4 or L_5 injection cases, labeled cells are found in the nucleus raphe magnus and nucleus raphe pallidus only (Figs. 6, 7), while only occasionally are labeled neurons found in the nucleus raphe obscurus. Neither in the cervical nor in the lumbar injection cases is the nucleus raphe pontis found labeled. Though the labeled raphe neurons stand out clearly under darkfield illumination, they are faintly stained under bright illumination; some even are barely visible. This is in sharp contrast with the labeling in the dorsal column nuclei, where the labeled cell bodies and their proximal dendrites are often so engorged with blue granules as to bear a resemblance to what was seen in Golgi preparations.

In order to analyze the distribution of the labeled neurons, we took the medium line of the base of the fourth ventricle or the central canal as the reference point and plotted the labeled neurons on a midsagittal plane according to their distance to it (Figs. 2. 2–7).

Since the normal distribution of cells in the raphe nuclei is not even, we worked out the distribution of cells in medullary raphe nuclei, taking cat $C_{11\text{-}11}$ as an example. The counterstained series were used and every 5th section was studied. As the counterstained series was made from every other section of the serial, 1/10 of the total cellular population was thus plotted, as shown in Fig. 2.1.

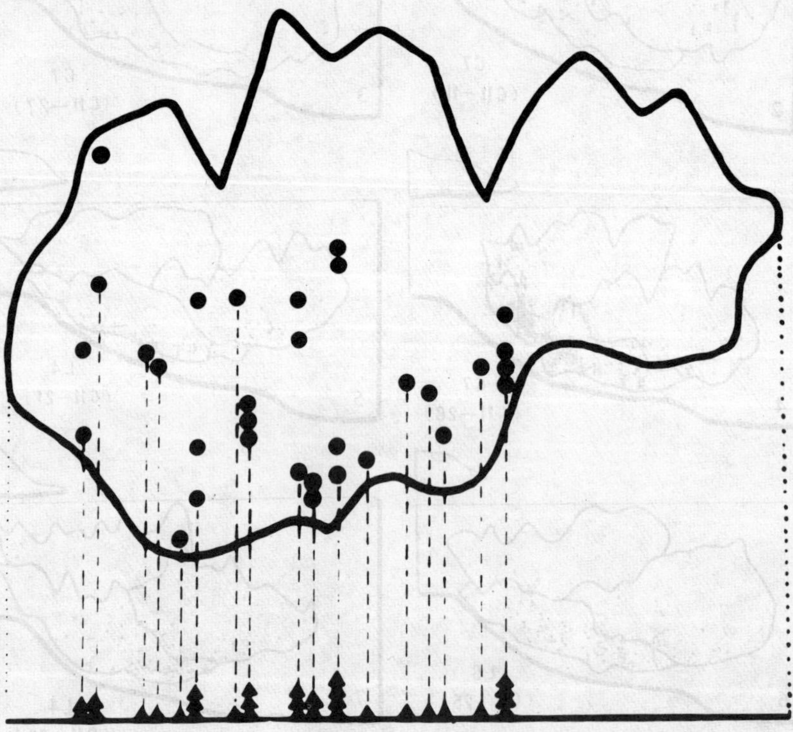

Fig. 3 Example of the projection of the labeled raphe neurons on a horizontal line, which represents the craniocaudal extent of the nucleus, the left end being its cranial pole. Triangles represent the labeled cells projected on the line.

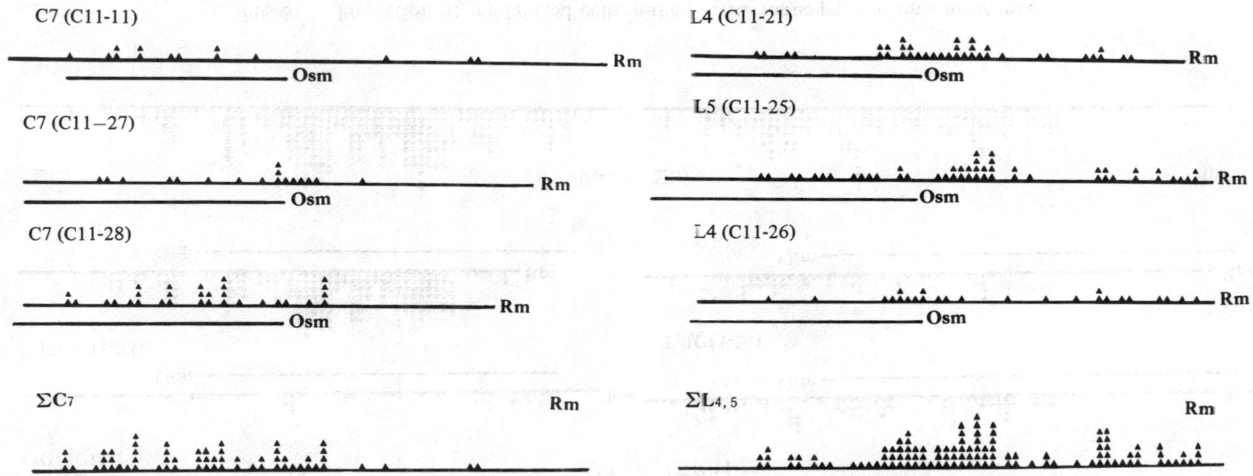

Fig. 4 Projection of the labeled cells in the nucleus raphe magnus on a horizantal line. Rm:nucleus raphe magnus. Osm:medial superior olivary nucleus. ΣC:3 cervical cases summed up. ΣL:3 lumbar cases summed up.

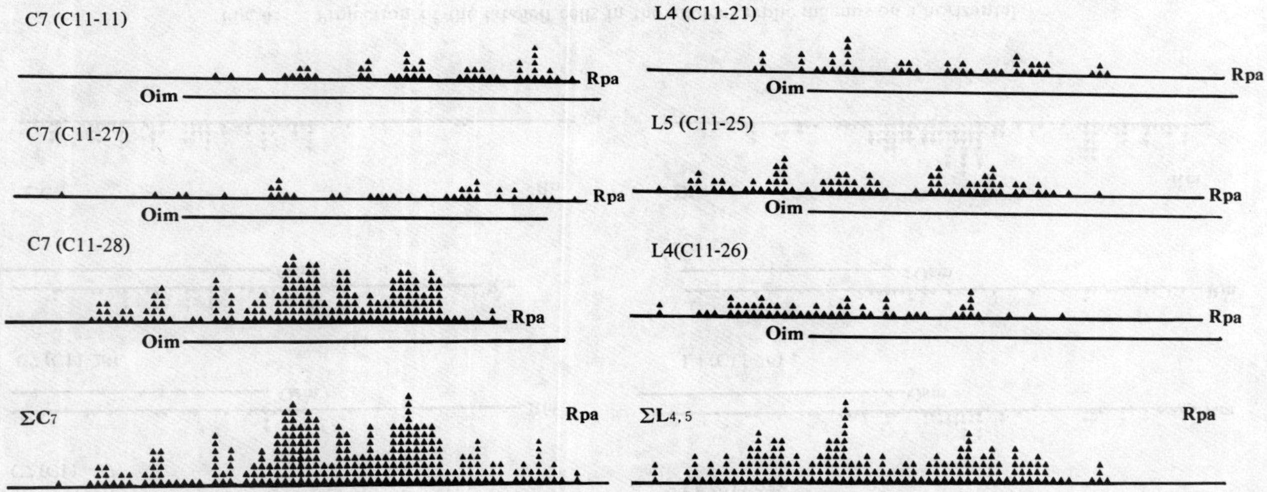

Fig. 5 Projection of the labeled cells in the nucleus raphe pallidus on a horizontal line. Rpan:nucleus raphe pallidus. Oim:medial accessory nucleus of the inferior olive. ΣC:3 cervical cases summed up. ΣL:3 lumbar cases summed up.

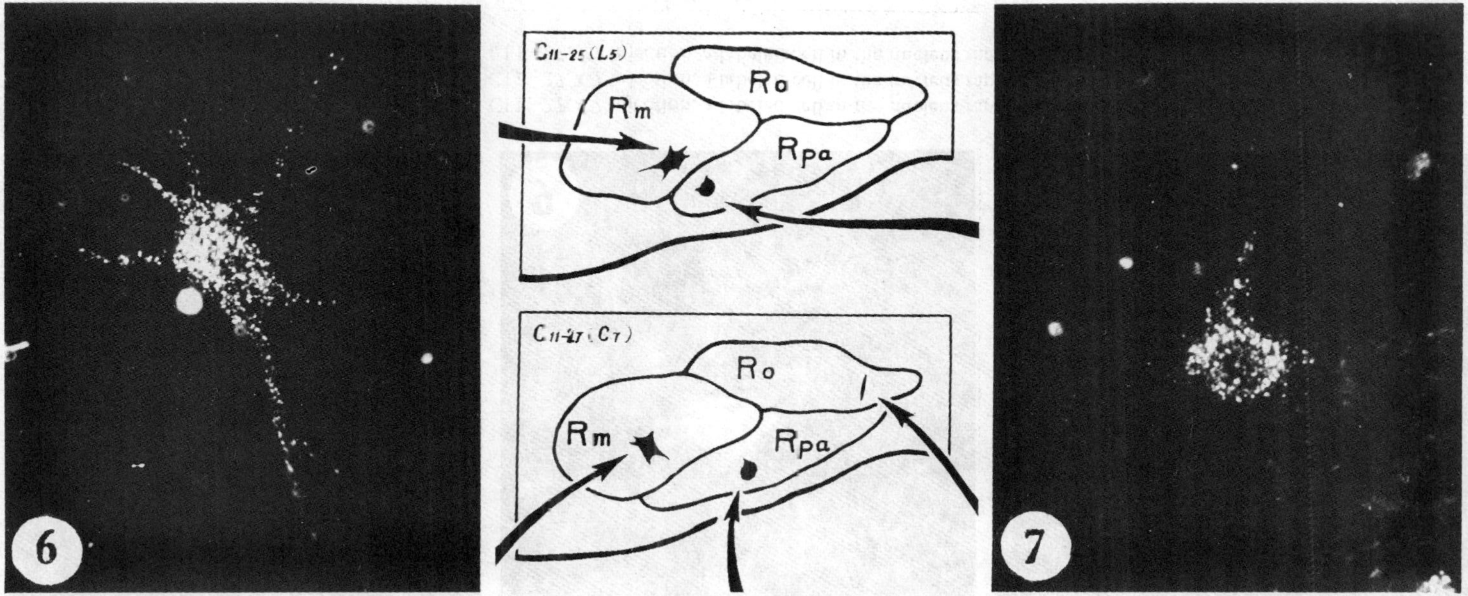

Fig. 6 C11−25 L5 injection, a labeled cell in the nucleus raphe magnus.
Fig. 7 C11−25, L5 injection, a labeled cell in the nucleus raphe pallidus.

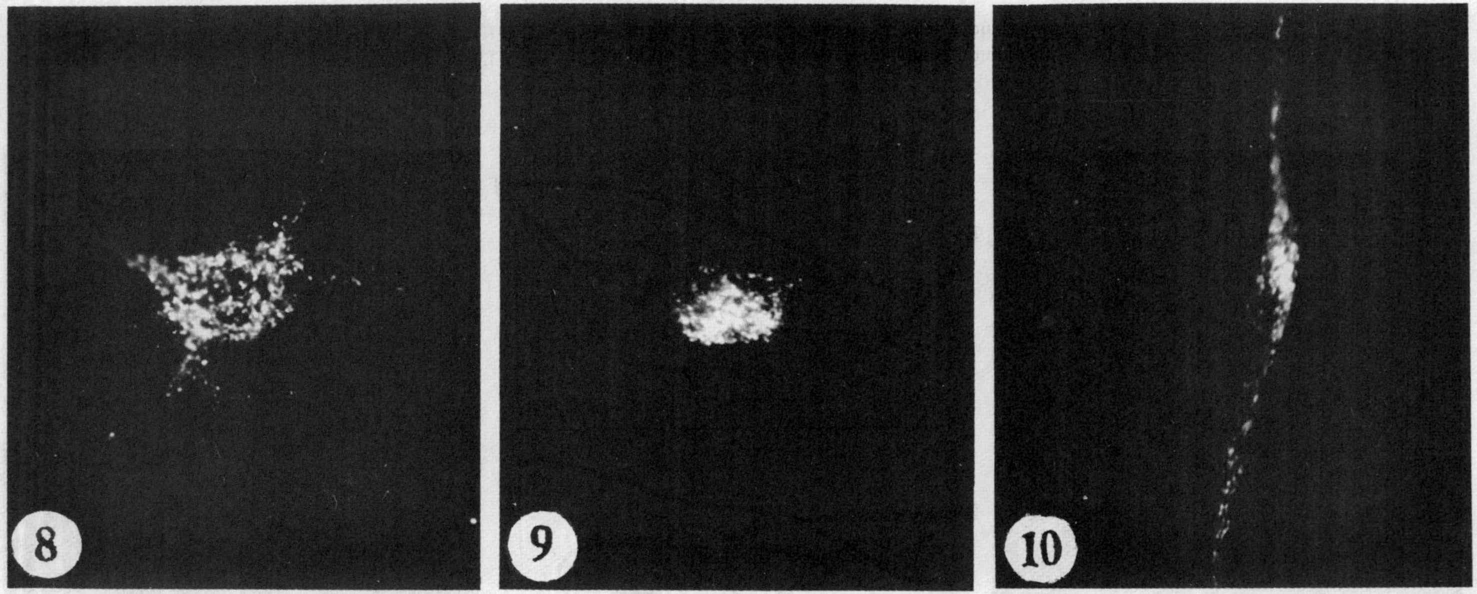

Fig. 8 C11–27, C7 injection, a labeled cell in the nucleus raphe magnus.
Fig. 9 C11–27, C7 injection, a labeled cell in the nucleus raphe pallidus.
Fig. 10 C11–27, C7 injection, a labeled cell in the nucleus raphe obscurus.

Fig. 6–10 are microphotographs under darkfield illumination, 790×. The locations of the labeled cells are shown in the schemeat the middle of the upper row. Rm: nucleus raphe magnus, Ro:nucleus raphe obscurus, Rpa:nucleus raphe pallidus.

From Fig. 2, it is evident that: (1) though the injection of HRP is limited to within one spinal segment, the distribution of labeled cells in the raphe nuclei is rather widespread; (2) the labeled cells are unevenly distributed and they tend to concentrate themselves on a certain region of the nucleus. This may partly be due to the normal uneven distribution of the raphe neurons. For example, there are more cells in the ventral part of the nucleus raphe magnus, where the labeled cells are also numerous. On the other hand, it is found to be closely related to the site of injection. By comparing Figs. 2.2–4 with 5–7, it is evident that the distribution differs in the cervical and in the lumbar cases after injection and the difference is shown mainly along the cranio-caudal axis.

To further analyze their cranio-caudal distribution, we plotted the labeled cells in the nucleus raphe magnus and nucleus raphe pallidus on horizontal lines as shown in Figs. 3,4, and 5. Since the cranial and caudal poles of the raphe nuclei may not always be clear cut, we marked out the extent of the medial superior olivary nucleus and the medial accessory nucleus of the inferior olive respectively for reference. We further summed up the cervical or lumbar cases (ΣC and ΣL in Figs. 4 and 5). By comparing ΣC with ΣL of either nucleus raphe magnus or nucleus raphe pallidus, it is clear that though the labeled cells, after a single spinal segment injection, are widely distributed, there remain, nevertheless, areas of relative concentration which differ in cervical and lumbar injection cases, though they overlap each other. In the nucleus raphe magnus, cells projecting to the cervical dorsal horn are located more cranially and those to the lumbar dorsal horn more caudally. On the contrary, in the nucleus raphe pallidus those projecting to the cervical dorsal horn are located more caudally while those to the lumbar cord more cranially.

III. DISCUSSION

(I) The Extent of Effective Uptake in Injection Areas

Opinions differ as to the extent of effective uptake of HRP by nerve terminals in the injection areas. Some maintain that the area of uptake fits well with the stained area[24]. Others, however, believe that only the center of injection was effective[25,26]. This is related to the length of the survival period. The clearing process starts almost immediately after HRP injection[25]. Haberly and Price[27] have reported that after 24 hrs, the extent of staining was definitely smaller than that after 6 hours survival. Besides, the technique of coloration also affects the result. Since different techniques differ in sensitivity, they give different extents of staining on the same material[23]. The survival periods in this study are 2.5–4.5 days, the stained areas are of course smaller than the original. But according to our observation, under our experimental conditions, even after 3 days of survival, when processed with Mesulam's method, the area of effective uptake fits largely with the central area of injection. The effective zones of uptake in the present study are thus estimated to be mainly in the dorsal horns.

(II) Somatotopic Localization of the Projection From the Nucleus Raphe Magnus

Our results show that the nucleus raphe magnus projects to the spinal dorsal horn rather diffusely. And yet, a certain degree of localization does exist, viz., cells projecting to the cervical cord are located more cranially and those to the lumbar more caudally.

The widely distributed projection fits well with the amount of the HRP granules found in the labeled cells. As mentioned above, the labeling of the raphe neurons is quite light, which contrasts sharply with the heavy labeling in the dorsal column nuclei. There can be two explanations for this: (1) the ability of the raphe neurons in taking up HRP may be weaker; (2) more likely, their axons are distributed to widely separated regions and a large part of the terminal arborization of a neuron may be outside of the sphere of injection, and the retrograde transport from the normal area dilutes the HRP transported from the injection area[28,29].

From the fact that the projection is widely distributed and at the same time somatotopically localized to a certain degree, it may be inferred that a focal stimulation of the nucleus raphe magnus may evoke analgesia of a wide region. In other words , the stimulation of a large area of the nucleus raphe magnus should be able to cause analgesia on the same body part. Meanwhile, the maximun analgesic effect should be somewhat somatotopically localized. Du et al.[17] have reported that the electrical stimulation of a large area in the nucleus raphe magnus tends to inhibit the discharges in the 11th intercostal nerve evoked by stimulating the greater splanchnic nerve (viscero-somatic reflex). From Fig. 4 it can be seen that the effective stimulating points in the nucleus raphe magnus are distributed at the level of facial nucleus and the caudal pole of the superior olivary nucleus, which happens to be an area between the labeled areas of our cervical and lumbar injection cases, but nearer to the latter.

During acupuncture analgesia, the effect of a specific acupuncture point is often rather widespread, but at the same time confined to definite body regions. Clinically, different prescriptions have been developed for operations on different parts of the body. Shirota et al.[20] had succeeded in evoking analgesia in different body regions by stimulating different acupuncture points electrically. When the stimulations were prolonged the analgesic areas expanded till they reached a certain limit, beyond which no further expansion was possible. The diffused but localized analgesic effect of acupuncture can of course be explained in different ways, but the descending projection from the nucleus raphe magnus has exactly the same features, thus supporting the hypothesis of the active role of the nucleus raphe magnus in acupuncture analgesia and providing a morphological explanation of the relative specificity of acupuncture points in their regions of analgesia.

(III) Somatotopic Projection From the Nucleus Raphe Pallidus to the Spinal Dorsal Horn

The nucleus raphe pallidus is also somatotopically localized. But, contrary to the nucleus raphe magnus, the cells projecting to the cervical cord are located more caudally while those to the lumbar more cranially. Brodal et al.[1] hemitransected the upper cervical cord of the cat and found the chromatolyzed cells located chiefly in the rostral part of the nucleus. At first glance, their result would seem to be contradictory to ours, but taking into consideration their findings that there were more chromotolyzed cells in the caudal part of the nucleus raphe magnus instead of in the cranial part, it became apparent that the areas where they found their chromatolyzed cells concentrated are exactly the areas where we found our labeled cells after lumbar injections. This naturally made us suspect their results to be limited by the method they used, viz., the modified Gudden's method. The degree of chromatolysis in a neuron is related to the proportion of the part cut off. When a cut is made at the upper cervical level, the part cut off in neurons projecting to the lumbar cord is evidently proportionally larger than that in neurons projecting to the cervical cord, and the former would then show more severe chromatolysis.

(IV) Spinal Projection From the Nucleus Raphe Obscurus and Nucleus Raphe Pontis

It has been mentioned in the literature[1,11] and confirmed by the present study that the nucleus raphe obscurus has efferent projection to the spinal cord. However, when the dorsal horn of the L4,5 spinal segment was injected with HRP, no labeled cells or occasionally only some were found in this nucleus (Figs. 2.5–7), while Martin et al.[11], after injecting HRP into the entire spinal grey at L6 in the cat, found large amounts of labeled cells in the nucleus raphe obscurus. It shows that in the lumbar spinal cord, the nucleus raphe obscurus may only project to the ventral part of the spinal cord. Martin et al.[11] found that, by cutting the different parts of the white matter at Th12-L1 level, the descending fibers from the nucleus raphe obscurus to the lumbar cord were seen to run mainly in the ventral funiculus. This is in accord with our inference. In our cervical injection cases, a certain amount of labeled cells were found in the nucleus raphe obscurus (Figs. 2.2–4 and 10). This was true in cat $C_{11\text{-}27}$ where the injection was entirely confined to the dorsal horn (Fig. 1). This proves that in the cervical cord the nucleus raphe obscurus has projection to the dorsal horn. This of course does not rule out the possibility that it may project more ventrally.

Brodal et al. ('60, cat)[1], Martin ('77, monkey)[6], and Martin et al. ('78, cat)[11] all found that the nucleus raphe pontis may project sparsely to the spinal cord. We could not demonstrate it in either the cervical or lumbar injection cases. This may be due to the sparseness of the projection and the small dosage in our injections as to escape detection. It is also possible that this projection terminates in areas outside of the spheres of our injections in the dorsal horn.

IV. SUMMARY

HRP was injected into the dorsal horn of the C7 or L4,5 spinal segment in cats and the labeled cells in the raphe nuclei were traced. In the cervical injection cases the nucleus raphe magnus, nucleus raphe pallidus and nucleus raphe obscurus were found labeled.

In the lumbar injection cases only the nucleus raphe magnus and nucleus raphe pallidus were labeled. The projections from the nucleus raphe magnus and nucleus raphe pallidus to the spinal cord are rather diffuse, and yet a certain degree of somatotopical localization exists, viz., the projection to the cervical dorsal horn originates from the more cranial part of the nucleus raphe magnus and the more caudal part of the nucleus raphe pallidus, while the projection to the lumbar dorsal horn, on the contrary, originates from the more caudal part of the nucleus raphe magnus and the more cranial part of the nucleus raphe pallidus.

This somatotopic relationship speaks in favor of the hypothesis of the role of descend-

---

Wang Xi-Lien took part in the technical work of this study.

ing inhibition from the raphe nuclei during acupuncture analgesia and it provides a morphological explanation of the relative specificity of acupuncture points in their regions of analgesia.

REFERENCES

[1] Brodal et al: *J. Comp Neur*, **114**:239, 1960.
[2] Dahlstrom A and Fuxe K: *Acta physiol scand*, **64**:suppl 247, 1965.
[3] Fuxe K: *Acta physiol scand*, **64**:suppl 247, 1965.
[4] Bobillier P et al: *Brain Res*, **113**:449, 1976.
[5] Kuypers HGJM and Maisky VA: *Brain Res*, **136**:159, 1977.
[6] Martin R: *Anat Rec*, 187:654, 1977.
[7] Castiglioni AJ et al: *Anat Rec*, **187**:547, 1977.
[8] Basbaum AI et al: *Proc Natl Acad Sci USA, 73*:4685, 1967.
[9] Basbaum AI et al: *J. Comp Neur*, **178**:209, 1978.
[10] Grutcher KA et al: *J. Comp Neur*, **79**:169, 1978.
[11] Martin RF et al: *J. Comp Neur*, **182**:77, 1978.
[12] Proudifit HK and Anderson EG: *Brain Res*, **98**:612, 1975.
[13] Beall JE et al: *Brain Res*, **114**:328, 1976.
[14] Field HL et al: *Brain Res*, **126**:441, 1977.
[15] Guilbaud G et al: *Brain Res*, **126**:355, 1977.
[16] Willis WD et al: *J. Neurophysiol*, **40**:968, 1977.
[17] 杜焕基等：生理学报，30：1，1978。
[18] 杜焕基及赵燕芳：中国科学（6）：631，1975。
[19] 张香桐：中国科学，（4）：465，1978。
[20] 代田文彦等：麻醉，22：73，1973。
[21] Graham RC Jr and Karnovsky MJ: *J. Histochem Cytochem*, **14**:291, 1966.
[22] Mesulam M-M: *J. Histochem Cytochem*, **24**:1273, 1976.
[23] 舒斯云，鞠躬：待发表。
[24] Hoddevik GH et al: *Brain Res*, **123**:209, 1977.
[25] La Vail JH: The Use of Axonal Transport for Studies of Neuronal Connectivity, p217, Elsevier, Amsterdam, 1975.
[26] Vanegas H et al: *J. Comp Neur*, **177**:193, 1978.
[27] Haberly LB and Price JL: *J. Comp Neur*, **178**:711, 1978.
[28] Nauta HJW et al: *Brain Res*, **67**:219, 1974.
[29] Mosko SS et al: *Brain Res*, **119**:269, 1977.

INFLUENCE OF ELECTROACUPUNCTURE ON ULTRASTRUCTURE OF SYNAPSES IN MEDIAL REGION OF RAT THALAMUS

Ai Minkang , Wu Zhongjing

(Department of Acupuncture Anesthesia Research, Wuhan Medical College)

Li Tongping

(Laboratory of Electron Microscopy, Wuhan Medical College)

It has been suggested that acupuncture analgesia is essentially a function of the central nervous system resulting from the inhibitory interaction between the afferent impulses arising from the point of acupuncture and those from the site of pain in the brain, especially in the thalamus[1]. The medial region of the thalamus may be the site receiving the impulse of pain[2,3,4].

Interneuronal transmission may take place at synapses and, in higher species, the transmission requires the release of a neurotransmitter from synaptic vesicles generally believed to be its storagesite. On this account, the medial region of the thalamus was chosen for observing the changes of the synaptic ultrastructure after electroacupuncture.

I. MATERIALS AND METHODS

10 rats were grouped in 5 pairs and each pair is made up of rats of the same sex and approximate weight. In the pairs, one was used for electroacupuncture and the other for a control. The pain threshold is taken according to the milliamperes required for irritating the vocalization of the rats. In the needled animals, besides the measurement of the basic pain threshold, electroacupuncture was given to the points "Renzhong" and "Chenjiang" for 30 minutes with a frequency of 200 per minute. The current intensity for needling was increased gradually from the beginning of the stimulation until the appearance of slight twitches of the limbs.

After postinduction, the pain threshold was measured and the animal was perfused through the left ventricle of the heart with cold 4% formaldehyde buffered with 0.1*M* sodium cacodylate (pH 7.2) for 15–20 minutes. After decapitation, the brain was rapidly removed. In accordance with the atlas in Craige's Neuroanatomy of Rat[5], a sheet of brain slice about 1 mm thick was cut along the A–A axis at the levels of A21 to A23 and was placed in the same perfusion fluid for 3 hours at 4°C. A tiny piece of the tissue (about 1 mm^2) directly ventral to the habenular nucleus from the thalamus of the right side of the brain slice was excised as material for ultrastructure study, while that of the left side was left intact. It was then put into Caulfield's osmic acid fluid (pH 7.4) for postfixating for 2 hours at 4°C. Afterwards, embedment with methacrylate, ultrasection, and staining with uranyl acetate or lead citrate were performed in succession before electron microscopy.

In order to make sure what nuclei were contained in the excised material, the following procedures were followed. First, the frozen section of the remaining brain slice after staining was examined under a light microscope, focusing especially on the corresponding region of the left side so as to deduce the nuclei in the excised material from the right thalamus. In addition, according to the cytological characteristics of the nuclei in the medial region of the thalamus[6,7] the nuclei were further identified in the thick sections from methacrylate block.

The presynaptic bag as well as the synaptic cleft in the electron micrograph were measured, and the actual area (μ^2), cleft width (Å) and the number of synaptic vesicles per μ^2 were also calculated.

II. OBSERVATIONS AND RESULTS

1. Pain threshold. It was found that the pain thresold was elevated after electroacupuncture ($P < 0.025$).

2. Synapses in control rat: From the observations of the methacrylate thick sections as well as the frozen sections of the brain slice under a light microscope, it was shown that the material removed for ultrastructure research contained Nuc. medialis, Nuc. parafascicularis, Nuc. paraventricularis and Nuc. parataenialis thalami.

Under electron microscopy, 218 synapses (113 synapses in the controls and 105 in the electroacupuncture group) were examined. Lots of synapses were found in the nuclei of the medial region of the thalamus. Among them, the axon-dendric type was predominant (Fig. 1) and axon-axonic and axonsomatic came next. The presynaptic bags with an average area of $0.513 \pm 0.201\ \mu^2$ contained different amounts of vesicles. In our formaldehyde-osmic acid fixed tissue the synaptic vesicles, mainly the clear type (without dense core) about 500Å in diameter (Figs.1,2,3,5,6) were well defined, while large granular vesicles, though also found in our preparations, were few in number. Electron microphotographs illustrate that the shape of the clear vesicles may vary; some are spherical and others ellipsoid or flat (Figs. 1,2). In the control group, the vesicles of oval or ellipsoid form are more obvious than those of round (Figs. 1,2,5).

3. Synapses in electroacupunctured rats. Accompanied with an elevation of the pain threshold after electro-acupuncture, there was an increase of clear synaptic vesicles especially those of the round shape (Fig. 3), while the vesicles of flat type appeared to have decreased. If the mean value of clear vesicles was taken as 100, the percentages of the different shapes of vesicles would show a similar tendency of ultrastructure changes (Table 1).

Besides this, the increase of vesicles and the elevation of pain threshold in needled rats were simultaneously accompanied by a widening of the synaptic cleft (Fig. 6). Fig.4 demonstrates that the synaptic cleft in the electroacupuncture group (133.14 ± 9.13 Å) is wider in comparison with that in the controls (110.05 ± 11.67 Å).

Provided the means of vesicle number (118.49) and the width of synaptic cleft (110.05) in the control group are taken as the standard value, the synapses examined can be classified

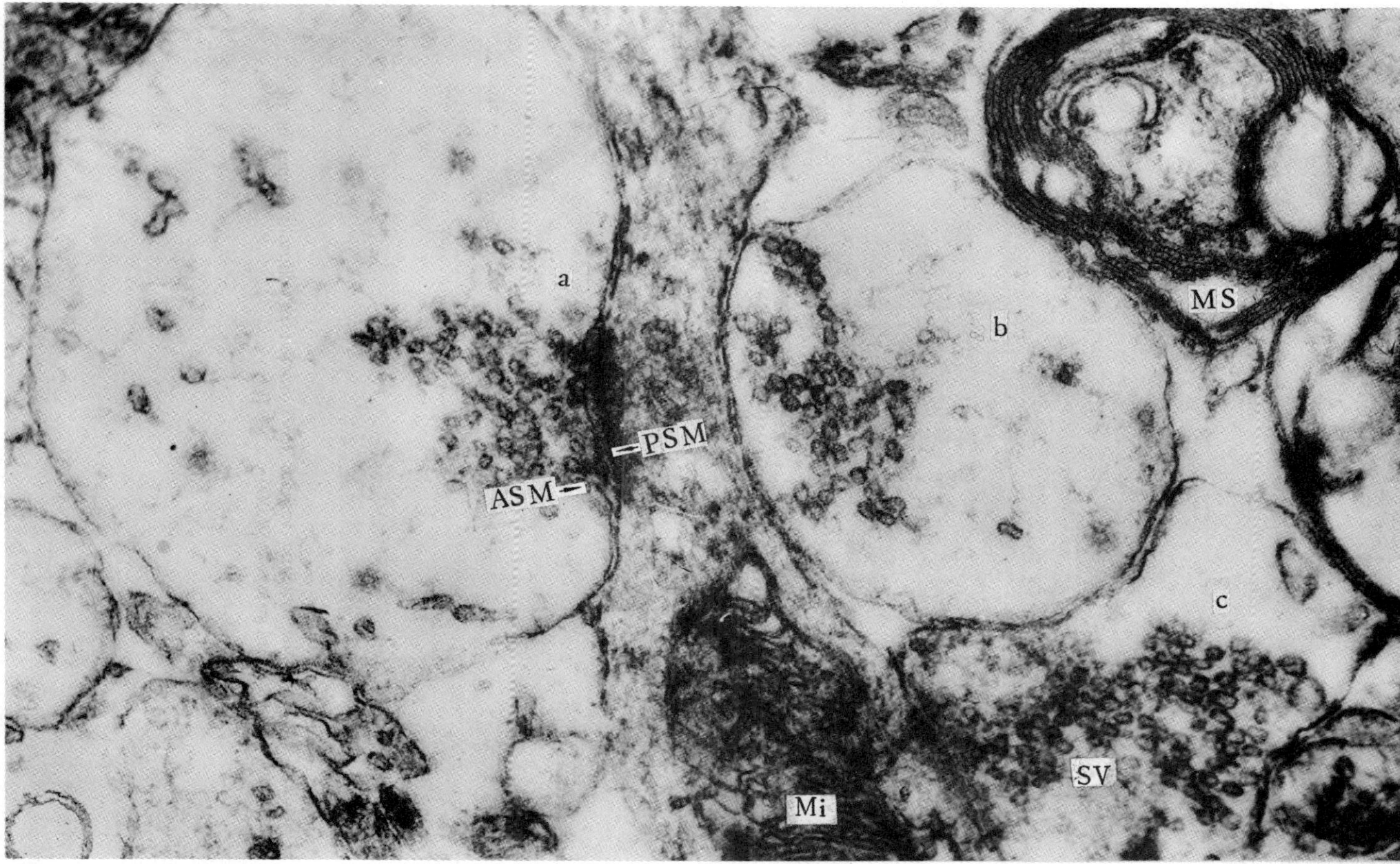

Fig. 1 Shows 3 presynaptic bags (a, b, c) of cont:ol rat. Each contains a small number of clear synaptic vesicles (SV), mainly of the ellipsoid shape. ASM: Presynaptic membranc; PSM: Postsynaptic membrane, Mi: Mitochondria, MS: Meylin sheath. × 63,140

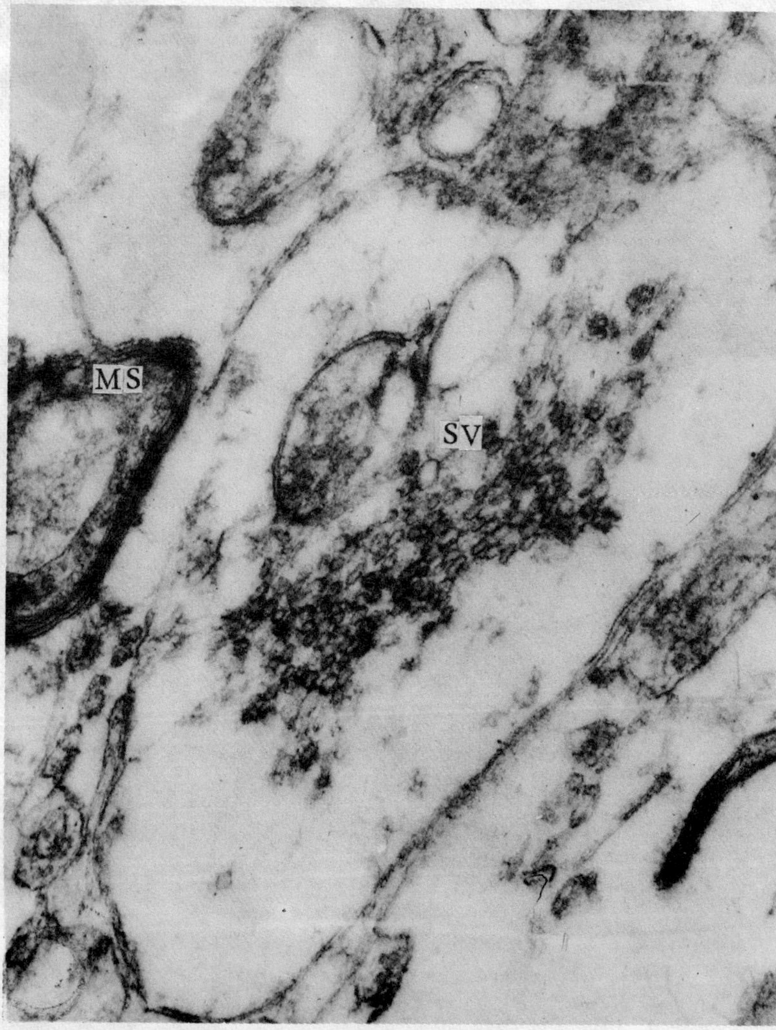

Fig. 2 Showing the synaptic vesicles (SV) of flat or ellipsoid shapes in the thalamus of the control group. × 57,000

Table 1. Changes of synaptic vesicles of different shapes after electroacupuncture

Synaptic Vesicle	Control Group		Electroacup. Group	
	Mean ± SD	%	Mean ± SD	%
Clear vesicle	118.49 + 26.30	100	198.63 + 65.21*	100
Round	11.98 + 5.28	10.1	42.05 + 19.08*	21.1
Ellipsoid	81.94 ± 23.31	69.2	138.03 +48.26	69.5
Flat	22.37 + 8.21	18.8	18.35 + 1.66	9.2

*P< 0.05

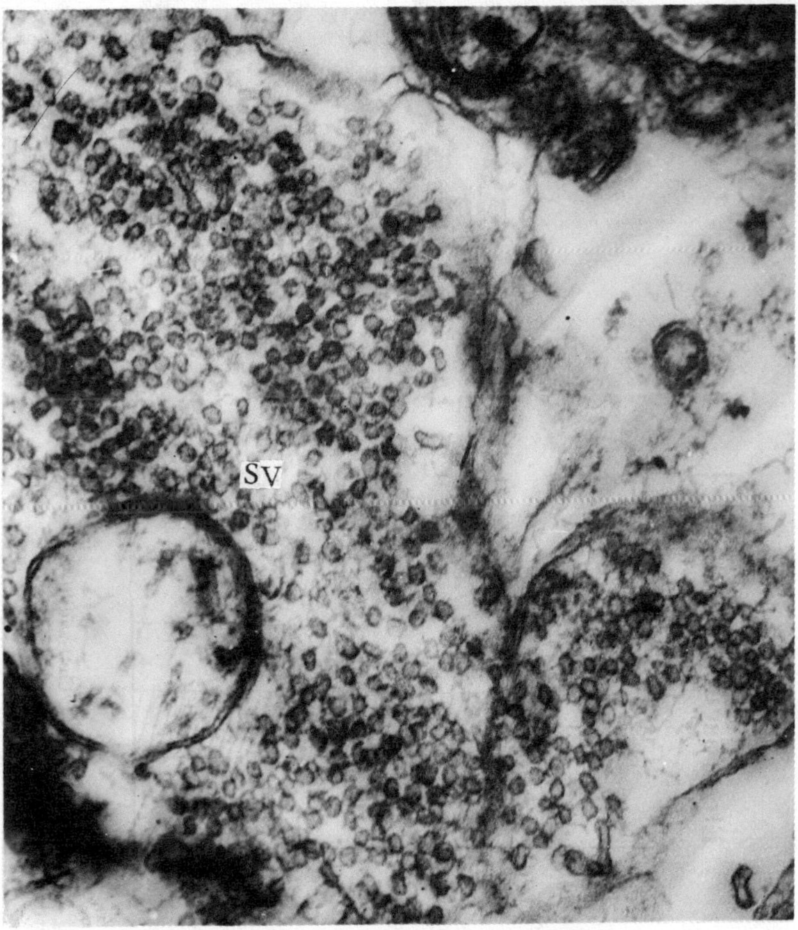

Fig. 3 Electron micrograph of the thalamus of an electroacupunctured rat. The presynaptic bag is crowded to its utmost capacity with numerous vesicles (SV), mainly of round shapes. × 87,000

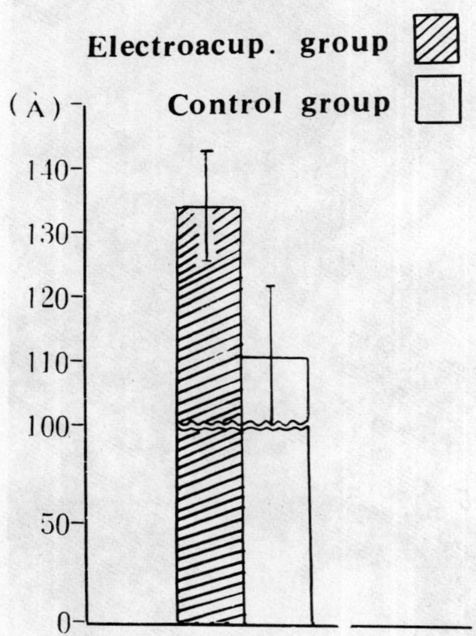

Fig. 4 Changes of Synaptic Cleft-width(Å) after Electroacupuncture
The vertical bars represent standard error.

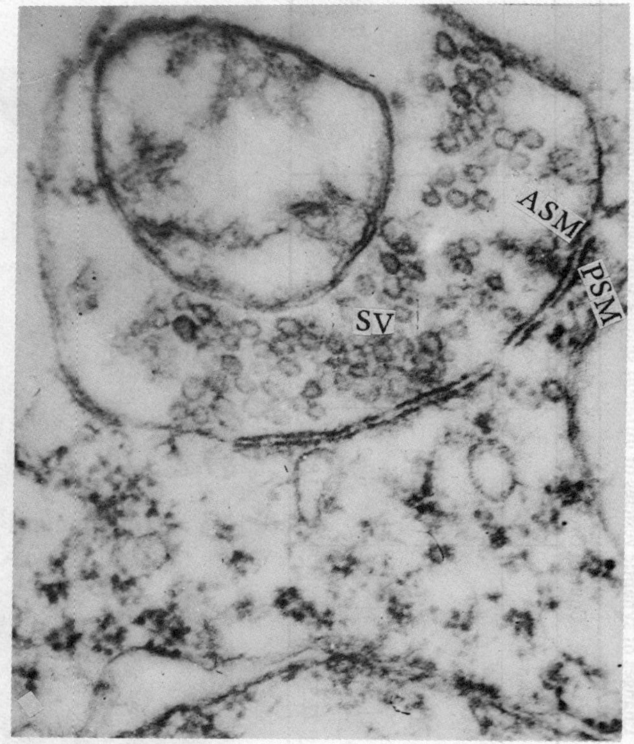

Fig. 5 Showing synapse with narrower synaptic cleft and fewer vesicles (SV) in a rat of the control group.
ASM: Presynaptic membrane.
PSM: Postsynaptic membrane.
× 72,500

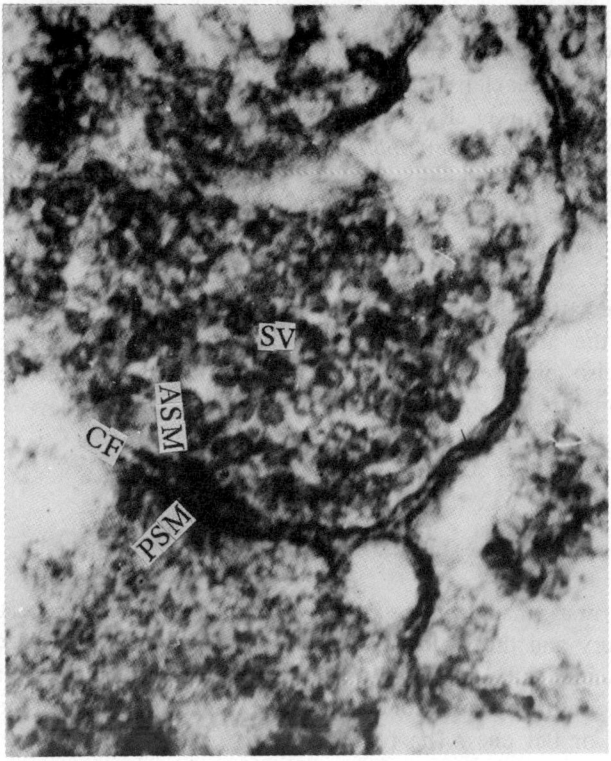

Fig. 6 Showing synapse with wider synaptic cleft (CF) and more vesicles (SV) in an electroacupunctured rat.
ASM: Presynaptic membrane.
PSM: Postsynaptic membrane.
× 78,400

Table 2. Changes of synaptic ultrastructure after electroacupuncture

	Synapses	Control Group (113)* %	Electroacup. Group (105)* %
A	With wider cleft & more vesicles	24.13	43.75**
B	With wider cleft & fewer vesicles	24.13	34.37
C	With narrower cleft & more vesicles	24.13	18.75
D	With narrower cleft & fewer vesicles	27.61	3.13**

* The number of synapses examined
** $P < 0.01$

into 4 types, namely:

(A) synapses with wider cleft and more vesicles;

(B) synapses with wider cleft and fewer vesicles;

(C) synapses with narrower cleft and more vesicles;

(D) synapses with narrower cleft and fewer vesicles.

There were 43.75% of synapses with wider cleft and more vesicles [type(A)] and only 3.13% synapses with narrower cleft and less vesicles [type(D)] in the electroacupuncture group, while the synapses of types (A) and (D) in the control group occupied 24.13% and 27.61% in sequence. Thus the percentage of synapses with wider cleft and more vesicles apparently increased after needling (Table 2).

In addition, the area of presynaptic bag and the electrodensity of the synaptic membrane were also observed; however, no significant statistical difference was found between the acupuncture and control groups.

III. DISCUSSION

(I) Synapses in the Medial Region of the Thalamus

It was shown that synapses in the central nervous system could be classified into two types, the excitatory and the inhibitory[8,9,10]. Studies made by Uchizono (1965)[11] also provided evidence that in the brain tissue fixed initially with aldehyde and followed by osmic acid, the excitatory synapse contained round clear vesicles, while the inhibitory one possessed ellipsoid or flat ones. The functional classification based on the morphology of the clear vesicle, though supported by some authors, has not been generally accepted. Bodian (1970)[12] noted that fixation by different fluids might influence the shapes of clear vesicles. Thus our data at present do not constitute sufficient evidence to suggest whether the existence of numerous vesicles of ellipsoid type (occuping almost 80% of clear vesicles) represents more inhibitory synapse in the medial region of the rat thalamus or whether the increase of spherical vesicles after electroacupuncture indicates an enhancement of the excitability of the synapse. The functional significance of the different shapes of clear vesicles in the medial region of the thalamus requires further studies.

(II) Clear Synaptic Vesicles

The synaptic vesicles may vary under different physiological conditions[13,14]. De Robertis[13] reported that under the influence of electro-stimulation, the vesicle amount was changed obviously. Hence the present findings with regard to the changes of synaptic vesicles in the thalamus after needling are not inexplicable. It has been generally considered that the acetylcholine (ACh) may be stored in the clear vesicles and in the central nervous system and a high concentration of ACh can be found in its fraction[15,16]. From this viewpoint the increase of clear vesicle ($P < 0.01$) (Tab. 1) found in this present experiment may indicate a rise of ACh content in the synapses of the thalamus following electroacupuncture, and this view is also supported by other studies[17] of our coworkers who, after an estimation of ACh concentration in the thalamus of an electro-needled rat with a microbioassay method, reported similar results.

It is worthy to note that an increase of synaptic vesicle in the medial region of the thalamus was accompanied by a rise of the pain threshold after electroacupuncture. Owing to evidence showing that the clear synaptic vesicle might be the storage site of ACh[15,16], and that the analgesic effect of acupuncture might be augmented by an intraventricular injection of ACh[18], the preceding data regarding the relationship of ACh with analgesia and synaptic vesicles can further indicate that the analgesic effect of electroacupuncture may be correlated with the changes of vesicles.

(III) Synaptic Cleft

From Table 2 and Figs.4 and 6 it is found that the synaptic cleft width and vesicle number were considerably increased simultaneously in the number of synapses during electroacupuncture; for example, in the acupuncture group, the percentage (43.75%) of type A synapse (more vesicles and wider cleft) (Table 2) is almost 14 times as much as that (3.13%) of Type B (less vesicle and narrower cleft) (Table 2). Since it was said that the synaptic cleft could be widened by the release of a larger amount of neurotransmitters, the widened cleft resulting from electro-needling seems to be a morphological basis for neurotransmitter release. From the above-mentioned results, however, whether the evidence of both the increase of vesicle amount and the enlargement of cleft width represent the acceleration of synthesis and the release of ACh after electroacupuncture remain to be a subject for further study.

Finally, it is emphasized that the influences of electroacupuncture applied to the points on the ultrastructure of the synapse were quite different from those of simple electron stimulation applied to nerves or neurons at the termination of which the synapses to be examined were located[19,20,21]. In the former case, the synaptic vesicles were increased after acupuncture, whereas in the latter the vesicles were remarkably reduced following electron stimulation[19,20,21]. Furthermore the different parameters used for electron stimulation are said to be another factor responsible for the changes of clear vesicle number[13].

IV. SUMMARY

10 rats were used and 218 synapses (113 in the control group, and 105 in the electroacupuncture group) were examined under an electron microscope. In the needled rats, besides the measurement of basic pain threshold, electroacupuncture was given to points "Ren-zhong" and "Chenjiang" for 30 minutes and postinduction pain threshold was then measured. After perfusion through the heart with formaldehyde, buffered with 0.1 M sod. cacodylate (pH 7.2), the medial region of the rat thalamus was removed and prepared by routine method for electro-microscopical research.

It was found that there were lots of synapses in the nuclei of the medial region of the thalamus, Among them, the axondendric type was predominant, and the axon-axonic and axonsomatic types came next. The clear synaptic vesicles (without dense core) were prominent, especially those of the ellipsoid shape which were much more in number than those of the round. Occasionally, a few granular vesicles were also found.

There was an increase of clear synaptic vesicles, especially those of the round type which were accompanied by a rise of the pain threshold after electroacupuncture. It is generally accepted that in the central nervous system, the clear synaptic vesicles contain a high concentration of ACh and can even be regarded as its storagesite. Thus the increase of vesicles after electroacupuncture may indicate the elevation of ACh level in the medial region of the thalamus. Besides this, an increase of vesicles and elevation of the pain threshold in needled rats were simultaneously accompanied by a widening of the synaptic cleft, which may be the morphological basis related to neurotransmitter release.

REFERENCES

[1] Chang HT.: *Scientia Sinica*, **16**:26, 1973.
[2] Albe-Fessard D et al: *J. Neurophysiol*, **25**:3, 1973.
[3] Kruger L and Albe-Fessard: *Exp Neurol*, 2:442, 1960.
[4] Poggio G P. and Mountcastle, V.B.: *Johns Hop. Hosp. Bull*, **106:266, 1960.**
[5] Craigie's Neuroanatomy of Rat, (Revised and Expanded by Zeman W.) Academic Press, New York, 1963.
[6] Gurdjian E. S.: *J. Comp. Neurol*, 43:1, 1927.
[7] Krieg, W. J. S.: *J. Com. Neurol*, 80:381, 1944.
[8] Eranko, O.: *Progress in Brain Res*, 34:149, 1971.
[9] Gray E. G.: *J. Anat.*, 93:420, 1959.
[10] Eccles, J.C.: The Inhibitory Pathways of the CNS, Thomas, Springfield, I11, 1969.
[11] Uchizono, K.: *Nature* 207:642, 1965.
[12] Bodian, D.: *J. Cell Biology*, **44**:115, 1970.
[13] De Robertis, E: *Expyl. Cell Res. Suppl.*, 5:347, 1958.
[14] Birks, R.I.: *J. Physiol*, 216:26P, 1971.
[15] De Robertis, E. *et al*: *Intern Rev. Cytol.*, 6:229, 1961.
[16] De Robertis, E. *et al*: *J. Neurochem*, 9:23, 1962.
[17] 武汉医学院针麻研究室：武汉医学院学报(增刊)，(2)：98，1976。
[18] 北京医学院生理组：中国科学，(1)：98，1974。
[19] Zimmermann, H. *et al*:*J. Neurochem*, **22**:1109, 1974.
[20] Zimmermann, H. *et al*: *J. Neurochem*, **22**:435, 1974.
[21] Cote, M. G. *et al*: *Rev. Canad, Biol*, **29**:111, 1970.

EFFECT OF PAIN ON ULTRASTRUCTURE OF INTERMEDIATE LOBE OF PITUITARY

Yuan Dexia, Huang Shansheng, Ying Guohua,
Li Xiangyin, Fu Zhiliang
(Hebei Medical College)

β-endorphin is a morphine-like substance produced mainly in the pituitary and has the properties of analgesia, hypnosis, euphoria and modified behavior. Under pain and stress the content of β-endorphin will be relatively altered in the serum. The morphine-like substance decreases in the rat's pituitary after electric stimulation with radioreceptoassays[1, 2]. After applying electric shock to a rat's foot[3], analgesia results and the level of β-endorphin in the serum increases five to six fold. The β-endorphin is secreted in large quantities during chronic pain and child delivery[4]. Acupuncture must be maintained for 20 min in order to obtain analgesia, because it needs time for the pituitary to release endorphin[5,6,7].

Recently, by utilizing the electronic microscopic immunohistochemical and unlabelled antibody technique in the study of the localization of β-endorphin, some investigators (Pelletier 1977[8], Guillmin 1977[9]) found that β-endorphin was present mainly in all the secretory cells of the intermediate lobe (in rat, sheep, pig and cow). Sequentially, many experiments had shown that β-endorphin, β-lipotropin, ACTH and β-MSH existed in the secretory granules of the same cell and all of them were secreted together under various conditions. On the basis of the localization of the β-endorphin and ACTH provided previously, the present experiment was performed to make a further observation on the changes in ultrastructure in the parenchymal cells and the secretory activities of the intermediate lobe during pain stimulation as well as to provide some data that may contribute to analyzing the mechanism of pain and acupuncture analgesia.

I. EXPERIMENTAL MATERIALS AND METHODS

Observation was made on twelve male rats, of which four were used for the control group, four for the experimental group of somatic pain, and four for visceral pain. Each of them weighed 200–300g. The animals were fed generally in the laboratory to adapt them to the surroundings for a week befor the experiment.

The animals of the control group were restrained inside a plexiglass cylinder fixing apparatus for 30 min, and were then decapitated at once.

(I) To obtain models of experimental pain

1. The experimental group of somatic pain. Two cotton enveloped platinic electrodes soaked in a 10% potassium chlorate solution were fixed near the radix of the rat's tail which was stimulated with 20 times/sec impulse. The stimulating strength used began with each time for 16v and the stimulation was carried out 10 sec with an interval of 1 min. If there was no respose, the stimulation was increased 2V progressively until the animal cried out and its extremities moved, which was taken as a pain threshold. When the stimulating strength th was increased sequentially the animal cried out continually and its whole body struggled; the point was taken as an endurable pain threshold. The pain threshold and the endurable pain threshold differed about 12V.

All the animals of the experimental groups of somatic pain were stimulated with the electric strength of the endurable pain threshold for 10 sec each time with an interval of 1 min. Stimulation was repeated and continued in this manner for 30 min.

2. The experimental groups of visceral pain. A rubber tube connected with a small air sac at its lower end was sent from the oral cavity to the stomach. A syringe used for pressurization was connected to the upper end of the tube, and a mercury pressure-gauge was connected to the middle of the tube to measure the pressure strength. When the pressure reached around 100 mmHg for 1–5 sec, the animal cried out and struggled; the point was taken as the criterion of pain threshold. Each of the animals of the experimental groups of visceral pain was stimulated with this stimulating strength of its pain threshold for 5 sec each time with an interval of 5 min, and the stimulation was repeated in this manner for 30 min. After the experiment, the animals were decapitated at once.

(II) The method of electronic microscope observation

After the decapitation of the experimental animals, the pituitary gland of each animal was taken out at once, and the anterior and posterior lobes of the pituitary were dissected. The intermediate lobes of the pituitary and the rostral zone were cut into fragments 1 mm in diameter and immersed into a 4% glutaraldehyde phosphate buffer (pH 7.2) separately. They were then fixed for 1.5 hours (in room temperature), washed by the buffer solution, post-fixed in 1% osmium tetroxide for 30 min, washed by the buffer solution once more, dehydrated by acetone (this procedure was carried on at 4°C), and imbedded in acrylic plastic "618". They were cut into ultrathin sections with "LKB" ultramicrotome. The sections were stained with uranyl acetate and lead citrate, and observed under a H–500 electronic microscope.

II. Observation

(I) Control groups

It was found that the intermediate lobes of rodents conjoined intimately with their neural lobes and both formed the posterior lobes of the pituitary. A cleft was found between the anterior and the posterior lobes of a pituitary. The posterior lobe was flat, ovoid in form and white in color while the anterior lobe, which enveloped the posterior lobe in semicircular form, was in front of the posterior lobe, showing dark red color in fresh preparation. The intermediate lobe combined with the anterior lobe to form the rostral zone in the pituitary stalk. Lothringer (1886) first suggested that the rostral zone belong to the intermediate lobe. The intermediate lobe was found to occupy 8% of the pituitary gland.

A layer of follicular cells was at the periphery of the intermediate lobe. Underneath this layer there was a thin layer of connective tissues which extended to the parenchyma of the intermediate lobe. The secretory substance could osmose into the capillaries situated among the connective tissues of the intermediate lobe, or litter down the blood sinus of the anterior lobe, but it usually osmosed into the capillaries of the posterior lobe. The secretory substance of the rostral zone could readily osmose into the capillaries because of the abundance of blood vessels and nerves in the zone.

The parenchymal cells of the intermediate lobe could be divided generally into two classes, the dark cells and the light cells. The dark cells with big cell-bodies were numerrous, and their cytoplasms were filled with a great number of secretory granules. The light cells with small cellbodies were relatively few in number as compared with the dark cells and their cytoplasms contained very few secretory granules.

1. Dark cells. They were found scattered in the parenchyma of the intermediate lobe. By form, they could be divided into the following types:

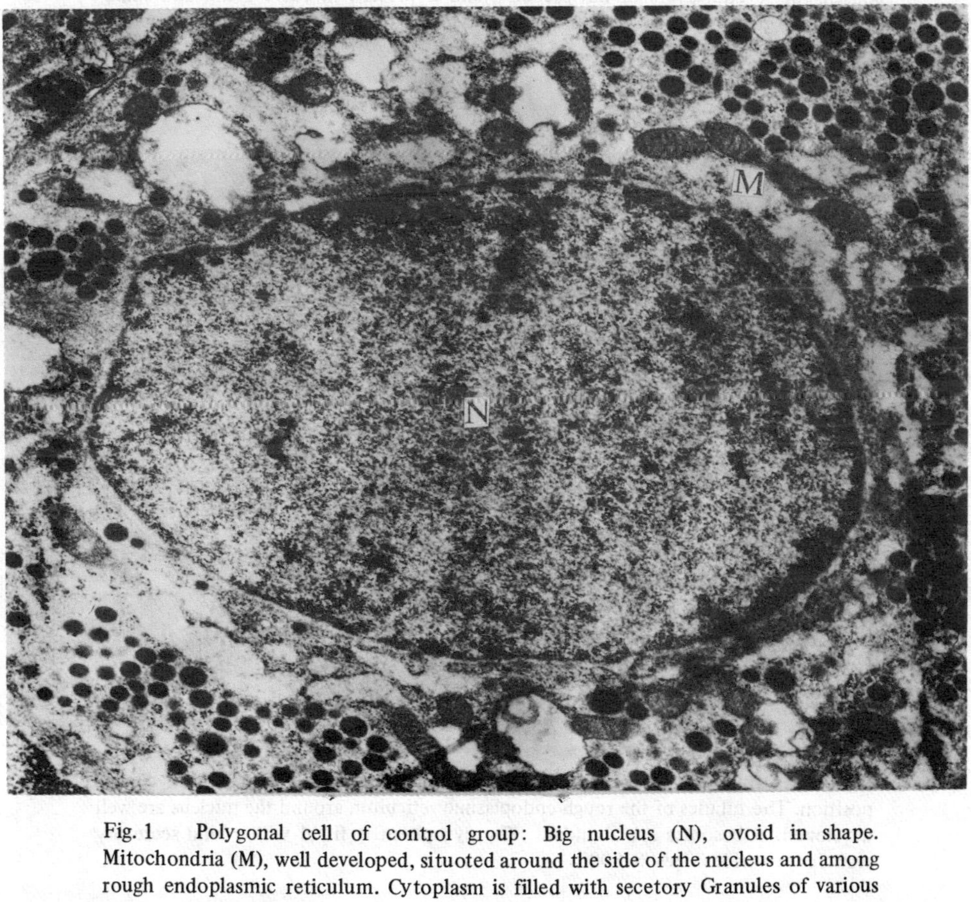

Fig. 1 Polygonal cell of control group: Big nucleus (N), ovoid in shape. Mitochondria (M), well developed, situoted around the side of the nucleus and among rough endoplasmic reticulum. Cytoplasm is filled with secetory Granules of various sizes. × 12,000

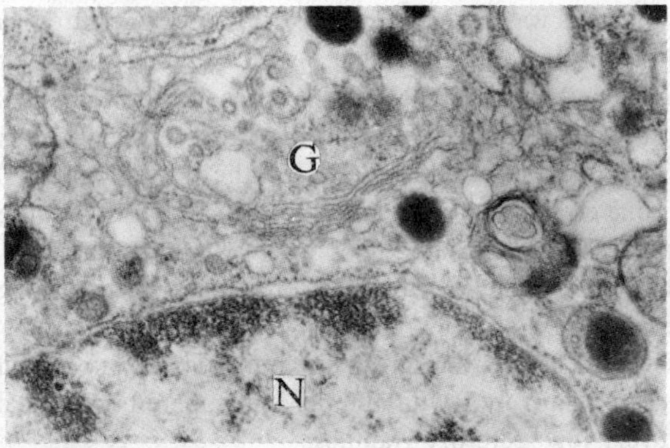

Fig. 2 Golgi complex (G) of polygonal cell in control group: the dictyosome consists of several layers of flat saccules, and is present in curve form, and some vesicles and new synthetic substance can be seen at the comcave surface. N=nucleus × 20700

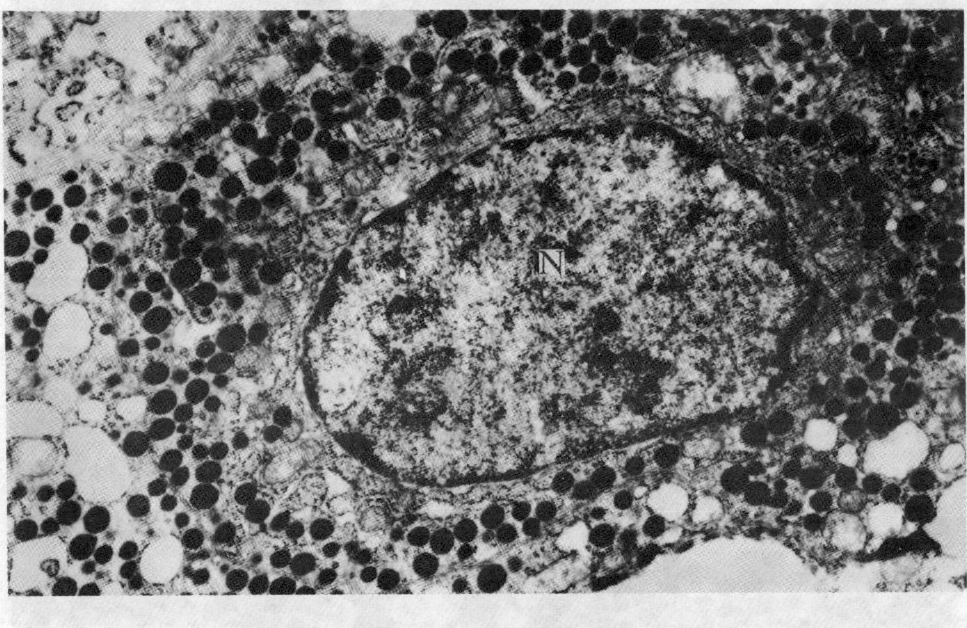

Fig. 3 Ovoid cell of contral group: A Large nucleus (N) situated in central position. The tubules of the rough endoplasmic reticulum around the nucleus are well developed. Ribosomes are abundant. The cytoplasm is filled with round secretory granules of various sizes. × 8000

Polygonal cell. The cell body of this cell was the largest in the intermediate lobe. These cells were arranged in groups or situated between light cells. The cell was found to contain a large ovoid nucleus in the center of its cytoplasm. Chromatin was scattered evenly in the nucleus. The cell abounded with round granules with high electronic density in the cytoplasm. The rough endoplasmic reticulum was moderately developed and contained few free ribosomes. The mitochondria were ovoid in shape with fine and very dense granules in their matrix. Their cristate portions which projected from the inner membrane in a right angle with the interior of the organelle were like plates and were orderly ranged (Fig.1). In some of these cells, dictyosome might be found near the nucleus. Dictyosome was a constituent and functional unit of the Golgi complex. The dictyosome consisted of several flattened saccules arrange in a parallel array and were often slightly curved (Fig.2). When the cells were in a state of relative rest, the dictyosomes were relatively few in number and smaller in figure.

Ovoid cell. The nucleus of this cell was central in position. The chromatin in the nucleus was present in a relatively low density. Rough endoplasmic reticulum was well developed

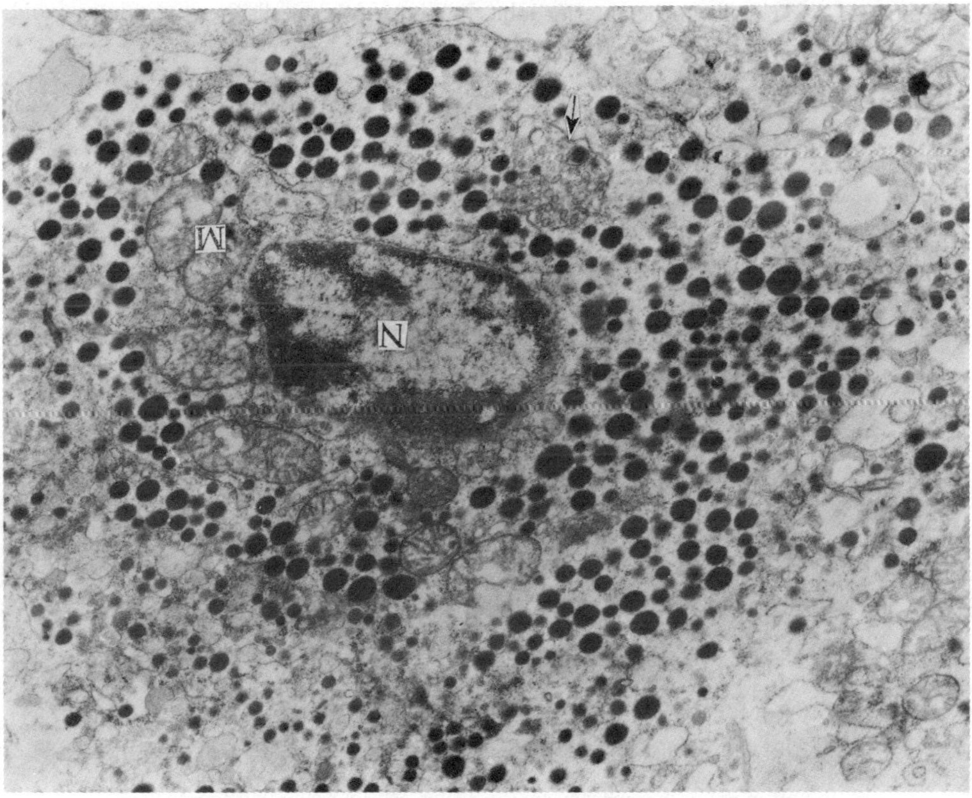

Fig. 4 Ovoid cell of control group: A small nucleus with high electronic density. The cytoplasm is sattered with secretory granules. The cell is clensely distributed with mitochondria. A small number of endoplasmic reticulum can be seen. The large multivesicular body is indicated by an arrow. × 10200

and contained abundant ribosomes on the flattened saccules. The secretory granules scattered in the cytoplasm were round, of homogenenous low density and of various sizes. The mitochondria were round or ovoid, and were present in medium quantity (Fig.3).

The ovoid cell situated in the rostral zone had a small nucleus. The chromatin in the nucleus exhibited high density; the heterochromatin at the periphery of the nucleus condensed in the shape of masses. The round secretory granules which filled the cytoplasm were of various sizes, and were homogeneous and of high density, and their exterior were covered by limit membranes. The round and ovoid mitochondria were concentrated generally on one side of the cytoplasm, and their cristate portions were dense (Fig. 4).

2. Light cells. These cells were small in size and number, with only few granules in their cytoplasms and a low density in their matrix. They could be divided into two classes.

ACTH cells. These cells were scattered mainly in the periphery of the intermediate lobe and in the rostral zone and only a few of them were found in the parenchyma of the intermediate lobe. The figure of these cells resembled the ACTH cells of the anterior lobe, but were smaller in size; the granules of them were smaller too, about 100–150 mm in the diameter of each. These cells were of a small stellate type with processes which were shorter than those of ACTH cells in the anterior lobe. In some of these cells there were large ovoid

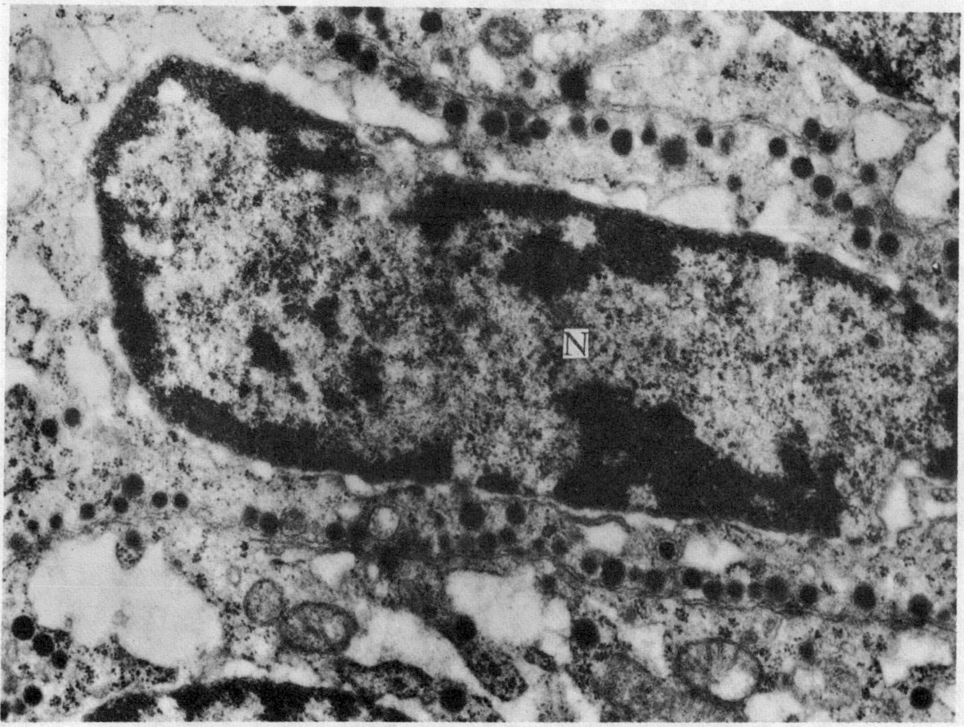

Fig. 5 ACTH cell of control group: It has a large nucleus which looks like an elongated ellipsoid and is situated in the centre. Its perinclear heterochromatin is dense. and its cytoplasms relatively few. The secretory granules are smaller in size and are ranged along the cell membrane, Endoplasmic reticulum well develop. × 17000

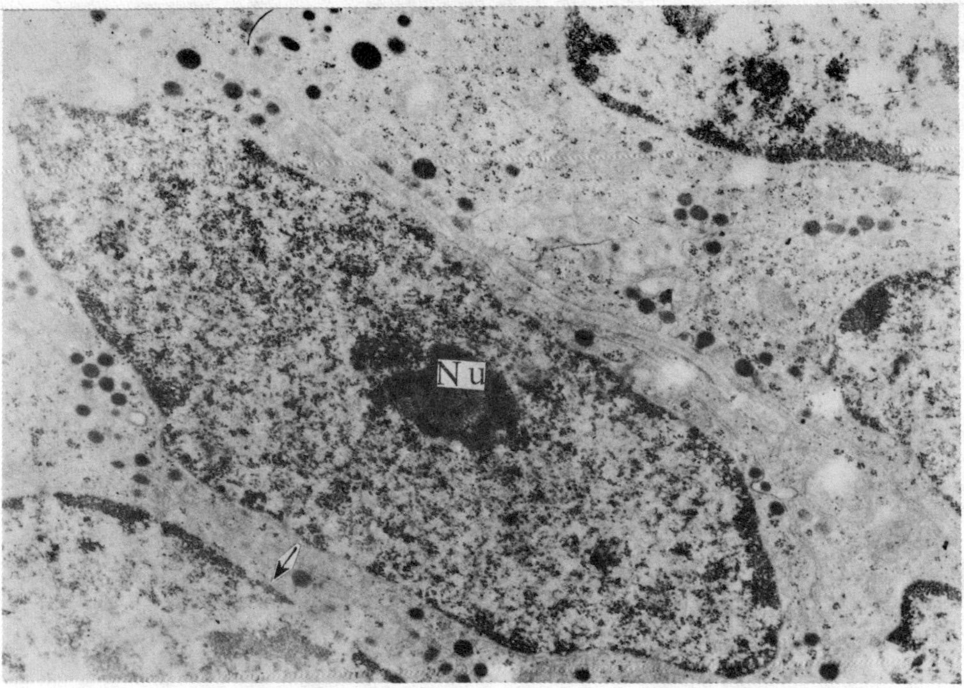

Fig. 6 Undifferentiated cell of control group: The cell body is ovoid. A large nucleus and a prominent nucleolus can be seen with little amount of cytoplasm and very few secretory granules. A small number of free ribosome and endoplasmic reticulum exist in the cytoplasm. × 15000

nuclei with dense chromatin which were present in diffuse small granules or condensed masses. The secretory granules ranged along the cell membrane in a single layer. The matrix of the secretory granules was homogeneous and of high density; there were also some of light density with empty halos. The rough endoplasmic reticulum was well developed, and the canalicular system widely dispersed, the canals of which were not arranged in parallel form (Fig. 5).

Undifferentiated cells: The cell was in spindle form with a large nucleus, prominent nucleolus, a small number of endoplasmic reticulum and small granules in its cytoplasm (Fig. 6).

(II) Experimental groups of pain

1. Experimental groups of somatic pain. The hypophyse was hypertrophied to about more than one third of its size and its intermediate lobe was hypertrophied too. Observation under an electronic microscope: Both the dark and light cells of the intermediate lobe increased in size; the nucleus was also bigger, the nucleolus prominent, the reticulum tissues between cells relaxed, the cleft enlarged, and the cavities of the capillary distended; the endothelial cells having projected into the cavities of bloodvessels, and the pores of the endothelium dilated. The changes of the various cells were as follows:

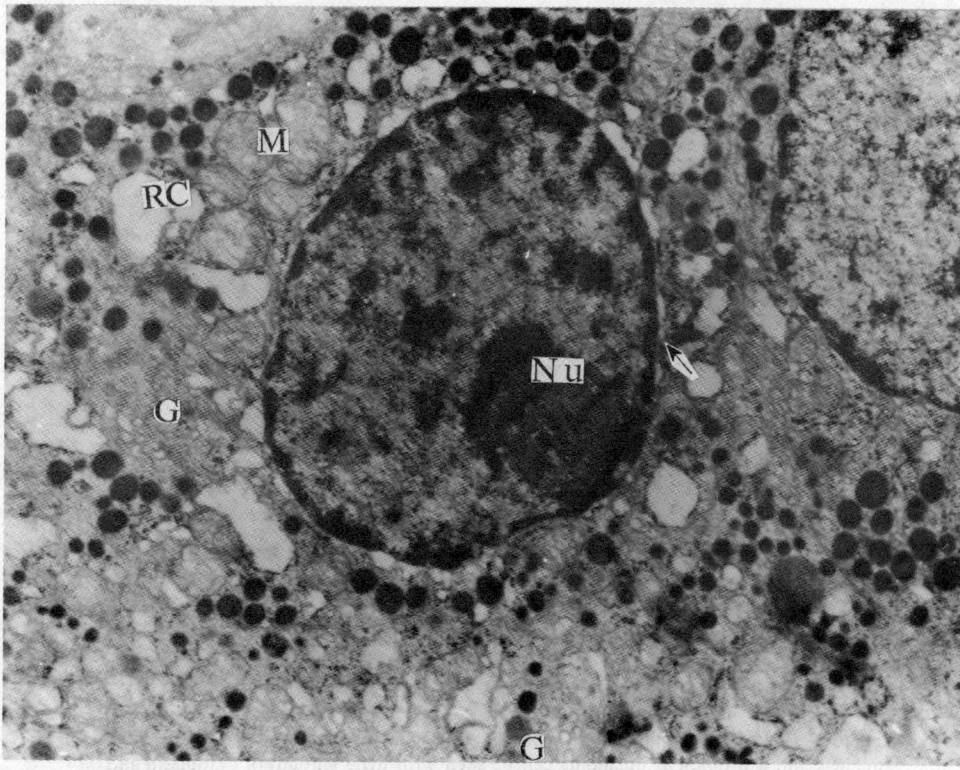

Fig. 7 Polygonal cell of the experimental group of somatic pain: The cell-body enlarges in irregular shape, several notches can be seen at the side of the nucleus. The nucleolus is prominent. A lot of saccules and vesicles can be seen of the Golgi complex near the nucleus. Mitochondria concentrate on one side. The endoplasmic reticulum distends to form the cisternae. Secretory granules move to the periphery of the cell body. The perinuclear space communicating the cisternae is indicated by an arrow. × 9000

Polygonal cell. The figure of this cell varied in round or irregular form when its cytoplasm increased. Some times, short processes from the cell-body can be seen extending among cells. The nucleus of the cell was hypertrophic with folds at its sides. The nucleolus was enlarged. The secretory granules of various sizes and different electronic density concentrated on the periphery of the cell. A lot of small granules with low density aligned along the cell membrane. The endoplasmic reticulum distended to form round, ovoid or irregular cisternae. Some of the cisternae were usually connected with the perinuclear space (Fig. 7). The number of dictyosome of the Golgi complex increased to 2–3 and the mitochondria which were usually concentrated among the granules increased too.

ACTH cells. The cell-bodies of these cells in the whole intermediate lobe became enlarged in different degrees. The nucleus hypertrophied or showed notches at its sides, the nuclei of some cells hypertrophied irregularly to form triangular or irregular shapes. Heterochromatin formed large granules which aligned along the membrane of the nucleus. The perinu-

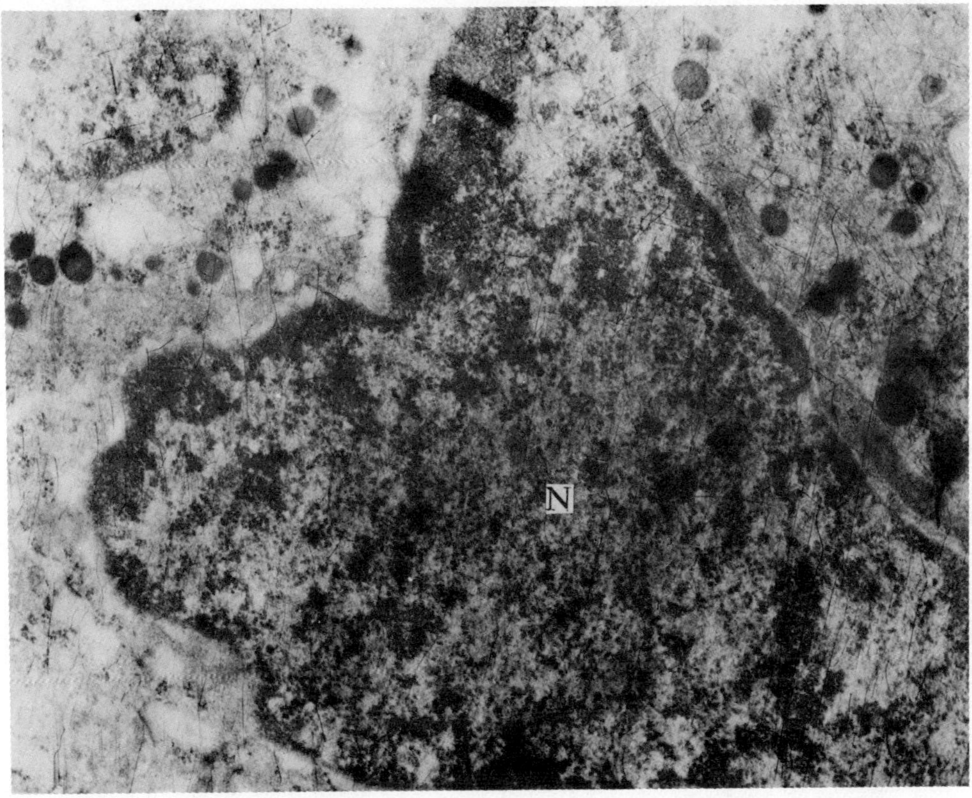

Fig. 8 ACTH cell of experimental group of somatic pain: It is a large nucleus in triangular form. The periphery of the nucleus is dense. The endoplasmic reticulum multiplies and the cisternae increases. Vacuoles of various size can be seen in the cytoplasm. The secretory granules with low electronic density still align along the cell membrane. × 20000

clear space distended to communicate with the cisternae of the endoplasmic reticulum. The polyribosome multiplied (Fig. 8).

The dictyosome of the ACTH cells in the rostral zone were well developed; the flat saccules of the dictyosome increased and formed into a group; and the newborn granules among the saccules were arrayed under the membrane of the cell (Fig.9). By the side of the ACTH cells, the nerve fibers extended to form hypothalamo-hypophyseal tract through the infundibular stem to the intermediate lobe. A great number of round nervous secretory granules filled the nerve ending.

2. Experimental groups of visceral pain. The changes of the cells of the intermediate lobe resulting from visceral pain were more striking than those of somatic pain. Almost all the cell-bodies of the cells in the intermediate lobe became enlarged. The large cisternae increased. The mitochondria became concentrated. The secretory granules decreased and the capillaries dilated.

Polygonal cell. The cell-body became enlarged to form an irregular shape. Short processes were seen projecting from the cytoplasm. The nucleus showed many small

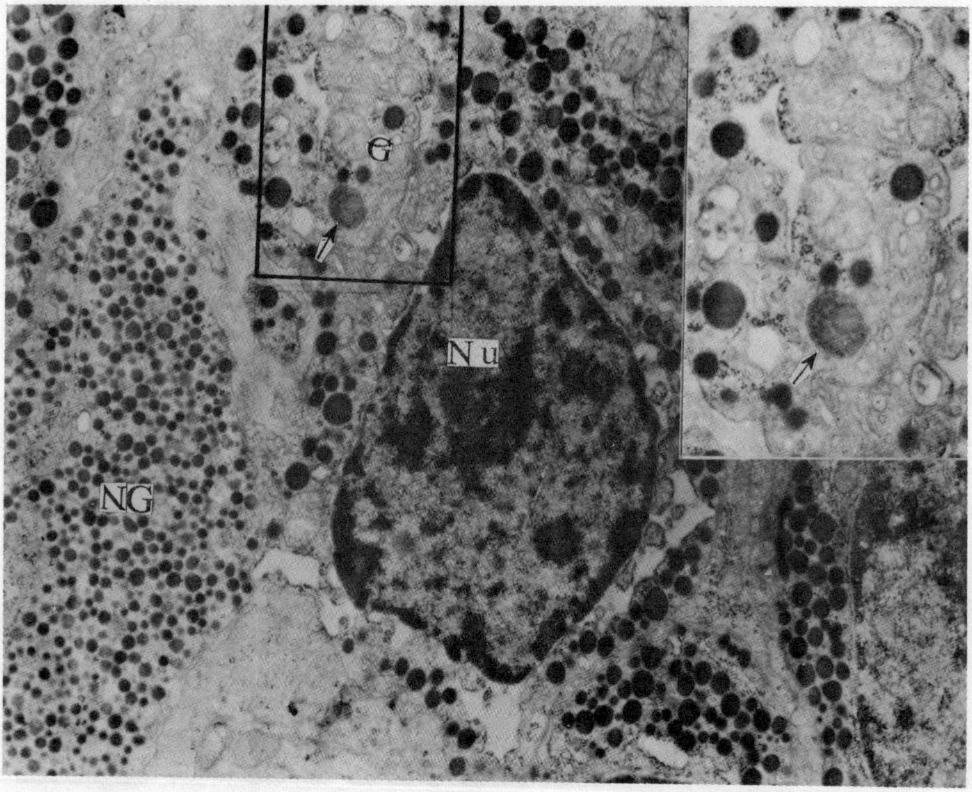

Fig. 9 ACTH cell of experimental group of somatic pain in the rostral zone: The cell body is small. Short processes project among neighbour cells. The nucleus is irregular in form and shows a nucleolus. The Golgi complex develops well and contains a great number of smooth saccules and vesicles. Secondary lysosomes can be seen among the granules (indicated by an arrow). Cisternae can be seen near the nucleus. Secretory granules align beneath the cell membrane. There is a nervous terminal from the nerve fibres of the hypothalamo-hypophyseal tract, and is filled with a lot of small round nervous secretory granules. × 12000
At the left corner, a magnified Golgi complex can be seen. × 16500

protuberances. The nucleolus was prominent. The rough endoplasmic reticulum multiplied and ranged in a parallel array. The tubules of them distended to form the cisternae and several cisternae combined with each other to form a large vacuole and contorted tube (Figs. 10, 12). Many microvillosity processes of the endoplasmic reticulum could be seen in the cavity of the contorted tube. At the outside of the tubules, ribosomes multiplied. The Golgi complex hypertrophied. Some vesicles with homogeneous substance gathered at the concave surface of the Golgi complex. The mitochondria with tubular cristae increased, hypertrophied and formed into a group. The matrix of them were of high density (Fig. 11). The secretory granules moved to the periphery of the cell-body and aligned themselves along the cell membrane, many of which were of light density.

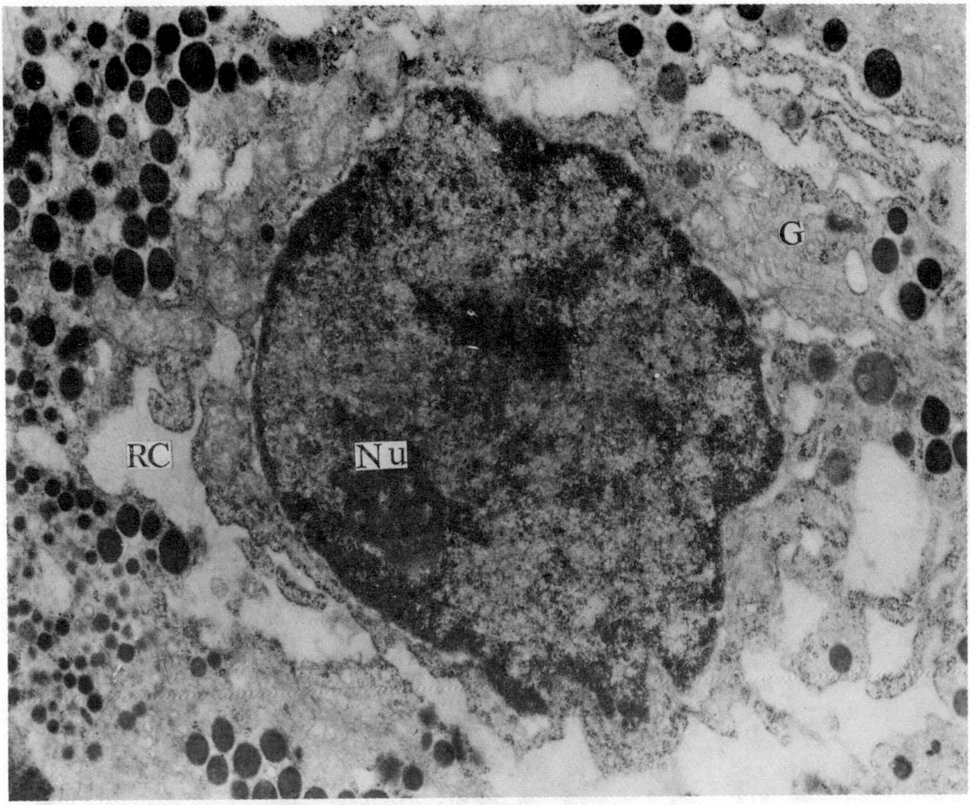

Fig. 10 Polygonal cell of the experimental group of visceral pain: The cell body is hypertrophic and the nuclear margin is in a zinzag manner. Its nucleolus (Nu) is prominent. The cisternae (c) of the endoplasmic reticulum multiply and the Golgi complex (g) is well-developed. The secretory granules move to the periphery of the cell body. × 13000

Ovoid cell. The cell-body became irregularly enlarged. Some of them projected laterally to configure a shape with two enlarged ends and a shrunken middle. The nucleus still occupied the central position, but was smaller. The density of the nucleus increased and its perinuclear space distended. The cisternae of the endoplasmic reticulum dilated and communicated with the perinuclear space to form vacuoles of various sizes. A large vacuole without any secretory substance could be seen at one side of the nucleus, and other smaller vacuoles were distributed in the cytoplasm (Fig. 13). The mitochondria converged on one side of the cytoplasm and the secretory granules moved to the periphery of the cytoplasm. The small secretory granules of light density contacted the cell membrane, which resembled making secretions. Some cellbodies distended to form round shaped ones; many large cisternae could be seen distributed in their cytoplasms; the free polyribosomes mutiplied and juxtanuclear dictyosomes with dilatant saccules were enlarged (Fig. 14).

ACTH cell. The cell-bodies hypertrophied more conspicuously than those caused by somatic pain. Many of these stellate cells enlarged to become round shaped cells, and some

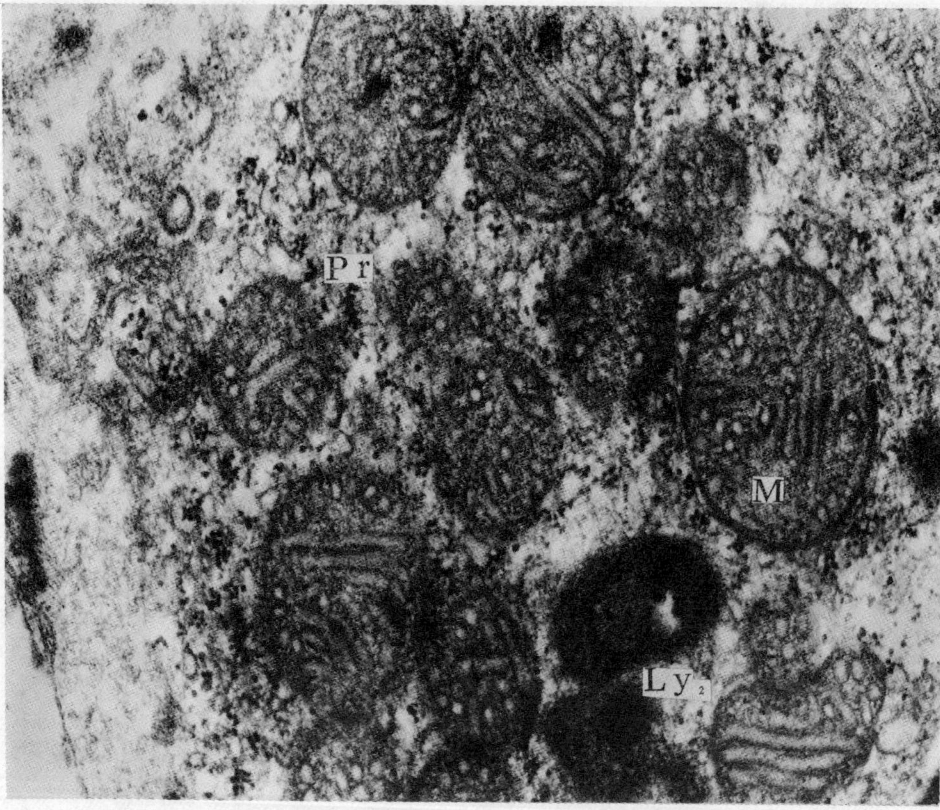

Fig. 11 Mitochondria of the polygonal cell in the experimental group of visceral pain: Mitochondria (M) gather into groups. Cristae distend to form tubular appearance. Polyribosome (pr) multply among the mitochondria. Secondary lysosomes (Ly_2) contain rough granules and vesicles. × 20,000

other cells became spindle-shaped cells with long processes extending among cells. The nucleus hypertrophied to become a large irregular nucleus with a zigzag margin and a low density. Endoplasmic reticulum increased and tubules formed dilative cisternae. Several cisternae combined with each other to configure a large straight tube. The secretory granules became smaller and their density increased, similar to newborn granules, and were ranged beneath the cell membrane. There were also some large secretory granules with low density. The mitochondria became enlarged and appeared in a round shape; the cristae of them became tubular and looked pale. The juxtanuclear dictyosome of the Golgi complex enlarged and saccules of them dilated. There were many smooth vesicles at the concave surface of the dictyosome showing signs of enhanced synthetic and secretory function (Fig. 15).

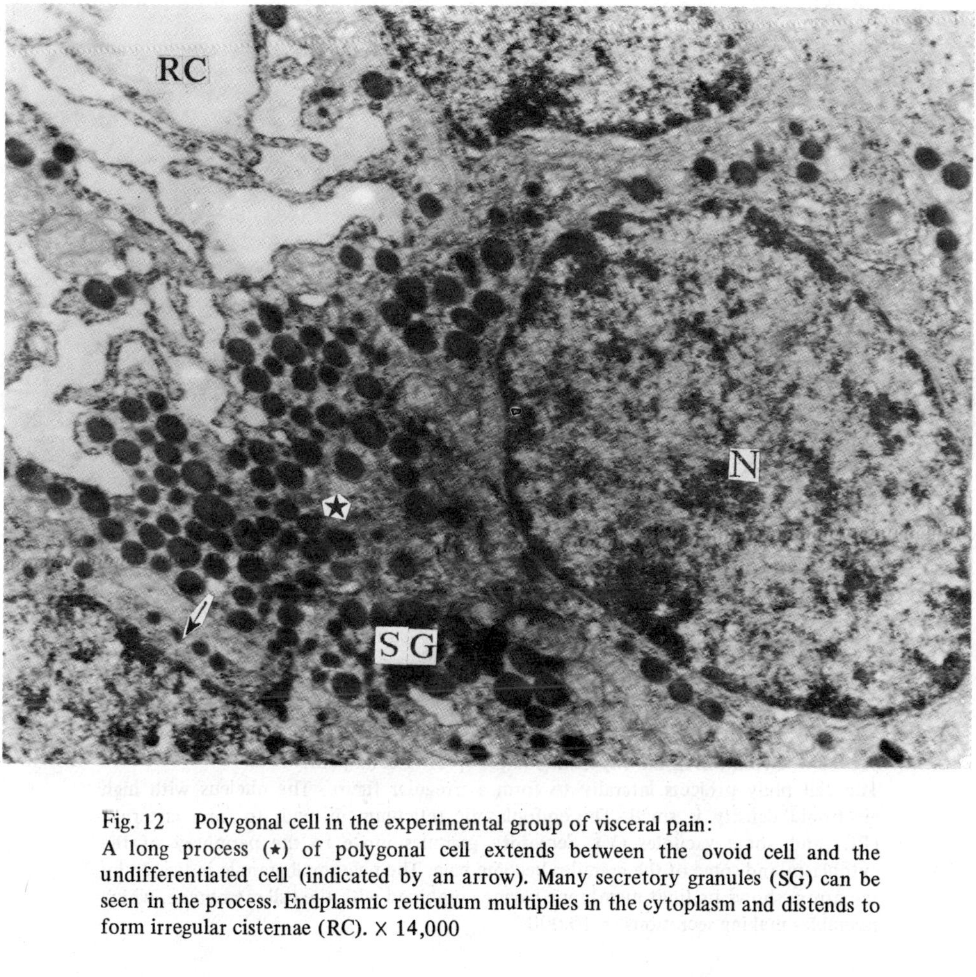

Fig. 12 Polygonal cell in the experimental group of visceral pain:
A long process (⋆) of polygonal cell extends between the ovoid cell and the undifferentiated cell (indicated by an arrow). Many secretory granules (SG) can be seen in the process. Endplasmic reticulum multiplies in the cytoplasm and distends to form irregular cisternae (RC). × 14,000

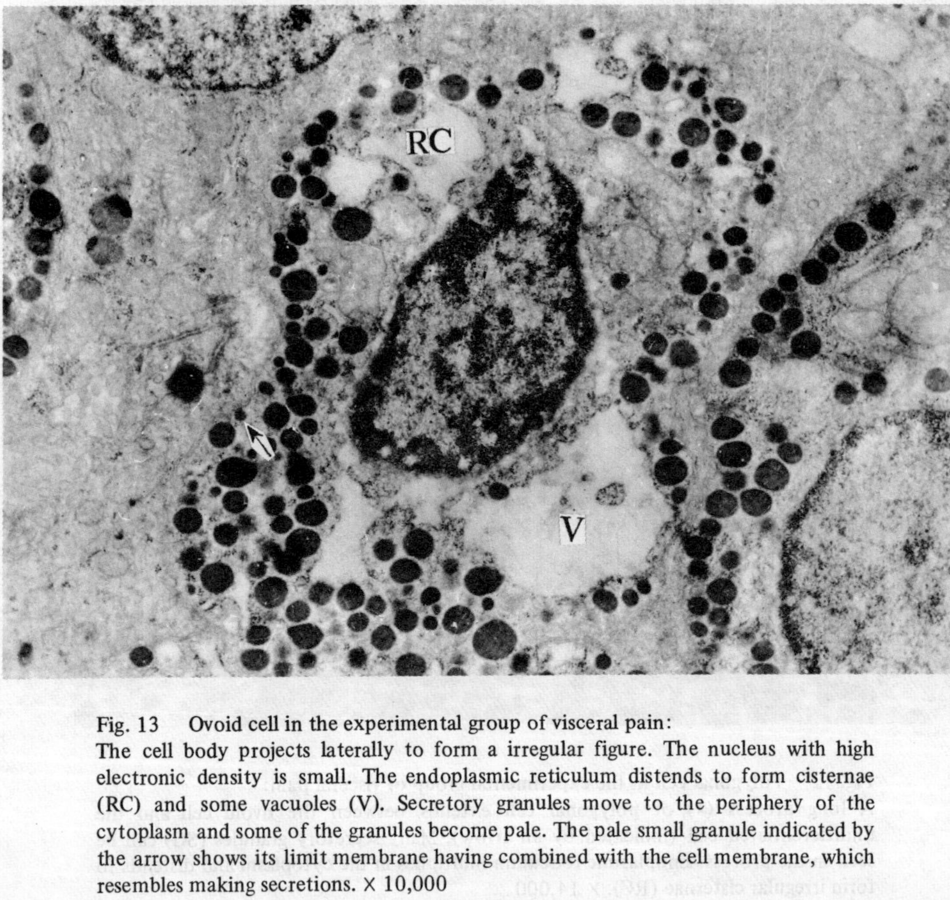

Fig. 13 Ovoid cell in the experimental group of visceral pain:
The cell body projects laterally to form a irregular figure. The nucleus with high electronic density is small. The endoplasmic reticulum distends to form cisternae (RC) and some vacuoles (V). Secretory granules move to the periphery of the cytoplasm and some of the granules become pale. The pale small granule indicated by the arrow shows its limit membrane having combined with the cell membrane, which resembles making secretions. × 10,000

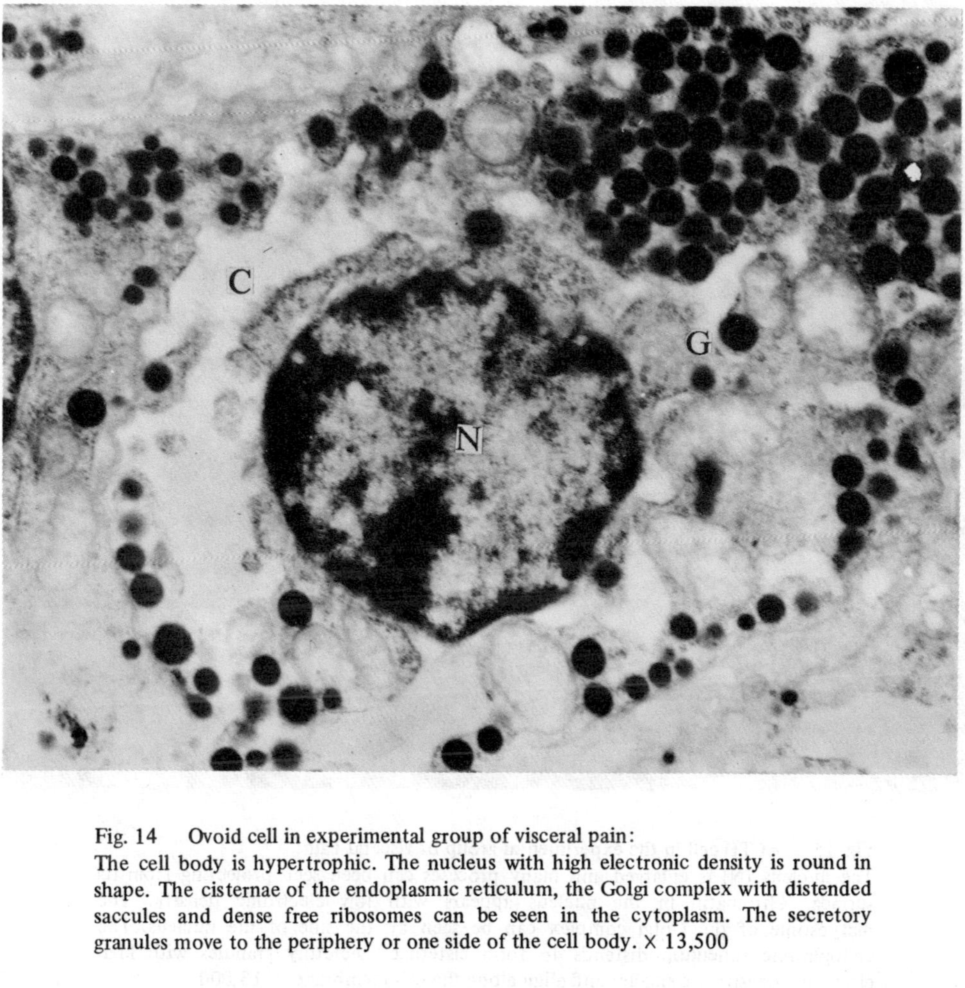

Fig. 14 Ovoid cell in experimental group of visceral pain:
The cell body is hypertrophic. The nucleus with high electronic density is round in shape. The cisternae of the endoplasmic reticulum, the Golgi complex with distended saccules and dense free ribosomes can be seen in the cytoplasm. The secretory granules move to the periphery or one side of the cell body. × 13,500

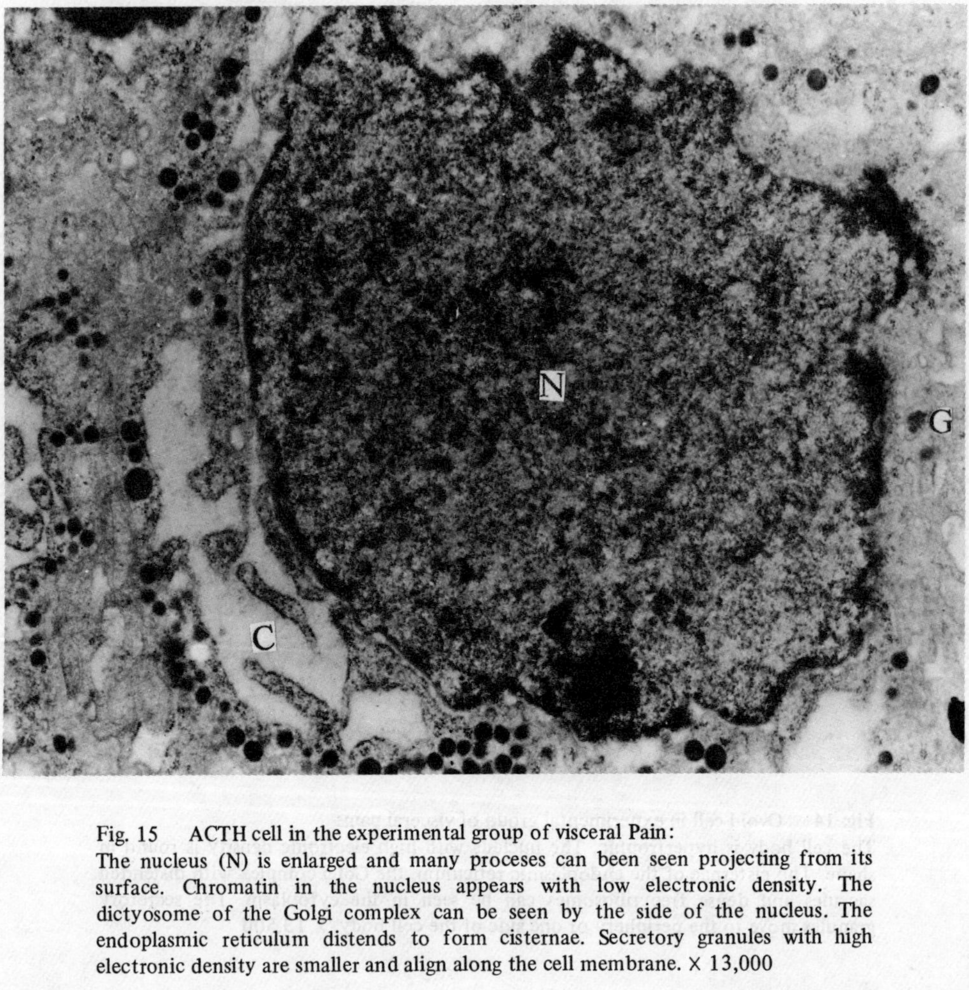

Fig. 15 ACTH cell in the experimental group of visceral Pain:
The nucleus (N) is enlarged and many proceses can been seen projecting from its surface. Chromatin in the nucleus appears with low electronic density. The dictyosome of the Golgi complex can be seen by the side of the nucleus. The endoplasmic reticulum distends to form cisternae. Secretory granules with high electronic density are smaller and align along the cell membrane. × 13,000

III. DISCUSSION

(I) Discussing the secretory substance of the intermediate lobe

The intermediate lobe was known in early times to contain MSH and ACTH. Recently, Moriarty(1973)[10] pointed out that lipotropic hormone (LPH) and ACTH were found to be present in all secretory cells of the intermediate lobe and ACTH cells of the anterior lobe in some mammalian animals. These two substances may be synchronously preserved in a cell and secreted concomitantly. These hormones are stored in the cisternae of the endoplasmic reticulum, the saccules of the Golgi complex and the secretory granules of the same cell. A little quantity of them is contained in the cytoplasm, but absent in the nucleus.

β-lipotropic hormone consists of 91 amino acids and is identified as a precursory morphine-like substance. β-endorphin is the c-terminal of 31 amino acid fragments of β-lipotropin. α-endorphin corresponds to β-LPH peptide linkage 61–76th segment; γ-endorphin, 61–77th segment; M-enkephalin, 61–65th segment. The activity of β-endorphin is the strongest among these morphine-like substances. β-LPH can dissolve lipoid and enhanced melanocyte to multiply granules. Recently, there has been a suggestion that it has a low analgesic effect. MSH may be divided into α-and β-MSH; β-MSH may be preserved in the intermediate lobe, while α-MSH is present in the arcuate nucleus of the hypothalamus. β-MSH corresponds to β-LPH peptide linkage 45–48th segment; therefore β-LPH is also the precursory substance of MSH.

Sequentially, Guillemin (1977)[9] discovered $ACTH^{1\text{-}39}$, β-LPH, γ-and β-endorphin present in the ACTH cells of the anterior and intermediate lobes and the secretory cells of the intermediate lobe. With the application of the calibrated filtration columns method, the content of β-LPH and β-endorphin had been measured it was found that β-endorphin was about 90% and β-LPH 10% in the extract of hypophyse. Therefore, the secretory quantity of β-endorphin may be larger than that of β-LPH.

ACTH which corresponds to β-LPH peptide linkage 1–39th segment may promote the suprarenal gland to secret cortisone and has the effect of MSH. $ACTH^{1\text{-}28}$ has been confirmed experimentally that it has an affinity to morphine receptor and that it produces the effect of analgesia. Jacquet (1978)[14] identified ACTH and β-endorphin as belonging to a part of the nervous regulative system, but their analgesic effect was mainly due to their combination with their corresponding receptors.

Rossier (1979)[15] with the immunocytochemical method discovered that a certain quantity of Leu-enkephalin was present in all the secretory cells of the intermediate lobe.

On the basis of the above data, it can be seen that there are β-LPH, β ξχλθ[ρκιχ'

On the basis of the above data, it can be seen that there are β-LPH, β-endorphin, β-MSH, ACTH, α-endorphin and Leuenkephalin, etc. in the intermediate lobe, but that the main secretory substances are ACTH and β-endorphin. Their responses in synthesis, maturity, secretion and regulation are identical; for example, if the extract of hypothalamus is put into a simple layer culture medium of hypophyse, ACTH and β-endorphin, etc. would be secreted concomitantly[9].

In the process of pain, these secretory substances are not sufficient in quantity to obtain an analgesic effect.

(II) The functional meaning of the results of this experimental observation

Pain can cause changes in the parenchyma of the intermediate lobe and significantly enlarge the cell bodies of most secretory cells; the nucleus and the nucleolus will become hypertrophic and the tubules of the endoplasmic reticulum will multiply and distend to become cisternae, and several cisternae combine to form vacuoles. In the cells of the experimental groups of visceral pain, the number of vacuoles and density of polyribosome increase in the cytoplasm. The Golgi complex enlarges and the number of dictyosome increases. All of these cytological changes as described above tend to indicate that the rate of synthesis is rising. The mature secretory granules of dark cells move to the periphery of the cell-body; the electronic density of some granules becomes pale and the number of granules decreases. In the visceral pain group, pale small granules are often seen arrayed on the cell membrane, and the boundary membrane of some granules combines with the cell membrane, showing the phenomenon of an increased exocytosis. Mitochondria are seen to converge and hypertrophy; their cristate portions distend to assume tubular form, but range regularly; the matrix appears dense. This suggests an acceleration of cell metabolism. During synthesis and the increase of exocytosis, mitochondria provide a large amount of energy.

IV. CONCLUSION

Pain to the point of tolerability was caused intermittently by electric stimulations on a rat's tail or by inserting a distended air sac in the rat's stomach for 30 min. The changes in the intermediate lobe are summarized as follows:

(1) The cell body, nucleus or nucleolus was hypertrophied. The number of rough endoplasmic reticulum, and particularly of its vesicular cisternae was increased. The Golgi complex became enlarged and the ribosomes multiplied. All these indicated that the activity of cells increased and the rate of synthesis was accelerated.

(2) Both the secretory granules which moved to the periphery of the cell body and some of those which showed pale density were interpreted as an increase in exocytosis.

(3) The mitochondria became enlarged and the cristate portions in them assumed tubular form. This suggested an acceleration of cell metabolism, which tended to provide a large amount of energy.

(4) There was no degenerative change.

(5) The cytological changes caused by visceral pain were similar to, but more striking than those caused by somatic pain.

(6) The secretions increased, among which β-endorphin and ACTH were known to be closely related to analgesia.

REFERENCES

[1] 邹 冈：内源性吗啡样物质和针刺镇痛(内部资料)，1977。

[2] 针刺镇痛作用的研究进展,针刺麻醉 (1)：1，1978。

[3] Rossier, J.: *Nature*, **270**: 619, 1977.

[4] Hughes, J.: *British medical Bullctin*, **33**: 157, 1977.

[5] Goldstein, A.: *Science*, **193**: 1081, 1976.

[6] Pomeranz, B.: *New Scientist*, **73**: 12, 1977.

[7] Norman, J.: *Brit. J. Anaesthesia*, **49**: 523, 1977.

[8] Pelletier, G. *et al*: *Endocrinology*, **100**: 770, 1977.

[9] Gullomin, R. *et al*: *Science*, **197**: 1367, 1977.

[10] Moriarty, G. C.: *J. Histochem. Cytochem.*, **21**: 855, 1973.

[11] Moon, H. P.: *Anat. Rec.*, **175**: 529, 1973.

[12] Moriasty, C. C.: *Anat. Rec.*, **172**: 374, 1972.

[13] Pelletier, G.: *Am. J. Anat.* **150**: 201, 1977.

[14] Jacquet, Y. F.: *Science*, **201**: 1032, 1978.

[15] Rossier, J.: *Nature*, **277**: 653, 1979.

[16] Wylic, V. *et al*: *Endocrinology*, **103**: 1910, 1978.

THE RELATION BETWEEN ACUPUNCTURE ANESTHESIA AND NEURO–TRANSMITTERS AND ENZYMES OF LOCUS COERULEUS AND RAPHE NUCLEUS

Ge Zi, Huang Weimin, Wang Zhiying, Song Wancheng

(Institute of Acupuncture and Moxibustion, Academy of Traditional Chinese Medicine)

Acupuncture anesthesia is a new method developed from acupuncture analgesia based on the channel theory of our traditional medicine. Recently the relations between acupuncture anesthesia and the central nervous system with its transmitters have attracted great attention[1-4]. This paper dwells on the influence of acupuncture anesthesia upon the neurotransmitters and enzymes of locus coeruleus and raphe nucleus. We selected these nuclei on account of their intimate relation with analgesia and the regulating function of the atomic autonomic nervous system[5-8].

The investigation of the reactions of Catecholamine (CA), Monoamine oxidase (MAO) and Acetylcholine esterase (AChE) of both nuclei under acupuncture anesthesia was intended to make clear the interrelationships between them.

I. MATERIALS AND METHODS

130 healthy, adult, and male rats were divided into two groups. Each of the rats of the acupunctured group was needled at Zusanli and Huantiao on one side, with an unloading voltage of 20–30 V; a frequency of 60–80 /sec; the electro-acupuncture time being 20 min. The control group was treated without electro-acupuncture. The influence of the different effects of electro-acupuncture was also studied with another 60 heathy, adult, male rats.

1. The value of the pain threshold was expressed by the latency (sec) of the rat flick response to 50°C water (Table 1). The pain thresholds of both groups were measured at the same time, before and after acupuncture.

Table 1 The influence of acupuncture upon the rats' pain threshold

Group	No. of animals	Pain threshold (sec.) Before acup.	After acup.	elevation %
Acup.	65	6.9	25.3	267%
Contr.	65	7.5	8.3	10%

After the administration of acupuncture anesthesia, the rats were conscious and active. The pain threshold of the electro-acupunctured was significantly elevated while that of the control group was not.

2. Histochemical reaction. After measuring the pain threshold, the rat was decapitated, and the whole brain was taken out immediately and put into the cryostat (−17.5°C–20°C) to be frozen for 15–20 minutes. The brain was divided into mes- and metencephalon (pons) by coronal sections, put on the prefrozen section stage plate, cut into 25 μ sections under −12°–20°C, and the following histochemical methods were then applied:

(1) Glyoxylic acid induced Monoamine histo-fluorescence method. We adopted the modified technique with cryostat sections[9] and also used reserpine as a tool drug for the further identification of catecholamine.

(2) Monoamine oxidase method. Fresh frozen sections, air-dried and incubated in Glenner's medium[10]; Nitro B. T. was used as hydrogen receptor for 1 hr and then the sections were mounted in glycerine jelly.

(3) Acetyl- and butyl cholinesterase method[11]. Fresh frozen sections were fixed in −4°C 10% neutral formalin for 15–60 minutes and incubated in acetyl- or butylthiocholine iodine medium for 3 hrs. In order to make further identification of the character of the enzymes, the following experiments were carried out. 1) Both nuclei presented negative reaction after the inhibition of 10^{-5} M eserine salicylate esterase upon cholin-esterase, indicating that within both nuclei, there were no noncholinergic enzymes at all. 2) The neurons of both nuclei presented negative reaction in butylcholinergic enzyme when the substrate-butyl thiocholine iodine was added in to the incubated medium. 3) When the strong nonspecific AChE inhibitor – ISO – OMPA was added to the AChE incubation medium it proved that both nuclei locus coeruleus and raphe nucleus dorsalis contained the real ChE – AChE. The chemical constituents of both nuclei were measured quantitatively with a microphotometer.

3. Results.

(1) The influence of electro-acupuncture upon the CA fluorescence of locus coeruleus. The locus coeruleus of 20 rats of both electro-acupuncture and control groups was observed with Fluorescent Microscope Leitz Ortholux (absorbing filter BG 38; exciting filter BG 12 and Blocking filter K530 mm.). In normal rats the locus coeruleus is found to be located at the ventro-lateral part of the gray matter of the floor of the 4th ventricle. It consists of many multi-polar neurons. There is a large amount of brilliant green fluorescent catecholamine granules in the perinuclear cytoplasm in the form of dots, streaks and strings in the neuropil. The nucleus is negative.

It was found that the fluorescence of the locus coeruleus of the electro-acupuncture animals was slightly weaker than that of the control.

Table 2 The influence of acupuncture upon MAO of locus coeraleus

Group	No. of animals	Transmission (T %) of MAO (mean value + S. E.)	P value
Acup.	20	21.85 + 2.79	<0.05
Contr.	20	28.23 + 2.81	

(2) The influence of electro-acupuncture upon the MAO of locus coeruleus and nuc. raphe.

The MAO reaction of locus coeruleus presents a strong blue violet coloration. There is a large amount of MAO positive granules in the perinuclear cytoplasm of the locus coeruleus (Table 2).

This experiment indicated that MAO reaction of the locus coeruleus of the electro-acupunctured group was stronger (Fig. 1) than that of the control group (Fig. 2). The transmittances of MAO of locus coeruleus of both groups were measured with the micropholometer, the results showed no statistical significance.

The MAO reaction of nuc. raphe dorsalis was not evident enough for us to make comparisons.

(3) The influence of electro-acupuncture upon the AChE of nuc. raphe dorsalis. The reactions of AChE of nuc. raphe dorsalis of the control group was not so prominent. There were only a few neurons scattered with a moderate degree of AChE positive granules (Fig.3). On the other hand, in the majority of the animals in the electro-acupuncture group, the neurons of nuc. raphe dorsalis were characterized by a reaction of moderate to strong brown color (Fig. 4). The average number of AChE positive neurons in 5 corresponding sections of nuc. raphe in both groups are listed in Table 3.

Our experiment showed that the number of AChE positive neurons in nuc. raphe dorsalis of the electro-acupunctured group was greater than that of the control group, and the difference was significant statistically. This phenomenon indicates that the activities of AChE of nuc. raphe increase under electro-acupuncture (Table 3).

(4) The influence of electro-acupuncture upon AChE reaction in locus coeruleus. The AChE of locus coeruleus of the control group presented a moderate to strong reaction whereas in the electroacupuncture group, the reaction became stronger. There was significant statistical difference between them, with the exception of only 2–3 animals.

High power microscopic observation. Locus coeruleus consisted of medium to small sized, multipolar, oval, spindlelike neurons. The reaction of AChE in perinuclear cytoplasm and neuropil ranged from moderate to strong dark brown color (Fig. 5). The processes of the neurons of locus coeruleus of the electro-acupuncture group seemed more prominent, some of them being stretched to the fourth ventriculum. There were more multipolar neurons in locus coeruleus of the electro-acupuncture group with stronger reaction in the perinuclear cytoplasm and the neuropil (Fig. 6) than that of the control group. The transmission of AChE of locus coeruleus of both groups was also determined with a microphotometer and treated statistically as the following (Table 4).

The results indicated that AChE activity of locus coeruleus in the electro-acupuncture group increased significantly than that of the control group (Figs. 5, 6). It showed less transmission, increased optic density and strong reaction which was in sharp contrast with those of the control group.

Moreover, the transmittal of the AChE in the individual neurons of locus coeruleus under electro-acupuncture was also determined by a microphotometer (Table 5).

Our data indicated that the AChE of individual neurons of locus coeruleus in the electro-acupuncture group increased significantly.

(5) The interrelationship between electro-acupuncture effects upon the AChE activity of locus coeruleus: 60 healthy, adult, male rats were selected for further investigation of the

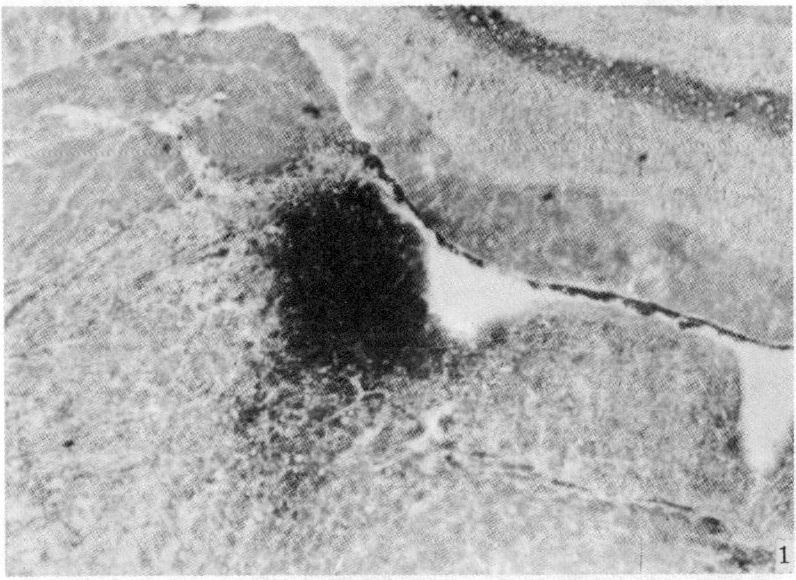

Fig. 1 MAO reaction in locus coeruleus of the acupuncture rat. 47.5 ×

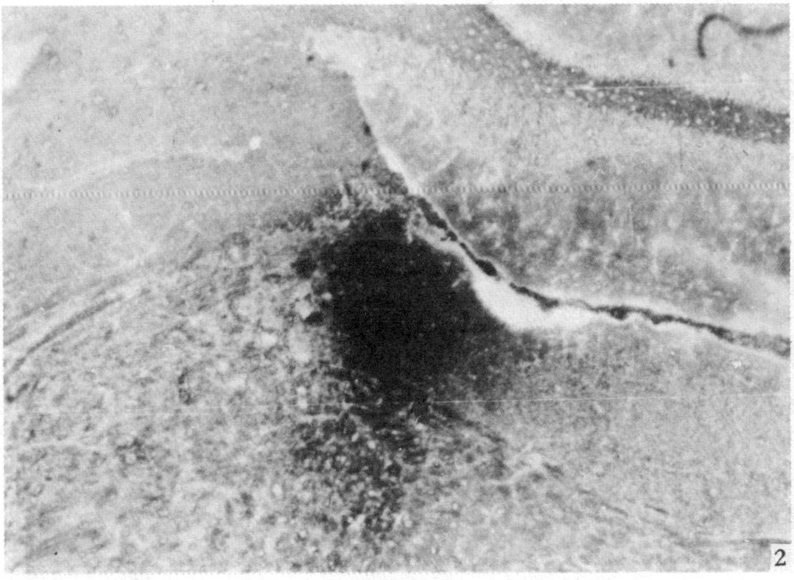

Fig. 2 MAO reaction in locus coeruleus of the control group. 47.5 ×

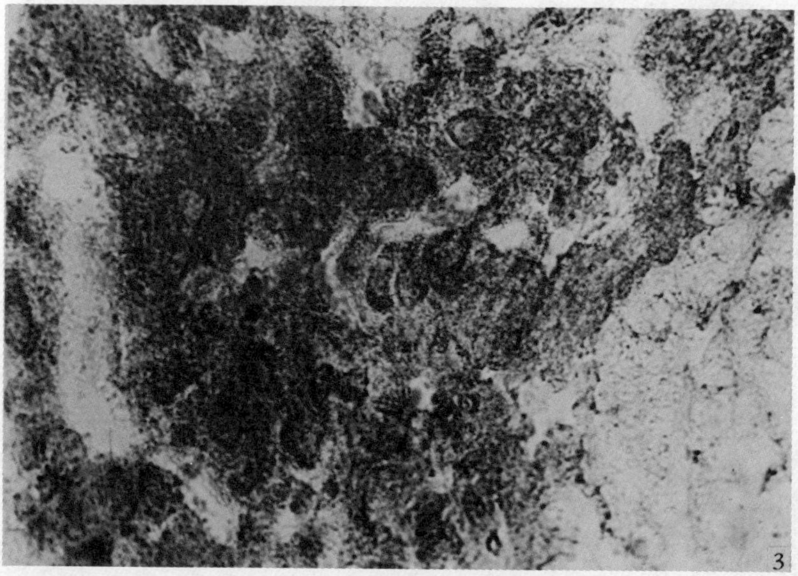

Fig. 3 AChE reaction in nucleus raphe dorsalis of the control group. 400 ×

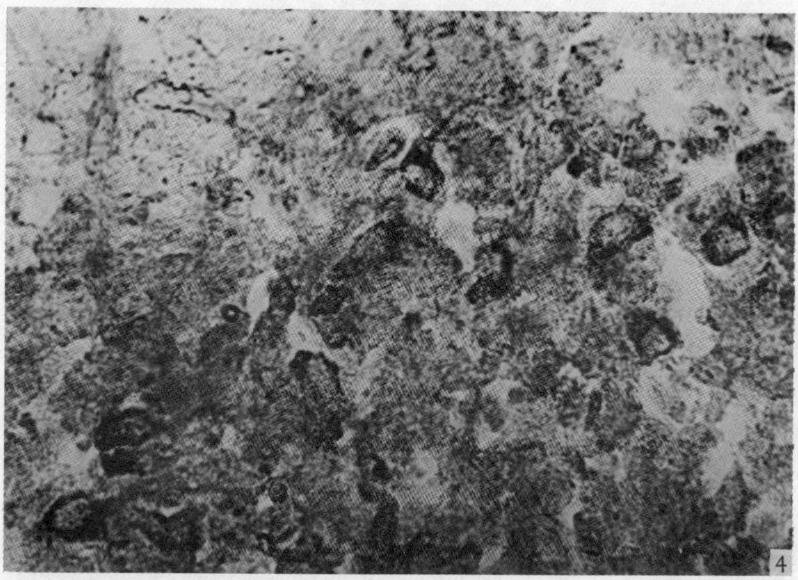

Fig. 4 AChE reaction in nucleus raphe dorsalis of an electro-acupunctured rat. 400 ×

Table 3 The influence of acupuncture upon the AChE positive neurons of nucleus raphe dorsalis

Group	No. of animals	No. of AChE positive neurons (Mean value + S.E.)	P value
Acup.	24	61.85 + 3.80	<0.001
Contr.	24	22.14 + 2.58	

Table 4 The influence of acupuncture upon AChE of locus coeruleus

Group	No. of animals	Transmission T% of AChE (Mean value + S. E.)	P value
Acup.	40	59.88 + 1.01	<0.001
Contr.	40	67.04 + 1.04	

Table 5 The influence of acupuncture upon AChE of individual cells of L.C.

Group	No. of animals	Transmittal T% of AChE (Mean value + S.E.)	P value
Acup.	22	14.95 + 0.32	<0.01
Contr.	22	20.09 + 0.53	

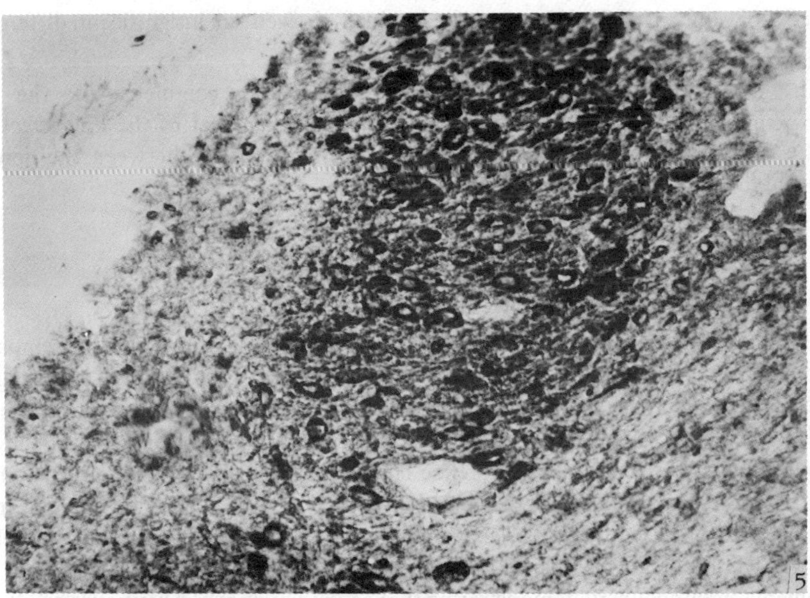

Fig. 5 AChE reaction in locus coeruleus in the control group. 180 X

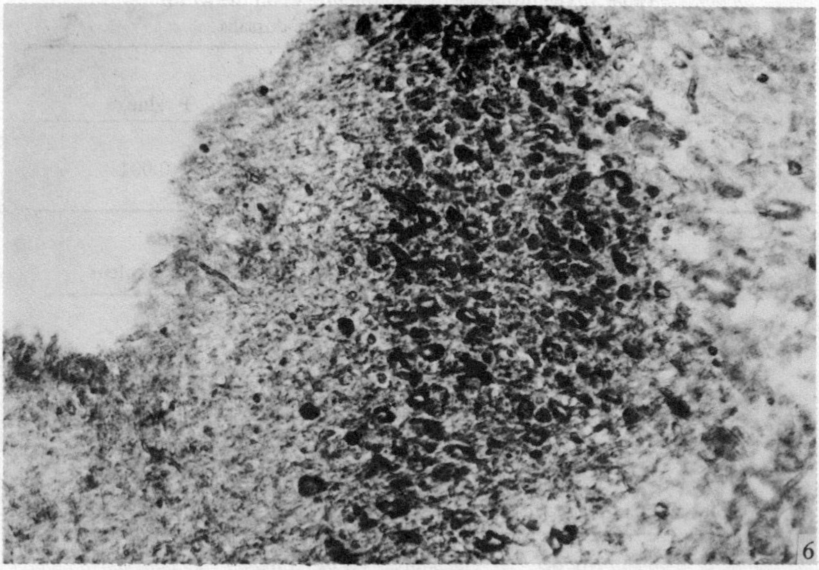

Fig. 6 AChE reaction in locus coeruleus in an electro-acupunctured rat. 180 ×

relationship between analgesia and AChE in locus coeruleus. Different voltages were used. The pain threhold was elevated 227% by a square wave voltage of 1.2 V; whereas it was elevated 20% only if 0.75 V was applied, which showed an insignificant difference with the control group (12%).

The results demonstrated that AChE in locus coeruleus of the effective electro-acupuncture group increased more significantly than that of the non-effective group and the control group, but there was no significant difference between the non-effective group and the control group (Table 6).

II. DISCUSSION

"A biological organism is a united integral system" is a viewpoint long emphasized in our ancient medical theory. It was recorded in the Canon of acupuncture as "using filiform-needle to open a channel and regulate the blood and vital energy", and "the twelve channels and 365 subsidiary channels with the blood and vital energy going up to the face and through the aperture and hollow". "These channels connect limbs and joints externally but belong to the internal organs internally." It was also recorded that vital energy came out of the brain. This indicated that these channels and the role of acupuncture were closely related with the whole organism, especially the central nervous system. There were a lot of experiments in our country demonstrating that acupuncture might have exerted an influence upon the functions of the central nervous system and that acupuncture analgesia and the regulation of body function were closely related with the central nervous system and its transmitters. Our experiments also demonstrated that acupuncture might activate certain transmitters and enzymes and regulate their circulation to taking active parts in acupuncture anesthesia. Now let us discuss briefly the few following problems.

1. The relationship between acupuncture analgesia and the regulation of noradrenalin and monoamine oxidase. The Research Group of Acupuncture Anesthesia in Peking Medical College used Reserpine to deplete monoamine and enhance the analgesic effect of finger puncture[2]. The Institute of Traditional Chinese Medicine in Shanxi province observed that the total amounts of monoamine of the whole brain of rats decreased significantly after acupuncture anesthesia[12]. NA of the metacephalon of rabbits decreased while its 5HT increased[13]. The catecholamine fluorescence of the locus coeruleus of acupunctured rats decreased, but not prominently[14]. M. Segal[15] discovered that when the catecholamine nuclei locus coeruleus and substance nigra were stimulated, analgesia was produced. Zhang Dexing et al.[16] took NA and locus coeruleus as an antagonist in acupuncture analgesia on account of the elevation of the pain threshold as expressed by vocalization after destroying locus coeruleus. Our research group of biochemistry observed no elevation of the pain threshold by using α methyl Tryptophan to deplete NE and DA to 50% and 80% respectively. After all, the relationship between locus coeruleus, NA and acupuncture analgesia is still debatable. We consider that locus coeruleus is a higher regulating center of the autonomic nervous system. It contains a great deal of MAO, AChE, oxydase, ACP, 5HT[17], P. substance, endohephalin and morphine receptors[18], and possesses a variety of functions. They might control the autonomic centrum, cerebrum, cerebellum cortex, hippocampus, hypothalamus and medulla spinallis. Its activities are closely related with respiration, pulsation, the state of being awake, sleep and muscle tonus[19]. The destruction of locus coeruleus will cause an imbalance of body functions, hematouresis, and myasthenia, and half of the experimental rats will die. So under such a situation, the use of vocalization and tail flick as an indicator of pain threshold is still a point open to question. Our experiments have demonstrated that under acupuncture analgesia, the catecholamine of locus coeruleus decreased a little. Monoamine oxidase increased slightly but both of them did not show any significant difference. So we suppose that a part of noradrenalin might have been released from locus coeruleus, though it did not play a decisive role.

2. The relationship among analgesia, the regulating function of acupuncture and AChE. The Research Group of Peking Medical College applied atropine to block cholinergic receptors, and the effect of finger puncture analgesia decreased[2]. Intraventricle infusion of Hemicholine to block 'the biosynthesis of ACh decreased the effect of acupuncture analgesia significantly[20]. It indicates that cholinergic nerve activities have taken part in acupuncture analgesia. The Acupuncture Anesthesia Group of Shanghai Medical College[21] demonstrated that when the pain threshold of the rabbit was elevated, the amount of ACh in the ventriculum also increased. Both electroacupuncture and stimulation of nucleus caudatus produced good results in a patient with severe pain at the late stadium of tumor of n. acusticus, the ACh in his liquid cerebro-spinalis having increased significantly. These experiments demonstrated that there was a close relationship between acupuncture and ACh. Besides, the pain threshold of morphine analgesia was often found to be parallel to the amount of ACh in the brain[22-24]. Although as yet, ACh can not be demonstrated histochemically, in general it is believed that there exists a great amount of AChE in both acetylcholinergic and acetylcholinceptive neurons, and AChE reaction also demonstrate the activities of the acetyl-

cholinergic neurons. Our experiments demonstrated that AChE of the acupunctured rats increased significantly which indicated that a substantial amount of AChE was closely related with acupuncture analgesia, and which could serve as one of the objective indicators of the effectiveness of acupuncture anesthesia. According to the research of ultrastructure [25], AChE was synthesized within the intracellular reticulum and transported through axon to the intersynapses site to take active roles. Thus, in all probability, the function of neurons would be activated and enzyme synthesis processes enhanced. If the needs are met, it would be effective, otherwise, ineffective. We held that acupuncture might promote the synthesis and activities of AChE in locus coeruleus and raphe nucleus and the roles of AChE (or/and ACh) might be more important than those of NA under acupuncture anesthesia. But the relationship between the ACh and NA in AChE positive neurons of locus coeruleus needs further investigation.

Numerous experiments have shown that acupuncture is closely related with raphe nuclei and 5–HT[3,12,13]. Shanghai Institute of Physiology demonstrated that 5–HT content in Raphe nuclei increased significantly in acupuncture analgesia[13]. Others also proved that 5–HT could produce an effect upon AChE to enhance the action of ACh[19]. Raphe nuclei are the main localization of 5–HT neurons. Excepting 5–HT and its metabolic products — 5HIHACL in these nuclei, no material concerning other neurotransmitters has been reported. Our experiments have demonstrated that the AChE reaction in raphe nuclei of the control was not prominent, though moderate AChE positive neurons increased significantly in the acupuncture group. Thus, we presumed that the neurons of nuc. raphe dorsalis might have possessed both 5–HT and ACh, and acupuncture could activate 5–HT of the raphe nuclei to enhance ACh in turn. They might be agonists in analgesia. It is also probable that in addition to 5 hydroxyl-tryptaminergic neurons, there might be acetyl cholinergic neurons in the same raphe nucleus, hence acupuncture might enhance the activities of both neurons, taking part in analgesia and regulating function. The interrelationship between 5HT and AChE in rephe nucleus dorsalis is a problem worth further investigation.

REFERENCES

[1] 湖南医学院针麻原理研究组：中华医学杂志，8：478，1973。

[2] 北京医学院基础部 针麻原理研究生理组：中国科学，1：98，1971。

[3] 中医研究院 针灸经络研究所生理组：新医药学杂志（3）：35，1976。

[4] 中医研究院 针灸经络研究所——生化组：新医药学杂志（3）：27，1975。

[5] Liebskind, J. C. et al: *Brain Res.* **50**:441, 1973.

[6] Mayer, D. J. : *Brain Res.* **68**:73, 1974.

[7] Russell, G. V.: *Tex. Reports on Biol. and Med.* **13**: 938, 1955.

[8] Moliner, E. R., et al: *Cell and Tissue Res.* **149** (2): 191, 1974.

[9] de la Torre J. C. and Surgeon J. W. : *Hustichemistry* **49**:81, 1976.

[10] Everson Pearse A. G.: Histochemistry, second edition, London, 1960.

[11] Almad El Badawi et al: *J. Histochem. and Cytochem.* **16** (10):586, 1968.

[12] 陕西中医研究所针麻研究组：针刺麻醉原理的探讨，人民卫生出版社，394 页，1974。

[13] 叶惟冷等：科学通报 22（8）：367，1977。

[14] 董新文等：生物化学生物物理学报，10（2）：109，1978。

[15] Segel M. and Sandberg D. : *Brain Res.* **134**(2): 359, 1977.

[16] 张德星等：科学通报 23（2）：117，1978。

[17] Sladek J. R. et al: *Brain Res.* **134(2):** 349, 1977.
[18] Guyenet P. G. and Aghajanian G. C. : *Brain Res.* **136:** 178, 1977.
[19] Jouvet M. : *Ergeb. der Physiol.* **64:** 168, 1972.
[20] 北京医学院针麻原理研究组　生理组：北京医学院学报，4：224，1975。
[21] 许绍芬等：科学通报　23 (9)：573，1978。
[22] Harris, L. S. : Fed. Proe. 29(l):28, 1970.
[23] Large, W. A. er al: *Brit. J. Pharmac.*, **38**:451, 1970.
[24] Dafny N. : *Neuropharmacology*, **15**:547, 1976.
[25] Ritter, J. et al: *Acta Histochem.*, **49**:176, 1974.
[26] Ungerstedt, U. : *Acta Physiol. Scand., Suppl.* **367**:1, 1971.

EFFECTS OF ELECTROACUPUNCTURE ON CELL-MEDIATED IMMUNITY IN HUMAN BODY

Wu Jinglan, Zong Anmin, Chai Xinmei, Cai Dehua, Luo Huimin, Kao Peiwen
(Research Group of Acupuncture Anesthesia, Henan Medical College)
Ren Zhichun
(Department of Histology, Henan Medical College)
Hu Zuofang
(Dept. of Biology, Henan Medical College)

According to traditional Chinese medicine, the functions of meridians are to link up the "outer" with the "inner", to regulate "Qì" and "Xiě", and to promote resistance against the evil. The effects of acupuncture on the enhancement of humoral immunity, of phagocytosis by leucocytes, and of the action of the mononuclear phagocyte system have been reported in man and animal[1,2,3]. However, few reports regarding the effects of acupuncture on cellmediated immunity (CMI) in man have hitherto been published.

E-rosette and lymphocyte transformation tests have been performed as the methods of detection of CMI in vitro. Whether there is any difference between the effects of acupuncture and drug anesthesia on CMI in man and how are the effects of electroacupuncture on CMI in comparision with those before acupuncture in patients are still unknown. The aim of the present investigation is to get an answer for the above-mentioned questions.

I. PATIENTS AND METHODS

70 patients, including 51 operated on under acupuncture anesthesia, 10 operated on under drug anesthesia (epidural), and the rest treated with electroacupuncture were observed. Acupuncture point Hegu or Zusanli was mainly used. Besides, CMI in patients before acupuncture was compared with that in healthy adults.

A small volume of blood (0.2–0.3 ml) was drawn from the ear lobes of patients before and 20 minutes after electroacupuncture (or drug anesthesia). 24 hours after the acupuncture, the blood of some of the patients was taken once again. Under identical conditions and/ or at the same time, the following tests on blood samples taken from each patient before and after acupuncture (or drug anesthesia) were performed.

(I) E-ROSETTE TESTS (60 cases observed)

1. Active E-Rosette Tests (47 cases observed). The procedure for the active E-rosette test described by Wybran and others[4,5,6] was improved by using a micromethod to purify lymphocytes on Ficoll-Hapaque and by supravital staining of the lymphocyte suspension mixed with sheep red cells immediately at room temperature. The percentage of rosette forming cells (RFC) was calculated in 47 cases, including 37 cases under acupuncture and 10 cases under drug anesthesia.

2. Nonactive E-Rosette Test (13 cases observed). According to Schaffer's method[7], the suspension of human lymphocytes and sheep red cells was placed in an ice bath (4°C) for 2–3 hours and fixed by glutaldehyde. RFC in both transient and permanent slide preparations were counted to take the average value of both.

(II) ASSAY FOR LYMPHOCYTE TRANSFORMATION

22 patients were observed. In 12 out of 22 cases, lymphocyte transformation and nonactive rosette formation were detected simultaneously.

The microtechnique of whole blood (0.1 ml) described by Yamada and others[8,9] was modified by preparing thick blood films, drop by drop, made of cultured blood with phytohemagglutinin (PHA) in vitro instead of smear. During fixation by Carnoy's fluid, the red cells were removed from the films. After the films were stained with methyl green-pyronin, the percentage of lymphocyte transformation was worked out under oil emersion.

II. RESULTS

(I) E-ROSETTE TESTS

1. Active Rosette Formation. The mean value of active RFC in healthy adults was 27.3 ± 0.58 in our laboratory, mostly in the range of 20–40%[6]. There were 31 patients with RFC < 40% before acupuncture; 20 minutes after the acupuncture, the increased mean value was 12.7 ± 1.43, P < 0.01 (Table 1). There were 6 patients with RFC > 41% before acupuncture; 20 minutes after the acupuncture, the decreased mean value in 5 cases was 6.8 ± 1.77, P < 0.05 (Table 1), except a slight increase in one case. After the acupuncture, the mean value of difference between the increased and decreased counts or total alteration

Table Effects of electroacupuncture (EA) or drug anesthesia on CMI

tests	active RFC %		nonactive RFC %	Lymphocyte transformation %	
mean values	20' after drug anesthesia	20' after EA	20' after EA	20' after EA	24 hrs. after EA
increased counts	2.3 ± 0.58 p < 0.05	12.7 ± 1.43 P < 0.01	13.0 ± 1.55 P < 0.01	12.7 ± 1.29 P < 0.01	15.3 ± 3.55 P < 0.01
decreased counts	5.0 ± 2.85 P > 0.05	6.8 ± 1.77 P > 0.05	7.5 ± 3.47 P > 0.05	7.0 ± 2.19 P > 0.05	0
total alteration	−1.35 ± 1.83 P > 0.05	9.82 ± 1.68 P < 0.01	8.30 ± 2.85 P < 0.05	7.61 ± 2.09 P < 0.01	

in the above-mentioned 37 cases was 9.82 ± 1.68, P < 0.01 (Table 1).

In 10 patients under drug anesthesia, the increased average value of active RFC in 5 cases was 2.3 ± 0.58, P < 0.05 (Table 1), and the decreased average value of that in the remaining 5 cases was 5.0 ± 2.85, P > 0.05 (Table 1). After drug anesthesia, the mean value of total alteration in the 10 cases was –1.35 ± 1.83, P > 0.05 (Table 1). The last two were of no statistical significance. Besides, there is a significant difference (P < 0.01) between the mean values of both groups enhanced under electroacupuncture (12.7 ± 1.43) and under drug anesthesia (2.3 ± 0.58).

2. Nonactive Rosette Formation. The nonactive rosette forming cells in permanent preparation are shown in Fig. 1.

The mean value of nonactive RFC in healthy adults was 61.1 ± 4.79 in our laboratory. After acupuncture the increased average value of nonactive RFC in 10 out of 13 cases was

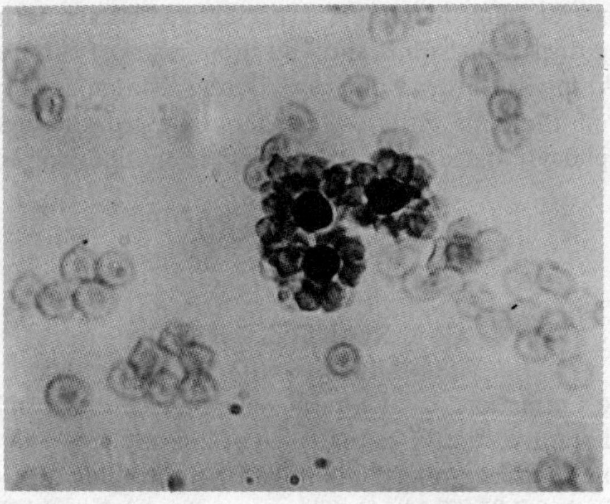

Fig. 1 Permanent Slide Preparation of three nonactive Rosette Forming Cells. Methly Green-Pyronin-Eosin stain. 950 X

13.0 ± 1.55, P<0.01 (Table 1). The decreased average value of that in the remaining 3 cases was 7.5 ± 3.47, P> 0.05 (Table 1). After acupuncture the mean value of total alteration in these 13 cases was 8.30 ± 2.85, P < 0.05 (Table 1).

(II) Lymphocyte Transformation

The transformed lymphocytes are shown in Fig. 2. The mean value of lymphocyte transformation in healthy adults was 56.7 ± 2.34. In 22 patients operated on under acupuncture anesthesia, the increased average value of lymphocyte transformation in 16 cases was 12.7 ± 1.29, P < 0.01 (Table 1); and the decreased average value of that in 5 cases was 7.0 ± 2.19, P < 0.05 (Table 1), except for only one case which had no alteration. After acupuncture, the mean value of total alteration in these 22 cases was 7.61 ± 2.09, P < 0.01 (Table 1).

The lymphocyte transformation in 7 out of 22 patients was investigated not only once

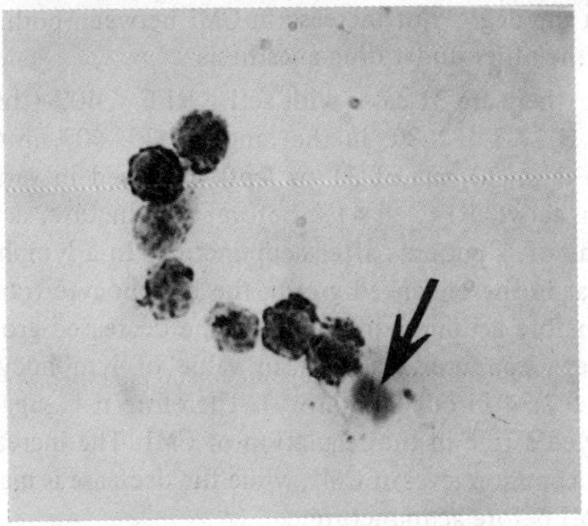

Fig. 2 Transformed Lymphocytes are larger and more irregular than nontransformed ones (Arrow points to two small cells on the right). The rest are the tronsformed cells with prominent nucleoli and abundant pyroninophil granules in cytoplasm Methyl Green-pyronin stain. 950 ×

after 20 minutes, but again at 24 hours after the acupuncture; the increased average value of lymphocyte transformation in both cases was 12.7 ± 1.29, $P < 0.01$ and 15.3 ± 3.55, $P<0.01$ (Table 1), respectively.

Both in the lymphocyte transformation and in the nonactive rosette formation tests, the results of increase or decrease ran parallel to each other in each of the 12 patients on whom both tests were carried out simultaneously.

III. DISCUSSION

In recent years, it has been demonstrated with various experiments by some authors that human T lymphocytes are characterized by bearing receptors of sheep red cells[10-12]. Addition of sheep red cells to human T cells in vitro causes clusterings around each T cell to form a spontaneous "rosette" (E–rosettes). It can be used to show the status of CMI in an organism. In an active rosette test, lymphocytes and sheep red cells are incubated together for a very short time, hence only the subpopulations of T cells are detected, and approximately 25% of human T lymphocytes form "active" rosettes. In a nonactive rosette test, human lymphocytes and sheep red cells are incubated together for a long period (mostly at 4°C), and approximately 50–80%[10] of T cells are detected. It has been postulated that the active rosettes are a better reflection of T cell competence than are nonactive ones[13, 5].

In the active rosette test, CMI in some cases (in decreased group) is reduced after electroacupuncture, while CMI in most cases (in enhanced group) markedly increased. On the whole, electroacupuncture plays a significant role in the enhancement of CMI. However, after drug anesthesia, CMI in some cases increased slightly (in enhanced group). On the whole, the effect of drug anesthesia on CMI is of no significance. Besides there is a significant difference in the degrees of increase in CMI between both enhanced groups, one under acupuncture and the other under drug anesthesia.

Before acupuncture, there are 31 cases with active RFC < 40% (the mean value of active RFC in healthy adults is 27.3 ± 0.89, in the range of 20–40% in our laboratory). After acupuncture, active RFC in 30 out of 31 patients increased in various degrees; whereas among 6 patients with active RFC > 41% before acupuncture, active RFC declined in various degrees in 5 out of 6 patients after acupuncture. In a lymphocyte transformation test, it is also found that in the enhanced group, the lymphocyte transformation rate in all cases is less than 60% before acupuncture, while in the decreased group it is in some cases more than 60% before acupuncture (the mean value of lymphocyte transformation in healthy adults is 56.7 ± 2.34 in our laboratory). Therefore it is suggested that electroacupuncture may have played a role in the regulation of CMI. The increase is found mainly in patients with a lower or common level of CMI, while the decrease is mainly found in patients with a higher level of CMI before acupuncture.

In active, nonactive rosette tests and assays for lymphocyte transformation, the mean values of enhancement are 12.7–13.0% after acupuncture. In the active rosette test and lymphocyte transformation test, the mean values of decrease are 6.8–7.0%. It shows that the effect of electroacupuncture on CMI in some patients increased, while in other cases decreased, with the ranges of increase or decrease in these tests basically in accord with each other. Moreover, the mean values of total alteration are 7.6–9.8% in these three tests. It demonstrates that, on the whole, electroacupuncture plays a significant role in the enhancement of CMI in patients.

E-rosette test not only measures the number of rosette forming cells, but also reflects the function of T cells. Especially active rosettes may represent the subpopulations with cytotoxic character among T cells[5]. It is well known that lymphocyte transformation also reflects the function of T cells. We consider that the combination of both tests is a better reflection of the status of CMI in an organism and of the alteration of CMI after electroacupuncture. 24 hours after the acupuncture, the lymphocyte transformation was seen to maintain the raised level similar to that 20 minutes after the acupuncture. It demonstrates that the effect of electroacupuncture on CMI can last 24 hours at least.

It has been reported that, with the addition of isolated lymphocytes from rabbit's peripheral blood to autoserum for cultivation separately both before and after acupuncture, the lymphocyte transformation in the electroacupuncture group will be much higher than that in the control one[14]. It indicates that under the influence of electroacupuncture, the enhancement of lymphocyte transformation is caused by the humoral factor in serum.

Good[15] reported the transplantation of fetal thymus to children with DiGeorge syndrome; the function of transformation of T cells in their peripheral blood was seen markedly improved in a few hours. Wybran[16] reported that when lymphocytes from the peripheral blood of normal adults and thymosin were incubated together for 1 hour in vitro, the active rosettes increased markedly. He postulated that thymosin tended to act on the subpopulations of T cells to make nonactive T cells become active ones. Wara[17] incubated thymosin together with lymphocytes from patients with immunodeficiency for 5 minutes at 37°C in vitro. He found that the E-rosettes increased in various degrees in patients, forecasting the different effects of treatment with thymosin on patients in vivo. Furthermore, the effects of the extracts of liver or spleen with a concentration 10 times that of thymosin on T cells turned out just the same as thymosin in vitro. At present,it is believed ed that thymosin may have influence over the differentiation and maturation of T cells; thymosin may act on T cells to make them become T_1 cells, and further develop from T_1 into T_2 cells, i.e., immunocompetent cells[16,17].

According to these data, we assumc that the mechanism of the effect of electroacupuncture on CMI may influence thymus, liver, spleen and so on to release a certain active substance similar to thymosin, and to make nonactive T cells become active ones through the regulation of the neuro-humoral system in an organism. In short, we assume that the effects of electroacupuncture on the activation of human T cells in peripheral blood may cause the alternative enumeration of E-rosette formation and lymphocyte transformation. The mechanism of electroacupuncture on CMI still remains to be shown.

In clinical practice, there is lower infection, better healing and more rapid convalescence in patients operated on under acupuncture than under drug anesthesia. This phenomenon may be related to the promotion of the resistance in an organism after acupuncture. It is found that electroacupuncture on "external" points in patients may have an influence on "internal" CMI reaction. This gives further evidence that meridians play a role in linking up the "outer" with the "inner". Besides, it may be observed that the major role of electroacupuncture is the enhancement of its effect on CMI; but it may also be observed that electroacupuncture also regulates CMI to a certain extent. This gives further evidence that the meridians play a role of promoting resistance and of regulation in an organism.

IV. CONCLUSION

1. Active E-rosette test is found to be a measurement of CMI in vitro. It is found that electroacupuncture plays a role in the regulation of CMI in some cases. On the whole, CMI is enhanced markedly under the influence of electroacupuncture with its effect able to last 24 hours. Under the influence of drug anesthesia, CMI is enhanced slightly in some cases. However, on the whole, the effect of drug anesthsia on CMI is of no significance. Besides, there is a significant difference in the enhancement between the two groups, the one under electroacupuncture and the one under drug anesthesia.

2. Active, nonactive rosettes and lymphocyte transformation are used as measurements of CMI in vitro. It is found that electroacupuncture plays a role in the regulation of CMI, and the ranges of increase or decrease run parallel to each other in these tests. The results of the total alteration in these tests indicate that under the influence of electroacupuncture, CMI is enhanced markedly.

3. This article provides data for the further understanding of the functions of meridians, such as the linking up of the "outer" with the "inner", the regulation of "Qì" and "Xiě" and the promotion of resistance.

REFERENCES

[1] 西安医学院针麻理论研究组：针刺麻醉原理的探讨，第 86 页，人民卫生出版社。

[2] 刘文琴等：陕西省中医研究资料汇编，第一辑，第 125 页，1964。

[3] 苏宝田等：安医学报 3 (23)：4，1960。

[4] Harris, F., Ukacjiofo. E. O.; *Lancetii* (7615):327, 1969.

[5] Wybran. J., Fudenberg H. H.: *New Eng. J. Med.*, 288:1072, 1973.

[6] 河南医学院组胚组、生物肿瘤科研组：河南卫生，288：1072，1973。

[7] Schaffer L. A. et al: *J. Immunological Methods*, 8(3): 241, 1975.

[8] 陈毓仙：免疫学讲义，中国医学科学院首都医院基础医学组，第 218 页，1975。

[9] 山田尚等：临床免疫 8 (10)：917，1976。

[10] Jondal. M: *J. Exp. Med.*, **136**(2):207, 1972.

[11] Yata. J. et al: *Clinical Exp. Immunol.*, **14**(3):319, 1973.

[12] Woritis. H. H. et al: *Nature New Biol.*, **243**(125):109, 1973.

[13] Wybran. J. Fudenberg H: *Ann. Intern. Med.*, 80(6):765, 1974.

[14] 细菌免疫学研究室：针麻资料汇编，北京市结核病研究所，第 105 页，1976。

[15] Good R. A. Bach F.H: *Clin. Immunobiology*, Volume II, Bach F. H. New York, Academic press., p. 71, 1974.

[16] Wybran J. et al: *Ann. N. Y. Acad. Sci.*, **249**:300, 1975.

[17] Wara. D. W., Ammann. A.J.: *Ann. N.Y. Acad. Sci.*, **249**:308, 1975.

PART II
RESEARCH ON CHANNEL–COLLATERALS AND POINTS

ADRENERGIC NERVE FIBERS — THE CHIEF FACTOR AFFECTING CHANGES OF ELECTRIC RESISTANCE OF RABBIT PINNA IN EXPERIMENTAL PEPTIC ULCER

Research Laboratory of the Mechanisms of Acupuncture Anesthesia, Morphology Group, Beijing Medical College

The meridian theory of the traditional Chinese medicine considers the meridians as channels connecting the internal visceral organs with the body surface. When any of the visceral organs is in a diseased condition, the corresponding meridian points on the body surface will respond to examination by lowering the electric resistance, producing a pain sensation on pressing, etc., and the diseased viscera will be treated by needling the corresponding meridian points. The purpose of the present research work is to study the validity of this viscero-body surface association and the nature of the connection between them.

First, a diseased condition in the visceral organs is induced by artificial means, then the change of the electric resistance of the skin of the rabbit's ear in the process of the disease is surveyed. The skin of the entire concave surface of the external ear of the rabbit is scanned with a high frequency (A.C, 550kC/sec) ohmmeter.

A solution of 40% glacial acetic acid was injected into the submucosa of the stomach wall of the rabbit and the animal developed a typical peptic ulcer lesion[1,2]. During the period of peptic ulcer many low electric resistance points (LERP) appeared on both ears of the animals, and the number gradually dropped down and became normal again when the animal recovered. The changes of the LERP on the ears corresponded to the development of the course of the disease.

Similiar results were obtained in two other models of experimental peritonitis[3] and infarct of the heart in the rabbits[4]. All of the three models show clearly that the change in the number of LERP is in response to the development of the diseased conditions of the visceral organs. It increases as the disease develops and decreases or returns to normal when the animal recovers from it. The viscero-body surface association of the traditional meridian theory is experimentally proved to exist. The next problem which is assigned to the present experiment is to search for the channel pathways of the viscero-body surface association.

I. MATERIAL AND METHODS

Twenty adult rabbits of both sexes with body weights between 2–3 kg, were divided into four groups. (1) The first group of ten animals had the right superior cervical sympathetic ganglion extirpated. (2) The second group of four animals had the branches of all the sensory nerves to the external ear, comprising the great auricular, the great occipital, the auriculotemporal and auricular branch of the vagus nerves severed, and, in addition, the right superior cervical sympathetic ganglion and a segment of the right common carotid artery were excised at the same time. (3) In the third group, 5 rabbits, only the branches of the sensory nerves to the right ear, as mentioned above, were severed. (4) Finally, one rabbit had a segment of its right common carotid artery, about 1 cm long, excised.

After the animals recovered from these operations, 40% glacial acetic acid was injected into the submucosa of the stomach according to the method reported in the previous work [2], in order to induce development of peptic ulcer in these animals.

Before and after the injection of acetic acid, the electric resistance of the concave surface of the rabbits' pinna were surveyed daily with a high frequency ohmmeter (made by Beihang, May-7 Factory with the cooperation of our group) following the procedure as mentioned in the previous works[2]. The values and locations where the LERP appeared on the concave surace of the rabbits' pinna, and those of the five selected points along the midline and in the vicinity of the inferior crus of the antihelix of the ear which served as controls were recorded daily.

The animals were killed 36–128 days after acetic acid injection. The scar formed by the ulcer on the stomach wall was confirmed, and the irides and the subcutaneous tissue of the ear were prepared as toto-mounts on slides. Parts of the preparations were processed with Falck-Hillarp's formaldehyde-induced-fluorescence (FIF) method for demonstrating adrenergic nerves[6], and the rest with Karnovsky-Roots method for acetylcholinesterase (AChE) positive nerves[7].

With the first method, the toto-mount preparations of the subcutaneous tissue or irides were dried by hot-air immediately and kept in a P_2O_5 desiccator for 24 hours. The reaction with formaldehyde vapor was carried out at 80°C, for 1.5 hrs in a well-sealed staining jar, containing about 1 g of paraformaldehyde powder already equilibrated with air of 60–70% relative humidity beforehand. The adrenergic nerve fibers were observed and photographed under a dark-field microscope with an HBO 200 lamp (Zeiss) and 2mm BG 12 filter as light source and OG 1 barrier filter for emission light. For AChE method, acetylthiocholine iodide was used as substrate and subcutaneous tissues or irides were incubated at 37°C, for 1.5 to 4 hrs. Tissues from the left and right ears or irides were prepared in the same reacting fluid and under the same conditions. Parts of the preparations were incubated with iso–OMPA ($3 \times 10^{-6} M$) as the inhibitor for the non-specific cholinesterases.

II. RESULTS

The results of the four experimental animal groups are as follows:

(1) Rabbits with extirpation of the right superior cervical symthetic ganglion (10 rabbits).

Peptic ulcer was induced 2–4 months after the extirpation of the right cervical ganglion. During the period of peptic ulcer (34 days), the results of daily survey of LERP are listed in Table 1. Eight out of ten rabbits showed little difference between the numbers of LERPs appearing on the left and right ears; in two rabbits, more points appeared on the right ear and in 6 rabbits, more on the left. With t-test, the difference between their daily average value of number of LERPs did not show any statistical significance (P>0.2–0.8 or more). In

Table 1. Comparison of LERP number and k Ω-value between left and right auicles during peptic ulcer after the extirpation of right superior cervical ganglion

Rabbit		No. of LERP*	daily average	δ	t-test	kΩ**	Daily average	δ	t-test
128	R	254	7.47	4.18	P<0.001	468.03	13.76	1.15	P<0.001
	L	461	13.55	6.71		417.81	12.28	0.83	
132	R	75	2.20	3.20	P>0.60	559.76	16.46	2.20	P>0.05
	L	93	2.73	3.83		530.88	15.61	1.44	
135	R	291	8.56	3.66	P>0.10	419.62	12.34	1.32	P>0.40
	L	341	10.03	4.46		395.70	11.63	1.22	
142	R	167	4.91	3.61	P>0.10	498.4	14.66	2.71	0.025<P<0.05
	L	229	6.73	5.01		458.6	13.49	1.80	
143	R	271	7.97	4.66	P>0.25	422.0	11.87	4.79	P>0.20
	L	272	8.00	4.21		403.5	12.41	1.42	
145	R	287	8.44	7.43	P>0.70	427.22	12.56	0.96	P>0.70
	L	273	8.02	4.25		423.74	12.46	1.87	
150	R	81	2.38	3.35	P<0.02	573.1	16.86	2.81	P<0.025
	L	181	5.32	6.14		501.7	14.76	4.37	
151	R	307	9.02	6.25	P>0.70	441.7	12.99	1.86	P>0.40
	L	327	9.61	6.51		428.7	12.61	2.10	
152	R	559	16.44	3.24	P>0.50	347.13	10.22	1.03	P>0.80
	L	539	15.85	4.70		348.91	10.26	0.85	
154	R	71	2.26	2.64	P>0.10	543.8	15.99	2.26	P>0.20
	L	111	3.26	3.39		520.6	15.31	2.60	

*Number of LERPs whose Ω values are lower than the lower limit of the average Ω value of the control points ABCDE.

**The sum of the KΩ-values of the ABCDE and the LERPs.

the remaining two rabbits (Nos. 128 and 150) the difference of the total number of LERPs between the two ears was greater, and the difference between their daily averages was statistically significant ($P<0.001$ for No. 128 and $P<0.002$ for No. 150).

The electric resistance of the concave surface of the pinna is expressed by the average ohm value of both of the LERP and ABCDE control points in kΩ. In five out of the ten rabbits this average value was greater in the right ear, and in two animals it was greater on the left. But this difference between the two ears was of no statistical significance ($P>0.05$–0.80). For the other three rabbits, the difference of the average electric resistance between the two ears was statistically significant ($P<0.001$–0.025). After excision of the right superior cervical sympathetic ganglion, in the course of peptic ulcer, the electric resistances of both ears, either expressed in the number of LERPs or in kΩ, showed no significant difference in the majority of the rabbits.

The animals were killed 78–195 days after the excision of the superior cervical sympathetic ganglion. The subcutaneous tissue was studied with the histochemical methods for AChE. The enzyme-positive nerve fibers were distributed in the external lamina of blood vessels and arteriovenule (A–V) anastomoses, in the sebaceous glands, around hair follicles and among the connective tissues. No apparent difference was observed between the two ears in distribution density and caliber of nerve fibers. A slight reduction of the enzyme-positive nerve fibers was observed in some animals (Figs. 3 and 4).

FIF reaction was carried out in 4 animals (Nos. 150, 151 152, and 154). Nerve fibers with rich green fluorescence were observed around the blood vessels and A–V anastomoses (Fig. 1). After the extirpation of the right cervical sympathetic ganglion, the right ear still showed an abundant network of the adrenergic nerve fibers around the blood vessels (Fig. 2). The FIF nerves of the irides of both eyes were compared; the distribution of FIF nerve fibers in the affected (right) side showed no apparent difference from that of the normal left side in two animals (Nos. 151 and 152). There were only a few networks of fine fibers observed in the right iris of the rabbit No. 150.

(2) Rabbits with complete severance of sensory nerves and excision of superior cervical sympathetic ganglion and a segment of the common carotid artery.

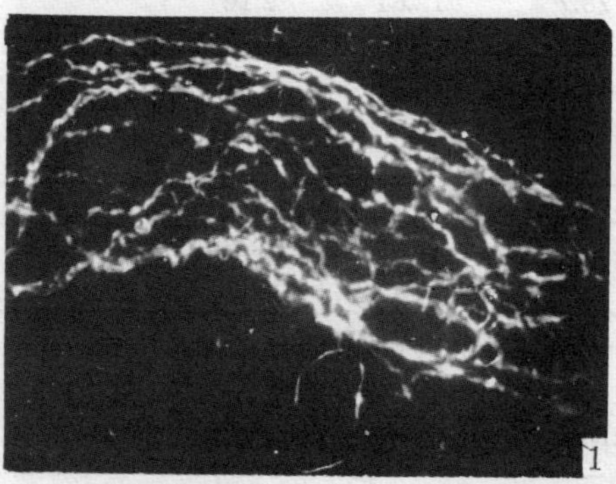

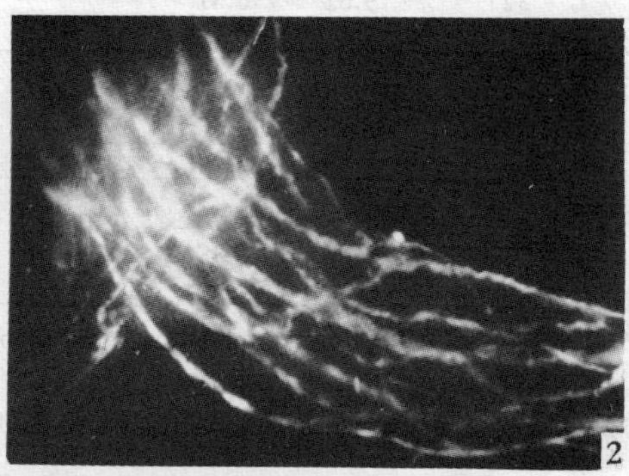

Figs. 1–2 Toto-mounts of subcutaneous tissue from the concave surfaces of Rabbit's (No. 154) ears, after extirpation of right cervical sympathetic ganglion. Falck-Hillarp's fromaldehyde-induced-fluorescence method to show the distribution of adrenergic nerve fibers. 5×, 10×.
Fig. 1: left ear. Fig. 2: right ear.

In the first experiment the adrenergic nerve fibers did not entirely disappear in the right ear of the rabbit after the extirpation of the right cervical sympathetic ganglion which showed that the supply of the adrenergic nerve fibers to the ear was not limited to the post-ganglionic fibers of the sympathetic ganglion. Therefore, in this experiment, besides the exptirpation of the right cervical sympathetic ganglion, all the sensory nerves to the right ear were severed and, in addition, one segment of the right common carotid artery was excised in order to cut off all possible sources of the adrenergic nerve fibers to the ear. In four rabbits of this group, after complete denervation, the electric resistances of both ears were surveyed for 35 days in the course of peptic ulcer. The number of LERPs appearing in the right ear during this period was reduced to only one half or even to one fourth of that in the normal left ear. Statistically, the difference between the daily average of either the number of LERPs or the kΩ values of both ears was highly significant (see Table 2). The result confirms those reported in the previous work[5]. To show the difference of the daily average numbers of LERPs in the two ears, a histogram is constructed with the results from the four rabbits in this group and the other nine from the former experiment[5] (Fig. 10).

On the 74–89th days after rest greater, the subcutaneous tissue and irides from the four rabbits were subjected to histochemical studies for FIF and AChE reactions. Under the fluorescence microscope adrenergic nerve fibers were absent in all of the 50 preparations from the right ears of the four rabbits; only two sites in the dorsal and concave surfaces of

Table 2. Comparison of the numbers and kΩ-values of the LERPs between the left and the right auricles during peptic ulcer (35 days) after the denervation of the right ear by complete severance of sensory nerves and extirpation of the superior cervical ganglion and a segment of the right common carotid artery

Rabbit No.		No. of LERP*	Daily average	δ	t-test	kΩ**	Daily average	δ	t-test
173	R	177	5.06	3.59	P<0.001	487.9	13.94	2.27	P<0.001
	L	374	10.69	3.91		416.9	11.89	1.01	
177	R	83	2.38	2.00	P<0.001	548.7	15.68	1.91	P<0.001
	L	382	10.91	4.32		413.4	11.81	1.52	
214	R	135	3.86	2.39	P<0.001	514.1	14.69	1.18	P<0.001
	L	217	6.20	4.09		466.6	13.33	1.81	
219	R	265	7.57	2.94	P<0.001	441.0	12.60	1.21	P<0.005
	L	430	12.29	7.50		405.4	11.58	1.75	

* See notes under Table I.

** See notes under Table I.

the ear of the rabbit No. 219 showed a few residual fibers. All the irides from the right eyes showed no fluorescent fibers. In contrast, the tissues from the left ears and left irides of the four rabbits possessed a very rich supply of green fluorescent nerve plexuses.

The AChE preparations of only one rabbit (No. 173) after a shorter incubation period of 1.5 hrs, showed weak reaction in the left ear and none in the right. In tissues from the other 3 rabbits, incubated for 3 hrs, dense enzyme-positive nerve plexuses were observed around the blood vessels and A–V anastomoses and among the connective tissues in the left ear, while they were relatively less in the corresponding locations of the right ear. (Figs. 5 and 6).

(3) Rabbits with the severance of the sensory nerve branches and intact cervical sympathetic ganglion.

In five rabbits the sensory nerves to the right ear, including the great auricular, the great occipital, the auriculotemporal and the auricular branches of vagus were severed. The numbers and kΩ values of LERPs that appeared during the period of peptic ulcer on both ears in 35 days are listed in Table 3.

The numbers of LERPs appearing on both ears differed slightly. In two rabbits there were more on the left ear and in three rabbits more on the right. Their difference was of no statistical significance. As to the average of kΩ values of the LERPs, the difference between

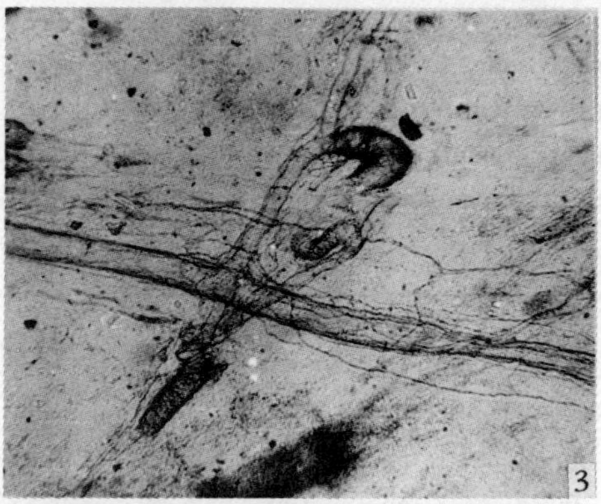

3

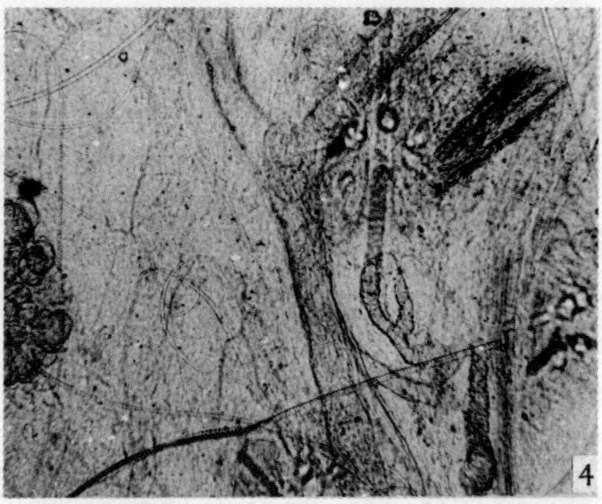

4

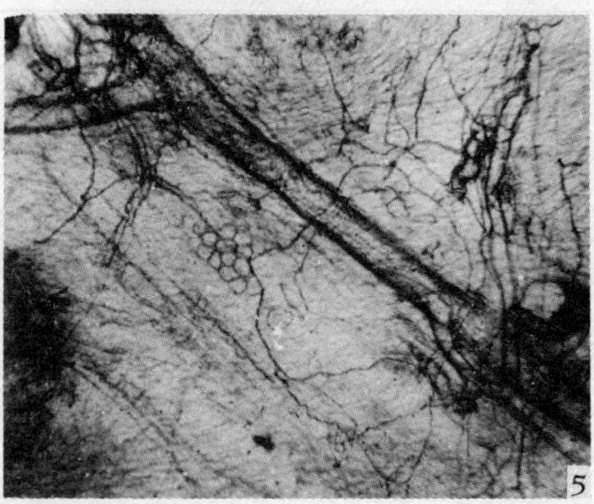

5

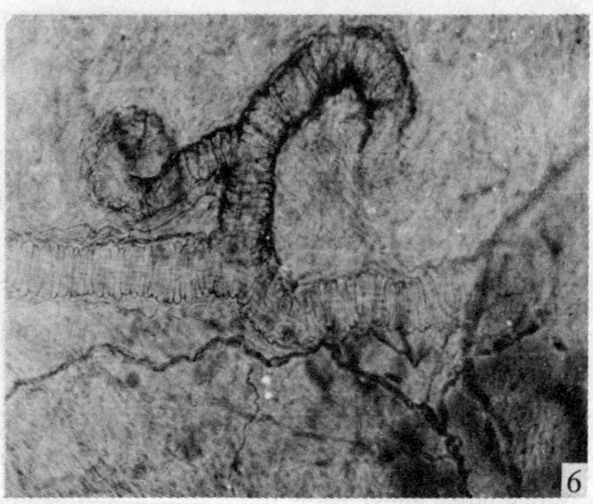

6

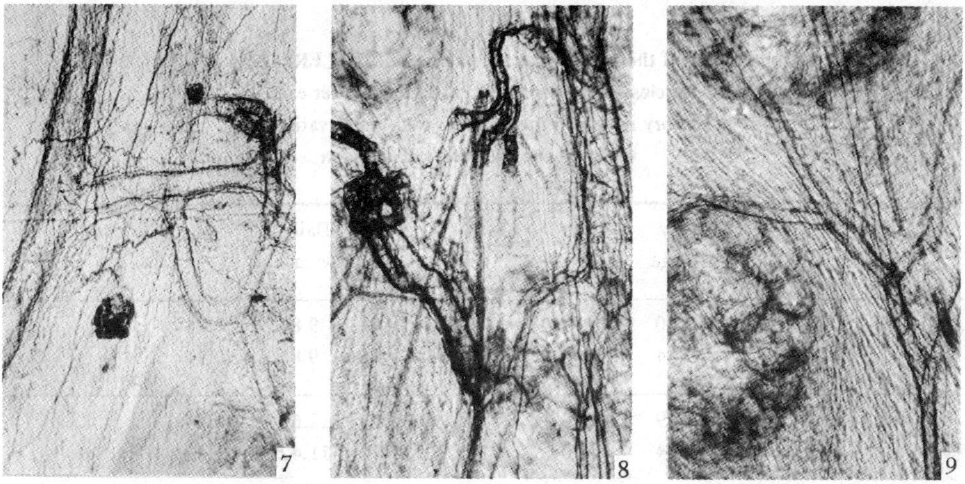

Figs. 3–9 Toto-mount of subcutaneous tissue from the concave surface of rabbit's ears. Karnovsky-Roots' method to show the distribution of ACHE-positive nerve fibers. 5×, 3.5×.
Fig. 3(left ear) and Fig. 4(right ear) from Rabbit No. 154 after extirpation of the right cervical sympathetic ganglion. Fig. 5(left ear) and Fig. 6(right ear) from Rabbit No. 219 after extirpation of right cervical sympathetic ganglion, excision of one segment of right common carotid artery and severance of the sensory nerves from the right ear. Fig. 7(left ear), Figs. 8 and 9(right ear) from Rabbit No. 207 after severance of the sensory nerves from the right ear.

the two ears was negligible. With t-test, only in one rabbit was the P-value less than 0.05, while in the rest greater than 0.80 or 0.90.

Histochemical study of the FIF and AChE reactions was made within 94–166 days after the severance of the sensory nerves to the right ear. The incubation period for AChE reaction was three hours. The adrenergic nerve fibers appearing on both ears were the same in distribution and fluorescence intensity in all the animals, while the AChE positive nerve fibers were nearly the same in distribution density in two rabbits (Nos. 207 and 242) or somewhat reduced in the other three (Nos. 216, 249 and 181) (Figs. 7,8,9).

(4) Rabbit with excision of one segment of the right common carotid artery.

Only one rabbit was subjected to this operation (No. 250). The purpose of this operation was to see whether the cut-off of blood supply from the common carotid artery and removal of the nerve plexus around its wall would affect the change of electric resistance of the right ear during peptic ulcer. The LERPs appearing on the concave surface of the right ear during peptic ulcer showed no change either in number or in kΩ values (Table 4), nor did the FIF and AChE reactions demonstrate any change of the adrenergic or AChE-positive nerve fibers in the affected side histochemically.

Table 3. Comparison of the numbers and k Ω-values of the LERPs between the left and the right auricles during peptic ulcer (35 days) after excision of the sensory nerves to the right ear with preservation of the right superior cervical ganglion

Rabbit No.		No. of LERP*	Daily average	δ	t-test	k Ω**	Daily average	δ	t-test
181	R	686	19.60	5.97		345.44	9.84	1.44	
	L	677	19.34	5.96		345.49	9.84	0.91	
216	R	332	9.49	6.53		443.21	12.66	1.84	
	L	404	11.54	6.90		399.70	11.42	1.72	
207	R	490	14.00	6.50		398.9	11.40	1.29	
	L	485	13.86	6.40		394.0	11.26	1.14	
242	R	315	9.00	3.49		429.60	12.28	0.83	
	L	316	9.03	3.83		426.80	12.20	0.94	
249	R	274	7.83	3.43		439.49	12.55	0.87	
	L	268	7.66	3.31		438.90	12.54	1.03	

* and ** See notes under Table I.

Table 4. Comparison of the numbers and KΩ-values of the LERPs between the left and the right auricles during peptic ulcer (35 days) after excision of the right common carotid artery

Rabbit No.		No. of LERP*	Daily average	δ	t-test	KΩ**	Daily average	δ	t-test
250	R	248	7.09	4.14		453.3	12.95	1.26	
	L	294	8.4	1.26		430.2	12.29	1.50	

* and ** See notes under Table I.

III. DISCUSSION

It is clear from the above experiments that only the second group of thc experiments showed that the association of viscera organs with the skin of the body was definitely affected by denervation. In the second group, after severance of all sensory nerves to the right ear, extirpation of the right cervical sympathetic ganglion and a section of the common carotid artery, the number of LERPs appearing on the right ear during peptic ulcer was greatly reduced, and histochemically all its adrenergic nerve fibers almost disappeared entirely. While in the other three groups, after only the right cervical sympathetic ganglion was extirpated, or only the sensory nerves were severed, or only one segment of the common carotid artery was excised, the LERPs appearing on both ears during peptic ulcer showed no marked difference in the majority of the animals and no apparent difference was found in the distribution density of the adrenergic nerve fibers on both ears. A parallel coincidence occurs in the results of both LERP survey and the demonstration of adrenergic nerve fibers.

The result of the distribution density of the AChE-positive nerve fibers in both ears of the experimental animals of these four groups differs from that of adrenergic fibers, either markedly or slightly reduced, or hard to discriminate from the normal in the affected ear. In the second group the survey of LERPs shows a definite difference between the two ears. In the rabbit No. 173, with an incubation period of 1.5 hours, AChE positive nerves occur sparsely in the left and none in the right ear, but by prolonging the incubation period to three hours in the other three rabbits, enzyme-positive fibers occur even in the completely denervated right ear, though less abundant than in the normal left. In the third group, the sensory nerves of the right ear were severed; the AChE positive nerve fibers still existed in various quantities. The existence or reduction of AChE positive fibers seems to play no important role in affecting the change of electric resistance of the ear. Thus, it is rather the adrenergic (sympathetic) nerve fibers in the ear which show an intimate relation with the reaction of the ear, expressed as the change of LERPs in response to the visceral disease, peptic ulcer. When these nerves are intact, the right ear is able to reflect the internal response to the disease in the organism, while in their absence, its reaction is weakened. The traditional Chinese medicine considers meridians as channels by which the visera organs and the external parts and skin of the body are linked up. In these experiments we have observed that the sympathetic nerve fibers play an important role in the channels of association between the viscera and the external parts skin of the body.

Abundant adrenergic nerve fibers were found in the right ear after the right superior cervical sympathetic ganglion was excised in the first group of the animals. Their presence indicates that the sympathetic nerves to the ear come from sources other than the cervical ganglion, e.g., from the nerve plexuses around the arteries, and from postganglionic neurons elsewhere out of the cervical ganglion. The postganglionic fibers from these sources can reach the right ear even after the extirpation of the right superior cervical ganglion. The abundant adrenergic nerve fibers could be derived or regenerate from those sources other than the superior cervical ganglion.

Kvirehishvili[8] found that an intramuscular injection of turpentine did not cause local changes (decrease in resistance) in the skin of the concha auriculae of the rabbits after bilateral sympathectomy (extirpation of bilateral superior cervical sympathetic ganglia), but he did not mention whether any residual adrenergic fibers still existed or not.

After division of the branches of the cerebral and spinal nerves of the right external ear (in the animals of the second and third groups), AChE positive fibers were still found on the right ear. The external ear of the rabbit is so large in size and with multiple nerve supplies, it is difficult to cut away all the nerves with naked eyes without leaving out any of their small branches. Part of the neurons in the cervical sympathetic ganglion are AChE positive[9], Naturally, some of these enzyme-positive nerve fibers could be their axons, and, in fact, the AChE positive fibers appeared to be more abundant in the animals of the third group in which the sympathetic ganglion is preserved than in those of the second group with the ganglion excised. Besides, the possibility of regeneration of nerve fibers can not be excluded in such a long span of time of 74–195 days after operation till the death of the animals.

In the first experiment of peritonitis[3] we discovered that the maximal number of LERPs appeared on the ear surface not during the serious crisis of the disease, but rather in the period when the animal began to recover. This suggested that the frequency curve of the daily change of the number of LERPs reflected the activity of the regulatory system against the damage in the organism during the period of the visceral disease. Afterwards, the same rule was observed in two other animal models of peptic ulcer[1] and infarct of the heart[4]. This regulatory system associates with the recovery process of the disease in the viscera on the one hand and with the change of electric resistance of the ear skin on the other. It con-

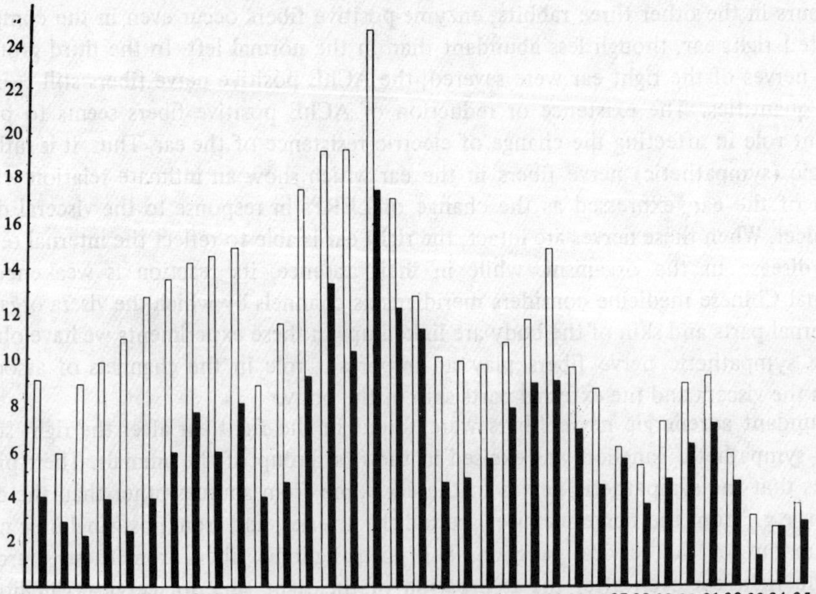

Fig. 10 Histogram to show the differences of the daily average number of LERPs on the two ears in contrast after complete denervation of the right ear.

co-ordinate: number of LERPs abscissa: number of days

left ear: □ right ear: ■

cretely proves the theme of the theory of meridians that they are channels connecting the viscera with external appendages. Thus we consider that the meridian is nothing but this regulatory system in the organism which links the viscera with the external parts of the body. This experiment may serve as evidence that the adrenergic nerve fibers are the chief factors affecting the change of electric resistance of the pinna in the process of peptic ulcer, hencc the important components of the visceral regulatory system of the body, i.e., the meridians. It further approves the validity of the hypothesis that meridian is a system of visceral regulations.

After complete denervation of the right ear, the number of LERPs appearing on the ear is reduced to about only one half of that of the left ear during peptic ulcer (Fig. 10). The remaining half of the LERPs on the right ear still keep the shape of the frequency curve. In this experiment it has been demonstrated that the adrenergic nerve fibers, rather than other sensory nerve fibers, are closely related with the reduction of the number of the LERPs. This fact may suggest that noradrenaline and its likes in the body fluid may be one of the factors to account for the residual half of the LERPs in the absence of adrenergic nerves.

Recently in a general survey of the phenomena of meridian conduction, red lines, white lines, and hypodermal hemorrgage, streaks etc., have been noted in some cases along the classical courses of different meridians on the body surface under acupuncture. Erection of hair, muscle fibrillation and sweating along the courses of meridians have also been reported. Based on these clinical observations, it is assumed that the autonomic nervous system may take part in the meridian conduction. Reports from abroad[10,11] have put forward a hypothesis holding that connection between the body surface and the internal viscera under acupuncture is made possible by vegetative nerves. These suggestions may be helpful to understand the nature of meridians. Our observations of three animal models provide objective evidence of the existence of the visceral regulatory system in the organism and its activity in the development of different disease processes and establish the role of the sympathetic nervous system in meridian conduction.

REFERENCES

[1] 北京医学院基础部针麻原理研究形态组 北京医学院学报，**1**: 12，1974。

[2] Acupuncture Anesthesia Research Goup, Morphology Unit, Peking Medical College: *Chin Med Jour:* **2**(6): 423, 1976.

[3] 李肇特等: 中华医学杂志 **7**: 428，1973。

[4] 北京医学院基础部针麻原理研究形态组，北京医学院学报，**2**: 75，1978。

[5] 北京医学院基础部针麻原理研究形态组，北京医学院学报，**3**: 147，1975。

[6] Falck, B.: *Acta physiol. scand. suppl.* **197** pp25, 1962.

[7] Baljet, B. and Durkker, J.: *Stain Technology* **50**:31, 1975.

[8] Kvirehishvili, V.I.: *Am. J. Acupuncture,* **2**:206, 1974.

[9] Yamauchi, A. and Lever J.d.: *J. Anat.* **110**(3): 435, 1971.

[10] Ionescu-Tirgoviste, C.: *Am. J. Acupuncture,* **3**: 199 1975.

[11] Ionescu-Tirgociste, C. *et al:* Revure *2*(6): 41, 1976.

EXPERIMENTAL STUDY OF THE AFFERENT PATHWAY IN FORMATION OF LOW-RESISTANCE POINTS ON THE AURICULAE OF RABBIT

Yin Huizhen, Zhou Shaoci, You Guofen

(Research Laboratory of Brain Function, The Biology Department, East China Normal University)

An important component part of the classic theory of medical science in our country is the view that the exterior of the human body is correlated with its viscera (the internal organs). And this has always been an important basis for clinical diagnosis. Since 1962, after the observations of the changes in the pain-pressing points on the auricles were made by Wu Wangyuan, Du Huanji and Shen Eh by injuring the limbs or any other part of an animal body, further work has been done in this field. It has been reported that a visceral disease or an injury, internal or external, inflicted on an animal, causes pain-pressing points, or the so-called pain-sensitive points or low resistance points on the auricles[1-7]. This phenomenon has been taken as a model for the study of the theory and principle of the traditional Chinese medicine that the exterior of the human body is correlated with its viscera. This methodology has several advantages. Corresponding to the changed conditions of the visceral disease, it might show a steady and more or less intuitive reflection on the surface of the body. Most of the diseases in the human body can increase the pain-pressing points on the auricles[4-5]. Since 1972 we have observed the increase of such pain-pressing points on the auricles. We found the increment was directly proportional to the degree and extent of the changes of the visceral disease. On the other hand, the experimental animal study, as a model confirmed the realization of correlation of the exterior of the human body with its viscera. Cooperating with the Morphological Research Group for the study of the principle of acupuncture anesthesia of Beijing Medical College[7], we[8] have recently concentrated our joint efforts on the study of the nervous pathway correlating the body surface with the viscera. It has been proved, not excluding the functions of other auricular nerves, that the activity of the sympathetic nerve fibers is of special significance for the formation of low resistance points on the auricles. But so far not much research work has been done on the afferent pathway that to links up the two phenomena. The present article deals with the method of prolonged implantation of electrodes to show that it is mainly the afferent impulse of the vagus nerve pathway that is responsible for the formation of low resistance points on the auricles.

I. METHODS

The experiments were made on 25 adult rabbits, irrespective of sex, weight from 2 to 3 kg. The operation was performed under sterilized conditions, using 2% procaine for local anesthesia. The skin incision was made on the left side, 2 cm below the xiphoid process. An abdominal opening was carefully cut, exposing the stomach, and separating the ventral gastric branch of the vagus nerves and also the sympathetic branch from celiac ganglion which is distributed along the right gastric artery forming periarterial plexus. The home-made micro-electrode made of non-poisonous silatic membrane and the multistrained teflon-coated silver wire (see Fig. 1) was then fixed on the ventral branch of the gastric vagus nerves or the gastric periarterial sympathetic plexus. For the construction of the electrode and its fixation, please read another article[9]. After operation, the animals were nursed (in the usual way). They were in normal condition – no marked change in digestion, circulation, or behavior observed. Nerve stimulation was carried out while the animal was confined in a wooden box (see Fig. 2), the frequency being from 80 to 100 cycles per second. The intensity for the vagus nerve was 20–25 V while that for the sympathetic nerve was only 1.5 to 2.0 volts. The stimulation was given uninterruptedly for 12 to 24 hours. During stimulation, the changes of the low resistance points on the auricle were carefully observed and determined every 2 to 4 hours. The method of determination and the equipment for it have been published before[6]. The control animals were in the same conditions as the experimental animals, except without stimulation of the visceral nerve.

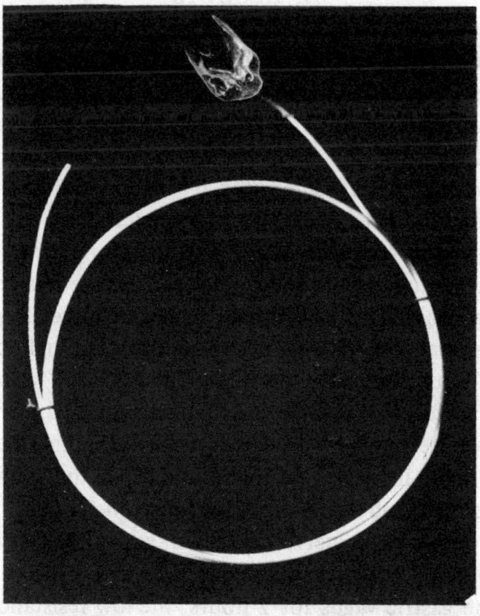

Fig. 1 The above picture shows the micro-electrode made of silatic membrane and multistranded, teflon-coated silver wire.

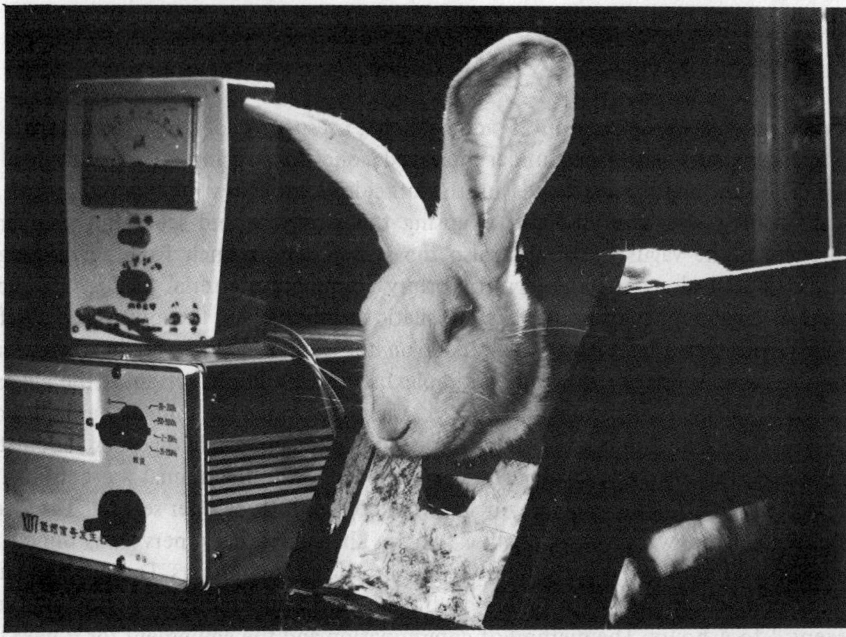

Fig. 2 The above picture shows a rabbit restricted in a wooden box and receiving stimulation of its visceral nerves.

II. RESULTS

1. There was no perceptible change in the heart rate of the animal when the ventral branch of the gastric vagus was stimulated by an uninterrupted galvanic current for as long as 12 hours. The number of beats before and after the excitation was around 275 per second, showing no distinct change. And there was no sign of any unusual change in the digestive function or behavior of the animal. The intensity of excitation for the vagus nerve was generally within the range of 20 to 25 V. When the excitation was beyond this range, the animal seemed to show signs of restlessness and even struggling for freedom.

The intensity for the stimulation of the sympathetic nerve was generally as low as 1.5 to 3.0 V. When the voltage was raised, the animal struggled to get free; it jumped and showed such signs of strong reaction of a defensive nature. Throughout the entire course of experimentation the galvanic intensity was kept around 1.5 V. Under this condition the animal seemed to be peaceful, showing no unusual behaviour. Under uninterrupted stimulation for 12 hours the average number of heartbeats of the animal went up from 235 to 250 per second, showing a slight increase. During stimulation, the animal could eat as before, having no unusual phenomenon about its digestive function.

2. The stimulation of the vagus nerve has a marked influence on the formation of low resistance points on the auricles. Our experiments have proved that after the stimulation of the ventral branch of the gastric vagus for 2 hours, the low resistance points on the auricles of the animal began to increase and after 4 hours the increase became even more remarkable. The mean number of such low resistance points generally was ten times greater than what it

had been before the stimulation. With the prolongation of the stimulating time, the rate of increase of such low resistance points continued to go up and after 12 hours the average became 700 times greater than that before stimulation. At this time, the low resistance points on the auricles appeared in large patches, widely distributed around the auricles. It was also observed that when the four rabbits were given an uninterrupted stimulation for 24 hours, the low resistance points spread to (or rather, appeared at) the helix, cavern conchae and the back of the ears. When the stimulation to the ventral branch of the gastric vagus was stopped, the number of the low resistance points on the auricles began to drop. Usually after 3 or 4 days the number returned to the original level. The changes in the number of the low resistance points, as mentioned above, seemed to take place on both auricles simultaneously. Fig. 3 shows the experimental results on 5 rabbits. The ordinate stands for the logarithmic values of low resistance points and the abscissa the time (in hours) of stimulation. It can be seen in the graph that the number of low resistance points on the auricles before stimulation was generally below 10. After stimulation started the number of low resistance points began to increase gradually, and after 12 hours of stimulation the average number of the low resistance points increased to 700 times of the original. There was no obvious change in the number of the low resistance points within 24 hours after the stoppage of stimulation. After that it began to full gradually, and in 4 days it nearly returned to its original level. The difference between the left and the right aruicles was not great during all these changes – the two auricles went rather side by side. The lower curves in Fig. 3 show the results of the experiment on the control animal which received no stimulation to its visceral nerves. It can be seen clearly from the curves that the average number of the low resistance points on the

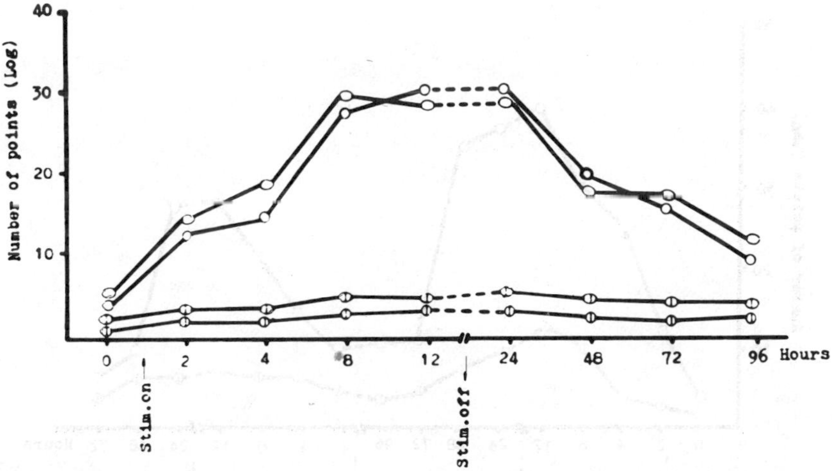

Fig. 3 In the graph as shown here the two curves above indicate the changing conditions of the mean of low resistance points on the left auricle (shown by the curve with oblong dots on it) and the right auricle (shown by the curve with circular dots on it) when the vagus nerves were being stimulated in one case, and when the stimulation was stopped in the other case.

The two curves below indicate the changing conditions of the mean of low resistance points on both the left and right auricles of control animals when the vagus nerves were not receiving any stimulation.

auricles during the entire process of its determination remained constantly steady, showing no perceptible change.

3. Our experiments in the past showed that the increase of low resistance points on the auricles caused by artificial gastric ulcer is correlated with the intactness of the sympathetic nerve innervating the auricles[8]. In order to know whether the increase in the low resistance points on the auricles caused by the stimulation of the ventral branch of the gastric vagus is also correlated with the sympathetic nerves innervating the auricles, we excised unilateral cervical sympathetic nerve on a part of the animals to observe whether there is any difference in the formation of low resistance points between both auricles when the gastric vagus was stimulated uninterruptedly. Experiments proved that the unilateral excision of the cervical sympathetic nerves had a distinct influence on the formation of the low resistance points on the ipsilateral auricles.

The curves in Fig. 4 represent the experimental results of the rabbits whose right cervical sympathetic nerves were excised. As soon as the ventral branch of the gastric vagus of a rabbit was stimulated, the number of the low resistance points on the left auricle began to increased and this increase continued with the time of stimulation, and after 12 hours, it reached its peak while the number of the low resistance points on the right auricule showed no change at all. After stimulation was terminated the number of the low resistance points on the left auricule dropped daily till it returned to its original level in 4 days. If stimulation of the ventral branch of the gastric vagus was resumed on the 5th day and continued for 12 hrs and then discontinued, the whole cycle of rise and fall would be repeated again.

4. No distinct change of the low resistance points on the auricles was observed when

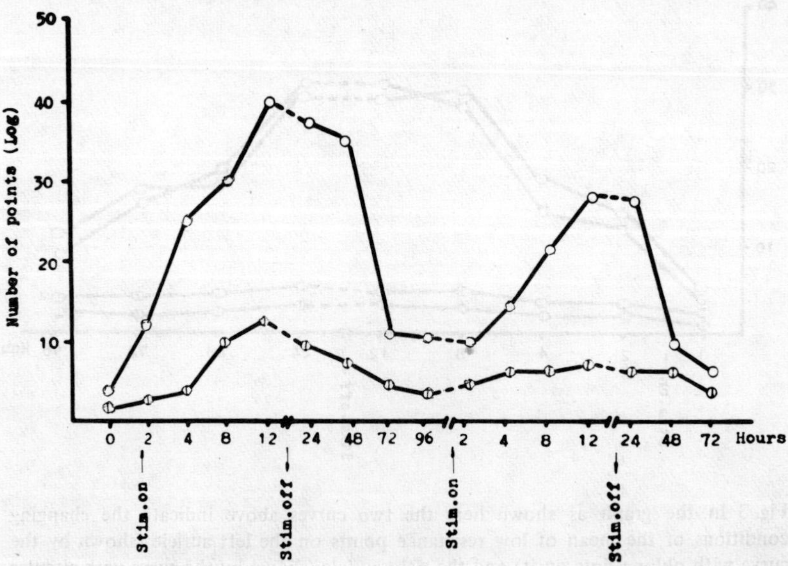

Fig. 4 The curves above show the comparative values of the changes of low resistance points on the left auricle (marked with plain circular dots, as shown on the curve above) and the right auricle (marked with circular dots with vertical crossings, as shown on the curve below) when the vagus nerves were being stimulated after the excision of the right cervical sympathetic nerves.

part of the animals were stimulated at the gastric periarterial sympathetic plexus uninterrupted for 8 hours duration. There was, however, a slight increase of the low resistance points for 12 hours stimulation. The unilateral increase of the points did not go beyond 8. This presents a striking contrast with the great increase of low resistance points on the auricles due to the stimulation of the vagus nerves. The graph in Fig. 5 shows the changes of the low resistance points on both auricles due to the stimulation of the sympathetic fibers in the gastric periarterial plexus. It can be seen from the curves that even after an uninterrupted stimulation for 8 hours, the number of the low resistance points did not show any marked increase. After 12 hours, however, the number increased to 12 from its original value, 4. And 48 hours after the termination of stimulation, it returned to its original level. The change of the number was, any case, within the normal range and did not have any special statistical significance.

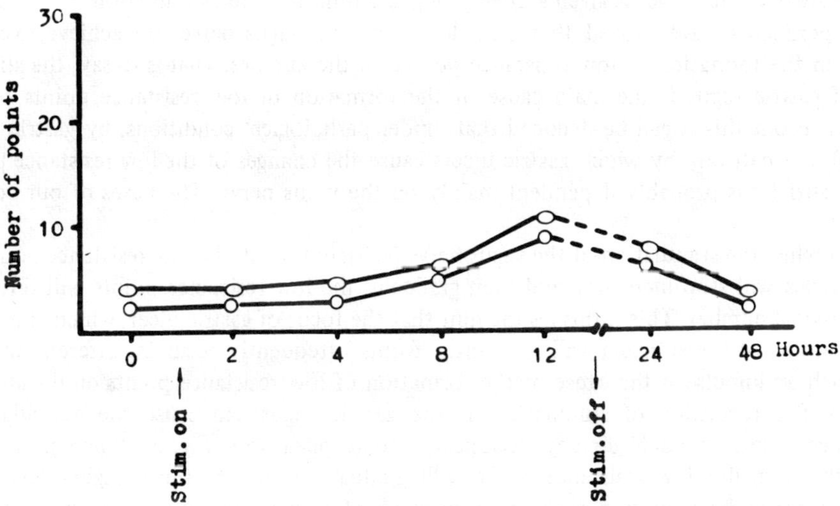

Fig. 5 The curves above indicate the changing values of the mean of low resistance points when the sympathetic fibres in the gastric periarterial plexus were being stimulated. The curve above with bigger oblong dots, shows the changing mean for the left auricle and the curve below with smaller circular dots, shows the mean for the right auricle.

III. DISCUSSION

Clinical observations show that the formation of low resistance points on the auricles is correlated with the surface area affected by the gastric ulcer. Experiments carried out on animals have confirmed that artificial gastric ulcer can affect the formation of low resistance points on both auricles of the rabbit, depending on the area affected by the ulceration. For instance, the gastitis mucosa produced by cauterizing the animal's gastric mucosa using 10% carbolic acid, can provoke a large-scale formation of low resistance points on both auricles of the animal in 18 hours. This quick growth is considered the result of the excitation of the receptors in the gastric mucosa and submucosa layers[6–8]. But the problem of what afferent pathways such an excitation affects the auricles through remains to be solved.

It is quite likely that different methods of experimentation will be used for solving this problem, such as the method of excision of the gastric vagus. But according to the data already available and our experimental observations, the excision of vagus nerves leads to such side effects as serious disorder of the digestive functions, hypotonia or atonia of the stomach, meteorismus or loss of appetite, and so on. Such complications constituted new additional factors in the observation of the formation of low resistance points on the auricles, and made the existing conditions more complicated and difficult to analyze. The method of stimulating the vagus nerve by the implantation of electrodes has fundamentally solved a series of such problems. We suppose that if the increase in the low resistance points on the auricles caused by gastric ulcer is the result of excitation of the receptors of the stomach wall through the afferent pathway, then under fairly steady physiological conditions the above-mentioned changes of the increase of low resistance points can be imitated when a stem of the nerves is given a direct, long and uninterrupted stimulation.

Experiments have proved that stimulation of the vagus nerve can achieve excellent results in the formation of low resistance points on the auricles. That is to say, the stimulation of gastric vagus is the main cause of the formation of low resistance points on the auricles. From this it can be deduced that, under pathological conditions, by gastric ulcer, the afferent pathway by which gastric ulcers cause the changes of the low resistance points on the auricles is probably dependent mainly on the vagus nerve. The bases of our conclusion are:

(1) When the stimulation of the vagus nerve is discontinued, the low resistance points on the auricles will stop increasing and then gradually the low resistance points will return to their original number. This furnishes the hint that the focus of gastric ulcer, which stimulates the receptors of the stomach wall constantly, forms a frequently occurring afferent impulse. And such an impulse is the cause of the formation of low resistance points on the auricles.

(2) The repetition of stimulation at the gastric vagus can cause the auricular low resistance points that had already disappeared to reappear (See Fig. 2). When stimulation ends, the auriculor low resistance points will gradually return to their original level. It is quite clear that the excitation of the vagus nerves is of primary importance for the formation and existence of low resistance points on the auricles.

(3) Lastly, the basis on which we consider the vagus nerve as the afferent pathway for the formation of low resistance points on the auricles is the evidence provided by the anatomy of the nerves and the research work on the receptors of the stomach wall. It is proved that the afferent fibers constitute the chief component of the vagus nerve[11–14], and that the various afferent fibers of the receptors located beneath the gastric mucosa and submucosa layers are intermingled within the vagus nerves as well. This naturally provides a firm basis from the anatomical point of view. Finally, our experiments have proved that the stimulation of the sympathetic nerve fibers in the gastric periarterial plexus does not affect the formation of low resistance points on the auricles so distinctly and effectively. The increase of low resistance points observed during the experimentation was only normal. Stimulation of long duration given to the sympathetic nerve fiber does not lead to any distinct increase in low resistance points on the auricles. This is an indirect way of demonstrating the important function of the vagus nerve in increasing low resistance points on the auricle. And then, according to published reports, chronic gastric mucositis can facilitate the formation of low resistance points on the auricles to a great number. As the terminals of the

sympathetic nerves are not in the mucosa and submucosa layers, therefore, it is quite reasonable to believe that they are in no way related to the afferent pathway for the formation of low resistance points on the auricles. Downama (1955) and Shen Eh (1974) regarded the overall reaction brought about by the stimulation of the major splanchnic nerve as a pain response[15,16]. We also noticed that when the stem of the sympathetic nerve was given a strong stimulation, the animal showed in many behaviors of a defensive nature, such as dilation of the pupils of the eyes and other reactions. This seemed to indicate once again that the sympathetic nerve fibers may mainly be the pathway causing visceralgia.

From the above experiment by employing implantation for a long duration, we may entertain the supposition that, under normal physiological conditions, not necessarily pathological, if the stimulation received by the visceral receptors is uninterrupted and with a definite degree of intensity, an increase of the low resistance points on the auricles can also be brought about reflexively through the responsive afferent pathway.

IV. SUMMARY

In concluding this article, we reiterate now its main points.

Two different results were obtained by using the method of long duration implantation of specially constructed microelectrodes to stimulate the ventral branch of the gastric vagus and the gastric periarterial sympathetic plexus uninterruptedly for 12 hours:

1. Following the time of stimulation of the vagus nerves, the low resistance points on both auricles were found to increase gradually, and also drop gradually when stimulation ended. When the vagus nerves were stimulated after the excision of unilateral cervical sympathetic nerve, the formation of low resistance points on the ipsilateral auricle was depressed, while the formation of low resistance points on the other auricle went up as usual. The low resistance points would disappear completely 120 hours after the stimulation ended, but when the ventral branch of the gastric vagus was stimulated again they would reappeared gradually.

2. There was no distinct change on any of the two auricles when the sympathetic nerve in the gastric periarterial plexus was stimulated. According to previous reports, artificial gastric ulcer can cause the formation of low resistance points in great number. The results of the present experiment have shown that, most probably, the afferent pathways that brought about the changes in the auricles are mainly the gastric vagus nerves themselves.

REFERENCES

[1] 南京部队某部«耳针»编写组：耳针，上海人民出版社，第 1 页，1972。

[2] 针刺麻醉编写小组：针刺麻醉，上海人民出版社，第 127 页 1972。

[3] 李肇特等：中华医学杂志，(7)：428，1973。

[4] 中国人民解放军总医院针麻组等单位：全国针麻学习班资料选编之二，人民卫生出版社，第 139 页，1974。

[5] 华东师范大学生物系等单位：针刺麻醉临床和原理研究资料选编，上海人民出版社，第 277 页，1977。

[6] 华东师范大学生物系等单位：针刺麻醉临床和原理研究资料选编，上海人民出版社，第 285 页，1977。

[7] 北京医学院基础部针麻研究形态组：针刺麻醉资料选编，人民出版社，第7页，1974。

[8] 华东师范大学生物系等单位：针刺麻醉临床和原理研究资料选编，上海人民出版社，第293页，1977。

[9] 殷慧镇等：内脏神经慢性埋藏电极的制备，第122页，华东师大学报，1980，第2期。

[10] Bell, G. H. *et al.*: Textbook of Physiology and Biochemistry, 4th ed. E. &S. Livingstone Ltd P. 225, 797–809, 1959.

[11] Hoffman, H. H. *et al.*: . Anat. Rec. **127**:551, 1957.

[12] Sharma, k. N. *et al*: Amer. J. *Physiol.* **202**:725, 1962.

[13] Sharma, K. N. : Handbook of Physiology, Sect. 6, Alimentary Canal. Washington, *Amer. Physiol.* Soc., P. 128, 1967.

[14] Leck, B. F.: Handbook of Sensory Physiology, Vol. 11, 1. Enterreceptors p. 113, Springer-verlag, N. Y., 1972.

[15] Downama C. B. :J. *Neurophysiol.* **18**:217, 1955.

[16] 沈 锷等：中华医学杂志，(54)：628，1974。

MORPHOLOGICAL STUDY OF SENSATIONS PRODUCED BY NEEDLING DIFFERENT POINTS

Pan Chaochong, Zhao Aifeng
(Institute of Acupunctural Anesthesia and Channels, Anhwei College of Traditional Chinese Medicine)

Acupuncture points are a constituent part of the theory of channels and are also the starting point of acupunctural effects. It was pointed out even in ancient times in traditional Chinese medicine that "the key point in acupuncture is that effectiveness is obtained only with the arrival of the vital energy" (Ling Shu: The Twelve Original Points of the Nine Needles). "Cure would be quick, if the arrival of the vital energy is quick, and there would be no cure, if the arrival of the vital energy is delayed" (You Biao Fu), and so forth. Acupuncture anesthesia and clinical treatment in acupuncture show that the effect of treatment is really dependent on needling sensations (sensations of soreness, numbness, distension, heaviness, etc.). For the unraveling of the nature of acupuncture anesthesia, the effectiveness of acupuncture and the nature of acupuncture channels, the work of studying the morphological mechanism of the production of needling sensations must be done. In order to clarify the problem of the morphological mechanism of needling sensations, many laboratories have done a large amount of work on human cadavers to study the anatomical structures according to cross sections or layers as well as histological examinations. They have accumulated a lot of valuable data. But owing to the limited scope of the objects investigated, these data could not reflect directly the nature of needling sensations. They could not show the internal relationship between needling sensations and the structural mechanism which produces the needling sensations. In recent years, different methods for labelling needling reactions have been devised in certain laboratories[1,2]. They investigated the structure-sensation relationship by studying the amputated limbs in certain operations[3]. Therefore, on the basis of our previous work on "Blue Point Method", we summarize further our studies on this site to bring forth the morphological basis for the study of needling sensations and to make some contribution to the early successful explanation of the nature of acupuncture anesthesia and the channels.

***Zusanli, Yanglingquan, Yinlingquan, Shangjuxu, Sanyinjiao, Xuanzhong, Neiguan, Yangchi, Shangqiu, Chongyang, Gongsun, Neiting, Neixiyan, Waixiyan**

I. MATERIAL AND METHOD

The patients' limbs (upper limb 2 cases, lower limb 31 cases, total 33 cases) to be amputated were utilized as the raw material for this study and 14 points* of needling sensation tissue (total 44 point-cases) were sectioned for histological examination. Before operation and anesthesia, the points were located by acupunctural needling sensations and labelled by the "Blue Point Method" devised by us. The detail of the method is as follows:

1. Generation of needling sensation. Before operation and anesthesia, needling was applied acupuncturally to the patient's limb to be amputated in order to locate the point of needling sensation tissue. A home-made concentric electrode (the stylet made of stainless steel wire with insulation coating could be freely taken out from and inserted into the trocar) was used instead of an acupuncture needle. By the acupuncture method this electrode was applied slowly with no twisting, no raising or inserting to avoid distorting nearby tissue till a needling sensation of soreness, numbness, distension or other was felt by the patient. Then the concentric electrode was held in situ.

2. Free ferric ion. The stylet of this electrode was connected to the anode and the trocar to the cathode of a 6-V battery. The switch was turned on and the current was adjusted to 30–50 μA for 30–60 seconds. Electrolysis occurred at the stylet with free ferric ion deposited in the tissue around the tip of the needle.

3. Prussian Blue Formation. After withdrawing the stylet from the trocar, sterilized 0.3% potassium ferrocyanide solution in saline 0.25 ml was injected into the tissue of sensation point so as to complete the Prussian Blue reaction. The sensation generation site was thus stained blue. After amputation a 1.2 mm thick of the blue-stained tissue of the amputated limb was excised immediately and fixed in glacial acetic acid-alcohol (glacial acetic acid 2 ml and 80% alcohol 98 ml). The tissue was impregnated with silver by the Cajal-Faworsky method and was embedded in paraffin; 15 μ thick sections were cut continously for 80 sections. Notes were taken on the sensation and the needling depth in detail.

Examinations were made on alternate tissue sections. Suggesting the circular area covered by the blue point as the center, within a radius of 1.8 mm it was observed as the main site for the sensation structure study, together with the nearby surrounding peripheral area (maximum radius less than 5 mm). The nearby structure area was considered to be involved in the needling sensation caused by raising, inserting and other acupuncture manipulations. Therefore all the observed receptors were noted and tabulated for examination supplement and reference.

II. RESULTS

44 points of needling sensation were observed. There were 11 different kinds of sensations such as soreness, numbness, distension, no-feeling and others (Table 1). The sensation points are located in muscles (Fig. 1), intermuscular connective tissues, tendons (Fig. 2), periosteum, synovial capsules, connective tissue inside the synovial capsules (Fig. 3), and the subcutaneous connective tissues. Prussian Blue was deposited on various fine structures. These fine structures existing in all were the blood vessels, nerve trunks and

Table1.

Points		Needling Sensations							
Name	Cases	Soreness	Numbness	Distension	Tingling	Soreness & Distension	Soreness & Numbness	Soreness & Tingling	Numbness & Distension
Zusali	10	3				3			1
Yanglingquan	2		1						
Yinlingquan	2					1			
Shangjuxu	5					1		1	
Sanyinjiao	6		1				2		
Xuanzhong	5	1			1		1	1	1
Neiguan	1					1			
Yangchi	1			1					
Shangqiu	1				1				
Chongyang	1	1							
Gongsun	6	1			1	1		1	
Neiying	2	1					1		
Neixiyan	1	1							
Waixiyan	1		1						
Total	44	13	1	6	3	7	2	5	2
	100%	29.5%	2.3%	13.4%	6.8%	15.9%	4.5%	11.3%	4.5%

Continued 1

Name	Distension & Tingling	Soreness Distension & Tingling	No Sansation	Accompanied with Propagated Sensation	Needling Depth: Depth (cm)	Needling Depth: Mean value (cm)	muscle	Inter muscular C.T.
Zusali				1	0.5–2.0	1.50	5	5
Yanglingquan	1				1.2–1.6	1.40	1	1
Yinlingquan	1			1	1.3–1.4	1.35	1	
Shangjuxu				1	1.9–3.2	2.28	3	2
Sanyinjiao				2	1.1–2.7	1.75	4	2
Xuanzhong	1				1.3–2.7	2.20	5	
Neiguan							1	
Yangchi								
Shangqiu					0.50	0.50		
Chongyang					0.70	0.70	1	
Gongsun	1		1	1	0.7–1.6	1.26	3	
Neiying					0.4–0.8	0.60		
Neixiyan					1.60	1.60		
Waixiyan					0.70	0.70		
Total	3	1	1	6			24	10
	4.5%	6.8%	2.3%	2.3%	13.4%			

Continued 2

Name	Hlue Point Area General Structure Tendon	Periosteum	Synovial Capsule	C.T. inside the Synovial Capsule	Subcutaneous C.T.	Blood vessele	Nerve	Free Nerve ending	Muscular spindle
Zusali						10	10	7	2
Yanglingquan						2	2	1	1
Yinlingquan	1					2	2		1
Shangjuxu						5	5	3	1
Sanyinjiao						6	6	3	4
Xuanzhong						5	5	4	1
Neiguan						1	1	1	
Yangchi	1					1	1	1	
Shangqiu					1	1	1		
Chongyang						1	1	1	
Gongsun		1			2	5	5	3	2
Neiying		1			1	2	2	1	
Neixiyan				1		1	1	1	
Waixiyan			1			1	1		
Total	2	2	1	1	4	43	43	26	12

Continued 3

Name	Receptors ofthe blue point peripheral area							
	Tendon spindle	Lamellar corpus-cle	Krause's bulbous corpusoles	Free nerve ending	Muscular spindle	Tendon spindle	Lamellar corpus-cles	Krause's bulbous corpuscles
Zusali			1	7	3	1	1	1
Yanglingquan				1	1			
Yinlingquan				1	2			
Shangjuxu		1		5	4	2		
Sanyinjiao			1	4	3		1	
Xuanzhong				4				
Neiguan	1			1				
Yangchi							1	
Shangqiu							1	
Chongyang				1	1	1		
Gongsun		2		5	4		2	
Neiying			1	1				1
Neixiyan				1				
Waixiyan								
Total	1	3	3	31	22	4	5	2

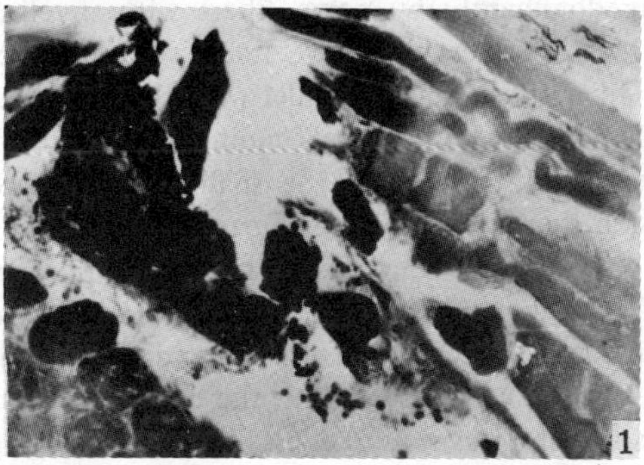

Fig. 1 Chongyang, Soreness, Showing the Blue Point located in the Muscle Tissues. (× 100)

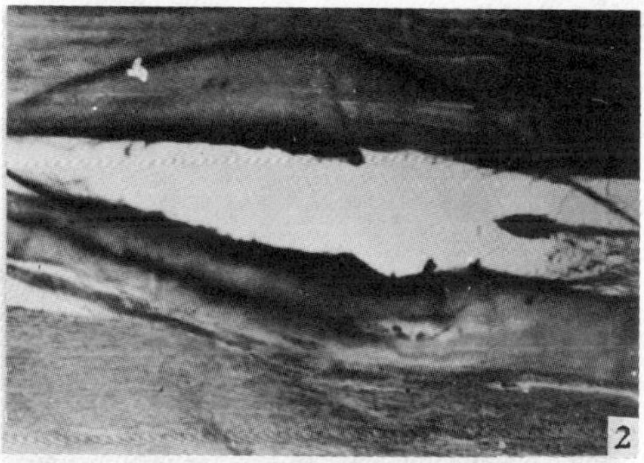

Fig. 2 Yangchi, Distension, Showing The Blue Point located in the Tendon. (× 40)

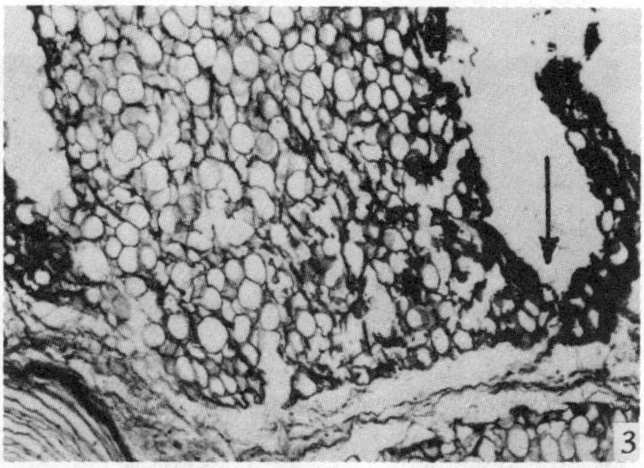

Fig. 3 Gongsun, Tingling, Showing The Blue Point located in the Subcutaneous Tissues. (× 40)

Some of the sensation points were mainly occupied by nerve trunks without myelin, while others points predominantly by nerve fibers with myelin (diameter of the latter ranged from 2.5 to 14 μ). Besides, the nerve tracts without myelin were also seen in the points. Some of these fiber tracts ran in parallel with the blood vessels, and some ramified into branches alongside with the blood vessels ending finally into the blood vessel walls. The observed sensory receptors distributed in the shallow layer were the free nerve endings principally. In hairy skin there were usually no capsule receptors, but corpuscles of Vater-Pacini were found in one case. In deep tissue there were free nerve endings (Figs. 4–6), muscle spindles (Fig. 7), tendon spindles (Fig. 8), corpuscles of Vater-Pacini, and end bulbs of Krause and synovial capsule recepters (free nerve endings). Taking sensation point-case as the standard unit for qualitative measurement, the point-case counting was made. In each pointcase the same structure was counted as one unit, no matter how many times it appeared.

Besides, the following 3 kinds of nerve apparatus were found.

1. Free nerve endings beside the blood vessels. They are located at the arteriole turning into capillary vessels and distributed between the blood vessels (Fig. 9).

2. Capsule receptors beside the blood vessels. They occurred in the vicinity of the arteriole, such as Krause's end bulbs type capsule sensory receptors (Fig. 10).

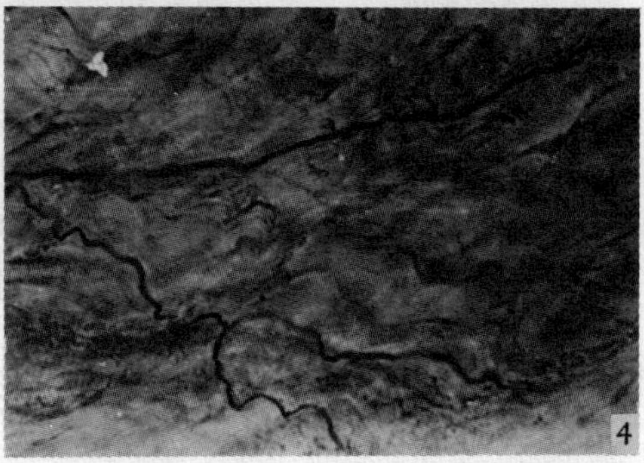

Fig. 4 Chongyang, Soreness, Showing Free Nerve Endings. (× 400)

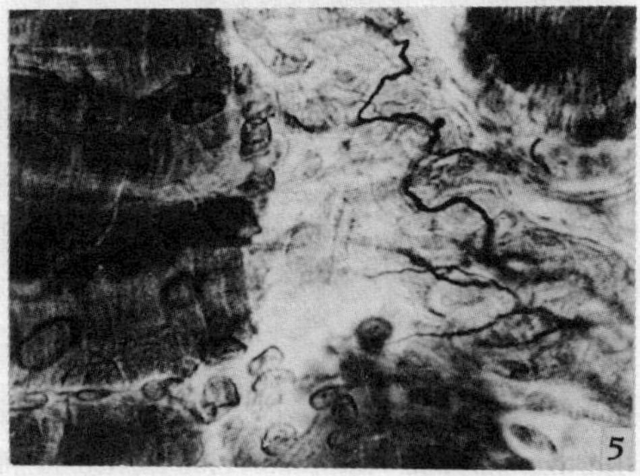

Fig. 5 Gongsun, Tingling, Showing Free Nerve Endings. (× 400)

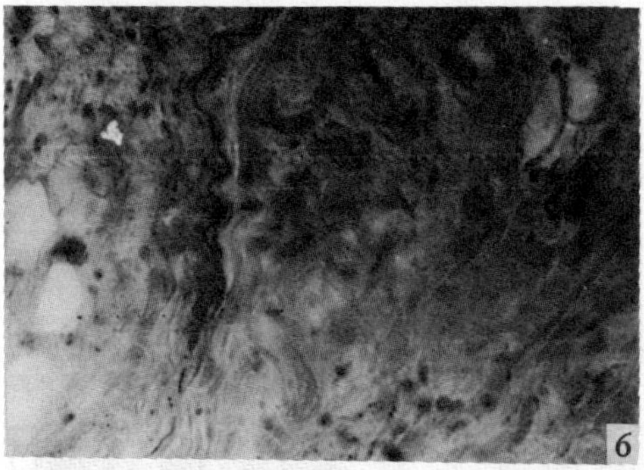
Fig. 6 Neixiyan, Soreness, Showing Free Nerve Endings. (× 400)

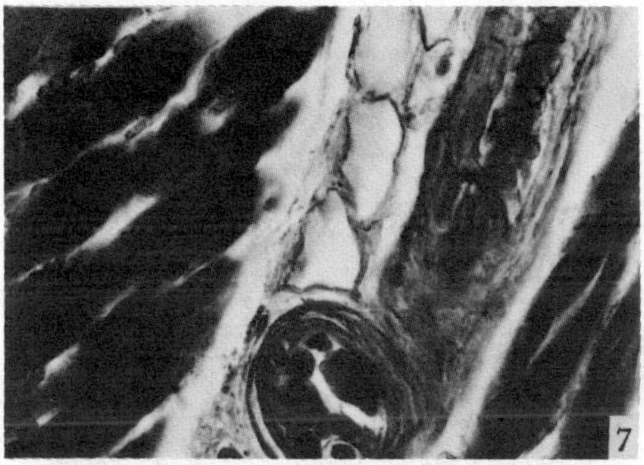
Fig. 7 Sanyinjiao, Sore and Tingling, Showing Muscular Spindle. (× 400)

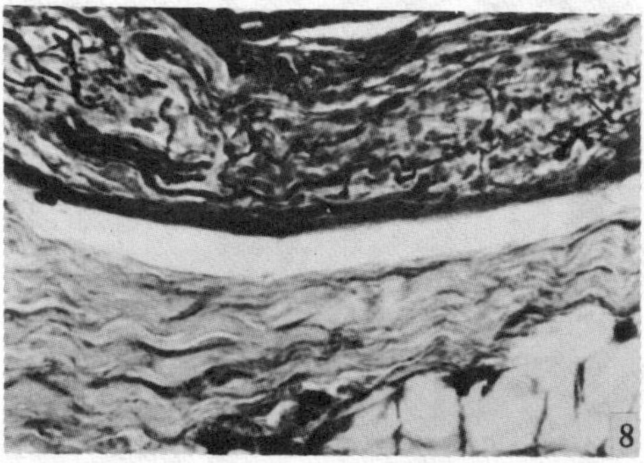
Fig. 8 Zisanli, Distension, Showing Tendon Spindle. (× 200)

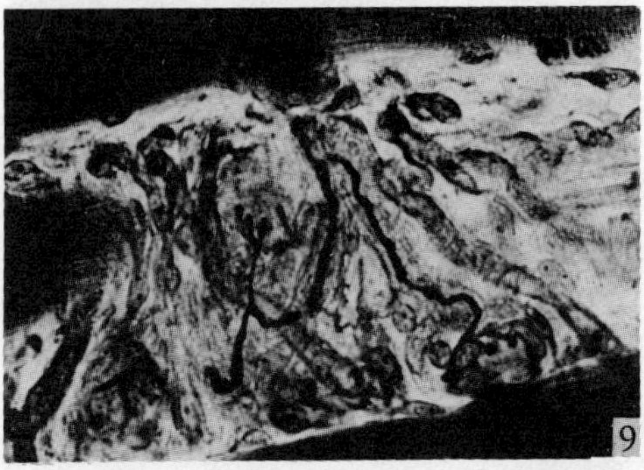

Fig. 9 Xuanzhong, Soreness and Numbness, Showing Free Nerve Endings beside Blood Vessels. (× 400)

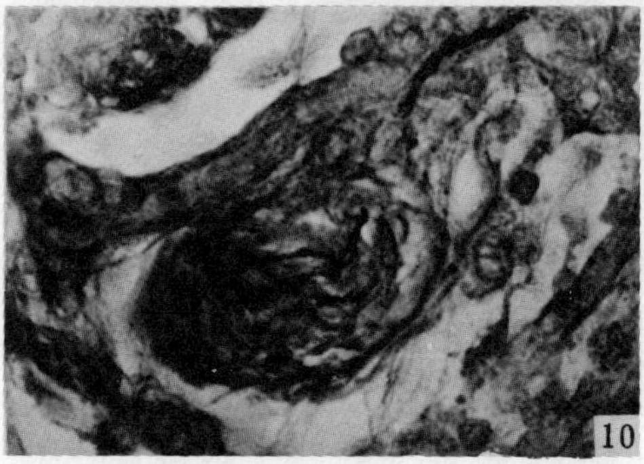

Fig. 10 Zusanli, Soreness, Showing Capsule Receptors beside Blood Vessels. (× 400)

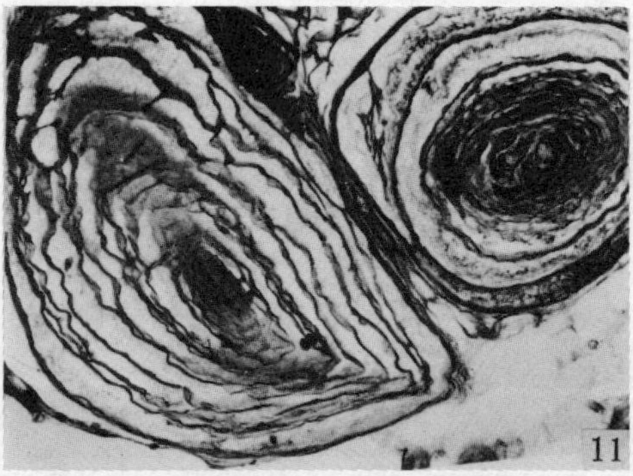

Fig. 11 Gongsun, Soreness and Tingling, Showing a Varied corpsule of Vater-Pacini. (× 100)

3. Varied corpuscles of Vater-Pacini. They are located in the intermuscular connective tissues and had lamellar structure. There were two forms of nerve apparatus (Fig. 11): one was formed by numerous fibers arranged in parallel, the other looked like tree-branches.

III. DISCUSSION

Concerning the locations of the needling sensation points of the human body and their morphological basis, the authors observed in 1974 in themselves bodily and in some channel sensitive people the needling sensation and the propagated sensation phenomenon by needle stimulation in layer-wise way. The authors discovered that the needling sensation and the propagated sensation are mainly generated in the deep layer tissues. Meanwhile many laboratories had also shown that the needling sensations are generated mostly in deep layer tissues in different ways[5–9]. The "Dual Structure Theory of Needling Sensation Receptors" was thus proposed[10]. But there are still many other explanations. Shanghai Institute of Traditional Chinese Medicine proposed that the blood vessel walls and their nerve apparatuses might effect the needling sensation. The nerve impulses from the nerve trunks and branches of the acupuncture points were coded into different forms conducted to the higher centers. These might be the cause of the needling sensations[11].

The Zoology Institute clainned that, excluding those free nerve endings, no other general "needling sensation receptors" ubiquitously distributed were found[12]. The following are the authors' conclusions based upon their observations on 44 point-cases of the 14 acupuncture points.

1. The Generation Sites of Needling Sensation

The needling sensations of the 14 points selected (stated in Table 1) are soreness, numbness, distension, tingling (disregarding the tingling caused by needle application on the surface of the skin), soreness and numbness, soreness and distension, soreness and tingling, distension and numbness, distension and tingling, soreness-distension-tingling, and no-feeling (Table 1). The majority of these are local sensations; the minority of them are accompanied with short distance propagated sensation (13.4%), a few of which arrived far beyond a bone joint. The depth of the point sensation tissue varied from 0.4 cm to 3.2 cm from the skin surface. The mean depth was 1.32 cm. There seemed to have some relation between the tissue depth of needling sensation and the location of the needling point: In the muscle-rich positions (Group 1 points in Table 2), the needling sensation points are deeper, while the needling points at the distal part of the extremities or near the joints (Group 2 points in Table 2) are more shallow. Based on the naked eye examination during sampling and depth measurements, all the needling sensation points of Group 1 are in the deep layer tissue, and one third of that of Group 2 are in the subcutaneous connective tissues.

According to the 44 blue-stained points, the points were found located in muscles, tendons, intermuscular connective tissues, periosteum, synovial capsules, connective tissue inside the synovial capsules and subcutaneous connective tissues (Table 2). From Table 2, it is apparent that the needling sensation may be generated by various tissues lying between the

Table 2. The Relationship between needling sensations and general structures

Groups	Needling Sensation / General Structure	Soreness	Numbness	Distension	Tingling	Sore Dis-tension	Sore Numbness	Sore Tingling	Numbness Distension	Distension Tingling	Sore Dis-Tension tingling	No Sensation	Total
Group 1 Points	Muscle	9		1	1	3	1	2	1	2			20
	Intermuscular C. T.			4		2		2	1		1		10
	Tendon					1							1
	Periosteum												
	Synovial capsule												
	C. T. inside the Synovial capsule						T.						
	Subcutaneous C. T.												
Group 2 Points	Muscle	1				1				1		1	4
	Intermuscular C. T.												
	Tendon			1									1
	Periosteum	1					1						2
	Synovial Capsule		1										1
	C.T. inside the Synovial capsule	1											1
	Subcutaneous C. T.	1			2			1					4

footnotes: Group 1 Points, total 31 point-cases, included Zusanli, Yanglingquan, Yinlingquan, Shangjuxu, Sanyinjiao, Xuanzhong, and Neiguan, etc.
Group 2 Points, total 13 point-cases, included Yangchi, Shangqiu, Chongyang, Gongsun, Neiting, Neixiyan, Waixiyan, etc.

skin and the periosteum. This indicates that these various tissues mentioned above exist the material basis for needling sensation (to be discussed in the following paragraph). But the blue-stained structures are mainly the deep layer tissues (approximately 91% of the total). This is in good agreement with the naked eye observation during the sampling. Therfore, the needling sensation seems to be generated in the deep layer tissues.

2. The Relationship between the Needling Sensation, the Nerve Trunks (or Branches) and the Blood Vessels

The needling sensation is also called "Needling Reaction". It is the content of the channels and collaterals theory. According to this theory, the channels have trunk routes and branches. They correlate with the viscerae internally and are distributed externally over the five organs, seven apertures*, four limbs and one hundred bones. They form the network in the whole body that carries the vital energy and the blood to the circulating inside of the body and to its skin by circulation. Therefore viewed as a whole this theory covers all the functions of the nerve and the circulation systems of modern medicine.

It has already been well-established and recognized in modern medicine that the nerve trunks and branches receive the various stimulations, conduct the nerve impulses to the higher centers and initiate the corresponding sensations. Thus it seems reasonable to suggest that the nerve trunks and their branches may initiate the needling sensation during needling. But whether it is the blood vessels (mainly the nerve apparatus of the blood vessel wall) that generate the needling sensation during needling is still an unsolved problem with controversy. T. A. Триторьва in her book "The Innervation of the Blood Vessels", pointed out that all the sensory apparatuses originate from the brain, the vertebral nerve ganglions or the neuron dendrites of the autonomic system distributed inside and outside the blood vessels, and the sensory nerve fibers in the blood vessels are not segmentarily distributed. The sensory nerve fibers of the blood vessels travel with the centripetal dendrites of the brain and the vetebral ganglions into the spinal cord and the brain stem. The nerve impulses from the blood vessels arrive at the cerebral cortex[13]. Therefore, theoretically speaking, the blood vessels may take part in the sequence events of the needling reaction process, and also may constitute the structural basis for the needling sensation.

The authors observed that on the walls of the blood vessels there are densely distributed free nerve endings (Fig. 16). At the sites of the arteriole branches there are free nerve endings (Fig. 9) and capsule sensory receptors (Fig. 10) beside the blood vessels. The non-myelinated nerve fiber bundles travel along and in company with the blood vessel walls. The blood vessel walls and the nerve trunks are directly blue-stained (Fig. 12, 13). From Tables 1 and 3, it is apparent that the blood vessels and the nerve trunks or branches are distributed widely over the various structures of all the needling sensation points both in Group 1 and Group 2. Their presence percentage is 100%. The results of the Table 4 and Graph 1 imply that in the 24 blue-stained needling sensation points in muscles, the presence rate of blood vessels and nerve trunks or branches are consistently in parallel with that of the needling sensation. On the basis of these results, the authors consider that the structures of the blood vessels and the nerve trunks or branches are closely related with the generation of needling

---

*The two eyes, the two nostrils, the mouth and the two ears.

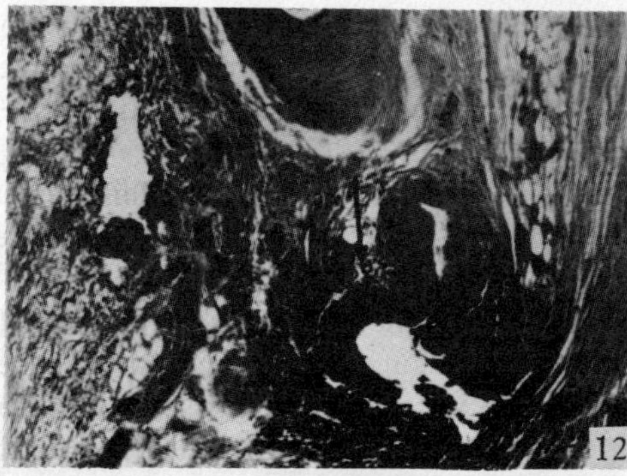

Fig. 12 Sanyinjiao, Sore and Tingling, Showing the Blue Point Located in the Wall of Blood vessels. (× 40)

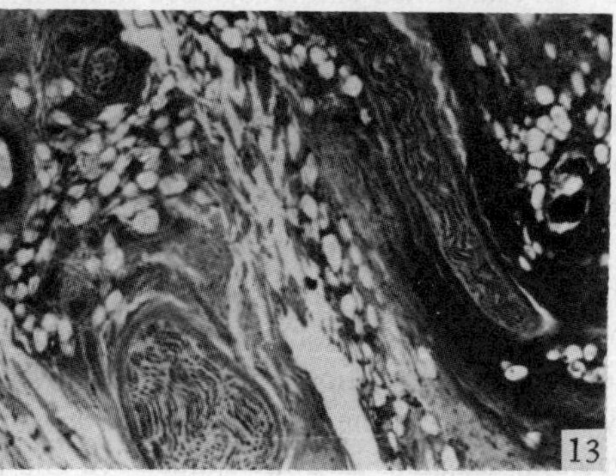

Fig. 13 Gongsun, Tingling, Showing the Blue Point Located in the Nerve Trunk. (× 40)

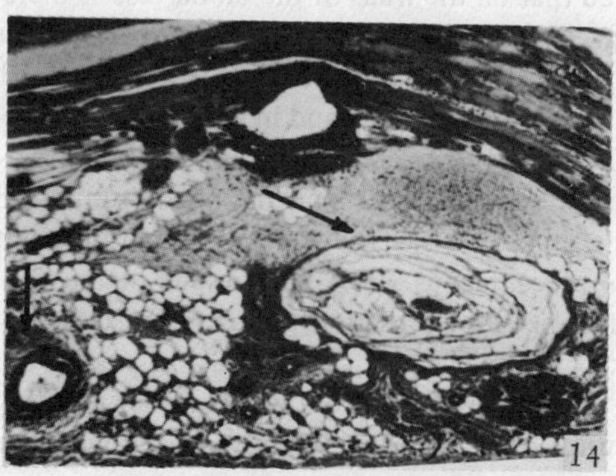

Fig. 14 Gongsun, No-Senation, Showing Blood Vessel (↓), Muscular Spindle (↘) Apparent Pathological Changes. (× 40)

Table 3. The Relationship Between Needlir g Sensations and Fine Structures

Groups	Needling Sensation / Fine Structure	Soreness	Numbness	Distension	Tingling	Sore-distension	Sore Numbness	Sore Tingling	Numbness Distension	Distension Tingling	Sore Dis-Tension Tingling	No-Sensation	Total
Group 1 Points	Blood Vessel	9		5	1	6	1	4	2	2	1		31 100%
	Nerve	9		5	1	6	1	4	2	2	1		31 100%
	Free Nerve Ending	6		2		4	1	3	2	1	1		20 64.5%
	Muscular Spindle	3		1				1		2	1		8 25.8%
	Tendon Spindle				1	1							2 6.4%
	Lamellar Corpuscles							1					1 3.2%
	Krauses Bulbous Corpuscles			1				1					2 6.4%
Group 2 Points	Blood Vessel	3	1	1	2	1	1	1		1		1	12 100%
	Nerve	3	1	1	2	1	1	1		1		1	12 100%
	Free Nerve Ending	2		1		1	1			1		1	7 60%
	Muscular Spindle					1						1	2 16.6%
	Tendon Spindle												
	Lamellar Corpuscles				1			1					2 16.6%
	Krause's Bulbous Corpuscles						1						1 8.3%

footnotes: In Group 2 Gong Sun point was blue – stained too dark to see the fine structure. This Point was not taken into account.

Table 4. The Needling Sensations and the Structure of the 24 Point Cases Located in the Muscles by Blue Point Method

Needling Sensation / Structure	Soreness	distension	Tingling	Sore Distension	Sore numb-	Sore Tingling	Distension numbness	Distension Tingling	No Sensation	Total
	10	1	1	4	1	2	1	3	1	24
Blood vessel	10 41.6	1 4.2	1 4.2	4 16.8	1 4.2	2 8.3	1 4.2	3 12.5	1 4.2	24 100%
nerve	10 41.6	1 4.2	1 4.2	4 16.8	1 4.2	2 8.3	1 4.2	3 12.5	1 4.2	24 100%
Free nerve ending	7 29.2			3 12.5	1 4.2	2 8.3	1 4.2	2 8.3	1 4.2	17 70.9%
Muscular spindle	3 12.5			2 8.3		1 4.2		2 8.3	2 4.2	9 37.5%
Tendon Spindle			1 4.2							1 4.2%
Lamellar corpuscles										
Kranse's bulbous corpuscles						1 4.2				1 4.2%

sensation. They seem to be the material basis of the needling sensation (Tables 3 & 4, Graph 1).

3. The Relation Between the Needling Sensation and the Sensory Receptors

Taking the blood vessels and the nerve trunks or branches as the morphological basis of needling sensation, the sensory receptors must have something to do in it. If there are not numerous sensory receptors of various types widely distributed everywhere in the whole body, the regulatory and certain other functions of the whole body could not be accomplished. Therefore, the sensory receptors are essential for the needling sensation generation and render active contribution to the point specificity.

At the location sites of acupuncture points, there are muscle spindles, tendon spindles, Vater-Pacini corpuscles, synovial capsule receptors (including the free nerve endings, Ruffini endings, Golgi endings) in the deep layer besides the ubiquitous existence of free nerve endings. In the shallow layer of unhaired skin are located the Meissner's corpuscles, Vater-Pacini corpuscles, Krause's end bulbs, Ruffini endings. In the haired skin there are the hair follicle receptors. All of these have been well-documented in histology[14–17]. The authors observed that the Krause's end bulb could only be seen in the deep layer and in the haired skin the Vater-Pacini corpuscles were seen in one specimen. The free nerve endings exhibit a wide variety of morphological forms in different sites (Figs. 4–6). But what role do these sensory receptors play in the needling sensation generation? Table 3 shows that among the sensory receptors the free nerve endings are the most abundant and are most widely distributed. Though the factors of staining, sectioning and counting made the number of free nerve endings appear much smaller than it actually was, the percentage of their existence in both Groups 1 and 2 was over 60%. Table 4 and Graph 1 indicate that in the 24 needling point-cases free nerve endings seem to coexist with needling sensations. It should be pointed out that the number of free nerve endings in the blood vessel walls are not counted in the tables and the graphs. If they are also taken into account, the existence percentage of free nerve endings would be 100%. In the process of blue-staining, the authors noted that during acupuncturing of the limbs, the first needling sensation was felt. At the time of electrolysis and the Prussian Blue formation a second, and even a third, needling sensation same as the first one was felt by the patient. This fact shows that the blue-stained points are the actual site producing needling sensation. At the same time this shows that the needling sensation tissues react to the mechanical, electric, and chemical stimulants. From the reactive function mentioned above it is reasonable to assume that the receptors receiving the needling might be these free nerve endings. Now the problem turns to the question of what part the muscle spindles act in the generation of needling sensation. Based on our observations, in the muscle-rich points the muscle spindle is also frequently the receptor present. Their presence rate is only lower than that of free nerve endings (Tables 3, 4). Basically there is a near paralellism between the needling sensation and the muscle spindle structure (Graph 1). So in the muscle-rich points the muscle spindle may play a certain role in the needling sensation generation. Limited by their distribution, the muscle spindles could not be considered as the structural basis of needling sensation in tissues other than muscles. The tendon spindles, Vater-Pacini corpuscles, Krause end bulbs and the others were seldom observed in this study.

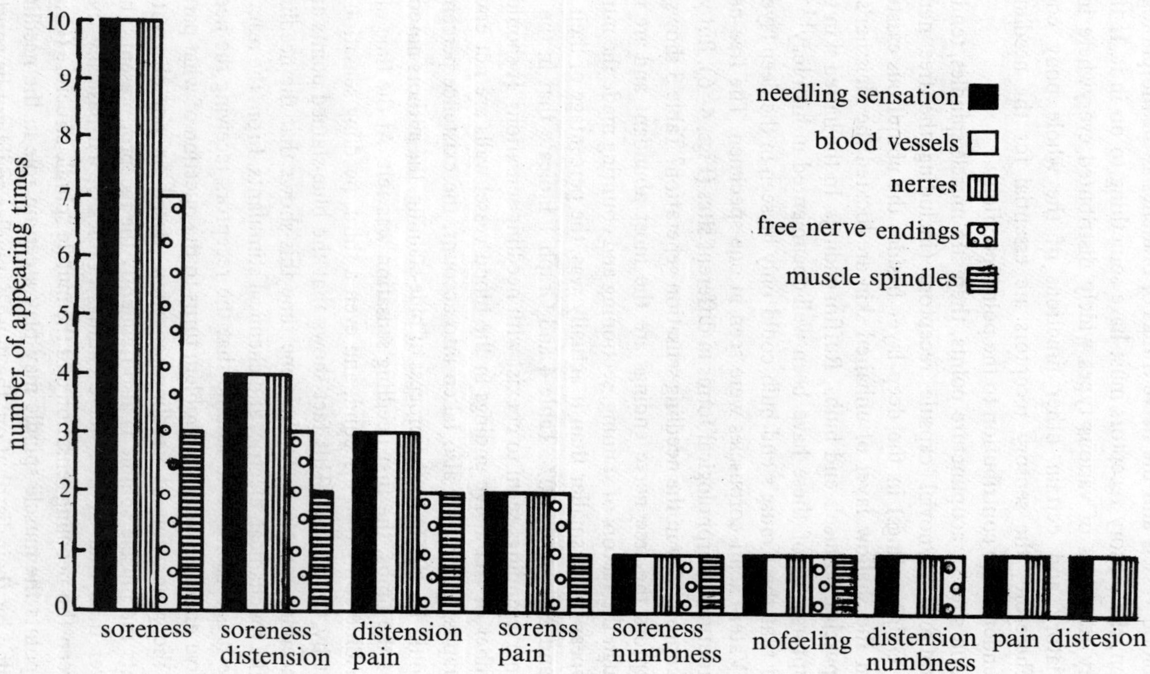

Graph 1. The Needling Sensation, The Bood Vessels and The Sensory Receptors.

They may be the morphological basis of needling sensation in certain points like the muscle spindles. For example, in the point Gongsun there are many Vater-Pacini corpuscles in the vicinity of the blue-stained point, and they are believed to probably take some part in the needling sensation. The authors also investigated the relationship between needling sensation and structure in two pathological cases. In one case the patient had no needling sensation during needling, but he felt a slight distension on needle twisting, raising and insertion. In histological examination of the tissue sections, pathological changes were clearly observed in the blood vessels, nerves, free nerve endings, and muscle spindles (Fig. 14). The muscle tissue was damaged slightly, and the connective tissue was proliferated. In the other case, good needling sensation was felt (distension). Under the microscope, there were no apparent pathological changes in the blood vessels, nerves and nerve endings, but the muscle tissues were almost completely displaced by the connective tissues, leaving only a trace of muscle tissues (Figs. 15, 16). These pathological findings imply that muscles and connective tissues are not the morphological basis of needling sensation, while the blood vessels, nerves and free nerve endings apparatus are.

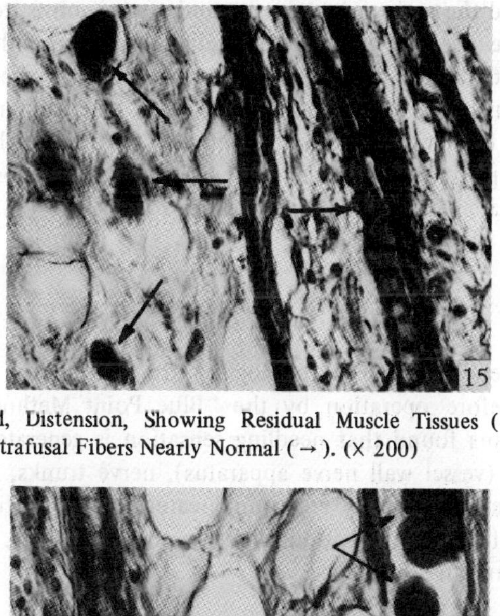

Fig. 15 Zusanli, Distension, Showing Residual Muscle Tissues (⇄), The Nerve apparatus of Intrafusal Fibers Nearly Normal (→). (× 200)

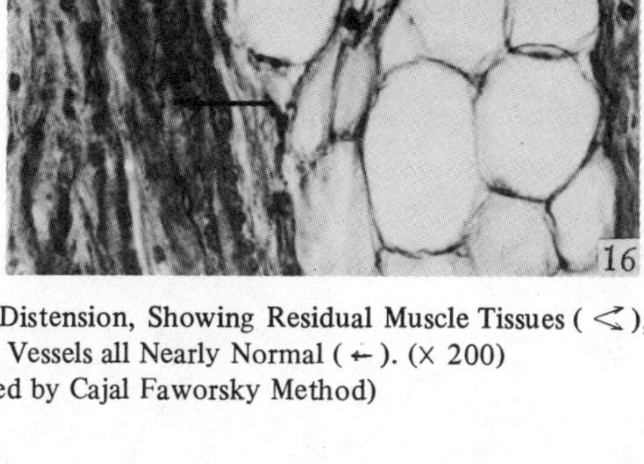

Fig. 16 Zusanli, Distension, Showing Residual Muscle Tissues (<), The Free Nerve Endings of Blood Vessels all Nearly Normal (←). (× 200)
(Fig. 1–16. stained by Cajal Faworsky Method)

4. Morphological Comparison Between Points With Propagated Sensation (P.S.) And Points Without P.S.

In this study, there were six patients who felt the needling sensation running back and forth for a certain distance, and even running beyond a joint. In order to investigate the difference between the points with P.S. and those without P.S., two control groups were formed: Group A with the same needling sensation, Group B with the same acupuncture points. The points were randomized. By our preliminary results, the structures shared by both groups are blood vessels, nerve trunks or branches and free nerve endings. No essential difference was found between them. Therefore it is believed that in ordinary people (excluding the channels-sensitive people) the P.S. generation may be related with needling manipulation, stimulation strength and the individuality of each patient.

Summing up the relationship between the distribution, quantity, presence rate of blood vessels (the nerve apparatus of the blood vessel wall), nerve trunks, nerve branches, free nerve endings and the main receptors situated at the points, together with the nearby sensory receptors, the needling sensation, together with the pathological considerations, the authors propose that these things constitute the morphological basis of the needling sensation. It is evident that owing to the limitation of the number of patients and the methods adopted in this study, the incompleteness of this conclusion is inevitable. The problems concerning point specificity and the role played by blood vessels and the nerve systems in acupunctural anesthesia still need further study.

IV. SUMMARY

This paper is a report on the morphological structures of the 44 points with needling sensations labelled before operation by the "Blue Point Method", in the limbs to be amputated. The authors found that needling sensation is generated mostly in deep layer tissues. Blood vessels (vessel wall nerve apparatus), nerve trunks, nerve branches, the free nerve endings, and the main sensory receptors located at acupuncture points constitute the morphological basis of needling sensation. Between points with P.S. and points without P.S., there is no essential structure difference.

REFERENCES

[1] Morphology Group, Schanghai Institute of Traditional Chinese Medicine: Histological Observations on Locations of Points "With Needling Sensation." *New Medicine*: **4**: 32–34, 1975.

[2] Sian College of Medicine, et al: Morphological Observations on Points with Needling Sensation. Acupuncture Anaesthesia Theory and Channels Research Data. p. 18–21, Anhwei College of Traditional Chinese Medicine (Ed.), 1976.

[3] Acupuncture Anaesthesia Group 1, Shanghai Institute of Traditional Chinese Medicine, et al: Morphological Observations on Point with Needling Sensation. Science Research Data, p. 1–4, Shanghai College of Traditional Chinese Medicine, Shanghai Institute of Traditional Chinese Medicine (Ed.), 1977.

[4] Acupuncture Anaesthesis and Channels Research Room, Anhwei College of Traditional Chinese Medicine: Modification of the Blue Point Method for the localization of Points with Needling Sensation. Acupuncture Anaesthesia Theory and Channels Research Data. p. 23–25, Anhwei College of Trnditional Chinese Medicine (Ed.), 1976.

[5] Acupuncture Anaesthesia Group, Department of Physiology, Chongqing College of Medicine: Preliminary Analysis of the Relationship between Needling Sensation and Nerve Systems. Reprint 1974.

[6] Jiang Zhen-yu et al.: The Peripheral Conduction Pathway Analysis Concerning Needling Abalgesia. *Scientia Sinica* **(2)** 157–161, 1973.

[7] Wei Ran-yu et al.: Observations of the Afferent Discharging by the certain deep Receptors during hindlimbs Needling of the Cats. *Kexue Tongbao* **(4)** 184–186 1974.

[8] Acupuncture Anaesthesia Group, Shanghai Institute of Physiology: The Electro-Myogram Activities during the needling locations "Point Reaction". *Chinese Medicine Journal* **(10)** 532–535, 1973

[9] The Basic Theory Research Group on Acupuncture Anaesthesia, Sian College of Medicine: The morphological Studies Concerning the Point Receptors at "He Gu" Point Area. *New Medicine of Shansi:* Nos. 1, 2 bound, 17–22, 1973

[10] Indem: The morphological Studies Concerning the Point Receptors at "HeGu" Point Area — On the Histological Structure of tye Needling Sensation Receptors. ibid. (5) 43–47, 1973

[11] Physiology Group, Shanghai Institute of Traditional Chinese Medicine: "Zusanli" — The Blood Vessel Factor in the Intestinal Peristalysis. *New Medicine Journal:* **(7)** 28, 1975

[12] Zoology Institute of the Chinese Science Academy: Observations on The Receptors of Acupuncture Point, Research on the Acupuncture Anaesthesis theory, p. 64 The Peoples' Health Publication, Beijing, 1974

[13] Риторьева Т. А.: Иннервация Кровеносных сосудов Медгиз, 1954 "血管的神经支配",王凤兰等译 226 页,科学出版社,北京, 1954。

[14] Bloom W. & Fawcett DW.: ATextbook of Histology, 10th. Ed. 362–365, W.B. Saunders Company Philadelphia, London, Toronto, 1975

[15] Rhodin JAG: Histology, A Text and Atlas, p. 294–305, Oxford University Press. New York, 1974

[16] Stacey M.J.: Free Eerve Endings in Skeletal Muscle of the Cat, *J. Anat.* **105**: 231–254, 1969

[17] Gardner E.: Nerves and Nerve Endings in Joints and Associated Structures of Monkey

RELATIVE REGULARITY BETWEEN JINGLUO POINTS AND SPINAL SEGMENTAL INNERVATION

Yang Feng, Ren Shizhen
(China Medical College)

In bringing to light the essential basis of Jingluo points, a variety of morphological methods have been employed by us, but so far we have neither found any specific structure in and round the Jingluo points, nor have we even noted any special tissues other than nerves and vessels along the Jingluo lines. As seen in the complete map of the Jingluo points, their distribution is characteristic. In the trunk, the distance between any two adjacent points whether in the upper or in the lower region is all the same and they are evenly spaced and symmetrically arranged[1] (Fig. 1). But in the limbs (also in the head and on the face), they are placed at irregular distances. Why is this so and how do we explain this phenomenon?

We believe that this has something to do with the segmental innervation. For in human beings as well as in vertebrates, there are segmental bony axle and symmetrical structures on both sides (Fig. 2). In the early stage of the embryonic period, the nerve segment sends out pairs of spinal nerves to either side to reach the trunk[2] (skin, muscle and bones).

A sketch copied from our anatomical specimen shows the parallelism of the nerve distribution on the ventral side of the trunk with the arrangement of the Jingluo points (Fig. 3).

The specimen was made in the following way: Points were selected on the skin surface of the trunk; needles were then inserted into the points and left there; then the whole chest and ventral wall was cut down and turned over. The nerve branches on the wall were dissected from the deep to the shallow surfaces and their relationship with the points was examined.

The result obtained shows that the points are located just where the nerves end and their arrangement coincides with the nerve distribution[3]

1. The points are equally, evenly and symmetrically distributed, identical to the regular arrangement of the nerve branches[4].

2. The points on both sides are all located between the neighbouring upper and lower nerve branches with smaller branches ending at the neighborhood of the points. The points on the midline are more typical[5] (Fig. 3a).

3. The subcutaneous nervous branches of the abdominal wall are shorter than those of the chest wall, and the Jingluo points on the former are arranged nearer to the midline than those of the latter. After repeated examination and comparison we got the impression that the above fact shows Jingluo points tend to function at the terminal ends of the nerves. This phenomenon is due to the fact that the horizontal width of the thorax, after the human

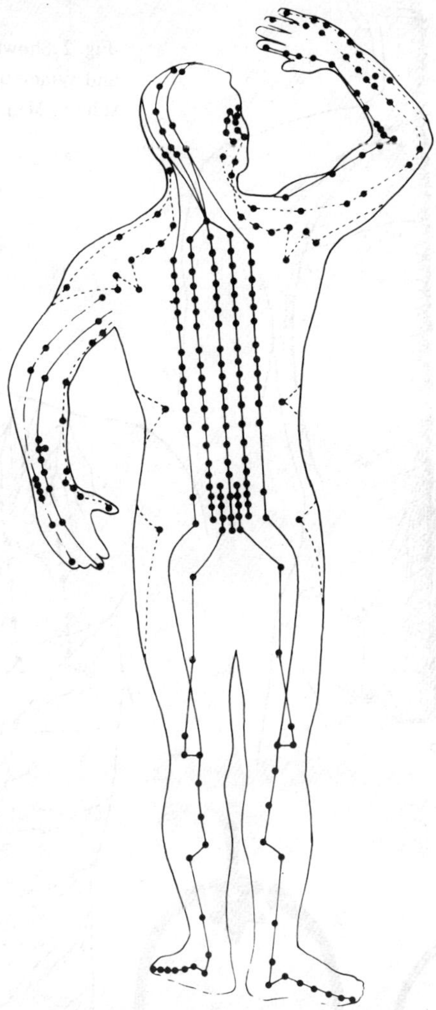

Fig. 1 The Panorama of the distribution of Jinlo Points.
in trunk: the Points are evenly arranged.
in limbs: the Points are irregular intervals.

body became erect during evolution, was widened (as compared with other mammalians[5] and the nerve branches in that part then spread out laterally. The above observation proves that the points on the trunk are all coincident with the segmental innervation. But it is different in the limbs; as a result of the development of its buds (Fig. 4) and the shift of the myotomes (Fig. 4), the nerve trunks are rearranged into nerve plexuses (Fig. 5), such as brachial plexus[7,8]. And these make up the ulnar nerve, radial nerve, median nerve[6], etc. We cannot say surely that there is any definite relationship between these nerves and the points merely on the basis of their innervation. Since they have lost the regularity of the segmental nature, we are not going carry out our investigations along this line.

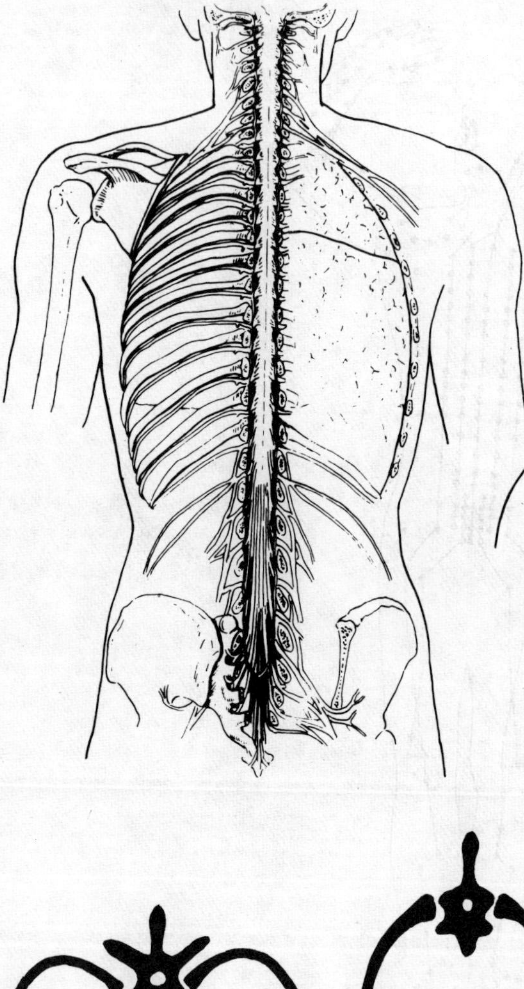

Fig. 2 Showing the segmental axle and symmetrical structures on both sides in Man. (Trunk, dorsal side).

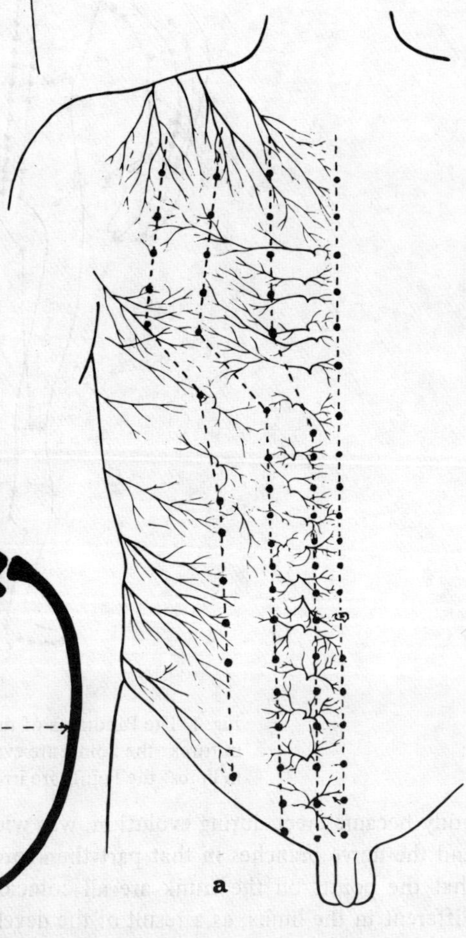

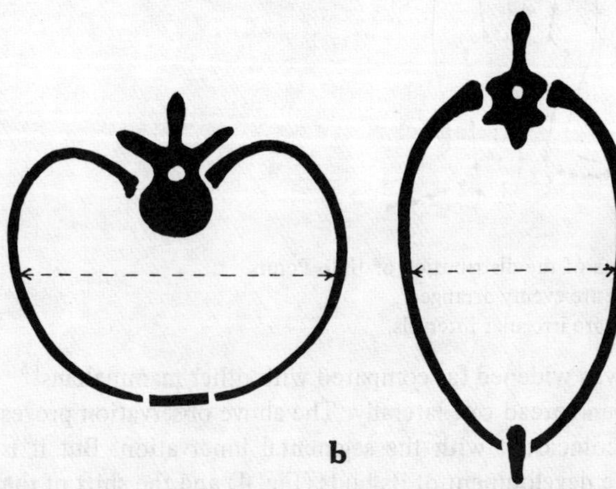

Fig. 3a A sketch copied from an anatomical specimen made by us, showing the agreement of the nerve distribution on the trunk with the arrangement of the Jinlo Points.

Fig. 3b A cross section of the thorax showing the transverse width.
left: Man   Right: generalizd Mammal.

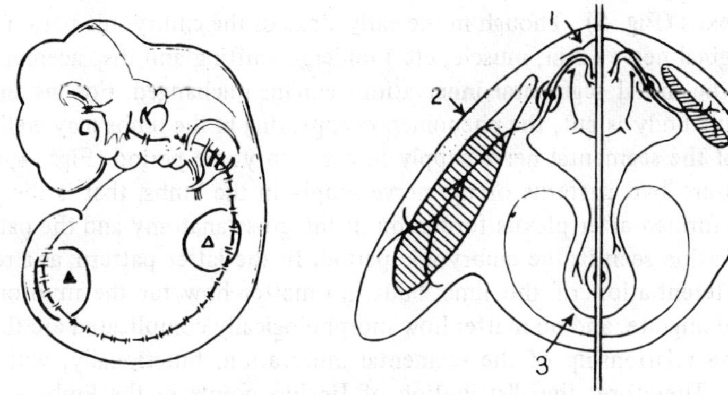

Fig 4a (left), a human embryo,
△ upper limb bud ▲ lower limb bud

Fig. 4b (Right) A cross section of the embryo in its early life. showing the growth of the limb bud and the shaft of the Dermatome and myotome with corresponding nerve innervation (2 →). 1. spinal sement. 3. splanchnic tube.

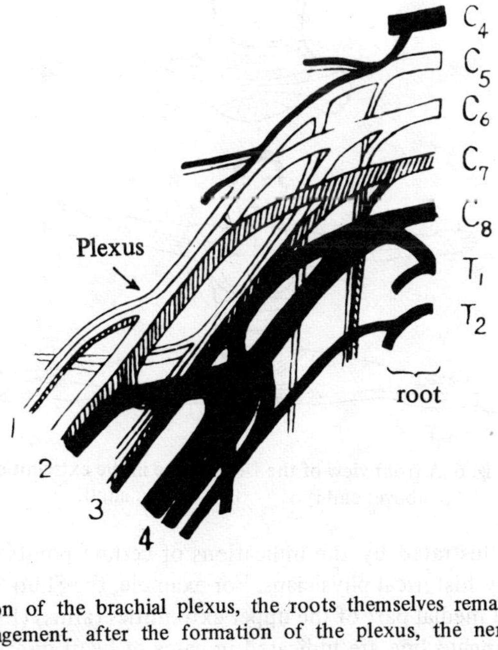

Fig. 5 Formation of the brachial plexus, the roots themselves remain the original segmental arrangement. after the formation of the plexus, the nerve roots have been disturbed.

1. The muscutocutaneous nerves,
2. The median nerves,
3. The radial nerves,
4. The ulnar nerves.

Functionally, however, it is still possible to see on the surface of the limbs the segmental innervation. The reason is that the nerve roots themselves are not changed before the formation of the plexus (Fig. 5). Though in the early stage of the embryonic period, tissues supplied by the original nerve (skin, muscle, etc.) undergo shifting and displacement along with the bud, and the initial segmental innervation remains unchanged. For instance, if a nerve root of an adult body is cut, the phenomenon appearing in the limbs may well reflect the characteristics of the segmental nerve supply in the embryonic period (Figs. 4, 6). For these reasons, there are two patterns of the nerve supply in the limbs, that is the pattern of the nerve supply formed after plexus formation in the gross anatomy and the pattern of the segmental innervation seen in the embryonic period. In the latter pattern, as a result of the growth and differentiation of the limb buds, no matter how far the myotome and dermatome shift and migrate, and no matter how morphologically complicated are the nerve plexuses formed, the relationship of the segmental innervation, functionally, will remain unchanged (Fig. 6). Therefore, the distribution of Jingluo points in the limbs is also in coincidence with the segmental innervation in the trunk[9].

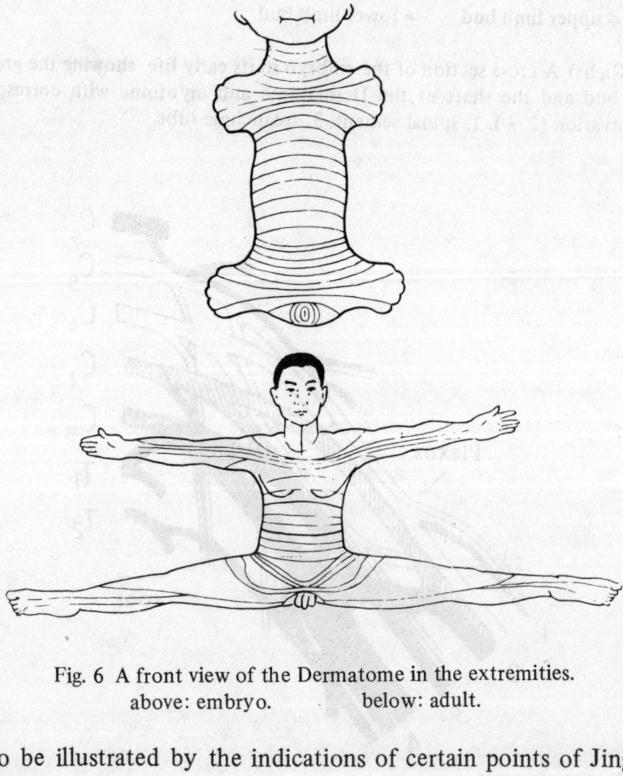

Fig. 6 A front view of the Dermatome in the extremities.
above: embryo. below: adult.

This can also be illustrated by the indications of certain points of Jingluo for certain diseases, experienced by historical physicians. For example, the Shuo Shao Yin Xin Jing line is distributed along the medial part of the upper extremities (arms) (Fig. 7). The majority of the points along this Jingluo line are indicated in cases of heart diseases[13]. However, the region through which this Jingluo line passes belongs to the dermatome, thoracic 1–3 (T_1-T_3) and the nerves serving this region are also the somatic nerves of T_1-T_3 segments

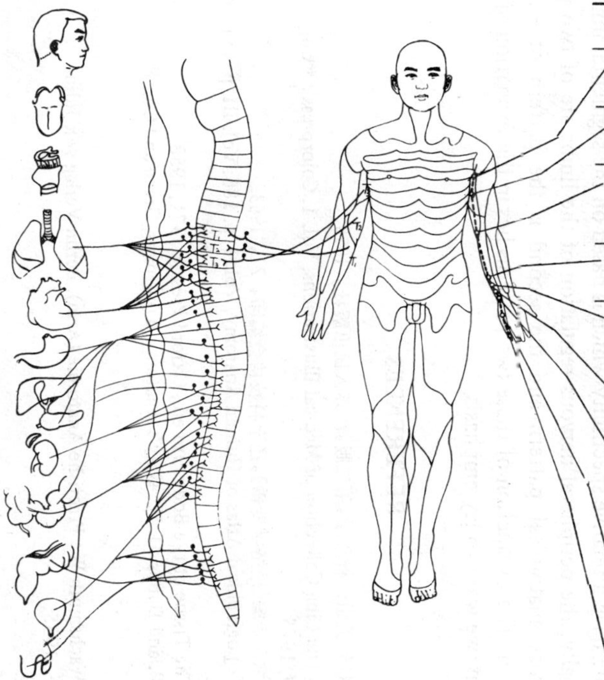

Fig. 7 The coincidence of the indications of the points along the Shou Shao Yin Xin Jin with the segmental innervation.

THE STATISTIC TABLE OF INDICATIONS ACCORDING TO DISTRIBUTIONS OF ACUPOINTS OF HEART CHANNEL OF HAND-SHAOYIN

Name of acupoint	Indications		
1 Jiquan	Heart pain, mental depression, hypochondriac pain	Cold pain of upper	Yellowish eyes, retching
2 Qingling	Heart pain	Difficult lifting of shoulder and arm	Headache, yellowish eyes
3 Shaohai	Heart pain, vomiting, mania forgetfulness, pain undder armpit	Numbness of arm, tremor of hands and spasm of elbow	Scrofula, headache and vertigo
4 Lingdao	Heart pain, fearfulness	Pain and spasm of elbow and upper arm	Sudden horseness of voice
5 Tongli	Palpitation, or constant and violent palpitation, febrile disorders	Pain of arm and wrist	Headache and vertigo, stiffness of tongue, painful throat
6 Yinxi	Heart pain, palpitation, hemoptysis		Epistaxis, night-sweating, aversion to cold
7 Shenmen	Heart pain, irritability, epilepsy dementia, amnesia, palpitation, insomnia, hypochondriac pain, asthms, fever and hemotemesis, hemoptysis		Yellowish eyes
8 Shaofu	Palptation, irritability, pain and fullness of chest	Hotness of palms, spasm of the little finger	Prolapse of uterus, vaginal itching, enuresis, dysuria, chronic malaria with chills
9Shaochong	Heart pain, fast heart beating, chest and hypochondriac pain, emotional lability, irritability due to fever		Emergency of wind-stroke
	Upper limb: chest and heart pain, mental disorders, febrile diseases		

(Fig. 7). At the same time the afferent nerves governing the heart enter the spinal cord via sympathetic nerves of the heart also by way of the posterior roots of the upper thoracic segments (T_1–T_5). Both nerves meet at the posterior horn of the spinal cord (possibly in the vicinity of the gelatinous substance)[12]. Consequently, the impulse produced by needling the points of this Jingluo enters the upper thoracic segments via the corresponding nerve and an influence is thus exerted upon the heart through the reflex connection of the corresponding somatic and splanchnic nerves[14]. That the majority of the points along this Jingluo line are indicated in cases of heart diseases possibly accounts for the fact mentioned above (Fig. 7). For the same reason the lower limbs, such as the points of Zusanli, may have an influence on the organs of the abdomen[11].

Although the points on the limbs are distributed irregularly, they also coincide with the regularity of segmental innervation. We have checked one by one all the points of the 14 Jingluo lines according to their indications, and found that most of them are fundamentally in conformity with segmental innervation. This common feature of regularity, whether in the trunk or in the limbs, coincides in the main with the segmental innervation. We think that the relative specificity of the acupuncture points and the Jingluo line through which the exterior and the interior are connected and unified lies in this, and the nerve connection is the essential basis of Jingluo.

SUMMARY

The report may be summarized in brief as follows:

1. The distribution of Jingluo points, whether on the trunk or on the limbs, conforms with the rules of segmental innervation.

2. Jingluo points have a relative specificity which is based on the segmental innervation.

3. Morphologically, the peripheral nervous regulation of the limbs are of two pattern; the first is the gross anatomical pattern and the second is the pattern of embryonic segmental innervation. The distinction of these two patterns lies in the formation of nervous plexus. On this point, we want to lay emphasis.

REFERENCES

[1] 江苏省中医学校针灸组：针灸学，第二版，江苏人民出版社，1958。

[2] Netter, F. H.: The Ciba Collection of Medical Illustrations, Vol. 1, Colorpress . *Co., New York, 49, 1975.

[3] 杨 枫：学术论文选编(经络学专辑)，辽宁科技协会编印，21，1963。

[4] Seiho Nishi: Topographical Atlas of Human Anatomy, Vol. 1, p. 186; Vol. III, p. 111, 1974.

[5] Clark L. G.: The Tissue of tye Body. 3rd ed., Oxford Press, p. 371, 1958

[6] Johnston, T. B. and Daires, D. V.: Gray's Anatomy, Longmans, Green and Co., P. 1155, 1958.

[7] Cf 4 Ref. 5.

[8] Lanz, T. und Wachsmuth W.: Practishe Anatomie (Arm), Berlin Verlag von Julius Springer, p. 28, 1935.

[9] Cf. 3 Ref. 3.

[10] House, E. L. and Pansky, B.: A Functional Approach to Neuroanatomy. McGraw-Hill Book Co., Inc. USA p. 188, 1960.
[11] 杨 枫 任进祯: 沈阳医学院科研资料汇编 (4): 21, 1963。
[12] 沈阳医生院针麻组(形态组): 中华医学杂志 (3): 144, 1973。
[13] 杨 枫,东北医学杂志 4 (8): 26, 1952。
[14] Лобшибянкин, А.К.: Физиол. Журнал 41:357, 1955.
[15] Hamilton, W. J.: Textbook of Human Anatomy, 2nd, MacMillan Press, London, 22, 1977.

RELATIONS BETWEEN CHANNELS AND LYMPHATIC SYSTEM

Gong Qihua, Cao Jiren
(Shanghai Institute of Acupuncture, Moxibustion and Meridians)

Whether or not the meridians possess their morphological base remains an interesting problem. Having analyzed the descriptions on acupuncture and meridians in "Lingshu", we see that the vessels are the morphological foundation of meridians[1] which include the channels and the collaterals. For example, in the book *Lingshu,* in the chapter on the origin of all diseases, it is said "when the Yang Collaterals are hurt, the blood extravasates outwardly, and when the Yin Collaterals are hurt, the blood extravasates inwardly." Here the collaterals mean the blood vessels. In the same book in the chapter on channels, it is said "when one drinks wine, the defensive vital energy first goes to the skin and flows into the collaterals. When all collaterals are full, the defensive vital energy will then be in an equilibrium and be still. Then the nutritional energy will be full, and the channels will be in a very energetic state." It seems that this description means that the channels and collaterals in the human body are closely related to the lymphatics and blood vessels. As is known to all, after a carbohydrate meal the sugar level in blood will rise rapidly, and that in the lymph will rise slowly; but soon an equilibrium will be established between the plasma and the lymph through the nutritive circulation in the blood capillaries. From this, we believe the channels may probably be related with the lymphatics.

I. The Distribution and Coordination Relation between the Channels and the Lymphatics

Using the characteristics of the lower electrical resistance at the points, we invented the electrophoretic method[2] for imaging the acupuncture points. Combining the electrophoretic imaging method of acupuncture points and the technique of X-ray microradiography, we observed the dilatation of blood capillaries and the convergence of arterioles under the electrophoretic point[3]. In lymphmicroangiography we can see some electrophoretic points situated at the lymphatic capillaries derived from the bundle of lymphatic vessels (see Fig. 1.). On a typical marked PSC person the electrophoretic image of the Stomach Channel on the leg seems to be in accordance with the distribution of the superficial group of superficial lymphatics of the leg (see Fig. 2.).

Therefore, we suggest the description of the channels may be partly based on the way of acute lymphangitis. In Fig. 3a we can see that the infected position concerns the point

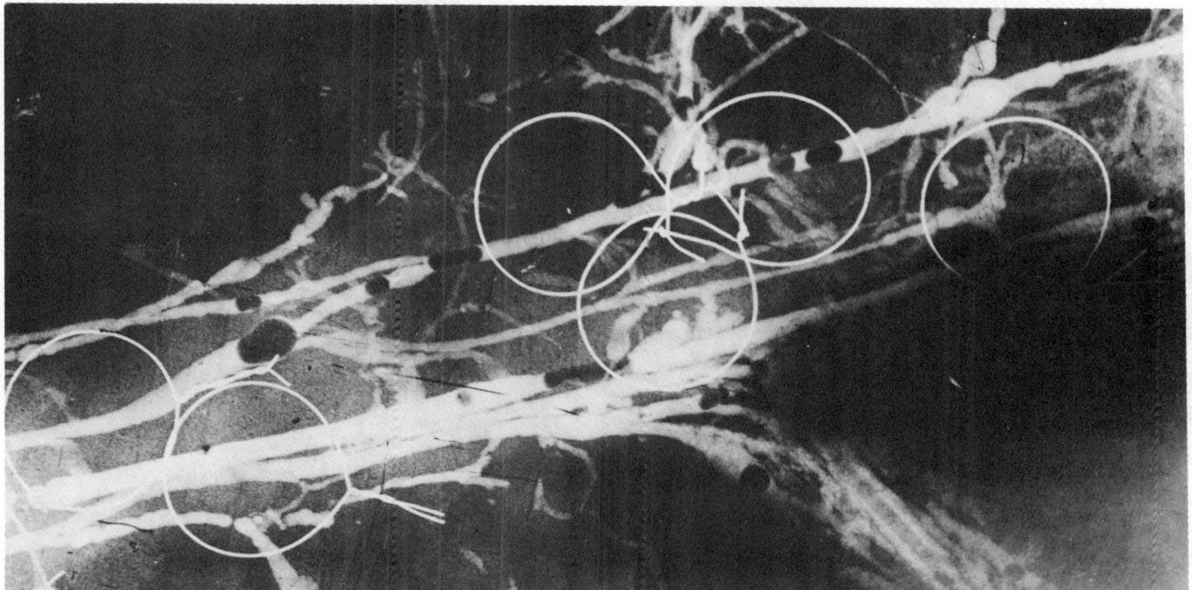

Fig. 1 The lymphmicroangiography (rabbit's pinna) showing some electrophoretic points (the white circles) situated at the lymphatic capillaries derived from the bundle of some lymphatic vessels.

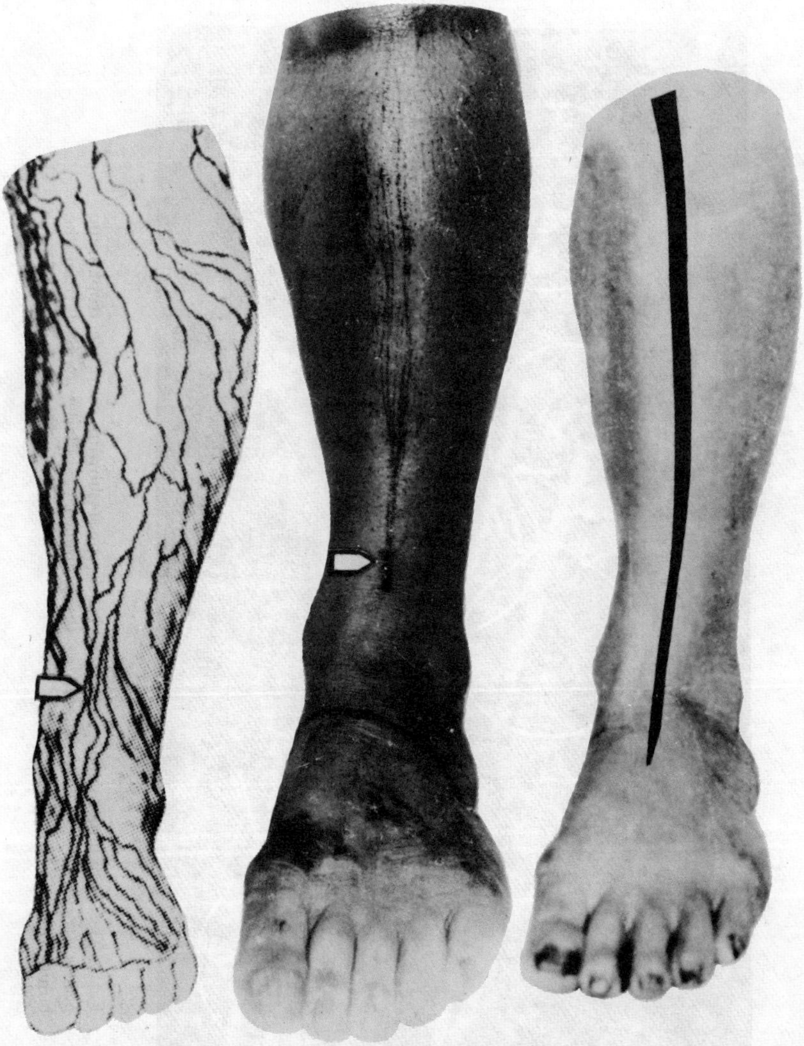

Fig. 2 A. The distribution of the superficial lymphatics of the leg (from Verge'-Brian).
B. A typical marked PSC person's electrophoretic image of the Stomach channel of the leg. C. The subjective feeling course during the examination of the person

Shaochong in the little finger, and the lymphangitis from the point of infection goes along the way of Heart Channel to Jiquan and extends up to the Pericardium Channel in the wrist. Fig. 3c shows an acute lymphangitis of a surgeon who suffered an accidental needle prick during an operation. In the figure we can see the place of needle prick on the thumb situated just at the Shaoshang point and the lymphangitis goes from the point of infection along the way of Lung Channel to the Yumen point where is located the tender part of the subclavian nodes.

We go further to compare the anatomical lymphatic system with the Channels. Fig. 4 is the distribution of the anterior meridians and the lymphatic system of the human body. In this figure we can see the distribution of Channels in the extremities, shoulder, neck and

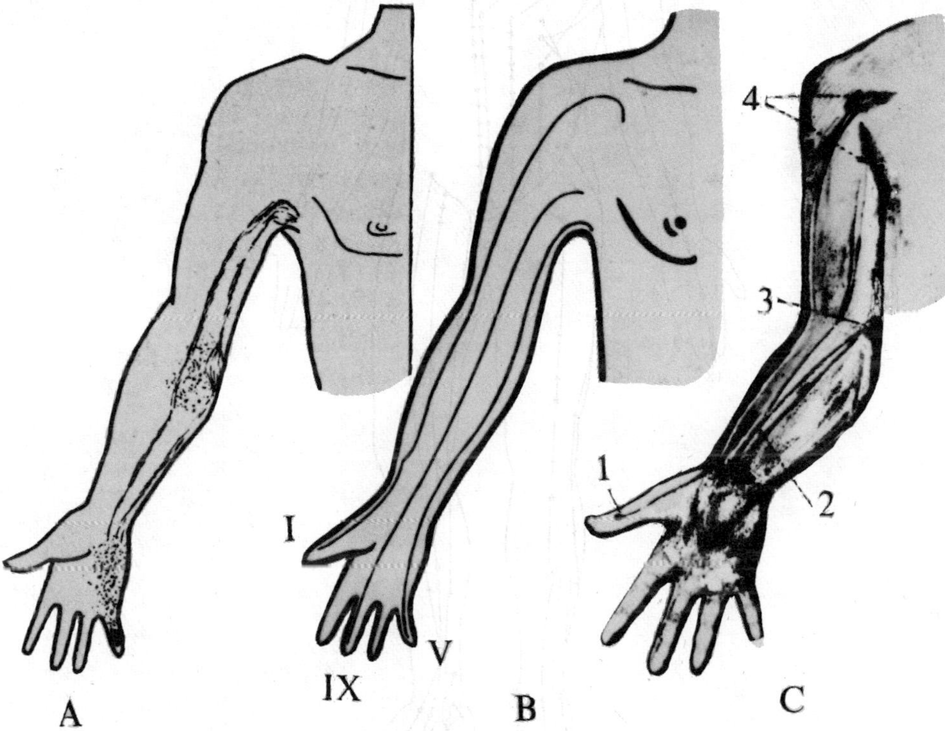

Fig. 3 A Comparison of the acute lymphangitis on upper extremity with the distribution of meridians.

A. The lymphangitis caused by the infec- of little finger (from Textbook of Surgery. F. Christopher).

B. Three Yin channels on upper extremity.

I–Lung channels IX–Pericardium channels V–Heart channel.

C. The lymphangitis caused by the infection of the place of the Shaoshang (From Babcok. Textbook of Surgery. W.B.Saunders)

1–Needle prick on thumb. 2–Irregular red streaks from point of infection. 3–Enlarged epitrochlear node 4–Tender axillary and subclavian nodes.

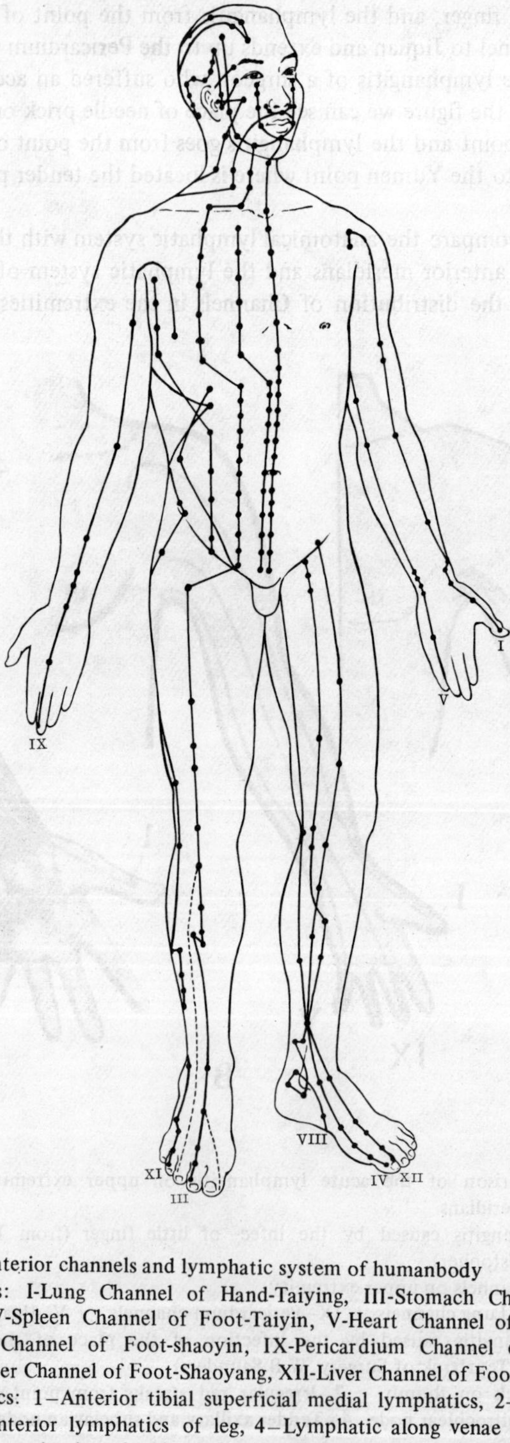

Fig. 4 The anterior channels and lymphatic system of humanbody

A. Meridians: I-Lung Channel of Hand-Taiying, III-Stomach Channel of Foot-Yangming IV-Spleen Channel of Foot-Taiyin, V-Heart Channel of Hand-Shaoyin. VIII-Kidney Channel of Foot-shaoyin, IX-Pericardium Channel of Hand Jueyin XI-Gall Bladder Channel of Foot-Shaoyang, XII-Liver Channel of Foot-Jueyin.

B. Lymphatics: 1–Anterior tibial superficial medial lymphatics, 2–Anterior tibial 3–Internal anterior lymphatics of leg, 4–Lymphatic along venae saphena magna, 5–Internal posterior lymphatics of leg, 6–Elbow ulnar lymphatics, 7–Elbow superficial lymph node, 8–Elbow cubital lymph node, 9–Delto-pectoral node,

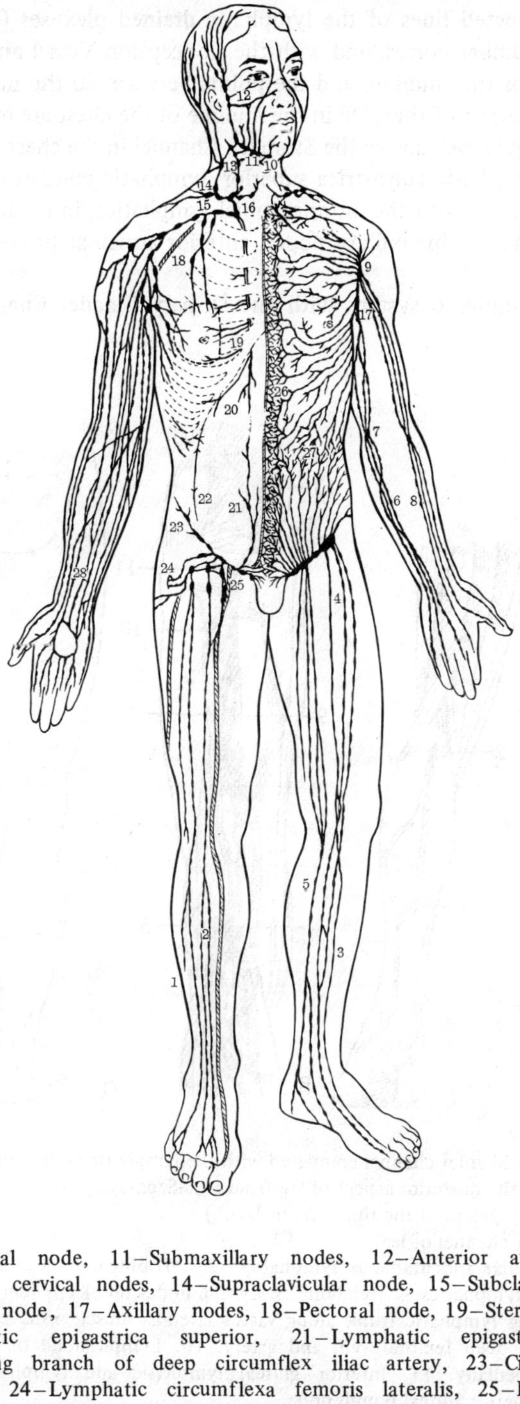

10–Submental node, 11–Submaxillary nodes, 12–Anterior auricular node, 13–Superior cervical nodes, 14–Supraclavicular node, 15–Subclavicular nodes, 16–Cervical node, 17–Axillary nodes, 18–Pectoral node, 19–Sternal lymphatics, 20–Lymphatic epigastrica superior, 21–Lymphatic epigastrica inferior, 22–Ascending branch of deep circumflex iliac artery, 23–Circumflex iliac lymphatics, 24–Lymphatic circumflexa femoris lateralis, 25–Inguinal nodes, 26–Lymphatic drained plexuses at the abdominal middle line, 27–The lymphatic drained plexuses at waist, 28–Lymphatic median cubitus.

head is nearly in accordance with the distribution of the channels. In the chest and abdomen it is clear that the connected lines of the lymphatic drained plexuses (LDP) right in the midline and round the lumbar correspond with the Conception Vessel and the Belt Vessel. There are 19–21 LDP in the midline, and the points here are 20 the number of both are nearly equal. The distribution of the LDP in the midline of the chest are more sparse, and so are the points. In the figure we can see the Stomach Channel in the chest and abdomen is in concordance with the lymphatic epigastrica superior, lymphatic epigastrica inferior and the sternal lymphatics, in the leg with the anterior tibial lymphatics, in the head and neck with the lymphatics derived from submaxillary nodes, anterior auricular nodes and subclavicular nodes.

We compare the lymphatic system with the Urinary Bladder Channel on the lower

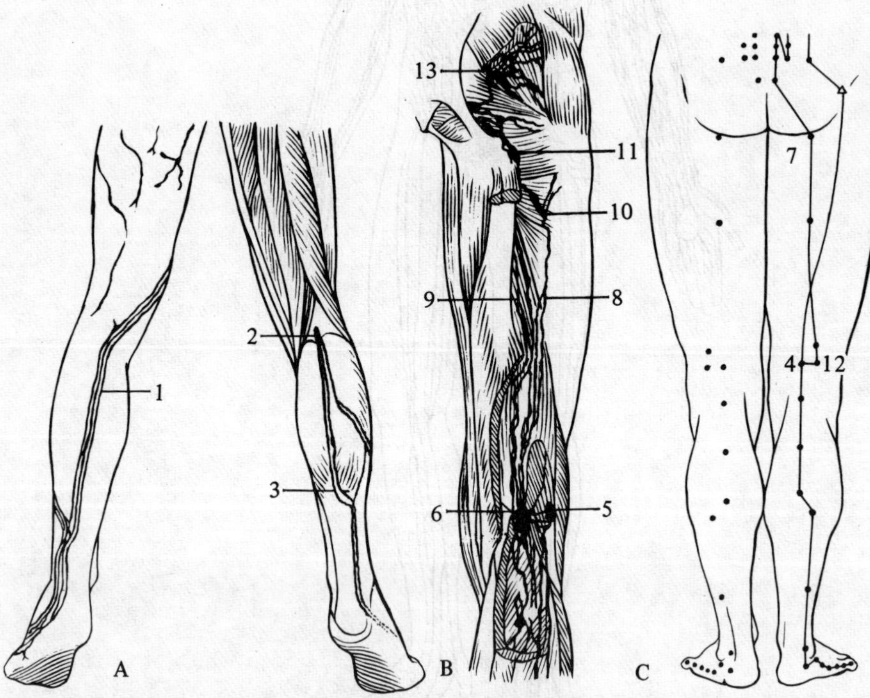

Fig. 5 The urinary bladder channel compared with the lymphatic system of leg.
A. Lymphatics of the posterior aspect of leg(from Kiss-Szentagothai)
B. Deep lymphatic system of the thigh (from Jacob).
C. Urinary bladder channel of leg.

1. Posterior fibular subcutaneous lymphatics. 2,6. Popliteal nodes. 3. Posterior fibular subfascia lymphatics. 4. Weizhong. 5. Lymph nodes on biceps femoris muscle. 7. Chengfu. 8. Big lymphatic trunk along vastus lateralis muscle runs upwards. 9. Lymphatic along deep femoral vein and artery. 10. Lymph node on lymphatic rotating thigh medially. 11. Interior gluteal lymphatic and lymph node. 12. Weizhong. 13. Superior gluteal lymph node.

extremity in Fig. 5. There are many agreements between them such as: Zhibian corresponds with the place of the superior gluteal lymph nodes, Chengfu with the inferior gluteal lymph nodes, Weiyang and Weizhong with the popliteal lymph nodes and the lymph nodes on biceps femoris muscle. Bladder Channel from popliteal lymph nodes downward to the lateral side of the tip of the small toe is in accordance with the posterior fibula subfacia lymphatics.

The description of the channels in most books of traditional Chinese medicine is often confined to the line of points, which is not entirely in accordance with those described in "Lingshu". According to the "Lingshu" the tibial branch of the Stomach Channel at Zusanli terminates in the lateral side of the middle toe, but in general descriptions the branch is often simplified to a line connecting Xiajuxu with Fenglong (see Fig. 4). Therefore, we consider the circle of the Kidney Channel near the interior ankle a result of the line formed by connecting the points situated in the lymphatics here (see Fig. 4). Fig. 6a shows that in general the three Yang Channels of the hand were described as from the shoulder to the neck without considering their passing through Point Quepen. In Fig. 6b shows the same three channels run from the shoulder to the neck through the Quepen point as described in "Lingshu". Of the two figures the second one is more true to the distribution of the lymphatics there. In fact the line connecting the points not only simplifies the channel branches but also in some parts adds to the main channel line some artificial connecting line, distorting thus the original line of the channel in some places. From this, we may infer that the three arcs at the head of the Gall Bladder Channel are the connecting line of points too (see Fig. 7) because in the figure we can see the Gall Bladder Channel runs parallel to the lymphatic system there except the three arcs (see Fig. 7).

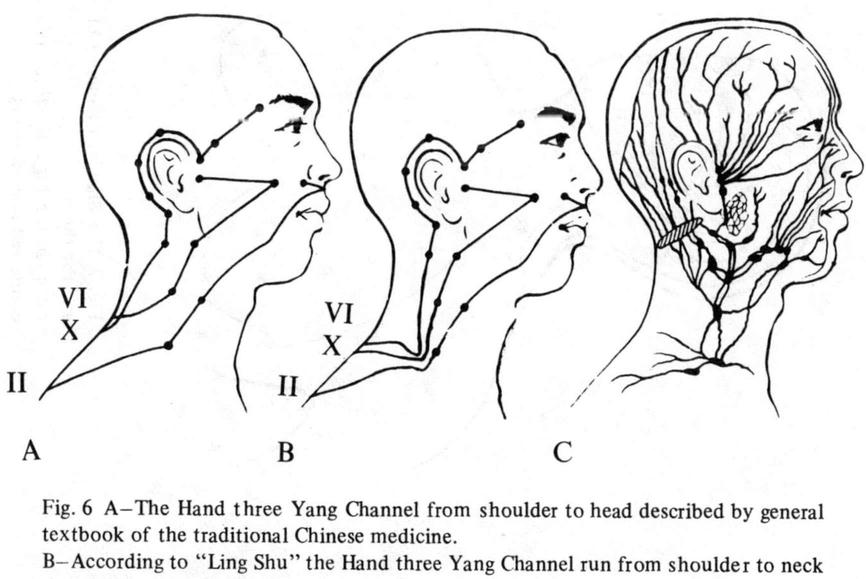

Fig. 6 A–The Hand three Yang Channel from shoulder to head described by general textbook of the traditional Chinese medicine.
B–According to "Ling Shu" the Hand three Yang Channel run from shoulder to neck through the Quepen point.
C–The lymphatic system there.

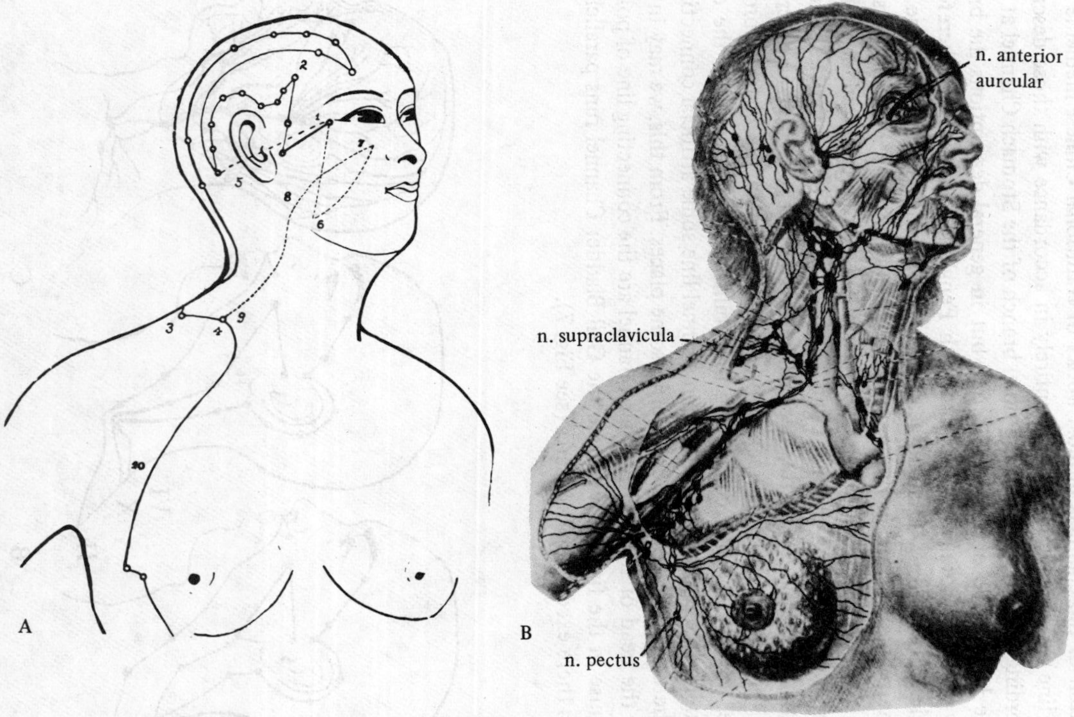

Fig. 7 The Bladder Channel (A) and the lymphatic system (B) at the head, the neck and the thorax.
Note: In the Fig.a the three arcs on the head of the Gall Bladder Channel may be the connected line of points.

II. IMPULSE CHANNEL AND THORACIC DUCT

The essential distribution of the description of the Impulse Channel described in the "Canon of Medicine" is shown briefly in Fig. 8. The Impulse Channel is the sea of 12 Channels, and it originates in the uterus (a) and below the kidney (b). Going downwards it emerges from the Chijie (c) and links up with all the viscera organs (d). Running upwards, the import of the channel energy starts at Dashu (e) and it comes out of the Hangsang of the nasal root (f). If we compare the Impulse Channel with the thoracic duct (Fig. 8b), it can be seen that the region from the lower part of the kidney to the uterus together with the inguinal portion is the region in which numerous lymph nodes are concentrated and from which the accumulated lymph is drained into the lumbar lymph trunks first and then into the thoracic duct. As the description in the literature shows[5], the abdominal portion of the thoracic duct is the place in which the three large lymph trunks (lumbar and intestinal trunks) terminate and from which the thoracic duct actually arises. The thoracic duct, from cisterna chyli to subclavian vein, links up all lymphatics of the viscera organs along the way, crossing the subclavian triangle obliquely and archwise joins the venous system in the venous angle where the junction corresponds relatively to the place of Dashu point (the right lymphatic connected venous at the right resemble position). And the Hangsang situated in

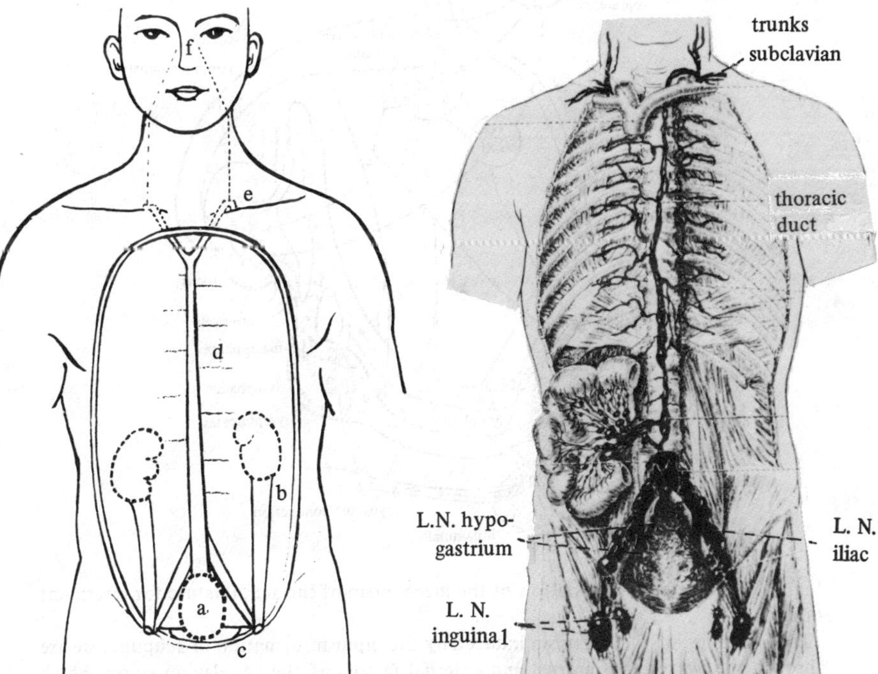

Fig. 8 Comparing the Impulse Channel (A) with the Thoracic duct (B).

the nose corresponds to the dense LDP of nose lymphatic.

Having compared the two figures we can see the distribution of the Impulse Channel and that of the thoracic duct are nearly coincident.

III. THE MECHANISM OF ACUPUNCTURE EFFECT

Edan[6] (1962) deemed that the lymphatic system plays a definite role in acupuncture effect. Kim[7] (1976) considered that the chemically active substances found in the lymph drained from the injured area might be the mediators of vascular reactions or inflammations. It seemed to him that these mediators are resposible for the action of acupuncture and will be called chemical or first mediators of acupuncture. We had demonstrated that an acu-

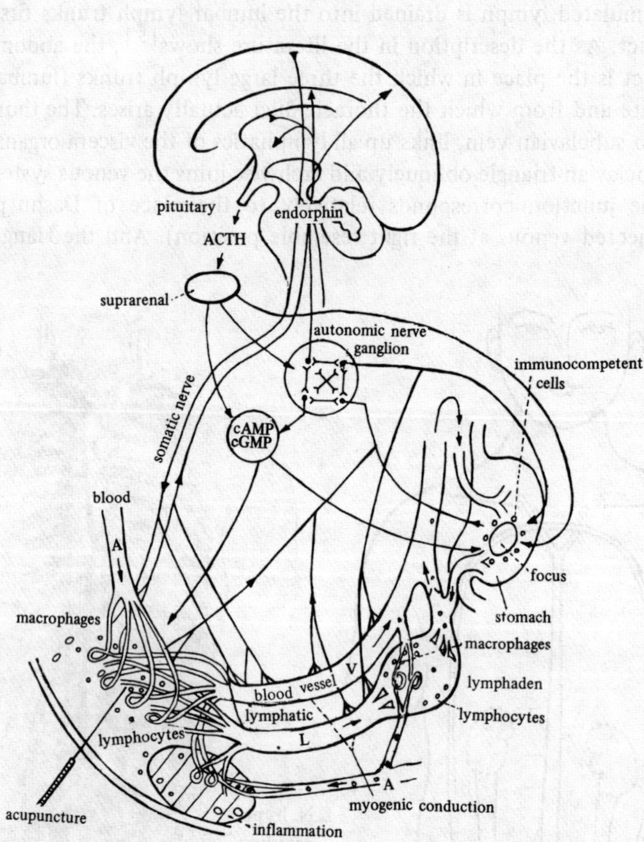

Fig. 9 The schematic illustration of the mechanism of the acupuncture for treatment of diseases.

The reactions of the organism induced by the input information of acupuncture are through the nerves and internal and external factors of the vessels and so on, which promote the activity of the body fluid and the immunocompetent cells, and maintain the organs in normal operation, relieve the inflammation of the nearby tissue or the focus of viscera, in the meantime, play a definite role in analgesia.

puncture point seems to be a spontaneus inflammatory area in which the blood capillaries and lymphatic capillaries are dilated.

The reaction of the organism is induced by the imput information of acupuncture to the nerves[8,9] (including the nerves distributed on the vascular vessels[10]) and to the internal [11] and external factors of the vessels. In the text we emphasizc that an important aspect of acupuncture therapy may probably be caused by the activation of organic defensive mechanism through the lymphatic system, especially the T lymphocyte[12] circulating within it. Besides these two main factors, the myogenic conduction of the vascular smooth muscle may have a definite effect in acupuncture[13]. According to the speed of myogenic conduction (10 cm/sec)[14], nearly equal the speed of needling sensation, we considered that the myogenic conduction may be one of the factors inducing needling sensation (see Fig. 9).

Acknowledgement

The a·ithors are indebted to Prof. Lu Yudao and Prof. Huang Xianming for their critical review of this manuscript.

REFERENCES

[1] 上海中医学院:〈针灸学〉，21，1974。

[2] 龚启华等：科学通报，(9): 425，1976。

[3] 龚启华等：中华医学杂志，(8): 476，1979。

[4] 中医研究院编：«针灸学简编»，43，1978。

[5] Rusznyak, I. et al.: Lymphatics and Lymph ciculation physiology and pathology (book), 75, 1960.

[6] Edam, K：针灸经络专辑，126，1965。

[7] Kim, S.S.: *Am. J.Acupuncture,* (1), p 25, 1976.

[8] Ionescu-Tirgovisle, C.: *Am. J.Acupuncture,* (3), p.199, 1975.

[9] 沈阳医学院针麻研究组：新医药学杂志，(8): 6，1973。

[10] 李仪奎等：上海中医药杂志，(11): 36，1964。

[11] 龚启华等：科学通报，(4): 187，1973。

[12] 曹及人等：待发表。

[13] 上海中医研究所：新医药学杂志，(7): 28，1975。

[14] Hilton, S.M.: *J. Physiol.,* 149, p.93, 1959.

AN OBSERVATION ON PHENOMENON OF PROPAGATED SENSATION ALONG THE CHANNELS

Academy of Traditional Chinese Medicine,
The PLA Hospital, No. 262 and
The People's Hospital of Jishan County of Shanxi Province

Various methods were applied to stimulate acupuncture points. Some subjects developed sensations such as soreness, tingling, distention or other peculiar feeling starting from the site of the stimulated points and spreading along the course of the classical channels. This phenomenon has been called "propagated sensation along the channel (PSC)." Scholars in ancient China already noticed such phenomena and recorded them in both 'Ling shu" and "Compendium of Acupuncture". These two books described "if the right point is punctured a sensation following the corresponding course will appear." It is very possible that such sensation was taken by ancient scholars as one of the important practical bases for the establishment of the channel theory. We considered that profound investigation upon PSC and exploration of its pattern of activity will be undoubtedly helpful for the elucidation of the mechanism of acupuncture and moxibustion and disclosure of the essence of the channel.

In recent years we have made some preliminary studies of PSC and the results are as follows.

I. RATE OF OCCURRENCE OF PSC PHENOMENON

Investigation of PSC was on 5,906 persons, of whom 2,618 were healthy individuals with low-frequency-pulse stimulation at Jing (well) points. It was found that 65 subjects (1.1%) of the whole had marked PSC, appearance of PSC being more than 3 channels. Six out of the 65 were normal, the percentage being 0.22 and the remaining 59 were patients with occurrence rate of 1.8%. The diseased was 7 times higher than that of the healthy. This fact indicates that the occurrence of PSC was closely related with diseases. [Though the number of marked PSC was small, a great deal of instances presenting one to two channels or propagating not too far were collected reaching a percentage 10 or 20.] These confirm that PSC phenomenon is not something strange but real.

II. THE EHARACTERISTICS AND PROPERTIES OF PSC

The nature of the PSC induced by pulse current was mostly tingling, flowing, jerking, warm, heat, or cold sensation; when elicited with conventional acupuncture or electro-acupuncture or point injection, it was soreness, distention, cold or heat in nature; when with moxibustion, it was warmth or heat. The sensory propagating tape was narrower on the extremities and wider on the trunk. It propagated bipolarly and the speed was rather slow (cm/sec), but the latter might be influenced by method and intensity of the stimulation.

The propagation of PSC might be affected or blocked by various factors. Mechanical pressure might cause complete blockage or change its pathway. Deep injection of procaine had the same blocking action, but injection of normal saline sometimes only produced slight blockage. Local application of heat accelerated the propagation and that of cold retarded it.

III. COMPARISON OF THE PATHWAYS OF PSC OVER THE BODY SURFACE WITH THE COURSES OF THE CLASSICAL CHANNELS

Comparison between pathways of PSC which had been induced by stimulating the Jing (well) Points of the twelve channels with low-frequency-pulse current or by stimulating the points of different channels on the limbs below the elbow or the knee joints with conventional acupuncture or electric acupuncture, and the courses of the classical channels described in the "Chapter on Channels", a chapter of the "Canon of the Internal Medicine", was made. According to the following criterion, PSC was classified into three types:

1. The pathway of PSC was in conformity with the courses of the classical channels described in the "Chapter on Channels" of the "Canon of Internal Medicine".
2. Part of the PSC pathway deviated from the classical channel course or did not travel the whole length of the traditional channel.
3. Most of the PSC pathways did not spread along their own classical channels, especially the termination was not within the scope of its own classical channel.

The above criteria were used for the study of the PSC of 102 cases who were sensitive to acupuncture. Eighty-eight channels of 9 cases were observed meticulously for 124 times. Among the 88 channels, 48 were Six-Hand-Channels, which were observed for 74 times; 40 were Six-Foot-Channels observed for 50 times. The results were listed in the following Table 1.

Table 1 shows that 81% of the PSC pathways are principally in conformity with the courses of the classical channels. The pathways of the PSC of Six-Hand-Channels as well as Foot-Channels of the extremities are basically identical with the classical channels, but deviations and fusions of channels are always present in the PSC of the trunk, and the abdomen. On the head and face, deviations are more frequent and even completely inconsistent with classical patterns.

Observations on other subjects showed similar results as mentioned above.

The proceeding results suggest that the courses of the channels described by the Chinese scholars of the ancient days were formed in practice. The phenomenon of PSC possibly is one of the important bases of the courses of the channels.

Table 1. The classified statistics of PSC of 12 channels of 9 marked PSC persons

	Channels	Type I	Type II	Type III	Total
Sin-hand-channel	Lung channel of hand-Taiyin	6	3	2	11
	Heart channel of hand-Shaoyin	5	0	0	5
	Pericardium channel of hand-Jueyin	5	2	2	9
	The large intestine channel of hand-Yangming	2	8	1	11
	The Sanjiao channel of hand-Shaoyang	1	3	2	6
	The small intestine channel of hand-Taiyang	0	4	2	6
Six-foot-channel	The urinary bladder channel of foot-Taiyang	0	4	1	5
	The stomach channel of foot-Shaoyang	1	6	2	9
	The gall bladder channel of foot-Shaoyang	0	6	1	7
	The spleen channel of foot-Taiyin	4	6	0	10
	The kidney channel of foot-Shaoyin	2	0	2	4
	The liver channel of foot-Jueyin	3	0	2	5
	Total	29	42	17	88
	Percentage	33	48	19	100

IV. CHANGES ALONG THE PROPAGATING COURSE AFTER APPEARANCE OF PSC

1. The raising of the pain and pain-toleration thresholds along the propagating zone.

Observation was made on 93 cases who had PSC. Most of them did not show obvious raising of pain threshold or pain-toleration threshold along the PSC zone and such phenomenon was found markedly only in a few of the instances. A typical case is now reported here.

Patient suffered from functional disorder of the mandibular joint and had phenomenon of PSC reaching the affected area. When point Xiajuxu of the Stomach Channel of Foot-Yangming was punctured, a sensory propagating band reached the region in front of the ear. The pain was measured by the following method.

Eight levels were marked out on the propagation band for determination. Beside the site of the lesion each level had been set 7 pain measuring points. The distance between every two points was 1–1.5 cm. The course of propagation band was within the range of the 3rd and the 5th points of each level. A 57–9A type potassium ion pain detector was used to produce pain. The pain tolerance threshold of each point was determined 15 minutes before and after insertion of the needle respectively. For avoidance of influence of any patient's subjective factors, the order of determination was arranged at random and the results were grouped based on the order number. The same ordinal number of different levels was set in same group, hence there were seven groups. Then the value of the average pain tolerance athreshold of each of the seven groups was obtained respectively.

Fig. 1 shows that: (a) before acupuncture, the average pain tolerance threshold of the seven groups, which was about 0.06 MA, was reciprocally similar; (b) the average values of all the 7 groups 15 minutes after the insertion of the needle increased from 0.2–0.5 MA; (c) among the increases the 4th, 5th and 6th groups were the most prominent ones, being about 7–9 times as that before acupuncture. These results indicate that there was presence of a pain insensitive band along the PSC zone due to elevation of the pain threshold.

The result of pain threshold with a spring prober was almost the same as measured with

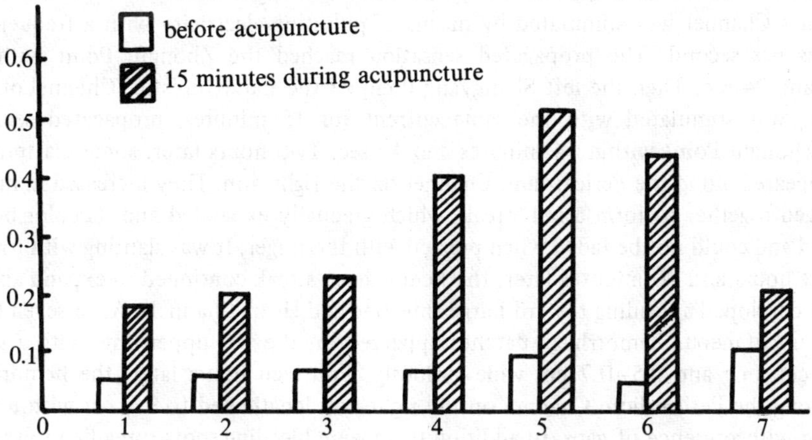

Fig. 1 The phenomena of the heightening of pain tolerance threshold.

potassium ion method and was also identical with the course of the PSC described by the patient himself, only the pain insensitive band was somewhat wider than the PSC since the latter was situated as an axon of the former.

2. Change of local blood flow on the PSC band.

The local blood flow of the channels themselves and their side-zone was measured by an OTE type recorder connected with a KR-Eα type amplifier. Thirty-four cases with PSC and 10 cases without PSC were examined. They were divided into 4 groups, the first three groups consisted of cases with PSC and the last one did not.

Group I, 14 cases — stimulating the Pericardium Channel;
Group II, 15 cases — stimulating the Heart Channel;
Group III, 5 cases — stimulating the Lung Channel; and
Group IV, 10 cases — control group.

The subjects were asked to rest for a few minutes in bed and then the local blood flow was measured as a control. Hereafter the Jing (well) point was stimulated by means of pulsating electricity, which was suitable in intensity with a frequency of 1–150 Hz to induce PSC. It was maintained for 10 minutes. The blood flow was immediately recorded after cessation of the stimulation. The results were listed in Tables 2 and 3.

[Table 2 shows after stimulation, the Ist and the increase of the wave amplitude and sharpening of angle of the main peak of RG with statistical significance upon Groups I and III and there was only sharpening of the main peak angle with statistical significance upon Group II.] No change was revealed upon Group IV.

Table 2 shows the local RG of the side-zone of the channel. No obvious change was found after stimulation in all the four groups. In Group I the difference of the changes of wave amplitude of the channel itself and the side-zone is statistically significant ($P < 0.001$). (Refer to Fig. 2).

The results show that there was a change of the local blood inflow in the corresponding channel when the propagated sensation was appearing along the channel.

3. The Appearance of Subcutaneous Hemorrhage Thread along the Course of the PSC.

Subcutaneous hemorrhage threads were noticed in a patient after stimulation of the Jing points in June 1975, in a general survey of PSC. The right Zhongchong Point of the Pericardium Channel was stimulated by means of pulsating electricity with a frequency of five times per second. The propagated sensation reached the Zhongfu Point within 14 minutes and 24 sec. Then the left Shangyang Point of the Large Intestine Channel of Hand Yangming was stimulated with the same current for 15 minutes; propagated sensation reached Zhongfu Point within 14 minutes and 40 sec. Two hours later, some scattered red rashes appeared along the Pericardium Channel on the right arm. They increased in number and merged together to form a red streak, which gradually expanded and its color became scarlet red and could not be faded when pressed with the finger. It was slanting with irregular edges. Six hours and 30 minutes later, the hemorrhage streak continued to expand and two new ones developed spreading toward Large Intestine and Heart Channels. After seven hours, 5 other subcutaneous hemorrhage patches appeared on the left upper limb with a size of 1.2–1.5 cm long and 0.5–0.7 cm wide variously. Fourteen hours later, the hemorrhagic thread along the Pericardium Channel on the right arm lengthened to 9.5 cm with a width of 1.2 cm with presence of gaps. In addition there were bleeding spots spreading toward the periphery and the number of patches of petechia strips on the left arm increased to eight,

Table 2. Changes of the RG of the channel itself after stimulating the Jing(well) point

Group	Wave amplitude (Ω)					The inflow period (ms)					The peak angle (degree)				
	Rise	No change	Descend	Average	P	Increase	No change	Decrease	Average	P	Increase	No crease	Decrease	Average	P
I	11	2	1	< 0.025	0.005	1	7	6	−10	> 0.4	1	1	12	−9.56	< 0.025
II	10	1	4	> 0.01	0.4	2	4	9	−10.1	> 0.5	1	5	9	−17.6	< 0.05
III	5	0	0	< 0.05	0.05	0	3	2	−8	> 0.1	0	1	4	−20	< 0.05
IV	5	1	4	> 0.011	0.5	1	3	6	−6	> 0.5	3	4	3	1.5	> 0.5

Table 3. Changes of the RG of the side-zone of the channel after stimulating the Jing (well) point

Group	Wave amplitude (Ω)					Blood inflow period (ms)					Peak angle (degree)				
	Rise	No change	Descend	Average	P	Increase	No change	Decrease	Average	P	Increase	No crease	Decrease	Average	P
I	7	4	3	0.012	> 0.2	2	7	5	10	< 0.5	3	3	8	–5.7	>0.1
II	11	1	3	0.019	>0.5	3	5	7	5.86	< 0.5	2	3	10	–5.66	>0.4
III	4	1	0	0.031	> 0.2	0	3	2	–32	> 0.2	1	1	3	–10	>0.1
IV	5	2	3	0.004	< 0.2	0	4	6	–30	< 0.05	4	0	6	–9.5	>0.1

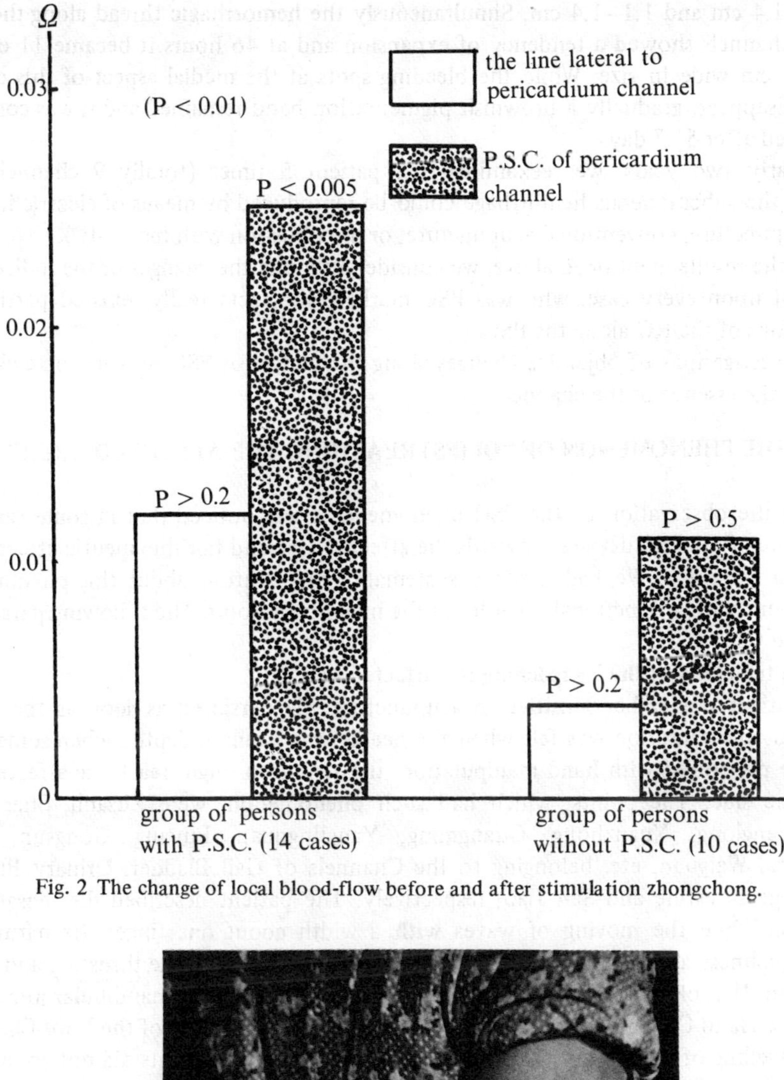

Fig. 2 The change of local blood-flow before and after stimulation zhongchong.

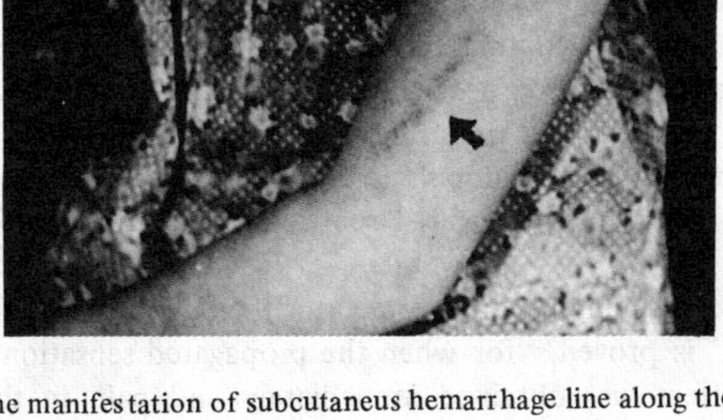

Fig. 3 The manifestation of subcutaneous hemarrhage line along the channel.

sized 2.3–1.4 cm and 1.1–1.4 cm. Simultaneously the hemorrhagic thread along the Large Intestine Channels showed a tendency of expansion and at 46 hours it became 11 cm long and 0.9–1 cm wide in size. While the bleeding spots at the medial aspect of this channel began to disappear, gradually a brownish pigmentation band remained and it was completely eliminated after 5–7 days.

In nearly two years, we reexamined the patient 5 times (totally 9 channel-times) and found the subcutaneous hemorrhage could be reproduced by means of electric impulse, electro-acupuncture, conventional acupuncture, or moxibustion with moxa stick.

From the results mentioned above, we consider although the changes of the indices were not present upon every case, who was PSC marked, the facts really, existed, particularly the alterations of the RG along the PSC.

The investigations of objective changes along the course of PSC provide some clues for research of the essence of the channel.

V. THE PHENOMENON OF "QI (PS) REACHING THE AFFECTED AREA"

During the observation of the PSC phenomena, it was noticed that in some cases the spreading line of the PSC deviated towards the affected area and fair therapeutic effect could be obtained instantly. We had made a systematic investigation about this phenomenon upon a patient with a functional disorder of the mandibular joint. The following paragraphs give the result.

1. The travelling of the PS reaching the affected area.

The patient was rather sensitive to acupuncture. He perspired as soon as the needle was inserted, and sensation was felt when the needle was 3 mm in depth; when some distal points were punctured with hand manipulation, the sensation might reach the affected area on the same side. The points, which had such phenomenon, were Zusanli, Shangjuxu, Xiajuxu, Fenglong, Xuanzhong, Guangming, Yanglingquan, Fuyang, Gongsun, Hegu, Zhongdu and Waiguan, etc. belonging to the Channels of Gall Bladder, Urinary Bladder, Spleen, Large Intestine and San Jiao, respectively. The patient described the sensation as going forward like the moving of waves with a width about one finger. Its nature was soreness, numbness and coolness, and the rythm was identical with the thrusting and lifting manipulation. It took about 3 minutes for the sensation to reach the mandibular joint when points of the Hand-Channels were punctured, and 5 minutes for those of the Foot-Channels.

The travelling of the needle sensation of the above mentioned points did not completely follow the classical course of the Twelve Channels, showing more conformity with those below the elbow and knee joints and less with those above them. The degree of deviation was different. The sensory course of the same point often took the same pathway of the same side at different times of acupuncture so that it was possible to reproduce.

Since the propagated sensation usually terminated at the adjacent parts of the shoulder and hip joints without arrival to the affected area when pulsating current was used for stimulation, we used mainly hand manipulation for treatment.

2. Relationship between "propagated sensation reaching the affected area" and therapeutic effect.

During treatment, the famous ancient record "therapeutic effect is attained only when Qi has been arriving" is proved, "for when the propagated sensation reached the affected area", therapeutic effect was obtained immediately and pain in that area disappeared.

His mouth could be opened much wider with a range from 2.5 to 5 cm and the deviation of the angle was corrected, and both occlusion and function of mastication were also improved.

After 3 months of treatment, the condition of the patient was markedly improved, his pain much relieved, and mastication recovered. Follow-up examination, done one month after discharge, showed that the therapeutic effect was steady.

3. Clinical observation of "Qi (PS) reaching the affected area".

(1) When propagated sensation reached the affected area, the functional state of the involved part could be improved.

When Zusanli which was ipsilateral to the lesion was punctured by hand manipulation for 15 minutes. the patient would feel sensation reaching the affected area. EMG of the masseter was then observed to determine the frequency of contraction and it was found five times more than that before acupuncture, and both the degree of mouth opening (the distance between the upper and lower incision teeth) and the pain threshold of the affected area were increased after acupuncture. Forty-five minutes after the withdrawal of the needle, the PS disappeared, the frequency of the EMG became markedly lowered, the opening of the mouth narrower and the pain threshold decreased (Table 4).

(2) Influence of therapeutic effect due to blocking of the propagated sensation to the affected area.

When PS was blocked to the affected area, EMG of the masseter showed no change. When Sanyinjiao was acupunctured, the propagated sensation was arrested after it had reached upward to the iliac region. The EMG was observed before, during and after acupuncture. The frequencies were 44/sec, 23/sec, and 33/sec, respectively, without any increase in the frequency of the EMG.

When the PS reaching the affected area was interrupted, change in frequency of EMG disappeared. When hand manipulated acupuncture was applied at Zusanli, ascending propagated sensation was elicited and then it was interrupted by heavy finger press on the course, a short distance above the site of needling. During the interruption the frequency

Table 4. Changes in the frequency of the EMG, pain threshold and the degree of mouth opening before and after acupuncture induced propagated sensation reaching the affected area

Item	Control (before acu.)	Acu. 15″	After withdrawal of needle (45″)
Frequency of EMG (time/sec)	48	295	111
Value of pain threshold (g)	85	155	80
Degree of mouth opening (cm)	0.7	1.5	0.8

Table 5. Influence on EMG, degree of mouth-opening and pain threshold during blocking of the PS with mechanical pressure

Item	Before blocking	During blocking	Removal of blocking
Frequency of EMG (time/sec)	33	34	295
Amplitude of EMG (low/high)	1:1.7	1:1.2	1:2.5
Degree of mouth opening (cm)	1	0.7	1.5
Value of pain threshold (g)	95	85	140

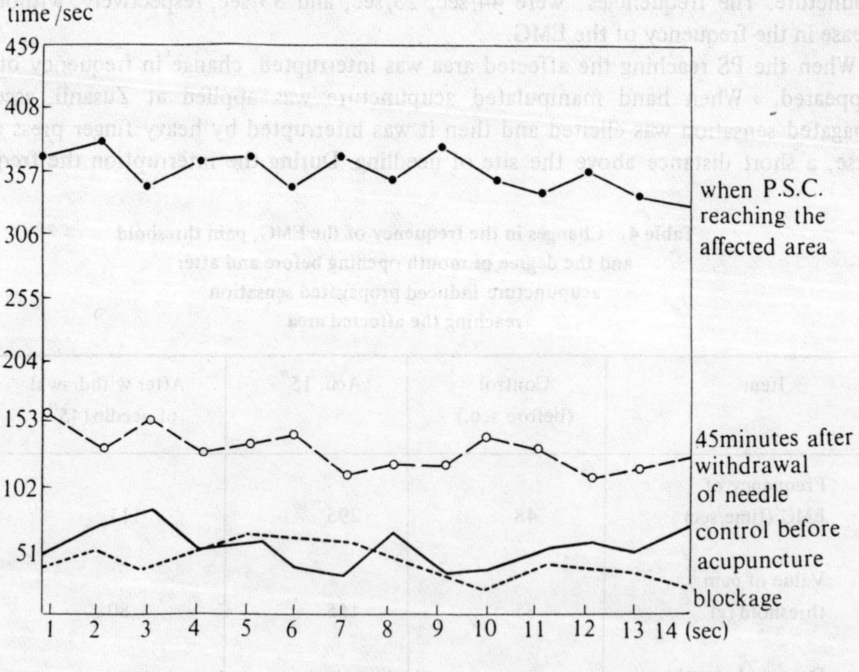

Fig. 4 Sequential distribution histogram of discharge of EMG.

and amplitude of masseter, the degree of mouth-opening, and the pain threshold showed no change at all. When pressure was released, the propagated sensation went upward again and finally reached the affected area, then all the frequency and amplitude of the EMG, the mouth-opening and the pain threshold raised (see Table 5, Fig. 4).

The above results show that "propagated sensation reaching the affected area" is closely related with the therapeutic effects. When PS was being interrupted by pressure or injection of procaine, the therapeutic effect on the inflicted organ was not significant by puncturing the distant point. This suggests that PSC has some interrelation with the connection of the acupuncture point and the viscera.

VI. THE COEXISTENT CHANGES OF FUNCTIONS OF THE INTERNAL ORGANS DURING THE OCCURRENCE OF PSC

In the observation of PSC it was noticed that some patients developed borborigmus when propagated sensation was induced by stimulation of the Jing (well) Point. Investigations were made upon six patients for 42 times. Results showed that when the patient complained of the developement of PSC over Gall Bladder, Stomach, Lung and Large Intestine Channels, changes upon density and amplitude of the borborigmus would take place. Such effect might be abolished by blocking of the PSC caused by mechanical press or other factors, but when the interference was removed the PSC reappeared and the effect would be present again. An electronic computer was used to treat the parameters of the borborigmus and it was proved that marked changes of the density of the borborigmus developed in existence of PSC and so was not the reverse. If blockage of the PSC was esta-

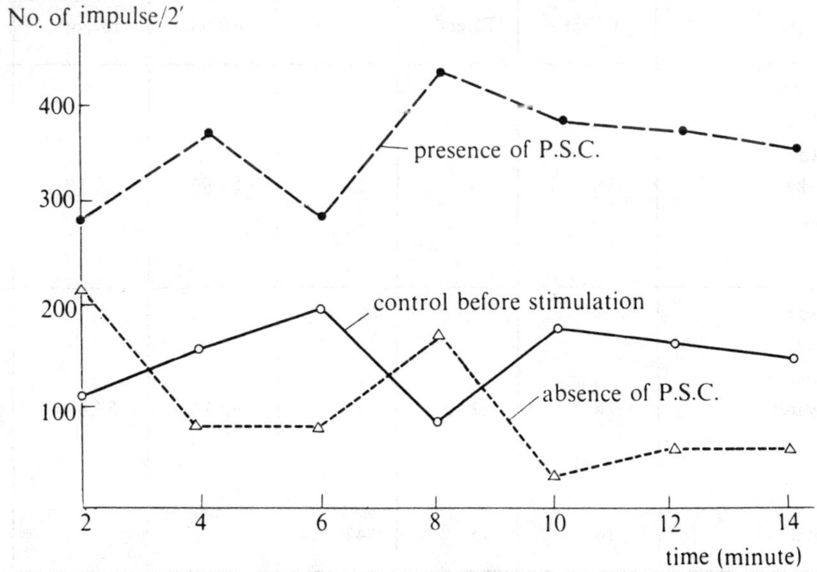

Fig. 5 Sequential distribution histogram of bowel sound when electro-stimulating the Jing-well point of the lung channel.

blished by mechanical pressure there was no marked difference in the density of borborigmus as compared with the basal parameters. (Fig. 5)

The above results show that during the presence of PSC, changes might take place not only over the PSC band, but also in the activities of some internal organs. These events reveal that acupuncture of points might cause corresponding changes upon the functional activity of the vegetative nervous system. Therefore the phenomenon of PSC may be the reflection of the moving process of connection between points and viscera. It is important upon investigation of PSC phenomena to pay more attention to this connection process to shed some light on the true nature of the channel.

VII. NEEDLING SENSATION, PROPAGATED SENSATION AND THERAPEUTIC EFFECT

The fact, [that the reaching of the PS to the affected area could cause the effect of the acupuncture,] led us to investigate the relationship between needling sensation and the effect of acupuncture upon 41 cases of perforation of peptic ulcer. All the patients were admitted on emergency and thoroughly examined including X-ray and abdominal puncture.

Table 6. Relationship between therapeutic effect and acupuncture sensation during acupuncture of zusanli and its adjacent tender points

	No. of Cases			Percentage (%)		
	Good Effect	Poor Effect	Total	Good Effect	Poor Effect	Total
Propagated sensation going towards the affected area	18	4	22	81.82	18.18	100.00
Local sensation or sensation downwards to the foot	8	11	19	42.11	57.89	100.00
Total	26	15	41			

Statistical result: $X^2 = 6.9290$

$P < 0.001$

During the first time of acupuncture with strong manipulation the patient was asked about the nature of needling sensation and the direction of spreading of the sensation. The patient did not understand the aim of the inquisition and the doctor could not anticipate what the therapeutic effect would be. This procedure was more or less the same as the double blind method. As a result, 22 (53.6%) out of the 41 cases, when treated by acupuncture Zusanli or its adjacent tender point, experienced needling sensation spreading proximally. Most of them Said the sensation went above to just the knee and a few to the affected area—the abdomen. The other 19 cases had no sensation propagated upward to the affected area, but around the site of acupuncture or spread downward to the foot. After needling for 1–3 times, with an interval of 4 hours between them, upon all the 41 cases, 26 showed good effect. The abdominal pain was relieved, the board-like abdominal wall softened, the peristalsis and bowel movement reappeared and the perforation healed. Hence the patients entered into the second stage of treatment and herbal drugs was administered. The remaining 15 cases, whose effect was poor, had no marked improvement but recurrence repeatedly. Therefore, operations had to be done. Statistical study of the relationship between needling sensation and effect showed that those patients who felt the needling sensation going towards the affected area had much better results than those who had only a local sensation or a sensation that went downwards to the foot (see Table 6).

The above results suggest that there might be an endogenic correlation between acupuncture sensation, PSC and the therapeutic effect.

VIII. DISCUSSION

1. The Channel theory is a component part of traditional Chinese medicine. It was used by ancient Chinese medical practitioners out of long-term medical practice to explain the physiological function and the pathological changes of the human body and the law of their special associations. It was asserted in Ling Shu: "The twelve channels connect with the viscera internally and the limbs and joints externally", and "Channels are passages in which vital energy and blood circulate to regulate Yin and Yang, nourish tendons and bones, and lubricate joints." In the Channel theory it is considered that channels are a network, running transversally and longitudinally to link up various parts of the body to made them an integral whole. They are distributed throughout the body. Internally they connect the viscera and externally the limbs and trunk and the organs of the five senses. If the normal motion of the vital energy through the channels is upset by the "six exogenous pathogenic factors" or "the 7 endogenous emotional factors", then pathological changes take place. Any derangement of the channel will affect the viscera and vice versa. Therefore, the function of the channel should be regulated when treating a disease, and the channel theory should be observed as instruction for clinical practice, especially in acupuncture therapy. It is pointed out in "Biaoyiu Fu" that "disregard of the theories of Channel and of Yinyang will made accidents in acupuncture unavoidable. If one wants to fina out whether the viscera are related to the nature of Xu or Shi, one must be find it from the channel. " In the early period of the Qing Dynasty, "Yu Jiayan" once said "any one who doesn't know the channel theory and the viscera, is bound to make blunders whatever he says or does." Such passages described vividly the relationship between the theory of channel and acupuncture practice.

PSC is one of the phenomena of the channel. From the great amount of research works done both at home and abroad, it is found that such a phenomenon exists in people regardless of nationality, race, sex, age, locality, profession, and there are some commun laws governing its occurrence. Thus, it is proved that PSC is a reality and is not a rare manifestation among patients. The courses of PSC over the body surface basically coincide with those of the classical channels, and some changes take place occasionally in the band of PSC in a few patients. Such evidence suggests that the classical channels described by ancient medical scholars actually exist. Besides, it substantiates the possibility that PSC is one of the bases on which the establishment of the courses of the Channels was made in the ancient days.

2. When PSC appears, changes of the functions of the viscera will occur. It suggests that research of PSC should not be limited to the PSC band alone. Channels are passages in which vital energy and blood circulate. Internally they connect with the internal organs, externally with the limbs and joints. They link up the points on the surface with the viscera, and the sense organs. Puncturing of these points would cause some changes in the functions of the internal organs, and during this process, PSC may appear. This suggests that PSC is a reflection of the connection between the points and the internal organs which is projected on the cerebral cortex. Though marked PSC only appears occasionally, the connection between the points and the internal organs is a common phenomenon in most people. The occurrence of marked PSC is not so common; probably it is related to the sensitiveness and constitution of the individual. It was reported that 60–70% of subjects had occult PSC. During breathing exercise and meditation, the percentage of appearance of PSC is much higher. Such a fact is also supports our belief that PSC is the result of the connecting process between the points and the internal organs projected on the cerebral cortex, and this is an important clue for the research of the existence of the channels.

IX. SUMMARY

1. Investigation of 5,906 subjects shows that the percentage of occurrence of PSC is higher in patients than in normal persons. Eighty-five percent of the pathways of PSC are in conformity with that of the classical channels described in the Treatise on Channels, Canon of Internal Medicine.

2. It was observed that some actual changes had taken place in the band of PSC. It is tentantively suggested that there is indirect evidence to confirm the existence of PSC.

3. It is very likely that there is a certain relation between the PSC phenomenon and the therapeutic effect of acupuncture.

4. The appearance of PSC may be accompanied by some changes in the functional activities of the distal effectors and the viscera.

5. PSC phenomenon may be a reflection of the connecting process between the acupuncture points and the viscera which is projected on the cerebral cortex. It is also possible that PSC substantiates the existence of the classical channels established by ancient Chinese medical scholars.

STUDIES OF PHENOMENON OF BLOCKING ACTIVITIES OF CHANNELS AND COLLATERALS

Research Group of Acupuncture Anesthesia,
Institute of Medicine and Pharmacology of
Fujian Province, et al.*

It is an outstanding characteristic that the propagated sensation along channels (PSC) can be blocked by some maneuvers. The earliest description about the controlling of "Qi" by mechanical compression was recorded in ancient books of traditional Chinese medicine such as "Jingzheng Fu" (Ballad on Gold Needles) and "Yixue Rumen" (Introduction to Medicine) and confirmed by some recent observations[1-4]. In the latest experiments the effects which can be blocked by mechanical compression and other factors are not confined to PSC alone, but all are related to it. These phenomena are collectively referred to as the blocking of the activities of the channels and collaterals. Hence, it is of great significance to make a thorough study of this phenomenon for further investigating the mechanism of acupuncture and elucidating the true nature of the channels and collaterals. There are two things to be reported in this paper: (1) factors that cause the blocking of PSC along channels (BPSC) and (2) characteristic influence of BPSC on the effect of acupuncture.

I. METHODS

37 subjects with marked PSC were put under observation, but some experiments were performed only on some of them. There were two principal methods used to bring out BPSC: (1) mechanical pressure exerted by a calibrated spring compressor on a point marked out for creating blocking; (2) local hypothermia, induced by setting a small ice bag on a point marked out for creating blocking (the contacting surface of the bag with the skin was 5×3 cm^2). The skin temperature and the point temperature of the marked spot (see below) were measured simultaneously.

Pain threshold, borborygmi and EMG were chosen as indices to evaluate the effect of acupuncture. Pain threshold was measured by means of a spring algometer, and digital plethysmogram was taken simultaneously in some cases. The regular decrease of the amplitude of pulse wave following noxious stimulation was designated as pain reaction. Borborygmi were picked up by a transducer wrapped on the right middle abdomen and recorded with a polygraph.

---

* Members of Fujian Cooperative Research Group on PSC took part in this research.

In two of the cases, the involuntary contraction of facial muscles was seen as PSC arrived at the face. If PSC was blocked, the muscle contraction disappeared instantly. A series of experiments were performed on one of them who had suffered from neurogenic deafness. Contraction of muscles in the preauricular region was visible as PSC reached there. The intensity of discharges was essentially proportional to the intensity of PSC perceived in the subject. In comparison with a series of control observations, it is evident that EMG, as mentioned above, is really a specifically evoked response to PSC. Therefore, it can be employed as an index indicating the arriving or variation of PSC, and the characteristics as well as the process of BPSC development have been studied objectively with it. EMG was led from zygomatic region by a pair of surface electrodes and recorded with a polygraph (Model RM–45) and a data recorder (Model DTR–1204) simultaneously.

In some experiments, action potential was recorded from the radial nerve in the upper arm for its course was relatively close to the path of the Large Intestine Channel which was observed in this experiment. The responses were averaged with an average response computer as Hegu was stimulated.

II. RESULTS

(I) The blocking effect of mechanical compression on PSC

For example, puncturing Hegu, PSC travelled upward along the Large Intestine Channel to Yingxiang. PSC could be blocked when Shousanli was compressed with a spring compressor. It disappeared completely above Shousanli, but remained unchanged or enhanced below Shousanli. After the removal of the pressure, PSC arrived at Yingxiang soon. The above results could be repeated time and again in a short interval. The results of observations on the 13 channels other than the Large Intestine Channel agreed fairly well with those obtained in the Large Intestine Channel. PSC could be completely blocked in 32 cases and partially blocked in 4 cases, it could not be blocked only in one of the 37 subjects under observation. However, in most of the subjects observed, the pressure had to be applied on the path of PSC in a direction perpendicular to the skin. There would be no effect on PSC when compression was applied on the sites apart from the path of PSC.

Fig. 1 is derived from the subject A-038. As PSC evoked by puncturing Guangming arrived in the preauricular region, an intensive EMG discharge occurred. Compressing Yanglingquan, PSC as well as associated muscle responses disappeared instantly. But no influences on either of them was observed when pressure was applied on the control spots 2 cm anterior or posterior to Yanglingquan, or when the skin of Yanglingquan was clamped under the same pressure.

PSC decreased gradually in accordance with the increase of the pressure applied till it disappeared eventually. The efficient pressure for blocking was varied in persons and averaged about 800 g /cm^2.

As shown in Fig. 2, puncturing Guangming, both PSC and EMG decreased step by step till they disappeared finally as graded pressure (600 g , 1000 g and 1400 g) was brought to bear on Yanglingquan. There was a direct relationship between PSC and EMG. Both of them changed in accordance with the increasing or decreasing of the pressure applied.

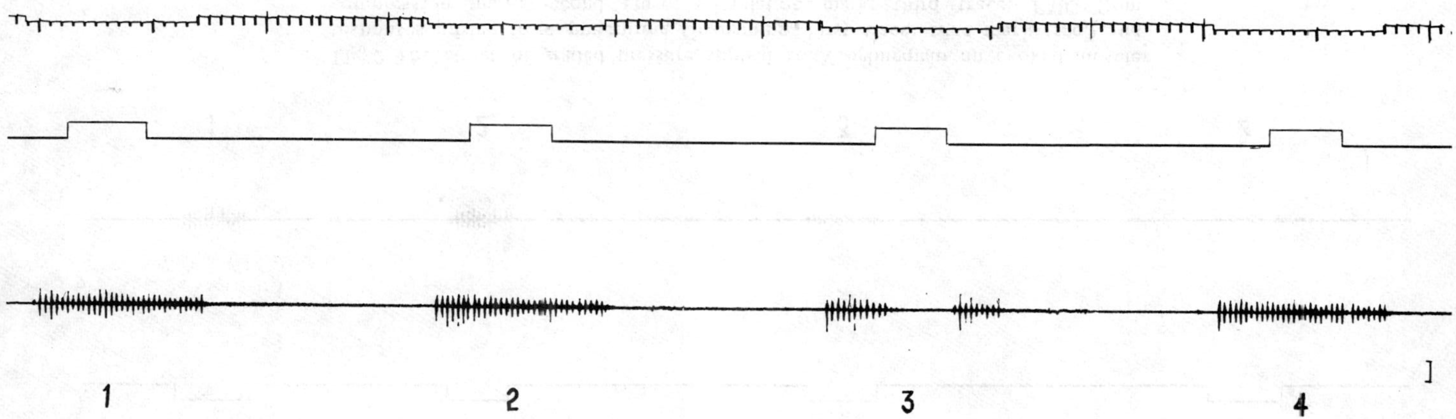

Fig. 1 The effect of compressing Yanglingquan and controls and clamping the skin of Yanglingquan on the evoked muscle response arising from puncturing Guangming.

First trace: time mark (sec.) and stimulation mark; second trace: compressing (1–3) and clamping (4) mark; third trace: EMG, calibration, $100\mu V$. 1–2, compressing the controls 2cm anterior and posterior to Yanglingquan respectively; 3, compressing Yanglingquan; 4, clamping the skin of Yanglingquan, the pressure applied in above four steps is exactly the same ($1500 gm/cm^2$). Puncturing point: Guangming.

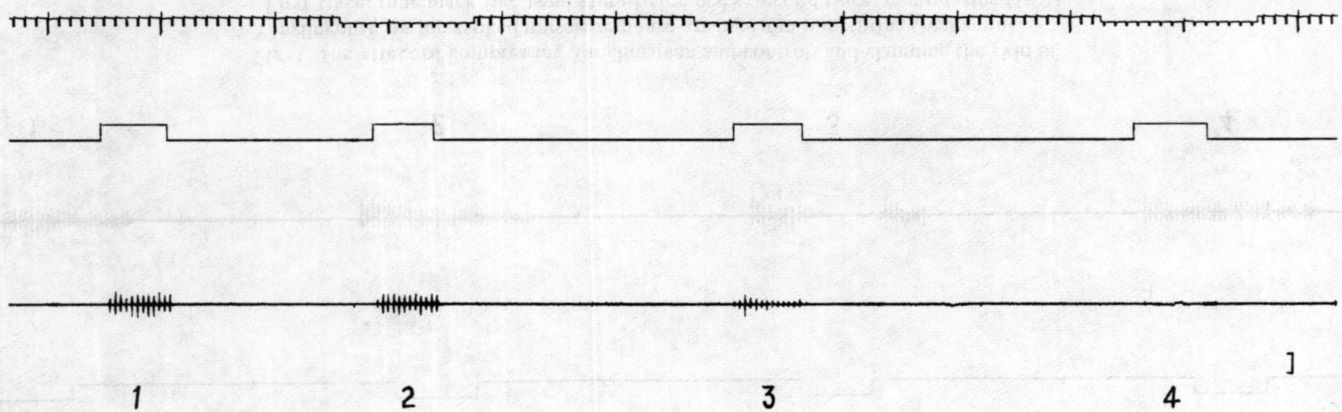

Fig. 2 The effect of graded pressure applied to Yanglingquan on evoked muscle responses arising from puncturing Guangming. First trace: time mark (sec.) and compression mark; second trace; stimulation mark; third trace: EMG from preauricular region, calibration, 100μV. 1, no compression; 2,3,4, compressions of 600gm, 1000gm and 1400gm respectively.

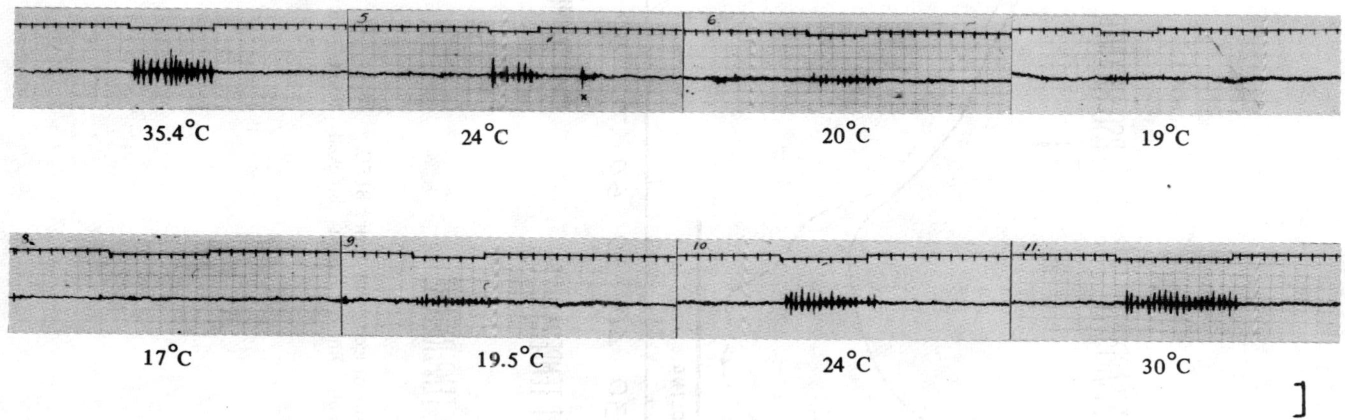

Fig. 3 Changes in evoked muscle potentials arising from puncturing Hegu in the process of cold-induced BPSC.

First trace: time mark (sec.) and stimulation mark;

Second trace: EMG, calibration 200μV, the datum below the trace indicating the point temperature of Shousanli Iced point: Shousanli.

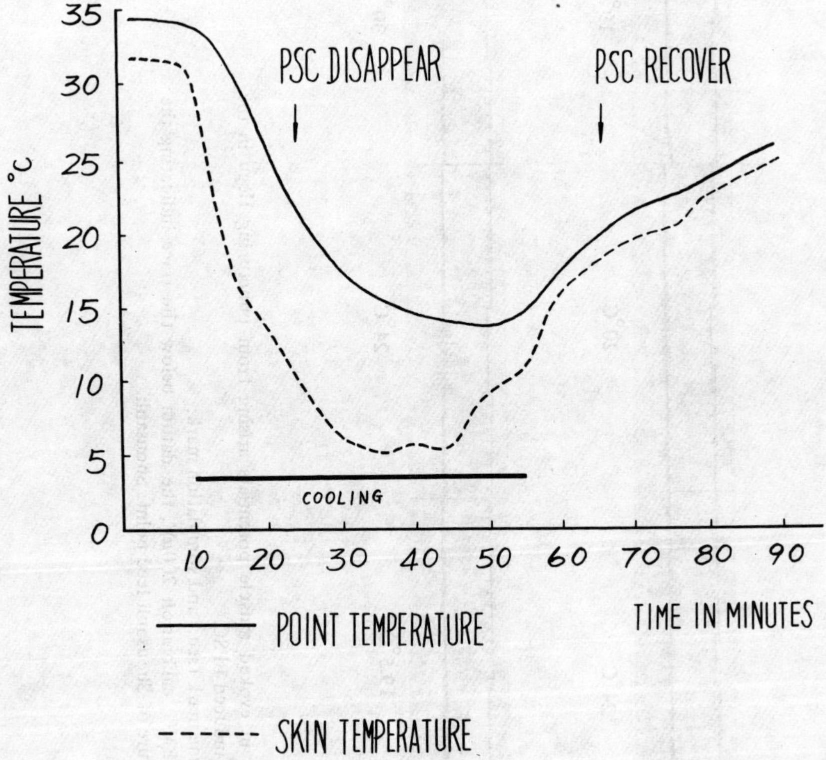

Fig. 4 Changes in the temperature of iced point during BPSC.
Yungxi Pianli Wenliu Wuli Binao Jianyu Blocked Points Unblocked Points

In some cases, PSC could be blocked with local administration of novocaine or normal saline in its path. The results of the two solutions were the same in all respects. It was suggested that BPSC, under both conditions, was brought about by the increasing of the local pressure in the deep tissue just as in the case of mechanical compression.

(II) The blocking effect of local hypothermia on PSC

PSC could be blocked by reduction of the temperature of the local deep tissue underneath the region chosen for blocking. The experiments were all carried out on the Large Intestine Channel. After a small ice bag was applied on Shousanli, PSC arising from puncturing Hegu decreased gradually and it disappeared eventually beyond Shousanli in about 20 minutes, but remained unchanged or enhanced below Shousanli. After the removal of the ice bag, PSC recovered step by step with the return of the tissue temperature. It was noted that both the development of BPSC and the recovery of PSC were progressing by degrees under the circumstances.

Fig. 3 is derived from the patient A–038. It shows that PSC and associated EMG both decreased gradually in keeping with the reduction of the point temperature of Shousanli and tended to disappear at 19°C. After the removal of the ice bag, PSC and EMG both recovered step by step with the recovery of the point temperature. It should be noted that there was a direct relationship between PSC and EMG in the development of BPSC and the recovery of PSC. Both of them varied with the variation of point temperature.

The results of 45 observations performed on 16 subjects were approximately the same. In some of them, the observation was repeated several times. It is safe to say that the results were reliable.

According to the results of 12 measurements performed on 9 subjects, the critical temperature of the deep tissue underneath the iced point for BPSC was 21.16±0.40°C. The depth of the needle inserted into the skin to induce PSC during puncturing Shousanli was about 2 cm. Therefore 2 cm was considered as the actual depth of Shousanli, and the tissue temperature measured here was designated as the point temperature.

Changes in the temperature of the iced point during BPSC in one of the measurements are shown in Fig. 4.

(III) Influence of BPSC on acupuncture analgesia

1. Before acupuncture; 2. During BPSC; 3. BPSC lifted. Data above the plethysmogram indicates the pain threshold (in hundreds of grams) in each measurement. Acupuncture point: Quchi. Compressing point: Shousanli.

Fig. 5 is one of the experimenting records. Before acupuncture, the pain thresholds from Yangxi to Jianyu were about 1100 g and the pain reactions appeared conspicuously on the plethysmogram. Puncturing Quchi, Shousanli was compressed at the same time. 30 minutes after Quchi had been stimulated, pain threshold increased sharply in Wuli, Binao and Jianyu where PSC had travelled; pain reaction disappeared from plethysmogram, but pain threshold had no conspicuous change in Yangxi, Pienli and Wenlu where PSC had been blocked, and pain reactions remained unchanged. After the lifting of the pressure, PSC

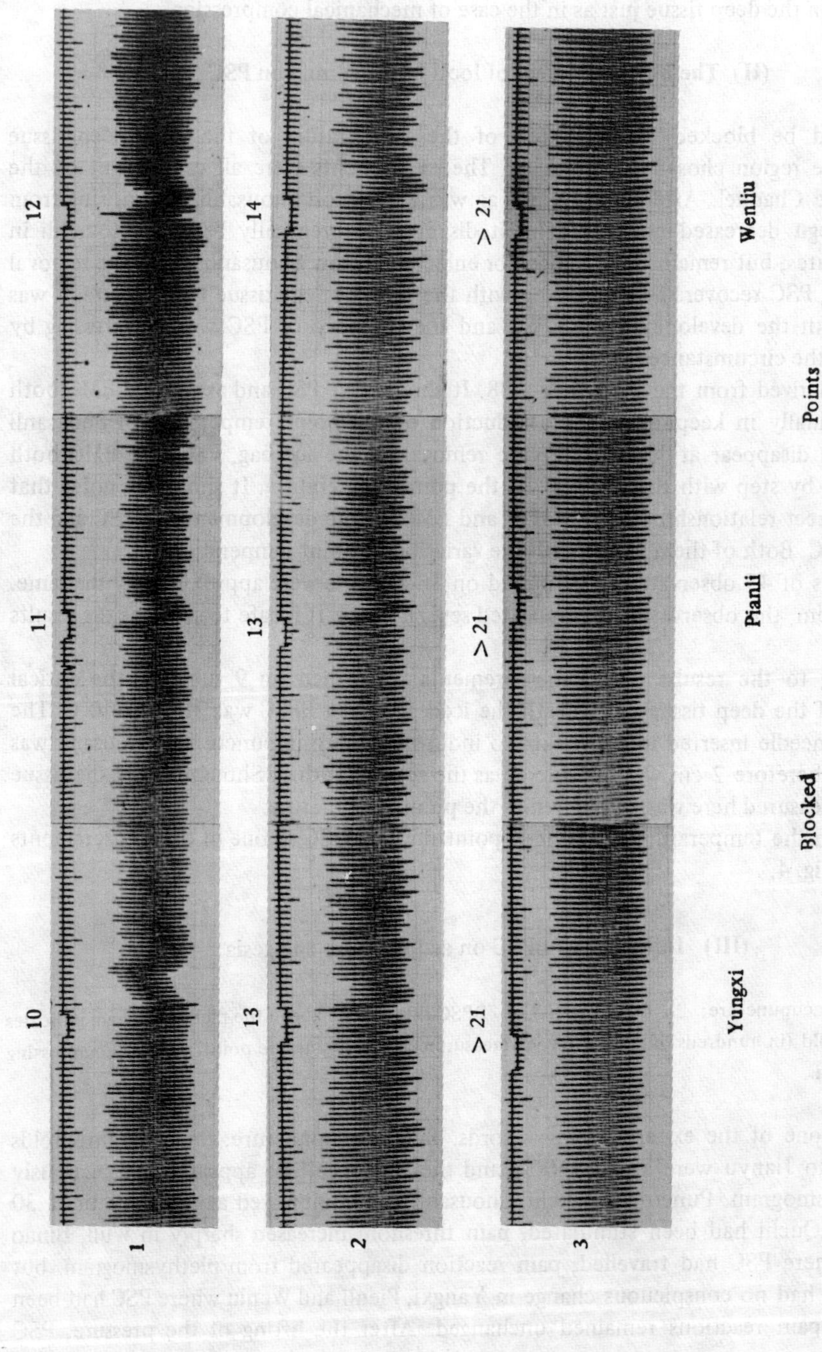
1
10
11
12
2
13
13
14
3
> 21
> 21
> 21
Yungxi
Blocked
Pianli
Points
Wenliu

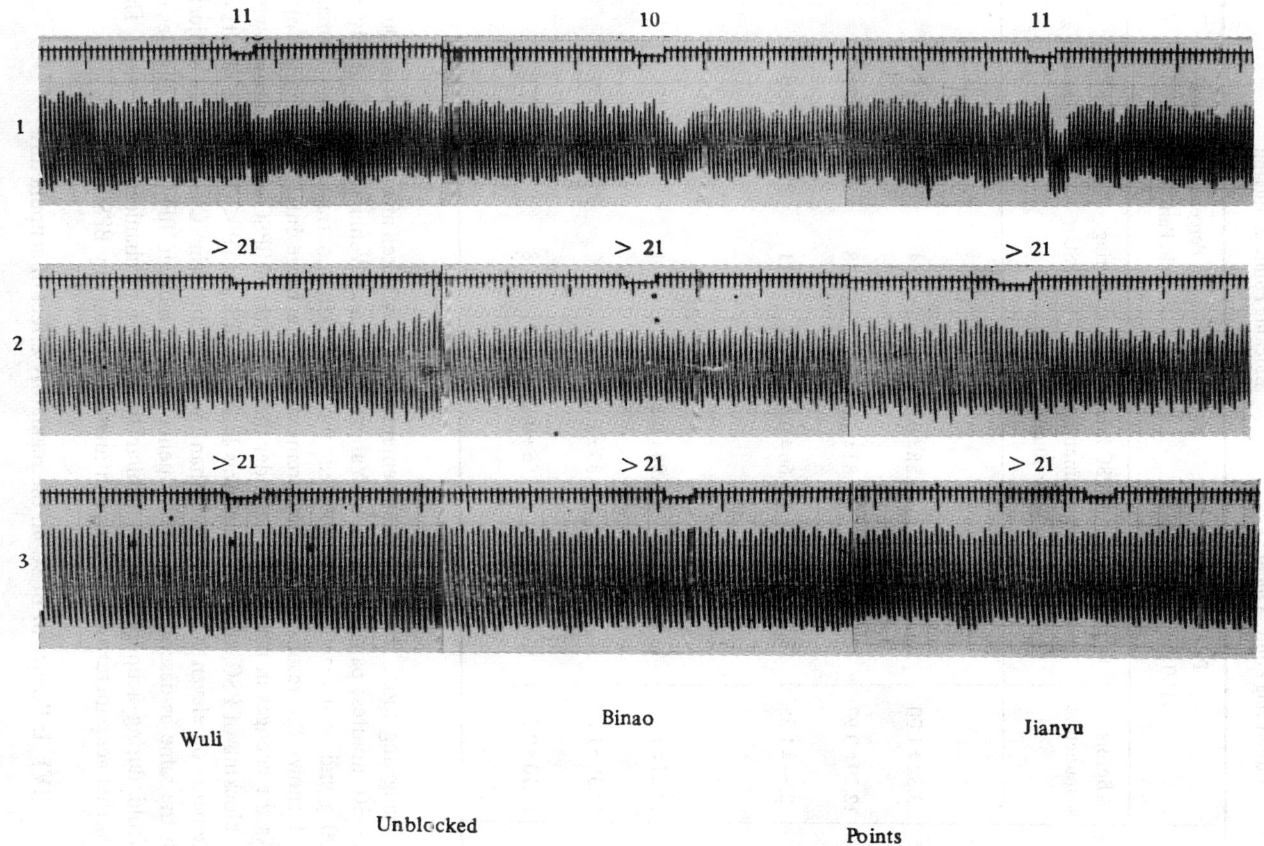

Fig. 5 The effect of BPSC on acupuncture analgesia

Table 1 The Effect of BPSC on the acupuncture analgesia

Puncturing Point: Quchi Blocking Point: Shousanli

Tested points	Pain tolerance (100 gm ; mean±S.E.)			Percentage increase in Pain tolerance (%)	
	Before acupuncture	During BPSC (puncturing for 30 min.)	BPSC lifted (puncturing for 60 min.)	During BPSC	BPSC lifted
Unblocked points					
Jianyu	13.32 ± 1.00	20.50 ± 0.33	20.88 ± 0.23	54	57
Binao	12.20 ± 0.97	20.55 ± 0.16	20.81 ± 0.25	68	71
Wuli	12.94 ± 1.25	18.56 ± 1.29	20.66 ± 0.43	43	60
Blocked points					
Pianli	13.27 ± 1.14	13.36 ± 1.22	20.94 ± 0.25	1	58
Yangxi	13.30 ± 1.29	14.18 ± 1.35	20.83 ± 1.55	7	57
Hegu	12.10 ± 0.72	13.01 ± 1.02	20.66 ± 0.35	8	71

arrived at Shangyang soon. The third measurements were then taken after stimulating Quchi for another 30 minutes; pain threshold of Yangxi, Pienli and Wenlu increased rapidly to above 2100 g and pain reactions disappeared, too. A striking contrast was then formed.

Table 1 shows the results of 19 measurements on the Large Intestine Channels of 6 subjects. As the changes in pain tolerance under the condition of BPSC were compared with that of no blocking of PSC, the difference was highly significant ($P < 0.01$). The results of 98 measurements on eleven channels other than the Large Intestine Channel of 11 subjects were much the same as described above. Influence of cold-induced BPSC on the changes of pain threshold during acupuncture was similar to that of mechanical compression. The results show that acupuncture analgesia was influenced seriously by BPSC indeed.

(IV) Influence of BPSC on the regulatory effect of acupuncture

Observations were made on 3 subjects with gastrointestinal sounds as an index indicating the movement of the gastrointestinal tract. The effect of puncturing Zusanli and Diji on the gastrointestinal sounds was observed at first. And then, the data obtained from the experiments under BPSC were compared with the former. The results of 26 observations show that the percent change in intensity index of gastrointestinal sounds (sum of the amplitudes in sound record in mm / time of recording in minutes) were 228% and 89%, respectively, following puncturing Diji and Zusanli. However, as PSC was blocked, they decreased to 22% and 29%, respectively. The difference was obvious. It reveals that the regulatory effect of acupuncture is markedly influenced by BPSC, too.

(V) Observations on the conduction of the sensory nerve that is connected with the acupuncture points during BPSC

The results show that the latency, duration and amplitude of the action potential of the radial nerve arising from stimulating Hegu did not show any change when PSC was blocked by mechanical compression at Shousanli. If 2% novocaine (2.5 ml) was injected at the point of Shousanli (for maintaining the blocked condition), the action potentials of the radial nerve arising from stimulating Hegu did not show any striking change, too. During cold-induced BPSC, there was also only a slight change in action potential.

Fig. 6 shows that PSC as well as associated EMG disappeared completely when Shousanli was iced for 20 minutes. However, only a slight change in amplitude and latency of the action potential appeared. After lifting of the BPSC, intensive discharges of the muscles reappeared. The action potentials were nearly the same under these three conditions.

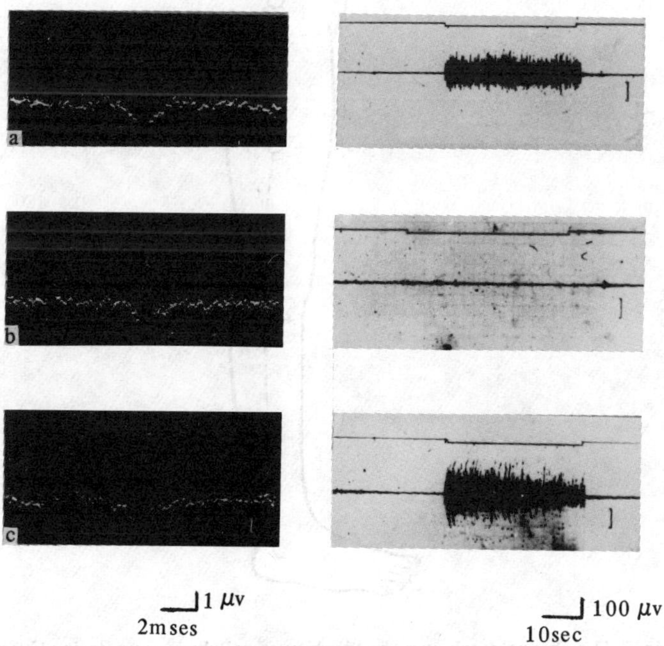

Fig. 6 Action potential of the radial nerve in the upper arm and the EMG from preauricular region during cold-induced BPSC.

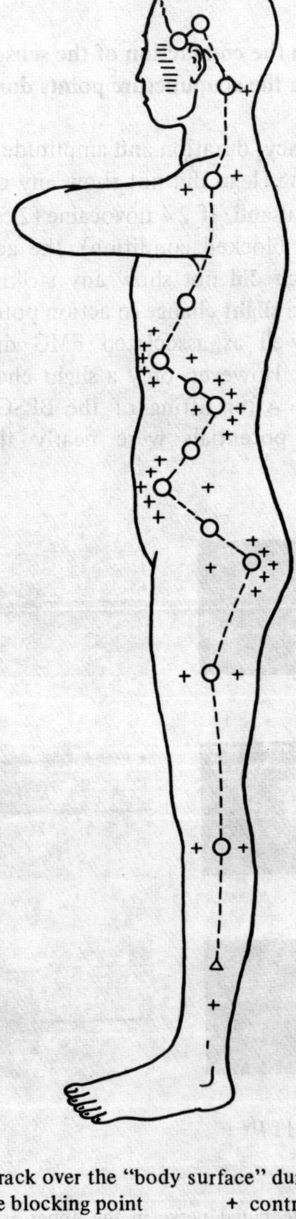

Fig. 7 The channel track over the "body surface" during puncturing Guangming.
o effective blocking point + control spot

It is evident that PSC (subjective sensation) and EMG (objective index) both changed sharply during BPSC, but the conduction of the radial nerve changed only slightly.

The results of 19 observations on 5 subjects with marked PSC were exactly alike. The results of control observations made on 10 subjects without marked PSC were nearly the same, too.

(VI) Mapping channel track on "body surface" by means of BPSC, with EMG as an indication of response of acupuncture

As mentioned above, on the subject A–038, PSC could be blocked immediately as any point on the path of PSC was compressed and the concomitant EMG discharges of muscles in the preauricular region also disappeared. However, mechanical compression applied on either side of the course of PSC or on other parts of the body manifested no influence on both PSC and EMG. Therfore, a series of blocking points could be found out by means of mechanical compression when EMG was employed as an indication of response to acupuncture. Thus, a track could be plotted out by connecting these effective blocking points.

The compressing points in mapping channel track during puncturing Guangming and the particular track obtained are shown in Fig. 7. When Guangming was punctured, intensive muscle discharges could be evoked. If one compressed one of the following 14 points: Yanglingquan, Fengshi, Huantiao, Juliao, Weidao, Daimai, Jingmen, midpoint from Jingmen to Riyue, Riyue, Zhejin, Jianjing, Fengchi, Shuaigu and Qubin, EMG discharges would disappear immediately, but no influence would occur when mechanical compression was applied on the control spots 2 cm apart from the above tested points or on the contralateral Yanglingquan and the Waiguan on both sides. Thus, a track as shown in Fig. 7 could be plotted out by connecting these 14 effective blocking points (actually it is an unbroken line linked point by point). This track not only bent forward and backward twice at the hypochondrium but also arrived at the preauricular region from the post auricular area, and its course coincided with the path of PSC and was nearly the same as the course of Gallbladder Channel. In the same way, a corresponding track could be mapped out as the points of other channels was punctured. Its existence is independent of the will of the subject. It reveals that PSC is not simply a phenomenon of sensation but also a reflection of a certain process proceeding over the "body surface" during acupuncture.

III. DISCUSSION

1. The evidence mentioned above demonstrates that PSC could be blocked by factors such as mechanical pressure and local hypothermia. The effect of acupuncture decreased markedly, and even sometimes disappeared completely, as PSC was blocked. In spite of the fact that the phenomenon of blocking of the activities of channels cannot yet be explained appropriately, its existence as well as its main characteristics have been confirmed by many other research groups[5]. In order to describe the phenomenon of BPSC objectively, we have cited a part of the records of the subject with evoked muscle response in the preauricular region in this paper. However, the characteristics of BPSC mentioned above are common to most of the subjects under observation.

2. What is the exact cause of the phenomenon of BPSC? The mechanism is not yet known, but some attempts have been made to elucidate it.

Since the conduction of the sensory nerve connected with the acupuncture point does not show any obvious changes during BPSC, and signals arising from puncturing point are still transmited to the CNS as readily as usual, it is evident that BPSC is not due to the dysfunction of the sensory nerve concerned. Up to now, there is yet no direct evidence to demonstrate whether the BPSC is caused by the mutual interference of the two afferent signals of acupuncture and compression (or cooling) in the CNS or by the blocking up of the channel path in the body surface by factors such as mechanical compression. Evidence from current research seems to favor the supposition of the "blocking up of the channel path". For example, PSC could be blocked by mechanical pressure applied to the path of PSC in a direction perpendicular to the skin, but no influence is observed when the skin of the same point is clamped. Both are mechanical pressure, however, there is a difference in direction in which the force of pressure is applied. In one the deep tissue is affected, but in the other, it is not. It seems that BPSC is not caused by mechanical compressing stimulation to cutaneous receptors. But owing to the complexity of the problem, further research is required.

3. Sufficient consideration should be given to the fact that the effect of acupuncture is markedly influenced by BPSC in further investigations on the exact cause of the phenomena of the blocking of the activities of the channels[4–10]. It follows that PSC is not simply a phenomenon of sensation but is closely related to the regulatory function of acupuncture. It cannot yet be explained satisfactorily with the medical knowledge available at present.

According to the theory of the channels and collaterals, "Xun Jing" (the progress of the functional activity in human being is closely related to channels) and "Qi Zhi" (effect is produced by the arrival of the vital energy) are two key factors in realizing the regulatory function of acupuncture. Since BPSC influences the effect of acupuncture strongly, it provides us with an efficient method for further investigation of this regulatory process. This is the basic reason why we pay so much attention to the investigation of BPSC.

IV. SUMMARY

The results of experiments performed on 37 subjects with marked PSC fully proved that the phenomenon of blocking the activities of channels surely exists. Its primary characteristics and possible causes which accounted for the phenomenon have been discussed.

Though the phenomenon of blocking the activities of channels so far cannot be explained satisfactorily, it is nevertheless an important clue in the investigation of the rule of PSC and the clarification of the nature of channels and collaterals. It should be studied thoroughly.

REFERENCES

[1] 胡翔龙等: 福建医学院学报，(3—4): 30，1961。

[2] 青岛医学院人体解剖教研组: 青岛医学院学报，(1): 76，1961。

[3] 中国人民解放军 309 医院等：针刺麻醉资料选编(二)，第 16 页，北京人民出版社，1973。
[4] 福建省医药研究所针麻原理研究组等：新医药学杂志，(4)：35，1976。
[5] 第二次全国经络感传经验交流会资料组：针刺麻醉，(2—3)：31，1977。
[6] Academy of Traditional chinese Medicine, et al : National Symposium on Acupuncture and Moxibustion and Acupuncture Anaesthesia, p.21, Beijing, 1979.
[7] Cheng Lianhu, et al : National Symposium on Acupuncture and Moxibustion and Acupuncture Anaesthesia, p.270, Beijing, 1979.
[8] Research Group on Acupuncture Anaesthesia and Channels, Guangxi College of Traditional Chinese Medicine: National Symposium on Acupuncture and Moxibustion and Acupuncture Anaesthesia, p.267, Beijing, 1979.
[9] Xiao Yongjian, et al : National Symposium on Acupuncture and Moxibustion and Acupuncture Anaesthesia, p.271, Beijing, 1979.
[10] 北京市中医院等：针刺麻醉，(2—3)：49，1977。

THE PHENOMENON OF PROPAGATED SENSATION ALONG CHANNELS(PSC) AND THE CEREBRAL CORTEX*

The use of acupuncture as a method for the examination of the function of parietal lobe and investigation of phantom limb

Xue Chongcheng**

(Department of Neuropsychiatry and Neurosurgery, The People's Hospital, Guanxi Zhuangzu Autonomous Region)

There are a lot of papers about the observation of PSC published in our own and foreign countries[1,2]. The PSC is a quite common phenomenon in the population[3] and there is no difference discovered in properties among races according to the observation of the author himself and other investigators[4]. It is still disputed as to its essence and the focus of contention is whether there exists a special tubular structure outside the nervous system or it is just a nervous function. However it is an important problem to decide.

In 1939 the author discovered that channel linear sense was present on a phantom limb when acupuncture applied to check a stump pain and a series of absences of limbs either congenital or acquired were further investigated after 1949 and the results were positive. Hereafter the author observed that PSC could occur spontaneously in patients who had intracranial stimulative lesions in the somatosensorimotor area and later on he studied the influence of development of PSC and the comparative changes of cortical sensation and PSC upon destructive cerebral lesions and positive results were also obtained. With the additional discovery of bilateral PSC induced by unilateral acupuncture, the results of clinical investigation of PSC are presented in four parts in this paper. From these results and those of modern neurological research, a preliminary idea of the basic nature of PSC has been formed and several views on it are presented here. The author considers that both in methodology and content, PSC advances forward many new things and problems for the clinical and fundamental studies of the nervous system. In some of these fields no progress has been made for several hundred years but acupuncture has done the first step. The biological significance of PSC is a very important subject worthy of serious further exploration and much attention should be given to it.

---

*Read at plenary session of the National Symposium on Acupuncture and Moxibustion and Acupuncture Anesthesia, Beijing June, 1979.

**The author's present address: Institute of Acupuncture and Moxibustion, Academy of Traditional Chinese Medicine,Beijing.

I. MATERIALS AND RESULTS

(I) Phantom limb and phantom PSC

Twenty-five patients with absence of limbs were studied. Twenty-two males and one female are acquired and two females are congenital. Their ages on observation ranged from twenty-four to fifty years old and the age of amputation (acquired only) was 17 to 41 years old. The interval between amputation and observation was from seven days to 24 years with the majority above 10 years. There are altogether 35 limbs missing, both acquired or born, including 6 left upper, nine right upper, 12 left lower and eight right lower. Eight cases are multiple absence. One of them had four limbs lost, two both upper limbs missing, four both lower limbs and one right upper and left lower. There were nine patients with 10 limbs missing over 50 cm. The longest of the absences is 70 cm and the shortest only as long as one segment of a finger and the rest are limited to between 10–50 cm. Except one acquired and two congenital that had never had experience of phantom limb before observation for 22 years and 24 years respectively, all the rest had it. The phantom was not felt upon every affected limb of the eight patients who had multiple absence. Therefore there were phantoms before observation upon 24 extremities only.

Phantom limbs of all the 25 patients were elicited by acupuncture and so were phantom channels except one congenital who refused to continue needling when the phantom limb began to develop because she was afraid of it. The phantom limb and phantom PSC were usually induced at the first time of acupuncture but this was not so when the case had never had phantom experience before. There were five cases with whom phantom limb did not occur at every acupuncture. The phantom limb and phantom PSC were felt either simultaneously as they were accompanying each other or the phantom limb prior to the phantom PSC. Though phantom limb might occur alone, there was never phantom PSC without prior phantom limb, no matter how transient.

Acupuncture could elicite phantom limb in patients who failed to get it by all other methods used previously. Phantom limbs induced by acupuncture were marked, vivid and complete, near the actual length and size of the original limbs. Furthermore they were obtained during the performance of needling and could be controlled by manipulation and the patients could tell or point out the location where the phantom was reaching.

It was found that phantom limb pain and stump pain of 16 limbs of 15 patients could be easily stopped or improved by acupuncture and no addiction was formed.

(II) Spontaneous PSC

Four patients, two male and two female, were observed. Their ages were from 20 to 69 years. Two of them suffered from intracranial tumor, one from head injury and the other had calcified spots on the skull films of unknown cause (Cases report, No. 2). All of the PSC manifested themselves in epileptic attacks. They might develop alone or as a prodromal symptom of a grand mal and they could be controlled with dilantin and relapsed when the drug was discontinued. In the case of parietal meningioma the leg of the opposite side of the lesion became paralyzed after operation, the PSC of that leg disappeared simultaneously and it reappeared again following the recovery of movement.

(III) Cortical sensation and PSC

Fifteen patients, nine male and six female, aged 11–70 years old were studied. Nine cases had space-occupying lesions such as tumour and abscess of the parietal lobe, two had frontoparietal injury, two had vascular accident of the internal capsule, and the nature of the other two was unknown although the involvement was localized at the frontoparietal region by apparent symptoms and signs. There were seven at right side, six left and two bilateral.

Four patients (two had operative destruction) had marked nervous symptoms and signs, but all the superficial, deep, acupuncture, cortical sensations and PSC were intact. Acupuncture sensation means senses such as soreness, numbness, and distension, etc., produced by acupuncture; it has been abbreviated as "acupuncture sense" and this term will be used in the following paragraphs.

Five patients' postcentral gyrus was damaged seriously by operation, but without effect on superficial, deep and acupuncture sensations; in three of them the cortical sensation was seriously decreased, but the PSC was slightly decreased, and in the other two patients both the cortical sensation and PSC were decreased.

One patient showed intact superficial, deep and acupuncture sensations while the cortical sensation and PSC were involved bilaterally, and the side opposite to the lesion was markedly decreased and the ipsilateral side was just decreased.

Two patients had no change in the superficial and acupuncture sensation. One of them revealed loss of deep sensation and the other was decreased. Their cortical sensation and PSC were lost. After regain of sensation, the deep sensation was returned to normal, the cortical sensation reappeared, accompanied by PSC correspondingly; one patient restored to decrease and the other one to normal.

Upon one cerebral injury of bilateral frontoparietal lobes, the cortical representation areas of both legs were more serious than the arm areas and the left side was more serious than the right, and the severity of disturbance of sensation was just the reverse of the severity of his trauma (details were described in Case report No. 3).

Upon one with bilateral lesions, the superficial and acupuncture sensations were not influenced while the deep sensation of the left upper limb was markedly decreased and lost over the left lower limb; it was normal over the right upper limb and decreased over the right lower. The cortical sensation was decreased over the left upper limb and the whole right side of the body and lost over the left lower limb. The PSC of the right extremities was normal and decreased markedly over the left upper limb and lost over the left lower.

One case with hemorrhage of the internal capsule lost all kinds of sensation including PSC at the early stage of the disease. During the reintegration of the sensations, the order of recovery was acupuncture sense, visual, vibration, superficial, PSC and cortical. Before the returning of PSC, the localization of superficial, deep and acupuncture sensation was incapable. When the recovery of cortical sensation was incomplete, the propagation of channel sensation was rather short and they regained their normal appearance almost proportionally.

From the results mentioned above it can be summarized that the location of changes of cortical sensation and the PSC are identical and the degrees of their disturbance and restoration are generally corresponding although they may be dissociated. The endurability of PSC against disease and injury showed to be stronger than that of the cortical sensation. The sore, numb and distending senses of acupuncture did not change with PSC and cortical sensation, but did so with superficial sensation.

(IV) Bilateral PSC induced by unilateral acupuncture

There were only two adult male patients. The site for eliciting bilateral PSC was restricted; one was located merely at both Tauwei points and the other at the points in the lower part of the body. During the occurrence of the bilateral PSC, neither of other sensations had bilateral reactions for their corresponding stimulation of a single side.

II. METHOD

All of the subjects of each group were mentally clear, cooperative, and communicative in language with the observer, and there was no auditory or verbal aphasia. They were approached by ordinary clinical contact and none was specialized for observation. Suggestion was avoided as much as possible.

The common filiform needle made of stainless steel was used. The manipulation for the first group varied according to the different concrete conditions of the subjects. The points acupunctured on the stump were those which were easier to get sensation. When comparison of the affected part and the healthy part was made in the same time of observation the affected part was acupunctured usually first and then the healthy part. Manipulation for the third group was of the slow rotation method for insertion and maintenance of the needle. The points used for observation were limited to the extremities only and the points of the trunk and head used for treatment were excluded. All points were acupunctured repeatedly.

The results of the third group were decided by means of the following criteria:

The duration of acupuncture of each point was limited to within 20 min each time. The longest length of PSC felt within the 20 min was used to judge the ability of its expression. It was considered as loss of PSC and acupuncture sensation if they did not occur within the 20 min allowed. The number of times of acupuncture for each patients was quite different. It would be small if it was easy to decide the presence of PSC and cortical sensation, and vice versa but it should not be less than 20 times. When counterrviews were taken about both sides, the points were symmetrically selected. Before each time of acupuncture, the superficial, deep and cortical sensations were checked. The period of observation was generally 15–30 days, but the longest one was over 10 years.

The cortical sensations consisted of steregnosis, barognosis, topesthesia, graphesthesia, and spatial discrimination and the steregnosis was the main one among them. The results were classified into five grades according to the location and other conditions of the body. A patient with ability of precise discrimination upon four of the above six senses would be rated as normal, and with none of them would be considered as loss of them. To be able to make out with difficulty only large and rough objects (which are easy to be distingushed) was considered as a serious derease in sense; to be able to do this without much difficulty was considered a marked decrease in sense. To be able to distingush surely large and bulky objects, but not closely similar things (such as the relief patterns on enamelware or socks made of similar fabrics like cotton and nylon) was regarded as a decrease in senses.

As the chief characteristic of PSC is propagation, it was used to determine whether the PSC of a patient is normal or not. Since the propagation rarely runs through the whole course of a channel as described in traditional Chinese medical literature by ordinary acupuncture in daily clinical work, the common ranges of propagation of some point were taken as the criterion for the graduation; for example, the range of propagation from above the knee down to the foot was considered to be normal for Zusanli, Sanyinjiao, Yinlingquan, and Yanglingquan, that from above the buttocks down to the foot for Fengshi, that from the shoulder down to the finger for Neiguan and Waiguan, etc. One hundred percent propagation within these ranges was considered as normal response of PSC; ¾ as decreased; ½ as markedly decreased; and ¼ as seriously decreased. It would not be regarded as completely lost as long as there is propagation, no matter how short it is. When there is no propagation sensation but only local sensation of soreness, numbness, or distention, the patient is said to have acupuncture sense but no PSC. The intensity of PSC and its maintenance time are not considered as main factors because they are not the most important properties. The assessment of the changes in superficial and deep sensations is made as it is done in ordinary clinical work but they are classified into five grades too and so are acupuncture sense.

The manual skill used for Group 4 was similar to that for Group 3 and the relay method was applied.

The propagative condition of PSC was described verbally by the patients and sometimes they showed the PSC course by drawing it on their body surface with their fingers.

III. CASE REPORT

Case 1. Male, aged 39 years. Amputation of both lower limbs was done in 1951 after injury. Immediately after the operation, he experienced uncomfortable phantom feeling and stump pain on the left side whenever the weather was turning cold. During such attacks he was unable to walk with the artificial limb. The right stump had no discomfort. He was investigated in March, 1964.

P. E. The right toes were all excised from the metatarsophangeal joints and the left was cut 13 cm below the lower border of the patella. The left leg was 27 cm shorter than the right one. The wound healed well without neuroma and the muscles were slightly atrophied. No phantom could be elicited by means of squeezing, vibration of tuning fork, pricking the skin or moving the stump. In the investigative period he received 12 times of acupuncture and five times of moxibustion, all of them induced phantom limb and PSC, and most of the latter were marked. The followings are instances.

On March 26, 1964, acupuncture of the right Yanglingquan produced numb and distending senses spreading like a thread upward through the lateral side of the thigh, the right side of the abdomen, and the chest, the right shoulder, the right side of the neck, the front of the right ear to the right fronto-temporal region. At the shoulder, a branch ramified to the right arm passing through the forearm along their dorsomedial aspect to the hand, then it divided into five branches, one to each finger. From the site of needling the linear sensation spreaded downwards through the lateral side of the leg to the dorsum of the foot and then it divided into five rami, one to each toe and the one to the great toe was more marked than the others.

Acupuncture of the left Yanglingquan, the spreading course of the linear sensation was similar to that on the right side while the upper end terminated at the shoulder.

Acupuncture of the left Yinlingquan, numb and distending linear sensation propagated upwards through the medial side of the thigh, the right side of the abdomen to the upper chest, then turned to the anterio-medial side of the left upper limb and ramified in the hand into five branches to the tips of the fingers, one for each. Simultaneously in the opposite direction the sensation travelled downwards along the medial side of the leg, the medial condyle, dorsum of the foot to the tips of the toes in the way as it does in the hand (Fig. 1).

Acupuncture of the right Yinlingquan produces the same result as that of the left side with the exception of the right arm.

Moxibustion of the right Yinlingquan produced warmth sensation spreading upwards and downwards just as the acupuncture does, but the ascending branch reaches only as far as the lower abdomen.

All of the limbs and PSC outside the stump are phantom.

Both insertion and maintenance of the needle were done by slow gentle rotating and twisting manipulation and mild moxibustion was practised. The patient has some local sensation at the site of acupuncture stimulation at the beginning and then the sensation propagated slowly and bipolarly upward and downward. Whenever the needle was twisted the sensation would be heavy, but when twisting stopped the sensation could be either light or lost completely. The intensity and speed of the propagation of the sensation in both directions were not always the same at different moments of stimulation. When sensation occurred, the phantom limb would appear first and then the PSC.

Case 2. Male, aged 32 years, married, a barefoot doctor in a village, right handed, was admitted on March 14, 1973, because of repeated attacks of convulsion for more than one year. The first seizure developed suddenly and afterwards it occurred irregularly, sometimes once in several months and sometimes many times in one day. At the beginning of each attack he had a numb feeling in the dorsal bifurcate region of the ring and the little fingers of the right hand and then the sensation would spread centrally throughout the dorsolateral surface of the hand, the middle line of the dorsum of the forearm and the lower and middle portions of the arm, and further upward it would turned slightly posteriorly in the upper portion of the arm, reaching the shoulder and the neck. It went to the face and the parietal region of the head just in front of the ear. Sometimes it branched along the upper edge of the auricle forwards to the outer canthus (Fig. 2). The intensity of the sensation and its speed of propagation of every attack were different but its nature was always the same sore, distending and numb pain. When the sensation was intense and its propagation was swift, then the convulsion would be violent, and conversely the weaker and slower the sensation the milder the convulsion would be. The patient had been a practitioner himself of acupuncture and moxibustion and once he blocked the spreading sensation by means of cone moxibustion and the convulsion was inhibited. Hereafter he always used this method to check his suffering and more often than not he was successful, especially when the sensation was weak and slow. If the spreading could not be blocked by one cone, another was given at a new site where the linear sensation was being felt. This might be repeated several times during each attack and sometimes he was triumphant at the suppression of the convulsion. It was difficult and impossible to stop the spreading when the sensation had arrived at the upper part of the middle one third of the arm. When the sensation reached the

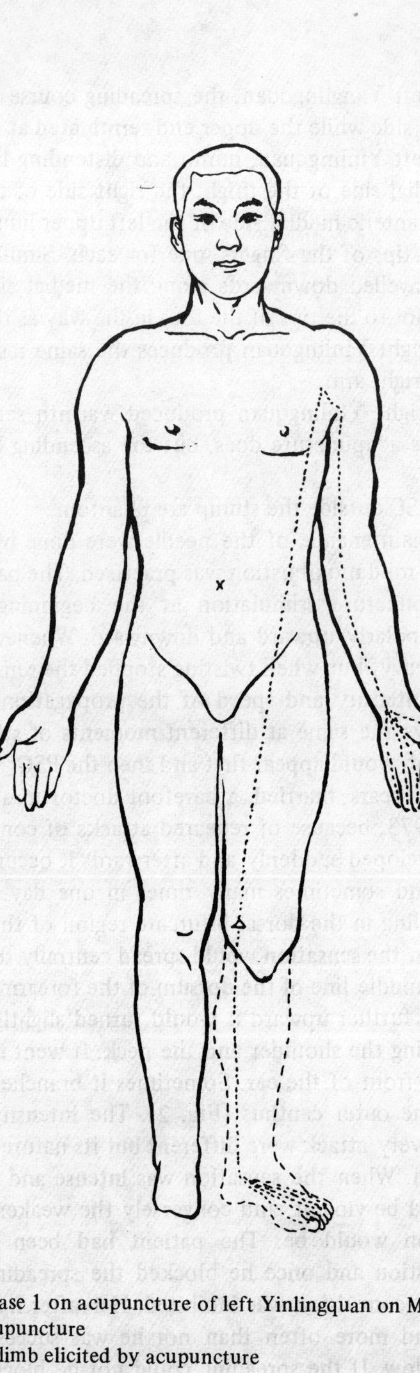

Fig. 1 The PSC of Case 1 on acupuncture of left Yinlingquan on March 26, 1964.

△ Site of acupuncture

–– Phantom limb elicited by acupuncture

. . . PSC during acupuncture

The course of the PSC manifested itself as connection of Foot Taiyin Spleen and Hand Shaoyin Heart Channels.

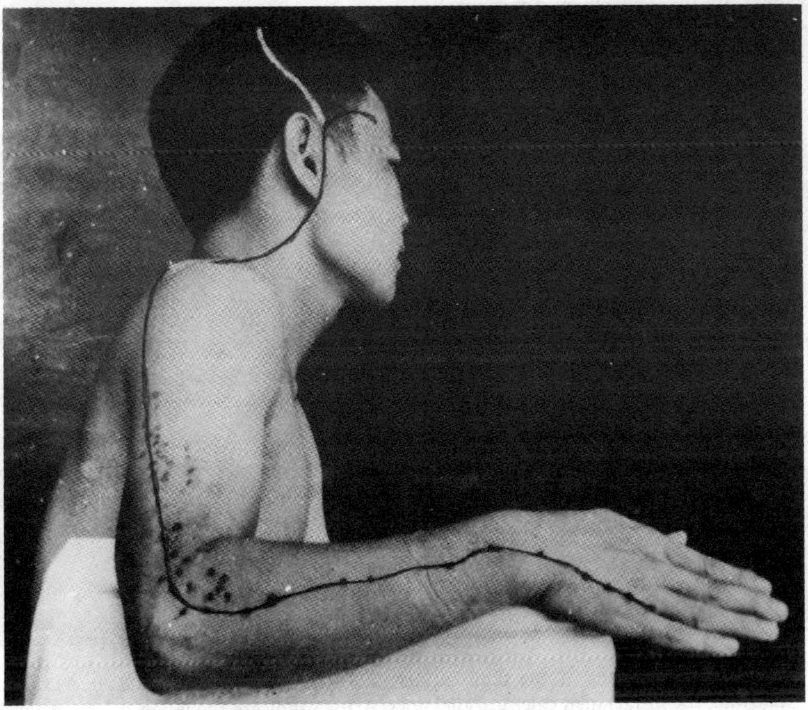

Fig. 2 The spontaneous PSC of Case 2 (black and white lines). The course of the PSC manifested itself as Hand Shaoyang Sanjiao Channel.
The black spots are the burning scars due to moxibustion applied by the patient himself in an attempt to cease the attack of convulsion.

face, his mind was still clear but he could no longer say what he wanted and he knew he was helpless. When it reached above the auricle, the involuntary movement would begin from the right arm, and his mouth would be twisted to the right. After this his whole body would be in convulsion and he lost consciousness. The effect of moxibustion was obtained when severe burning pain was just occurring. A lot of drugs were tried without success except dilantin which would check both the attack of convulsion and the occurrence of the linear sensation.

There was nothing unusual in both his personal and his family's histories.

General and neurological examinations showed no pathological findings except many burn scars, sized 0.5 cm in diameter over the dorsal side of the arm around the elbow joint (Fig. 2). The numb sensation elicited by acupuncture was the same as the natural one and for fear of inducing attack of convulsion no attempt was made to produce PSC. X-ray films of the skull showed a patch of calcification spots behind the middle and lower portions of the coronary suture of the left side with a total area of about 2.5 × 3 square cm. The bone around the spots was denser than other part (Fig. 3, 4). The EEG, cerebral arteriograms and lumbar puncture were all normal. He was diagnosed as symptomatic epilepsy correlated to the calcifications and discharged with the suggestion of continuous administration of dilantin. One and half years later he was reexamined and found normal in all respects. The

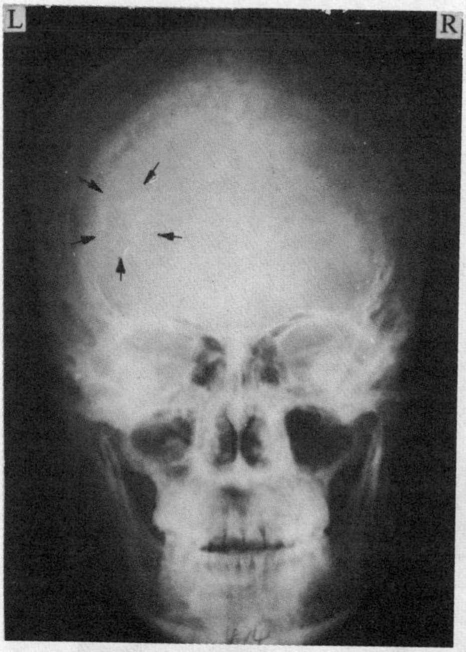

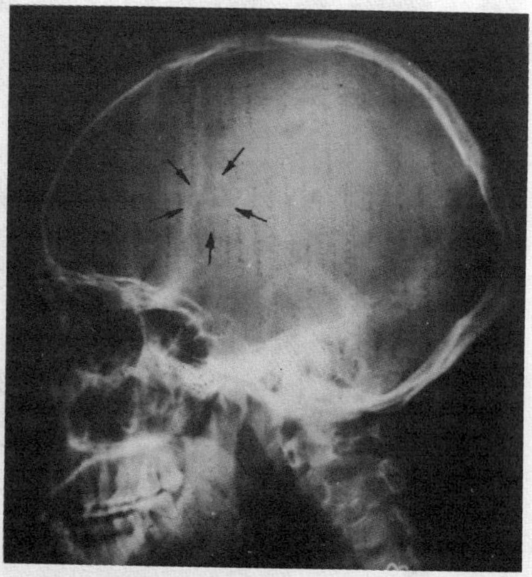

Fig. 3 & 4 The films of the skull of Case 2. P–A (Fig. 3) and lateral (Fig. 4) views. Showing the intracranial calcification spots. Arrows indicate the lesion.

epilepsy recurred occasionally but it would be effectively controlled with dilantin and it would return as soon as the taking of the drug was discontinued.

Case 3. Male, 44 years old, suffered from head injury in a gunshot accident in 1951 and lay unconscious for four days. When he regained his mind, his four limbs had been paralyzed and he was also suffering from retention of urine and stool. A little bone and brain tissue were sectioned for removal of foreign bodies from the wound. After operation he lost control of urine and was as paralyzed as before but no aphasia was developed. Three months after the operation, incontinence of urine disappeared gradually, and after 15-17 months his left and right hands gradually became moveable one after the other and after two years his both legs also began to be able to move.

From the date of injury till 1962, the patient had only sense of pain below the neck, and all other sensations such as texture, size, form, hardness, and weight were all lost. Even right and left and the position of the body and the limbs could not be distinguished. When he saw a familiar object he could name it, describe its nature and usage and how to use it but he could not make those out by his hands and feet. He actually had tactile agnosis and autotopagnosis. Only after 1962 did these sensations began to appear first in the two hands but merely for the simple and coarsest objects.

Since 1958 he had received acupuncture and moxibustion therapy for five years, and the total number of times of needling was about 5,000– about 1,000 for each of the four limbs and one thousand for the trunk. In the first six months, there was only pain sensation from acupuncture and in the second six months, the sensation became numb pain and one year later, it became gradually numbness and distension. After 1960, linear sensation began to occur in the left upper limb occasionally and later in the right arm and after 1961 also occasionally in both legs. However the spreading of the sensation did not go far and could not last long in the early stage and as time went on the sensation went further and further so that in the left side of the body it went from the arm to the finger. During the five years the total number of appearance of PSC was less than 20 times in the upper limbs and less than 8 in the lower ones and most of these only occurred in the last stage of the treatment.

Physical examination on March 28, 1964 showed the sagittal distance from the external occipital protuberance to the middle of the two eyebrows was 36 cm long. The defect of the skull was prismatic in shape with a length 12 cm long, perpendicular to the sagittal line. It was 7 cm long on the left side of the middle line and 5 cm on its right. The widest part of the defect was 6 cm located right on the middle line. The posterior edge of the widest part was 12 cm above the external occipital protuberance and the anterior edge was 18 cm to the middle of the eyebrows. Cerebral pulsation was palpable at the defect. The cranial nerves were normal. The upper limbs had a muscular force of Grade V and the legs, IV, the right limbs being weaker than the left ones. The right hand and both legs were seriously deformed and he could not walk. Both legs showed crippling muscular atrophy due to uselessness and were hypertonicity of the clasp knife type. The knees were extended and the legs crossed each other. All the tendon reflexes of the four limbs were exaggerated and ankle clonus was sustained on both sides. The abdominal reflex of the left side was next to nothing and that on right side was totally lost. Cremesteric reflex was lost on both sides. Both hands had pathological reflexes and all types of plantar reflex were also pathological.

Superficial and acupuncture sensations of the whole body were normal. The deep sensation of the arms was normal, but that of the legs was seriously decreased. The cortical sensation of the upper limbs was normal (e. g., the two-point discrimination was 42 mm) and that of the both legs had decreased seriously (e. g., the two-point discrimination was 180 mm). The PSC of both arms was normal and that of both legs had seriously decreased. Reexamination in April 1974, showed that superficial and deep sensation and acupuncture sensation were all normal. The cortical sensation of the left arm had seriously decreased and that of all the rest limbs was completely lost. PSC was decreased in the left upper limb and seiously decreased in the left lower limb and that in both the right limbs was totally lost.

A comparison of the number of occurrences of PSC and the number of times of acupuncture may also show the severity of disturbance of the PSC; therefore they are listed in the following table. The number of times of acupuncture is given in parenthesis.

Limbs	Left		Right	
	Upper	Lower	Upper	Lower
1964	5(6)	1(5)	5(6)	2(15)
1974	4(6)	2(15)	0(6)	0(15)
Total	9(12)	3(30)	5(12)	2(30)

Case 4. Male, 23 years old. His third lumbar vertebra was broken comminutedly on Dec. 20, 1958 and laminectomy was performed immediately for decompression. After the

operation both paraplegia and incontinence of urine remained without improvement.

Physical examination on March 26, 1964, found that both legs showed complete flaccid paralysis and all tendon reflexes were completely lost. Marked myatrophy occurred below the waist and there was no pathological reflex. Periodic reflex micturition appeared once about every 15 min. Below the level of L2, no corresponding sensation except numbness could be induced by the various means of stimulation used in such physical examination even when knocked with a percussion hammer. Sensations above this level were normal. No bilateral reaction was discovered when classical sensory stimulations were applied unilaterally.

Acupuncture of the left Zusanli made the patient feel tightness, distention, numbness and pulsation at beginning and then spreading linearly and quickly upward through the medial side of the thigh to the left testicle. With the arrival of the sensation at the testicle, a tight-pressing linear sensation developed over the right testicle, and spread downward along the medial side of the right thigh and lateral side of the leg, the dorsum and the sole of the foot to the five toes. The right Zusanli was then acupunctured and the sensory phenomenon was just a repeat of the above. Acupuncture of Quchi produced only unilateral PSC. Because of the presence of paresthesia on the lower part of his body, the observation was discontinued.

In April of 1974, the patient was examined again. All sensations were lost below the 12th thoracic segment except vibration. No paresthesia disclosed. Other symptoms and signs were the same as 10 years ago.

Acupuncture of left Zusanli, produced numb and distending sensations first at the site of stimulation. Then the sensations propagated bipolarly as a line ascending to the knee where it stopped for a little while and then continued to go upward along the lateral side of the thigh to the anterior part of the iliac region where it had a very transient second intermission and then passed through the abdomen and stopped at the left Tianshu. When an addition of needling of Tianshu was taken the propagation extended again from the point upwards to the left costal margin where it ceased again. The patient felt very uncomfortable because of the occurrence of severe peristaltic gurgles in the abdomen when the Tianshu point was acupunctured; therefore no relay was given at the terminal of the sensation. The descending portion of the propagation went to the second toe along the leg anterio-laterally. When the travelling of the PSC reached the foot and the middle of the left thigh there was a numb and distending sensation developed over the right Zusanli spontaneously and then propagated like a thread both upward and downward. The ascending propagation reached the right Tianshu where it stopped and when the left Tianshu was read it went on again to the costal margin. The descending branch went on the right foot. The course of propagation downward and upward was the same as that on the left side. The intensity of the right PSC was reinforced when the stimulation of the left side was strengthened but somewhat less than that on the left side. The sensations remained for several hours after withdrawal of the two needles on the left side.

On the next day when the right Zusanli was acupunctured, the same happened on the left side as the day before, but the occurrence of PSC of the contralateral sied was 15 min behind that on the right side. To avoid excessive peristalsis that made the patient very uncomfortable, no additional acupuncture was done at Tianshu. On the same day the left Neiquan and Sibai were acupunctured and PSC appeared at both points but the response was limited to the left side. There was no response on the opposite side. Hereafter points such as Xuanzhong, Fengshi, Futu, Sanyinjiao and Yinlingquan and so on were acupuncture repeatedly for 18 times upon each side. Thirty-one out of the 36 (17 upon left and 14 right) developed bilateral PSC by unilateral acupuncture, but acupuncture of points of the face and the upper limbs for 25 times never produced any bilateral PSC.

IV. DISCUSSION

PSC cannot be used as evidence of the existence of a tube structure of channel or meridian because it is a kind of sensation, and this concept has been reinforced after the discovery of phantom PSC.

Hecaen and Penfield[5] declared that phantom limb could be elicited by stimulating the parietal lobe and abolished by excision of the posterior central gyrus. These events lend support to the belief that the cerebral cortex is the material foundation of phantom sensation. From this it can be inferred that PSC should also have a material foundation as the phantom limbs have. Cases presented in this paper show that spontanecus PSC could be induced by stimulative lesions on the cortex without any peripheral needling; the PSC manifested itself as epileptic attack and it could be controlled by administration of dilantin; on the other hand no PSC could be elicited by peripheral acupuncture in presence of destructive lesions on the cortex even by persistent stimulation and the intimate relationship of the corresponding changes of the cortical sensation and PSC in intracranial diseases, etc. All of these are further evidence verifying the above viewpoint.

The study of phantom limbs has a history of over four hundred years. It was thought that the phantom limb was the result of the engram of body schema on the cortex due to the long and repeated stimulation of the limb, and the schema would not disappear even when the limb no longer exists, and the phantom would be experienced whenever suitable stimulation, either physical or chemical, on the cortex occurred. This is the body schema engram theory of phantom limb.

Weinstern and Sersen[6] discovered the phantom limb of congenital absence of limbs and they explained that the body schema had its origin in the gene. This genetic theory has not been extensively accepted because the number of cases is still too small, the phantoms of the congenitals are too vague, the occurrence is very infrequent in the whole life of the patients and the duration of each occurrence is also too short. Discovery of phantom PSC makes the genetic theory seem more hopeful. Since PSC can appear on phantom and it is not engramed by long standing stimulation of a limb and it occurs on the phantoms of congenital and normals too, so it supports the genetic theory favorably. Simultaneously these facts indicate the genetic origin of the PSC itself too. It can be present in different length of propagation for everyone under certain conditions without any variation in character among races and its important therapeutic actions are also in support of this viewpoint. It is evident that the specific spreading along channel pattern in the cerebrum had been developed by phylogenesis and evolution.

However PSC is a kind of sensation and the author had called it channel or meridan sensation. Sensation is not delivered at the peripheral site where stimulation is applied but in the cerebrum, especially its cortex. When some part of the cortical body representation area is stimulated or impulse reaches it, sensation develops and is felt at the corresponding peripheral part by projection. Reversely, sensation propagated along certain course like a thread or a band over a peripheral part of the body must have impulse spreading along a phylogenetic channel specific pattern over the part of the corresponding body representation area of the cortex.

Some corresponding points of the peripheral acupoint on the specific channel pattern of the cortex initiates propagation easily as a trigger does. It may be the cause of sensitivity of some peripheral points and the so called marked PSC person may be the result of presence of extensive sensitive points on the cortex.

Recognition of PSC must be at Brodmann's areas 3, 1, 2, because it has properties of awareness of localization, direction, size, nature and intensity, etc., so it is a kind of discriminative sensation. However, it can be dissociated from cortical sensation and manifest itself bilaterally when stimulation is applied unilaterally, and furthermore its spreading condition such as speed is disproportional to the size of the respective body representation areas of the sensory area I (SI), and the order of spreading of the PSC from the originating point outward or vice versa is not entirely identical with the order of the arrangement of the sensory homunculus of the SI even in thalamus. Therefore it may be closely related to SI, but it is not produced entirely there; the spreading is rather likely to be in other sensory areas such as sensory area II (SII). Hence the author thinks that the specific spreading pattern may be at other sensory areas, e.g., SII, and the completion of recognization is at SI. It is accomplished in two steps (Fig. 5). Thus the clinical phenomena such as the approximate identification in the changes of cortical sensation and PSC, their dissociation from each other and the bilateral projections of PSC, could be explained by this two-step viewpoint. Based on the characteristics of PSC it has been considered that there might be meridian centers in the cerebral cortex. The area where the impulses spread may be named as Meridian Center I (MI) and where recognition of PSC takes place as Meridian Center II (MII). The bilateral PSC induced by unilateral stimulation may be expounded as bilateral projections of fibers of the propagative area as SII to the SI of both sides and it has no connection with other sensations.

The results reveal that the disturbance of PSC in some cases was milder than that of the cortical sensation. This phenomenon makes the author think that the strength of resistance of PSC against diseases and injury may be greater than that of the cortical sensation. Viewed from phylognesis, this means PSC is older than cortical sensation. This two-step viewpoint of the formation of PSC lends support to the theory that SI is newer than the other sensory areas such as SII.

In accordance with the changes of various kinds of sensations produced by acupuncture upon patients with cortical destructive lesions, the PSC changed with the cortical sensation, but the changes of the acupuncture sensations such as soreness, numbness and distension, were accompanied closely with the superficial sensation. Therefore it may be considered that the PSC gets into consciousness at the cortex and the acupuncture sensations may be percepted in the subcortical centers.

Actually the spontaneous PSC of the stimultive cortical lesion is a kind of epilepsy and it is further confirmed by the fact that dilantin could control it and it would break out again as soon as the drug is discontinued. To the author's knowledge there was no description about this type of epilepsy both in the foreign and our own medical literature. Really it introduces a new attack type of epilepsy and the author has called it meridian sensory epilepsy or sensory epilepsy of the meridian attack type.

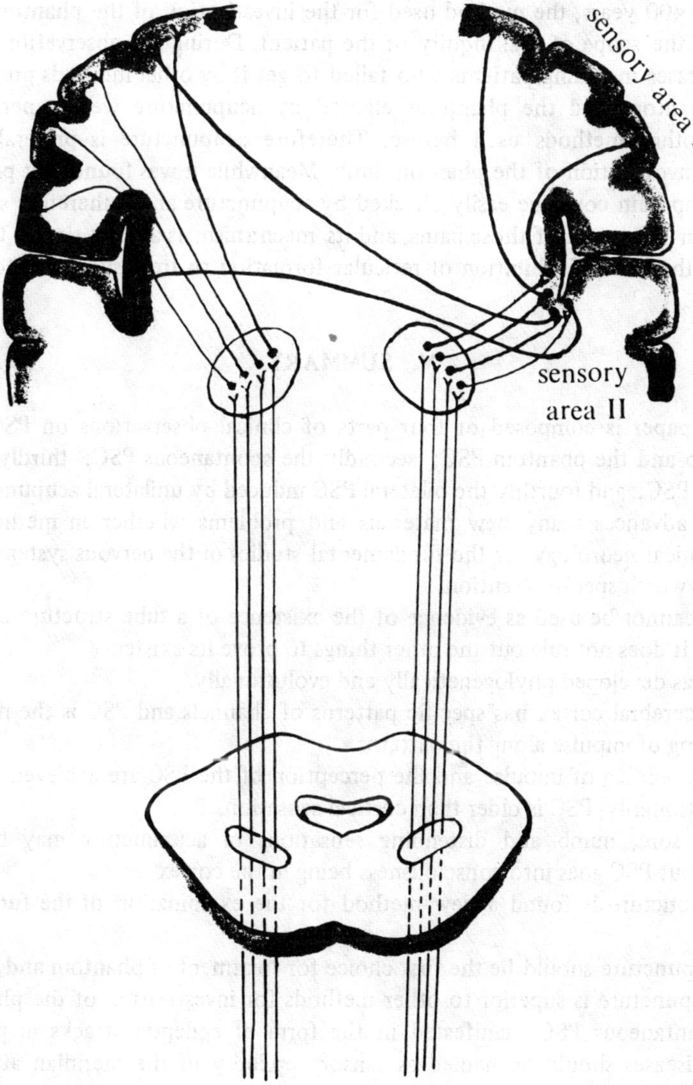

Fig. 5 The presumptive conduction course of PSC (right side) and the conduction course of cortical sensation (left side). Pons below omitted.

As PSC is an expression of the function of the parietal lobe, therefore it is possible to examine the function of that lobe by observing the PSC with use of acupuncture. The clinical experiences related in this paper also prove the feasibility of this method. It would be a new technique for the clinical examination of the parietal lobe since the recommendation of bilateral simultaneous stimulation made by Bender in 1952.

For over 400 years, the method used for the investigation of the phantom limb never went beyond the scope of oral inquiry of the patient. During the observation of phantom channels, all cases including patients who failed to get it by other methods previously used, developed phantom and the phantoms elicited by acupuncture were superior to those induced by other methods used before. Therefore acupuncture is preferable to other methods for investigation of the phantom limb. Meanwhile it was found that phantom limb pain and stump pain could be easily checked by acupuncture and it therefore should be the first choice for treatment of those pains, and its mechanism is at least similar to the theory of increasing the level of inhibition of reticular formation to treat such phantom pains[7].

V. SUMMARY

1. This paper is composed of four parts of clinical observations on PSC, firstly the phantom limb and the pbantom PSC; secondly the spontaneous PSC; thirdly the cortical sensation and PSC; and fourthly the bilateral PSC induced by unilateral acupuncture.

2. PSC advances many new materials and problems whether in methodology, the essence of clinical neurology, or the fundamental studies of the nervous system. Its biologic significance is worth special attention.

3. PSC cannot be used as evidence of the existence of a tube structure of channel or meridian, but it does not rule out the other things to prove its existence.

4. PSC has developed phylogenetically and evolutionally.

5. The cerebral cortex has specific patterns of channels and PSC is the manifestation of the spreading of impulse along the patterns.

6. The spreading of impulse and the perception of the PSC are achieved in two steps.

7. Evolutionarily, PSC is older than cortical sensation.

8. The sore, numb and distending sensations of acupuncture may be percepted subcortically but PSC goes into consciousness being in the cortex.

9. Acupuncture is found a new method for the examination of the function of the parietal lobe.

10. Acupuncture should be the first choice for treatment of phantom and stump pains.

11. Acupuncture is superior to other methods for investigation of the phantom limb.

12. Spontaneous PSC manifested in the form of epileptic attacks in patients with intracranial diseases should be named as sensory epilepsy of the meridian attack type or meridian sensory epilepsy.

REFERENCES

[1] Shanxi Traditional Chinese Medical College: "A Review of the Studies of the Essence of Channel in China since 1958, "*The Review of Acupuncture Anesthesia,* Vol. I, pp.28–67, The People's Healthy Publishing House, Beijing, 1973.

[2] Nagahama Y. et al.: *The Study of Channel* (translated by Cheng Danan). Qian Qing Tang Press, Shanghai, 1955.

[3] Cooperative Group of Investigation of PSC: "A Survey of Occurrence of the Phenomenon of Propagated Sensation along Channels (PSC) in the Mass and its Basic Properties, "*National Symposium of Acupuncture and Moxibustion and Acupuncture Anaesthesia*, p. 260, Beijing, 1979.

[4] Li Baining: A survey of propagated sensation along channel phenomenon of 203 Mozambicans. *National Symposium of Acupuncture and Moxibustion and Acupuncture Anaesthesia*, p. 263, Beijing, 1979.

[5] Hecaen H., Penfield W. et al.: "The Syndrome of Apractognosis Due to Lesions of the Minor Cerebral Hemisphere, "*Arch. Neurol. and Psychiatr.*, **75**: 400–434, 1956.

[6] Weinstern, S. and Sersen E.A.: "Phantoms in Cases of Congenital Absence of Limbs," *Neurology*, **11**: 905–911, 1961.

[7] Melzack R.: "Phantom Limb Pain: Implications for Treatment of Pathologic Pain," *Anesthesiology*, **35**: 409–419, 1971.

STUDY OF OBJECTIVE PARAMETERS IN PHENOMENON OF PROPAGATED SENSATION ALONG CHANNELS

Wu Sihong, Sheng Lingling, Gu Peikun,
Yang Hongying, Tie Shuangyu
(Research Department of Acupuncture Anesthesia and Xinhua Hospital, Shanghai Second Medical College)

A pressing problem in the study of the phenomenon of propagated sensation along channels (PSC) is how to record the dynamic changes of PS – a subjective feeling – by some objective parameters. Many Chinese authors have attempted to work in this field. From Jan. 1977 to Oct. 1978, taking rheogram, ECG, urinary volume and 3',5' – cAMP excretion as parameters, we studied the changes along the sensory conduction lines and of the corresponding viscera during the process of PSC. The following is a brief account of our work.

I. METHOD

1. Subjects studied. Twenty-four subjects with positive PSC above the elbow and/or knee including five subjects with marked PSC (channel sensitive ones) were studied.

2. Parameters.

a. Rheographic changes on the Stomach Channel during the process of PS.

b. Changes in heart rate during the process of PS along the Pericardium Channel.

c. Changes in urinary volume and 3', 5' – cAMP excretion after PS along the Kidney and Bladder Channels.

3. Procedure.

(1) Electro-pulse-stimulator was used to elicit PS by stimulation of the twelve Jing (well) points at the frequency of 200Hz with the intensity adjusted to the tolerance of each subject.

(2) The nature of the test was explained in detail to the subjects to avoid any possible apprehension. They were told to lie down quietly for at least fifteen minutes before the test started. The feeling of the subject was inquired about from time to time.

(3) Control studies were done for each parameter.

(I) Rheographic changes on the Stomach Channel during the process of PS

Rheogram was taken with a bridge-type rheostat; the signals were introduced into a

ECG machine and recorded on standard Lead II. The electrode used was a 1mm thick circular lead plate with a diameter of 2cm. Electrodes were placed on the points of Jiexi and Zusanli of the Stomach Channel of Foot – Yangming.

1. Grouping.

Group I: Nineteen individuals with post-poliomyelitic sequelue, having positive PS along the Stomach Channel.

Group II: Eighteen individuals with post-poliomyelitic sequelue, without positive PS along the Stomach Channel.

Group III: Eight healthy children, without PS.

Changes in the systolic wave amplitude and index of peripheral resistance on the rheogram were noted before and during the process of PS and also ten minutes after the stimulation.

2. Analysis of data. (see Tables 1, 2)

Table 1. Rheographic changes after PS along the Stomach Channel

Parameter / Result / Progress of PS	Systolic wave amplitud P value	Index of peripheral resistance P value
Jiexi	<0.05	< 0.05
Zusanli	>0.05	> 0.05
Regression of PS	0.05 <	0.05 <
10 minutes after stimulation	0.05 >	0.05 >

Table 2. Rheographic changes in the controls

Group	Procedure	T-value	P-value
Subgroup I	Stimulation for 5 minutes	1.6001	>0.05
(no PS)	Stimulation for 10 minutes	0.2052	>0.05
Subgroup II	Stimulation for 5 minutes	0.1455	>0.05
(healthy children)	Stimulation for 10 minutes	0.087	> 0.05

The result showed that in the PS positive group, after stimulation of the Jing point on the Stomach Channel, the systolic wave amplitude and index of peripheral resistance on the rheogram changed correspondingly with the dynamic process of PS. As the PS passed in between the points of Jiexi and Zusanli, the wave amplitude and index were both markedly increased. Right after the stimulation, the PS rapidly regressed; the wave amplitude and index of peripheral resistance were then significantly and very significantly increased, respectively. Ten minutes after the stimulation, both parameters were restored to the basal level. In the control group, no statistically significant differences were observed after stimulations for five and ten minutes. The test clearly demonstrates that there are definite and specific changes along the channels during the process of PS.

(II) Change of heart rate during the process of PS along the Pericardium Channel

The heart rate was recorded on standard Lead II with a SJ–41 physiologic recorder and the mean value in five seconds was taken. The subjects tested were four "Channel sensitive" ones. Changes in heart rate were observed during PS along the Left Pericardium, Stomach and Large Intestine Channels. The test was done nine times on the Pericardium Channel, four times on the Stomach Channel and one time on the Large Intestine Channel. On the same individual, repeated observations were made several days apart. The results are as follows.

From Table 3 we see that when the PS along the Pericardium Channel passed to the chest region, there were invariably transient increases in heart rate; the increment was: below five, once; five – ten, four times; ten – twenty, twice and over thirty, twice. Ten minutes after the stimulation, the heart rate remained increased in only one test and dropped back to or even below the basal level in all the other occasions. For the Stomach and Large Intestine Channels, the PS also crossed the chest region, but the increments were usually below five. The test shows that there are dynamic changes in heart rate accompanying the PS process along the Pericardium Channel, the changes being channel specific.

(III) Changes in urinary volume and 3', 5' – cAMP excretion after PS had passed along the Kidney and Urinary Bladder Channels

The subjects tested were four "Channel sensitive" ones. Changes in urinary volume and 3', 5' – cAMP excretion were observed after positive PS had passed along the Kidney and Urinary Bladder Channels. Control studies were done four times with PS running along Stomach and Spleen Channels.

The subjects tested were given regular diet but with restricted fluid intake. Sample of urine was taken ten times during 24 hours and measured separately. Urinary 3', 5' – cAMP excretion was determined by the method of saturation analysis of conjugated protein.

Besides the increase of urinary volume and 3', 5' –cAMP excretion an obvious peak output of the urinary volume was observed one to three hours after PS was obtained along either the Kidney or the Urinary Bladder Channels. With the exception of a single case, there were also transient peaks in urinary 3', 5' – cAMP excretion corresponding to those of

Table 3. Changes of heart rate (beat/minute) during the process of PS

Subject tested	Pericardium channel			Stomach channles			Large intestine Channel		
	Before PS	PS to chest	10 miuntes after stimulation	Before PS	PS to chest	10 minutes after stimulation	Before PS	PS to chest	10minutes after stimulation
Liu	82.8	87.6	88.8	84	86.4	85.4	80.4	86.4	84.2
Liu	74.4	90.0	79.2	86.4	88.8	97.2			
Liu	75.6	85.2	80						
Hu	88.8	103.0	85.0	87.6	94.5	86.4			
Hu	96.0	104.8	91.2	79.2	80.4	74.4			
Hu	79.2	85.8	84						
Ho	90	99	75						
Hsu	78	108	76						
Hsu	72	104	78						

Table 4. Changes in urinary volume and 3'5' – cAMP excretion after PS along the Kidney, Urinary Bladder Channels and the Stomach, Spleen Channels

Channels studied	Subject tested	Urinary volume	Urinary 3'5' – cAMP excretion
PS on the	Ho	+++	+++
Kidney and	Liu	+++	+
Urinary Bladder	Hu	+++	+++
Channels	Li	+++	–
PS on the	Ho	+	–
	Liu	–	–
Stomach and	Hu	–	–
Spleen Channels	Li	++	++

+++: increased significantly after PS
++ : increased after PS
+ : slightly increased after PS
– : no marked difference

Table 5. Changes in 24-hour urine volume (in ml)

	Ho	Liu	Hu	Li
Kidney and urinary bladder channels	3163	705	651	1455
Stomach and spleen channels	960	305	495	991
% increased	229	132	31	46

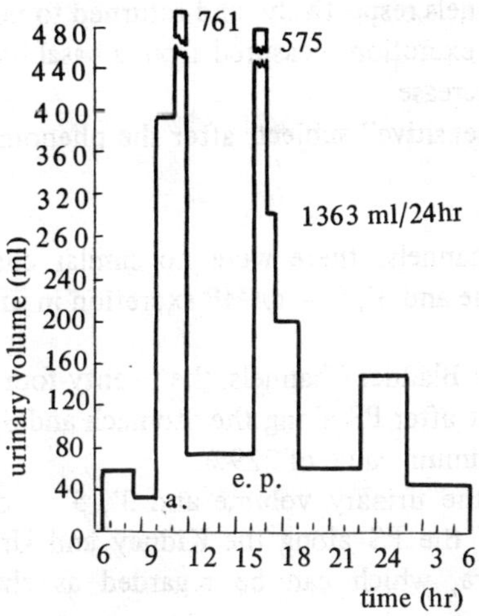

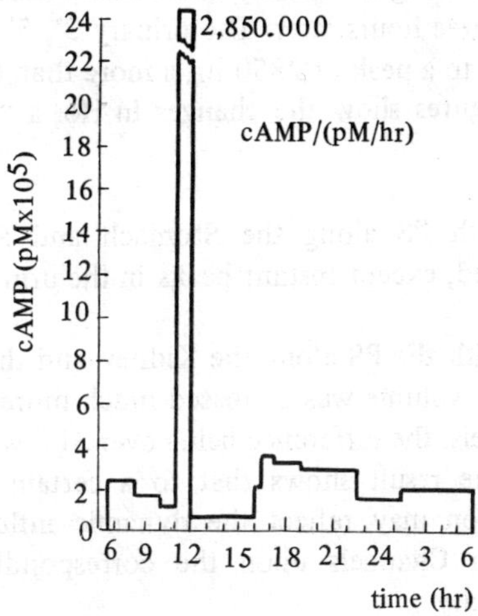

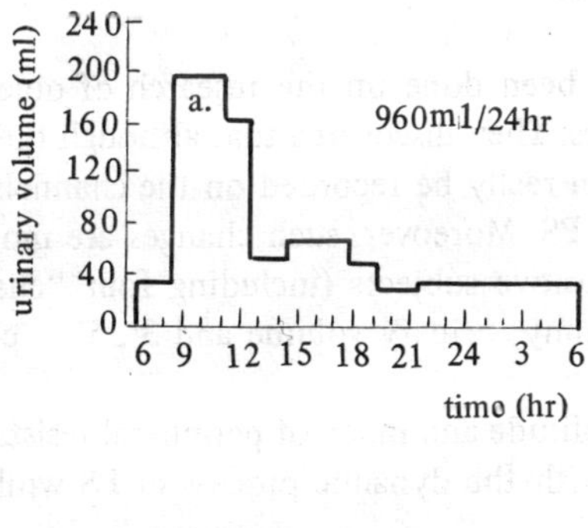

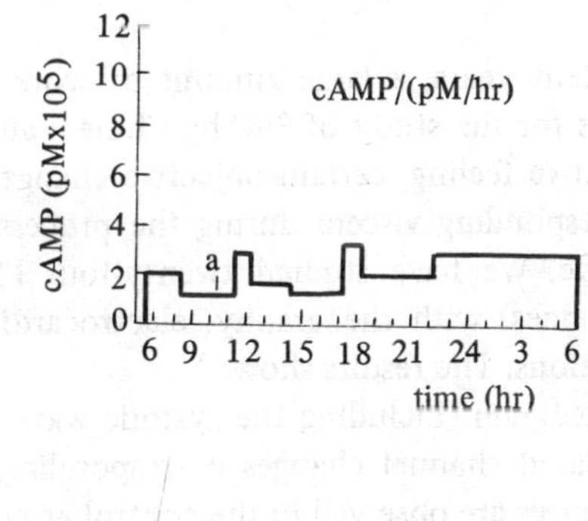

Fig. 1 Changes of the urinary volume after Stimulation of the Kidney and Uninary Bladder Channels.

Fig. 2 Changes of the urinary 3′5′-cAMP after Stimulations of the Kidney and Urinary Bladder Channels.

Fig. 3 Changes of the Urinary Volume after the Stimulation of the Spleen and Stomach Channels.

Fig. 4 Changes of the Urinary 3′5′-cAMP after the stimulation of the Spleen and Stomach Channels.

urinary volume in the remaining three subjects. The changes in subject Ho were most marked: urinary volume increased from 36 ml/hr to 400 ml/hr and 761 ml/hr after PS was elicited along the Kidney and Urinary Bladder Channels respectively, and returned to normal level three hours later. The urinary 3', 5' – cAMP excretion measured from a basal level of 173/hr to a peak of 2850/hr, a more than tenfold increase.

Figures show the changes in Ho, a "channel sensitive" subject, after the phenomenon of PS

With PS along the Stomach and Spleen Channels, there were no similar changes observed, except instant peaks in the urinary volume and 3', 5' – cAMP excretion in subject Li.

With the PS along the Kidney and the Urinary Bladder Channels, the twenty-four hour urinary volume was increased much more than that after PS along the Stomach and Spleen Channels, the difference being over 31% with a maximum value of 229%.

The result shows that to a certain extent, the urinary volume and 3', 5' – cAMP excretion may reflect the dynamic influences of the PS along the Kidney and Urinary Bladder Channels upon the corresponding viscera, which can be regarded as channel specificity.

II. DISCUSSION

In recent years, a large amount of work has been done on the research of objective parameters for the study of PSC by Chinese authors. They discovered that although the PSC is a subjective feeling, certain objective changes can really be recorded on the channels and their corresponding viscera during the process of PS. Moreover, such changes are more or less specific. We have studied twenty-four PS positive subjects (including four "channel sensitive" ones) with rheography, electrocardiography, urinary volume and 3', 5' – cAMP determinations. The results show:

1. The rheogram (including the systolic wave amplitude and index of peripheral resistance) on the related channel changes correspondingly with the dynamic process of PS while no similar changes are observed in the control group.
2. As the PS along the Pericardium Channel passes to the chest region, the heart rate is markedly increased and it changes with the dynamic process of PS. The PS along the Stomach and Large Intestine Channels also crosses the chest region but there are no corresponding changes.
3. After PS is elicited along the Kidney and Urinary Bladder Channels, the urinary volume and 3', 5' – cAMP excretion are markedly increased. One to three hours after PS is obtained, there are also transient peaks in these two parameters. With the Spleen and Stomach Channels, there are no similar changes except in one case. The twenty-four hour urinary volume is much increased after PS along the Kidney and Urinary Bladder Channels.

These results of the test demonstrate that both on the channels and their corresponding viscera, there are specific changes of the various parameters. This suggests that there actually exist certain changes during the process of PS which effect the changes in the objective parameters. Such changes are channel specificities.

Ancient literature of Chinese traditional medicine points out "there are vessels in all of the twelve channels" and the channels "are the thoroughfares of the vessels. This means that the circulation of Qi and blood is closely related to blood vessels and this circulation is one of the important functions of channels. We applied the rheogram to study the circulation of Qi and blood on the channels during the process of PS and discovered that the systolic wave amplitude and index of peripheral resistance on the rheogram change with the dynamic process. This illustrates that during the process of PS, change of Qi and blood along the channel can induce corresponding changes in the blood vessel capacity and elasticity. In the PS negative group, possibly due to the inconspicuous changes in Qi and blood, the rheographic changes are much less. Thus rheograms are of definite value in reflecting the changes in Qi and blood during the process of PS.

Besides, changes in heart rate, urinary volume and 3', 5' – cAMP excretion are obviously channel specificities. To those channel sensitive ones, these specific changes are reproducible. Hence, these parameters are of definite significance in the study of the phenomenon of PSC.

III. SUMMARY

This article is a report on the result of our study of objective parameters of PSC in twenty-four subjects. It is discovered that during the process of PS along the Stomach Channel, the systolic wave amplitude and index of peripheral resistance on the rheogram were markedly increased. Ten minutes after the stimulation was over they all returned to their respective normal levels. In the control group, no similar changes were observed. After stimulation of the Pericardium, Kidney and Urinary Bladder Channels, the heart rate, urinary volume and 3', 5' – cAMP excretions were significantly and specifically increased in most cases. There were also no such changes after stimulation of the channels of the Spleen and the Stomach of the controls. Hence, to a certain extent, the above-mentioned parameters can reflect the dynamic process of the phenomenon of PSC and can be used to study this phenomenon objectively.

REFERENCES

[1] 经络感传现象专题研究交流会议资料组：经络感传现象的研究(初稿) 1975。

[2] 一年来经络感传现象研究的概况，针刺麻醉 (2—3)：31 1977。

[3] «难经・一难»。

[4] 针灸大成，卷 4。

PROPAGATED SENSATION ALONG CHANNELS (PSC) INDUCED BY STIMULATION OF EAR POINTS

Research Group of Acupuncture Anesthesia and Channels,
Guangxi College of Traditional Chinese Medicine

In order to investigate the underlying mechanism of ear-acupuncture, we made some observations on the rheodigitogram, electromyogram and pain threshold along the propagating courses of the PSC induced by stimulating visceral points of the auricle of normally marked PSC adults with low frequency current impulses. The results are presented below.

I. MATERIAL AND METHODS

The main experimental subjects were two male normal adults with marked PSC who had demonstrated elevated pain threshold along the propagating course of ordinary PSC. One of them, No. 7, was Yao, carpenter, aged 33 and a man of minority nationality; the other, No. 12, was a retired PLA man, 24 years old. Some of the observations, mainly of the fist part of the experiment, were also made on nine other PSC adults in addition.

1. Method of stimulation. Continuous pulse waves with a frequency of 10C/sec were applied with a pulse generator G 6805. The intensity of the pulse was adjusted to what the subjects under experiment could endure. A silver-coated round plate, 2 mm in diameter, served as the stimulating electrode and the indifferent electrode, a 4X7 cm. plate made of silver chloride, was placed on the opposite lower leg.

Election of stimulating point on the auricle:

In the "visceral" area of the auricle designated to be stimulated, the point corresponding to a certain PSC course was decided by testing. The stimulating electrode was fixed onto the point with adhesive paper and the site for the leading electrode of myoelectricity and that for blocking the channel course were marked out.

2. Method of blcoking. The pressure intensity of the pressing block was 350 g/cm^2 and a soft brush brushing circularly at the blocking spot once per second served as brushing block with force not big enough to distort the surface of the skin. The spots for blocking, except that for testing pain threshold, were all separated away from the areas to be observed by at least the distance between two adjacent joints along the channel courses, and the control blocking spots were spaced at the same distance from the channel courses.

3. Method of testing the rheodigitogram. Rheodigitogram was obtained with a Jilin-made rheogram, Model TX 74—A, connected to a Shanghai-made electrocardiograph Model XDH-2, and the standard technique was used.

Two lead-strips of 1 cm in breadth each were fixed on the finger, at which the propagated sensation was expected to arrive, the distance between the two electrodes being 2 cm.

Monitored with an electrocardioscope, the rheodigitogram before stimulation, at the arrival of the propagated sensation at the Jing point 3—5minutes after the arrival, blocking and de-blocking, and finally after the disappearance of the propagated sensation, were all recorded respectively from both the experiment finger and the control finger. The control experiment was performed simultaneously with the hand on the same side or on the opposite side and with the same channel of the same person under the same experiment condition.

4. Method of testing the myoelectricity. Myoelectricity was conducted by mono-podial homocentric electrodes switched in a Shanghai-made polygraph with four leads.

Recording parameters: 30Hz, 0.1 second and 100 microvolt/cm. The leading electrode was inserted into the central portion of the musculus extensor digitorum longus of the leg along the Gall Bladder Channel and the reference electrode into that of the musculus soleus along the Spleen Channel, the indifferent electrode being 10 cm apart from the leading electrode.

The person undergoing the experiment was asked to lie down in a supine position. The myoelectricities before stimulation, at the arrival of the propagated sensation at the Jing point, during the process of propagation, on the appearance of muscular twitchings along the channel as well as that both before and after blocking and control blocking were recorded respectively.

5. Method of testing the pain threshold. Pain threshold was tested with an Anhui-made algometer Model K^+—4, with quantitative adjustment. The subject was asked to turn off the starting switch as soon as he definitely felt pain. The current control button was not turned or only slightly turned within a definite period of time in the course of the experiment to see if any subjective factors had come in. The pain threshold was expressed in milliamperes. The painless areas mapped out on both sides of the points selected on the propagating channel course by pricking with a mm acupuncture needle are called the painless zones. The breadth of these zones is expressed in cm.

Pain threshold-test was made in the leg, taking the acupuncture points Yang, Xiajuxu, Zusanli, Futu, Tienshu, Burong, and Yingchuang in the thoracico-abdominal region along the Stomach Channel of Yangming, and for the control test, places 5cm away from the three points Zusanli, Futu and Tienshu on the external side were selected.

The blocking point was above Zusanli and the point 5 cm on the external side on the same level was taken as the control.

Order of testings. The subject was made to lie in a supine position. Pain threshold at each selected point of the Stomach Channel was tested three times, beginning from the foot upward, and the points of the control were similarly tested and the results were the control value. Then, a low frequency impulse current was applied and the pain threshold and the breadth of the numb zone, 30 minutes and an hour after the propagated sensation along the ear Stomach Channel reached the Litui point, were measured and those of the control were measured at the same time. The propagating channel course as well as the control line was then pressed and brushed respectively for 20 minutes and the pain threshold at each point was measured in the same way.

II. RESULTS

1. PSC induced by stimulation of ear points. 104 examinations were made on subjects including Nos. 7 and 12 as well as other PSC adults; the courses of 90 induced PSC which had special correspondence with the stimulating sites of the auricle (86.0%). Those of the remaining 14 examinations (13.46%) were uncertain, their propagating course being either along the same-named channel, or the exterior or interior, and even irrelevant channels.

The PSC induced by stimulation of ear points was often centrifugal. It either began from around the auricle, travelled along a certain course to the start or end point of the corresponding channel and then propagated throughout the whole length of the channel, or circulated through a certain course within the auricle first and then travelled out of the auricle to connect with the start or end point of the related channel or, rarely, it might start directly from the centripetal end of the related channel and propagate to the Jing Point. Areas capable of inducing PSC along the Ren and the Du Channels by stimulation were also found on the auricle. Stimulation of a definite visceral point might evoke a PSC of either the corresponding channel or an irrelevant one and conversely, the same PSC might be elicited by stimulation of different points of the auricle.

The characteristics of PSC evoked by auricular stimulation such as sensation propagation velocity, its special connection with the five sense organs and the viscera, capability for blocking, focal-taxis and assembling phenomenon were all similar to ordinary PSC.

2. Rheodigitogram. According to the extents of the changes induced when the PSC reached the finger, the changes of the wave form of the rheodigitogram might be classified into the following four degrees:

I. Remarkable: The wave form changed remarkably.

II. Mild: only slight changes occurred.

III. Doubtable: changes in wave form occurred on both the tested and the control fingers.

IV. No change: the wave form did not change at all.

The results of the tests are summarized in Table 1.

The rate of positive wave form changes along the channels was 63.6% (11+10/33), that of doubtable changes, 18.2% (6/33), and that of no change, 18.2% (6/33).

The wave of rheodigitogram changed mostly from steep wave to triple-peak, turning or dome-formed wave for fingers where PSC has reached, suggesting preliminarily that there might be changes in the tonisity of the blood vessels on the arrival of PSC. There are also changes in the arrival inflow time and the ascending angle of the PSC compared with those before the arrival of PSC at the fingers tested ($P < 0.05$). No significant change was noticed with the control finger of the same person.

Table 1. Results of rheodigitogam test after induction of PSC by stimulation of ear points

Subject	Degrees				Total No. rested
	I	II	III	IV	
007	7	1	2	5	15
012	4	9	4	1	18
Total	11	10	6	6	33
No. Tested					

No wave form changes were noticed when control experiment was carried out with a non-PSC including point.

The wave form in one of the subjects, No. 7, returned to that before the induction of PSC on blocking the channel activity by pressing after changes in wave form had occurred on arrival of PSC. The test was repeated once with similar results. Only mild changes occurred with brushing and no change was observed in control experiment of blocking (Fig. 1).

3. **Myoelectricity.** In subject No. 7, there appeared muscular twitching or trembling of limbs 25 times along the course of PSC mostly one hour or so after stimulation; the frequency of muscular twitching or trembling was different from that of the stimulating impulse. Muscular twitching continued for another 0.5–3 minutes after electric stimulation had stopped.

In 6 out of the 7 experiments performed with the Gall Bladder Channel, marked muscular twitching along the Gall Bladder Channel was observed with the naked eye with the limb in a state of rest. The strength and intensity of the twitching gradually increased to such a degree that the gastrocnemius and the soleus muscles were eventually affected Fig. 2–1 (1).

Observation records of myoelectricity: Myoelectricity was in static state before stimulation. Small monophasic or biphasic waves of low voltage on the Gall Bladder Channel were recorded twice on the arrival of the PSC at the Jing point before the appearance of muscular twitching. Changes in myoelectricity could always be recorded on the Gall Bladder Channel with the appearance of muscular twitching. These changes were quite marked for three times; for another three times, simultaneous myoelectric changes were also observed on the control channel. No muscular twitching appeared throughout the entire process of propagation in another test, but changes in myoelectricity were recorded on the Gall Bladder Channel but not on the control channel.

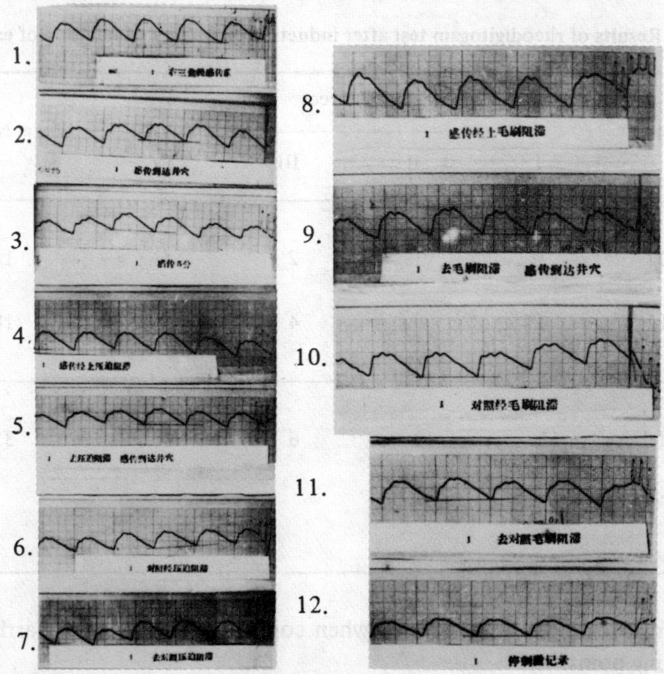

Fig. 1 (No. 7) changes in the rheodigitogram of the right hand ring finger on blocking by prissing and brushing respectively before and after the arrival of PSC induced by stimulation of Sanjiao point of the right auricle and in that of the control blocking:

1. Turning wave of the Sanjiao Channel before the arrival of propagated sensation.
2. The wave form changed to that of an ascending triplepeak one on arrival of PSC at the Jing Point.
3. Five minutes afterwards, still the ascending tripepeak form.
4. The wave returned to ascending form on disappearance of the propagated sensation when the channel was pressed one "Cun" (Chinese equivalent of the inck) above the sidu point.
5. Blockage removed, propagated sensation reached the Jing point once more and the wave resumed the ascending triplepeak form again.
6. No apparent effect produced onto the propagating channel when control blocking (pressing) was applied at "Cun" above the Kongzui point of the Lung Channel.
7. Control pressing removed, still no apparent effect observed.
8. No definited propagated sensation felt below the region blocked with brushing Cun above the Sidu Point of the prooagating channel, waves being of ascending or ascending triple-peak form respectively.
9. Brushing removed, the wave again changed back to ascending triple-peak form after the propagating line had been cleared up.
10. No. change of wave form on the propagating channel occurred on the application of control brushing one Cun above the Kongzui Point of the Lung Channel.
11. After the removal of the control brushing being, no change of wave form on the propagating channel occurred.
12. On the stoppaged of stimulation the wave form, partially returned to its original ascending form and partially retained its triple-peak ascending form pro-Propagation disappeard.

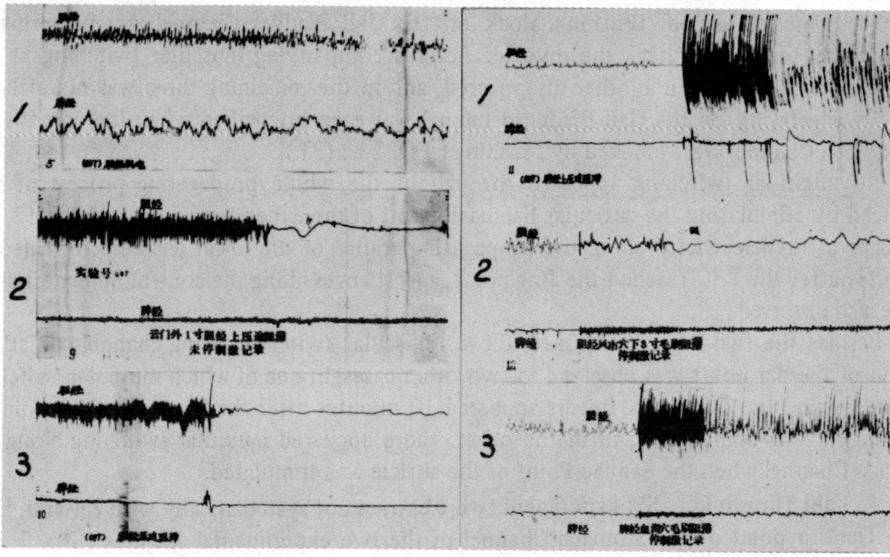

Fig. 2–1 (No. 7), myoelectricity on Gall Bladder Channel induced by stimulation of the Gall Bladder Point of the ear and effects of blocking of the channel activities by mechanical pressing:

(1) Muscular twitching along the Gall Bladder Channel followed by trembling of the lower leg appeared in a certain period by stimulation of the auricular Gall Bladder Point. Myoelectricity appeared from the Gall Bladder Channel during the trembling of the leg. The control Spleen Channel was also affected.

(2) Myoelectricity of the Gall Bladder Channel disappeared as it's acticity was blocked by pressing at the level of Yunmen Point of the thorax.

(3) The myoelectricity of the Spleen Channel disappeared earlier than that of the Gall Bladder Channel when the a activies of the Gall Bladder Channel below Fengsi Point were blocked.

Fig. 2–2 (No. 7), changes in myoeledtricity induced by different methods of blocking:

(1) Myoelectricity on the Gall Bladder Channel was not affected when the control Spleen Channel was blocked by pressing.

(2) Effects on the Myoelectricity of the Gall Bladder Channel when It's activity was block by pressing below Fengsi Point.

(3) The original myoelectricities on the Gall Bladder and the Spleen Channel were not affected when the activity of the latter, which served as control, was blocked by brushing.

Local muscular twitching and trembling of the limb of subject No. 7, disappeared for 13 out of 15 blocking experiments performed by pressing Fengsi point or the area slightly lateral to Yunmen point of the Gall Bladder Channel. Myoelectricity along the channel also disappeared or dropped markedly (Fig. 2–1 (2)). Myoelectricity lead from the Spleen Channel was also affected simultaneously for 7 times, in two of which, even were affected earlier than that of the Gall Bladder Channel (Fig. 2–1 (3)). Myoelectricity of the Gall Bladder Channel was not affected in 6 out of the 8 control experiments of pressing block performed on the Spleen Channel (Fig. 2–2 (1)), with that of one impaired and that of another even intensified. Brushing block on the Gall Bladder Channel was performed 5 times with the result that the myoelectricity accompanying muscular twitching in one dropped Fig. 2–2 (1), in another disappeared, and in the remaining three was not affected; the myoelectricity on the Gall Bladder Channel was even intensified when the activities of the Spleen Channel were blocked by brushing (Fig. 2–2 (3)).

No muscular twitching appeared throughout the whole propagating process of PSC induced by stimulating the auricular Stomach point of the experimental subject No. 12, but changes in myoelectricity along the propagating course of the lower leg were recorded 37 minutes after the PSC reached the Jing point, and changes along the control Spleen Channel were also observed.

Besides the two cases mentioned above, muscular twitching along channels on stimulation of the ear point was observed in two other cases, in one of which muscular twitching of the lip and the two index fingers appeared 10 minutes after the Large Intestine point of the auricle was stimulated and in the other, there appeared muscular twitching along the Sanjiao Channel when the Sanjiao Point of the auricle was stimulated.

4. Pain Threshold. Six experiments were carried out systematically with Zusanli, Futu and Tienshu point of the Stomach Channel of the two experimental subjects (No. 7 and No. 12).
The results were as follows:

There was a remarkably significant elevation of pain threshold an hour after stimulation as compared with the basal value ($P < 0.005$). Numb zone of different widths (maximum 15 cm, mean: 8.78 cm for that at the level of Zusanli point and for that at Tianshu point maximum 17.5 cm, mean: 8.89 cm) appeared. As a result of lateral extension of the numbness, the pain threshold on the control point (5 cm laterally to the same-named point of the propagating channel) was only slightly elevated with no statistical significance ($P > 0.05$) (Table 2).

The pain threshold on the Stomach Channel below the point of pressing was markedly lowered with much significance as evaluated with t-test ($P < 0.005$), and that below the spot of brushing was also lowered with much significance ($P < 0.05$). No significant change of pain threshold appeared on the Stomach Channel when the control point was pressed or brushed ($P > 0.05$) (Tables 3, 4). The normal range of pain threshold among the Chinese was ±40–60% as reported by some authors[1, 2]. The pain threshold of the two subjects in our experiments elevated 6.9 times one hour after propagation of PSC. These results are of much statistical significance.

III. DISCUSSION

1. That PSC may be induced by stimulation of the Jing or Yuan point has already been reported by many Chinese as well as foreign acupuncture medical workers[3, 5], but the present paper shows it might also be induced by stimulation of the ear point. As a preliminary result of our observation, it seems that PSC of the ear point follows the general rules followed by the PSC of other acupuncture points of the body in spite of certain specificities it possesses. There were certain changes in the rheodigitogram, myoelectricity

Table 2.Comparison of pain threshold one hour after the propagation of PSC with the basal values on both the point on the propagating channel and the control point

Point on the propagating Channel				Control Poin			
Point	BPT* (mA)	PT* 1 hr. after propagation (mA)	P	Point	BPT* (mA)	Pt* 1 hr. after propagation (mA)	
Zusanli	1.00	4.83		5 cm Lat* to Zusanli	0.63	1.25	
Futu	0.71	4.74	0.005	5 cm Lat* to Futu	0.64	1.25	0.05
Tianshu	0.77	5.05		5 cm Lat* to Tianshu	0.60	1.13	

*BPT = basal pain threshold
PT = pain threshold
Lat. = lateral-wards

and pain threshold along the propagating channel after the induction of the PSC by ear point excitation and the changes might be blocked with mechanical pressing. These demonstrate the objective existence of PSC induced by ear point and some its rules of action,

Table 3. Changes in pain threshold (P–T) after the activity of the propagating (Pr) course was blocked by pressing and brushing respectively

Points	P–T ! hr. after Pr. (mA)	P–T on 20 minutes Pressing (mA)	P	P–T 1 hr. after Pr. (mA)	P–T on 20 Minutes Brushing (mA)	
Chungyang	3.99	1.81		3.39	2.14	
Xiajuxu	4.63	1.49	0.005	4.58	2.42	0.05
Zusanli	5.02	1.93		4.64	2.62	

suggesting the existence of certain connections between the auricle and the human organism as a whole – the viscera, the sense organs and the acupuncture points of the body- and thus providing additional evidence for the old theory in traditional Chinese medicine that "the ear is a point on which all channels are converged" and "there are points with corresponding channels on the ear."

2. There may be, on the propagating courses, multiple functional activities of PSC, as certain changes were observed in all of the three objective indices in the experiments presented in this paper. The rheodigitogram slightly changed. Part of the myoelectricity was impaired and the pain threshold was markedly lowered on application of brushing block onto the propagating channel. Brushing block has definite influence upon the effects of PSC as shown by our experiments, indicating the central nervous system participates to a certain extent in the propagating effects.

It has been proposed that different effects produced by pressing block upon the channel course was due to the fact that pressure excites the deep acceptor and thus interferes with the propagating process of PSC in the central nervous system and lowers the central reflexive function in response to the peripheral effectors[3], but this hypothesis couldn't sufficiently explain why no blocking effect is induced when pressure of the same intensity is applied onto the nonpropagating channel of the same limb.

It deserves further investigation as to whether the centrifugal direction of the propagating course of the ear along the classical channels can be explained by the central diffusing course of excitation progressing in an order of an arrangement corresponding to that of the dermatome.

Table 4. Effects upon the painthreshold (P–T) on the propagating (Pr.) channel on blocking the control point by pressing and brushing respectively

Points on the Pr. Channel	P–T 1 hr. after Pr. (mA)	P–T on 20 minutes Pressing (mA)	P	P–T hr. after Pr. (mA)	P–T on 20 minutes Brushing (mA)	P
Chongyang (5 cm Lat*)	3.99	4.07		3.39	3.94	
Xiajuxu (5 cm Lat*)	4.63	4.57	0.05	4.58	4.56	0.05
Zusanli (5 cm Lat*)	5.02	4.91		4.64	5.01	

* Lat = lateral-wards

It has been reported that the PSC phenomena of patients with sequelae of poliomyelitis disappeared, shortened or changed in propagating courses post-operatively in 55.5% of the cases[6]. Similar phenomena of gradual disappearance of PSC after thyroid operation in cases who were originally PSC individuals was also observed in Hospital No. 2 of our college.

In conclusion, we think it possible that the function of the channels is connected with the peripheral nervous, humoral, central as well as certain physical functions[7].

Whether the fact that stimulation of different areas induces PSC along the same channel is due to some kind of integrating effect of the central nervous system deserves consideration.

3. The occasional absence of changes in the wave form of rheodigitogram on repetition of the experiment for the second or third time after the disappearance of the propagated sensation induced in the first experiment might probably be due to the fact that the original functional state of the organism did not recover shortly after the disapparance of the PSC already induced. Slight changes that appeared in 18.2% of the control channel might be related to displacement of channels of PSC or extension of the numb zone. The absence of changes in myoelectricity in the remaining 18.2% might be due to the fact that the intensity of the propagation was too low to produce any changes in the function of the blood vessels of the finger.

4. The myoelectricity evoked represents the electric activity of the motive units of the voluntary muscles. The localized muscular twitching appearing along the channels on the myoelectricity might be blocked by the application of mechanical pressing onto the channel course, suggesting certain internal association between the muscular twitching and the changes in myoectricity appearing during the propagation of the PSC induced by ear points and the specific propagation along the channels.

In another experimental subject, although no muscular twitching appeared along the channels, changes in myoelectricity were recorded in a certain period after the arrival of the PSC at the Jing point, suggesting the possibility of taking myoelectricity as an objective index for studying PSC.

5. Blockability is, at present, considered as one of the important characteristics of PSC and has been observed in all of the three objective indices. There are, however, still some problems deserving further study, such as the occasional occurrence of muscular twitching along the control Spleen Channel during its appearance along the Gall Bladder Channel. Although this might be explained by certain association between the Gall Bladder Channel and the soleus muscle through the Urinary Bladder Channel at Huantiao point, the fact that myoelectricity along the Spleen Channel was often lowered after the application of a pressing block onto the spot below Fengshi point of the Gall Bladder Channel, and that sometimes the myoelectricity was even affected earlier than that along the Gall Bladder Channel is not likely to be explained by this supposition. The fact that at times no effect could be observed by pressing block also deserves further investigation.

6. The pain threshold on the region distal to the pressing or brushing spots was lowered significantly, and the phenomenon was just the opposite of that reported by other authors[8] that only the PSC itself but not the concomitant effects of it was blocked by brushing. It is also in contradiction with the observation of Hillman and Wall[9] who on the basis of their experiments proposed that relevant cells of the posterior horn of the spinal cord and thus the afferent process of pain sensation might be depressed by exciting the larger afferent nerve fibers by pressing or touching of the body surface. It remains to be further investigated whether these disagreements were due to the possibility that the PSC induced by stimulation of the ear with low frequency current impulses has changed the functional state of the relevant cells in the posterior horn of the spinal cord or some other special mechanism that has taken place.

Although there are certain limits to the three indices, and subjective constituents from the experimental subject were impossible to be excluded, the recorded changes in rheodigitogram, myoelectricity and pain threshold mentioned above along the propagating course of the PSC induced by stimulation of the auricle of the two subjects No. 7 and 12 provide valuable information for further specialized studies in this field.

In view of the fact that observations of the propagating process of PSC are still mainly based on subjective descriptions and the number of experiments performed is small, these preliminary results still have to be verified and confirmed by further investigation.

PHENOMENON OF PROPAGATED SENSATION ALONG THE CHANNELS INDUCED BY LIMITATION OF SPONTANEOUS CONSCIOUS ACTIVITY (ENTERING QUIESCENT CONDITION)

Wang Buxiong, Cui Lihua, Chu Weizhong
(Shanghai Institute of Traditional Chinese Medicine)

The phenomenon of propagated sensation along the channels (PSC) is as important clue to the explanation of the nature of channels. However, the rate of occurrence of PSC among the people is rather low and typical cases are especially rare. To study the way of inducing PSC in persons originally without PSC, it is not only significant to find more subjects for investigation, but the study itself should be relevant to the understanding of the nature of PSC.

Beginning from 1977, the method of entering-quiescence (EQ) inducement in combination with point-pressing has been adopted to bring about PSC, and the result obtained is just as expected.

I. PLANNING OF THE EXPERIMENTS

The symbol of PSC is a most fundamental and marvellous one and can denote spreading as well as the reverse action "back flow". Dissemination and concentration of both stimulus and inhibition are the basic processes of higher nervous activities. In Jacksonian epilepsy, the attack of a tic occurring at certain part of the body may spread from proximal to distal, while its cease is just the reverse, i.e., from distal to proximal. A direct electric stimulus to the somatosensory area (S_1) may arouse a tactile formication on the counterlateral of the body. Some connections may be found between these phenomena and the basic process of PSC.

In the training of breathing exercise, the phenomenon of PSC appears during EQ inducement and "concentrating mind within Dantian point" without stimulating any peripheral points. To stimulate the limb stump left by amputation or due to congenital malformation, the induced PSC can be transmitted to the nonexistent part of the limb. The spreading process of PSC mentioned here is obviously in the CNS and not in the periphery.

Recent physiological research shows that the cell columns of the somatosensory area exist in the form of linear arrays. These correspond to the linear pathways of the peripheral receptive field in "dermatomal trajectory". The neuron-combination in cerebral somatosensory and motor areas, cerebellar cortex, thalamic ventrobasal complex, nucleus of trigeminal nervous spinal tract, nucleus of gracile fascicule and nucleus of cuneate fascicule has an organization of the "body region" type, i.e., corresponding to different peripheral parts with an obvious functional localization. Probably, in these body representations, the linear array (channel array) corresponds to the spatial distribution of the peripheral channel routes. The channel system, which exists as an entity, should have its pedigree developed from the periphery to the centre, from the lower rank to the higher rank. It is manifested anatomically in our country that almost all the channel points are related to the cutaneous nerves. In this way, the linear array of the receptor might probably be one of the manifestations of the peripheral "channel array".

The basic process of PSC might be the projection of the spreading excitation in the cortical "channel array" to the periphery being accompanied by a series of complicated processes, including the corresponding changes of the effector.

The reason why the phenomenon of PSC appears less in normal conditions might probably be that, under the action of numerous stimuli from the external and internal environments of the human body, numerous interacting excitatory and inhibitory points are "mosaicked" on the cortex, so that the spreading excitation within the cortical "Channel array" might be pinned or weakened down. [Likewise, due to the decrease of afferent impulses, which "purifies" the "mosaic" background around the "Channel array" to make the process of the spreading excitation relatively strengthened], the appearing rate of PSC is far higher in various sensory, motor disturbance cases such as paraplegia, hemiplegia, deafmutism and infantile paralysis, etc. than in normal persons.

The reason why the phenomenon of PSC appears less in normal condition might probably be that, under the action of numerous stimuli from the external and internal environments of the human body, numerous interacting excitatory and inhibitory points are "mosaicked" on the cortex, so that the spreading excitation within the cortical "Channel array" might be pinned or weakened down. Likewise, due to the decrease of afferent impulses, which "purifies" the "mosaic" background around the "Channel array" to make the process of the spreading excitation relatively strengthened. The appearing rate of PSC is far higher in various sensory, motor disturbance cases such as paraplegia, hemiplegia, deafmute and infantile paralysis, etc. than in normal persons.

The inducement of EQ in breathing exercise makes the cortex remain in a sleep-like inhibitory state. This would be a similar process of purification, and the "mind-concentrating point" would mobilize the spreading excitation on such a "purifying" background, so that the phenomenon of PSC is induced.

Our design of EQ inducement is based on the above hypothesis with reference to the ancient breathing exercise treatment. But both self-inducing and mind-concentrating within the Dantian point are subjective experiences which take a lot of time and their effect cannot be always expected. Therefore the method — an experimenter's conducting advice instead of self-inducing and a given "starting signal" in combination with point-pressing instead of self mind-concentrating — is adopted.

The so called "starting signal" is simply a "motor" idea transferred to the experimental subject through lingual relation. This is to ask the subject to experience the "moving" sensation at the pressed point, without involving any hints concerning the nature and characteristic of PSC.

Due to the help of "conducting advice", an "excitatory alarm focus" with a selective response to the experimenter's language would be set up in the cortical auri-analysor at the time of EQ. This excitatory focus would occupy a superior status on the inhibitory background. When the "starting signal" is imported and the afferent impulses induced by point-pressing reach the cortical receptive point, the excitement process concentrates at this point and begins to spread at once. If the excitement spreads among the neurons of the "channel array", the expectant PSC route which projects to the periphery shall take the form of channel distribution.

II. ANALYSIS OF 118 INVESTIGATED CASES

In April and May 1977, preparatory experiments were performed. They were carried out upon 26 cases in the condition of EQ. As a result, 18 cases succeeded in the inducement of PSC. Among them 9 cases coincided with the marked type. It was observed that the nature and characteristics of the induced PSC were in concordance with those investigated in the past. In adults, a parallel relation existed between the degree of EQ and the rate of success and rate of transforming into the marked type.

Thereafter from June 1978, we improved the experimental procedure, strictly controlled the experimental conditions and accomplished the experiments on 118 cases according to plan. The following is a report on these experiments.

1. Subjects. Of the 118 cases there were 22 soldiers, 35 middle school students, 56 primary school pupils and 5 patients. 80 cases were male, 38 female.

In order to make sure that no PSC was present primarily, all the subjects were checked in advance, before inducement was performed. 12 Jing (well) points on the upper limbs of the subjects were pressed. None of the subjects had any knowledge of channel or PSC.

In students and pupils the inducement was made at random, but in soldiers and patients the inducement was carried out on those with a better condition of EQ.

2. Method.

(1) Inducement of EQ. The subject was asked to sit down and relax, close his (or her) eyes and listen to the "conducting advice". The experimenter covered the subject's ears with palms and flicked 20 strokes or so at bilateral occipital regions of the subject (beating the heavenly drum). Meanwhile the subject was asked to count the number of strokes by memory. Then he (or she) was ordered to count his (or her) respirations for 30 – 50 times by memory, and advised to get rid of all disturbing wild thoughts and maintain absolute quietness. Once the subject came into the state of EQ, inducement of PSC would begin.

(2) Inducement of PSC. At first, give the subject a "starting signal", and ask him (or her) to point out the changing part of the sensation and then press the point with the tip of a match-stick. If PSC was started, the subject would point out the direction and route of the PSC automatically. Then he (or she) was further interrogated about the experience of the sensation and all the answers would be taken down as notes.

(3) Re-examination after coming to. After PSC was induced, the subject would come to at once (to come out of the EQ state) and he or she was re-examined under consciousness to observe the aftereffect of the transformation by EQ. For the sake of avoiding "track response" of EQ, a new point on another limb should be taken in the re-examination. The

nature and characteristic of PSC induced during re-examination should likewise be interrogated and recorded in detail for comparison purposes.

(4) Follow-up studies of indefinite period. After long intervals (of weeks, months or even a year or years, similar examination was done by pressing the points under ordinary consciousness. The points stimulated in follow-up studies included those not adopted previously. This was to observe the long term aftereffect in the transformation by EQ.

III. ANALYSIS OF THE RESULTS

Of 118 cases, PSC was successfully induced in 101. The success rate reached 85.89% (without applying the method of "relaying"). 72 cases were of the marked type, constituting 71.29% of total PSC cases. The rate of transformation to the marked type of 118 cases was 61.01%

1. Relation between degree of EQ and result of inducement. The degrees of EQ could be classified into 3 types, among which there were transitional ones not clearly distinguishable.

(1) Light degree: calm, relaxed, with no desire to move, with an expression of light sleep, spontaneous consciousness activity reduced, but response to external stimulation (such as sound, light) as well as voluntary movement still existing.

(2) Moderate degree: with expressionless face, very little voluntary movement, response to external stimulation markedly reduced, muscular tension slightly increased (brady-kinesia), slow of movement, conscious activity inhibited.

(3) Heavy degree: with conscious activity markedly reduced, even vague in time and / or spatial conception, almost no response to external stimulation (loss or slowing of ciliary reflex), but response to experimenter's "conducting advice" prompt and accurate.

Out of 22 cases of soldier-subjects, 13 cases were of light degree, 7 cases moderate degree and 2 cases heavy degree. In 5 cases of low degree, marked PSC appeared with 2. In all 9 cases of moderate and high degree PSC appeared in the form of the marked 0 type. It could be clearly seen that the degree of EQ and the results of inducement were closely related. 83 among the 91 pupils and students who served as subjects experienced PSC, a high success rate of 91.21%. The relation between the degree of EQ and its rate of success was unclear, but the degree of EQ and the rate of the marked type transformation were obviously parallel according to statistics (see Tables 1 & 2).

2. Integral effect of EQ transformation. In the process of inducement, if one point succeeded in inducing PSC, the corresponding PSC could basically be induced at any points by simply pressing the point without repeating the "starting signal". This just showed that EQ inducement has an integral effect in transformation. In 101 successful cases, 468 points were pressed in EQ state, and PSC appeared in 450 of them, a percentage of 96.15.

3. Sustained effect of EQ transformation.

(1) Re-examination after coming out of EQ state: According to the analysis of 97 cases, after the EQ state was over, it was still possible to bring out PSC by simply pressing points alone (including the new points not adopted previously) without repeating the

Table 1. Relation between the degree of EQ and the rate of success (pupil and student subjects)

Degree	Light	Moderate	Heavy	Total
No. of induced cases	55	19	17	91
No. of PSC cases	49	17	17	83
Rate of success (%)	89.10	89.47	100	91.21

Table 2. Relation between the degree of EQ and the rate of transformation into the marked type (pupil and student subjects)

Degree	Light	Moderate	Heavy	Total
No. of induced cases	55	19	17	91
No. of cases of the marked type	29	13	17	59
Rate of transformation into the marked type	52.73	68.42	100	64.84
X^2 test	$P < 0.005$			

Table 3. Comparison of examination during EQ with that after it

	No. of points pressed	No. of points PSC induced	Appearance rate of PSC
Entering quiescence	356	338	94.95
After coming out of quiescence	333	326	97.90

"starting signall". This showed that after the disappearance of EQ, the integral effect of EQ transformation was still sustained (see Table 3).

(2) Re-examination at indefinite termed intervals: After weeks, months, even more than a year, we re-examined at random 42 cases, among which 40 cases succeeded in inducing PSC (31 were the marked type), 2 cases failed (PSC not reaching the joint of elbow and/or knee). Re-examinations were carried on out under ordinary conscious condition by pressing two points. One was used previously; the other was a new point.

The result was: in 39 cases out of the 40 successful cases, corresponding PSC appeared; among the 39, 2 cases were transformed into the marked type from the nonmarked type; 2 failed cases were transformed into successful cases due to the extension of the PSC route.

This showed that the aftereffect of EQ transformation was sustained basically for a long duration.

4. Nature and characteristics of induced PSC. They were in concordance with the results of investigations by ancient medical doctors. As to the similarities between the two, it is not necessary to go into detail in this paper. We report now only what may be helpful in future investigations.

(1) Nature of PSC as shown in Table 4.

Table 4. Nature of PSC

Nature of PSC	Sensation like running-water		Numbness	Sourness	Formication or Ltch	Distension	Throbbing	Other sensations	Total
	Hot	Cold							
No. of cases	35	6	16	14	12	9	3	6	101
%	34.65	5.94	15.84	13.86	11.88	8.91	2.97	5.94	100

Table 5. Width of PSC

Nature of PSC	Thin Thread (hair)	Thick thread (woolen Threâd)	Rope (chopstick or little finger	Belt of 1.5–6 cm Width	Unknown	Total
No. of cases	16	48	29	6	2	101
%	15.84	47.53	28.71	5.94	1.98	100

(2) Width of PSC (Table 5).

When PSC was **progressing**, the width of its path was not uniform throughout the course. They might appear like a thread or a belt or appear in these forms alternatively. A distinct center line was experienced within the belt-shaped PSC in 4 cases. When the subjects were interrogated in detail during re-examination, most of them who originally had a thread – or a rope-like PSC-primarily, experienced now a weak induced belt from 0.5 – 3 cm in width on both sides of the PSC.

(3) Depth of PSC.

In 68 cases out of 101 the route of PSC ran superficially in muscleless parts and deeply in muscle-rich parts. When the PSC route passed the chest or the abdomen, according to the observations made on 36 cases, in 30 of them the PSC route ran deeply in the thoracic and abdominal cavities, in 6 cases the PSC route ran superficially on the chest and the abdominal wall.

(4) PSC changes when point-stimulation was suspended. (Table 6) was made of observations on 88 cases.

(5) Blocking PSC by finger press (based on observations on 87 cases) (see Table 7).

Among 68 cases with blocked PSC, 51 cases claimed that the sensation of PSC route adjacent to the finger-pressed point increased (75%), in 13 cases it decreased (19.12%), in 2 cases it remained unchanged (2.9%), and only in 1 case it disappeared completely (1.47%).

Table 6. PSC changes when point-stimulation was suspended

PSC changes	Reflux	Disapearance in situs	Running the whole course	Total
No. of Cases	54	24	10	88
%	61.36	27.28	11.36	100

Note: "Disapearance in situ" means that as soon as stimulation was suspended, PSC stopped on the spot, or went on running a little while (4–5 cm. generally), before disappeared entirely.

Table 7. Finger-press Block of Induced PSC

Press on the paths of PSC with the finger	Blocked	Unblocked	Total
No. of cases	68	19	87
%	78.20	21.80	100

(6) Some peculiar phenomena of PSC.

a. Fluctuation. When PSC runs forward along its route, it goes up and down like a tidal wave. The peak occurs in the superficial part under the skin, the trough sinks deeply into the muscle and the channel points are always distributed along the trough. For example, points Yuji, Taiyuan, Jingqu, Kongzui, Chize, Xiabai, and Tianfu, etc. exist along the trough of PS of the Lung Channel. The above phenomenon was manifested in 3 cases out of 101.

b. Conjugation. All PSC run toward counter-laterals along their symmetrical channel routes through a common intermediate zone (conjugating zone), which is mostly located in the anterior or posterior portion of the ears, the parieto- frontal region or the upper portion of the chest. This phenomenon is manifested in 17 cases out of 101.

c. Propagating in endless circle. When PSC finishes running within its proper channel, if point stimulation continues, it would go on running through many other channels. Finally, it would go round and round along a definite route. So long as the point stimulation continues, PSC would go on running without stop uninterr uptedly. This phenomenon was manifested in 23 of 101 cases.

There are two types of circles. One is the circles connected by the channels other than the proper channel. The other is circles including the proper channel passing through the stimulation point. Of the 23 cases, 13 were of the former, 10 were of the latter.

d. Projecting. Once PSC is started, it flows off like an arrow leaving the bowstring and rushes forward without turning back. Even if point-stimulation has stopped, it would not stop until the whole course is completed. Even if its route is pressed with finger heavily or met head-on, the PSC would still be going through without difficulty and could not be blockaded, though heavy pressing might setback the drive and slow down the speed. This phenomenon was seen in 10 out of 101 cases.

IV. CLINICAL APPLICATION

Two cases successfully transformed into the marked type of PSC at the beginning of our investigation were attacked by asthma. Acupuncture treatment was applied with a Di needle at Shaoshang point. As soon as the PS along the Lung Channel reached the chest, the patients felt hot within, and immediately heavy breath and fullness of chest were relieved. Another patient suffered from toothache. When the induced PS reached the ached tooth along the Large Intestine Channel, the pain was alleviated. In another nervous deafness patient, after PSC was induced, his hearing was evidently improved (20db increased).

At present, stress is laid upon PSC inducement by EQ. At present clinical applications are confined to a few cases. More systematic observations have to be made hereafter.

PRELIMINARY STUDY OF EXCITATION OF PROPAGATED SENSATION ALONG CHANNELS

Zhang Jin, Liu Wancheng
(Heilongjiang Institute of Traditional Chinese Medicine)

Wang Tong, Cheng Keming
(Wannan Medical College)

Yu Shuzhuang, Zhang Ruxin
(Beijing Hospital of Traditional Chinese Medicine)

A large number of studies and investigations[1] have shown that the distribution of propagated sensation along channels (PSC) in the population is not isolated but rather very widespread, but the frequency of occurrence of this phenomenon is quite uneven. This is considered to be connected with the constitutional differences between individuals and is thus a relatively permanent thing.

The important aim of the manipulation of traditional acupuncture is to achieve "exciting Jingqi (vital energy of the channel) ". In light of this doctrine and on the basis of former studies of the characteristics of PSC of points commonly used at acupuncture clinics and the control of its nature and orientation[2–5], we have undertaken another study to investigate further the PSC phenomenon. It has been found that the frequency of occurrence of PSC is closely correlated with the method, intensity and amount of stimulation. Multiple short-course relays of stimulation can significantly enhance the frequency of induced PSC.

The relay method of short-course stimulation at the points or change of the environmental conditions both inside and outside the body so as to evoke PSC and increase its length and intensity, thus making it possible for PSC to reach the affected area, has been given the term "excitation of PSC". We have been studying the excitation phenomenon since 1975. The data accumulated during the past four years are presented and analyzed in the present paper.

I. METHOD OF EXCITATION AND SELECTION OF CASES

The three different methods of stimulation were used in different cases and their effects were observed.

(I) Electric Di-needle Method

Electric Di-needle method is a method of stimulation with the needle connected to an electrode. In ordinary electric needle stimulation, the electrode is connected to the filiform needle. In the electric Di-needle stimulation, the electrode is connected to the Di-needle. The Di-needle we use is a pencil-like needle that is easy to manipulate. Di-needle is one of the nine needles mentioned in the book "Nei Jing" (Internal Channel). The use of this needle is "to press the channel to get to the Qi (vital energy) without puncturing it. The tip of the needle is like a milletgrain and is used to press the point, but not to insert into the skin. It is required that the angle between the needle and the skin be 15 degrees when the points are stimulated and that the tip of the needle is oriented to the direction in which the PSC should propagate. After PSC appears the spot where it stops is to be noted and marked so as to continue stimulation in relays until the PSC would go no further. Generally, each point is stimulated no less than 2 minutes. The current used for stimulation is mainly pulse-wave current and partially sound-wave current, i.e., sound waves converted into corresponding current[6].

34 deaf-mute students from the 5th grade were randomized as subjects for observation. In combination with treatment of cases we studied the excitation of propagated sensation along the Sanjiao and the Large Intestine Channels. Stimulation was started from the Jing (well) point and then all the related relay points were stimulated one by one. The stimulating parameters were different with different individuals and were regulated flexibly according to need. Stimulation was performed once a day. 15 consecutive stimulations make a course of treatment. A complete course of treatment usually consisted of 3–5 such separate courses with an interval of 5–10 days in between as needed.

(II) Electric Di-needle combined with Heating of the Channel Course

A rubber tube, with a diameter of 0.8 cm and a total length of more than three large joints of the patient, is placed on the skin along the channel to be tested and is fixed with adhesive plaster. Both ends of the rubber tube are connected to a specially made warm water bottle. The temperature of the water in the bottle is kept at about 40″C. It is required that the water in the warm bottle be circulated through the rubber tube continuously, thus exerting heat stimulation effect on the channel course. Then two filiform needles are inserted, one at the starting point and the other at the termination point of the heated section of the channel course. The needles inserted at the two points are connected to a pulse wave current ; meanwhile the regions near the main points are stimulated with the Di-needle. After 30 minutes, analysis of the PSC lengths before and after excitation is made.

One hundred outpatients have been randomly selected as subjects for observation. In combination with treatment, the excitation of PSC along seven main channels– the Lung, Large Intestine, Small Intestine, Kidney, Stomach, Spleen and Urinary Bladder channels– has been studied.

In order to further ascertain the relationship between temperature and PSC, we have also studied the influence of hot bath and high fever of the patients on PSC.

(III) Method of Stimulation with Filiform Needle

A point was selected at the distal end and a filiform needle was inserted at it. After needling sensation appeared the needle was withdrawn and pushed in continually like a piston while being twirled. The range of twirling was about 150 degrees; the frequency of the up and down movements of the needle was about 80–120 times/per minute. The needle was left in the point for 30 minutes and the changes in PSC were observed.

The subjects for observation were 28 randomly selected patients with facial paralysis and / or spasm, and observations were made in close combination with treatment.

II. RESULTS OF EXCITATION AND ITS ANALYSIS

(I) The Effects of Stimulation with Electric Di-needle and its Analysis

1. The results of excitation of Sanjiao Channel are shown in Tables 1 and 2. In the process of excitation, the number of relay stimulations for the PSC to reach the ear from the Jing point tended to become less and less. Before excitation, relay stimulations were required for all cases, but by the end of excitation, there were 19 cases (82.6%) in which PSC could reach the ear without relay. The average number of stimulations before excitation was 9.2; in the middle of it, (20 times of excitation) it fell to 3.6; by the end of it (40 times of excitation) it was only 1.2 . Since all cases in this series were hearing impairment, PSC reaching the ear could be considered as a manifestation of "Qi (energy) reaching the affected area." In 31 cases, the average number of stimulations for excitation is 38.6 . In the process

Table 1. Change of the numbers of relay stimulations required in the process of excitation of the sanjiao channel

	Total number of cases	The number of cases in groups requiring different number of relay stimulations (mean value)					
		without relay	1–2 times	3–5 times	6–9 times	more than 10	no PSC
Initial stage	23	0	1	1	10	8	3
Middle stage	23	2	9	8	4	0	0
Last stage	23	19	1	0	2	1	0

of excitation, the number of times of PSC reaching the ear accounts for 91.8% of the total number of stimulations for excitation. This indicates that in deaf-mutes, excitation of propagated sensation along the Sanjiao channel had made the manifestation of "Qi (energy) reaching the affected area" very markedly. As is shown in Tables 1 and 2 , with accumulation of the number of excitation stimulations, the percentage of PSC reaching the ear by only one stimulation (without relay) tends to increase significantly.

Table 2. The average number of excitation stimulations of the sanjiao channel and the incidence of PSC reaching the ear

Number of cases	Total number of excitation stimulations	The average number of excitation stimulations in each person	The incidence of PSC reaching the ear in the process of excitation			
			PSC reaching the ear		PSC not reaching the ear	
			the number of times	%	the number of times	%
31	1173	38.3	1077	91.8	96	8.2

2. The results of excitation of the Large Intestine Channel are similar to those described above. In the whole process of excitation, the number of relay stimulations required for PSC reaching the ear from the Jing point tends to decrease in a progressive manner (Table 3). The difference is that the PSC of the Large Intestine Channel is better than that of the Sanjiao Channel from the very beginning of excitation. Considering the fact that the excitation of the Large Intestine is done after the excitation of the Sanjiao Channel and is, in most cases, for treatment of illnesses of the same individual, it is postulated that this difference is due to the influence of excitation of the Sanjiao Channel on the PSC of the Large Intestine Channel. We had the same experience in our past practice. The comparison of figures shown in Table 4 supports this speculation.

After excitation of the Large Intestine Channel, the incidence of PSCs reaching the ear by one stimulation was significantly enhanced, up to 90% and more.

3. PSC originating from any channel tends to cease temporarily in the areas near the ear before reaching it. These areas are mostly consistent with the positions of the points along the channel. The highest frequency of cessation is in the area of Tinggong point of the Small Intestine Channel. The next is in the areas of the points Ermen and Yifeng of the Sanjiao Channel. These are those points which are commonly used at acupuncture clinics in the treatment of ear diseases. In fact, similar temporary cessation of PSC is also seen in other regions. This phenomenon has been given the term "Shu-point phenomenon" of PSC. A detailed description of this phenomenon is given in another article devoted exclusively to this subject[7].

After PSC reaches the ear, most patients feel a thunder in the ear or distension and numbness or the creeping of some insect. The data obtained from tests of 65 ears showed that in the case of PSC not reaching the ear such effect could also be felt, but it was far less marked.

Table 3. Change in the number of relay stimulations required in the process of excitation of the large intestinal channel

Stage of excitation	Total number of cases	The number of cases in groups requiring diffcrent number of relay stimulations (mean value)					
		Without relay stimulations	1–2 times	3–5 times	6–9 times	more than 10	no PSC
Initial Stage	34	22	2	4	4	2	0
Mid-stage	34	26	2	3	2	1	0
Last-stage	34	31	1	1	0	1	0

Table 4. Comparison of PSC of the sanjiao channel and the large intestinel channel before and after excitation in the same individual in 13 cases

	The average number of relay stimulations during investigation	The average number of relay stimulations in the beginning of excitation	The average number of excitation before PSC reaching the ear by one stimulations
Sanjiao channel	11.8	10.1	15.8
Large intestinel channel	11.2	3.2	3.3

In the whole process of excitation, the speed of PSC is relatively stable. The progressively increased speed is not seen[8]. For example, the time for PSC of the Large Intestine Channel to reach the ear from the Jing (well) point is generally stabilized at about 8 minutes and 27 seconds.

From the viewpoint of immediate effect and the number of relay stimulations required, the effect of sound-wave electric Di-needle used for excitation of PSC is superior to that of pulse-wave electric Di-needle. In the process of excitation, the decrease in the number of relay stimulations in the pulse-wave electric Di-needle group is not so stable as in the sound-wave electric Di-needle group, and from the fourth week of excitation there is a tendency to increase again.

The effect of excitation has a certain relationship with the constitution of the patients. In weak individuals the number of stimulations required for excitation is less and the incidence of "reaching the affected area" is higher.

(II) The Effect of Excitation of Electric Di-needle Combined with Heating and its Analysis

The method of excitation with electric Di-needle combined with heating of the channel course can also enhance the incidence of PSC significantly. The detailed results are shown in figures. There is no exception to the seven channels observed. The average enhancement is 35.8%. The most prominent one is that of the Spleen Channel. The difference between incidences before and after excitation is 60%.

In order to exclude any possible effect of hint that may be aroused by the rubber tube placed along the channel and to further assess the relation of PSC to temperature, we selected randomly 100 patients after a hot bath and 100 febrile patients to make a comparative study. The results show that the incidence increases and decreases with the increase and decrease of the skin temperature. Of the 100 patients who had taken a hot bath, there were 14 with skin temperature at 32°C and in 4 of them PSC developed, an incidence rate of 28.6%. There were 62 with skin temperature at 34°C and in 41 of them PSC developed, an incidence rate of 66.1%. There were 24 with skin temperature at 36°C and in 21 of them PSC developed, an incidence rate of 87.5%. In the febrile group, the incidence rate of PSC was 42% in patients with temperature at about 37°C; 55.9% in patients with temperature at about 38°C; 88.9% in the patients with temperature at about

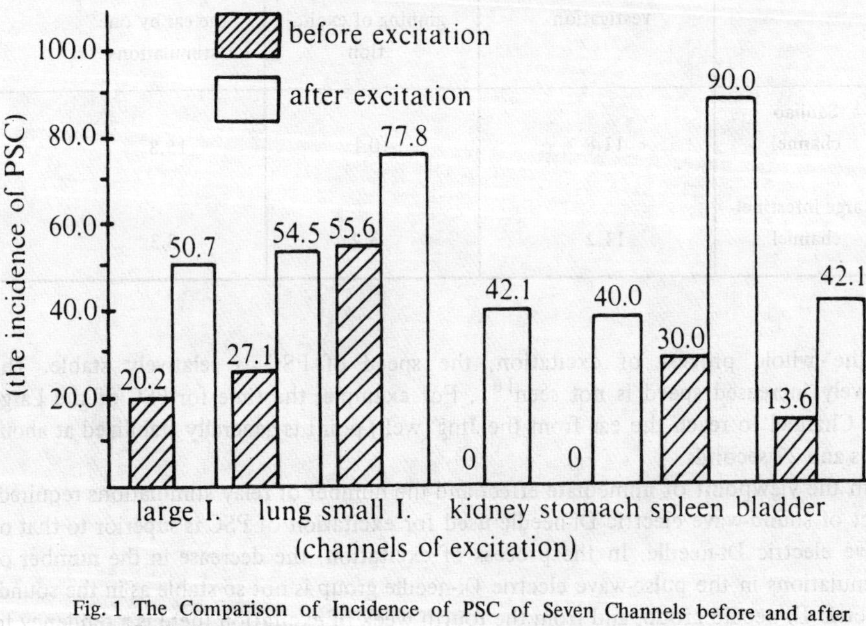

Fig. 1 The Comparison of Incidence of PSC of Seven Channels before and after Excitation

Table 5. The results of Eexcitation of PSC with filiform needle

Stage of excitation	The development of PSC				
	Regional	within 1 large joint	within 2 large joints	within 3 large joints	beyond 3 large joints
Initial stage	7	2	11	5	3
Middle stage	1	2	6	5	14
Final stage	1	1	2	5	19

39°C; 94.4% in the patients with temperature at about 40°C. When the 66 patients in whom PSC had developed were re-examined after the temperature has returned to normal, it was found that PSC had disappeared in 29 of them (43.9%).

(III) The Effect of Excitation with Insertion of Filiform Needle and its Analysis

Practice has shown that the method of excitation of PSC with insertion of filiform needle also enhances the incidence of PSC (Table 5). In the beginning of excitation, PSC is mostly restricted within the region of stimulation, and out of 28 cases studied only 3 had PSC reaching beyond 3 large joints. In the middle stage, PSC in most cases went to the distal end, and half of the cases (14 cases) had PSC reaching beyond 3 large joints. By the end of excitation, this tendency became more evident. In the last stage, there are 19 cases (67.8%) that had PSC reaching beyond three large joints. The effect of treatment increases significantly with the incidence and development of PSC.

III. DISCUSSION

1. The PSC phenomenon is one of the commonest channel phenomena. Research on PSC phenomenon is a key link in disclosing the true nature of the channels. In recent years, the attention of many researchers and investigators has been focused on this problem; as a result, a large amount of data has been accumulated.

Although PSC phenomenon is a subjective sensation, it has, however, an objective existence. This has been confirmed by the large amount of data accumulated and extensive experimental studies. The contention that the classic theory of channel course is an imaginary and artificially connected line apparently does not correspond to objective reality. It is obvious that the classic theory of channel course is to a great extent consistent with the PSC course observed by modern researchers[9].

PSC phenomenon is quite common in the population. This is not only confirmed by the data accumulated in the country, but also by that collected in other countries[10]. However, its distribution in the population is not even. Some hold that it only develops in minority peoples, especially sensitive people[11]. Others, that PSC phenomenon is related with the different stages of some diseases[12]. Our own data show that the PSC phenomenon is characterized by its existence in the entire population[13]. It is by no means a rare, occasional phenomenon. Its appearance or development is determined by a number of conditions. PSC develops if all the necessary conditions are satisfied; otherwise it would not. The conditions include a great number of factors, internal and external. Examination by the same method of stimulation in different groups of people produces different results. This is because the internal factors are different. When different stimulation conditions are given to individuals of the same group of people, the incidence of PSC could also be different. This is because external factors are different. The method of stimulation used in the present study is to change the internal factors by means of external factors to thus increase the incidence of PSC. All the three methods described above have achieved significant results of excitation. They differ from the EQ method used by Wang Poxiong[14]. Phenomenon of PSC induced by the EQ method is a result of direct change of internal factors. The fact that PSC can be successfully excited has disclosed an important objective attribute of PSC, i.e., excitability. Excitability of PSC indicates that it is completely possible to control and utilize PSC freely in numerous ways for many purposes if we understand it better and deeper. Theoretically it is not only very important for clinical acupuncture treatment but also for elucidation of the rationale of the effect of acupuncture treatment and anesthesia and for disclosing the true nature of the channels.

2. In excitation of PSC, the method used is in itself an important condition. In our opinion the development of the PSC phenomenon first of all depends on the condition of the functions in the body, the internal basis, while the excitation stimulation of PSC is an external condition. However, in the absence of external condition the PSC phenomenon would not manifest itself even if the internal basis exists. It is not known, at present, what kind of stimulation is by far the most efficient. All the three methods mentioned above have the effect of excitation. We do not know exactly, however, which one is better because we have not made sufficient comparative study of them. It can be said with certainty that in the process of excitation, attention must be paid to the way the stimulation is given. Before excitation, the means of stimulation must be selected according to the individual condition of the patient. During excitation, the amount of stimulation must be adjusted properly according to the physical reaction of the patient, and the parameters must be regulated in time. In doing so, optimal stimulation conditions can be created. In a word, the art of manipulation and its flexibility are of great importance.

Temperature is another important condition. Our practice has shown that, generally, in patients with skin temperature below 20°C, PSC will not develop. In cases when some regions of body surface are heated or in patients with fever, the positive rate of PSC is significantly enhanced. The effect of electric Di-needle combined with heating is better than that of electric Di-needle alone. In Shanghai, Zhang Jianqui's method of excitation with moxibustion had produced some PSC phenomena that could not be brought about by needle stimulation[15]. It is not surprising that in the silkbook dug out from the Mawangdui Han grave No. 3, the moxibustion method is in many parts of the book together with the channels.

In the future it is not only necessary but also possible to search for better methods of excitation on the basis of accumulated experience.

3. The excitability of PSC phenomenon has put forward an interesting academic problem, i.e., before PSC is excited, is there any latent PSC exciting or not? This also reminds us of the problem of why sometimes at acupuncture clinics, effects of treatment can be obtained without PSC? Why does interruption occur in the PSC course? Why in some cases does PSC sometimes appears, and sometimes not?

Putting all the above together, we conjecture that PSC may exist in latent form. The line between latent PSC and manifested PSC is not absolute. Possibly they are converted into each other under certain conditions. Recently our work has confirmed this hypothesis. Knocking on skin surface, we are able to trace out the track of latent PSC. However, in the field of latent PSC, there remain many aspects of it to be explored in the future. If the existence of latent PSC can be demonstrated, then the problem of excitation of PSC is just to convert the latent PSC into a manifested one and thereby many vague understandings in the past will be clarified.

IV. CONCLUSION

The present paper reported for the first time a new concept of excitation of the PSC phenomenon and described several methods the authors developed in their acupuncture practition. Excitation can significantly enhance the incidence of PSC. The fact that PSC phenomenon can be excited has demonstrated an important objective attribute of the PSC phenomenon, excitability. Recognition of the excitability of PSC will help to disclose the process of motion of the PSC phenomenon. Development of PSC as a result of excitation may be a conversion or continuation of latent PSC. In order to establish the objective existence of latent PSC, further study of the problem must be made.

REFERENCES

[1] 循径感传现象调查协作组：全国针炙针麻学术讨论会论文摘要(一)，第 199 页，北京，1979。

[2] 裴廷辅：哈尔滨中医 (4)：67，1960。

[3] 夏玉卿：黑龙江中医药研究 (1)：16，1963。

[4] 张缙：同 [3]。

[5] 张缙：同 [3]。

[6] 裴廷辅等：声电波针刺麻醉。同 [1]，第 158 页。

[7] 赵淑敏等：同 [1]，第 266 页。

[8] 裴廷辅等：中医药研究 20-31，1976。

[9] 孟昭威等：十四经感传路线的研究。内部资料，1979。

[10] 李伯宁：同 [1]，第 263 页。

[11] 中国人民解放军 309 医院：针刺麻醉原理探讨(第一册)，第 20 页，人民卫生出版社，1974。

[12] 各地经络感传现象研究汇报资料摘要 (内部资料)，1975。

[13] 张缙等：同 [1]，第 263 页。

[14] 王卜雄：同 [1]，第 278 页。

[15] 张缙等：热电镘针在激发感传中的应用（内部资料），1979。
[16] 张剑秋等：灸法在测查循经感传现象中的应用（内部资料），1979。
[17] 于书庄等：同 [1]，第 276 页。

STUDIES OF PHENOMENON OF LATENT PROPAGATED SENSATION ALONG THE CHANNELS

I. THE DISCOVERY OF A LATENT PSC AND PRELIMINARY STUDY OF ITS SKIN ELECTRICAL CONDUCTANCE

Zhu Zongxiang, Yan Zhiqiang
(Institute of Biophysics, Academia Sinica)

Yu Shuzhuang, Zhang Ruxin, Wang Juyi
(Beijing Hospital of Traditional Chinese Medicine)

Liu Yiming
(Beijing College of Aviation)

Hao Jinkai
(Hospital of District of Yanan)

Zhang Xuliany, Yu Shuling
(Institute of prevention and Public Health of Neimenggu)

He Qingnian
(Institute of Traditional Chinese Medicine of Beijing)

Meng Zhaowei
(Anhui College of Traditional Chinese Medicine)

Propagated sensation along the channel means that, during stimulation at an acupuncture point, a phenomenon of sensation starts from the site of stimulation and propagates along the course of the channel. A typical "meridian sensitive" subject is able to point out the line, the speed and the nature of such a sensation accurately. Since 1972[1], a large amount of general investigation work in this country[2] has shown that about one percent of the people have this typical propagated sensation and about 19 percent behave moderately sensitive to PSC. As to the rest of the people (80 percent), no such PSC could be elicited anyway.

However, clinical experience shows that patients with good curative effects from acupuncture or acupuncture analgesia are not necessarily PSC-sensitive. On the other hand, according to the theory of traditional Chinese medicine, the meridian system is essential to the "Orbiting of the Qi (vital energy) and the blood and the balancing of the 'Yin' and 'Yang', and it decides life or death and manages all kinds of diseases." In other words, life cannot be maintained without the regulatory function of the meridian system. Thus, if PSC is really a significant phenomenon of the meridian, there must not be any hard drawn line between the people with sensitive PSC and those without it that is insuperable. Typical PSC may just be a particular reflection of the general phenomena of meridian, under certain definite conditions.

This paper deals with the discovery of another latent propagated sensation along the channel (LPSC) in 1976 among subjects not sensitive to PSC. Furthermore, it has been evidenced preliminarily recently that the line of LPSC has the characteristic of high electrical conductance (or low resistance) with respect to its surrounding areas.

I. METHOD

(I) Discovery of the lines of LPSC

1. Subjects: Experiments were carried out on 10 patients at an acupuncture clinic. Among these, 5 patients were found to develop PSC to a certain degree during needling. According to the electric impulse stimulation method[1], 4 cases were found to have mild PSC, and 1 case moderate PSC. In other words, they were dominant PSC. The other 5 cases were found unable to develop PSC both by needling and by the electric pulse stimulation method. Therefore, they were negative in dominant PSC.

2. Excitation of the channels: Determinations of LPSC were conducted on the Yangming Channels of hand and foot. The subject was asked to keep quiet, and lie down in bed for 5 minutes. The room temperature was maintained at 23–25°C. Then the channel was excited electrically as follows: The Jing (well) point (e.g., Shangyang for hand Yangming Channel) was cleaned with alcohol and was fastened with a stimulating electrode by a nylon knot. The stimulating electrode was a 2.5X2.5 mm silver plate, wrapped up in gauze saturated with saline. The reference electrode was also saturated with saline and fixed on the opposite leg. As the current was turned on, the impulsive stimulation, generated from a 57–6 Type stimulator, acted at the Jing point with a frequency of 10 times per second. The current intensity was increased gradually until the subject got a local feeling of numbness or distension without pain.

3. Determination of the lines of LPSC: After 5 minutes impulsive stimulation at the Jing point, with a small plexor (made by a small rubber stopper of about 2 grams with a ground tip of 2 mm in diameter, which will touch the skin during knocking), light knocks were made on the skin along lines perpendicular to the channel and crossing over it from the medial side to lateral side at a speed of about 2 times per second. The first line of knocking may be selected at the (original) point of the channel (e.g., Hegu of the Large Intestine Channel). At each knocking, the subject was asked to tell his sensation and what it is like. In general, after 2 to 3 rounds along the same line, the subject would be able to tell objectively and actively the numbness and distention he felt when the plexor hit the channel. This is positive knocking response, and the point that produces the strongest sensation is called the positive reaction point (PRP).

After the PRP on the first knocking line has been located, the second line of knocking might be chosen at the level of another acupuncture point of the channel nearby and proximate to the first one, e.g., Yangxi in case of the Large Intestine Channel. From then on, the 3rd, 4th and other lines may be conducted at the levels of Wenliu, Quchi, etc. until PRP could no longer be elicited. By linking up these PRPs, an imaginary line coinciding with the classical channel line would be formed. This line is what we call the line of "latent propagated sensation along the channel (LPSC)", because, unless through knocking, no marked sensation of propagation along this line could be felt.

After the length of the line of LPSC has been determined, electrical stimulation at the Jing point should be turned off to eliminate effects of the excited Qi (vital energy) of the channel. Five minutes later, as a control test, the above PRPs were knocked again and the sensations produced were recorded to see the result of the removal of channel excitation.

For patient with marked PSC, a line of LPSC might also be elicited through knocking without impulse stimulation at the Jing point.

Determinations of LPSC were made along with actual acupuncture therapy. Determinations were done on the same patient at intervals of several days, and generally such dertermination was repeated 4 times.

(II) Determination of the cutaneous conductance of the line of LPSC

Experiments were performed on 10 subjects with marked LPSC in a quiet environment at 23–25°C. After a quieting down period of 10 minutes, the subject was asked to lie down on a bed face upward with his right arm folded up 90° at the elbow with the palm facing his head. Then the line of LPSC of the Large Intestine Channel, lying between Hegu and Shouwuli, including such acupuncture points as Pianli, Wenliu, Xialian, Shousanli and Shou wuli and also the PRPs of certain nonacupuncture points, was determined. Cutaneous conductance of LPSC line can be determined if after 3 days' repeated determination, the locations of the PRPs are basically stable within 0.5 cm.

For skin conductance determination, the skin surface was acted upon by a stream of bipolar electric impulses at a frequency of 1000 Hz through a probe. The current was adjusted to be monopolar through a full wave rectifying circuit and was measured through a 200 μA meter. The current intensity of the pulse generator was so designed that it could be adjusted from 0 to 100 volts. The probe was a rod of 3 mm in diameter with a round tip. The reference electrode was 2 cm in diameter. All were made of copper with chromium-plating. While testing, the subject held the reference electrode in his left hand and the tester held the probe and swept the skin with it along one of the lines perpendicular to the line of LPSC at a speed of about one centimeter per second. Sweeping started from one side and ended at the other side, 1 cm apart from the line of LPSC. The pressure applied to the skin should be handled lightly and evenly without making any wrinkles. The intensity of current began from 30 V and increased step by step (10 V for each step) until it reached a voltage (60–80 V in general) at which the subject began to feel a sharp numb or sore sensation at a certain point on the line of sweeping. This point was named electrical sensitive point (ESP). From then on, the voltage was lowered gradually until the sensation at the ESP became much weakened but still felt during sweeping. Then the electric conductance of an ESP was determined by setting the probe on the point and taking the reading on a 200

μA meter. As control, readings were also taken at the sites 1 cm apart from the ESP bilaterally. Likewise, the electrical conductance at the other PRPs along the line of LPSC was determined. The PRPs, however, might or might not be acupuncture points of the channel as mentioned above. The experiment on every patient was made twice in 2 days in an air-conditioned room in summer or autumn to determine its reproducibility.

II. RESULT

(I) LPSC on subjects with dominant PSC

5 subjects with dominant PSC of different degrees were capable of developing both dominant and latent PSCs in all of the 51 experiments on them on different days without exception. The rules of the results could be generalized as follows:

1. After impulsive stimulation for 5 minutes at Jing (well) point, a propagated feeling was evoked from the Jing points to a certain distance along the channel (dominant PSC); to the elbow or knee joints in 4 cases of mild PSC; to the shoulder or iliac joint in one case of moderate PSC.

2. While knocking the lines perpendicular to the channels but above the level of the dominant PSC, PRPs were always elicited above the shoulder or the iliac joint and in some cases, throughout the whole channel concerned. These are the characteristics of PRPs:

(1) Subjects would not feel them unless through knocking.

(2) The feeling at these points is quite different from that of the other sites of the knocking line in that it is an apparent conductive numbness and distention travelling quickly towards the stimulated Jing points.

(3) All PRPs are located basically on the pathways of the classical channels. Consequently, an imaginary line linking up these PRPs would just be the courses of these channels.

(4) The imaginary line, named as "the line of latent propagated sensation along the channel (LPSC)" is always the continuation of the line of the dominant or marked PSC.

Fig. 1 shows one of the experiments. Patient Yang XX was found to be a mild PSC case by the method described previously[1]. After impulsive stimulation for 5 minutes at the Jing (well) point Lidui of the Stomach Channel, he complained of a feeling of numbness travelling like a thread along the channel and ending at the knee joint (Dubi point), above which there was no more sensation felt. However, knocking along the lines perpendicular to the channel at the levels of Liangqiu, Futu, Biguan, Qichong, Tianshu, Ruzhong, Kufang, etc., PRPs were always elicited just at these points marked by a numb feeling going quickly to the Jing point under electrical stimulation, except at the Ruzhong point where the PRP deviated slightly toward inside of the classical point. Consequently, by linking up these PRPs with an imaginary line, a latent line of PSC which coincided basically with the classical Stomach Channel was formed. After the impulsive stimulation at the Jing point was turned off for 5 minutes, a weakened positive reaction still remained along the channel between the points Chongyang (foot) and Futu (thigh) as shown by knocking.

Besides, a shorter line of LPSC could also be elicited on this subject before electric excitation was applied at the Jing point by knocking and linking up the points of weak PRPs.

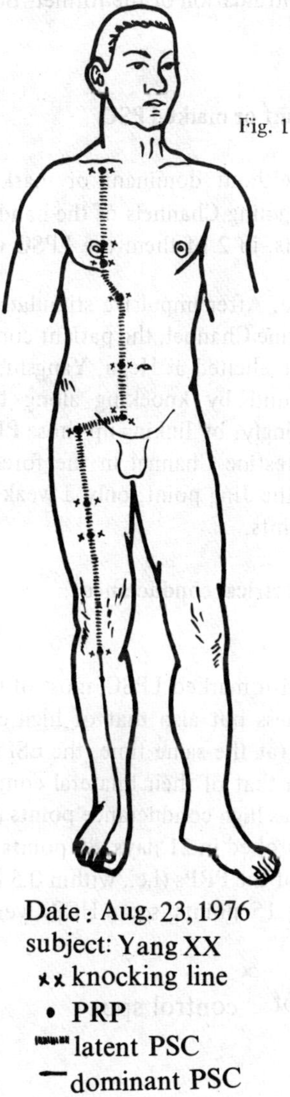

Fig. 1 The Line of LPSC of a subject with dominant or marked PSC

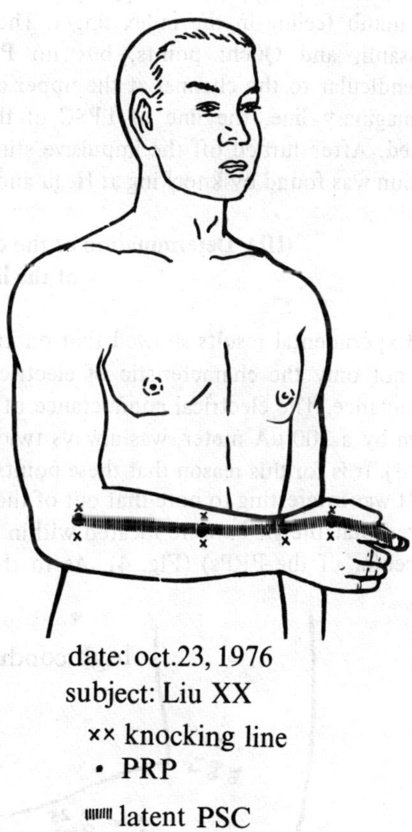

Fig. 2 Line of LPSC of subject without dominant PSC

Thus it can be seen that in addition to the line of dominant or marked PSC, there exists another latent line of PSC. The latter is generally the continuation of the former. Both lines belong to the same channel system.

(II) LPSC on subjects without dominant or marked PSC

20 experiments were conducted on 5 subjects without dominant or marked PSC. Positive latent lines of PSC were elicited along the Yangming Channels of the hand and the foot in 17 experiments. Of the remaining 3 experiments, in 2 of them the LPSC were not obvious, and in 1 the result was negative.

Fig. 2 shows one of the experiments on patient Liu. After impulsive stimulation for 5 minutes at the Jing point Shangyang of the Large Intestine Channel, the patient complained of a numb feeling in the index finger. Then PRPs were elicited at Hegu, Yangshi, Wenliu, Shousanli, and Quchi points, but no PRP was found by knocking along the lines perpendicular to the channel at the upper arm. Accordingly, by linking up those PRPs with an imaginary line, the line of LPSC of the Large Intestine Channel in the forearm was formed. After turned off the impulsive stimulation at the Jing point, only a weak positive reaction was found by knocking at Hegu and Yangshi points.

(III) Determination of the cutaneous electrical conductance of the line of LPSC

Experimental results showed that on 10 subjects with marked LPSC, most of the PRPs bore not only the characteristic of electrical sensitiveness but also that of high electrical conductance. The electrical conductance of these PRPs (at the same time, the ESPs too) as shown by a 200 μA meter, was always twice more than that of their bilateral control sites (Fig. 3). It is for this reason that these points are known as high conductance points (HCPs).

It was interesting to note that out of the 95 points probed in 21 days, 80 points (84.2%) showed that the HCPs were located within the sphere of the PRPs (i.e., within 0.5 cm from the center of the PRPs) (Fig. 4). As to the remaining 15 points, some HCPs were found

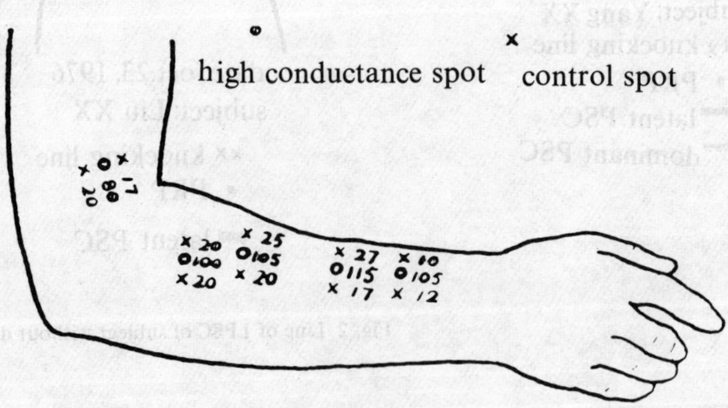

Fig. 3 High conductance spots of the line of PSC

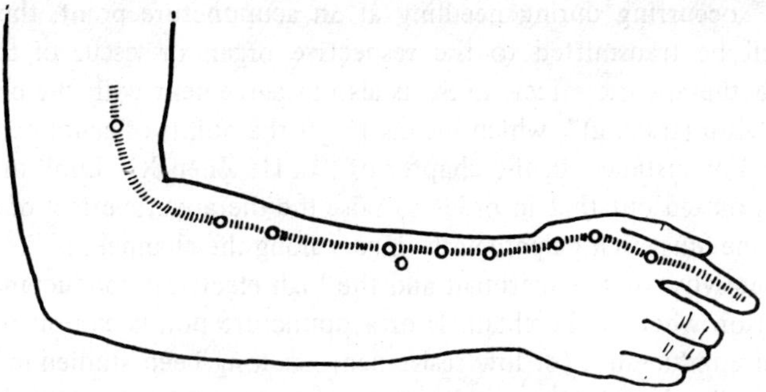

Fig. 4 Line of LPSC and high conductance points

outside the area (diameter 0.5cm) of LPSC, and there were some ESPs, but their high conductance is not significant.

Thus it can be seen that most of the PRPs on the line of LPSC, in addition to their hyperesthesia to mechanical (knocking) as well as electrical stimulation, are characterized by marked high electrical conductance (low resistance) as compared with the adjacent areas. Owing to the fact that the PRPs of the latent line includes both acupuncture and nonacupuncture points, it seems reasonable to assume that the entire line of LPSC bears high electrical conductance. Moreover, it may be also reasonable to consider that the lines of the classieal channels also bear high electrical conductance inasmuch as they coincide with the lines of LPSCs.

III. DISCUSSION

1. The universality of the phenomenon of PSC. By integrating an electrical impulsive stimulation with a mechanical one (knocking), subjects insensitive to PSC may manifest another type of PSC and those with mild PSC may develop a much longer line of LPSC. These facts show that the phenomenon of meridian is not confined to a few sensitive people, but is a general rule with the majority of people.

It is noteworthy that dominant as well as the latent PSC belongs to the same channel system described in the classical literature 2,000 years ago. On the other hand, the line of PSC is usually the pathway of the sensation induced by knocking at points on the line of LPSC. Besides, we have observed on many occasions that the distance of the line of PSC was elongated gradually during the course of acupuncture treatment. All these evidences prove that a specific functional orbit system of the channels for transmitting various information does really exist all over the body surface. In general, this system lies dormant, but under stimulation under certain conditions, it will show itself and become dominant and be thus recognized by the cerebral cortex.

The discovery of the latent PSC provides strong evidence in the principle of "selection of points according to channel" in acupuncture and acupuncture anesthesia practice. Owing to the existence of the latent orbit system, it is reasonable to consider that even though there is no PSC occurring during needling at an acupuncture point, the information of needling can still be transmitted to the respective organ or viscus of the channel, thus bringing about a therapeutic effect. LPSC is also in agreement with the classical theory of the method of "Xun (tracing)", which means to get the points of acupuncture by following up the channels. For instance, in the chapter of "Li He Zhen Xie Lun" in the "Cannon of Medicine", it is pointed out that in order to raise the therapeutic effect of acupuncture "to find the points, one must first palpate with fingers along the channel . . .".

2. The objectivity of the meridian and the high electrical conductance of the line of LPSC. The question whether the channels or acupuncture points exhibit the characteristics of high electrical conductance (or low resistance) has long been studied in this country and abroad. In the fifties, Nagatani[5] and Niboyet[6] reported separately the low resistance property of the acupuncture points. Since then, a lot of work has been done by Chinese physiologists and acupuncturists with an affirmative but not unanimous conclusion[7]. Since the seventies, and especially after China made acupuncture anesthesia public to the world , this question again aroused the interest of international medical scholars. Recently, a series of papers by Niboyet[8], Voll[9], Dumitrescu[10], Reichmanis[11], etc. showed that the low resistance property at acupuncture points can be accepted generally, although this assertion is still challenged by some authorities such as Noordergraaf[12] and others.

Using a low frequency skin conductance detector to study the electrophysiological characteristics of the channel, the authors of the present work show preliminarily that not only acupuncture points but also the entire line of LPSC exhibits an increased electrical skin conductance (or decreased resistance). Obviously, this fact provides the evidence that the existence of the channels can be substantiated both subjectively by the sensation in the central nervous system and objectively by the high electrical conductance at the periphery (skin). It is hoped that this preliminary work will be useful in the further study of the biophysical and biochemical characteristics as well as the nature of the meridian system.

REFERENCES

[1] 中国人民解放军 309 医院，中国科学院生物物理研究所，北京大学生物系：针麻资料选编(二)，北京人民出版社，16 页，1973。

[2] 经络感传现象专题座谈会资料组；中医药研究参考，(9)： 45—54，1975。

[3] Zhu Zongxiang, *et al.*: National symposia of acupuncture and moxibstion and acupuncture anaesthesia (Beijing), p. 288, 1979.

[4] 唐、王冰；黄帝内经素问，卷八，离合真邪论第二十七，商务印书馆、151 页，1955。

[5] 中谷义雄：汉方の临床，3 (7)： 54，1956。

[6] Niboyet JEH: Essai sur 1' acupuncture Chinoise, Paris, Wapler, 358, 1951.

[7] 陕西中医学院；医药资料选编 (经络研究专辑)，陕西中医学院，1975。

[8] Niboyet JEH: *Traited' acupuncture, IT: 121-345, 1970.*

[9] Voll R: *Am J Acupunct* **6**(1): 6, 1978.

[10] Dumitrescu LFI *et al*: International congress of scientific acupunct. & applied technology (Abst) Bucarest: 20, 1977.

[11] Reichmanis M *et al.*: *Comp. Med, East West* **5**(3–4): 289, 1977.

[12] Noordergraaf A *et al.*: *IEEE Trans. Biomed, Eng. BME* **20**: 364, 1973.

STUDIES OF PHENOMENON OF LATENT PROPAGATED SENSATION ALONG THE CHANNELS

II. INVESTIGATION OF THE LINES OF LPSC IN THE 12 MAIN CHANNELS

Yu Shuzhuang, Zhang Min, An Suqi, Yang Shuying, Zhang Shuyuan

(Beijing Hospital of Traditional Chinese Medicine)

Zhu Zongxiang

(Institute of Biophysics, Academia Sinica)

He Qingnian

(Institute of Traditional Chinese Medicine of Beijing)

It was proved in the previous papers[1,2,3] that by combining an electrical impulsive stimulation with a mechanical one, most patients at the acupuncture clinic bore a series of specific points along the Yangming Channels of the hand and the foot. By linking up these specific points, an imaginary line coinciding with the classical channel could be traced out. This line was named the line of latent propagated sensation along the channel (LPSC), because unless knocked at points along it, the subjects could not feel its existence.

LPSC, unlike marked or dominant PSC which can be evoked in a few sensitive people only, seems to be a general phenomenon in most of the subjects examined. This is significant in providing a theoretical basis for the universality of the curative effects of acupuncture and acupuncture anesthesia.

Chinese traditional theory of meridians points out that the channels of the body are not isolated but are mutually dependent and interrelated. For instances, between the channels there exist relationships of "Ying-Yang", and "exterior-interior" and also that of "interflowing". Consequently, it is reasonable to predict the existence of lines of LPSC of the Taiyin channels of hand and foot inasmuch as that of the corresponding channels, the Yangming channels of hand and foot, have been found. As all the channels are mutually connected, if LPSC exists between any two of them, it must also exist between all of them.

This paper deals with our investigation of the lines of LPSC of the 10 main channels besides the two channels of Yangming of hand and foot[2].

I. METHOD

(I) Subjects

Subjects for LPSC examination were selected randomly from patients at our acupuncture clinic with clear consciousness, normal reflexes to stimuli and accurate expression. However, patients with cerebral-vascular accident, dysfunctions in sensation and movement of the extremities, or with acute pains were excluded. Investigations were conducted on 200 patients, 79 male and 121 female. They ranged from 10 to 60 years old. For each channel, 10 subjects were examined at least twice in 2 days. The Yangming channels were excluded because they had been examined on 100 cases and the result had been reported elsewhere[2].

(II) Determination of the lines of LPSC

Methods of determination have been described in detail in previous papers[1,3]. The Jing (well) points at which electric impulsive stimulation was applied were: Shangyang and Lidui for hand or foot Yangming respectively; Guanchong and Qiaoyin for hand and foot Shaoyang respectively; Shaoze and Zhiyin for hand and foot Taiyang respectively; Shaoshang and Yinbai for hand and foot Taiyin respectively; Zhongchong and Dadun for hand and foot Jueyin respectively; Shaochong and Yongquan for hand and foot Shaoyin respectively. Determinations were generally conducted on the right channels except for particular reasons.

(III) Criteria of determination

Each patient was examined for one channel. At least two experiments were made in 2 days. Further examination was required if the results of the 2 tests were inconsistent. Results of each patient were analyzed as follows:

1. **Positive LPSC.** Subjects were determined to be LPSC positive according to the following 3 criteria:

(1) In one day's experiment, by knocking along the lines at various levels perpendicular to the channel, more than 3 positive reaction points (PRP) were elicited along the channel. The last of these points should be on the wrist or ankle joint. Each PRP could be well duplicated. These would constitute one positive LPSC experiment.

(2) Subjects were finally diagnosed to be LPSC positive if the 2 days' results were all positive. A third examination should be taken in case inconsistent results occurred. Then, the subject would be diagnosed to be positive LPSC if there were 2 positive results in the 3 days' experiments.

(3) The PRP was symbolized by sensations of numbness and distension radiating quickly towards the Jing points during knockings. After the stoppage of the impulsive stimulation at Jing points, such sensations became weakened or even disappeared.

2. **Negative LPSC.** In one day's experiment, a negative result meant there were no more than 3 PRPs elicited along the channel. Such a subject would be finally diagnosed to be LPSC negative by 2 negative results in 2 days' experiments.

3. Labile type of LPSC. Patients were diagnosed to be of the labile type of LPSC in one of the following conditions:

(1) There were one positive and 2 negative results in the 3 days' experiments.

(2) In the 2 days' examinations, although there were more than 3 PRPs elicited along the channel, the points were not well duplicated or stable in position so that the continuation of the linking line was disturbed to some extent by PRPs of the neighboring channels.

II. RESULTS

(I) Rate of occurrence of the lines of LPSC

Investigations on the 12 main channels on 200 cases (each case for 1 channel) in 416 examinations showed that there were 137 cases (of 68.5%) of positive LPSC, 19 cases (or 9.0%) of the labile type and 45 cases (or 22.5%) of negative PSC (see Table 1). If the cases of the labile type were also counted as positive, the total rate of occurrence would be 77.5%.

It is noteworthy that among the 12 main channels, except those of the Spleen and the Liver, almost all of which are of positive LPSC, the rates of occurrence of the other 10 main channels, i.e., the Lung, the Large Intestine, the Stomach, the Heart, the Small Intestine, the Urinary Bladder, the Kidney, the Pericardium, the Sanjiao and the Gall Bladder, were quite

Table 1. Rate of occurrence of LPSC of the 12 main channels

Channels	Cases	Positive	Labile	Negative
Lu.	10	8	1	1
L. I.	50	34	7	9
St.	50	31	6	13
Sp.	10	9	0	1
H.	10	5	2	3
S. I.	10	6	0	4
U.B.	10	7	0	3
K.	10	7	0	3
P. C.	10	8	0	2
S. J.	10	7	0	3
C.B.	10	6	1	3
Liv.	10	9	1	0
Total	200	137	18	45
%	100	68.5	9.0	22.5

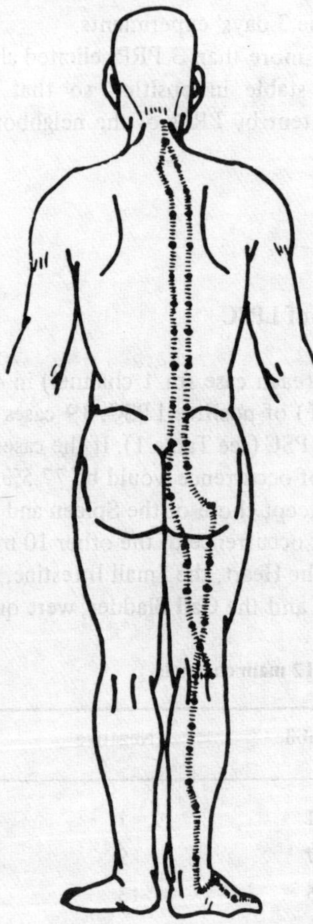

Fig. 2 Line of the LPSC of the Urinary bladder.

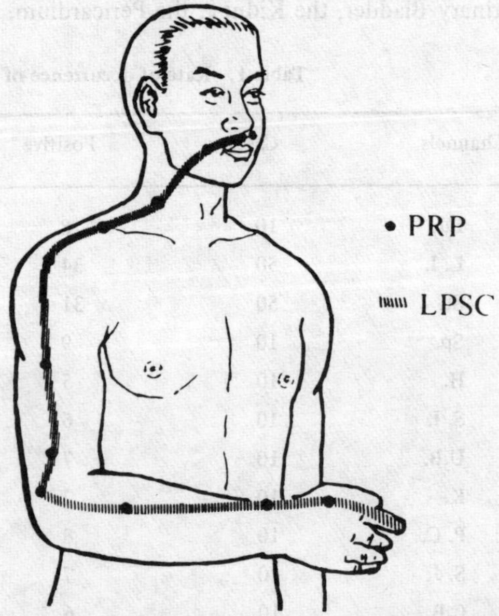

Fig. 1 Line of the LPSC of the arge intestine.

close to each other. Thus it can be seen that the line of LPSC of any channel could be elicited in most of the patients at the acupuncture clinic.

(II) The length of the lines of LPSC

Of the 133 cases with LPSC but without PSC, after 5 minutes of impulsive stimulation at Jing (well) points, the lines of LPSC of 106 cases (79.6%) could be traced out above the elbow or the knee joint, 57 cases (42.8%) above the shoulder or the iliac joint, and 29 cases (21.8%) throughout the whole channel. Fig. 1 showed a typical case of the line of LPSC of the Large Intestine and Fig. 2 of that of the Urinary Bladder.

It is interesting to note the parallelism between the lines of LPSC and the courses of the classical channels, especially the two branches of the Urinary Bladder Channel on the back and the intersecting lines from the right and the left on the face of the Large Intestine Channel.

The above results showed that most patients were able to manifest lines of LPSC from the tips of the extremities to the elbow or the knee joints, near 50 percent above the shoulder or the iliac joints, and about one fourth throughout whole channels. Thus, the objectivity and necessity of the occurrence of the lines of LPSC was substantiated.

(III) The sensations of the PRP

During impulsive stimulation at Jing points, subjects reflected different sensations in response to knocking at the PRPs. Numbness, distention and vibration occurred usually. There were also sensations of soreness, heaviness, numbness, pain, cold, hot, etc., which might appear singly or together. Sometimes the sensations were confined to the points of knocking, and sometimes they were propagated quickly to the stimulated Jing points. Among the 137 cases with positive LPSC, 60 cases (44%) complained of a propagated sensation to the Jing points and as a result, an intensification of the sensation at the Jing points occurred. This was more frequently met with in cases of marked LPSC. For instance, knocking at the Yingxian, the last acupuncture point of the Large Intestine Channel, an intensified feeling of numbness appeared instantly at the Shangyang (the Jing point). It was also true of the Dadun (the Jing point of the Liver Channel) when knocking was made at the Qimen point. Obviously, such an entire channel propagated sensation was quite similar to that of dominant PSC.

(IV) The reactions of the lines of LPSC before and after electrical impulsive stimulation

As control tests for comparison, knocking along perpendicular lines across the channels at different levels was also conducted on the 200 subjects before electrical impulsive stimulation at the Jing points. Results showed that in 29 cases (14.5%) PRPs were also elicited, but in the remaining 171 cases (85.5%) no PRP was elicited.

On the 137 cases with positive LPSC and 18 cases with labile LPSC, knocking at the same PRPs after the impulsive stimulation had been cut off for 5 minutes elicited weakened or no sensation at the PRPs in 109 cases (70%), no response in 39 cases (25%), and intensified sensation in 8 cases (5%).

The above facts showed that firstly, for some patients, it is not necessary to apply electric impulsive stimulation at the Jing points in order to bring out the lines of LPSC, because there is an inherent tactile hyperesthesia along these lines. Secondly, for most patients, impulsive stimulation will indeed stimulate the channels and enhance their hyperesthesia. Thirdly, there is an aftereffect of excitation of the channels following the cessation of electrical impulsive stimulation.

(V) The relative specificity of the lines of LPSC

If the effect of knocking at points in one line of LPSC reaches a neighboring channel, some weak PRPs may also be elicited along that line. This means that the specificity of the lines of LPSC induced by stimulation at the Jing points of a channel is only relative.

III. DISCUSSION

By combining electric impulsive excitation and knocking, we have shown that on any one of the 12 main channels, in most patients at the acupuncture clinic, a series of latent orbits coinciding with the courses of the Chiness traditional channels could be elicited. This fact cannot but arouse our great interest and close attention, because, up to the present, it is still an unsolved international problem as to whether the meridians exist, and whether they exist universally. However, this work provides further evidence that the existence of the meridian phenomenon is not limited to a few sensitive people, but is an objective universal one.

Recently, works done by other medical organizations have proved that even dominant PSC is not confined to a few sensitive people. Zhang Jin et al.[4] showed that it is possible to transform subjects of LPSC to subjects of dominant PSC by various means. Wang et al.[5] succeeded in enhancing the rate of dominant PSC in people by the EQ method (see the previous paper). All these valuable studies fully proved that the distribution of the meridian phenomenon is a very common one. To sum up, owing to the facts that the lines of LPSC of the 12 main channels have been established and that the orbits of the dominant and the latent PSC are identical and interconvertible, it can be assumed that the universal existence of the phenomenon of PSC has been substantiated by experimentation.

It was of interest to note the relationships between the latent and the dominant PSC. They belong to the same classical channels and are interconvertible. In some cases, the lines of LPSC are always the continuations of the dominant ones and the sensation evoked by knocking at the PRPs propagated just along the dominant PSC lines; this means that the two lines of PSC form an information system on the body surface, which might play a significant role in maintaining the homeostasis of the body.

Localizability seems to be one of the distinguishing features of the line of LPSC. It is much apparent in cases with a line of LPSC covering the entire length of a channel. In such cases, the subjects are able to differentiate a PRP within a limit of 0.5 centimeter from the bilateral tissue during knocking. In other words, the width of the lines of LPSC is confined to 0.5 centimeter. This width, however, differs from that of the dominant PSC which, according to various acupuncture workers[6,7], may appear as a band 1 to 3 centimeters wide. Obviously, the localization is beneficial to further the studies on the nature as well as the biophysical and biochemical characteristics of the lines of PSC.

Another distinguishing feature of the lines of LPSC is their independent character. As it has shown above, in spite of the application of impulsive stimulation at the Jing points, subjects with dominant PSC or LPSC may also develop lines of LPSC simply through knocking. It means that the traces of LPSC are inherent on the body surface, and excitation of the channels has but an enhancing effect. The independent character of hyperesthesia of the traces seems to be a physiological basis of the existence of the meridians which is distributed at least partially on the body surface.

REFERENCES

[1] 北京中医医院，中国科学院生物物理研究所等：针刺麻醉，(2—3)：50，1977。

[2] 北京中医医院，中国科学院生物物理研究所等：中医药研究参考（1）：1—4，1978。

[3] Zhu Zongxiang *et al.*: National Symposia on Acupuncture and Moxibustion and Acupuncture Anaesthesia (Beijing). p. 275, 1979.

[4] Zhang Jin *et al.*: ibid. p. 277.

[5] Wang Boxiong *et al.*: ibid. p. 278.

[6] 中国人民解放军 309 医院，中国科学院生物物理研究所、北京大学生物系：针麻资料选编(二)：北京人民出版社，16 页，1973。

[7] 福建省医药研究所针麻原理研究组等：医药研究资料选编——经络感传现象研究专辑，2：福建省医药研究所出版，9 页，1976。

PRELIMINARY INVESTIGATION OF PHENOMENON OF SENSORY CONDUCTION ALONG THE CHANNELS IN PATIENTS WITH POLIOMYELITIC SEQUELAE

Sheng Lingling, Wu Sihong, Gu Peikun, Tie Shuangyu, Yang Hongying

(Research Section of Acupuncture Anesthesia and Xinhua Hospital, Shanghai Second Medical College.)

The meridian Channels Theory is one of the important articles in the treasure house of traditional Chinese medicine. Two thousand years have elapsed since the formal establishment of the theory. But we are still not quite clear about its true nature, so it is an urgent task to investigate the nature of the Channels. The phenomenon of the Channels was already vividly described in the classical medical work"Nai Jing". Thus it is said in the book "when a bole of Qi or vital energy is hit, the needle moves freely in a broad Channel ··· just like the birds, flying freely. " This means "Qi" (the vital energy) can be reached by acupuncture only when it is done on some definite line. This is the phenomenon of propagated sensation.

On the basis of a general survey of the propagated sensation along channels, observations on the PSC of poliomyelitic patients and the influence orthopedic operation on propagated sensation were carried out in our hospital. Three hundred and seventy-seven child patients ranging from 5 to 12 years old were studied. One hundred and twenty-nine normal children and 100 cases suffering from various nonpolio ailments were used as controls.

I. METHOD OF INVESTIGATION

According to the nationwide standard, those with propagated sensation reaching upward to the elbow and downward to the knee are considered as of "+", while those with PS reaching upward to the shoulder and downward to the hip as of "++". The apparatus used was an "NA-57-6" stimulator.

1. Result. Among the 377 post-poliomyelitic patients studied, eighty-three patients showed propagated sensation, a percentage of 22. No PS was observed in the 129 normal children, and only two cases with it were found in the 100 cases with nonpolio ailments. Therefore there was a higher incidence of PS in post- poliomyelitis patients. The rate of PS occurrence of each of the twelve channels is different from those of the others and they are listed in Table 1.

Comparison of PS rate of affected limb and that of normal limb: Among 708 channels

Table 1. **Rate of PS occurrence of each of the twelve channels (Total no. 662)**

Channel	No. of propagated sensation	percentage
Lung	25	3.7
Large intestine	27	4.1
Pericardium	25	3.7
Small intestine	23	3.4
Sanjiao	24	3.6
Heart	23	3.4
Liver	84	12.7
Spleen	92	13.8
Stomach	98	14.8
Gall bladder	81	12.2
Kidney	81	12.2
Urinary bladder	79	11.9

in the lower limbs of 59 PS sensitive patients, there were 289 channels with PS in affected limbs for a percentage of 40.8, while 96 channels in normal limbs developed PS, a percentage of 13.6. The rate of the former was three times higher than that of the latter. This shows very obvious statistical significance ($P<0.01$).

There were 662 channels in 83 subjects showing the phenomenon of propagated sensation, the incidence rate of the six channels in the lower limbs being higher than that of the six channels of the upper limbs. The PS rate of 98 Stomach Channels was 14.8 per cent. It seems that channels rich in "blood" and "vital energy" give higher PS incidence rate. Spleen Channel was the next, with 92 PS channels, amounting to 13.8 per cent. The Small Intestine and Heart Channels had the least number of PS channels, being each with only 23 such channels (3.4%).

II. CHANGE IN PSC BEFORE AND AFTER OPERATION

1. **Method.** A few days prior to operation, the twelve Jing (well) points of the lower limb were tested 2–3 times to see whether they were stable in PSC. If PS occurred in the affected limb, it would be noted down for comparison after operation. Measurement was carried out 2–3 times within one week postoperatively. Occasionally patients were followed up one to six months after operation, the longest being two years.

2. **Result.** Thirty eight cases of 7–12 years old were investigated; 25 were male and 13 female. There were eight cases having two operations, totalling 46. The common operations were tendon lengthening of the Achilles tendon, replacement of the quadratus femoris and supracondylar ostectomy of the femur.

Table 2 shows that of 234 channels in 38 cases, 160 did not run through the operative field, and the other 174 channels passed through the incisional area. One hundred thirteen channels (65%) showed changes postoperatively, 61 showed no change and 66 lost propagated sensation completely. The PS of 23 channels was reduced from "++" to "+", Twenty

Table 2. Changes in PSC of affected limbs before and after operation

PSC	Stomach	Spleen	Urinary bladder	Kidney	Gall bladder	Liver	Total
Lost	11	9	15	10	13	8	66
Reduced	5	4	2	5	4	3	23
Route changes	2	4	6	4	4	4	24
No change	12	12	7	9	8	13	61
Unaffected	10	13	6	8	8	15	60
Total	40	42	36	36	37	43	234

Table 3. The changes in PSC in patients of "++" before and after operation

		Stomach	Spleen	Urinary bladder	Kidney	Gall bladder	Lung
Peng	Before op	++	++	++	++	++	++
	After op	++	++	++*	++*	++*	++
Shao	Before op	++	++	++	++	++	++
	After op	++	++	++	++	++	++
Liu	Before op	++	++	++	++	++	++
	After op	++	++	++	++	++*	++*
Wang	Before op	++	++	++	++	++	++
	After op	++*	++	++	++	++	++
Liu	Before op	++	++	++	++	++	++
	After op	++	++	++*	++*	++	++
Tao	Before op	++	++	++	++	++	++
	After op	+	+	++	+	+	+
Li	Before op	++	++	++	++	++	++
	After op	–	–	–	–	–	-

* Channels of PSC changed or bypassed.

five channels showed changes of routes of PS, deviated either to the inner or to the outer side or from the posterior to the dorsum of the foot.

Changes in six channels of the lower limbs were the greatest along the Urinary Bladder (76.6%), the next being that of the Gall Bladder Channel.

One fact deserves further notice, that is, among the 21 cases there were seven of "++" before operation. After the operation, five of the seven showed no change in PSC in the cephalic direction but their PSC courses were altered or bypassed. One had its PSC reduced and one had its PSC course shortened after operation. The follow-up after one to six months showed no change from the state in which the patient was discharged.

III. DISCUSSION

Our observation shows that the incidence of PSC of post-poliomyelitic patients could be as high as 22 per cent, the highest being those along the Stomach and Spleen Channels.

The PSC phenomenon varies with internal and external changes, but it is relatively stable. In order to eliminate the influence of other factors, we checked the PSC 2–3 times before operation. The postoperative investigation was only commenced on those cases with relative stability for comparison. The result showed that 113 channels out of 174 channels related to operations either disappeared, were lost, detoured or shortened to some extent.

Though the PSC phenomenon shows some variance, yet those of "++" are not likely to lose it turbed. For example, of the seven cases of "++" the PSCs of five cases only altered or bypassed their original courses, but none of the seven disappeared.

These changes of the PSC have a certain relationship with the "twelve tendonous channels" and the "twelve cutaneous areas". Therefore, all the twelve channels have cutaneous areas. They are the interrelated circulation system of the muscles and skin located in the superficial surface and outside the twelve channels. They all have definite regions of distribution and rely on the twelve channels for moistening and nourishment. According to our investigation PSC usually occurs over the surface of the subcutaneous, musculous layer, and therefore it can be stopped or blocked by simply pressing the skin above it. Operation itself would only damage the skin, muscles, and tendons, but not the large vessels and nerves. But the majority of senses can be damaged, so PSC can be influenced by operation. That is why it will not recover even after the healing of the wound; the damaged PSC can never be recovered again. But the PSC of persons of "++" or more cannot be easily destroyed by operation. That is because, we believe, it is rooted in the deeper part of the twelve channels and is connected with the viscera.

IV. SUMMARY

1. PSC rate is higher in patients with post-poliomyelitic sequelae than in normal children, the incidence being 22 per cent.
2. The majority of cases (65.0%) showed changes in PSC after operation. Therefore, they must have been caused by the damage of the skin, muscles and tendons by operation.
3. Our investigation of seven cases of "++" PS in the six channels of the lower limbs showed that the phenomenon of PSC is not likely to be damaged by operation because it is rooted in the deeper part of the twelve channels.

PRELIMINARY OBSERVATIONS ON PROPAGATED SENSATION ALONG CHANNELS (PSC) IN 102 CASES OF SPINAL CORD TRANSECTION

Fu Zhaoming, Li Boning, Xiao Zhijiang

(Research Group of Acupuncture and Channels, Chengdu College of Traditional Chinese Medicine, Sichuan)

A large amount of data hasindicated that PSC is an objective phenomenon and it has received great attention both in clinical acupuncture treatment and the research for principles of acupuncture anesthesia. How this particular sensation of stimulation finds its way into the brain center is a problem that has aroused the deep interest of a vast number of medical workers. Though investigations have been made on PSC in patients with either damage or disease in the spinal cord by some institutions, yet reports on the results are not unanimous. We have also carried out some investigation on PSC in 102 cases of traumatic paraplegia and the following are our results.

I. METHOD

(I) Selection of cases

The group of patients with traumatic spinal cord transections were all in a clear state of mind, with normal I. Q and able to give a clear account of the phenomenon of PSC.

(II) The diagnostic bases

1. Cases history. The patients had immediate disturbance of sensation, movement and reflex below the damaged segment after traumatic injury of the vertebral column.

2 X-ray examination. All the patients in the group went through X-ray examination of the vertebral column. The films revealed vertebral fracture, dislocation and deformity of angulation, etc. in most cases.

3. Operative findings. Of the 102 cases, 67 went through laminectomy, and damage of varying degrees was found in the spinal cord during the operation.

4. Objective signs. Every patient was given a thorough check-up of the nervous system. The degree and plane of the spinal cord damage were ascertained according to the actual findings.

(III) Apparatus and method of examination

Model I Huiwei 6.26 General Purpose Transistor Medical Therapeutic Apparatus was used and dense wave applied for the test, the electrode for stimulation being a silver-coated plate with a diameter of 0.5 cm and the insignificant pole being a copper plate. It was attached to the inner side of the calf, conduction paste being applied on some parts of the skin. The stimulating frequency was 100 cycles per second, and the intensity was just enough to induce a distinct stimulating sensation and at the same time be endurable by the patient. After the Jing (well) points along the channels on the upper limbs and the lower limbs were both examined, records were made as the patient was asked to give an account of his or her sensation without any hints given.

II. GENERAL DATA

Of the 102 cases, 64(62.75%) had complete spinal cord transections and 38(37.25%) had incomplete transections. The shortest history of the injury was 2 months, and the longest 18 years. Six cases had a history of less than one year, 33 cases from 1–5 years, 36 from 5–10 years, 22 from 10–15 years and 5 over 15 years. According to the localization of clinical diagnosis, the highest plane of the spinal cord damage, 10 cases (9.8%) were damaged at the cervical spinal cord, 54(52.9%) at the thoracic spinal cord, and 38(37.3%) at the lumbar spinal cord.

III. RESULT

(I) The criteria of the reaction of stimulating channels

1. **Negative reaction:** No subjective sensation whatever following stimulation.
2. **Positive reaction:** (1) Localized sensation of stimulation. Following the stimulation, only localized sensation occurred, either with or without propagation going not beyond the wrist or the ankle. (2) PSC localized sensation of stimulation occurred with propagation along or basically along the channels going beyond the wrist or the ankle.
3. **False-positive reaction:** The occurrance of positive reaction caused by other factors under no direct stimulation of the channels.

(II). Results

1. **The reaction of stimulating the channels in the upper and lower limbs of paraplegic patients.** The results of stimulating the Jing (well) points or Yuan points along the channels on both the upper and lower limbs of the 102 cases are in Table 1.

It is obvious from Table 1 that there was a marked difference between the upper and lower limbs of paraplegic patients in the rate of occurrence of PSC.

2. **The reaction of stimulating the channels in the upper limbs of paraplegic patients.** The results of stimulating the Jing (well) points or Yuan points along the channels in the

upper limbs in the group of patients with complete transections and in another group with incomplete transections are in table 2.

It is obvious from Table 2 that there was no marked difference between the two groups of patients with complete transection and incomplete transection in the rate of occurrence of PSC in the upper limbs.

3. The reaction of stimulating the channels in the lower limbs of paraplegic patients.

The results of stimulating the channels in the lower limbs in the groups of patient with complete and incomplete spinal cord transections are in table 3.

It is obvious from Table 3 that no PSC was found in the 768 channels in the lower limbs of patients in the complete transection group, whereas PSC occurred in 42 (9.21%) channels of the 456 tested in the lower limbs of patients in the incomplete transection group. There was marked statistical difference between the 2 groups in the rate of occurrence of PSC in the lower limbs.

IV. DISCUSSION

(I) The role of spinal cord in the occurrence of PSC

Except for 10 cases (9.8%) damaged at the cervical spinal cord, all the rest of the 92 cases (90.2%) were damaged at the thoracolumbar segments of the spinal cord. It was therefore significant to demonstrate the role of the spinal cord in the occurrence of PSC between the upper and lower limbs, which, as a result showed a marked difference. The positive PSC rate was 25.25% in the upper limbs and only 3.43% in the lower limbs, the former obviously higher than the latter. Then by comparing the seriousness of the spinal cord damage, it was found that in the upper limbs. whatever the damage of the thoracolumbar segments of the spinal cord might be, either complete or incomplete transection, the occurrence rates of PSC between them would be close to each other, being 25.65 and 24.56 respectively. There was no marked statistical difference. But in the lower limbs, the PSC occurrence varied with the seriousness of damage in the spinal cord. No PSC occurred in any of the cases of the complete transection group while the rate of PSC occurrence was 9.21% in the incomplete transection group. These facts showed that the spinal cord transection had a considerable effect on the occurrence of PSC, thus lending support to the view that the spinal cord was essential to the occurrence of PSC.

(II) False-positive reaction

Following the stimulation of channels in the lower limbs of the 102 cases of paraplegia, false-positive reaction occurred in 64 of the channels, 24 (3.12% of the channels in the lower limbs) of them were of the complete transection group and 40 (8.77% of the channels in the lower limbs) were of the incomplete transection group. Patients with false positive reaction generally complained of:

(1) A feeling of intensive stimulation;

(2) A feeling of propagation either along or not along the channels; and

(3) Discomfort in the chest and abdomen. Sweating and frowning occurred in a few

Table 1. The results of stimulating the channels in the upper and lower limbs of paraplegic patients

		Upper limbs		Lower limbs		X^2 test
		Channels tested		Channels tested		
		No.	%	No.	%	
Negative reaction		12	0.98	879	71.81	P<0.01
Positive reaction	Localized sensation	903	73.77	239	19.53	P<0.001
	PSC	309	25.25	42	3.43	P<0.01
False-positive reaction		0	0	64	5.23	
Total		1224	100	1224	100	

Table 2. The result of stimulating the channels in the upper limbs of paraplegic patients

		Complete transection group		Incomplete transection group		X^2 test
		Channels tested		Channels tested		
		No.	%	No.	%	
Negative reaction		6	0.78	6	1.32	P>0.05
Positive reaction	Localized sensation	565	73.57	338	74.12	P>0.05
	PSC	197	25.65	112	24.56	P>0.05
Total		768	100	456	100	

Table 3. The result of stimulating the channels in the upper limbs of paraplegic patients

		Complete transection group		Incomplete transection group		X^2 test
		Channels tested		Channels tested		
		No.	%	No.	%	
Negative reaction		741	96.49	138	30.26	P<0.01
Positive reaction	Localized sensation	3	0.39	236	51.76	P<0.01
	PSC	0	0	42	9.21	P<0.01
False-positive reaction		24	3.12	40	8.77	
Total		768	100	456	100	

cases. The case of false-positive reaction of PSC reguires further studies. It might be associated with the following factors:

1. **Conditioned reflex**: Having been treated with acupuncture-moxibustion and electro-needling many times, these patients would have an intensive feeling of stimulation in the lower limbs on being stimulated with the same kind of medical apparatus, which had turned into conditioned reflex in the patients.

2. **Spinal defense reflex**: Intensive muscle contraction might occur in the limbs of some paraplegic patients when they were stimulated. Thus indirectly drawing the structure concerned above the damaged segment of the trunk, and causing a feeling far down, the patient would mistake such a feeling of vague, uncertain location for PSC . The examiner may thus draw an erroneous conclusion. Yet it would not be hard for us to understand the patients' visceral reactions, such as discomfort and sweating, if we took into consideration Riddoch Mass reflex, which in certain conditions, presents abdominal muscle contraction, evacuation of the urinary bladder and rectum, hair erection and sweating on stimulating the lower limbs of paraplegic patients.

3. **Illusions caused by limb pain or phantom limb pain.** Ordinarily a number of patients felt pain, numbness and all sorts of discomfort in the lower limbs, in fact, some of which were caused by phantom limb pain. These sorts of discomfort, when mixed up, might be taken for PSC in the test, so great attention must be paid to false-positive reaction of PSC in the research. The characteristics of such reaction were that it occurred in a vague and uncertain location before the channels had been effectively stimulated, and it differed from the positive reaction normally induced by stimulating the channels of the limbs in often not presenting the typical sensations of soreness numbness and distention. It would be quite possible to distinguish the positive reaction from the false one in some cases by starting the test in the upper limbs and letting the patient experience the characteristics of normal positive reaction of channel stimulation, and some of them might learn to distinguish the true from the false PSC in time.

V. SUMMARY

1. Preliminary observations on the phenomenon of PSC were made on 102 cases of patients.
2. The PSC rate of occurrence was higher in the upper limbs than in the lower limbs of paraplegic patients.
3. The damage and disease at the thoracolumbar segments in the spinal cord had no effect on the PSC rate of occurrence in the upper limbs of paraplegic patients. But in the lower limbs, the PSC rate of occurrence was obviously higher in the incomplete transection group than in the complete transection group. No PSC was found in the latter.
4. Discussions were held on the role of the spinal cord in PSC occurrence, the cause of false-positive reaction and the way for avoiding it.

STUDIES OF RELATION BETWEEN PROPAGATED SENSATION ALONG CHANNELS AND EFFECTIVENESS OF CLINICAL ACUPUNCTURE ANALGESIA

Cooperative Group in Research of PSC, Fujian Province

Acupuncture anesthesia is originated from acupuncture relief of pain. Thus, it is of great significance to investigate the peculiarity of acupuncture analgesia and to summarize the rich experience in acupuncture analgesia contributed by the practitioner of Chinese medicine for further improvement of the efficacy of acupuncture anesthesia as well as elucidation of its intimate mechanisms. The theoretical basis guiding the acupuncture therapy is the theory of channels and collaterals. Since ancient times, the importance of "selection of acupuncture points along the channel related to the affected region", "waiting for 'Qi'", "mobilizing 'Qi'" and "conducting it to the affected region" have been emphasized by the physicians of traditional Chinese medicine. There are many reports about the relief of pain or improvement in patient's condition immediately as the propagated sensation along channels (PSC) arrived at the affected site in acupuncture clinics[1–13]. In 1973, according to these clinical experience and the phenomenon of distribution of acupuncture analgesic region along its channel, we proposed that to select puncturing points along the channels related with the affected region on the basis of Bian-Zheng (i.e, analyzing the illness and the patient's condition by type differentiation on the theory of traditional Chinese medicine) and to make PSC reach the affected or operated region might be an effective approach for further improvement of the efficacy of acupuncture analgesia as well as acupuncture anesthesia[14]. In order to clarify the relationship between PSC and efficacy of acupuncture analgesia and to examine the reliability of the above supposition, some investigations on this problem have been carried out in recent years.

I. SUBJECTS AND METHODS

One thousand, one hundred and six outpatients and inpatients suffering from pain in the head, neck, chest, back, abdomen and lumbar were taken at random for observation. The patients were clear-minded and could cooperated with the observers. Six hundred and seventy-seven of them were male (61.21%) and 429 female (38.79%). The youngest was 6 years old and the eldest 83 years old. The majority of them were in the age group of 20–59 years old. Most of them (89.90%) were workers and cardres.

According to the principles of selection of the puncture points along the channels related to the affected region, one or two points below the elbow or the knee joint of the related channel were chosen. No local point was added. Every effort was made during treatment to make PSC reach the affected region as near as possible.

PSC was divided into grades according to the distance which PSC travelled from puncturing point to pain region.

Grade I : PSC arrived at the pain region. In other word, 'Qi' reached the affected site.

Grade II : PSC travelled over half the distance between the puncturing point and pain region.

Grade III: PSC travelled less than half the distance.

Grade IV: Without PSC.

Grade V : PSC travelled in the opposite direction of the pain region.

The effectiveness of acupuncture analgesia was evaluated as following:

Excellent: Pain and other symptoms disappeared more or less completely.

Good: Pain was relieved to a large extent and the patient's condition was improving.

Fair: Pain was relieved in some degree, the improvement of the patient's condition was not satisfactory.

Poor: No pain relief was achieved. Other treatment has to be used.

II. RESULTS

(I) Analysis on the Relationship Between the Grade of PSC and the Effectiveness of Acupuncture Analgesia

The results obtained from 1,106 patients are presented in Table 1. It reveals that the more marked the centripetal PSC is, the better the effectiveness of acupuncture analgesia will be. For example, there were 84 cases (54%) of excellent results out of 155 patients with Grade I PSC, while there were only 10 excellent cases (4.16%) out of 215 patients with Grade IV PSC.

Fig. 1 is made from the values listed in Table 1. It shows that the percentage of excellent results decreases step by step as PSC goes from Grade I to Grade IV. It was highest in patients of Grade I PSC and lowest in patients without PSC. Though the percentage of excellent results increases slightly again in Grade V, it is still far lower than those of Grades I–II. It seems that the direction of PSC is important. If the rates of excellent and good results instead of excellent are compared, the result will be nearly the same. The difference of effectiveness of acupuncture analgesia between the patients with different grades of PSC is clear.

The characteristics of acupuncture analgesia in patients with different grades PSC are summarized in Fig. 2. It shows that the peaks of effectiveness of acupuncture analgesia in patients of Grades II–V PSC fall in the class of good results and the rate of fair and poor results gradually increases as PSC passes from Grade II to Grade V. However, the case of patients with Grade I PSC is different from those of the others. Its peak falls on the excellent results and the rate of fair to poor results is very low. It reveals that distinct effect is always achieved when PSC does arrived at the affected region.

The difference in the effectiveness of acupuncture analgesia between the patients with marked centripetal PSC (Grades I–II) and those without (Grades III–V), as shown in

Table 2, is highly significant ($P<0.001$). It is clear that a close relationship between PSC and effectiveness of acupuncture analgesia really exists.

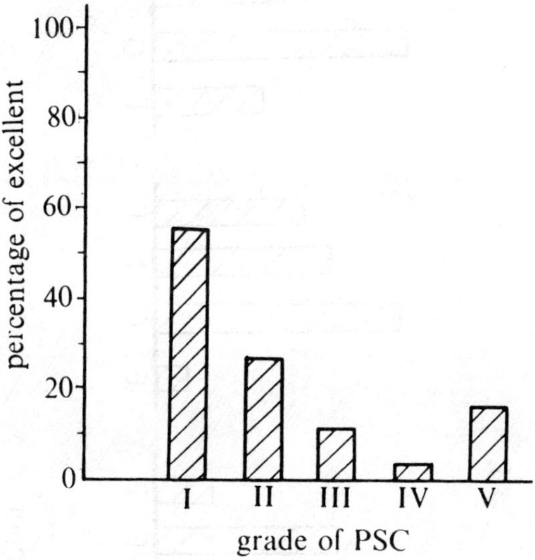

Fig. 1 Comparison of rate of excellent results of acupuncture analgesia in patients with different grades of PSC.

(II) Relationship between effectiveness of acupuncture analgesia and PSC grade in different affected regions

As shown in Table 3, if the 1,106 patients are divided into groups according to the affected regions such as head, neck, chest-back, abdomen and lumbar, the tendency of the effectiveness decreases as PSC goes from Grade I to Grade V is also obvious for every group of patients. The best result is achieved in patients with Grade I PSC no matter where is the affected region.

If the effectiveness of acupuncture analgesia in the above-mentioned five groups of patients is analyzed statistically on the basis of the rate of excellent to good results, there is no significant difference between them ($P>0.2$). The results clearly demonstrate that the effectiveness of acupuncture analgesia bears no relation to the affected region. The Grade of PSC is the principal factor for the realization of analgesia.

(III) Observations on patients of cholecystitis-cholelithiasis and acute sprain of the lumbar region

In order to avoid the effectiveness of acupuncture analgesia being cancelled out by different diseases in patients, 112 cases of cholecystitis-cholelithiasis and 192 cases of acute sprain of lumbar region were analyzed separately. The results are shown in Fig. 3 and Fig.4 respectively.

Though the pain from cholecystitis-cholelithiasis and that from acute sprain of lumbar

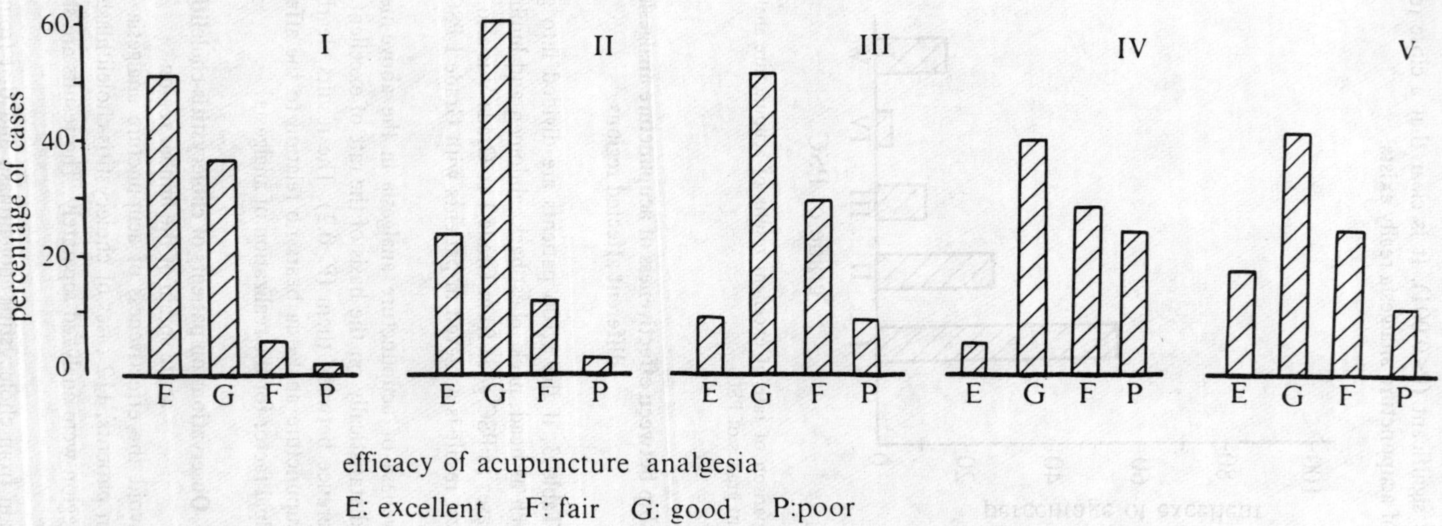

Fig. 2 The relationship between grade of PSC and efficacy of acupuncture analgesia.

region are different in nature, the former belongs to visceralgia and the latter to deep pain, but the results are the same as those mentioned above.

If the effectiveness of acupuncture analgesia between the patients with marked centripetal PSC and those without it are compared in each group of patients, the difference is highly significant ($P<0.001$) between the two groups.

Table 1. Relationship between grade of PSC and effectiveness of acupuncture analgesia

Grades of PSC	Effectiveness of acupuncture analgesia				
	Excellent	Good	Fair	Poor	Total
I	84	60	10	1	155
II	47	116	24	3	190
III	28	145	82	22	277
IV	10	90	64	51	215
V	48	119	69	33	269
Total	217	530	249	110	1,106

Table 2. Comparison of effectiveness of acupuncture analgesia in patient with and without marked PSC

Patients	No. of cases	Excellent to good results	Rate of excellent to good results (%)	P
With marked PSC (Grades I–II)	345	307	88.90	
Without marked PSC (Grades III–V)	761	440	57.82	<0.001
Total	1,106	747	67.54	

Table 3. Relationship between grade of PSC and effectiveness of acupuncture analgesia in different pain regions

Grades of PSC	Effectiveness of acupuncture analgesia (No. of Cases)																			
	Head				Neck				Chest-Back				Abdomen				Lumbar			
	E	G	F	P	E	G	F	P	E	G	F	P	E	G	F	P	E	G	F	P
I	13	19	3	0	13	3	1	0	4	5	1	0	30	11	3	0	24	22	2	1
II	17	39	10	0	1	13	2	0	6	11	2	2	18	28	2	0	5	25	8	1
III	6	48	25	6	2	15	4	3	2	10	3	3	15	33	23	5	3	39	27	5
IV	4	31	19	14	1	6	6	9	1	4	4	1	2	19	11	9	2	30	24	18
V	7	17	8	7	2	4	5	1	1	2	2	0	37	55	34	17	1	41	20	8

E: excellent G: good F: fair P: poor

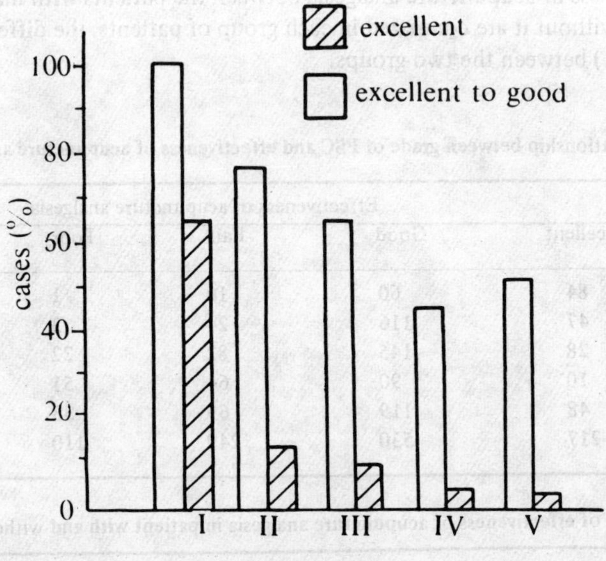

Fig. 3 Comparison of efficacy of acupuncture analgesia in patients with different Grades of PSC. (acute sprain of lumbar region)

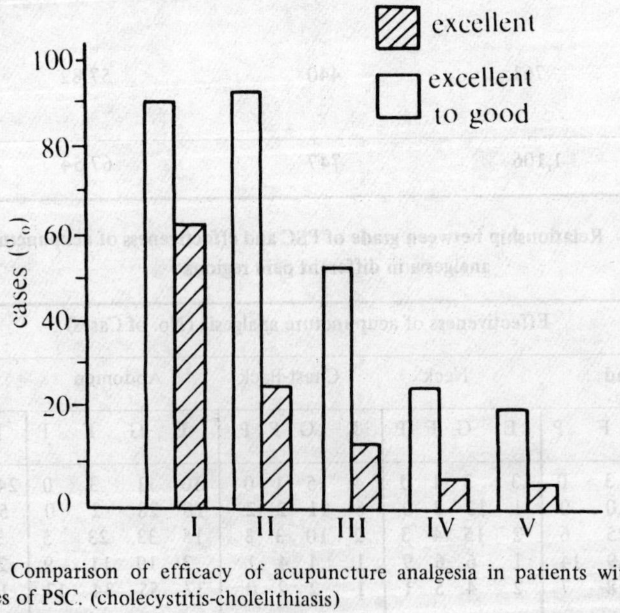

Fig. 4 Comparison of efficacy of acupuncture analgesia in patients with different Grades of PSC. (cholecystitis-cholelithiasis)

III. DISCUSSION

1. The results of the observation on 1,106 patients suffering from pain demonstrate that a close relationship certainly exists between PSC and the effectiveness of clinical acupuncture analgesia. The more marked the centripetal PSC is, the better will be the effectiveness of acupuncture analgesia; the distinct effect is always achieved when PSC does arrive at the affected region. Though many treatments were used for some of the patients who had been suffering from sharp pain for a long time, the pain remained still. However, the great pain was relieved instantly as soon as PSC reached the affected region during acupuncture. The results of observations on this problem of various reports were the similar[15-18].

2. Fig.2 and Table 3 show that in patients with Grades II–V PSC, the peaks of the effect of acupuncture analgesia all fall on "good" result and the percentage of "fair to poor" results increases as PSC passes from Grade II to Grade V. However, in patients with Grade I PSC, the peak fall on excellent result and the percentage of "fair to poor" results is very low. If cases are analyzed in groups according to the affected regions such as the head, neck, chest-back, abdomen and lumbar, the tendency of the efficacy of acupuncture analgesia to decrease as PSC goes down from Grade I to Grade V is also clear. The same results were obtained when the 112 cases of cholecystitis-cholelithiasis and the 192 cases of acute sprain of lumbar region were counted seperately.

The above results indicate that the more marked the centripetal PSC is, the better the efficacy of acupuncture analgesia will be. Such a relationship may be universal. It bears no relation to the affected region and the kind of disease. The distribution of the efficacy of acupuncture analgesia in the patients with Greade II–V PSC is nearly the same. The "good" results were achieved in most of the patients of all the four groups. However, the characteristics of the patients with Grade I PSC were entirely different from those of all the others with Grade II–V PSC. The excellent rate was as high as 54.19%, and the poor result was 0.65% only. This reveals that the characteristics manifested in the phenomenon of " 'Qi' (PSC) travelling to the affected region" were apparent, and PSC played an important role in the realization of acupuncture analgesia. The ancient physicians's emphasis on the importance of making the "Qi" (vital energy) to flow to the pain region by acupuncture is based on rich experience from practice experience[19]. It is important for us to earnestly study the characteristics of the phenomenon of " 'Qi' coursing to the affected region" and to search by analysis the reason why distinct effect is always achieved when "Qi" reaches the affected region for further elucidating of the mechanisms of acupuncture anesthesia.

3. The pain in acute sprain of lumbar region belongs to deep pain caused by the damage of muscles, ligaments, etc., while the pain in cholecystitis-cholelithiasis belongs to visceralgia. Though they are different in nature, nevertheless they all can be relieved by acupuncture. Furthermore, with both of them, the efficacy of acupuncture analgesia is closely related to the grade of PSC. This suggests that investigation of PSC not only can lessen the pain caused by the damage of deep tissues, but is also conducive to further overcoming the traction response of the viscera and visceralgia during operation under acupuncture anesthesia.

4. The results mentioned above show that there surely exists a close relationship between PSC and the efficacy of acupuncture analgesia; whether the 1,106 patients are

analyzed in groups according to the affected region or the kind of disease, the results are exactly the same. It is clear that such relationship may be universal. The difference in the effectiveness of acupuncture analgesia between the patients with marked centripetal PSC and those without it is highly significant.

One of the main characteristics of PSC is that it runs both in centripetal and centrifugal directions simultaneously or in centripetal direction at a rather slow speed. The centrifugal needling sensation is characterized by its speedy radiation accompanied by a sensation of electrical shock in nature. It might be the projection of sensation caused by stimulating a nerve trunk (or its branches) and is different from PSC. As mentioned above the acupuncture analgesic effect in patients with centrifugal PSC is somewhat better than that in patients without PSC. This suggests that though a measure of analgesic effect could be achieved as a nerve trunk is stimulated, but it falls much short of that of patients with marked centripetal PSC.

The mastering of PSC was considered by physicians in all the past ages as the key to the improvement of the efficacy of acupuncture, from the fabulous medical doctor Hua Tuo to Yang Ji-Zhou of the Ming Dynasty. It has been pointed out in the medical literature of the Ming Dynasty (such as 《 Zheng Jiu Da Cheng 》 and 《 Jin Zheng Fu 》) that it is necessary not only to select the acupuncture points along the related channel, but also to make the "Qi" to reach the affected region in acupuncture treatment. Many manipulation techniques for controlling the "Qi" were collected in these medical works. Yang Ji-Zhou had dealt at length the great significance of "selection of the acupuncture points along the related channel and the driving the 'Qi' to the affected region". He put his main points in such aphorisms: Rather lose the points than the channel, and the opportune moment than the "Qi"[20]. This is an important advance in the art of acupuncture therapy made by the physicians of the Jin and Ming Dynasties. Great attention should be paid to learning from them and to exploring the rich content of these invaluable legacies in the investigation of the mechanisms of acupuncture.

Evidently, "selection of the acupuncture points along the related channel and guiding the 'Qi' to the affected region" may be an effective approach to enhance the efficacy of acupuncture therapy and acupuncture anesthesia. The fact that there is a close relationship between PSC and efficacy of acupuncture is a favorable condition for further studies in this respect. Provided some effective measures for controlling and enhancing PSC could be found and PSC could be made to reach the affected site in most cases, the effectiveness of acupuncture therapy and acupuncture anesthesia can surely be improved to a great extent.

IV. SUMMARY

1. The results of observation on 1,106 patients suffering from pain show that there is a close relationship between PSC and the effectiveness of acupuncture analgesia. The more marked the centripetal PSC is, the better the effectiveness of acupuncture analgesia will be. The difference in the effectiveness of acupuncture analgesia between patients with marked centripetal PSC and those without it is highly significant ($P<0.001$).

2. It is evident that selection of acupuncture points along the related channels on the ground of "Bian-Zheng" and guidance of PSC to the pain region is a reliable approach to

improve the effectiveness of acupuncture analgesia and is worth while to study seriously.

(Written by the Research Group of Acupuncture Anesthesia, Institute of Medicine and Pharmacology of Fujian Province.)

REFERENCES

[1] 焦勉斋：山东省中医经络针灸学术经验交流会议资料选编，7页，山东省卫生厅，1960。

[2] 杨其寿：中医临床经验汇编(第一辑)，126页，云南省卫生厅，1957。

[3] 邓慕石：中医杂志，(4)：205，1957。

[4] 徐立孙：中医杂志，(8)：551，1958。

[5] 朱天洪：江苏中医，(3)：29，1952。

[6] 中山医学院口腔科教研组：中山医学院科学论文集(第一辑)，针灸研究专辑，下册，121页，1960。

[7] 黄教崴：中医杂志，(8)：437，1957。

[8] 金忠恩：浙江中医杂志，(4)：5，1958。

[9] 西安中医门诊部：西安市医药卫生资料选编79页，西安市卫生局，1959。

[10] 施震：浙江中医杂志，(4)：35，1958。

[11] 萧应干：现代针灸资料选集(第4集)，169页，人民卫生出版社，1960。

[12] 王品三：中医杂志，(1)：40，1958。

[13] 保定地区中医院等：针刺麻醉资料选编(2)，82页，北京人民出版社，1973。

[14] 福建省医药研究所针麻原理研究组：医药资料选编(2)，6页，福建省医药研究所，1973。

[15] 吉林医科大学第四临床学院经络感传研究组：针刺麻醉(2-3)：73，1977。

[16] 江苏省经络研究协作组：针刺麻醉(2-3)：66，1977。

[17] 河南中医研究所临床组：中医药研究资料，65页，河南中医学院编，1976。

[18] 皖南医学院临床针麻组：皖南医学(3)：6，1975。

[19] 明·高武纂集：针灸聚英，262页，上海科学技术出版社，1961。

[20] 明·杨继洲：针灸大成，46页，人民卫生出版社，1959。

EXISTENCE OF CHANNEL SYSTEM AS EVIDENCED BY 93 CASES OF SKIN DISEASES APPEARING ALONG THE CHANNELS

Li Dingzhong
(Beijing Sixth Hospital)

The channel theory is an important component of the theoretical system of the traditional Chinese medicine. Treatment of diseases by acupuncture and operations performed under acupuncture anesthesia are all based upon the channel theory. Therefore, studies on the existence of the channel system and its nature have become a principal subject in this field.

Since 1954, with a clinical experience of twenty odd years, we have been able to observe objectively the existence of channel lines by studying 12 kinds of channel phenomena. These included changes appearing along the channel lines, such as skin diseases, pains, low electro-resistance points, body surface sensory changes (of visceral diseases, brain traumas and those with marked PSC), sweating, angioneurotic functional changes, three kinds of PSC (physiologic, pathologic and autonomic) and the so-called "excitation" points of the channels. We have, thus far, acquired only a preliminary knowledge about the features and rules of channels.

Investigations on channels are now being undertaken in many countries of the world. Owing to the dynamic nature and instable objective indices of PSC, it is sometimes difficult to carry out the experiment more objectively to ascertain the existence of PSC. There is controversy about the existence of PSC. But the skin diseases appearing along the channels showed quite a different pattern. Once the lesions appeared they remained there steadily and showed histomorphological changes. Acquired lesions might remain for a few days to as long as several years; congenital cases might persist for life. Such lesions suggest strongly the existence of the channels. Among various kinds of skin diseases, linear lesions appear most commonly along the channel lines.

Ninety-three patients suffering from 13 kinds of skin diseases were studied. There were III skin lesions of these diseases found along the channels. There were cases with histological changes of epidermis and dermal papillae, such as pigmented nevus, verrucoid nevus, dermatrophia, eczema, neurodermatitis, psoriasis and lichen planus; cases with histological changes of vascular dilatation, avasculosis, hemorrhage and collagenous degeneration, such as bright red macular nevus, nevus anemicus, purpura and scleroderma; and cases with histological changes of the skin appendages, such as nevus sebaceus and porokeratosis. Of the III channel lines on which skin lesions appeared, 42 lines (37.84%) were lesions of congenital cases and 69 (62.16%) were acquired ones (see Table 1).

As shown in Table 1, most of them were various kinds of congenital nevi, while neurodermatitis and lichen planus constituted the majority of acquired cases. They are discussed in the following in three parts.

Table 1. **Skin diseases found along the 111 channels**

Congenital Skin Diseases						
Naevus verrucosus	Naevus pigmentosus	Naevus anemicus	Naevus flammeus	Naevus sebaceus	Porokeratosis	Atrophoderma
14	5	10	1	6	5	1

Acquired Skin Diseases					
Neurodermatitis	Lichen planus	Eczema	Scleroderma	Purpura	Psoriasis
34	20	6	5	2	2

I. RULE OF CHANNELS

Although different skin diseases take different forms, as a rule, they are all distributed on channel lines which basically coincide with the classical channels. The following is considered as an important rule: No matter where they come out and along which channel, cutaneous eruptions are always identical in clinical appearance as well as in histological changes. In the case of nevus anemicus the changes were always located in the blood vessels of dermal papillae, and in that of nevus sebaceous the changes were found in the sebaceous glands. In neurodermatitis, inflammatory infiltration surrounding the blood capillaries of the dermal papillae with subsequent epidermal changes is seen. This shows that the site and nature of the pathological changes as well as the histomorphological changes are also identical. It also reflects the internal relations and the disease specific nature of the channels.

(I) Eruptions appearing on a single channel line

1. Pericardium Channel. As recorded in "Lingshu Jing", the Pericardium Channel of hand Jueyin begins from the mid-thorax, passes along Naonei via antecubital space to tip of the middle finger.

Case 1. Neurodermatitis. Huang X X, female, 8 years old, first visited our clinic on Aug. 18, 1955. She had suffered from neurodermatitis along the Pericardium Channel for 8 years. On examination, a band lesion with lichenification was noticed on the inside medial aspects of the left and arm. The eruptions were grey in color and elevated slightly above the skin surface. Shortly afterwards, a brown verruciform hyperplasia developed on the medial aspect of the carpus and the lateral aspects of the palms and fingers. The diagnosis of

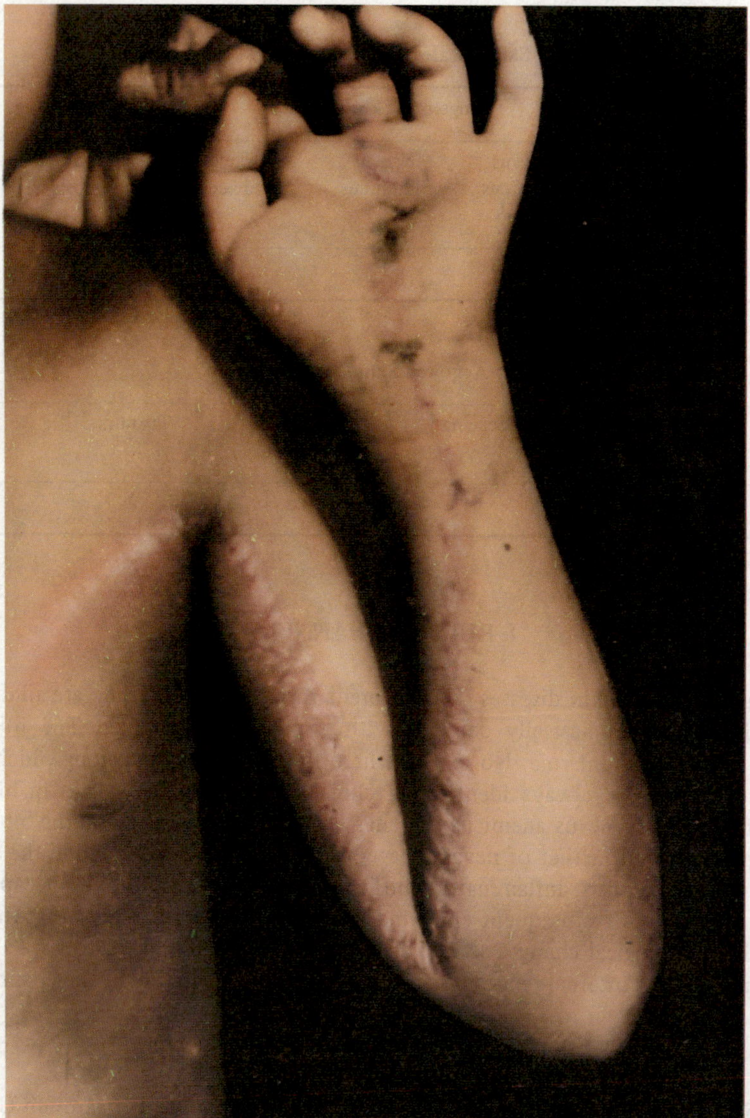

Fig. 1

Huang ××, Female, 8, Neurodermatitis appeared along left pericardium channel neurodermatitis was confirmed by biopsy. The distribution of the lesions was basically along the course of the Pericardium channel as that described in the "Lingshu Jing" (see Fig. 1).

2. **Liver Channel.** As recorded in the "Lingshu Jing", the Liver Channel of foot Jueyin begins from hallux, passes the medial knee and the perineum, and stops at the lower abdomen (Qimen).

Case 2. Lichen planus. Patient Du X X, male, 30 years old, first visited our clinic on Sept. 28, 1971. Red flat papules with smooth surface appeared on the medial aspect of the left thigh for 6 years. The lesions extended rapidly down to the leg in the form of a band, 0.5–0.7cm wide. The distribution of the lesion was basically along the Liver Channel as recorded in the "Lingshu Jing" (see Fig. 2).

3. **Urinary Bladder Channel'** As recorded in "Lingshu Jing", the Urinary Bladder Channel of foot Taiyang begins from the inner canthus, runs along the buttock to the popliteal fossa and ends in the dorsum of the little toe via outer-ankle.

Case 3. Neurodermatitis. Yang X X, male, 6 years old, first visited our clinic on April 24, 1971. The lesions started as an erythematous infiltration with marked itching on the right popliteal fossa for 6 months. Increased lichenification was noticed after scratching. They extended upwards and downwards in band form, measuring0.8– 1.0cm wide. Their distribution along the Urinary Bladder Channel, ranging from Chengfu, Weizhong to the outer-ankle, coincided with that described in the "Lingshu Jing" (see Fig. 3).

The above typical cases show that the distribution of lesions is closely in accord with the courses of channels. This is not a mere coincidence. It reflects the actual existence of the channels. The problem is discussed further as follows.

(II) Different skin diseases appearing on the same channel line

The above 3 patients suffered from different kinds of skin diseases (congenital or acquired) with skin lesions all distributed along the Kidney Channel.

Case 4. Nevus anemicus. Peng X X, male, 45 years old, first visited our clinic on Aug. 10, 1970. A white band, 0.5– 0.9cm wide, was noticed on the medial thigh shortly after birth. The surface of the lesions was smooth and nonindurated. No hyperkeratosis except a slight atrophy was observed. No subjective symptoms were complained of by the patient. The diagnosis was confirmed by biopsy. It should be noted that the band lesion appeared along the Kidney channel, beginning from Shuiquan and stopping at the perineum (see Fig. 4).

Case 5. Neurodermatitis. Wang X X, male, 35 years old, first visited our clinic on Aug. 25, 1973. An itchy, lichenoid band lesion, 0.5–0.8cm wide, appeared on the right buttock 4 months ago. Two days ago, it extended suddenly downwards along the course of Kidney Channel, i.e., from the posterior aspect of the right thigh via Yingu to Shuiquan (see Fig. 5). The patient had some mental disturbance before the onset of eruptions.

Case 6. Scleroderma. Sun X X, male, 31 years old, visited our clinic in 1963. Brown band lesions, 1cm wide, appeared on the postero-medial aspects of the left thigh 2 years ago. The lesions were firm, smooth and well demarcated. No marked atrophy was noticed. They distributed along the course of Kidney Channel, i.e., from Shuiquan to Shenshu and joined with lesions on the Daimai Channel at the left side of the lower abdomen, and ended in the neighborhood of Yu Point.

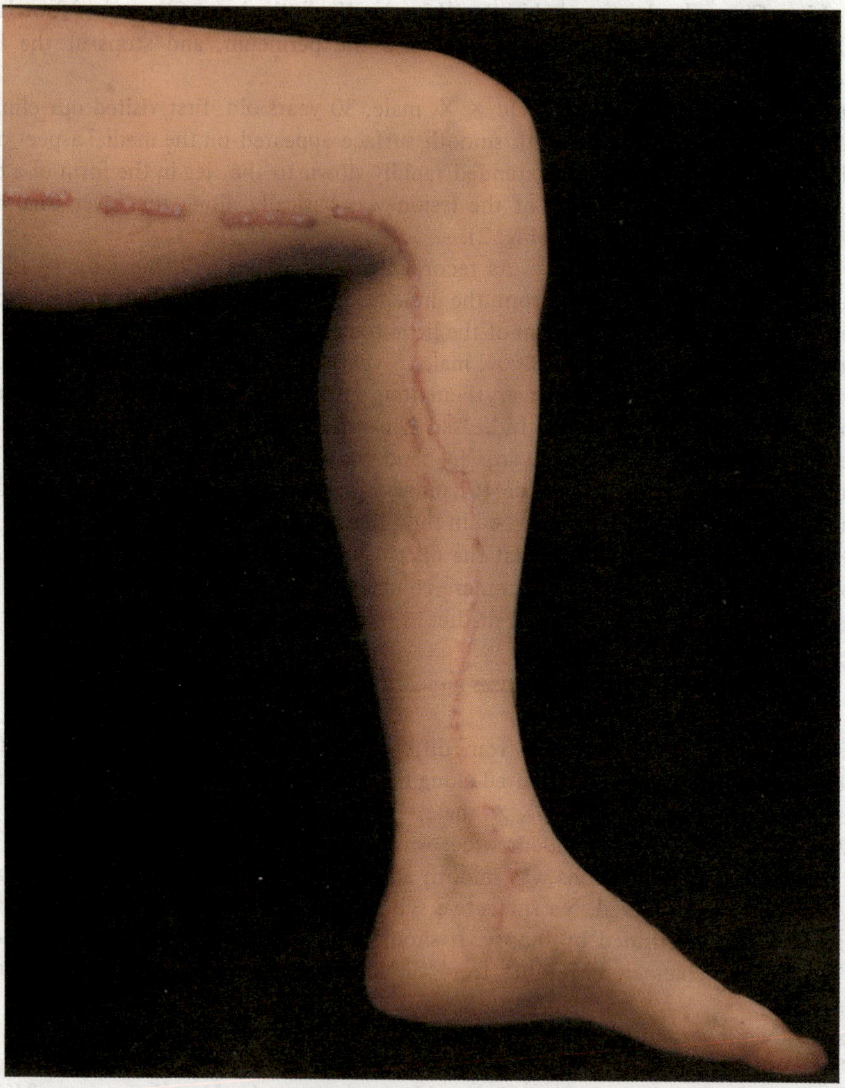

Fig. 2

Tu××, male, 30 years old, with lichen planus related to the left liver channel

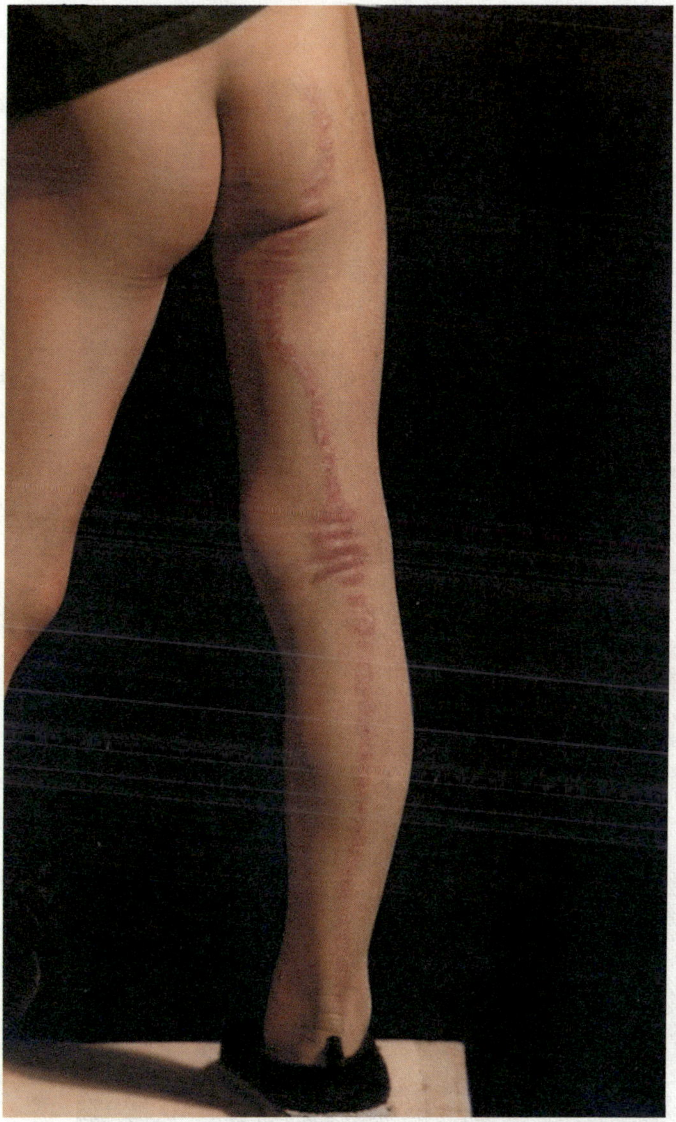

Fig. 3

Yang××,male, 6 years old, with neurodermatitis related to the right urinary bladder channel

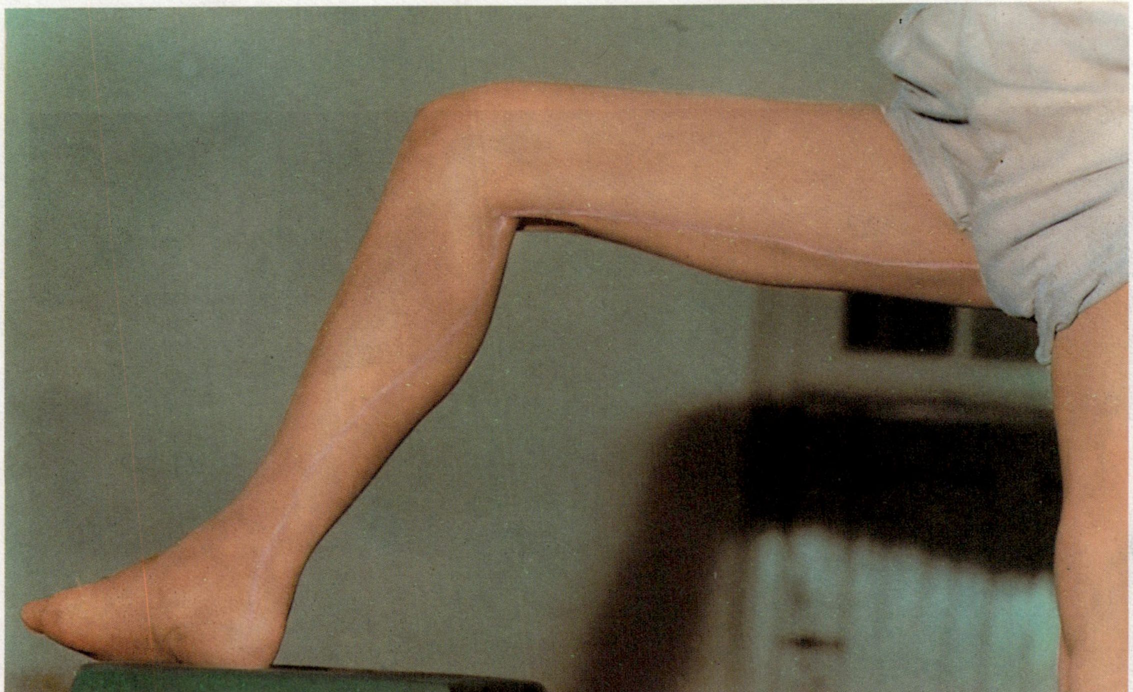

Fig. 4

Peng××,male, 45 years old, with nevus anemicus related to the kidney channel

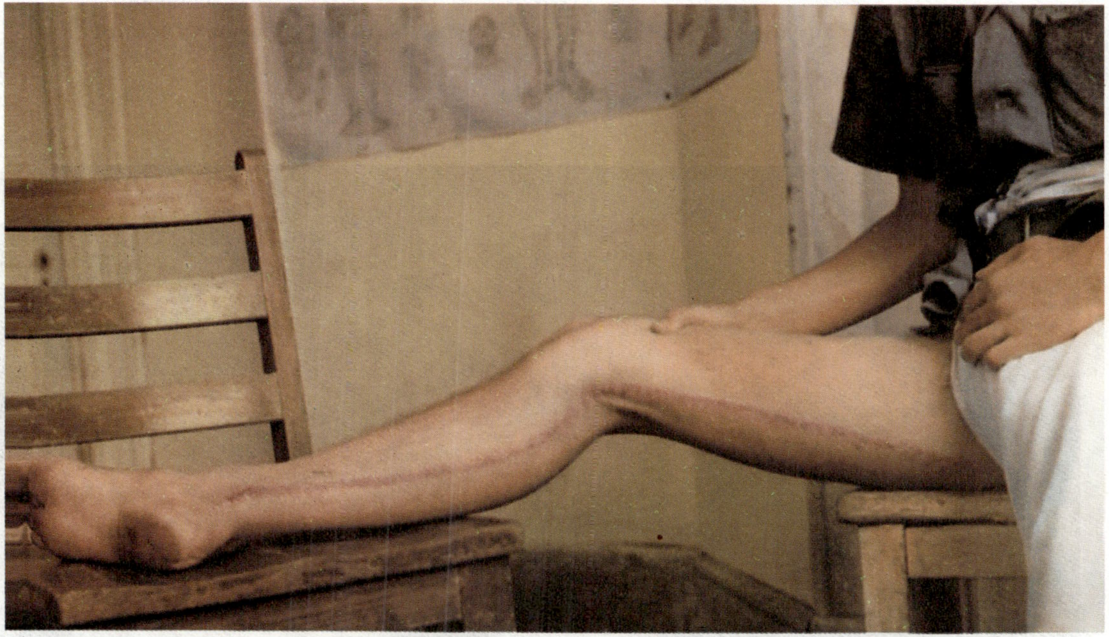

Fig. 5

Wang××, male, 35 years old, with neurodermatitis related to the right kidney channel

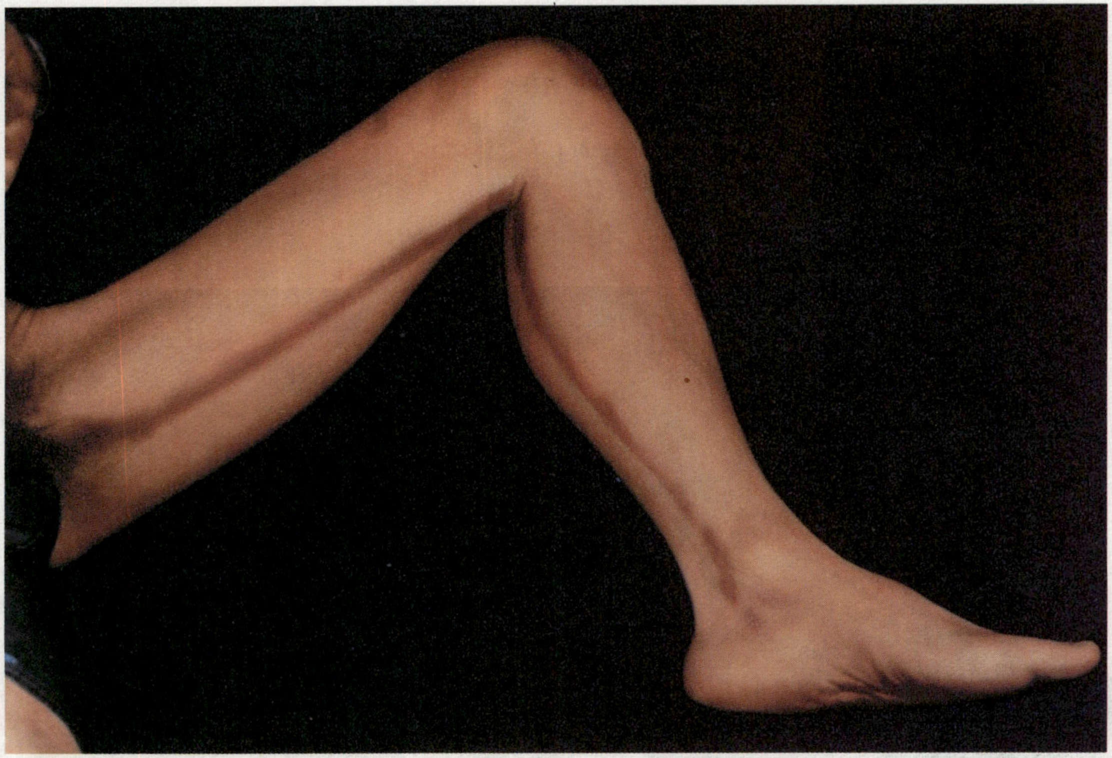

Fig. 6

Sun××, male, 31 years, with scleroderma related to the left kidney channel

The above cases showed that different skin diseases in different patients had appeared along the same channel line. That was quite consistent with the Kidney Channel recorded in the "Lingshu Jing".

(III) Skin diseases appearing on several channel lines in one patient

Skin lesions appeared not only on a single channel line but also on two or more channel lines of the same patient. In patient Shi, the lesions of lichen planus appeared concurrently on the Large Intestine and the Pericardium Channels. In patient Cheng, lesions of nevus anemicus appeared on three channel lines, namely the Pericardium, Liver and Gall-bladder Channels. In patient Dong, lesions of porokeratosis appeared on 4 channel lines, namely the Large Intestine, Pericardium, Heart and Kidney Channels. In patient Han, a case of nevus sebaceus, the lesion appeared concurrently on five channel lines, namely the Heart, Large Intestine, Lung, Kidney and the Daimai Channels. This last patient was a girl of 17, whose first visit to our clinic was on Jun. 20, 1976. She complained of some brownish eruptions over the scalp, face and the neck since birth. It was less prominent on the extremities. After the onset of menstruation at age 13, the eruptions developed into villiform hyperplasia with some lipid secretions. Part of the eruptions over the scalp and face turned into verruciform lesions and coalesced gradually with lesions on the chest and the extremities into band forms. Histological sections confirmed the diagnosis of nevus sebaceus (see Figures below).

Fig. 7. Nevus sebaceus along the right Heart Channel. The lesions started from the mid-thorax, passed Shaohai via axilla and stopped at the palm.

Fig. 8. Nevus sebaceus along the left Lung Channel. The lesions started from the upper mid-thorax, passed the upper limb via the left axilla and stopped at the left thumb, deviated to the Pericardium Channel at Neiguan and Jianshi.

Fig. 9. Nevus sebaceus along the left Large Intestine Channel. The lesions started from the space between the left thumb and the index finger, passed Jianyu via Hogu and Quchi, and stopped at Dazhui. They divided into two branches at the cervical region, one branch ran upwards toward the head and the other to the mouth corners.

The distribution of nevus sebaceus lesions along the different channels shown in the above figures are basically the same as the courses of these channels described in the "Lingshu Jing".

From the above cases, it is quite clear that the character and basic rule of the channel may be reflected objectively by skin diseases. We believe, therefore, that it is not a mere coincidence.

II. VARIATION PHENOMENA OF CHANNELS– SIX KINDS OF VARIATION PHENOMENA HAVE BEEN OBSERVED

1. The spreading-contracting phenomenon: Lesions along the lines show irregularity of width.

2. The bending phenomenon: Lesions turn in midway to a neighboring channel and then return to the original one.

3. The channel crossing phenomenon: Lesions on one channel run into another one.

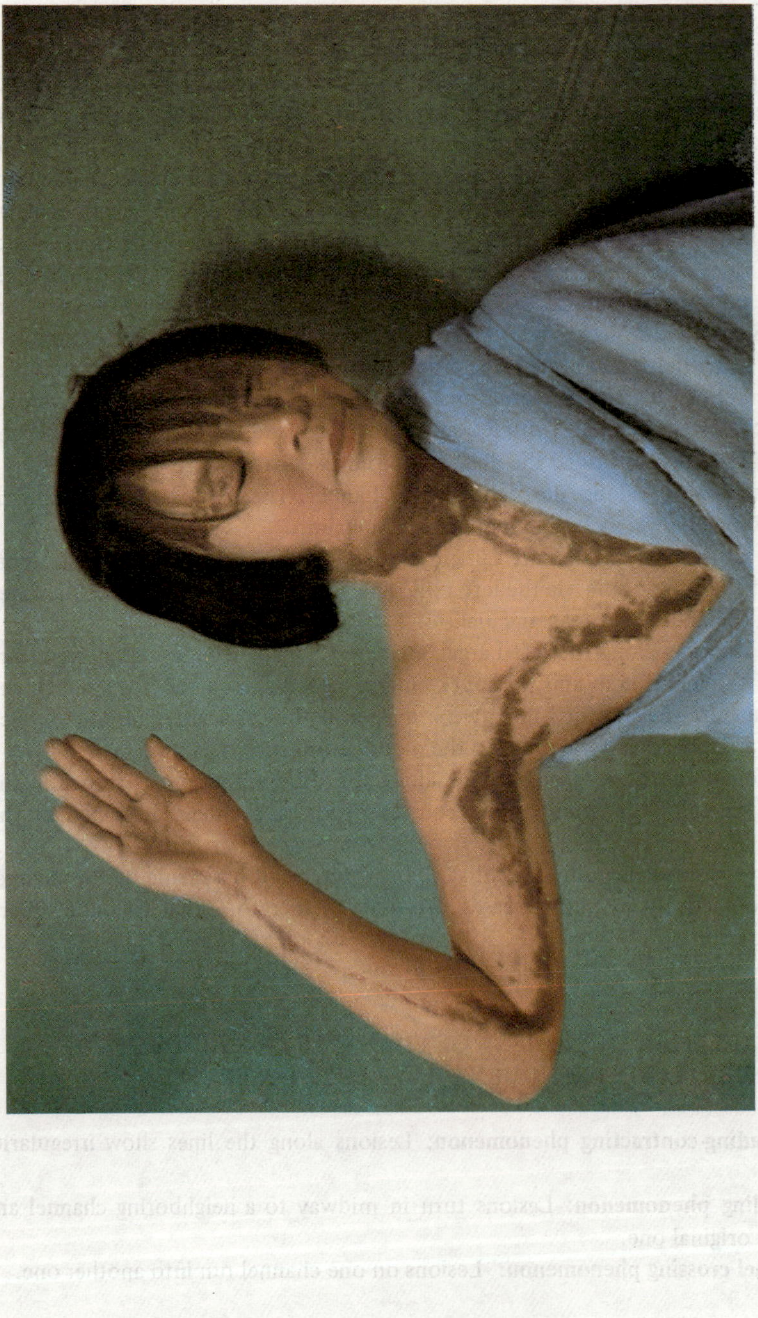

Fig. 7

Han × ×, Female 20 Nevus sebaceus appeared along the right heart channel

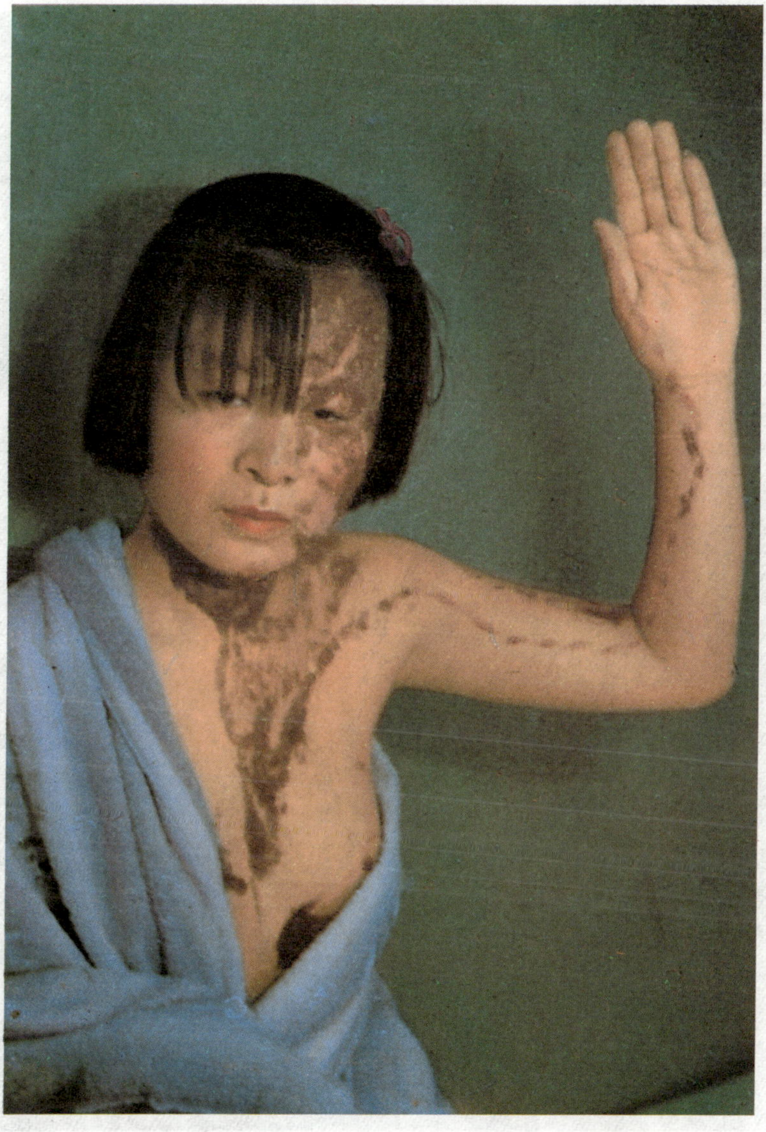

Fig. 8

Han × ×, Female 20 Nevus sebaceus appeared along the left lung channel

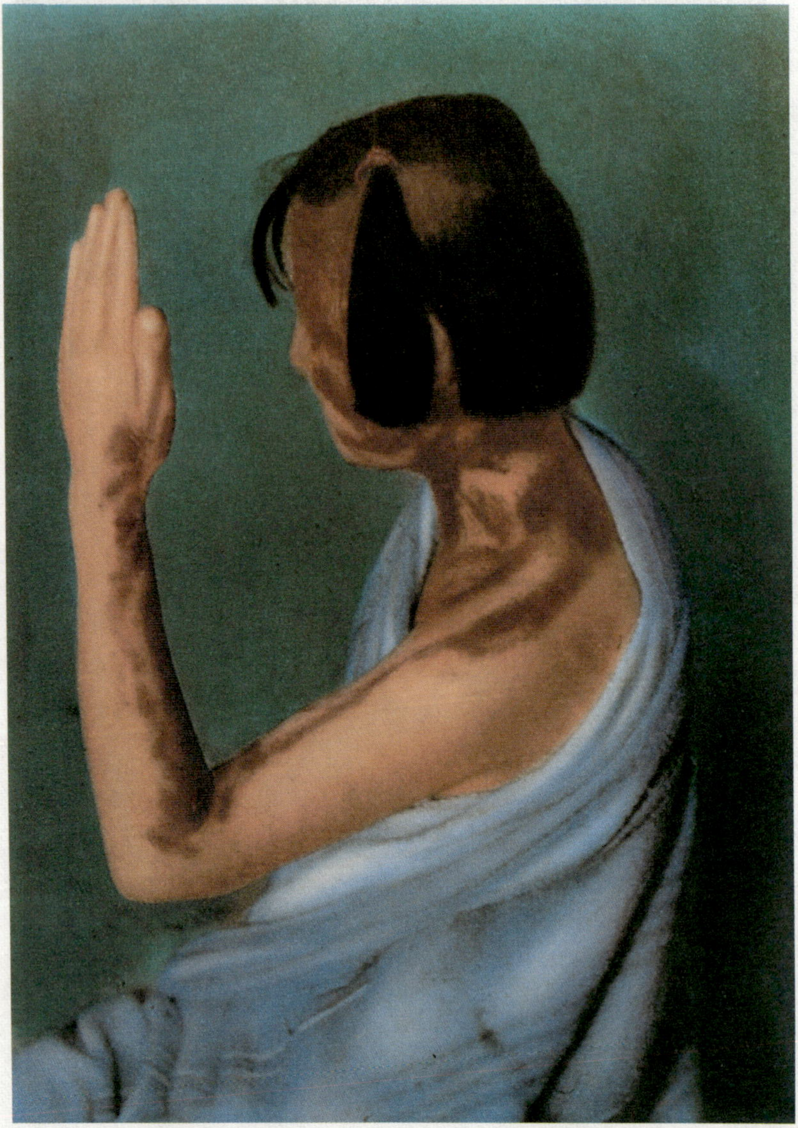

Fig. 9

Han × ×, Female 20 Nevus sebaceus appeared along the left large intestine channel

4. The branching phenomenon: Lesions divided into branches at the end of a channel line (see Fig. 10).

5. The confluent phenomenon: Lesions of one channel line coalesce with those of two neighboring channels (see Fig. 11).

6. Phenomenon of association with neural segments: This was exemplified in patient Liu, a case of bright red macular nevus. The lesions distributed primarily along the Lung Channel with partial involvement of the Pericardium Channel. The location of the lesions over the chest was within the range of the cervical 3,4,5 and the thoracic 2,3,4 spinal segmental innervation. The lesions over the chest may be related to the spinal segments while those distributed along the extremities may be related to the channels. This phenomenon cannot be explained singly by segmental innervation. We presume there is an association of the channels with nerve segments.

Based upon these variation phenomena, we believe that the channel is not an unchanged pathway. It changes according to its own rules.

III. TREATMENT OF SKIN DISEASES WITH ACUPUNCTURE AND CHANNEL POINT INJECTION

No systematic observations on this subject have taken place yet, but treatments of selected cases have shown satisfactory results.

Case 1. Chou X X, male, 54 years old, suffered from neurodermatitis along the Kidney Channel with a history of 10 years. Marked hyperkeratosis was noticed on examination. More recently the lesions aggravated with generalized eruptions spread all over the body accompanied by itching. Subcutaneous injections of oxygen in both Shenshu points were given every other day. The itching improved after 3 injections and continued to improve after 6 injections. The eruptions also showed marked improvement. They subsided entirely after 12 injections. However, the lesions along the Kidney Channel became thinner without noticeable itching. After 25 injections they were arrested and even disappeared in some parts.

Case 2. Liang X X, male, 29 years old, suffered from eczema along the Liver Channel for one year. Dense papules and erythematous infiltration with erosions of the epidermis were noted on the inguinal region, extending down to the medial aspect of left toe. Acupuncture treatment by using the Taichong, Zhongdu and Yinbao points was given daily. Only the points of the diseased side were used during the first week, which resulted in a subsidence of only 1/3 of the lesions as well as some improvement of the pruritus. When points of both sides were used during the following week, the lesions disappeared in 5 days.

Case 3. Zhang X X, female, 28 years old, suffered from neurodermatitis along the left Small Intestine Channel (see Fig. 12). The lesions started from the cervical region and progressed along the Small Intestine Channel to Wangu. She had suffered from the disease for one year. Neither the rash nor the pruritus had had any improvement following treatments by acupuncture, electro-acupuncture and channel point injections of Vit. B-12 on the affected side. At the pain pressure point near Weizhong of the unaffected side, one single injection of Vit. B-12 improved the pruritus remarkably. The lesions disappeared entirely after one week's treatment.

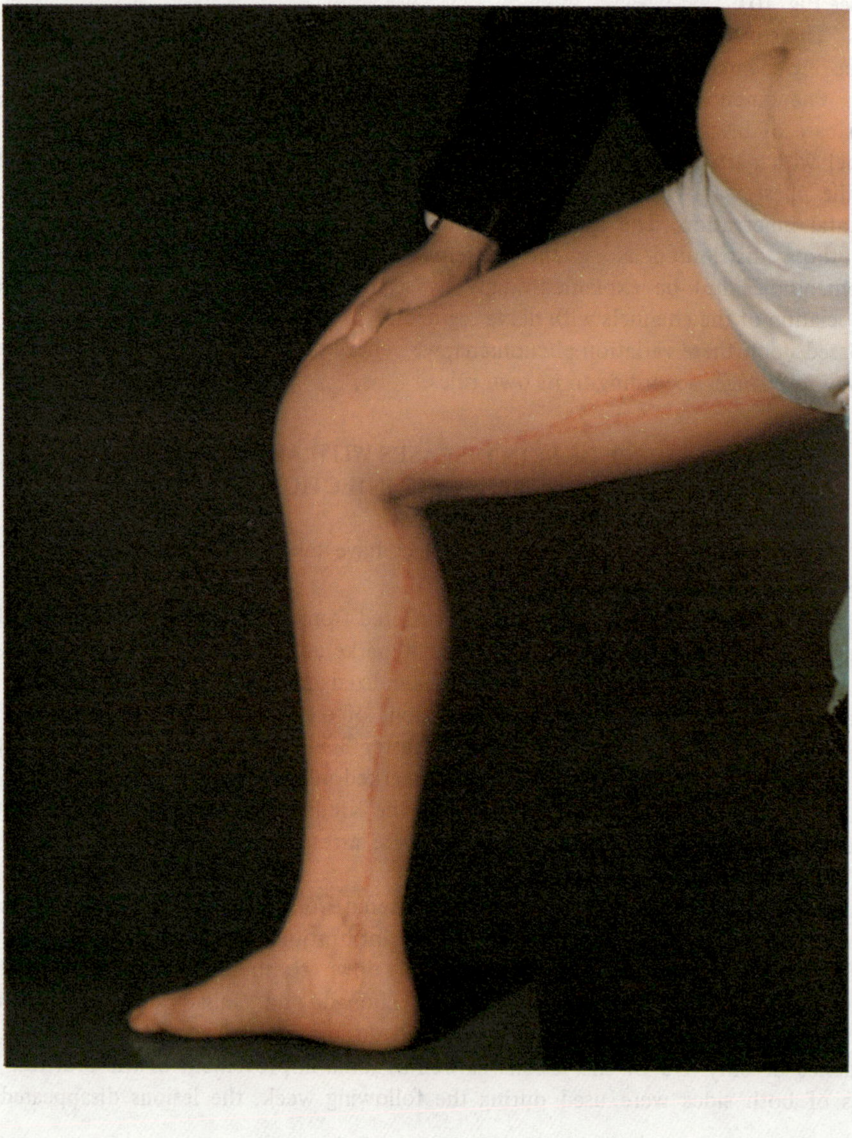

Fig. 10

Sheng X X, Female 27 Neurodermatitis appeared along the right kidney channel

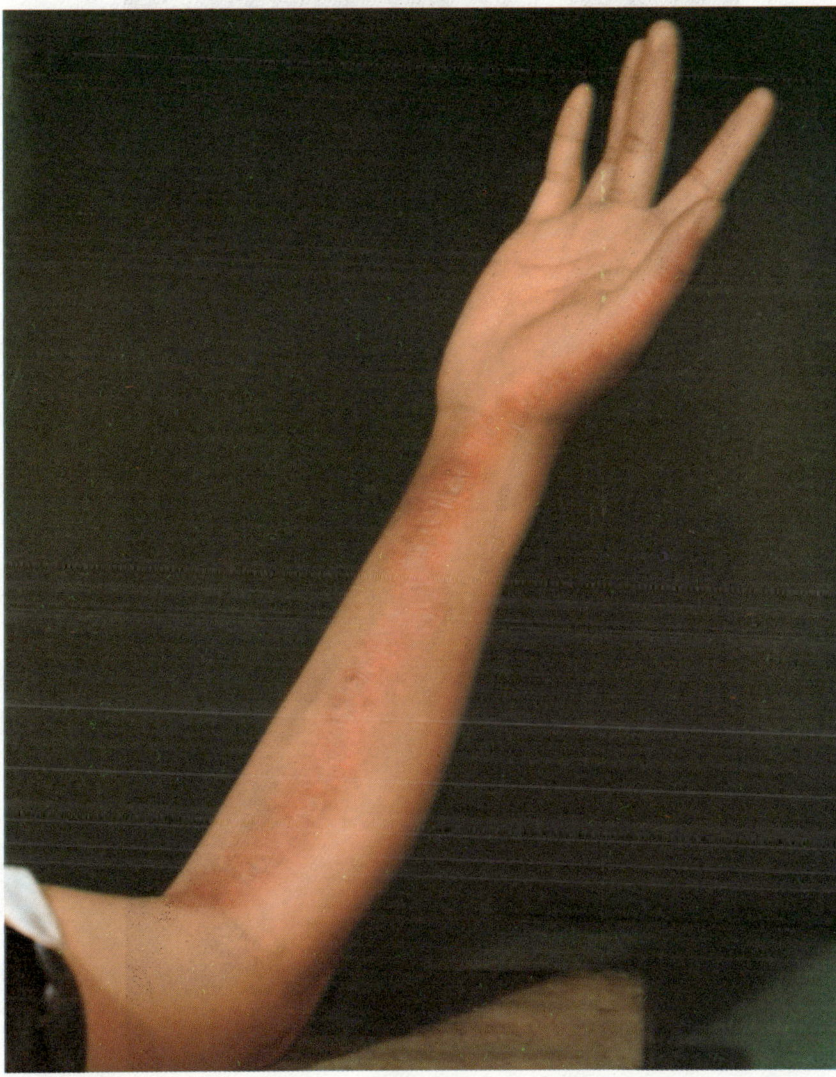

Fig.11

Zhang ×× , Female 21 Neurodermatitis appeared along the lung & pericardium Channels

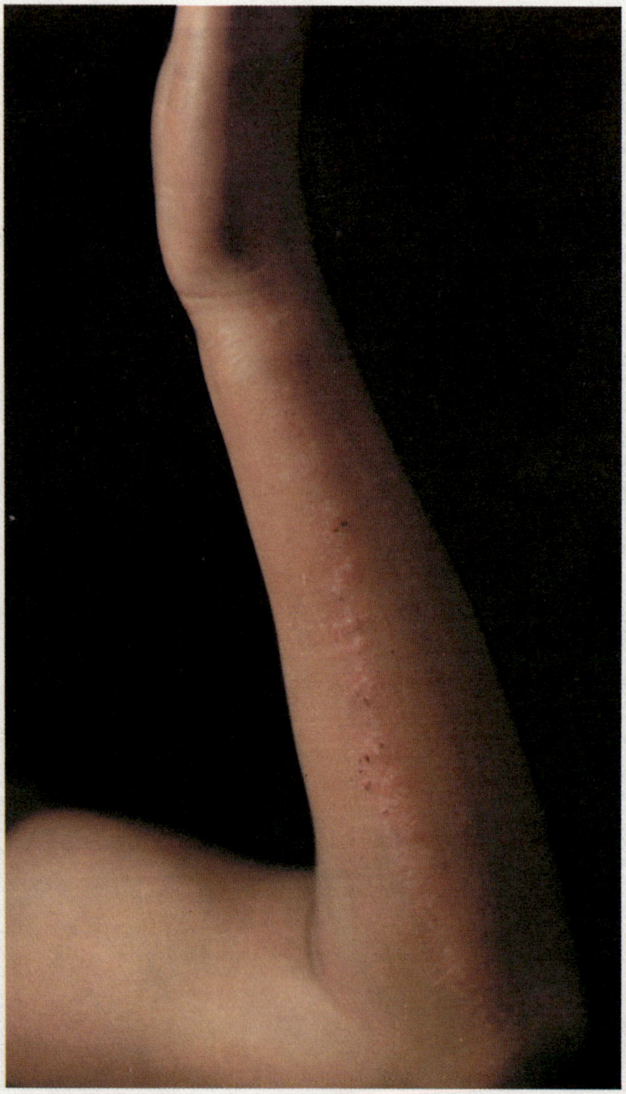

Fig.12

Zhang××, female, 28 years old, with neurodermatitis related to the left small intestinal channel

Case 4. Sheng X X, female, 27 years old, suffered from neurodermatitis along the right Kidney Channel for 2 months (see Fig. 10). The pruritus improved after one acupuncture of the pain pressure point on the left Heart Channel. The lesions receded after 3 treatments and cleared away within 2 weeks.

Case 5. Yu X X, male, 42 years old, suffered from neurodermatitis along the right Kidney Channel for 2 months. By needling the pain pressure points opposite to the right Kidney and left Heart Channels of the diseased site, the lesions were cured in 2 weeks.

The satisfactory results from the treatment of skin diseases along the channels by acupuncture, especially by needling the pain pressure points of the unaffected side, revealed that there is an association of the diseases with the channels. It should be pointed out that only some kinds of skin diseases could be cured by acupuncture. In cases of congenital skin diseases and scleroderma, the results were unsatisfactory.

In addition, we have found that some skin disorders along the channels occurred during the attack of certain internal troubles, and with a remission of the latter, the skin lesions disappeared dramatically. Conversely, the appearance of a skin disorder may also inhibit an episode of some internal symptoms. We presume, therefore, that some regulatory and inhibitory interactions exist between the viscerae and the channels.

The histopathological changes of skin diseases appearing along channels failed to show any special structures. However, most of them are vascular changes as well as epidermal changes.

To sum up, the skin diseases described above manifested themselves in four prominent features. (1) They appeared along the channel lines; some occurred along the whole line while others occurred only on a part of them. These were observed on all the 14 channels and the Daimai. They appeared more often on the Kidney and Large Intestine Channels and less often on the Lung and Pericardium Channels. (2) The pathologic changes were mainly at the upper dermis and the epidermis. (3) 66.65% of 93 cases were under 15 years of age (including the congenital cases). (4) Most of the acquired cases were neurodermatitis and lichen planus which are closely related with the autonomic nerve system. Further studies are necessary to elucidate their pathogenesis.

IV. CONCLUSION

The existence of the Channel system has been proved by skin diseases occurring along channel lines. On the basis of the 12 kinds of channel phenomena, the author suggests that the channels are an active phenomenon of life closely related to the neuro-humoral mechanism. They change according to their own rules. They seem to be a sensory conducting system, a disease reflecting system, and a functional regulating system as well as a disease repairing system.

ALGESTHESIA AND PARESTHESIA PROPAGATED ALONG THE CHANNELS
(Report of 80 Cases)

Liu Chengzhong*
(Medical University of China)

The disease in the present paper is characterized by a sort of paroxysmal morbid feelings which spread along the channels on the body surface.

If it is a painful feeling, it is called "algesthesia propagated along the Channels" (APC). If it is of various other abnormal feelings, it is called "paresthesia propagated along the Channels " (PPC). "APC" and "PP" may together be termed "Sensory Disease propagated along the Channels" or "Disease Sensation propagated along the Channels" or "Disease-SPC"[1,2] .

Eighty cases of the disease collected between 1974–1978 are presented here.

I. CLINICAL DATA

1. Sex, age and clinical history. Of the 80 cases, 45 were male and 35 female. Their ages ranged from 11–60 years. The shortest clinical history was 3 days and the longest 10 years, with the majority of them under 3 years (72 cases, 90.0%).

2. Distribution of APC and PPC. Of the 80 cases, 43 were APC and 37 PPC. Their sensory characters are listed in Table 1.

3. Width, length and speed. The width of APC or PPC is usually between 1.5–3.0cm. In a few cases the propagation may penetrate the body cavity; if so, it is rather widely spread in this part.

When considering the length of APC and PPC, we analyzed only those cases with distance longer than one long bone of the body. There were 49 cases (61.2%) with APC or PPC propagated along the whole course of the Channels.

In calculating the speed of APC or PPC, patients who could remember clearly were asked to point out it on their body surface. In 6 cases tested, the speed was 10–40 cm/sec.

4. The course of propagation. The 119 courses of propagation of the 80 cases were conformed to those mentioned in Chinese traditional medicine on the courses of the "Channel (Meridian)". Those propagated along the Urinary Bladder, Stomach, Large Intestine, Gall Bladder, Pericardium, Ren (Front Midline) and Du (Back Middle) Channels, totalled 101 times (84.9%) (Table 2). In 2 cases, the propagation joined with another

*** Present address: Dalian Medical College.**

Table 1. Sensory characteristics of APC and PPC

Name of disease	Sensory character	Cases	Total
APC	Pain	43	43
PPC	Numbness	21	37
	Sensation of warmth	4	
	Pulsatory sensation	4	
	Feeling of wind	2	
	Feeling of waterflowing	2	
	Cold feeling	2	
	Ache and itch	2	

Table 2. Distribution of the 119 times of APC and PPC in 80 cases

Times	Name of the channels		Times
39	Urinary bladder C.	Dai Mai	6
14	Stomach C.	Spleen C.	3
12	Large Intestine C.	Kidney C.	3
11	The Du(Back Middle) B.	Sanjiao C.	2
10	Gall Bladder C.	Chong Mai	2
8	The Ren (Front Midline) C.	Small Intestine C.	1
7	Pericardium C.	Yinchiao Mai	1
Total 101 times (84.9%)		Total 18 times (15.1%)	

Channel of the same name, as the Hand-Yangming with the Foot-Yangming, the Hand-Shaoyang with the Foot-Shaoyang.

5. Characteristics of attacks. Both APC and PPC are characterized by attacks. They usually occur 2–6 times/day, but may be as many as 10 times/day or once every few days or every few months.

Attacks always began at a fixed point on the body surface, which is called "The Starting Point". After an attack had propagated along the Channel for a definite distance, it might either stay there or disappear for a while and then reappear in a pulsational state. Each attack might last 3–5 minutes or 2–3 hours. There were only 2 cases that lasted 1–3 days.

In a few cases, the attacks were accompanied by mental and emotional disturbances, visceral crises, local venous hyperemia, sweating along the Channel, vomiting, congestion of conjunctiva, epistaxis and involuntary incoordinate movement of the limb. One case fell asleep after the attack, one case had ptosis of the eyelid;after each attack on the homolateral side (left), two cases were followed by paresis of the limb of the homolateral side. All these symptoms remained 3–4 hours after the attack and then disappeared.

6. Relations with other physical diseases. All the 80 cases complained of some illness at the time when they were chosen for the study or had some form of illness before. They totalled 38 kinds of diseases, including 17 cases (21.25%) of concussion of the brain. In 21 cases, small localized foci were found at the starting point of APC or PPC. In 21 cases, small localized foci were found along courses of the channels. These two kinds of cases totaled 62.50%. These small localized foci included small nodules on the body surface or in the deeper tissues, scars, bone spurs or calluses. In 3 cases, the localized foci were found in some internal organs (chronic cholecystitis, polyp of the urinary bladder, localized pulmonary tuberculosis), and these foci were right under the starting point, and all their attacks presented a picture of crisis of internal organs. They were occasionally misdiagnosed as acute abdomen or spontaneous pneumothorax. One should also watch out for cerebral disease, gastric ulcer or chronic disease of the gall bladder.

When suffering from concussion of brain, the course of the propagation is related with the site of injury. When suffering from diseases of the other part of the body, the course of the propagation is related with the location of the foci, for example, cholecystitis with the Gall Bladder Channel, gastric ulcer with the Stomach Channel, and diseases of genito-urinary system with the Kidney Channel or the Ren (Front Midline) Channel. Usually, the sensory character of APC or PPC can reflect the character of the stimulating foci. For example, APC is usually related with painful stimulating foci; numbness propagated along the Channel usually occurred in pressing localized stimulating foci and sensation of heat propagated along the Channel usually occurred with inflammatory stimulating foci.

7. **Artificial stopping of the attacks**. After the onset of APC or PPC attacks, 55 cases (68.8%) could be stopped by means of applying pressure on the courses of propagation.

If an attack starts from one point and spreads along two courses, the pressure applied at one of them might drive the pain or paresthesia from this course to the other. In certain patients, the pressure applied usually by himself to stop pain often formed a traumatic wound or scar at the site of pressure. One patient, who was suffering pain starting from a point on the leg, must have somebody sit on his thigh in order to apply pressure to stop the attack.

8. **Dysesthesia after attack**. After an attack, 47 cases (58.8%) might had hypoesthesia or anesthesia over the body surface. It might be either of 2 types: dysesthesia propagated along the Channels or polysegmental dysesthesia.

(1) Dysesthesia propagated along the Channels: It is characterized by a band-like distribution of the course of APC or PPC. Its width was a little wider than that of the course of the primary attack but its length might be shorter than the primary. This type of dysesthesia propagated along the Channel may be called: "Hypoesthesia-PC" or "Anesthesia-PC". The 29 cases of dysesthesia propagated along the Channel observed by the author of this article were mostly located in the Stomach Channel, Gall Bladder Channel and the Urinary Bladder Channel (62.1%). The rest were distributed among the other Channels.

(2) Polysegmental dysesthesia: It is formed by the uniting of multiple skin segments into various forms of zones of hypoesthesia. The 31 zones presented in this article were of the whole body form, half body form, whole jacket form, half jacket form, lower part of the body form, whole saddle form and half saddle form, etc.

In all types of one-sided dysesthesia, their boundaries did not cross the middle line of the body. Sometimes, the Anesthesia-PC might be distributed on the background of the corresponding polysegmental hypoesthesia. For example, the anesthesia propagated along the Pericardium Channel was distributed in the area of homolateral hypoesthesia of the half jacket form.

Dysesthesia of these two types might last from a few hours to a few months or even years, the longest seen being 5 years. Some of the patients were still having attacks quite recently.

9. Duplication of SPC and dysesthesia-PC. All the APC or PPC attacks started spontaneously. But during the interval phase, in 76 cases abnormal feelings propagated along the Channels, "Sensation Propagated along the Channels" or "SPC" might be artificially induced by applying pressure at the course of Channel. The author believes that the basis of this phenomenon is a sensory reflex, i.e., "Sensory Reflex-PC" or "Reflex-SPC"[3].

By the use of this "Test of SPC", 158 times of SPC were induced artificially, a number much more than that seen in the preceding APC and PPC (119 times).

In 18 cases, tests were made to duplicate bands of dysesthesia-PC and zones of polysegmental dysesthesia. Having attained artificial induction of SPC, continuing the stimulation for another 5–15 minutes, a dysestheia band distributed along the Channel might be obtained. By prolonging the stimulation, the dysesthesia band would gradually become wider or develop into a half jacket, half body or whole body form of dysesthesia. They might last for 1–3 hours.

10. Changes of electroencephalography. Electroencephalograms were examined on 13 patients during the interval of attacks. Of 9 cases, the results of examination were normal. In 2 cases, there were quite a number of slow waves (3–7 cycles per second) distributed in the frontal, Parietal and occipital lobes. The electroencephalogram as a whole was of moderate wide spread abnormality. Another case was diagnosed as slow wave foci of the left fronto-temporal area. No examinations were made during attacks.

II. ILLUSTRATIVE CASES

Case 1. Yu, female, age 19, was hit on the left neck and left cheek with a spade. She developed coma and asphyxia for a short duration after the accident. During the 5 days before being seen, there were many paroxysmal attacks of pain. Starting from a little below the left clavicle, one branch spread upward through the inner canthus to the vertex of the head; another branch propagated downward along the inner side of the breast, abdomen, thigh, along the internal aspect of the leg and finally to the big toe. This course is identical with that of the Yinchiao Channel. If pressure is applied above the starting point, the pain would be propagating only downwards and the head was clear. There was tenderness of the deep part of the hyoid bone at the left side. The patient could not protrude her tongue. There was also hypokinesia and hypoesthesia of the left side of the body. SPC test (+). After taking librium (Chlordiazepoxidum) for 15 days and blocking the start point of the APC with 2 cc of 2% procaine hydrochloridum, APC did not recur. Movement and sensation of the left half side of the body recovered. All symptoms of SPC disappeared 60 days later.

Case 2. Gu, male, age 41, paroxysmal attacks of severe pain starting from a little below the left costal margin for 1 year. One branch propagated along the Gall Bladder Channel upward, crossing the back of the neck to the Gall Bladder Channel of the opposite side and then propagated downward to the lateral aspect of the right breast. Another branch propagated to the back diagonally upward to enter the Urinary Bladder Channel, and finally propagated to the neck to unite with the first branch. The attack at first occurred once a month, but later developed to several per day. The patient suffered from severe pain during the attacks, with sense of distention of the left eye and discomfort of the thoracic and abdominal organs, and was erroneously diagnosed as acute abdomen illness twice. There was a history of sprain of the left lumbar region and complaint of dislike of rich food since onset of illness. During attack, test of pancreatoamylase was normal; ECG showed low voltage. Half jacket form of hypoesthesia following attack lasted several days. After applying electric acupuncture to the course of the Pericardium Channel or the Gall Bladder Channel for 20 minutes, there might appear a band- like dysesthesia distributed along these Channels. The width was 1 cm, gradually increasing to 3 cm and finally to a half jacket form or half body form of anesthesia, lasting altogether 65 minutes. X-ray film showed proliferation and hyperporosis of the lumber vertebrae, pyelography normal, barium meal showed incomplete filling of the duodenal bulb, the barium meal passing rather rapidly. Cholecystogram showed the gall bladder did not shrink after taking rich food, with no shadow of calculus, and chronic cholecystitis was diagnosed. After taking phenytonium natrium and blocking the starting point of the APC, the result was remarkable. Finally after inducing Anesthesia-PC and burying of catgut (no anesthetic was used, but the patient felt no pain) the attacks of APC ceased immediately. No recurrence found in 3 years of follow-up.

Case 3. Lu, male, age 38, had an operation on a nasal polyp of the right side 8 years before. The pedicle arose from the base of the right middle turbinate. Soon afterwards, starting from a point on the skin surface of that region, a paroxysmal numbness propagated along the lateral side of the nose, round the mouth, then downward to below the lower lip. Three years later, numbness propagated upwards; one branch propagated from the inner canthus up to the vertex, and another branch propagated round the eye laterally to the vertex, conforming to the head-face part of the Stomach Channels. Attacks occurred frequently. There was an interval of 5–10 days after two weeks of attacks. Simultaneously, the right eye lost its sensation to wind and sand stimulation. Conjunctivitis and corneal ulcer occured frequently. The reflex of the right cornea and conjunctiva was slow. SPC test (+). The anesthetic band of the above propagation course might be found with a width of 2–3 cm. After blocking the starting point at the skin surface of the nose 3 times and blocking of the right middle turbinate 2 times, the attacks of PPC ceased. When followed up 2 weeks later, there was a quick response of corneal and conjunctival reflex. Dysesthesia of the right side of the head and face disappeared.

Case 4. Jiang, female, age 26, 11 days before the right hand was injured by a needle. There was pain and swelling for 1 day, forming a crust afterwards. Eight days later, there appeared a paroxysmal type of intense itching starting from the crust, propagated along the Pericardium Channel, upward to the chest, entered the Ren (Front Midline) Channel, downward to the ensiform process, then across to the under surface of the homolateral breast. The attack occurred 3–4 times every day, accompanied by an inexpressibly intense itching of the right chest cavity. The face turned pale and twitching of extremities occurred during severe attacks. Repeated pressure on the point at the center of the sternum to retard the symptoms caused the forming of blister and crust at that site. Right sided half jacket form of hypoesthesia might be found. SPC test (+). After stimulating Neiguan (Neikuan, P. 6) point of the right side by electroacupuncture for 20 minutes, there appeared a dysesthesia band of the Pericardium Channel propagated to the crust at the center of the sternum, with a width of 2.5cm. It might persist for 3 hours. Examination after 3 hours showed that dermatographia might be induced throughout the whole course of the Channel, rapidly fusing together to form a "urticarious band" propagated along the Channel. After taking phenytonium natrium for 5 days, the PPC attacks ceased.

III. DIAGNOSTIC CRITERIA

1. Over the body surface, there are painful feelings or other abnormal feelings spontaneously propagated along the "Channel" or "Meridian", as described in literature of traditional medicine of China.

2. Cyclical or noncyclical attacks, a fixed "starting point", a suffering sensation, even crises of the internal organs or sensory organs appearing during the attacks and the possibility of stopping the attacks by means of pressure on the course of APC and PPC.

3. After an attack, there remained an band-like dysesthesia-PC or a polysegmental dysesthesia zone. Occasionally there remained a dyskinesia of the corresponding extremities.

Besides a past history of concussion of the brain, the presence of deep or shallow lesions distributed along the Channels, SPC test (+), and changes of the electroencephalography, etc. may all be helpful in the diagnosis.

IV. DISCUSSION

Since 1959, 16 cases of this disease had been reported in China under different names[4–11]. Only one case was PPC (reported by Chen Keqin, in 1964); the rest were APC (Table 3).

All the above reports only concentrated on the state of the propagation of algesthesia or paresthesia, but did not mention the various diagnostic criteria mentioned in this article.

As far back as 2,000 years ago, "pain propagated along the whole course of the Channel" and "diseases produced automatically in the Channel" were recorded in various books of canons of traditional Chinese medicine, such as "Huandi Nei Jing · Ling Shu Jing". The words "Iao" (malaria) and "Jue" (crises) in these books of canons probably mean the cyclical or noncyclical state of the attacks. That was the earliest historical record on APC.

In modern medicine, there is a so called "localized sensory epilepsy" or "Jackson's sensory epilepsy" characterized by an attack and propagation of the localized painful sensation or various other abnormal sensations on the body surface, accompanied by involuntary movements of the extremities. Moreover, transient anesthesia on the old site of

Table 3. Cases of APC and PPC reported in China

Year	Author	Name used	Cases
1959	Xiao Youshan et al.	Spasmalgia-PC	2
1964	Chen Keqin et al.	Phenomenon of channel	2
1974	Xiao Yongjian et al.	Hypoesthesia-PC	1
1976	Jiao Guorui et al.	Paroxysmal causalgia-PC	2
	Chen Keqin	Phenomenon-SPC	9

attacks may exist for a few hours after an attack[12]. Each attack started from a fixed point on the skin surface, which is an inportant characteristic of this type of epilepsy.

As to the sensory epilepsy, there are accounts of using sensory stimulation to control its attack. In 1881 Gowers repeatedly used ligation of the elbow to cease sensory attacks propagating upward from the hand. He also pointed out that as early as 1772, Lysons, by ligating the knee, controlled the attacks starting from the foot[13].

Clinically, there is also the so-called "reflex epilepsy". It is due to the presence of the persistent stimulation of a diseased foci which sent impulses continuously to the cerebral cortex causing an inert excitation. It is also maintained that history of brain injury is an important cause of this type of epilepsy[14]. Reflex epilepsy may also present itself in the form of sensory attack, i.e., "reflex sensory epilepsy".

According to Wilkinson and Fine, the electroencephalograms of the patients who are ill with sensory epilepsy have not the stimulative electric activity. They have only slow waves[15].

If one compares the APC and PPC with the two types of epilepsy mentioned above, one will find that there is much similarity between them. Therefore, the disease reported in this article may be a kind of sensory epilepsy whose propagation along the Channels may have a dual character—local epilepsy and reflex epilepsy, i.e., "Sensory Epilepsy propagated along the Channels" or "Epilepsy-SPC".

The discovery of this disease strengthens the belief that in the human cerebral cortex there may exist a set of functional pathways of propagation along the Channel.

All 80 cases were treated with phenytonium natrium and librium. Thirty one cases were also treated by blocking with drugs along the course of the Channels or burying catgut at the starting point. Except for 18 cases not followed up, the rest all recovered.

V. CONCLUSION

This article presents a cyclical or noncyclical paroxysmal type of disease which is charactarized by the propagation of pain or other paresthesia with a definite width, speed and route starting from a fixed point on the body surface. Its route of propagation is conformed to the Channels described in literature traditional Chinese medicine. From observations on 80 cases, the basis clinical characteristics have beens found and the disease is named "algesthesia propagated along the Channels" and "paresthesia propagated along the Channels". After reviewing the literature on this subject, it is concluded that this disease belongs to the "disease produced automatically" in the syndrome of Channel. In modern medicine, it may be a type of "sensory epilepsy propagated along the Channels".

REFERENCES

[1] Qian Xinzhong: Progress in Scientific Research on Acupuncture, Moxibustion and Acupuncture Anesthesia by Integration of Traditional Chinese and Western Medicine. Monograph Published in National Symposium on Acupuncture and Moxibustion and Acupuncture Anesthesia (June 1–5, 1979). Page 17 of this book.

[2] 刘澄中：针刺麻醉 (2—3)：59，1977。

[3] 刘澄中：中国医科大学学报（1）：55，1975。
[4] 肖友三：中国杂志（8）：66，1959。
[5] 北京中医院针灸教研组：北京中医学院学报（1）：56，1959。
[6] 陈克勤：中医杂志（5）：22，1964。
[7] 袁善堂等：武汉医学杂志（6）：470，1964。
[8] 肖永俭等：山东医药（3）：28，1974。
[9] 长春中医学院针麻经络研究组：新中医（2）：37，1976。
[10] 焦国瑞：新中医（2）：39，1976。
[11] 陈克勤：陕西新医药（4）：29，1976。
[12] Bing, R.: Bing's diagnosis in neurological diseases, 中译本，曹天祥译，177页，科技卫生出版社，1958。
[13] Eforn, R.: *Brain,* **80**: 251–262, 1957.
[14] Гопова Ю.Г.: Жур.Невр.и псих 65 (9): 1351, 1965.
[15] Wilkinson H.A.: *Neurology* **23**(5): 518, 1973.

PART III
CLINICAL RESEARCH ON ACUPUNCTURE AND MOXIBUSTION

RESEARCH ON THE ORIGIN AND DEVELOPMENT OF CHINESE ACUPUNCTURE AND MOXIBUSTION

Wang Xuetai

(*Institute of Acupuncture and Moxibustion,*
Academy of Traditional Chinese Medicine)

Acupuncture and moxibustion are important medical inventions of the Chinese nation. At first, these were only essential means for medical treatment, but the have developed gradually as into a branch of medical knowledge wyich includes the basic theory of channels as its main content, and various kinds of manpiulating methods and rich experiences of applying the treatment according to the differentiation of the symptom-complex.

Acupuncture and moxibustion have always been major component parts of the great treasures of traditional Chinese medicine and pharmacology. Today it has become the common medical property of people all over the world.

I. THE ORIGIN OF ACUPUNCTURE AND MOXIBUSTION

Human beings probably first appeared in the vast land of China about 1.7 million years ago. About 600,000 years ago the Beijing man began to use stone implements and fire. From the remote past to the twenty first century B.C., our ancestors went through the different stages of primitive society, creating a primitive agriculture and a system of animal husbandry, a handicraft industry, and primitive artistic and, cultural works. Keeping steps with these developments, acupuncture and moxibustion also, gradually, took form.

(I) The Primitive Acupuncture Tool-----The Bian Stone

The treatment of diseases with stone implements is mentioned in many ancieant books, appearing from the 6th century B.C. to the 1st century A.D., such as "Zuozhuan" (Commentary on the Spring and Autumn Annals), "Shanhaijing" (Classics of the Mountains and Seas), "Guanzi" (Master Guan), "Zhanguoce" (Tactics of the Warring States), "Hanfeizi" (Master Hanfei), "Suwen" (The Plain Question), "Lingshu" (Canon of Acupuncture), "Shiji" (Historical Records), "Hanshu" (汉书 Book of the Han Dynasty), "Huainanzi" (Master Huai Nan), "Shuoyuan" (Garden of Arguments), "Hanshi Waizhuan" (Legends of Han Poems), "Yantielun" (Essays on Iron and Salt) and "Mai Fa" (Methods of Pulse Diagnosis)[1] and "Wushier Bingfang" (Prescriptions for Fifty-two Kinds of Diseases). These books are inscribed on the silk scrolls excavated from the Han Tombs of Mawangdui at Changsha in Hunan Province in 1974. In recent years, other archaeological findings have also proved that ancient medical stone implements were used for cauterization, massage, percussion and tapping on the body surface, incising and pricking boils or abscesses and for blood-letting[3]. The "Bian Stone" was one of these implements. The "Shuowen Jiezi" (Analytical Dictionary of Characters) of the 2nd century detines the word "bian" as "a sharp stone used to prick at the body surface in order to cure diseases". In the "Yifa Fangyi Lun" (On Different Methods and Prescriptions for Suitability of District), a chapter entitled "Suwen" (The Plain Question), describes the origin of the "bian stone" in the following way: "In the eastern lands. ... most common illnesses are boils and ulcers; they should be treated with bian stone". This showed that the pointed "stone needle" was originally used for incising sores and abscesses. It gradually developed into the stone needles used for acupuncture treatment. Wang Sengru who lived around the 5th or 6th century A.D. pointed out that "ancient people used needles of stone not of iron"[4]. One of his contemporaries, Quan Yuanqi also said: "Bian stone, is an ancient method of external treatment and was known by three names: 1. Needle stone; 2. Bian stone; 3. Arrow-headed stone. In fact, they are the same thing because there was no iron casting in the ancient times, therefore they used stone for the needle"[5]. All these historical records show that the art of treatment with stone needles originated in the Stone Age.

In the Old Stone Age (from the remote past to 10,000 years ago), there were no special medical instruments. Scrapers and other sharp work tools were used for incising abscesses, draining pus and letting blood out so they were the predecessors of the bian stone. In the New Stone Age (10,000–4,000 years ago) because of improvements in the techniques of carving and shaping stone, the ancient people were able to make different shaped stone instruments. The bian stone was developed, specially shaped for medical use. Since the founding of new China, archaeologists have discovered examples of the bian stone. Most of these were made during a period extending from the New Stone Age to the Spring and Autumn Period (770–221 B.C.). These bian stones were obviously prototypes of the metal needles which were used later. For instance, in 1963, a bian stone 4.5 cm. long was discovered in ruins in Toudao Valley, in the Duolun District of Inner Mongolia which date from the New Stone Age (Fig.1)[7]. At one end, it is oval-shaped with a smei-circular edge used for incising boils and abcesses; at the other end, it is cone-shaped with a blunted tip used for acupuncture. The middle of the stone is 4-sided, and this is where it was held. The size and shape of this bian stone needle are very similar to that of a bronze bian stone needle found in Inner Mongolia![8] This needle also has the same type of square handle as a golden needle excavated from a Han Tomb in Mancheng, Hebei. Moreover, in 1972 a bian stone, made before the 3rd century B.C., was discovered in the ruins of an old city of the Shang and Zheng States in Xin Zheng County of the Henan Province. This stone needle which is oval at one end for massage and three-edged at the other for letting blood, resembls the round-headed needle mentioned in the "Canon of Internal Medicine"[9] (Fig. 2).

(II) Ancient Books Recording the Origin of Acupuncture Therapy

The "Diwang Shiji" (The Emperors Centuries), edited by Huangfu Mi in the 3rd century mentions that Fuxi "tasted a hundred kinds of herbs and created 9 kinds of needles"[10]

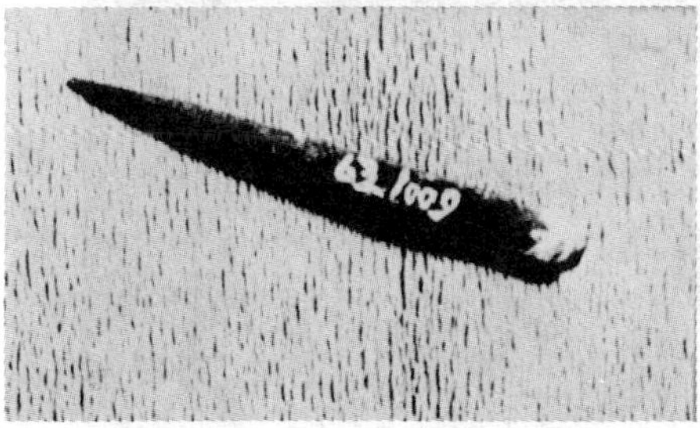

Fig. 1 The bian stone (found in Inner Mongolia).

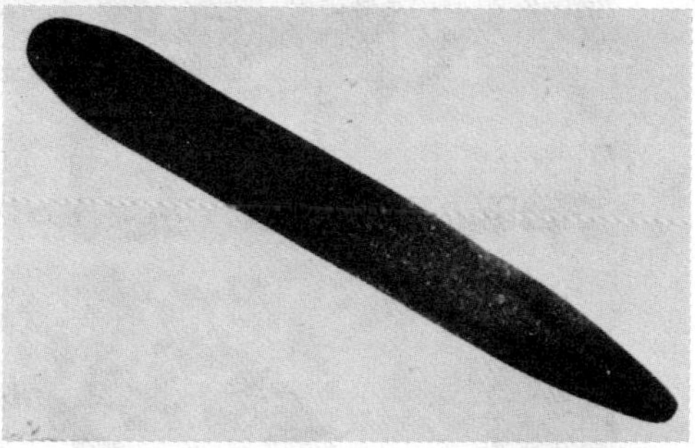

Fig. 2 The bian stone (found in Henan).

In the preface of "Zhenjiu Jiayi Jing" (The Classic of Acupuncture and Moxibustion) Huangfu Mi again said: "Emperor Huangdi visited Qi Bo, Bo Gao, Shao Yu and held discussions with them; therefore the art of acupuncture came into being." In the 7th century, Sun Simiao in the preface of "Qian Jin Fang" (The Thousand Golden Prescriptions) stated that "the Emperor Huangdi gave orders to manufacture nine kinds of needles". In the 12th century, a book called "Lu Shi" (The History of Roads), written by Luo Mi appeared, which was famous for its historical legends. It contained a story about "Tai Hao-Fu Xi tasting all kinds of herbs and making a bian stone to treat the diseases of the people". These recorded legends about the origin of acupuncture all point to it beginning during the period of the primitive society.

"Fu Xi and Tai Hao" have often been taken to be different names for the same person, but some have disagreed with this. It was said that Tai Hao was the chieftain of the Yi tribe in Shandong Province in Eastern China during the period of the primitive society[11]. There is a passage in "Yifa Fangyi Lun" (On the Different Methods and Prescriptions for Suitability of District) which says that "the bian stone originated in the East". In "The Dongshan Jing" (The Classics of the East Mountains) from "The Classics of the Mountains and Seas", it is said that "on the top of the Gao's Mountain there is much jade, and at its foot, there are many stone needles". Guo Pu in the Jin Dynasty explained that "these stone needles may be the bian stones"[12]. The Gao's Mountain is in the Eastern part of China and this story confirms the legend that Tai Hao made the bian stone needles.

Recently, four tablets of the Han Dynasty were unearthed in the Liangcheng Mountain, Weishan County of the Shandong Province, on which was carved a supernatural half-man, half-bird being holding a large needle and trying to puncture the body of a patient[13] (Fig. 3). Obviously this comes from the mythical legend of totem worship in primitive society. This is further proof that the treatment of diseases with bian stones probably originated in the regions of the east coast and was later introduced to the other parts of the country.

(III) The Origin of Moxibustion

In the "Yifa Fangyi Lun" (On the different Methods and Prescriptions for Treating Diseases) from the "Suwen" (The Plain Questions), there is a description of the origin of moxibustion which says "Moxibustion originated in the North, because the Northern

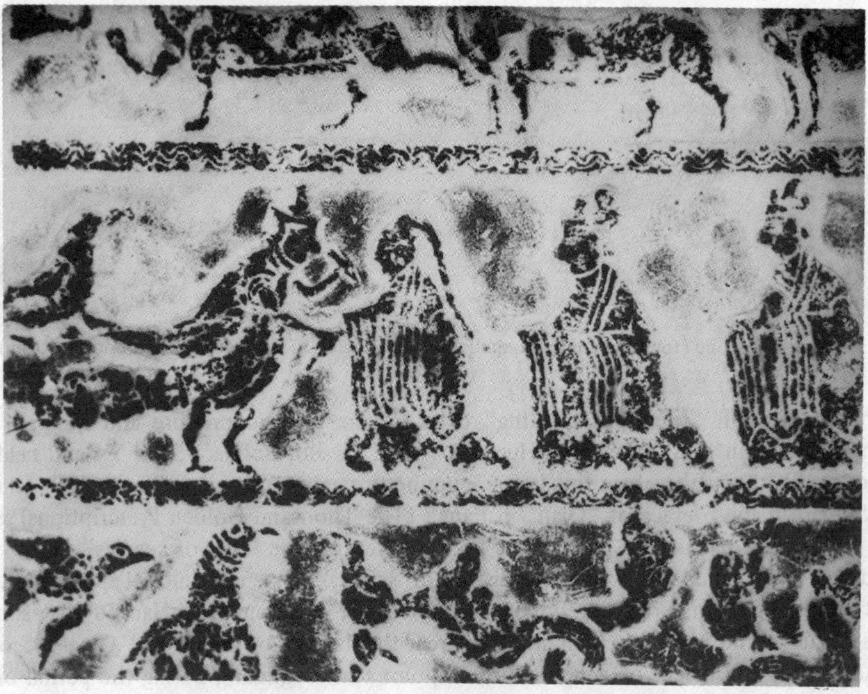

Fig. 3 Tabblet engraved with picture of practicing acupuncture.

parts are shut off from heaven and earth, they are situated at a high altitude, and are freguently attacked by piercing cold wind and surrounded by seething ice. Its inhabitants live in camps and subsist on milk. The accumulated cold easily produces diseases, and so they should be treated by moxibustion. That is why moxibustion originated in the North". This brief account reveals that the discovery of moxibustion was closely related to the cold environment. In the primitive society, when people warmed themselves by fire, they accidentally discovered that applying heat to or scorching the abdominal region sometimes relieved abdominal pain, distention and fullness. Based on such experiences, heat packs and moxibustion methods were developed and applied to the treatment of many illnesses and pains. Such an explanation is in complete conformity with the laws of natural development. In the Tang Dynasty, Wangbing produced an annotation to the "Yifa Fangyi Lun" (The Treatise on the Different Methods and Prescriptions for Different Diseases) in which it mentioned that in the 8th century, Northern people were still using methods of moxibustion.

II. THE FORMATION OF THE THEORETICAL SYSTEM OF ACUPUNCTURE

It was approximately in the 21st century B.C. that our ancestors forned a slave society. Division of mental and manual labour, the manufacture and the usage of bronze wares, the appearance and development of inscriptions on bones and tortoise shells and the invention of astronomy and a calendar provided favourable conditions for the development of medicine and pharmacology. During the time leading up to the Spring and Autumn Periods (770–476 B.C.) and the Warring States (475–221 B.C.), the social system of China grew from a slave society into a feudal society. This great social change promoted rapid development in medicine and pharmacology.

In the period of the Warring States, Chinese medicine and pharmacology experienced a great consolidation. From the time of Warring States to the 1st century B.C., the "Huangdi Nei Jing" (Canon of Internal Medicine), was gradually completed, and is the representative work of this great consolidation. This book consists of two parts: "Suwen" (The Plain Questions) and "Lingshu" (Canon of Acupuncture). Its main content is composed of Yin-Yang, Five Elements, Zang-Fu, Channels and Collaterals, mentality and spirit and Qi (vital-energy) and blood, etc. It explained the physiology and pathology of the human body, the principle of diagnosis and the prevention and treatment of diseases from the perspective of an integral whole, of development and change, and of the human body adapting to nature. This book provided the theoretical foundation of Chinese medicine and pharmacology, including acupuncture and moxibustion (Fig.4).

From the Han Dynasty (206 B.C. to 220 A.D.) to the period of the Three Kingdoms (220–265 A.D.) Chinese medicine and pharmacology were further summarized and the theoretical system became more complete.

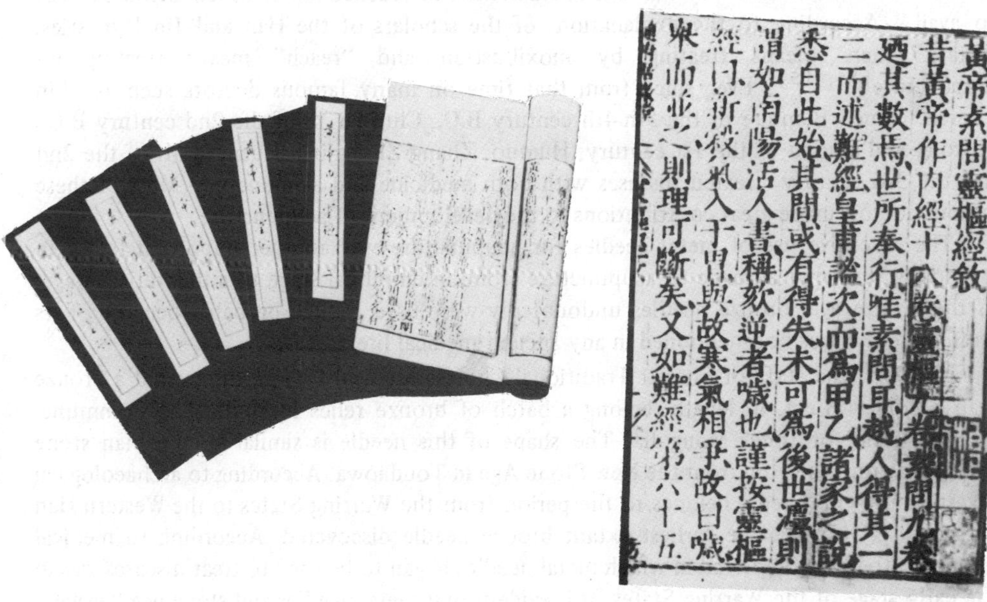

Fig. 4 Lingshu

In 256–260 A.D. Huangfu Mi compiled "The Zhenjiu Jiayi Jing" (The Classic of Acupuncture and Moxibustion), which was a summary of the development acupuncture techniques. In this book, he collected all the acupuncture materials from the ancient books such as the "Canon of Internal Medicine" and "The Mingtang Kongxue Zhenjiu Zhiyao" (The Chart of Essential Points of Acupuncture and Moxibustion). He edited and arranged the materials according to the following order: the theories of the Zang-Fu, Qi (vital-energy) and blood, channels and collaterals, points, the pulse diagnosis, acupuncture and moxibustion technique and the clinical practice of various branches of traditional Chinese medicine. This is the earliest specialized book on acupuncture which is both systematic and relatively integrated.

(I) The Principal Factors Which Promoted the Formation of the Theoretical System of Acupuncture and Moxibustion

In the Spring and Autumn period (770–476 B.C.) following the crumbling of the slave system, medicine and pharmacology were freed from the fetters of the religious superstitions of the wizards of the slave-owing class and won independent positions. Professional doctors came into being. This was the principal factor which accelerated the development and improvement of Chinese medicine and pharmacology.

There is a passage in the "Zuozhuan" (Commentary on the Spring and Autumn Annals) mentioning a famous doctor named Yi Huan, who lived in the Spring and Autumn Period and gave medical treatment to Emperor Jin in 581 B.C. He pointed out the location of the emperor's disease by saying, "the disease had gone deep above the Huang and below the Gao" (probably the place situated between the diaphragm and the pericardium). He continved, "There was no way out as it could neither be reached nor attacked. Medicine is of no avail." According to the explanations of the scholars of the Han and Jin Dynasties, "attack" here means treating by moxibustion and "reach" means treating by acupuncture[14, 15]. Ever since from that time on many famous doctors such as Chin Yueren, named Bianque of the 5th-4th century B.C., Chunyu Yi of the 2nd century B.C., Fuwong and Guoyu of the 1st century, Huatuo, Zhang Zhongjing, Huangfu Mi of the 2nd and the 3rd century treated diseases with both medicine and acupuncture. Most of these famous doctors made great contributions to the development of acupuncture.

The extensive use of metal needles for acupuncture was another important factor in promoting the rapid advance of acupuncture from an empirical stage to a theoretical stage. In the bronze age, bronze needles undoubtedly were used though probably because of its limited use this was not mentioned in any ancient medical literatures.

In 1978, the staff of Shanxi Traditional Chinese Medical College discovered a bronze bian needle, 4.6 cm. in length, among a batch of bronze relics in Shulinzhao Commune, Dalati District of Inner Mongolia. The shape of this needle is similar to the bian stone excavated from the ruin from the New Stone Age in Toudaowa. According to archaeological investigation, this needle belongs to the period from the Warring States to the Western Han Dynasty[16]. This is the earliest extant bronze needle discovered. According to medical literature, the specific period in which metal needles began to be used to treat diseases was in the early stage of the Warring States. It is evident that metal needles and stone needles were used simultaneously. This was the time when China was just entering the Iron Age. It shows that there was a direct connection between the development of metallurgical technique and the popularization of acupuncture. In the "Canon of Internal Medicine", nine kinds of metallic needles are mentioned. These include the cutting needle for operating on abscesses, the arrow-headed needle for dispersing heat, the sharp needle for blood letting, the round-headed needle for massaging, the pressing needle for pressing on the points, the large needle, the long needle, the round-sharp needle and the filiform needle used for acupuncture treatment.

In 1968, in Mancheng County, Hebei Province, the ancient tomb of Liu Shen, of the Western Han Dynasty who was buried in 113 B.C., was excavated. Among the relics, there were four golden needles which were as sharp as when they were new and five damaged silver ones. These discoveries demonstrate the original shapes of the ancient round-needle, the filiform needle, the sharp needle and the pressing needle[18] (Fig.5). The discovery of thse nine kinds of needles broadened our understanding the of the ancient acupuncture practice and provided a deeper understanding of the theory of acupuncture.

Since the Spring and Autumn Periods, the ancient philosophic theories of Yin-Yang and Wuxing (the Five Elements) had been used extensively to analyse and explain various natural phenomena. These helped people to observe the objective laws of matter from the perspective of the unity of opposites, and of change and correlation. Such perspectives contributed to the summarization of the theory of acupuncture, and helped organize it into a system of knowledge.

(II) The Core of the Theory of Acupuncture: The Theory of the Channels and Collaterals

The theory of acupuncture is a component part of the theories of traditional Chinese medicine. The theory of the channels and collaterals is the core of the theory of acupuncture.

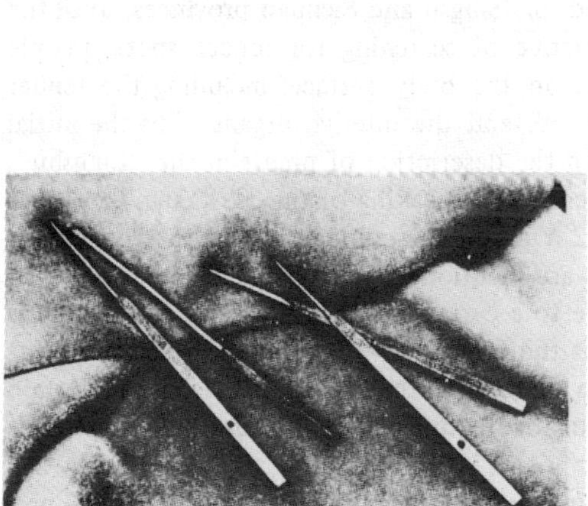

Fig. 5 The ancient golden needles.

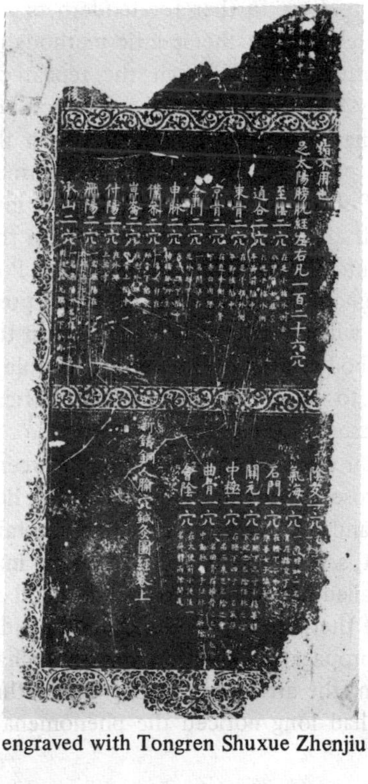

Fig. 6 Tablet engraved with Tongren Shuxue Zhenjiu Tujing.

During long-term medical practice, channels and points were discovered gradually. During the period of the Warring States, the theory of the Channels was formed. Bianque mentioned "channels" and "collaterals", "Yin mai" (yin channel) and "yang mai" (yang channel) at the beginning of this period. He cured Prince Guo (who was said to be Prince of the Zhao in the book 'Shuoyuan) of syncope by needling the three yangs (channels) and the five shus ('shu' means points)[19, 20]. "Jingmai" were mentioned in a silk scroll volume written around the time of the period of the Warring States, which was discovered in the excavation of the Han Tomb No.III at Mawangdui, Hunan Province. This volume roughly describes the pathways of eleven channels and their indications, reflecting the early theory of the channels[21]. The concept of the theory of channels had been completed when the "Canon of Internal Medicine" came into being, which recorded that the channels were internally connected with the viscera and externally connected with the limbs and joints[22]. The channels are the passages through which the vital energy and blood circulate to nourish every part of the body. They form a network joining the upper part with the lower part, the left side with the right side, the internal part with the external part of the body. Each of the channels and each of large collaterals follows its own course, linking its related points. If any disorder occurs along its course, then a corresponding symptom-complex will appear.

At first people did not know that there were acupuncture points. On the basis of the experience of using bian stones to incise and prick abcesses and ulcers, practice gradually developed that "where the pain is, there is the point"[23]. So where the pain and disease was located, acupuncture and moxibustion or blood letting be was applied. Later, people learned to look further for tenderness and applied acupuncture or moxibustion to these areas. Such ancient therapeutic methods lasted, in Jiangsu and Sichuan provinces, until the 7th century[24]. Through the repeated practice of searching for tender spots, people gradually discovered that the reaction-points on the body surface, including the tender points, had a definite connection with the trunk and the internal organs. This the initial concept of acupuncture points was formed. In the description of points in the "Lingshu", some of them are reaction-points. For instance, when speaking of the 12 "Yuan" (source) points, it claims "there are reactions in the 12 Yuan-source points when the internal organs are afflicted"[25]. When the Back-shu Points are mentioned, it says that "if one wishes to have a good therapeutic result, apply pressure to a certain spot on the back; if the pain is relieved when that area is pressed, then that is the point"[26]. Besides the reaction points on the body surface, the ancient people also discovered that to cause bleeding in certain areas or to stimulate certain spots is efficacious for treating certain disorders. All these were predecessors of the acupuncture points.

After discovering the relation between points and the various parts of the body, the problem arose of finding the lines which linked the points together. Although people could understand the correlation between certain areas of the body through observation of radiating pain, sensory abnormality, sensory impairment or motor impairment in certain diseases, the detailed courses of the channels and collaterals had not yet been defined. The determination of the pathway of the channels and collaterals is closely related with the phenomenon of the propagated sensation along the channels (PSC) during acupuncture, moxibustion and Dao Yin (the art of conducting the Qi through the consciousness of breathing). The ancient people had long noticed the phenomena of propagated sensation along the channels. For example, during the 2nd century, the famous doctor Hua Tuo pointed out that before he inserted the needle the, "Sensation should reach a certain area" and "when the patient says 'the sensation is present', the needle is then withdrawn"[27]. In the 13th century, there was a book entitled "Beiji Jiufa" (Moxibustion for Emergencies), in which there is a passage saying that when moxibustion is applied to the back a heat sensation might reach the sacrococcygeal area, the testis, and then flow down to the point Yongquan (K.1). In the "Canon of Internal Medicine" the propagated sensation along the channels is described as the phenomenon of "deqi" (needling sensation). This book mentions that there is "slipping vital energy" and "hesitating vital energy"[28]. When the reinforcing method is applied, "if the local Qi is not lost, the distal Qi will arrive"[29]. Due to "individual differences of blood and Qi of the human body", there might be the phenomena either of "awareness of the arrival of Qi before insertion of the needle due to the activity of spirit," or of an awareness that "as soon as the needle is inserted, it works together with the Qi" or of an awareness that "Qi works alone after the needle is withdrawn"[30]. In recent years, researchers in China have investigated the phenomenon of P.S.C. from various angles and the results conform with the classic courses of the channels and collaterals. The speed of P.S.C. may differ in channels and times in various persons. The speed usually ranges from 0.5cm. to over 10cm. per second but is usually a few centimeters per second. This proves to be in conformity with the "Canon of Internal Medicine", which says the speed of the sencsation propagated along the channels is 6 "cun" (a unit of length, one 'cun' equals one tenth of a 'chi'—Chinese foot) in a normal breath[31]. Moreover, the propagated sensation along the channels also appeared in the Dao Yin (precursor of the Breathing Exercise) cone by the ancients as well as in the Breathing Exercise of the present day. Such phenomena not only had been described in ancient literature but also proved in recent practice[32]. The art of Dao Yin originated in very early days, as it was very popular already in the Spring and Autumn Period of the Warring States. Both the book "Zhuangzi" (Master Zhuang) and the "Canon of Internal Medicine" mentioned it. When explaining his philosophy of health, Zhuangzi in his book "On Health" said that "one should always keep an upright posture using the Du (midline channel) as a criterion." On the silk scroll discovered in the Han Tomb No. III at Mawangdui, Hunan Province, there is a diagram on which the description of channels and collaterals is placed between the essay on "Quegu Shiqi" Fasting and Taking Breathing Exercise) and the "Daoyin Tu" (The Dao Yin Illustration)[33]. All these witness that the ancient people had noticed the phenomena of channels and collaterals during the Exercise of Dao Yin.

During the process of discovery of the pathways of the channels, the ancient people were obliged to search for the material basis of them. Since the Spring and Autumn Period, medical men had attached great importance to human anatomy. For instance, in "Jingshui" (Channel Fluid) the chapter from "Lingshi" of "The Canon of Emperor's Internal Medicine", it is said that "a human being, 8 'chi' (a unit of length) tall with flesh and skin can be measured and touched only externally, but after his death, he can be anatomized for observation." Through anatomy, people discovered that the blood vessels could communicate with every part of the whole body, and their distributions had a certain relation with propagated sensation along various channels. Moreover, when pulse diagnosis became more advanced, they came to know that different forms of pulse reflected different conditions of the viscera. So it was concluded that the blood vessels were the substantial ground for the channels and collaterals. That is the reason why these channels and collaterals were known as Mai (Vessel) in the ancient days.

As mentioned above, the points and their indications which were discovered during acupuncture treatment, the phenomenon of propagated sensation along the channels which were discovered during Dao Yin, the symptoms and signs which were linked up with individual channels through diagnosis, and the blood vessels which were discovered in anatomy were all correlated, although their discoveries were made from different angles. The theory of the channels and collaterals was a summarization of all these discoveries.

III. THE DEVELOPMENT OF ACUPUNCTURE AND MOXIBUSTION

In the middle of the 3rd century, the book "Zhenjiu Jiayijing" (The Classic of Acupuncture and Moxibustion) appeared. The development of acupuncture and moxibustion continued along the established theoretic system described above, right up to 1840, when the Opium War broke out. During this time therapeutic experiences were being enriched, the manipulation methods became more and more proficient and theoretic knowledge was greatly substantiated.

(I) The Increase and Revision of Acupuncture Points

There are two main groups of points: the points on the 14 channels and points that are not on the 14 channels which are known as the extra points. The former ones are the acupuncture sites distributed along the channels. According to "The Classic of Acupuncture and Moxibustion" there are altogether 349 points with designations. The "Zhenjiu Fengyuan" (The Source of Acupuncture and Moxibustion) written by Li Xuechuan in 1817 lists 361 points. The number of points outside the channels are called extra points and these, which are quite effective for treating diseases, are increasing continvasly. They have become more nomerous than the total number of the points of the 14 regular channels[34].

In the process of the development of acupuncture, there was some confusion of the names and locations of some points due to the appearance of many different schools of acupuncturists with their own experiences and theories. For instance, there was a lack of clearness concerning the location of point Xinshu (U.B. 15) and, it was stated that this point corresponded with the 3rd, 5th, 6th or 7th vertebra. Even before the Tang Dynasty, people were at a loss to determine the precise location of the point[35]. To solve this confusion, the Tang Government, in the years around the time of Zhenguan (The title of the reign of one Emperor of Tang Dynasty (627–649), ordered the famous doctor, Zhenquan, and three other doctors to revise the locations of the points, the acupuncture books and the diagrams[36]. About 400 years later, the Song Government ordered Wang Weiyi to check and revise the location and to make amendment to the indications of each point again. In 1026, he wrote "Tongren Shuxue Zhenjiu Tujing" (Illustrated Manual of the Points for Acupuncture and Moxibustion Marked on the Bronze Figure) which was published by the government[37]. Such supports for the revision of the points given by the governments of the Tang and Song Dynasties greatly promoted the uniformity of the acupuncture points.

(II) The Development of Acupuncture Technique

After the publication of "The Classic of Acupuncture and Moxibustion", acupuncture gradually became specialized. In the 7th century, it was recognized as a special field of medicine.

As medicine was meticulously divided into various departments, the 9 kinds of needles in acupuncture were also attributed to different departments according to their usage. The cutting needle was attributed to the surgery department and the round-headed needle to the massage department; while the filiform needle was gaiving more significance among the equipment used for acupuncture. Acupuncture techniques then also became very complicated.

As early as the time of the "Canon of Internal Medicine" and the "Nan Jing" (The Classic of Reply to Difficulties Questions), acupuncture techniques were already very elaborate. They consisted of the direction and depth of the needle insertion, the speed of entering and withdrawing the needle, retaining of the needle, the coordination of the left hand with the right hand, the reinforcing and the reducing method, etc. Later, acupuncture techniques were further developed along these lines. From the 13th to 16th century, the technique for using the filiform needle became very elaborate. According to such books as the "Zhenjiu Daquan" (A Complete Manual of Acupuncture and Moxibustion, 15th century). "Zhenjiu Wendui" (Questions and Answers Concerning Acupuncture and Moxibustion, 1530). "Gujin Yitong" (Ancient and Modern Medical Systems, 1556), and "Zhenjiu Dacheng" (The Compendium of Acupuncture and Moxibustion, 1601), there were more than 10 types of basic manipulation methods, over 20 types of combined methods and seven or eight types of finger-pressing methods. All these techniques were mainly for insertion and withdrawal of the needle, inducing needle reaction, evoking the propagated sensation along the channels, and producing the effect of reducing or reinforcing. As for the manipulation method of reducing and reinforcing, it was further divided into the methods of lifting and thrusting of the needle, twirling of the needle, opening and closing of the acupuncture hole, exhalation and inhalation, choosing the direction of the needle, and of determining the speed, etc.

(III) The Development of Moxibustion

Books devoted to moxibustion appeared as early as in the 3rd century, such as "Chaoshi Jiufang" (The Chao's Method of Moxibustion)[38]. In the 4th century, Bao Gu, the wife of the famous doctor Ge Hong, was well known for her skill in moxibustion. After the 7th century, moxibustion became very popular. At that time not only did professional moxibustion doctors appear but also books on this subject, such as the "Guzheng Bing Jiufang" (Moxibustion Method for Consumptive Diseases) of the Tang Dynasty, "Waike Jiufa Luncui Xinshu" (The New Essential Methods for Surgical Moxibustion) of the Song Dynasty, "Gaohuang Shuxue Jiufa" (Moxibustion on the Point Gaohuang) and "Beiji Jiufa" (Moxibustion for Emergency), etc.

The materials used for moxibustion treatment not only incloded mugwort (moxa or Artemesia Vulgaris), but many other substances such as sulphur, rush (lampwick), mulberry twigs, peach twigs, wax, and some special medical troche, etc.

Techniques for moxibustion were becoming more and more embellished. It had developed from direct cautery of the skin to indirect cautery. Materials used for application between the igniting substance and the skin were garlic, ginger, scallion, leek, salted soybean, Sichuan peper, aconitum, Allium Chinense G. Don., Phylolacca Acinsa Roxb, Lepidium Apetalum Willd, sword bean, honey locust, salt, soya sauce, yellow earth, feces of earthworm, grubs, toad, etc[39].

In the ancient days, moxibustion was very popular. It was mentioned as a means to alleviate pain from burnts, in "Bian Que Xinshu" (Experiences of Bian Que, 1146), which also mentioned that the flower of dutura was used for general anesthesia. In "Gujin Yijian" (The Medical Warnings of Ancient and Present, 1589) it was mentioned that "rubbing the skin with medicated paper will numb the skin and flesh."

The earliest use of moxa stick was in the 14th century in "Shouyu Shenfang" (The Magic Remedies of Longevity). "Taiyi Shenzhen and Leihuo Shenzhen" (Taiyi Magic Acupuncture Stick and Thunder and Fire Magic Acupuncture).

(IV) The Enrichment of the Theory of Acupuncture and Moxibustion

Chinese physicians of various historical periods and different dynasties arduously worked on the compilation and revision of the theory of channels on the basis of "Canon of Internal Medicine" and "Nan Jing" (The Classic of Reply to Difficulties). The attribution and arrangement of 361 points of the channels were established. In "The Classic of Acupuncture and Moxibustion) points were arranged and marked in lines according to different areas of the body and most were traced to definite channels, but still some of them were left out. In the early 7th century, Yang Shangshan compiled the "Huangdi Neijing Mingtang Leicheng" (Classification of the Points on the Chart in Canon of Internal Medicine) in which he says that, "each of the twelve channels was composed of one volume, and the eight extraordinary channels were composed of one volume"[40]. Yang Shangshan marked the points according to each individual channel, which makes him the forerunner of the practice of locating the points along channels. Unfortunately most of these volumes have been lost and it is now impossible for us to know his entire view. In 752, A.D. Wang Tao compiled and wrote "Waitai Miyao" (The Secret Recipe of the Outer Library) in which the points are illustrated by using 12 human figures and are arranged according to the pertinent connecting Zang-Fu organs (internal organs). There were, however,differences in the attribution of points to the channels when compared with those of later periods. In 1026, the "Tongren Shuxue Zhenjiu Tujing" (The Illustrated Manual on the Points for Acupuncture and Moxibustion Marked on the Bronze Figure) appeared, in which points were clearly arranged according to the 12 channels and the Du and Ren channels. In 1341, "Shisijing Fahui" (The Enlargement of the Fourteen Channels) written by Hua Shou was published. In this book the channels known as the 14 channels points and so the auangement according to the channels was further established.

As to the technique of acupuncture, the principle of the reinforcing and reducing methods had further advanced after the Song Dynasty. In the 11th century, the famous writer, Su Shi pointed out that the "tip of the needle is like the awn of wheat, while the vitalenergy has the function of the axis of a wheel"[41]. In the 16th century, Gao Wu an acupuncturist, explained the meaning of reinforcement and reduction with a simile. He said that "It is just like a balloon; if there is no air in it, it will become flat and not able to bounce, but if air is blown into it through a hole, then it will be become inflated. This is what is known as reinforcement. On the other hand if the cap of the little hole is removed, air will escape and the balloon will become flat again. This is known as reducing"[42].

(V) The Advance of Acupuncture Education

In ancient days, acupuncture training was mainly through apprenticeship to a master or through inheritance of family skill. In the 7th century during the Tang Dynasty, a large scale imperial medical college was established, in which the special field of acupuncture and moxibustion were included. In the department of acupuncture, "there was one with a degree of doctor of acupuncture, one assistant instructor, 10 professors, 20 technicians and 20 students. The professor was to give lectures on the theory of the channels and collaterals, on the points, on the differentiation of the four main types of pulse (floating, sinking, hesitant and rolling) and on acupuncture methods of reinforcing and reducing performed by the nine kinds of needles"[43].

In the 11th century, during the Song Dynasty, the Imperial Medical College had nine departments and acupuncture and moxibustion were again included. The knowledge of the internal organs, channels and points was being taught. For visual teaching, in 1027 Wang Weiyi purposely designed and cast two bronze figures, with the internal organs set inside and the channels and points engraved on the surface[44]. The book "Illustrated Manual on the Points for Acupuncture and Moxibustion Found on the Bronze Figure" was inscribed on stone tablets to ensure that the contents of this book could be preserved. Several years ago five fragments of these tablets were discovered in Beijing[45] (Fig.6).

(VI) Publications of Books on Acupuncture and Moxibustion

After the publication of "The Classic of Acupuncture and Moxibustion," books devoted to this subject appeared continuoysly, especially after the invention of the printing technique. These books were widely circulated. The earliest blockprinted edition of acupuncture and moxibustion which has been found is "Xinji Beiji Jiu" (A New Collection of Moxibustion for Emergency) [46]. It appeared in the year 862. According to the author's statistical estimation there are some 300 kinds of books on acupuncture and moxibustion listed in historic literature and bibliographies VP until the end of Qing Dynasty (1911); some of them have academic value. For an instance the "Zhenjiu Dacheng" (The compendium of Acupuncture and Moxibustion) compiled by Yang Jizhou was a collection of acupuncture achievements of all periods and dynasties. This was a gigantic work and it exerted great influence on later generations (Fig.7).

Besides the publication of books on acupuncture and moxibustion, there were quite a number of charts of channels and points, such as the "Yance Tu" (Lateral Recumbent Diagram)[47] of the 4th century, and the "Mingtang Sanren Tu" (Diagrams of the Three Figures) designed and made by Sun Simiao in the 7th century. In this book "the 12 channels were illustrated in colours and the eight extraordinary channels were in green. There were

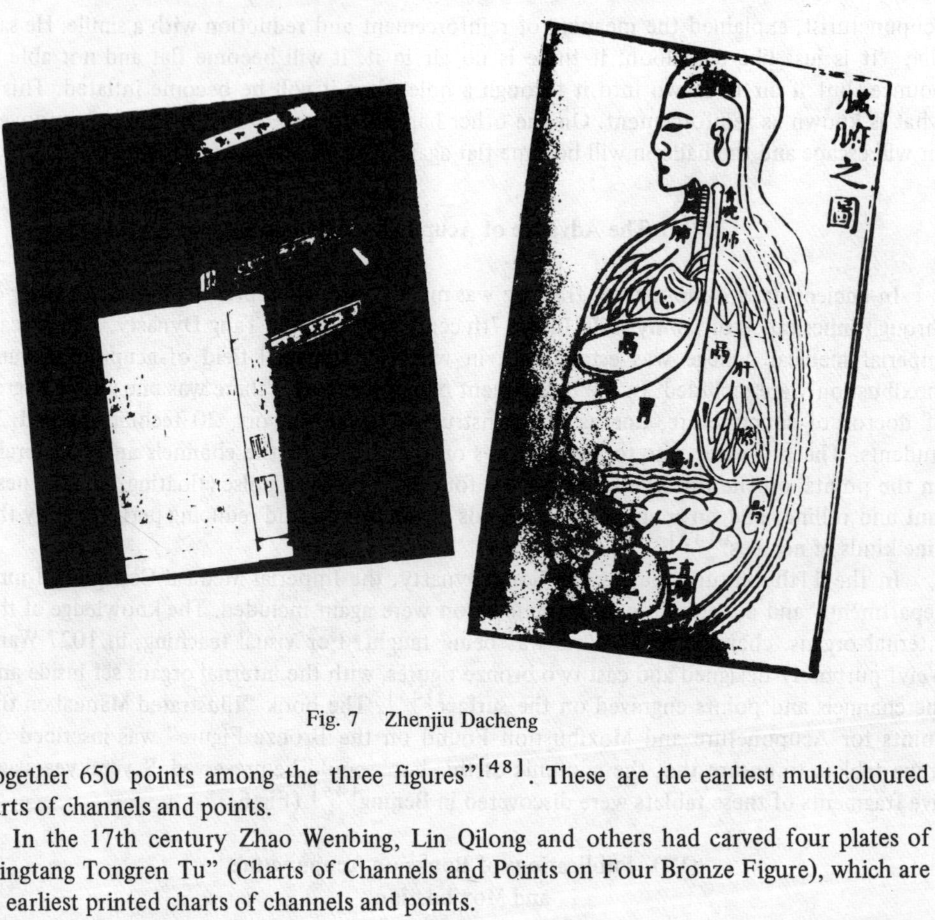

Fig. 7 Zhenjiu Dacheng

altogether 650 points among the three figures"[48]. These are the earliest multicoloured charts of channels and points.

In the 17th century Zhao Wenbing, Lin Qilong and others had carved four plates of "Mingtang Tongren Tu" (Charts of Channels and Points on Four Bronze Figure), which are the earliest printed charts of channels and points.

In the 11th century there was the "Liuzhu Zhiwei Fu (A Verse on Direction of the Circulation of Vital-energy and Blood) written by He Rouyu. From that time on poems and rhymes on the theme of acupuncture and moxibustion appeared continuously. In the 18th century, the "Yizong Jinjian. Cijiu Xinfa Yaojue" (Rhyme of Essential Acupuncture and Moxibustion Technique–a Chapter of Golden Mirror of Medicine) appeared.

IV. DECLINE AND RENAISSANCE OF ACUPUNCTURE AND MOXIBUSTION

At the beginning of the 19th century, the feudal society of China was shaken with crises as the court of the Qing Dynasty became more and more corrupt and was in the final stage of dissolution. In 1822, the authority of Qing Dynasty is sued an order abolishing the department of acupuncture and moxibustion at the imperial Medical College permanently because "acupuncture and moxibustion are not suitable to be applied to the emperor"[49]. Since that time acupuncture has effen been discriminated against. Following the Opium War in 1840, China fell into a semi-feudal and semi-colonial society. The masses of the Chinese people were in deep distress and acupuncture and moxibustion, too, were being trampled.

Later, western medicine was introduced to China. This would have been a welcome development but the imperialists used it as an aggression measure. They brazenly claimed: "western medicine is the vanguard of Christianity and Christianity is the forerunner of promotion of sales of goods"[50]. With this a purpose in mind the imperialists denounced and smashed Chinese traditional medicine brutally. Some people even defamed acupuncture and moxibustion as "instruments of professional torture" and called the acupuncture needle the "deadly needle"[51]. Form 1941 on, the reactionary government of China was continuously called on to ban traditional medicine and a series of measures were adopted to restrict its development. This caused in the decline of all Chinese traditional medicine including acupuncture and moxibustion.

Many acupuncture doctors made unrelenting efforts to protect and develop this great medical legacy by founding acupuncture associations, publishing books and journals on acupuncture, and launching correspondance courses to teach acupuncture. Above all, they made efforts to explaining the theory of acupuncture and moxibustion using the knowledge of modern science. In 1899, Liu Zhongheng wrote "Zhongxi Huican Tongren Tushuo" (Illustration of the Bronze Figure With Chinese and Western Medicine), paving the way for the study of acupuncture through a combination of traditional Chinese and western medicine. In 1934 "The Technique and Principles of Electroacupuncture"[52] and the "Study of Electro-acupuncture"[53] written by Tang Shicheng first introduced firstly the use of electro-acupuncture into China.

Since the founding of the People's Republic of China in 1949, acupuncture and moxibustion have gained its new life. The Chinese Communist Party and the Chinese Government called on all the medical workers of the traditional and western schools to unite, which is an important policy. In addition doctors with western trainine have been encouraged to study traditional medicine. Since 1951 acupuncture institutes have been established, one after another. Institutes and colleges of traditional Chinese medicine on the central, provincial and municipal levels have put great efforts into developing acupuncture in the fields of research, treatment and teaching. As a result acupuncture is thriving. Answering Chairman Mao's teaching that "Chinese medicine and pharmacology are a great treasure house, and efforts should be made to explore them and raise them to a higher level", medical workers have systematzed, and have condvcted research on acupuncture and moxibustion using modern scientitic methods. Theretore quite a lot of significant work has been done. From 1949 to 1977, 8,000 articles on acupuncture and moxibustion were published in various medical journals and newspapers. This is 27 times the total number (300 articles) published during the 40 years before 1949[54, 55, 56].

There are various methods of the manipulation of acupuncture such as the ancient firing needle, warming needle, cutaneous needle, blunt needle, finger "needle", blood letting needle and various methods of moxibustion. The extra long filiform needles, the stitching method and incising therapeutic method, etc. were discovered among the the common people.

There are also many newly created methods such as the scalp needle, hydroacupuncture, thread imbedding therapy, point ligating, point radiating and point electroexcitation therapy, etc. In addition, there are the electro-acupuncture, ear-acupuncture, point-magnetic therapy technigves which were developed from traditional Chinese medicine and intormntion learned from the experiences of methods used in foreign countries[57, 58].

There are 300 kinds of diseases that can be treated with acupuncture and moxibustion. Among them, about 100 kinds may obtain marked therapeutic results[59].

Acupuncture analgesia was created as a the method of relieving pain by needling. At present, there are the simple acupuncture analgesia, electro-acupuncture analgesia, hydroacupuncture analgesia and finger pressing analgesia, etc. As early as the 17th century, a book appeared entitled "Shoushi Baoyuan" (Health Care for Longevity), in which a passage says: "Before moxibustion is applied, press the point hard" so as to suppress the pain during moxibustion[60]. This is the earliest record of finger pressing analgesia.

At present all the medical workers of the country engaged in the study, clinical application and teaching of acupuncture and moxibustion are determined to follow the road of integrating traditional Chinese medicine with western medicine so that they may make greater contribution to the creation of a new school of medicine and pharmacology.

REFERENCES

[1] 马王堆汉墓帛书整理小组：文物（6）：1，1975。

[2] 马王堆汉墓帛书整理小组：文物（9）：35，1975。

[3] 马继兴 周世荣：文物（11）：80，1978。

[4] 李延寿：南史·王僧孺传。

[5] 素 问·宝命全形论，新校正引全元起旧注。

[6] 马继兴 周世荣：文物（11）：80，1978。

[7] 耿鉴庭：学术资料（手稿）。

[8] 张厚墉：关于内蒙古地区医学史中几个问题的考察，陕西中医学院资料，1979。

[9] 永 寿：新中医（2）：59，1976。

[10] 李 昉等：太平御览，卷七二一。

[11] 范文澜：中国通史简编，修订本，第一编，第一章，人民出版社，1964。

[12] 李延寿：南史，王僧孺传。

[13] 刘敦愿：文物（6）：47，1972。

[14] 荀 悦：申鉴

[15] 干 宝：搜神记

[16] 张厚墉：关于内蒙古地区医学史中几个问题的考察，陕西中医学院资料，1979。

[17] 司马迁：史记·扁鹊仓公列传。

[18] 钟依研：考古（3）：49，1972。

[19] 司马迁：史记·扁鹊仓公列传。

[20] 刘 问：说苑·辨物。

[21] 马王堆汉墓帛书整理小组：文物（6）：1，1975。

[22] 灵 枢·海论。

[23] 灵 枢·经筋

[24] 孙思邈: 千金要方,卷二十九,灸例。
[25] 灵 枢 · 九针十二原。
[26] 灵 枢 · 背腧。
[27] 陈 寿: 三国志 · 华佗传。
[28] 灵 枢 · 根结。
[29] 素 问 · 调经论
[30] 灵 枢 · 行针。
[31] 灵 枢 · 五十营。
[32] 上海气功疗养所,全国中医经络针灸学术座谈会资料选编,1959。
[33] 唐兰: 文物 (6): 14, 1975。
[34] 郝金凯: 针灸经外奇穴图谱, 1963。
[35] 丹波康赖: 医心方,卷二,诸家取背腧法。
[36] 孙思邈: 千金翼方,卷二十六,取孔穴法。
[37] 夏 竦: 铜人腧穴针灸图径 · 序。
[38] 尹继善 黄之駕: 江南通志,卷一九二,艺文志。
[39] 王雪苔: 黑龙江中医药研究资料汇刊, (1): 21, 1964。
[40] 黄帝内经明堂 · 杨上善自序。
[41] 苏 轼: 东坡集,卷十五,赠眼医王生彦若。
[42] 高 武: 针灸聚英 · 附辨。
[43] 刘 昫: 唐书 · 职官志。
[44] 夏 竦: 铜人腧穴针灸图径 · 序
[45] 于 柯: 考古 (6): 18, 1972。
[46] 姜亮夫: 敦煌, 1956。
[47] 葛 洪: 抱扑子内篇 · 杂应。
[48] 孙思邈: 千金要方,卷二十九,明堂三人图。
[49] 任锡庚: 太医院志。
[50] 王吉民: 医史杂志 (3): 1, 1951。
[51] Jefferys, W.H. and Maxwell J.L.: Diseases of China, Phiadelphia, 1910.
[52] 重庆科学针灸研究所: 针灸研究所概况, 1934。
[53] 李善初 陈浩彬: 五十年来针灸文献(中文)索引,上海科学技术出版社, 1960。
[54] 李善初 陈浩彬: 五十年来针灸文献(中文)索引,上海科学技术出版社, 1960。
[55] 上海中医学院医史博物馆: 针灸文献索引, 1966。
[56] 中医研究院针灸研究所: 针灸针麻题目索引(未发表稿)。
[57] 王雪苔: 针灸学手册,修订第二版,人民卫生出版社。
[58] 上海中医学院: 针灸学,人民卫生出版社, 1974,
[59] 焦国瑞: 针灸临床经验辑要(未发表稿)。
[60] 龚廷贤: 寿世保元,第十卷。

ACUPUNCTURE IN COMBINATION WITH X-RAY EXAMINATION FOR DIAGNOSIS OF GASTROINTESTINAL DISEASES

Zhang Fachu, Li Shuchin, Wang Siaoya,
Ying Ruchun, Qu Chunshui, Ying Chaoti,
Xie Ruiling, Ching Shaoqi
*(Department of Radiology and Department of Acupuncture,
Yangpu District Central Hospital, Shanghai)*

Acupuncture of vital points has been widely practised not only for treatment and analgesia, but also as a reliable and applicable auxiliary method of increasing the accuracy rate in roentgen diagnosis. Owing to the fact that the channels and collaterals are connected internally with viscera and externally with the body surface, acupuncture of the extremities has an effect on the function of the visceral organs.

Since 1959, we have used X-ray examination to observe the effect of needling points over the body surface on the motility of normal gastro-intestinal tract, and later to assist in diagnosing chronic appendicitis, scirrhous carcinoma of pyloric antrum and intestinal adhesions. The results are quite encouraging. The present study will be given under the following four headings.

I. OBSERVATION OF THE EFFECT OF ACUPUNCTURE ON THE MOTILITY OF A NORMAL APPENDIX, STOMACH AND SMALL INTESTINE

The effect of acupuncture on the motility of the appendix, stomach and small intestine was observed by X-ray examination in 100, 120 and 10 normal healthy adults respectively. We found that acupuncture of the "appendical" point would increase the motility of the appendix; acupuncture of the Zusanli point would influence the function of the stomach markedly; and acupuncture of the "small intestinal" point would increase the motility of the small intestine. These vital points are located in the lower extremities of the same gastric channels as shown in Fig. 1.

1. Subjects Examined: All the persons in this series were normal healthy adults without any gastro-intestinal diseases.

2. Groups for Observation: The subjects were divided into the following groups for observation:

A. Subjects for acupuncture at points of the gastric channels: The acupuncture points were the "appendical" point, the Zusanli point and the "small intestinal" point respectively which show the effect of acupuncture on gastro-intestinal motility.

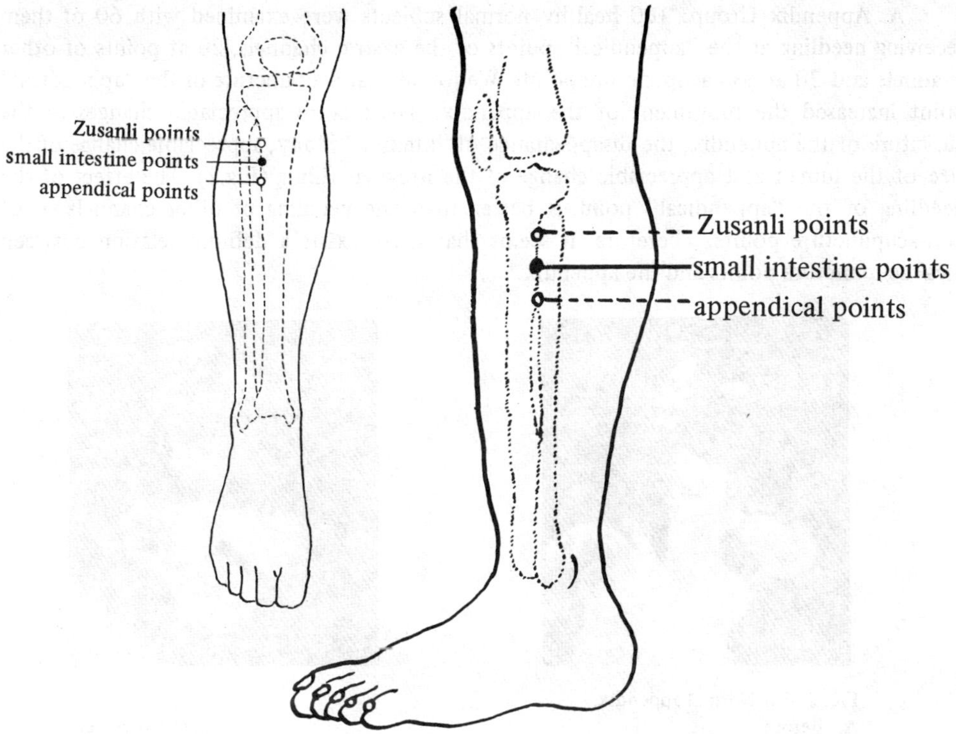

Fig. 1 The location of zusanli Zoint, "appendical" point and "small intestinal" point.

The Zusanli point is located at 3 cun below the knee, the "appendical" point at 2 cun below the Zusanli point, and the "small intestinal" point at the mid-point between the Zusanli and the "appendical" points. No matter whether the subject is tall or short, fat or thin, the length from the knee to ankle is 16 cun, and the "small intestinal" point is at its upper 1/4.

B. Subjects for acupuncture at points of other channels.

C. Subjects for acupuncture at non-acupuncture points.

D. Control group.

3. Methods of Acupuncture: We used filiform needles. The depth of needling was about 1.5 "inches". this produced a feeling of soreness, numbness, distention and heaviness. Needle insertion was done swiftly with a needle retention of about 5 minutes. The needle was withdrawn after twirling manually.

4. The Procedure of Observation: 4 radiograms were taken 5 minutes immediately before acupuncture, directly following acupuncture and 5 minutes after acupuncture respectively.

5. Preparation Before Examination: The preparation of the subject for examination and barium meal used were practically the same as in the routine examination of the gastro-intestinal tract. For examination of the appendix, 15 c.c. of 50% Magnesim sulphate was administered 2 hours after the barium meal in order to have a better filling or visualization of the appendix.

6. Results:

A. Appendix Group: 100 healthy normal subjects were examined with 60 of them receiving needling at the "appendical" points of the gastric channels, 20 at points of other channels and 20 at non-acupuncture points. We found that acupuncture of the "appendical" point increased the movement of the appendix. There were appreciable changes of the curvature of the appendix, the disappearance of "kinking" if any, appreciable change of the size of the lumen and appreciable change of the irregular filling (Fig.2). The effect of the needling of the "appendical" point is better than the needling of other channels or of non-acupuncture points. Therefore, it seems that there exists a definite relation between dical acupuncture points and the appendix.

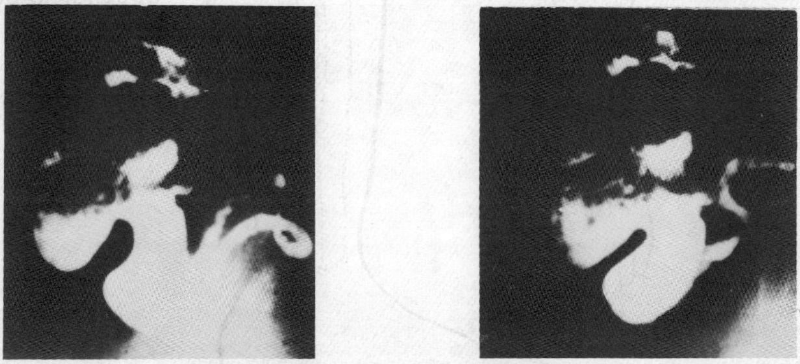

Fig. 2–1 Normal appendix.
A. Before acupuncture.
B. After acupuncture showing disappearance of the "kinking", appreciable

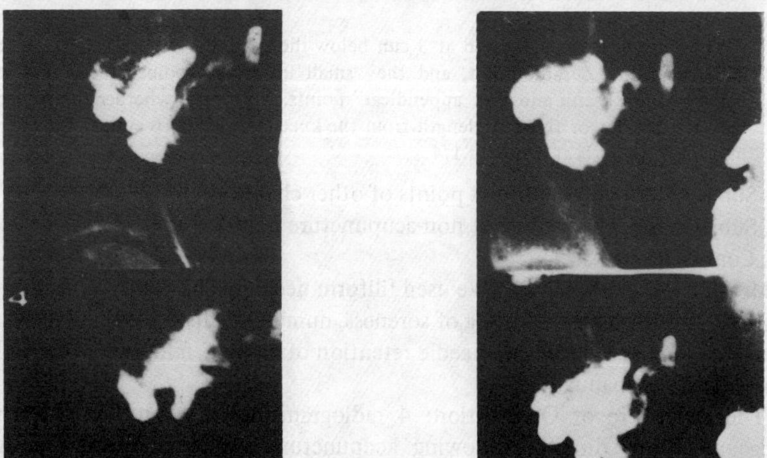

Fig.2–2 Chronic appendieitis.
A & B. Before acupuncture.
C & D. After acupuncture showing no appreciable change of the kinking, angulation, irreguiar filling and size the lumen of the appendix.
Operative and histopathological findings and the follow-up observation confirm the diagnosis of chronic appendicitis.

B. Stomach Goup: Altogether 210 examinations were performed in 120 persons comprising 120 cases of needling at the Zusanli point of the gastric, 35 cases of needling at points of other channels and 45 of needling at non-acupuncture points. In addition, 50 cases were observed as a control to learn the emptying time of normal stomach without acupuncture. We found:

(A) Acupuncture at Point Zusanli can regulate the function of the stomach. When peristalsis is too weak, acupuncture can strengthen it. On the other hand, when peristalsis is too strong, acupuncture can also reduce it and can relieve the spasms (Fig.3).

(B) The effect on the function of the stomach of acupuncture of the other channels or at non-acupuncture points is not remarkable.

(C) In most cases, acupuncture at Point Zusanli can shorten the emptying time of the stomach.

C. Small Intestine Group: Altogether 20 examinations were performed in healthy normal subjects comprising 10 cases of needling at "small intestinal" points of the gastric channels, 5 of needling at of the other channels and 5 at non-acupuncture points. We found that acupuncture at "small intestinal" point could increase the motility of the small intestine, while acupuncture at points of the other channels or at non-acupuncture points was less effective.

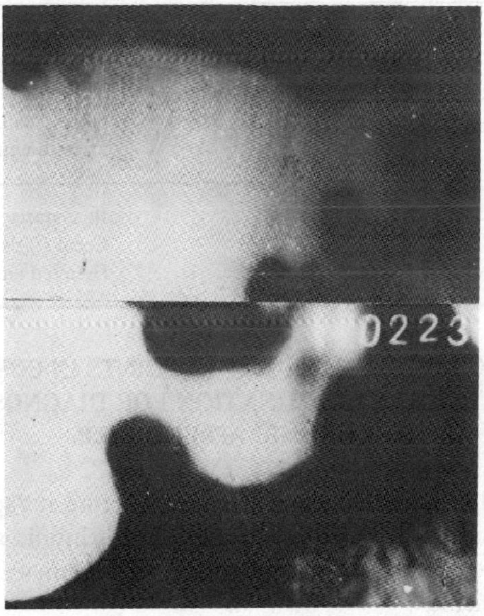

Fig. 3–1 Narrowed lumen and irregular contour of the pyloric antrum.
A. Before acupuncture.
N.. Aftre acupuncture. The radiogram demonstrates disappearance of saw-toothed like irregularities along the greater curvature side and a small niche is present along the lesser curvature side of the proximal portion of pyloric antrum. Thus, a benign ulcer is accordingly made.
Operative and histopathological findings confirm the roentgen diagnosis.

Table 1. Roentgen images of a normal appendix and an appendix with chronic appendicitis

Roentgen images / Reliability	Normal appendix	Appendix with chronic appendicitis
Reliable roentgen images	After acupuncture, appreciable change of the appendical curvature	After acupuncture, no change of the appendical curvature
	After acupuncture, appreciable change of the size of the appendical lumen	After acupuncture, no change of the size of the appendical lumen
	After acupuncture, appreciable change of the appendical irregular filling	After acupuncture, no change of the appendical irregular filling
	After acupuncture, disappearance of the "kinking," if any	After acupuncture, no change of the kinking, if any
	After acupuncture, the existence of a tender point not directly over the appendix	After acupuncture, the existence of a tender point directly over the appendix
Suspicious images		Delayed emptying of the appendix, even after acupuncture
		Non-visualization of the appendix after after magnesium mixture
Unreliable and unwarranted roentgen images		Ileal stasis Cecal stasis Delayed emptying of the stomach

II. ACUPUNCTURE OF APPENDICAL POINTS IN COMBIINATION WITH X-RAY EXAMINATION FOR DIAGNOSIS OF CHRONIC APPENDICITIS

A comparison of radiograms before and after acupuncture at "appendical" points in 100 healthy normal adults and 300 patients suffering from chronic appendicitis respectively showed that acupuncture could increase the motility of a normal appendix, but not that of one with chronic appendicitis.

From experience in practice we have found a new criterion for roentgen diagnosis of chronic appendicitis as shown in Table 1.

When the roentgen findings were compared with the findings of operative and pathological examinations, the correctness of the roentgen diagnosis was increased from 84.7% in routine examination to 100% when combined with acupuncture; when the roentgen diagnosis was checked with the result following the appendectomy, the accuracy of roentgen diagnosis was increased from 61.1% in routine method to 91.7% when combined with acupuncture (an analysis of 60 cases).

III. ACUPUNCTURE OF ZUSANLI POINT IN COMBINATION WITH X-RAY EXAMINATION FOR DIAGNOSIS OF SCIRRHOUS CARCINOMA OF PYLORIC ANTRUM

A comparison of radiograms before and after acupuncture of Zusanli points in 120 normal adults and 250 patients suffering from pyloric stenosis and irregular contour of pyloric antrum showed that acupuncture can regulate the function of normal pyloric antrum. This is lessened to a small degree when there are benign lestions in the antrum, and it hardly occurs in the scirrhous carcinoma of pyloric antrum (Fig.3). Through experience, we have found that the characteristic features of the scirrhous carcinoma of pyloric antrum are:

1. After acupuncture, the contraction and rigidity of the gastric lumen remain unchanged, displaying a lessened flexibility of the pyloric antrum due to the malignant infiltration.

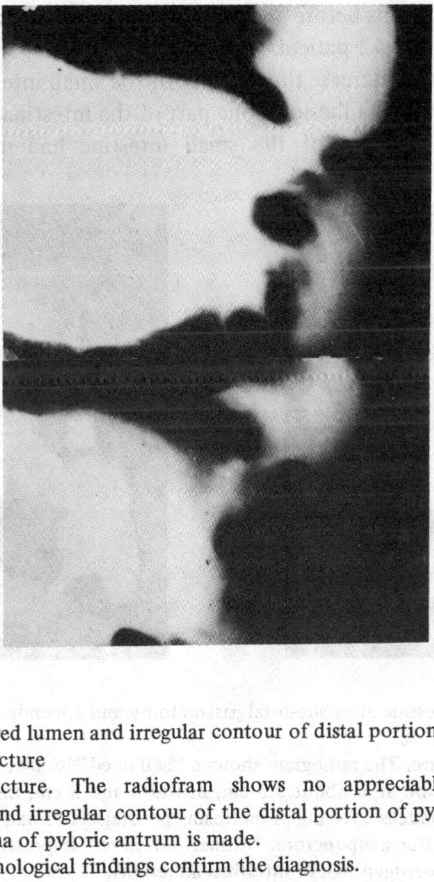

Fig. 3–2 Narrowed lumen and irregular contour of distal portion of pyloric antrum.
A. Before acupuncture
B. After acupuncture. The radiofram shows no appreciable change of the narrowed lumen and irregular contour of the distal portion of pyloric antrum. Thus, scirrhous carcinoma of pyloric antrum is made.
Operative and pathological findings confirm the diagnosis.

2. After acupuncture, there is still a lack of peristaltic activity in the antrum or aperistalsis.

3. After acupuncture, there are no appreciable changes of the irregular, disordered and interrupted mucosal relief pattern.

4. After acupuncture the narrowed pyloric antrum remains unchanged, indicating a lessened expansion of the pyloric antrum.

5. After acupuncture, the narrowed lumen and irregular contour remain constant in shape or no appreciable change of the contour.

The correctness of X-ray diagnosis checked with operative and pathological findings was found to increase from 80.4% in routine examination (an analysis of 46 cases) to 90.7% when combined with acupuncture (an analysis of 54 cases).

IV. ACUPUNCTURE OF "SMALL INTESTINAL" POINT IN COMBINATION WITH X-RAY EXAMINATION FOR DIAGNOSIS OF INTESTINAL ADHESIONS

A comparison of radiograms before and after acupuncture of "small intestinal" points in 10 healthy normal adults and 42 patients suffering from post-operative intestinal adhesions showed that acupuncture can increase the motility of the small intestine. On the other hand, in cases of early small intestinal adhesions, one part of the intestinal loops showed a fixation or no movement, while the rest of the small intestine had movement (Fig.4). Thus,

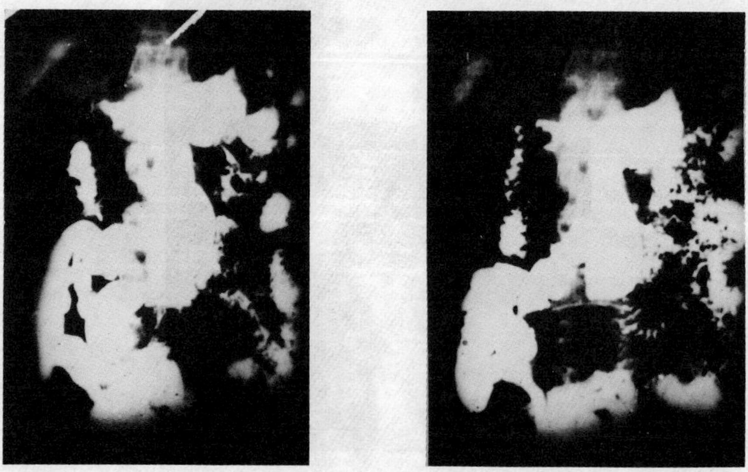

Fig. 4–1 Small intestine after sub-total gastroctomy and appendectomy.
A. Before acupuncture
B. After acupuncture. The radiogram shows a "ball-oned" loop at the distal portion of ileum. It is about 3.5 cm, in width and 5 cm, in length. Clinically, the patient produces a feeling of increasing peristalsis of small intestine immediately after acupuncture. Normal movement is present in the intestine indicating no roentgen sign of intestinal adhesions.

acupuncture can help to diagnose comparatively early cases of intestinal adhesions by radiograms. From experience, we found that the cardinal X-ray diagnostic features are:

1. After acupuncture, a part of the intestinal loop and/or one loop with abnormal contour have no appreciable change in contour and arrangement, while the rest of the small intestine have movement with change of contour and arrangement.

2. After acupuncture, one part of the intestinal loops remains unchanged in a saw-tooth like shape.

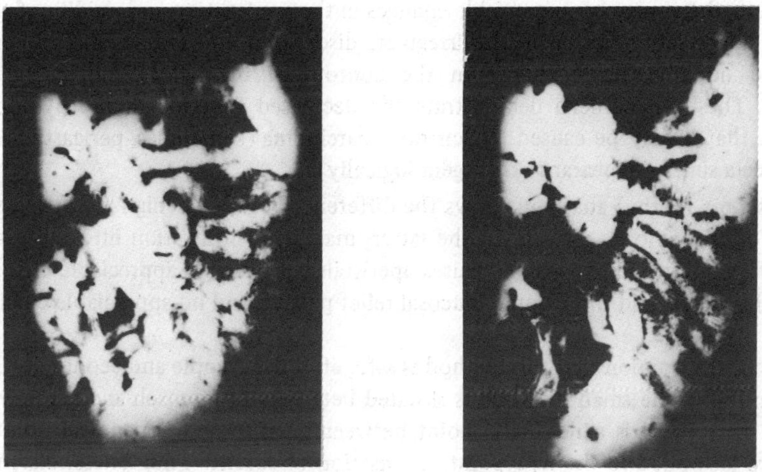

Fig. 4–2 Intestinal adhesions after exploratory
A. Before acupuncture
B. After acupuncture. The radiogram shows no approciable change of the dilated and rigid loops of the proximal portion of ileum (marked with arrow) indicating intestinal adhesions. Normal movement is present in the rest of small intestine.

3. After acupuncture, one part of the intestinal loops remains unchanged in abnormal segmentation.

V. DISCUSSION

In the fluoroscopic observation and radiographic study of the appendix, we observed two phenomena. One is that the disappearance of the "kinking" if any, the appreciable change of the size of the appendical lumen and the irregular filling after acupuncture of "appendical" point. The other one is that after acupuncture, there is no change of the appendical curvature, no change of the kinking, if any, and no change of the size of the appendical lumen and their irregular filling. This suggests that the appendix is in a non-functional state or is diseased.

Macroscopic morbid anatomy shows the difference between the normal appendix and the appendix with the chronic appendicitis. The latter undergoes fibrous and inflammatory changes which lead to a thickened wall, kinking, angulation, irregular filling, fixation, delayed emptying and adhesion to adjacent structures.

Similarly, on screen examination and in the radiograms of the narrowed and irregular contour of the gastric pyloric antrum, two kinds of phenomena could be observed. One was that after acupuncture of Zusanli point, there was an appreciable change in the size of antral lumen displaying the function of contraction and expansion as a peristaltic wave, appreciable change in the irregular, disordered and interrupted mucosal relief pattern and appreciable change in the contour of the pyloric antrum. Another one was that after acupuncture of Zusanli point, there were no appreciable changes in the contraction and rigidity of the antral lumen, no appreciable change in the irregular, disordered and interrupted mucosal relief pattern and no appreciable change in the contour of the pyloric antrum, which was aperistaltic. These phenomena demonstrate the decreased function of the pyloric antrum and suggest that it may be caused by scirrhous carcinoma (sometimes, perigastric adhesions may produce a similar appearance roentgenologically).

Macroscopic morbid anatomy shows the difference between benign lesion and scirrhous carcinoma of the pyloric antrum. In the latter, malignant infiltration into the gastric wall lessens its flexibility and expansion, causes aperistalsis, causes no appreciable change in the irregular, disordered and interrupted mucosal relief pattern and no appreciable change in the contour.

We are of the opinion that this method is safe, effective, simple and economical.

Anatomically, the small intestine is situated between the stomach and the appendix, so we assume that there is a new vital point between Zusanli and appendical points. When acupuncture is applied to the new point, a sensation of soreness, numbness, distension and burning is felt all the way that goes downw to the foot. In addition, some patients felt an increase of peristalsis of the small intestine immediately after acupuncture or after the insertion of the needle or during its retention. Such feeling ended with a comfortable sensation after the expelling of the "gas". The sensation of "gas" caused by needling is shown in the radiogram. We name the new vital point as the "small intestinal" point. Its anatomical location is shown in Fig. 1.

When acupuncture was applied to the "small intestinal" point of post-abdominal surgery patients, similarly, two kinds of phenomena were observed on the examination screen and in the radiograms. One was that part of the intestinal loops and/or one loop with abnormal contour had no appreciable change in contour and arrangement: part retained the saw-tooth like shape or abnormal segmentation. This suggest the fixation or lessened movement of one part of the intestinal loops. The other one was that the loops of the small intestine changed their contour and arrangement. It suggests that the motility of the small intestine is normal.

Consideration of the macroscopic morbid anatomy will indicate the difference between the normal loops of the small intestine and intestinal adhesions. In the latter, it signifies that one part of the intestinal loops has adhered to an adjacent structure, which leads to fixation and abnormal contour of the involved intestinal loops.

VI. CONCLUSION

The writers' opinion is that X-ray examination in combination with acupuncture affords a reliable and applicable method for increasing the accuracy rate in roentgen diagnosis for chronic appendicitis, scirrhous carcinoma of the pyloric antrum and intestinal adhesions. Because this is a promising method for accurate diagnosis of these diseases, it is worthwhile to report our study.

STUDIES OF VERSION BY MOXIBUSTION ON ZHIYIN POINTS

Cooperative Research Group of Moxibustion
Version of Jiangxi Province*

Version of abnormal fetal position by moxibustion of Zhiyin points was recorded in many Chinese medical books for generations and this method was widely used by the common people[1–5]. In two decades, its therapeutic effect has been proven through wide clinical observations in our country[6–9]. With a view toward realizing the principles of treatment governing moxibustion version and the effects of the moxibustion on maternal physiological functions, a number of patients with abnormalities in fetal position were admitted for observation, and at the same time a preliminary study was made with experiments on animals.

I. CLINICAL INVESTIGATIONS

(I) Objects to be observed

One hundred and eleven patients with various abnormalities in position of their fetuses were admitted and no treatment was given in the first two days after admission as a control. This was done to rule out the cases of spontaneous version, and 11 cases were found to be such, of which 9 had been pregnant to a period of under 34 weeks. The remaining 100 patients were given moxibustion therapy. Most of the patients, aged 23–28 (80%) had been pregnant for 30–38 weeks. Among them 45 were primipara; 32 already had given birth to one child and 23 were the mothers of two or more children. 93 fetuses were in breech position. and 7 transverse. 6 cases were given other treatments without success before admission, of which 3 had practiced knee-chest position, 2 combined kneechest position with self-applying moxibustion and the other, in addition to the above treatments, had taken a concoction of Chinese herbal medicine.

* Cooperative units: Jiangxi Medical College; Jiangxi college of Traditional Chinese Medicine; Nanchang First Hospital; Jiangxi Maternity Health Hospital

(II) Methods

The patients were given moxibustion in the supine position the first time in order to record the physiological parameters. The rest of moxibustion treatments were given with the patients sitting and leaning against the back of the chair so as to relax the abdominal wall. According to the conventional methods, the Zhiyin point is located 1 Fen (3mm) lateral to the nail root of minimus pedes. Moxibustion was performed by the indirect method, with the distance between each point and the moxa-stick being ajusted from time to time to keep the local skin temperature around 40°C (using semiconductor thermodetector), the highest temperature tolerated. Moxibustion was applied to the points once a day for 20 minutes, and a complete course of treatment consisted of 9 days. During the course of treatment, daily activities and sleeping posture of the patients were not specified or restrained.

(III) Diagnosis of the fetal position and criterion of short-term therapeutic effect

The fetal position before and after moxibustion was diagnosed by experienced obstetricians with the Leopold maneuver, combined with intravaginal examination if necessary. Consultations were held for difficult cases. Examinations were made every 6–8 hours after moxibustion and observations were recorded schematically and compared with those before moxibustion therapy in order to know the process of cephalic version.

The effectiveness of moxibustion was studied in a therapeutic course of 9 days. It was considered successful if cephalic version was acheived without recurrence. If the fetal position was not corrected within 9 days, or, though corrected within 9 days the abnormal position recurred in the course of treatment, it was considered a failure.

(IV) Results

In the course of therapy, the fetal position in 71 cases was corrected and in 29 cases the position was not corrected. This includs 7 cases in which the position was corrected after moxibustion but in which an abnormal position recurred. The majority of the successful cases were corrected after 1–3 applications of moxibustion. There were 24 cases in which the fetal position was corrected with 1 application, 17 cases with 2, 13 cases with 3, 9 cases with 4–5, 5 cases with 6–7 and 3 cases with 8–9 applications.

Among the 100 cases, there were 93 with breech presentation in which 68 were corrected and 25 were not. In the 7 cases with transverse presentation 3 proved successful and 4 failed. 29 of the 45 primipara (64.4%) and 42 of the 55 multiparous (to 76.4%) patients proved successful. No significant difference between the two groups was shown statistically (x^2=1.707, p>0.1), indicating that the therapeutic rate was not related to the number of parity. It was also shown that the therapeutic rate was not related to the number of weeks of pregnancy, (Table 1).

Table 1. Relationship between weeks of pregnancy and therapeutic rate of moxibustion

Weeks of pregnancy	28	29	30	31	32	33	34	35	36	37	38	39	Total
Number of cases	4	2	9	9	18	9	8	9	13	8	8	3	100
Success	3	2	7	8	13	7	6	5	9	5	4	2	71
Failure	1	0	2	1	5	2	2	4	4	3	4	1	29

II. THE EFFECTS OF MOXIBUSTION APPLIED TO ZHIYIN POINTS ON SOME MATERNAL PHYSIOLOGICAL FUNCTIONS AND FETAL ACTIVITIES

(I) Methods

Of 41 cases with abnormal fetal position several physiological parameters were simultaneously recorded just at 10 minutes before (pre-), after start of (mid-, the whole period of moxibustion being 20 minutes) and after (post-) moxibustion respectively. The thoracic respiratory movements, digital (index finger) photoelectric plethysmogram and galvanic skin between the palm and dorsum of the hand were recorded with a polygraph. The digital skin temperature was determined with a semiconductor thermodetector and the brachial blood pressure and fetal heart rate were determined by auscultation. Blood smears were simultaneously taken from 30 cases of the 41 for differential white blood count.

(II) Results

1. Respiratory activity. It was demonstrated that in the course of moxibustion the rate, rhythm and amplitude of respiration didn't change obviously (Fig.1). But under certain circumstances when local burning pain was induced by overheating, change in respiration might appear.

2. Digital plethysmogram. The amplitude of pulse wave was 20.44 ±2.43 mm (mean SE) during pre-moxibustion. At mid-moxibustion it increased by 1.02±1.25 mm. It was insignificant statistically. The amplitude kept on increasing by 4.76±1.69 mm post-moxibustion. This increase was remarkable ($P<0.01$).

3. Galvanic skin: Spontaneous variation of the galvanic skin was usually present during pre-moxibustion. At mid-moxibustion and post-moxibustion it became more active and inhibition was not observed generally (see Fig.1).

4. Digital skin temperature. The digital skin temperature during mid- and post-moxibustion was much higher than during pre-moxibustion. On the average it was 30.02±0.84°C pre-moxibustion, increasing by 1.95±0.35°C mid-moxibustion and by 3.26±0.59°C post-moxibustion, with $P<0.001$ in all cases.

5. Arterial blood pressure. The systolic and diastolic pressure had no marked changes with only the systolic pressure somewhat lower during post-moxibustion (Table 2).

Table 2. Variations in systolic and diastolic pressure (mmHg) mid- and post-moxibustion

Arterial blood pressure	Pre-moxibustion (mean±SE)	Difference between pre- and mid-moxibustion (mean±SE)	Difference between pre- and post-moxibustion (mean±SE)
Systolic pressure	109.3±2.20	1.22±1.11(P>0.05)	−3.46±1.07(P<0.01)
Diastolic pressure	72.3±0.88	0.54±0.97(P>0.05)	−0.88±0.86(P>0.05)

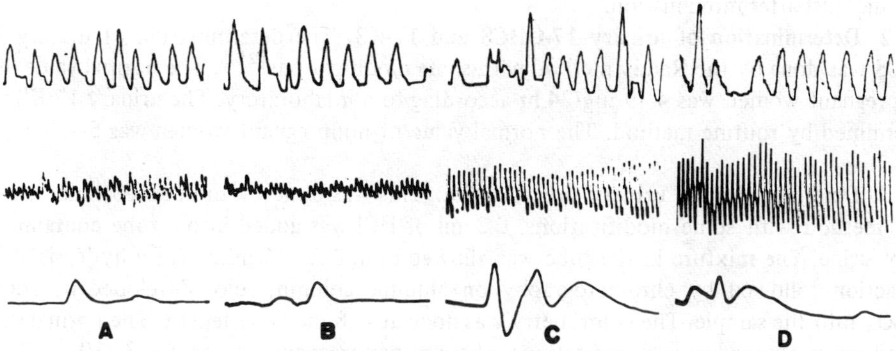

Fig. 1 The effects of moxibustion on respiratory activity (upper), digital plethysmogram (middle) and galvanic skin (lower).
A. Before moxibustion (pre-moxibustion).
B. At start of moxibustion.
C. In the middle of moxibustion (10 minutes after start, mid moxibustion).
D. After moxibustion (post-moxibustion).

6. **Differential white blood count**. The percentage of neutrophil and lymphocytes during both mid- and post-moxibustion revealed no obvious change as compared with pre-moxibustion. The percentage of neutrophil during pre-moxibustion was 74.8±1.21 and that of lymphocytes was 25.1±0.72, while the percentage during mid- and post-moxibustion increased by 1.00±1.29 and 2.37±1.44 for neutrophil and 1.73±6.93 and 1.77±1.32 for lymphocytes respectively, P>0.05 in all cases.

7. **Maternal heart rate**. There was no apparent change in maternal heart rate during mid- and post-moxibustion. The average heart rate was 80.7±1.56/min. It increased by 0.34± 0.79/min mid-moxibustion and decreased by 0.41±1.05/min post-moxibustion, P>0.05.

8. **Fetal heart rate**: The fetal heart beats increased measorably evidently during moxibustion and the increase was still prominant 10 minutes after moxibustion. The fetal heart rate was 137± 3.13/min pre-moxibustion, increased by 7.37±0.98/min mid-moxibustion and by 4.37± 1.23/min post-moxibustion on the average. All were statistically significant (P<0.001).

III. THE EFFECTS OF MOXIBUSTION APPLIED TO ZHIYIN POINTS ON SOME ENDOCRINE ACTIVITIES

(I) Material and methods

1. Collection of samples: 24-hour urine samples were collected before and immediately after moxibustion for the determination of urinary 17-hydroxycorticosteroids (17-OHCS), 17-ketosteroids (17-KS) and pregnanediol. 1 ml of blood taken from the median cubital vein was heparinized and centrifuged for determinating free plasma cortisol. Blood samples were taken between 8:00–9:00 in the morning just before moxibustion and at the same time on next day just after moxibustion.

2. Determination of urinary 17-OHCS and 17-KS. The determination of urinary 17-OHCS was done by the Raddy method with some modifications[20]. The normal value of 20 nonpregnant women was 4–9 mg/24 hr according to our laboratory. The urinary 17-KS was determined by routine method. The normal value of nonpregnant women was 5–10 mg/24 hr.

3. Determination of urinary pregnanediol. This was done by the conventional laboratory method with some modifications. 0.3 ml of HCl was added into a tube containing 5 ml of urine. The mixture in the tube was allowed to boil for 15 minutes for hydrosis. After extraction followed by chromatography on alumine column, color developed by adding H_2SO_4 into the sample. The colorimetry was done at 448 mμ wave length. The normal value of urinary pregnanediol in progestational phase of nonpregnant women was 3–10 mg/24 hr. In the 3rd trimester of pregnancy, it might rise to 30–50 mg/24 hr.

4. Determination of free plasma cortisol. Plasma obtained from the centrifuge was extracted with dichloromethane. Cortisol in plasma extract was determined by radioimmunoassay. The reagents used were supplied by Beijing Chemical Plant. The normal value of free plasma cortisol of nonpregnant women was in general less than 20μg/100 ml.

Table 3. Variations in the value of adrenocortical hormones and pregnanediol in pregnant urine and plasma before and after moxibustion therapy

Hormones	Number	Pre-moxibustion (mean±SE)	Post-moxibustion (mean±SE)	P
Urinary 17–OHCS (mg/24hr)	33	11.9±1.07	16.8±1.06	<0.01
Urinary 17–KS (mg/24hr)	33	15.03±1.19	20.05±0.88	<0.01
Urinary pregnanediol (mg/24hr)	20	32.98±2.05	33.95±1.73	>0.5
Plasma free cortisol (μg/100ml)	20	57.19±14.6	152.49±22.55	<0.01

(II) Results

The figures obtained were given in Table 3. It was found that before moxibustion the value of urinary 17-OHCS and 17-KS of the pregnant women was higher than that of non-pregnant women. This was in accord with the physiological variations of pregnancy. After moxibustion to Zhiyin points, the excretion of these hormones increased significantly ($P<0.01$). Pre- and post-moxibustion values of free plasma corticosterone showed similar variations. The excretion of pregnanediol didn't show any change (Table 3).

IV. THE EFFECTS OF ACUPUNCTURE OR MOXIBUSTION APPLIED TO ZHIYIN POINTS ON THE MOTILITY OF THE RABBIT UTERUS

(I) Methods

15 female rabbits weighing 1.8–3.0 Kg anesthetized with urethane (lg/Kg body weight) were laparotomized to expose the uterus. A thread was fastened to one horn of the uterus and connected to a strain resistance transducer of the physiological monitor by means of a glass uterine conduit. This allowed the uterine activity to be recorded on an auto-balance recorder to which the signal from the transducer was fed.

Acupuncture or moxibustion was applied to the points on both hind feet corresponding with the Zhiyin points in human being. During moxibustion the moxa-stick was directed to the "point" at a distance of 1.5–2.0 cm from the "point". The application of moxibustion lasted for 25 or 30 minutes.

Electroacupuncture was performed by a Model G6805 electrophore with a sparse-dense wave. The electricity was to be intense enough to induce a slight slaking of the rabbit's hind foot. The electric stimulation started 5 minutes after insertion of the needle and lasted for 15 or 20 minutes.

(II) Results

1. The effects of moxibustion applied to bilateral "Zhiyin Points". After moxibustion, an increase of both the activity and the tension of the uterus was found in the majority of the experimental rabbits. The latent period of response was comparatively long. Generally, the increase in activity of the uterus appeared several minutes after moxibustion (Fig. 2).

2. The effects of electroacupuncture of "Zhiyin Points". It was found that electric stimulation induced an increase in uterine activity and tension (Fig. 3).

V. DISCUSSION

1. The possibility of spontaneous version of abnormal fetal position had been analyzed by foreign authors[21]. Breech presentation was found to be 7.2% by the end of the 34th

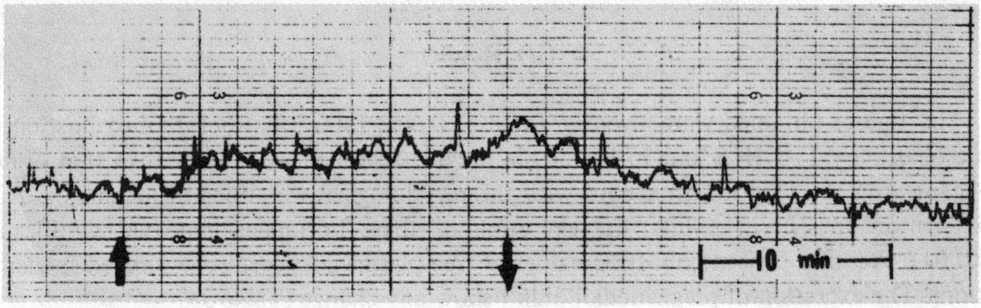

Fig. 2 The effects of moxibustion applied to "Zhiyin Points" on uterine activity of the rabbit.

↑ – Start. ↓ – Stop.

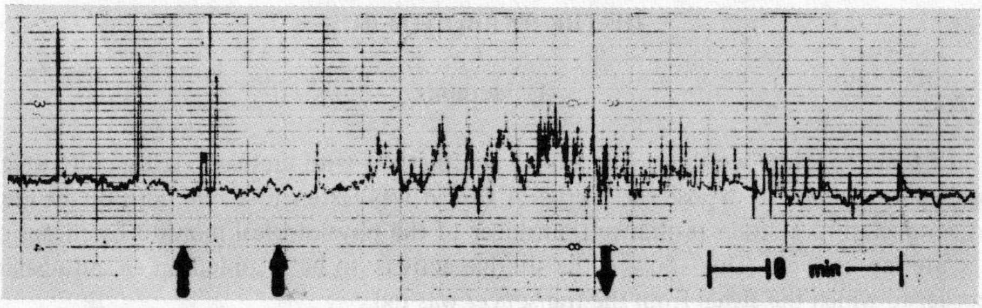

Fig. 3 The effects of electric stimulation of "Zhiyin Points" on uterine activity of the rabbit.

–Insertion of the needles,

–Current on,

–current off; withdrawal of the needles.

week of pregnancy and was just a little over 3% at term. This shows that the rate of spontaneous cephalic version was over 90% before 34 weeks of pregnancy. It also suggests that about 60% of the cases with breech presentation might spontaneously convert into vertex presentation in the last 6 weeks of pregnancy.

Of 100 cases with abnormal fetal position treated with moxibustion 71 were corrected in a course of 9 days. In 41 patients with pregnancy over 34 weeks 25 (61%) were successful. In the 71 successful cases 24 were cured with 1 application of moxibustion, which amounted to 33.8% and 54 cases (76% of the successful cases) were cured with 1–3 applications. These results coincided with data recently reported in China. Therefore, though spontaneous cephalic version would take place in some cases, the high rate of correction in so short a period of moxibustion treatment can hardly be explained by spontaneous version. Moxibustion must have promoted the version of the fetal position. This presumption was strengthened by the fact that of the 6 cases in which the subjects had practiced knee-chest position or other treatments with no effect, 5 were cured with moxibustion therapy they received after admission. The facts mentioned above suggest that moxibustion therapy has good effects on correcting abnormal fetal position.

In this series 29 were unsuccessful. The causes of the failures might be various, including the short umbilical cord the coiling of the cord around the baby's neck which restricts the motion and descending fixation of the fetus, the fetal head being fixed in the hypochondriac region or the abnormal presentation being already engaged to disturb the version of the fetal position. There were 7 cases in which the fetal position had been corrected with moxibustion but in which the abnormal position recurred in the course of therapy due to the high floating of the fetus or other factors.

No definite relationship was found between the therapeutic effect and the number of parity or weeks of pregnancy. In most of the successful cases the fetal movements increased after moxibustion and the patients had an average abdominal wall tension.

2. Several physiological parameters were recorded simultaneously. It was demonstrated that in the course of moxibustion the maternal cutaneous blood vessels kept dilated (shown by the fact that the amplitude of the pulse wave increased and the digital skin temperature rose), the heart rate did not increase, the blood pressure did not go up (the systolic pressure even fell somewhat) and the percentage of the neutrophil did not increase. These data suggest that the activities of the sympatho-adrenomedullary system were low then. Moxibustion of Zhiyin points was different from ordinary noxious stimulations in that its action was mild and would not result in measurable responses from the sympatho-adrenomedullary system.

The galvanic skin kept active, indicating that the related sympatho-cholinergic system was in a relatively active stage and suggesting that the response of this system to moxibustion was different from that of the sympatho-adrenomedullary system which controlled the cardiovascular activity. The functions of these two systems might be separated.

3. It was found that after moxibustion the excretion of pregnanediol in urine had no significant variations while that of 17-OHCS and 17-KS and the level of free plasma cortisol increased significantly. These data show that moxibustion could stimulate the secretion of the adrenal cortex. It has been demonstrated that cortisol stimulated placental production of estrogen[22], and that dexamethasone increased the concentration of prostaglandin(PG) in the maternal placenta. This may have been brought about by corticosteroids increasing the synthesis of estrogen, with the latter then stimulating PG production[22–26]. It was well known that estrogen increased the sensibility of the myometrium, while PG stimulated contraction of the myometrium. From this it was presumed that moxibustion stimulated the hypophysial-adrenocortical system and secretion of the adrenal cortex, and enhanced the tension and activity of the uterus through estrogen-PG links. The fetal movements were then reinforced and consequently the version of fetal position resulted.

The observation on experimental animals demonstrated that moxibustion or acupuncture on the points of anesthetized rabbit which correpond to the Zhiyin points in human being could increase the tension and contraction rate of the uterus. According to its characteristic responses, it was shown that the latent period was relatively long and it was unlikely to be a simple nervous reflex but a might be mediated via some humoral or other links.

It was found in clinical investigations that the enhancement of fetal movement could be felt within a few minutes after moxibustion and would continue for several hours, but version usually took place several hours or even agreat many hours after moxibustion. This lag of version indicated that the response of uterine activity induced by moxibustion had two phases, i.e. the immediate and the delayed effects. It also suggested that the effects of moxibustion might be mediated by a humoral link.

During moxibustion the increase of heart rate of the fetus was evident but it didn't coincide with that of the mother. It might be presumed that moxibustion enhanced the uterine tension and contraction which disturbed the blood supply of the fetus and resulted in the reinforcement of the fetal movement and the increase of the fetal heart rate.

VI. SUMMARY

100 cases of abnormal fetal position were treated by applying moxibustion to the bilateral Zhiyin points. Through a therapeutic course of 9 days there were definite results for version with a success rate of 71% after admission.

During the treatment, it was revealed that the maternal cutaneous blood vessels remained dilated, the heart beats didn't accelerate, the blood pressure didn't go up and the differential counts of WBC remained unchanged. The heart beats of the fetuses, however, accelerated significantly.

Based on the above results, it was suggested that moxibustion caused no obvious stimulaation to the sympatho-adrenomedullary system and that the great increase of fetal heart rate might be brought about by some unknown mechanism.

Moxibustion applied to Zhiyin points raised the value of free plasma cortisol and increased the excretion of 17-hydroxycorticosteroid and 17-ketosteroid which demonstrated that there was a stimulation effect of moxibustion on the hypophysial-adrenocortical system. Recent reports indicate that the hormones of the adrenal cortex stimulate the uterine activity indirectly, hence, it was presumed that the increased secretion of adrenocortical hormone during moxibustion therapy might result in the same effects. In the experimental anesthetized rabbits, acupuncture and moxibustion applied to Zhiyin points increased the tension and the contraction of the uterus. These facts gave support to the above presumption.

According to available physiological and biochemical materials, it was presumed that when moxibustion were applied to Zhiyin points, the secretions of adrenocortical hormones were increased, the activities of the uterus were enhanced, and the movements of the fetuses were also increased.

These three factors may have a cause and effect relationship with each other in turn, while the latter two might be the dynamic factors responsible for the spontaneous version of the fetal position.

REFERENCES

[1] 王执中(宋): 铖灸资法经，卷七，第 30 页，上海科学技术出版社，1959。

[2] 孙炬卿(宋): 备急灸法，第 11 页，罗嘉杰(清)重刻版。

[3] 杨继洲(明): 针灸大成，第 300 页，人民卫生出版社，1963。

[4] 张介宾(明): 类经图翼，第 155 页，人民卫生出版社，1973。

[5] 吴　谦等(清): 医宗金鉴，第五分册，第 180 页，人民卫生出版社，1973。

[6] 俞寿亲：浙江中医杂志（12）：48，1959。
[7] 魏凝瑞：中华妇产科杂志（1）：17，1960。
[8] 广州市第三人民医院妇产科：中华妇产科杂志（3）：189，1960。
[9] 王文石　郑毅伟：中华妇产科杂志（3）：193，1960。
[10] 天津工人医院针灸科、妇产科：天津医药杂志（12）：890，1960。
[11] 张纪云：哈尔滨中医（7）：82，1960。
[12] 沈阳市产科医院：辽宁医学杂志（8）：39，1960。
[13] 伍书辉等：江西中医药（9）：38，1960。
[14] 刘佩贤：广东中医（4）：152，1961。
[15] 雷　杰：江西医药（12）：20，1962。
[16] 高琪瑜等：福建中医药（1）：36，1964。
[17] 吴子亚：广东医学(祖国医学版)（4）：23，1965。
[18] 龚彩玲、汤　均：浙江中医药（3）：14，1965。
[19] 王文石：针灸杂志（1）：14，1965。
[20] 江西中医学院生理教研组：关于尿中 17-羟皮质类固醇测定方法的一点改进(未发表资料)。
[21] White, A.J.: *Obstet. Gynaec. Brit. Emp.* **63**:706, 1956.
[22] Liggins, G.C. *et al.*: *Rec. Prog. Horm. Res.* **29**:111, 1973.
[23] Liggins, G.C. *et al.*: *J. Endocrinol.* **42**:323, 1968.
[24] Liggins, G.C. *et al.*: *Biol. Reprod.* **16**:39, 1977.
[25] Flint, A.P.F. *et al.*: *J. Endocrinol.* **63**:67, 1974.
[26] Umo, I. *et al.*: *J. Endocrinol.* **68**:383, 1976.

CLINICAL INVESTIGATION OF TREATING PATIENTS WITH ACUTE BACILLARY DYSENTERY BY ACUPUNCTURE

Qiu Maoliang, Sheng Canruo, Li Naiying,
Wang Junmei
(*The Affiliated Hospital of Nanjing College of Traditional Chinese Medicine*)

Wang Jinsheng
(The *PLA 8lst Hospital*)

Xu Bingqing, Lu Zhenchu, Deng Guogang, Zhang Wanwen

(*Jiangsu Institute of Traditional Chinese Medicine*)

Bacillary dysentery, commonly seen in summer and autumn, is an infectious disease caused by dysenteric bacilli. Traditional Chinese medicine recognized it in very early times and records concerning it can be found in Chinese ancient medical literature, such as Neijin (i.e., Canon of Medicine, written in the period of the 5th-3rd century B.C.) and Jinkui Yaolue (i.e., Treasured Medical Essays of the Golden Cabinet), written in the Han Dynasty. In these classic books it was called respectively "disorders of the bowels" and " diarrhea". Later, it was referred to as "intestinal catarrh". Not until the Jin Dynasty was it described as "dysentery". A careful study of the ancient records of dysentery reveais that what was referred to as dysentry must also have includes such intestinal diseases as amebic dysentery, allergic enteritis, dysfunction of intestines, etc. In other words, it doesn't refer only to bacillary dysentery. However, in the period of Song (Sung) Dynasty (460–1279 A.D.) and Yuan Dynasty (1279–1368 A.D.), it was known as "pestilential dysentery", namely, "an infectious disease which will infect all the members of a family or the people of the same district". It shows that its infectivity is similar to that of acute bacillary dysentery.

The method for treating dysentery by acupuncture was recorded in Jiayijing (A Treatise on Acupuncture, written in the Jin Dynasty, 265 A.D.), in which there are prescriptions for treating intestinal disease with bloody and purulent stools, such as Qianjinfang (Prescriptions Worth A Thousand Pieces of Gold) of the Tang Dynasty, Zishengjing of the Song (Sung) Dynasty and Zhenjiu Dacheng (Compendium of Acupuncture and Moxibustion) of the Ming Dynasty. Through these rich experience was accumulated. However, because of historical limitations at that time, systematic observation and enunciation were impossible. In order to inherit and carry forward the heritage of traditional Chinese medicine and study the principle governing the treatment of this disease by acupuncture, we have treated many cases of bacillary dysentery by applying only acupuncture and then systematically systematically recording observations. These experiments have been conducted by doctors of both Chinese and western medicines. The following is an analysis of 645 cases with positive tests of bacteria in stool cultures.

I. CRITERIA FOR SELECTION OF CASES:

1. With typical symptoms and signs of acute bacillary dysentery;
2. With positive tests of bacteria in stool culture;
3. Not having been medicated by antibacillary drugs;
4. Length of time of disease not more than 3 days.

II. ANALYSIS OF CASES

For admission, all patients must have typical symptoms and signs of acute bacillary dysentery. The results of various examinations are shown in the following Tables 1–3:

From the above tables, it can be seen that in this group, there were 576 cases with fever, mostly 38–39°C, the highest being 40.2°C. Among them 445 cases had more than 10 defecations a day and the severest ones had more than 30. Under observation with the naked eye, the stools of 417 cases were found to be purely pus and blood. Stool cultures revealed that most of the cases 478 in number–had Shigella Plexneri, accounting for 74.1%. Among them 131 cases were examined with sigmoidscope to observe pathological changes of the intestinal tract. The result was that 117 cases were of the catarrhal type, 8 cases of the ulcerative type and 6 cases of the erosive type.

III. METHOD OF TREATMENT

The method of treatment is determined according to the theories of traditional Chinese medicine. It is considered, in traditional Chinese medicine, that the causative factors of dysentery are mainly irregular food intake and the invasion of toxicant damp-heat which injures the stomach and intestines and cause dysfunction of the two organs in reception and transmission. The affliction of damp-heat and the stagnation of the *qi* and the blood, injure the mucosa and the blood vessels of the intestinal tract, eliciting symptoms of fever, abdominal pain, tenesmus, and purulent and bloody stools. So the principle of treatment is to eliminate the heat, dispel the damp, clear away the stasis and restore the normal circulation of the *qi* and blood. The points for acupuncture are selected accordingly. At the beginning, about ten pairs of points were used for the above purposes. This not only made the procedure complicated, but also added to the suffering of the patient. After repeated practice, we gradually grasped the law of treating the disease. Points were sifted again and again and finally the following prescription was formulated.

(I) Main points: Tianshu (St. 25), Qihai (Ren 6), Shangjuxu (St. 37)

Tianshu (St. 25) and Shangjuxu (St. 37) are points of the Stomach Channel. The form-

Table 1. Cardinal symptoms and signs in 645 cases at admission

	Abdominal pain		Tenesmus		Fever (°C)					Abdominal tenderness	
	Present	absent	Present	absent	<37	<38	<39	<40	>40	Present	absent
No. of Cases	633	12	623	22	43	215	213	148	26	617	28
%	98.1	1.9	96.5	3.5	6.7	33.3	33.0	23.1	4.0	95.7	4.3

Table 2. Stool character and its laboratorial tests in 645 cases at admission

			No. of cases	%
Visual Gross Observation	Pus & blood		417	64.7
	Mucous pus & blood		104	16.1
	Pus-like		5	0.8
	Mucus		90	13.9
	Loose and paste-like		29	4.4
Microscopic cxamination	Phagocyte	Present	447	69.3
		Absent	198	30.7
	Red blood cell	Absent	10	1.5
		Small amount	55	8.5
		+	121	18.9
		++	159	24.6
		+++	234	36.2
		++++	66	10.2
	Pus cell	Absent	10	1.5
		Small amount	12	2.0
		+	47	7.2
		++	180	27.9
		+++	264	49.3
		++++	132	20.6

Table 3. Distribution of types of bacteria in stool culture of 645 cases

	Shigella flexneri								Shigella sonnei	Shigella boydii	Shigella schmitz
	Undifferentiated	I_a	I_b	II_a	II_b	III	IV_a	IV			
No. of Cases	128	146	27	82	17	8	61	9	121	10	36
		478									
%		74.1							18.7	1.5	5.5

er is Front-Mu point of the large intestine and the latter the lower He-Sea point of the large intestine. So they exert actions on both organs and are important points in dispelling damp-heat, clearing away stasis and restoring the normal functions of the two organs. This coinciqes with the ancient experience of treating diseases of the *fu* organs (i.e. stomach, large intestine, small intestine, gall bladder, urinary bladder and *sanjiao*) by using Front-Mu and He-Sea Points. Qihai (Ren 6) has the effect of regulating the *qi*; it can not only stop pain, but also relieve tenesmus.

Method of addition and omission of points:

1. In cases in which heat is predominant, add Quchi (L.I. 11) and Hegu (L.I. 4) to clear away the heat in the Yangming Channels.

2. In cases in which damp ness is predominant, add Yinlingquan (Sp. 9) to regulate the spleen and resolve damp.

In application of the prescription, points should be added or reduced according to the condition of the disease. Severe abdominal pain and diarrhea mean serious accumulation of damp-heat in the stomach and intestines. Since it is a matter of urgency to eliminate the heat, dispel the damp ness and clear away the stasis, all the main points should be used. When bowel movements are decreased to 5–6 times a day and abdominal pain is alleviated, Qihai (Ren 6) may be omitted. When the frequency of the movements return to normal and all the symptoms disappear but the stool culture, remain positive, only Shangjuxu (St. 37) is needed. Quchi (L.I. 11) and Hegu (L.I. 4) are used when the body temperature is above 38°C, and omitted when fever subsides. For cases with poor appetite, scanty urine and sticky tongue, Yinlingquan (Sp. 9) is added to eliminate damp ness.

(II) Manipulation method

Bacillary dysentery is a heat syndrome of the *shi* (real) type. According to the principle of "reducing in case of *shi*", a reducing manipulation method should be used, i.e. rapid insertion of the needle, deep puncture (generally 1.5–2 *cun*–Chinese inch, for adults), and, after the needling sensation is obtained, swift lifting and gentle thrusting should be combined with the twisting of the needle. Needles should be manipulated repeatedly so as to enhance the needling sensation. It is required that for points on the abdomen, the needling sensation should diffuse in all directions, and for those on the extremities, it should go upwardly or downward. Thus the symptoms can be controlled rapidly. Special attention should be paid to the lst and 2nd treatments, on which success or failure hinges, so that the seriousness of the disease can be abated. After that, with the remission of the symptoms, the stimulation to be given and the depth of puncture may both be reduced. Needles are generally retained for 30 minutes, and 60 minutes for severe cases. During retention of needles, if the patient wants to defecate, manipulation of the needles may cause the feeling to disappear, so it will not be necessary to take out the needles. On the first few days after admission or for severe cases, treatment is given twice a day or even once every 8 hours. After the symptoms are improved, treatment may be given once daily until 3 successive negative stool cultures are prodred. 10 treatments make a course of treatment. Cases which fail to recover completely after a course of treatment is completed should be transferred to other groups for treatment. For cases with marked dehydration due to high fever and repeated vomiting and diarrhea, infusion of fluid is necessary so as to normalize electrolyte disorders.

IV. OBSERVATION OF THERAPEUTIC EFFECT

(1). Observation with the naked eye of the character of the stool at least once a day;

(2). When making the gross observation of the character of the stool every morning, take the most marked portion of it as a sample for microscopic examination daily, until 3 successive negative are produced;

(3). Stool culture of bacteria daily in addition to routine stool examination until 3 successive negatives are produced;

(4). Inquire about the state of the patient at least twice a day and write down the most marked changes;

(5). In case no improvement of clinical symptoms occurs following 2–5 days of acupuncture treatment, the patient should be discharged for other treatment. Cases in which symptoms disappear after a course of treatment but stool culture remains positive are considered failures.

V. CRITERIA OF A THERAPEUTIC CURE

(1). Total disappearance of all clinical manifestations;

(2). Normal stool, less than 2 defecations per day;

(3). Normal appearance of stool on gross observation, no R.B.C. and pus cells under microscopic examination;

(4). No growth of bacteria in 3 successive stool cultures.

VI. ANALYSIS OF THERAPEUTIC EFFECT

(1). After a course of treatment, 596 cases reached the above criteria of therapeutic

Table 4. Days for the cardinal symptoms to disappear and for stools to return to normal under microscopic examination

	Total Cases	Time for recovery (Days)										Mean days for recovery
		0–1		2–3		4–5		6–7		8–10		
		No. of Cases	%	No. of Cases	%	No. of Cases	%	No. of Cases	%	No. of Cases	%	
Fever	489	252	51.5	203	41.5	30	6.1	4	0.8			1.88
Abdominal pain	595	171	28.7	248	41.6	110	18.4	49	8.4	17	2.8	2.95
Tenesmus	584	309	52.9	170	29.1	84	14.3	16	2.7	5	0.9	2.15
Diarrhea	596	151	25.3	185	31.0	151	25.3	96	16.2	13	2.2	3.40
Character of stool	596	165	27.7	192	32.2	184	30.9	41	6.8	14	2.3	3.11
Stool microscopic finding	596	102	17.1	185	31.0	154	25.8	131	21.9	24	4.0	3.90

cure, amounting to 92.4%.

(2). Among the 596 cured cases, the days it took for the cardinal symptoms to disappear and the laboratorial tests to return normal are shown as follows (Table 4):

During the treatment, it was observed that the body temperature of those cases with fever generally began to go down 4 hours after the antipyretic points were used, and the mean time for the temperature to return to normal was 1.88 days. During retention of the needles, abdominal pain was markedly alleviated and sometimes disappear. Generally the character of stool was improved before the frequency of bowel movements was brought under control. On the average, the latter returned to normal in 3.40 days (Table 5).

From Tables 4 and 5, it can be seen that the improvement of the clinical manifestations coincides with the negative results of the laboratoriy tests. This conforms to the general law of the curing of bacillary dysentery.

Table 5. General picture of negative returns of stool bacteria culture in 596 cases

Days for negative return	1	2 3	4 5	6 7	8 9 10
No. of Cases	23	68 88	99 89	63 56	49 35 26
Cumulation percentage	3.7	29.8	61.0	81.5	100.0
Mean time	5.12				

VII. COMPARISON OF THERAPEUTIC EFFECTS

The following two tables (Tables 6 and 7) show a comparison of therapeutic effects between the acupuncture group and the drug group. The latter was composed of 281 cases of bacillary dysentery cured by oral administration of furoxone.

From Table 5, it can be seen that on the average, tenesmus, abdominal pain and diarrhea disappeared earlier in the acupuncture group than in the drug group ($P<0.05$).

Table 7 shows that the total rate of negative results and the rate of negative results above 7 days are higher in the drug group ($P<0.05$), and the rate of negative results within 7 days is higher in the acupuncture group ($P<0.05$).

Table 6. Means number of days of disappearance of symptoms in the acupuncture and drug groups

	No. of cases	Fever	Tenesmus	Abdominal pain	Diarrhea
Drug group	281	1.8	4.3	5.3	5.5
Acu. group	596	1.88	2.15	2.95	3.4

Table 7. Comparison of the time for negative results of stool cultures in the acupuncture and drug groups

	No. of positive cases	No. of negative return cases	Rate of negative return (%)	Mean time for negative return	Within 7 days		Above 7 days	
					No. of negative returns	%	No. of negative returns	%
Drug group	281	276	98.2	4.3	205	74.2	71	25.6
Acu. group	645	596	92.4	5.12	486	81.5	110	18.4

VIII. FOLLOW-UP

In 268 cases, in which the pafients were checkes more than half a year after they were cured and discharged from the hospital, a recurrence of symptoms and positive findings in stool culture occurred in 33 cases, amounting to 12.3%.

IX. DISCUSSION

(1). Practice has proven that in treating bacillary dysentery by acupuncture, not only can the symptoms of fever, abdominal pain and tenesmus be brought under control rapidly, but the microscopic findings and bacteria culture of stools also turn negative rapidly. Judging from either the average number of days for the symptoms to disappear and the bacteria culture to turn to negative or from the rate at which pafients are cured, this therapy is by no means inferior to treatment with antibacillary drugs. Therapeutic effect can be confirmed so this therapy is worthy of being popularized.

Through our observation in clinical treatment during these years, we have found that the therapeutic effect of treating bacillary dysentery by acupuncture depends upon the synthetic action of channels, points and manipulation methods In other words to first select channels in line with the particular disease; secondly, to formulate a prescription according to the action of points; finally, to apply different manipulation methods in accordance with the *xu* (apparent) or *shi* (real) condition of the disease.

We also tried acupuncture treatment on 40 cases of bacillary dysentery by using points which had no relation to the stomach and intestines with the intention of observing and comparing the effects. The result was that most of the treatments failed. This shows the importance of correct selection of channels and points. The manipulation method is another question worthy of discussion. Proper manipulation of needles often plays a decisive role in the treatment of this disease. For instance, for cases of bacillary dysentery with high fever, puncturing the antipyretic points with the proper manipulation will soon cause sweating and the dropping of body temperature; for cases with abdominal pain, the pain will be brought under control. On the contrary, improper manipulation will markedly weaken the effect or yield no effect at all. Therefore, emphasis should be placed on the organic combination of channels, points and manipulation methods which are of great significance in raising the therapeutic effect. The same is also true of treatment of all other diseases.

(2). In our clinical work, we found that in treating the same disease with the same points and manipulation method, different therapeutic effects might result. Some cases were cured soon and others not. Why is it so? Our preliminary understanding is that the therapeutic effects are related to the pathological changes of the intestinal tract, clinical manifestations and the season of occurrence. Among the 131 cases subjected to sigmoidoscopy, 108 of the 117 cases which were of the catarrhal type were cured, while 6 of the 14 cases which were of the ulcerative and erosive types failed. This shows a certain relation between the severity of pathological change of the intestinal tract and the therapeutic effects. 155 cases were differentiated into three types according to traditional Chinese medicine, i.e. the type of severe heat with mild damp ness, the type of severe damp ness with mild heat and the type of cold-damp ness. The treatment was given to observe the effects. It was found that acupuncture produced more rapid effects and needed a shorter course of treatment in cases of the severe-heat-mild-damp ness type which were characterized by high fever, frequent mooements, red mucus in stools, thirst and yellow sticky tongue coating than in those of the severe-damp-mild-heat type. Which are characterized by mild fever, stuffiness of chest, lassitude, white mucus in stools, no thirst and yellowish sticky tongue coating. The conditions of the latter cases were mild in comparison with those of the former, but their therapeutic effects were not so good as those of the former. Explained by traditional Chinese medicine, this is because "heat is a non-substantial pathogenic factor which is easy to be dispelled, while damp ness is a pathogenic factor characterized by stickiness which is difficult to resolve." From clinical observation during these years, we have also found that generally the therapeutic effects are not so good and a comparatively long course of treatment is needed in treating cases occurring in late autumn. The same is true of cases treated with drugs, and so far no satisfactory explanation has been given to this phenomenon by modern medicine. However, the theories in traditional Chinese medicine concerning seasonal meteorological factors and the attack of summer pathogenic factors late in autumn are worthy of consideration. These explanations follow from what has happened in clinical practice, but they remain to be further expounded on by the studies of modern science. As to the types of bacteria, no marked difference in the therapeutic effect has been observed when treating this disease by acupuncture.

(3) According to what was recorded in *Neijing*, acupuncture can treat malaria, cholera, leprosy and various acute febrile diseases. This shows that as far back as two thousand years ago, acupuncture was widely used to treat infectious diseases. The scope of acupuncture treatment was further developed by physicians of the later generations. Treatment of bacillary dysentery by acupuncture is one of the methods handed down from ancient times. How can a fine needle cure a disease caused by bacteria or a virus? Surely it is incomprehensible that acupuncture could directly act upon bacteria. In traditional Chinese medicine, it is thought that acupuncture may yield the effect of readjusting *yin* and *yang*, activating and regulating the *qi* and the blood, reinforcing the apparent (*xu*) and reducing the real (*shi*), so as to reach the aim of curing the disease by strengthening the anti-pathogenic factors (i.e. the active factors and immune functions of the body*) and eliminating the pathogenic factors. This may be used as an explaination of the reasons for treating bacillary dysentery by acupuncture. We have made experiments on the effect of needling serum protein

electrophoresis in rabbits and in patients with bacillary dysentery and observed the changes of various immune functions during acupuncture treatment of bacillary dysentery. All the results obtained have proved that acupuncture exerts influence on the various immune functions in many ways. It can promote the activity of the reticuloendothelial system, cause the specific and non-specific antibodies to increase, enhance the defensive forces of the body, and thus overcome the disease. These experiments have provided powerful evidence for the theory of "strengthening the anti-pathogenic factors to eliminate the pathogenic factors." Therefore, this theory may serve as guidance in a wide range of clinical treatments.

In addition to its close relation with immunity, the mechanism of treating bacillary dysentery by acupuncture also has effects on the subsidence of fever, alleviation of pain and regulation of the functions of the stomach and intestines. If it should be clarified, the mechanism of acupuncture treatment of diseases will be clarified to a certain degree. Therefore, gaining a clear theoreticall idea of why acupuncture can cure bacillary dysentery in such a short period of time is of great importance to both the development of our traditional medicine and to the creation of a new medicine.

EXPERIMENTAL STUDY OF ACUPUNCTURE TREATMENT OF ACUTE BACILLARY DYSENTERY

ROLE OF HUMORAL IMMUNE MECHANISM

Xu Bingqing, Lu Zhenchu*

(Biochemical Laboratory, Jiangsu Institute of Traditional Chinese Medicine)

Deng Guogang, Zhang Wanwen

(Physiological Laboratory, Jiangsu Institute of Traditional Chinese Medicine)

Li Naiying, Wang Junmei

(Clinical Laboratory, Hospital Affiliated withe the Nanjing College of Traditional Chinese Medicine)

Qiu Maoliang, Sheng Chuanruo

(Department of Acupuncture, Hospital Affiliated with the Nanjing College of Traditional Chinese Medicine)

Wang Jinsheng, Wu Defu

(Department of Infectious Diseases, the PLA 81st Hospital)

Acupuncture treatment of acute bacillary dysentery (simply written ABD in the following) has proved effective in clinical practice. But the mechanism of this treatment is still not well understood. Since 1974 we have made a preliminary study of some humoral immune functions during the course of acupuncture treatment of ABD in 50 human cases and also in experimental animals. The results are summarized as follows:

I. MATERIALS AND METHODS

(I) Objects of Observation and Sources of Specimens

1. Men: (1) Selection of cases and method of treatment: same as in the clinical observation.

---

*Compiled by Lu Zhenchu

(2) Collection of blood and stool specimens in acupuncture treatment group: from those patients admitted to the hospital for observation.

(3) Collection of blood and stool specimens in normal control group: from students of the medical school and staff members of our hospital.

2. Animals: Rabbits with the same feeding conditions and similar body weight were selected. They were divided into 3 groups:

(1) Electroacupuncture group: banding plus electroacupuncture (needling of points corresponding to "Shangjuxu" and "Tianshu" points in man)

(2) Control group: banding without electroacupuncture.

(3) Blank: no banding and no electroacupuncture.

(II) Methods

Serum protein electrophoresis[1], total serum complement[2], serum immunoglobulins (Ig G, Ig A, Ig M)[3,4], plasma bactericidal power[5], serum specific antibodies[6,7], secretory immunoglobulin A(SIg A) in stool[8, 9, 10], serum lysozyme[2] and phagocytic activity of liver reticulo-endothelial system (RES)[11, 12] were determined by the usual methods for these examination and tests with only minor modification in some cases.

II. RESULTS

(I) Effect of Acupuncture on the Nonspecific Humoral Immunization of the Body

1. Effect of electroacupuncture of serum protein electrophoresis in rabbits. Blood samples were taken from the 3 groups mentioned above for serum protein paper electrophoresis on the 1st, 6th, 10th, 15th and 20th days respectively. In comparison with the control, it was found that on the 6th day following acupuncture, the albumin(A) and α_1, α_2 globulins were markedly depressed, while the β and γ globulins were elevated markedly. The albumin was reduced by 4.2% ($P<0.01$) and γ globulin increased by 28.3%, both significantly differed from the statisfics for the control values ($P<0.05$).

2. The changes of serum albumin electrophoresis before and after acupuncture treatment in patients of ABD. 33 cases of the hospitalized patients were subjected to a dynamic study of the serum protein electrophoresis by taking blood samples before treatment and on the 3rd, 6th, and 9th day following treatment. It was found that on the 6th day the albumin was depressed significantly in comparison with the control, being reduced by 5.6% ($P<0.01$). The 4 other globulins however produced an augmenting tendency to various extents in which the elevation of α and β globulins was conducive to strengthening the phagocytic activity of white cells, and the increase of γ globulin was closely related to the formation of antibodies. This indicated that acupuncture actually may strengthen the defensive immune activity of the patients.

3. The changes of the total serum complement content before and after acupuncture in patients with ABD. 35 patients and 11 healthy persons (needling of bilateral "Shangjuxu" points successively for 12 days) were studied for determination of total serum complement content Blood samples were taken before acupuncture and on the 3rd, 7th and 12th days respectively. The total serum complement content of patients before acupuncture treatment was found to be 162±28 unit/ml (SE) on the average, which was lower than that of a normal person's 178±7.59 units/ml (SE). However, following successive acupuncture treatment for 3 days, there was a marked increase in the total serum complement contents in both the patients and the normal persons, which still persisted on the 7th to the 12th days following acupuncture.

4. Changes of the serum immunoglobulins (Ig G, Ig A, Ig M) **content before and after acupuncture**. In 50 patients and 11 normal persons blood samples were taken before acupuncture and on the 3rd, 7th, 12th day after acupuncture for determination of serum immunoglobulins (Ig G, Ig A, Ig M). The results were:

Ig G: in patients it increased by 11%, 12% and 23% on the 3rd, 7th and 12th days respectively, following acupuncture. This differed sisnificantly from the control before acupuncture ($P<0.01$).

Ig A: in healthy persons it increased by 9%, 20% and 19% on the 3rd, 7th and 12th days respectively, following acupuncture where as in patients it increased by 19%, 33% and 43% on the same days respectively following acupuncture. The groups showed parallel and significant variations under the influence of acupuncture ($P<0.01$), but in the patient group the increase of Ig A was found to be more marked.

Ig M: in patients it increased by 33% on the 3rd day in comparison with the level before acupuncture ($P<0.01$), and it declined gradually afterward,. Thus it presented a pattern of early onset and rapid subsidevce in the bactericidal activity in the early stage of the disease.

5. Influence of electroacupuncture of "Shangjuxu" and "Tianshu" points on plasma bactericidal power in rabbits. 22 animals were used which were divided into electroacupuncture, control and blank groups. Blood samples were taken before experimentation and this was repeated 30 minutes and 3 hours after the successive applications of electroacupuncture respectively in order to α determine the plasma bactericidal power. 6 applications of electroacupuncture at 4 hours intervals were administered within 24 hours.

It was found that the bactericidal power of the body was increased markedly 30 minutes to 3 hours after electroacupuncture, while no change was observed in the blank group. It is noteworthy that a similar change was also observed in the control group, though much attenuated. This is thought to be due to the immobilization imposed on the animals by banding.

6. Effect of acupuncture on the bactericidal power of the patients' blood. In 37 cases of ABD, blood samples were taken before acupuncture and 30 minutes after the 2nd trial of acupuncture respectively to determine the plasma bactericidal power. It was found that in these 37 cases the number of colonies, on the average, 434±76 (SD) was reduced to 235±40 (SD) following acupuncture. This difference is very significant statistically ($P<0.01$).

The animal experimental results and the clinical laboratory findings mentioned above all demonstrate that acupuncture may strengthen the plasma bactericidal power against dysentery bacilli. But, owing to the complex constituents of plasma, it is still obscure which factors are responsible for this mechanism. For this purpose we subjected the blood samples to heating at 56°C for 30 minutes, to see whether heat-labile factors were involved in the bactericidal activity.

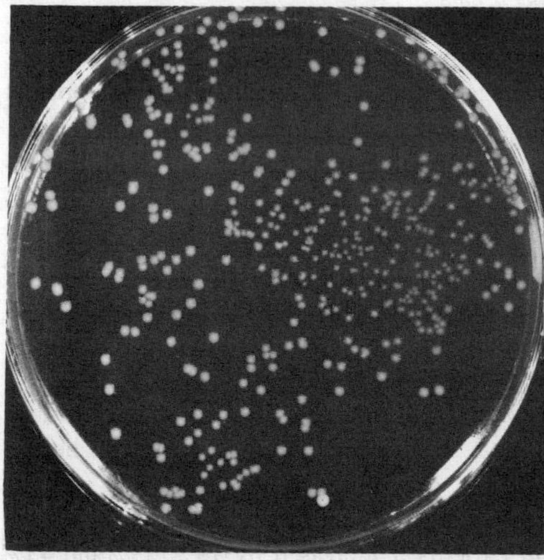

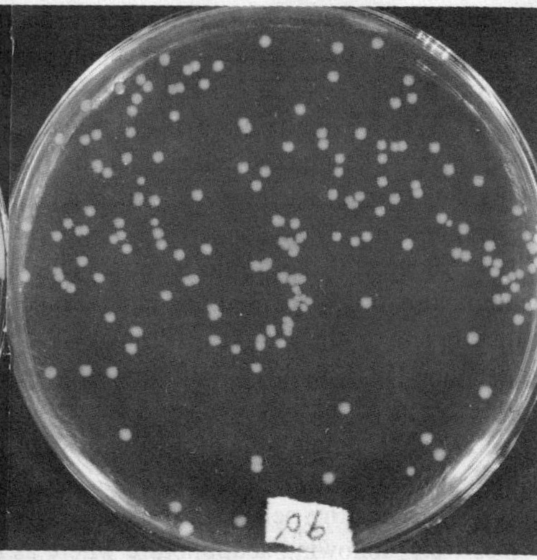

Fig. 1 No. colonies before needling. Fig. 2 No. colonies after needling

It was found that in the non-heated group, the number of colonies was obviously reduced following acupuncture, while in the beated group the number of colonies was much greater than that of the non-heated group, both before and after acupuncture. The difference is very significant ($P<0.01$). It indicates that certain bactericidal substances originally present in the normal plasma may exert their bactericidal actions more powerfully under the influence of acupuncture. These substances, probably complements, complement-bond antibodies, and other heat-labile materials, are entirely inactivated after heating.

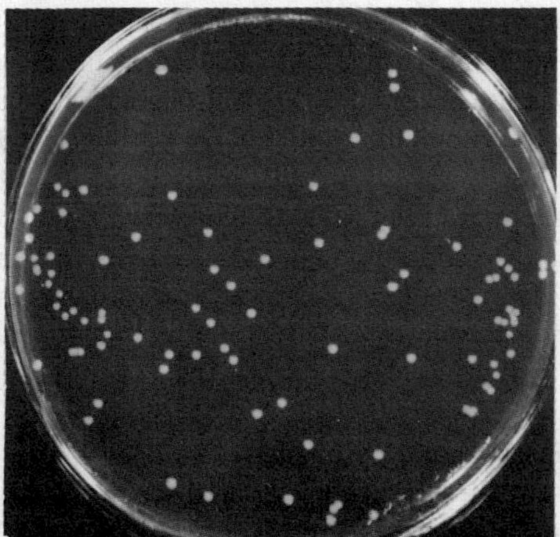

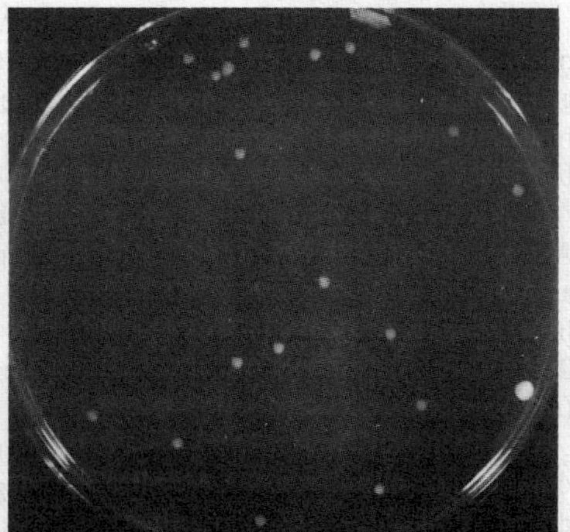

Fig. 3 No. colonies 56°C/30′ inactivation. Fig. 4 No. colonies Activation.

(II) Effect of Acupuncture on the Specific Humoral Immunity of the Body

1. Observation of the specific antibodies before and after acupuncture in ABD patients. In: 39 of the cases we observed, specific antibodies were determined by means of an indirect blood agglutination test between the blood samples and the de-activated medium of dysentery bacilli elaborated from the stool culture. The results being compared with those of healthy persons (50 cases).

The results revealed that the serum antibodies titer of ABD patients before acupuncture was 1:82±1.6 on the average, which was lower than that of normal persons (1:88). This is thought to be a result of the depression of immune functions during the severe infectious stage. On successive acupuncture treatments, the titer was raised rapidly, reaching the value of 1:349±3 on the 5th-7th day following acupuncture treatment.

2. Effect of acupuncture on the content of secretory immunoglobulin A (S Ig A) in stools of ABD patients. In 36 patients, stool specimens were collected over a 24 hour period on the 1st, 3rd, 5th, 7th and 12th day following acupuncture treatment in order to determine the S Ig A content.

Two groups were divided according to whether or not pus and blood were present in stool under gross observation on admission.

Group A: no pus and blood.

Group B: with pus and blood.

In 12 cases from group A, the stool S Ig A content on the 1st day was 23.92±3.32 (SE) mg%/24 hrs, and it rose to 44.15±8.48 (SE)mg%/24 hrs on the 3rd day. The variation was significant ($P<0.05$). It gradually declined to the normal level again after the 5th day in accordance with the convalescent tendency in clinical manifestation.

In 24 cases of group B, the stool S Ig A content on the 1st day was 55.4±8.88 (SE) mg%/24 hrs, which was obviously higher than the normal value. This is considered to be due to the admixture of pus and blood from the local lesions into the stool. Thus the actual stool S Ig A level could hardly be manifested reliably by the specimens taken on the 1st day. But owing to the fact that the S Ig A content still remained higher than normal on the 3rd day during which pus and blood could no longer be observed on gross examination in the majority of the cases, the opinion that acupuncture may potentiate the local immunity mechanism is substantiated. A similar declining tendency of S Ig A was also observed after the 5th day, as stated in group A.

(III) Changes of Serum Lysozyme Content Before and After Acupuncture Treatment in ABD Patients

The lysozyme content was determined in 46 cases of ABD which was compared with that of 22 healthy persons. It was found that the mean content of lysozyme before acupuncture in these 46 cases of ABD was 52.2μg/ml, which was higher than the normal value (27μg/ml), indicating that lysozyme takes an active part in the bacteriolytic mechanism in the early stage of ABD. On the 3rd day following acupuncture, it rose to the level of 89μg/ml, then subsided after the 7th day and with the clinical convalescence and the negative turn of stool culture, it declined to the level of normal persons on the 12th day.

(IV) Effect of Electroacupuncture of "Shangjuxu" and "Tianshu" Points on the Phagocytic Activity of Liver Reticulo-endothelial System(RES)

The liver RES phagocytic activity on the 1st day after acupuncture treatment which was higher than that of the control group by 7.5% rose to 49% on the 6th day and 63% on the 10th day ($P<0.01$). In addition to the observations of the effect of needling "Shangjuxu" and "Tianshu" points on serum protein mentioned above, it is noted that the period in which the phagocytic activity showed most marked potentiation coincides with the moment of elevation of the serum globulins.

III. DISCUSSION

(I) Acupuncture May Activate and Potentiate the Humoral Immune Function of ABD Patients

The fact that acupuncture may potentiate the body defensive function has been proved by numerous reports, but few of them have touched on ABD cases. From the experimental results mentioned above we have confirmed the marked increases of serum immunoglobulins, total complements, plasma bactericidal power, specific antibodies, lysozyme and local stool antibodies under the influence of acupuncture. However, whether such potentiation of humoral immunity is really initiated by the action of acupuncture or whether it is simply a manfestation of spontaneous immunization induced by the disease itself is still a problem which must be clarified. Obviously, we can not just form the purpose of study, deny some patients treatment so they may be used as controls. The only thing we can do is to compare the various items before and after acupuncture in patients and explain the results by comparing them with those of animal experiments and the obseivation of healthy persons.

The clinical manifestation of all the patients on admission showed that they all presented a typical picture of ABD. Thus, the patients are considered to be in the acute stage of the disease. Determination of various humoral immune items from the blood samples taken in this stage revealed that the mean value of total serum complement was lower than that of healthy persons, 162±28u/ml versus 178±7.59u/ml, and it increased markedly on the 3rd day of acupuncture treatment in both groups. The serum Ig G content in patient and healthy groups before acupuncture were similar, being 1000±87(SD)mg% and 1000±117(SD)mg% respectively. The Ig A content of patients and healthy persons was 158±57(SD)mg% and 196±85(SD)mg% respectively being lower in patient group. On the 3rd day of acupuncture treatment, both in healthy persons and in patients, the serum Ig G and Ig A both increased markedly. It is noteworthy that Ig A increased by 19% on the 3rd day which presented a tendency of an even greater increase on the 12th day. On the contrary, in healthy persons, no further increase was observed on the 7th day of acupuncture treatment. As to the content of serum specific antibodies, the level of patients was slightly lower than that of healthy persons (1:83 versus 1:88) before acupuncture treatment. This increased rapidly to

1:349 on the 5-7th day folowing treatment with the rise of this factor being faster and earlier than those reported elsewhere in the medical literature of foreign coontries[16]. In addition, it was observed from animal experiments and blood sampling in patients that the plasma bactericidal power was also markedly increased following acupuncture. All these data indicate that in the acute severe infectious stage, some humoral immune activities which are depressed may be activated and potentiated under the influence of acupuncture.

(II) Humoral Immune Functions Are the Important Material Basis of Acupuncture Treatment for ABD

Based upon clinical and epidemiological data, it is considered that during the infection of ABD the nonspecific defensive factors of the body are put into action. In this aspect the majority of authors have emphasized the potentiation of phagocytic activity of white cells in peripheral blood against the dysentery bacilli, but have paid less attention to the nonspecific humoral defensive factors involved in ABD.

In recent years, numerous data have proved that in the defensive mechanism against infections, the white cells and phagocytes usually exert their actions in combination with mutual activation, facilitation and reinforcing of the humoral immune factors, such as complements and immunoglobulins.

As mentioned above, on needling of "Shangjuxu" and "Tianshu" points in rabbits, the liver RES phagocytosis was enhanced and was accompanied by a rise of serum γ globulins. In accordance with this, on needling of "Shangjuxu" and "Tianshu" points in patients during the course of treatment, the three main immunoglobulins (Ig G, Ig A, Ig M), total complements, lysozyme and bactericidal power of plasma all were raised in the same time period as animal experiment. The number of colonies which survived before and after acupuncture were 434±76 and 235±40 respectively. The difference being very significant. It is also suggested that the bactericidal factors involved are probably related to the complements and complement-bond antibodies[13, 14, 17, 18, 19], which are widely known to have definite bactericidal actions. Considering the interrelationship between these substances, the increase of Ig G is conducive to neutralization of toxins and activation of complements,[13, 15, 19] according to some authors,[20] and the increase of Ig A may also activate the complements. The rise of total serum complement content reveals that it plays a key role in bacteriolysis and bactericidal activities[13, 21, 22]. The rapid increase of Ig M also manifests its early participation in the bactericidal action of bond complements.

As to the problem of the determination of the pathway through which the humoral immune function is mobilized by acupuncture and the question of how the potentiated humoral immune function kills the dysentery bacilli, further studies are required.

REFERENCE

[1] Maore, D.H.: *J. of Bio. Chem.* Vol. 161 No. 1:21, 1945.

[2] The Capital Hospital of Chinese Academy of Medical Science: Collection of Methods of Experiment on Chronic Bronchitis. The People's Health Press 1973.

[3] TeachingR esearch Group of Microbiology of Beijing Medical College: Acta of Beijing Medical Colloge 1976.

[4] Mancini, G. *et al.*: *Immunochemistry* **2**:235, 1965.

[5] Weijingshuen *et al.*: Collection of Data From Research Work on Tradition Chinese Medicine in Shanxi (I) 121, 125, 1964
[6] Ni Ben *et al.*: Acta Microbiologica Sinica 1:31, 1955.
[7] Zhong Qui Zhen *et al.*: Research on Mechanism of Acupuncture Anesthesia (Channels) 1972.
[8] Beijing Medical College: Lecture Sheets of Immunology 1976.
[9] Preer, J. R.: The J. of Immunology 1:52, 1956.
[10] 前田修一: 医学のあゆみ 99:196, 1976.
[11] Rawls, W.B. *et al.*: *J. Lab. Clini.* **4**:512, 1954.
[12] Benelerrof, B. and Delafresuaye, J.F. : Physiopathology of the Reticulo-Endothel System 80:431, 1957.
[13] Jiangran: The Basic Knowledge of Immunology, Press Jiangsu Medical Association 1977.
[14] Shanghi Medical Information Station: The Inter-Changes of Medical Information 8, 1975.
[15] Liu Xanmin: Reference Material of Foreign Medical Information (The Volume of Eqidemic Disease and Infectious Disease) 2:4, 1976.
[16] 宫田义人: 感染症学雑誌(日文) 8:431，1970。
[17] Ballow, M. *et al.*: *J. Immunol.* **103:944, 1969.**
[18] Ward, P. A. *et al.*: *J. Immunol.* **102**:331, 1969.
[19] Hensen, P. M.: *J. Immunol.* **111**:300, 1970.
[20] Lihui,: Acta of Medicine and Pharmacology, Shantong Medical College 2:78, 1977.
[21] White, A. *et al.*: *Principles of Biochem.* **58**:37, 1959.
[22] Lituock, G.: Proç. Sec. P. Biol. Led. 89:401, 1976.
[23] Research Group of Biochemistry of Jiangsu New Medical College : Outline of Complement, 1976.

CLINICAL RESEARCH ON ACUPUNCTURE TREATMENT OF MALARIA

Group of Acupuncture Treatment on Malaria, Institute of Acupuncture and Moxibustion, Academy of Traditional Chinese Medicine

Acupuncture treatment of malaria has a time-honored history. The method for treating malaria with acupuncture is described in detail in Ci Yue Pian on Acupuncture Treatment, a chapter of the book Su Wen which is one of the earliest traditional Chinese medical books. The effectiveness of the treatment has been confirmed by Chinese doctors today[1-5]. However, its effectiveness in treating malaria of immigrants from highly endemic malarial districts has still to be proved. In order to solve this problem, the therapeutic effect of acupuncture on malaria in such malarial districts has been studied for three consecutive years and the relationship between acupuncture and non-specific immunity of malaria has been further investigated.

I. CLINICAL OBSERVATIONS ON THERAPEUTIC EFFECT

(I) Method and Subjects

1. Cases selected. All the cases were selected from the local inhibitants of highly endemic malarial districts, who were born or have settled there permanently, or immigrants who have immigrated there from lower endemic malarial districts according to the following conditions:

With typical clinical manifestation, with positive blood smear showing plasmodia; no medication of any antimalarial drugs during the half month before the present attack; no medication with Chinese or occidental antimalarial drugs, antibiotics or sulfa drugs after the onset of the present attack; number of attacks have not exceeded 3 times; and without other chronic disease.

2. Methods of observation. Thick and thin blood smears were made once a day after the beginning of treatment, and the number of plasmodia in every cubic millimeter was determined by means of white blood cell count technique in some patients. The development of the illness was watched closely.

3. Points selected. Dazhui, Taodao, Ganshu and Geshu were used as the main points. Points on extremities were added according to symptoms. The prescription of those points was also varied with different persons and with different types of malaria. These points were divided into two groups and the two groups were taken alternately day after day.

(1) Various types of malaria in immigrants and malignant malaria in local inhabitants.

The first group: Dazhui, Ganshu (bilateral), Geshu (bilateral), Quchi (bilateral), and Zusanli (bilateral).

The second group: Taodao, 1.5 cun lateral to the lower border of the spinous process of the 8th thoracic vertebra (bilateral), Danshu (bilateral), Neiguan (bilateral) and Yinlingquan (bilateral).

(2) Tertian malaria of local inhabitants.

The first group: Dazhui, Geshu (bilateral) and Zusanli (bilateral).

The second group: Taodao, 1.5 cun lateral to the lower border of the spinous process of the 8th thoracic vertebra (bilateral) and Quchi (bilateral).

4. Manipulation method and depth of needling. Generally, it is suitable to insert the needle at the points Dazhui and Taodao to a depth of about 1 cun, to get a feeling of soreness, distention, numbness or wondering sensation, and it should be emphasized that the needle must not touch the spinal cord. As soon as the patient has a needling sensation, the needle must at once be withdrawn to a depth where the sensation disappears. Twirling of a needle in deep tissues is strictly forbidden. The needle was retained at the proper depth for 15 minutes.

The depth insertion of the needle at the Shu points of the back depends on how thin or fat the patients are. Depth puncture or slanting needling towards the spinal column must be avoided. Lifting, thrusting, twisting and twirling of the needle were manipulated alternatively several times after a needle sensation was attained during the retaining of the needle, which was limited to 15 minutes.

For points on extremities the same manipulations were applied. Lifting, thrusting, twisting and twirling of the needle were often manipulated alternately to keep the needling sensation for the 15 minutes duration of the acupuncture.

5. The time for treatment. Generally speaking, the time of malaria attack is related to the patient's life habits: usually it occurs around noon. Therefore treatment is to be applied in the morning or 2–3 hours before the attack, once a day. 5–7 trials constituted one course of treatment.

6. Criteria of therapeutic effect. Clinical cure: clinical symptoms disappear within 3 days after acupuncture treatment begun; tests of malarial parasites turn to negative within 6 days; and negative findings in 3 successive smears.

Improvement: Clinical manifestations are eliminated within 3 days; number of plasmodia markedly reduced but not turned to negative in blood tests within 6 days after treatment.

No improvement: The symptoms persist within 3 days and the counts of plasmodia in the blood remain unchanged or even increased.

(II) Results

1. Therapeutic effect. 242 cases were divided into the immigrant group and the local inhabitant group. There were 200 cases in the former group and 42 cases in the latter. Contrast of their therapeutic effect is shown in Table 1.

Table 1. The therapeutic effect of acupuncture on 242 cases of malaria

Type of Malaria		No. of Cases				Percentage(%)			
		Cured	Improvement	No improvement	Total	Cured	Improvement	No improvement	Total
Local inhabitants	Maligant malaria	18	9	3	30	60	30	10	100
	Tertian malaria	3	7		10	30	70		100
	Mixture malaria	1	1		2	50	50		100
Lmmigrants	Malignant malaria	8	2	38	48	17	4	79	100
	Tertian malaria	23	48	64	135	17	36	47	100
	Mixture		1	16	17		6	94	100
Total		53	68	121	242		$X^2 = 82.764$	P <	0.001

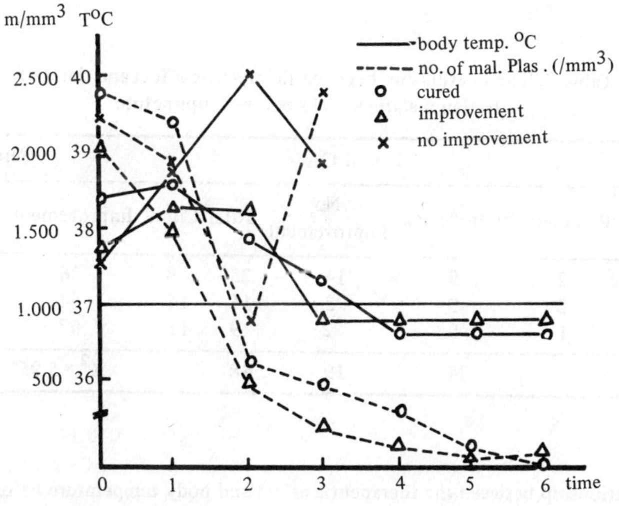

Fig. 1 The relationship between the therapeutic effect of acupuncture treatment on tertian malaria with fever and the number of plasmodia (average value) on 18 patients of immigrants

As seen in Table 1, the effective rate of local inhabitants for malignant malaria was 90%, of which the cured rate was 60%; but the effective rate of the immigrants was only 21%. The therapeutic effect of acupuncture treatment on tertian malaria was also better in local inhabitants, $X^2 = 82.764$, $P<0.001$. It shows that there is a very significant difference between the two groups, i.e., the therapeutic effect of various types of malaria is better among the

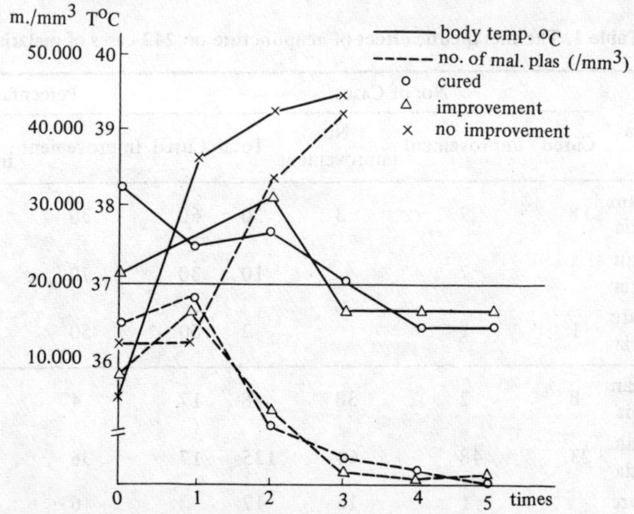

Fig. 2 The relationship between the therapeutic effect of acupuncture treatment on subtertian malaria with fever and the number of plasmodia on loca inhabitants

Table 2. The relationship between therapeutic effect and times of tertian malaria attacks before acupuncture

Times of malaria Attacks Before Acup.	No. of Cases: Cured	No. of Cases: Improvement	No. of Cases: No improvement	No. of Cases: Total	Percentage(%): Cured	Percentage(%): Improvement	Percentage(%): No improvement	Percentage(%): Total
1	2	9	14	25	8	36	56	100
2	2	9	3	14	14	64	22	100
3	1	6	2	9	11	67	22	100
Total	5	24	19	48		$X^2 = 5.952$	$P > 0.2$	

Table 3. The relationship between the therapeutic effect and body temperature before acupuncture

Body Temp. Before Acupuncture (°C)	No. of Cases: Cured	No. of Cases: Improvement	No. of Cases: No improvement	No. of Cases: Total	Percentage(%): Cured	Percentage(%): Improvement	Percentage(%): No improvement	Percentage(%): Total
38	4	7	8	19	21	37	42	100
39	3	15	5	23	13	65	22	100
40	3	8	16	27	11	30	59	100
Total	10	30	29	69		$X^2 = 8.8596$	$0.1 > P > 0.05$	

local inhabitants than among the immigrants.

2. The relationship between the therapeutic effect of acupuncture and the body temperature and counts of plasmodia. The results of analysis of 18 cases of immigrants suffering from tertian malaria are given in Fig. 1.

As shown in Fig. 1, in the cured cases, both the average temperature and the average counts of plasmodia went down day by day. Generally, fever was controlled within 48 hours and test of plasmodia in the blood became negative within 6 days. In cases with improvement, despite the return to normal of body temperature, tests of plasmodia in the blood were still positive. In cases with no improvement, fever persisted and the counts of plasmodia increased obviously.

Similarly, the analysis results of cases of malignant malaria among the local inhabitants are given in Fig. 2.

3. The factors influencing therapeutic effect of acupuncture treatment on tertian malaria among immigrants.

(1) The relationship between the therapeutic effect and the number of malaria attacks before acupuncture among immigrants with tertian malaria.

Based on the number of tertian malaria attacks before acupuncture in 48 cases of immigrants, they were divided into 3 groups for comparison (Table 2).

There was no therapeutic effect difference of statistical significance observed between the three groups.

(2) The relationship between the therapeutic effect and the strength (strong or moderate) of manipulation of the needle. 51 cases of immigrants suffering from tertian malaria were treated by acupuncture with various manipulations. In 42 cases, manipulation with strong stimulation was applied; their total effective rate was 62%. 9 cases were manipulated with moderate or weak stimulation; their total effective rate was 44%. It seems that better therapeutic effect may be obtained under strong stimulation, but the conclusion has still to be further confirmed as the number involved in the present case is not sufficient.

(3) The relationship between the therapeutic effect and the body temperature before acupuncture. 69 cases with tertian malaria were divided into 3 groups according to their temperature (Table 3).

From Table 3, it can be seen that the total effective rate was 78% in the 39°C group, 58% in the 38°C group and 40% in the 40°C group. $X^2 = 8.8596$, $0.1 > P > 0.05$. There was no significant difference among the three groups.

Table 4. The relationship between the therapeutic effect and the number of plasmodia in the blood before acupuncture

No. of Plasmodia Before Acup. (/mm^3)	No. of Cases: Cured	Improvement	No improvement	Total	Percentage(%): Cured	Improvement	No improvement	Total
500– 1,000	1	2	10	13	8	15	77	100
1,000–10,000	8	22	18	48	17	46	37	100
10,000–50,000	1	6	1	8	13	75	12	100
Total	10	30	29	69		$X^2 = 10.5984$	$P < 0.05$	

(4) The relationship between the therapeutic effect and the number of plasmodia/mm^3 before acupuncture. 69 cases of tertian malaria were divided into 3 groups according to the number of plasmodia in the erythrocytic stage (Table 4).

The total effective rate was 88% in the 10,000–50,000/mm^3 group of the erythrocytic stage, 63% in the 1,000–10,000/mm^3 group, but only 23% in the 500–1,000/mm^3 group. $X^2 = 10.5984$, $P<0.05$, indicating marked statistical significance in the difference between the three groups. This shows that the number of plasmodia in the blood stream before acupuncture is closely related to the therapeutic effect.

II. EXPERIMENTAL STUDY

The value of serocomplement was used as an index to observe the relationship between the therapeutic effect of acupuncture and serocomplement.

(I) Method and Material

0.2 ml of serum sample were diluted with normal saline solution to 1:10, 1:20, 1:30, 1:40, 1:50, 1:60, 1:80 and 1:100 separately, and then were placed into 8 test-tubes respectively. The amount of solution in each test-tube was 0.5 ml and 2 units of hemolysin and 1 ml of 1% sensitive erythrocytic solution of sheep were added. Each test-tube was placed in a bath of 37°C constant temperature water for 30 minutes. Its half-hemolysis unit was determined according to the contrast with half-hemolysis comparison tube after centrifuge[6].

A half-hemolysis comparison tube was 0.5 ml of 2 units of hemolysin and 1% sensitive erythrocytic solution of sheep, adding 1 ml of normal saline solution after it was hemolysised with saponin. All measurements of serocomplement were accomplished within 12 hours after the collection of samples.

(II) Results

1. A comparison of serocomplement values between normal subjects and patients. The values of serocomplement of 20 normal subjects and 46 patients with malaria were measur-

Table 5. Change of serocomplement value pre- and posttreatment with acupuncture or chloroquine

	48 hr After Acup. (Drugs)				72 hr After Acup. (Drugs)			
Group	No. of cases	$\overline{X} \pm S_{\overline{X}}$	P	Comp. among groups, P	No. of cases	$\overline{X} \pm S_{\overline{X}}$	P	Comp. among groups, P
Chloroquine	8	3.7 ±3.2	> 0.2		5	4.0 ±4.0	> 0.3	
Effective	5	8.0 ±7.3	> 0.2	> 0.4	9	26.7 ±7.6	< 0.01	> 0.05
Ineffective	5	2.0 ±10.2	> 0.2	> 0.1	7	–2.9 ±7.7	> 0.5	< 0.05

ed. The average value of serocomplement in normal subjects was 73.5 half-hemolysis units and 64.6 half-hemolysis units in patients. The average value of serocomplement in normal subjects was higher than that in the patients but through t-test, $t = 1.74$, $P > 0.05$. So there was no statistical significance.

2. The change of serocomplement value pre- and post-treatment with acupuncture or chloroquine. Serocomplement value increased gradually, being most evident 72 hours after acupuncture in the effective group; on the contrary, it rather decreased in the ineffective group. There is no change in the chloroquine group. The results are shown in Table 5.

Table 5 illustrates a comparison between various groups. There is no marked difference among the 3 groups at the 48th hour after acupuncture or taking of drugs. But there was obvious difference at the 72nd hour after acupuncture or drug treatment between the effective group and the ineffective group.

III. DISCUSSION

As 242 cases with various types of malaria were treated with acupuncture, certain therapeutic effects were obtained. The effective rate of malignant malaria in local inhabitants was 90%, similar to the rate obtained by the Acupuncture Research Group of the Guangdong Area[7]. There were some therapeutic effects on malignant malaria in immigrants who had settled in the area for more than 10 years and acquired some immunity against malaria. So it is supposed that acupuncture therapy may produce some therapeutic action on chloroquine-resistant malaria patients.

The time for treatment. In Ci Yue Pian, a chapter of Su Wen[8], it was said "malaria is treated with acupuncture just at the time needed for cooking a meal before its attack; the first needling would make the patient feel relaxed, the second one would reduce the symptoms obviously and the third one would make the patient feel cured." This practical experience of the ancient acupuncturists has obtained scientific demonstration now by the fact that better therapeutic effect is obtained with patients whose number of plasmodia in the erythrocytic stage were high before acupuncture, because the schizogenous cycle of plasmodia is closely related with malarial attack. As mature schizonts released merozoites into the blood circulation, symptoms of attack are induced. Merozoites are very active during the period of time needed for cooking a meal before the malarial attack, and at this time their resistance is relatively low so that they are easily killed or inhibited by external factors. Therefore better therapeutic effect may be obtained by acupuncture treatment at about 2 hours before malarial attack.

On the therapeutic effect of acupuncture treatment on tertian malaria some authors commented "it is the natural rule of tertian malaria itself that is responsible for the effectiveness."[9] All our patients under treatment were new immigrants in the highly endemic malaria district; these cases of infection were severe, and their immunity ability was poor. Their number of malarial attacks was not more than 3 times before acupuncture. So we do not consider that the therapeutic effect of acupuncture treatment on tertian malaria in their cases was brought about by the natural rule of the disease itself.

Owing to the relation of the therapeutic effect of acupuncture treatment on malaria with immunity of organism[10], we investigated the relation between serocomplement and the therapeutic effect of acupuncture treatment. Better therapeutic effect was obtained in patients with increasing serocomplement after acupuncture; otherwise, it was poor. It is possible that the anti-plasmodia ability of the patients was raised by acupuncture. Hence it becomes one of the effective factors in the cure of this disease.

IV. SUMMARY

242 cases of various types of malaria among immigrants and local inhabitants were treated by acupuncture in the highly endemic malarial district for three years. It demonstrated that the therapeutic effect on various types of malaria among the local inhabitants was higher than that of the immigrants. There was some therapeutic effect on malignant malaria of immigrants who had lived in the highly endemic malarial district for a long time.

In order to raise the therapeutic effect of acupuncture treatment on immigrant victims of malaria, the factors affecting it were investigated. It was found that the number of plasmodia in the peripheral blood of the patients before acupuncture treatment had a definite influence on the therapeutic effect, indicating the importance of the time of treatment.

The experimental result demonstrates that the therapeutic effect of acupuncture treatment on malaria is definitely correlated with the titers of serocomplement, its value being increased markedly at the 72nd hours following acupuncture in the effective group which corresponds to the time of disappearance of clinical symptoms. Therefore we believe that on the basis of the acquired immunity of the patient, acupuncture increases the anti-plasmodia ability of the body, and by repeatedly increasing this anti-plasmodia ability, malaria is finally cured. This is the mechanism of the curing of various types of malaria by acupuncture as we can learn from our studies today and it provides us with a theoretical foundation for acupuncture treatment of malaria.

REFERENCE

[1] 周志明 韩世荫：中华内科杂志 8：634，1956。

[2] 谢锡亮：中医杂志 3：202，1958。

[3] 马亦林：中医杂志 4：30，1959。

[4] 孙心楚等：浙江中医杂志 8：5，1958。

[5] 陈巩荪等：全国针灸针麻学术讨论会论文摘要(一)，第31页，1979年。

[6] 仲涛等：中华医学杂志 48(10)：623，1962。

[7] 广东地区针灸研究组：寄生虫病防治资料汇编(内部资料)，1971。

[8] 黄帝内径素问

[9] 张家壎等：中华内科杂志 4：213，1962。

[10] 广东中医学院疟疾防治组：疟疾研究(内部资料)，1973。

ACUPUNCTURE TREATMENT OF 209 CASES OF CEREBRAL THROMBOSIS AND OBSERVATION OF EFFECT ON RHEOENCEPHALOGRAM AND ELECTROMYOGRAM

Department of Neurology and Department of Physiological Research No. 2,
Institute of Acupuncture and Moxibustion, Academy
of Traditional Chinese Medicine

We have treated 209 cases of cerebral thrombosis and its convalescents mainly by acupuncture. The effect of acupuncture on the rheoencephalogram and amplitude of electromyogram of normal subjects as well as patients both before and after acupuncture was observed. The results are as follows:

I. OBSERVATION ON THE THERAPEUTIC EFFECT OF ACUPUNCTURE

(I) The General Condition of the Patients

All the 209 cases were clinically diagnosed as cerebral thrombosis or such convalescents. Among the 209 cases, 136 were male and 73 female. Their ages ranged from 20 to 83. 10 of them are 20–40 years old, 122 of them are 41–60 years old and 77 of them are 61–83 years old. Among 209 cases, there were 99 who had suffered from the illness for less than one month; 25 for 1–3 months and 85 for over 3 months.

The majority of the patients asked for acupuncture treatment after they found that both traditional Chinese and Western drugs produced no improvement in them.

(II) Method of Acupuncture Treatment

Points were selected along the channels and the points chosen were Jianyu, Quchi, Hegu, Huantiao, Zusanli and Juegu on the affected side. For some patients points on the head such as Baihui, Zhengying and Xuanlu were selected and needling of these points was twisted rapidly. For the other points, the even re-inforcing and even reducing manipulation methods were applied daily for 15 minutes each time. Ten times of treatment were considered as one course. A rest of 5–7 days then followed after each course.

(III) Criteria of the Therapeutic Effect

Basically cured. The subjective symptoms basically disappeared. The movement of the affected limbs was recovered or approximately recovered. The muscular strength was restored to the 4th–5th degree. Speech was clear and the patient could take care of himself.

Marked improvement. The subjective symptoms were greatly reduced and the movement of the affected limbs were markedly improved and the muscular strength was restored to the 3rd–4th degree.

Improvement. The subjective symptoms reduced and the movement of the affected limbs was restored to some degree.

No effect. No reduction of the subjective symptoms and no restoration of the movement of the affected limbs at all.

(IV) Analysis of the Therapeutic Effect

Among the 209 cases treated by acupuncture, 34 cases (16.3%) were basically cured, 49 cases (23.5%) had marked improvement, 99 cases (47.3%) had improvement and 27 cases had no improvement whatsoever. The total effective rate was 87.1% and the markedly effective rate 39.8%.

Comparison of the therapeutic effects between the groups treated only with acupuncture and those with acupuncture cum drugs.

The 209 cases were divided at random into 2 groups: one group receiving acupuncture only and the other receiving acupuncture cum drugs. The second group had 143 cases, all treated with nicotinic acid or Ginseng Zaizao wan, of which 63 were basically cured or had marked improvement, 64 had improvement and 16 showed no improvement; the effective rate as a whole was 88.8% with a markedly effective rate of 44.1%. The first group had 66 cases, of which 20 cases were basically cured or had marked improvement, 35 showed improvement and 11 showed no improvement; the effective rate was 83.3% with a markedly effective rate of 30.3%. There is no significant difference in the therapeutic effects ($P>0.05$) of the two groups. It shows that the therapeutic effect of acupuncture only group is almost equivalent to that of acupuncture cum drugs.

The relation between the duration of illness and the therapeutic effect.

Among the 209 cases, 124 cases had been ill for less than 3 months and 85 cases over 3 months. Their therapeutic effect is shown in Table 1.

From Table 1, it is shown that the difference in the therapeutic effect between the two groups of cases is very significant. Comparison of the markedly effective rates and the total effective rates of these two groups shows that P values are less than 0.001. It shows that acupuncture is more effective for cases under 3 months of illness than cases over 3 months.

Among the 209 cases, 84 cases were given 1–2 courses of treatment; 53 cases 2–3 courses; 41 cases 3–4 courses; and 31 cases more than 4 courses. Their therapeutic effects are given in Table 2.

From Table 2, it is shown that both the effective rate and the markedly effective rate obtained by 2–4 courses of acupuncture treatment are higher than those for the other number of courses.

In addition, we observed that therapeutic effect was better in young patients and patients with sensitivity to needling sensations.

Table 1. Comparison between the time of illness and therapeutic effect

Time of Illness	No. of Cases	Basically or Marked Improvement	Improvement	No Effect	Markedly Effective Rate (%)	Total Effective Rate (%)
Under 3 months	124	64	53	7	51.6	94.4
Over 3 months	85	19	46	20	22.4 P<0.001	76.5 P<0.001

Table 2. The relation between therapeutic effect and the number of courses of treatment

No. of Courses of Treatment	No. of Cases	Basically Cured	Marked Improvement	Improvement	No Effect	Markedly Effective Rate (%)	Total Effective Rate (%)
1–2	84	14	13	42	15	32.2	82.1
2–3	53	11	16	22	4	50.9	92.5
3–4	41	7	14	16	4	51.1	90.2
>4	31	2	6	19	4	25.8	87.1

II. THE EFFECT OF ACUPUNCTURE ON RHEOENCEPHALOGRAM (REG)

Observations were made on 21 cases of cerebral convalescents and 10 normal subjects, to whom acupuncture was only given at the points of the head. The home-made rheoencephalograph Type BD-II made by ourselves was used and the frontal-mastoid channels were applied. The signal of the cerebral blood flow was input to the 40 channel physiological recorder, RM-150, and 10 waves in REG were taken at random and averaged with Signal Processor 7S06. Then the photographic recording was made.

Table 3. Comparison of parameters of REG between normal and hemiplegic patients after needling on points of head

Item	Normal Subjects					Hemiplegic Patients					
	No. of cases	During acup.		Post acup.		No. of cases	During-acup.		No. of cases	Post-acup.	
		$\overline{X}$	P	$\overline{X}$	P		$\overline{X}$	P		$\overline{X}$	P
Relative height of the dicrotic wave (ohm)	10	0.0051	>0.4	0.0012	>0.5	21	0.0016	<0.001	20	–0.0002	>0.5
Vascular resistant index	10	–0.07	>0.4	0.096	>0.1	21	0.078	>0.1	20	0.137	<0.01
Out-flowing time (sec.)	10	–0.05	<0.02	0.012	>0.7	21	0.0106	>0.8	20	–0.0124	>0.3
Inflow speed (ohm/sec.)	10	–0.062	>0.2	0.094	>0.5	21	0.0596	>0.4	20	–0.012	<0.05

The changes of eight parameters in REG were observed, in which the height of the contracted wave, the height of rapid inflow segment, the inflow time and the extensional time of the rebound wave were not changed obviously in normal subjects or hemiplegics after acupuncture. There were some changes in the relative height of the dicrotic wave, the index of the vascular resistance, out-flow time and inflow speed. These changed parameters are listed in Table 3.

From Table 3, it is seen that needling at points of the head had no marked effects upon the cerebral hemodynamics of the normal subjects. But the arterioles might be dilated and the outflow of the blood might be sped up during the retaining of the needle (outflow time: $P<0.02$). This effect would disappear after the withdrawal of the needle. The effects of acupuncture at head points on the REG of the hemiplegic patients were greater than on that of the normal subjects. During the retaining of the needle, the cerebral blood flow of the hemiplegic patients was increased and the peripheral resistance (the relative height of dicrotic wave: $P<0.001$) was decreased. However, within 5 minutes after withdrawal of the needle , the small vessel resistance increased (the index of the vascular resistance; $P<0.01$). It needs further investigation to determine whether this is a temporary effect or not.

III. THE EFFECT OF ACUPUNCTURE ON THE AMPLITUDE OF ELECTROMYOGRAM (EMG)

The electromyograph DISA 14A20 was used in the test, in which the EMG of the hypothenar muscle was recorded by giving a single electrical pulse at the sulcus of the ulnar nerve on the upper extremities of normal subjects but on the affected one of patients. The amplitude of EMG before acupuncture was used as a control. Then under the same conditions the EMG was recorded at 5 min and 15 min during the retaining of the needle and at 5 min, 15 min, 25 min and 35 min immediately after acupuncture, respectively; for patients another was taken at 45 min after acupuncture. The EMG of the control group without acupuncture was induced and recorded at the same intervals and sequences as in the test group.

(I) The Effect of Acupuncture on the Amplitude of EMG in Normal Subjects

Electromyographic observations were made 29 times on 24 normal subjects, 10 times for the control group and 19 times for the acupuncture group.

Points of the head were used only.

Fig. 1 shows the results of observation on the control and the acupuncture groups.

From Fig. 1, it is shown that the amplitude of EMG was elevated in both groups of the normal subjects. There is a statistical significance between them shown by "variance analysis" and "least significant difference" analysis.

It demonstrates that needling the points of the head could markedly increase the EMG amplitude of normal subjects ($P<0.05$); this increase started 15 min after twisting the needle, and lasted for 35 min after the needle was withdrawn.

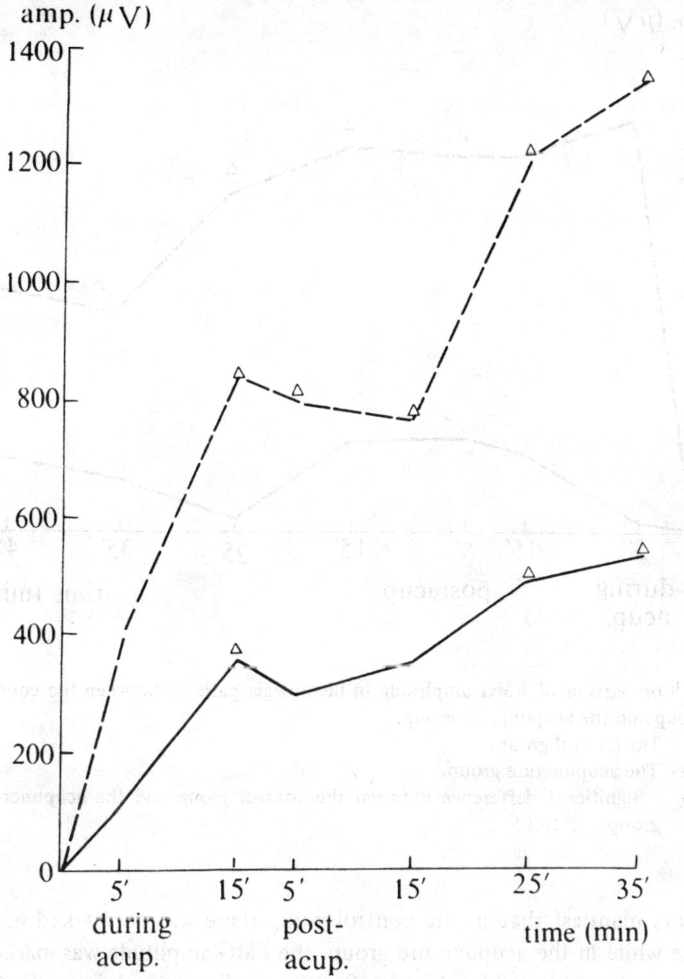

Fig. 1 Comparison of EMG amplitude in normal subjects between the control group and the acupuncture group.
—— The control group.
- - - The acupuncture group.
Δ Significant defference between the control group and the acupuncture group. $P<0.05$

(II) The Effect of Acupuncture on the EMG Amplitude of Hemiplegics

Observations were made 20 times on the affected upper limb of 14 convalescents of cerebral thrombosis, 10 times for the control group and 10 times for the acupuncture group. The test results in the control group and the acupuncture group were analyzed statistically (see Fig. 2).

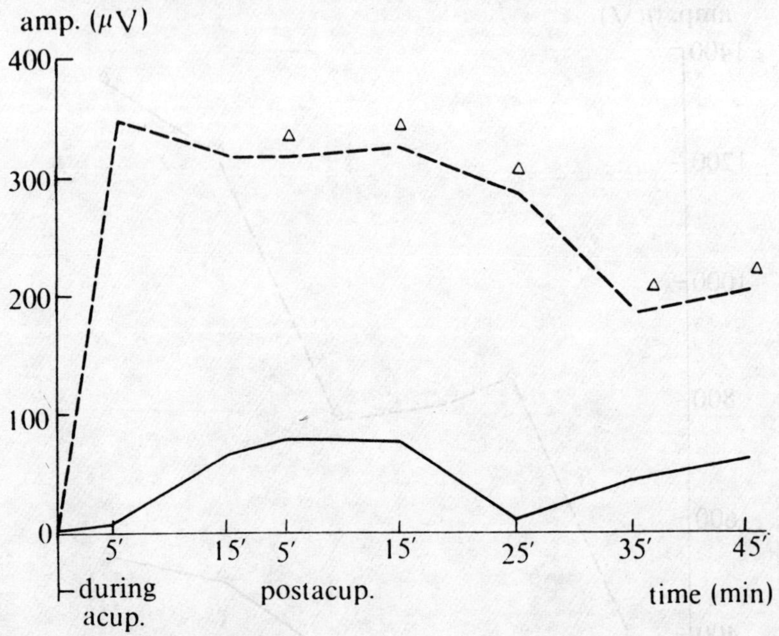

Fig. 2 Comparison of EMG amplitude in hemiplegia patients between the control group and the acupuncture group.
—— The control group.
- - - The acupuncture group.
Δ Significant defference between the control group and the acupuncture group. $P<0.05$

These results manifest that in the control group there was no marked increase of the EMG amplitude while in the acupuncture group, the EMG amplitude was markedly raised 5 min after acupuncture and lasted for 45 min after the needle was withdrawn ($P<0.05$).

The above-mentioned results demonstrate that the motor function of the hemiplegic patients may be raised and the recovery of muscular strength may be promoted by acupuncture.

IV. CONCLUSION

1. The effective rate of acupuncture treatment in 209 cases suffering from cerebral thrombosis and such convalescents is 87.1% with a markedly effective rate of 39.8%.

2. Acupuncture may improve the function of brain blood circulation of the hemiplegic patients.

3. Acupuncture may increase the muscular strength of both normal subjects and hemiplegic patients, and promote the recovery of the motor function of the patients.

ELECTROACUPUNCTURE AND MAGNESIUM SULFATE ADMINISTRATION FOR CHOLELITHIASIS

CLINICAL INVESTIGATION OF 522 CASES AND PRELIMINARY CONSIDERATION OF FEATURES OF STONE-EXCRETION

Zhao Shiduo, Song Xieen, Pan Guishan,
Lin Zhihua, Wang Shanmin, Wang Laixiu, Sun Huafeng
(Group for Treating Cholelithiasis with Acupuncture, Department of Surgery, Wendeng Hospital, Yantai, Shandong)

Cholelithiasis is a commonly encountered disease with the characteristics of acute onset, protractedness and frequent recurrence. They form a great menace to the patient and bring untold sufferings. Up to the present medical workers both in China and abroad have considered that the key to successful treatment of this illness is to remove the stones, and traditionally, the removal of stones by surgical operation is regarded as a positive measure, and the excretion of the stones by non-operative method as only wishful thinking. Nevertheless, there are still some doctors who do not lose hope in the non-operative method. In the 16th century,Fallopins and Sholzius described the symptoms of cholelithialsis and the excretion of gallstones[1]. In the early years of the 20th century, it was reported that emetics, mineral water, etc., could promote stone excretion, and stones were actually recovered in the stools by the cleansing method[2]. Iwamura recommended (1975) a composite method to facilitate the stone-excretion of the patient, but at last he concluded that the labor consumed was far greater than the effect obtained[3]. Thus, it is obvious that not much attention is now being paid to non-operative methods. Although acupuncture treatment of gallstone disease had been proposed in the early 1920s[4], and clinical reports began to appear in 1959 in China[5], owing to the small number of cases reported and the large number of acupuncture points, medical workers have not been attaching much importance to this method. So even right now acupuncture treatment of cholelithiasis is still merely a supplementary measure. In order to take the matter seriously, a great amount of clinical application is needed to test and verify its effectiveness. This article presents 522 cases treated by electro-acupuncture of the right Riyue and the right Qimen in points in the period from January 1975 to November 1978 with the stones of 409 cases excreted (rate of stone-excretion, 78.4%), and 74 cases treated simply by magnesium sulfate administration in the period from March 1977 to November 1978 with the stones of 20 cases excreted (rate of stone-excretion, 27.2%). Criteria of diagnosis are the same and their results are compared. Here is a brief review summary of our clinical data and a preliminary view on the rule of stone-excretion is put forth.

I. DIAGNOSTIC BASIS[6] AND TYPE DIFFERENTIATION

1. The acute onset type. History: Recurrent upper right quadrant abdominal pain accompanied with chills, fever, jaundice, or choledocholithotomy had been performed with radiographically demonstrated choledocholithiasis.

Physical signs: Body temperature around 38.5°C, jaundiced sclera, Pain on percussion in the hepatic field, right epigastric tenderness of various degrees and distention of the gallbladder, etc.

Laboratory data: Increased icterus index with direct reaction to van den Bergh test and slightly increased serum transaminase. No significant changes in all other liver functions tests.

Peripheral hemogram: WBC count increased very much above 10,000–20,000/mm^3. In a very few cases, whose WBC count did not increase, there was a shift to the left of different degrees in the differential count. Neutrophil granulocytes>80%. Rod-like granulocytes increased.

2. The shock type. In addition to the history of remarkable acute onset, physical signs, and laboratory data, the blood pressure was below 80/60 mm Hg, and the heart rate about 120/min.

3. The stable type. History of recurrent acute onset, but on admission, symptoms not remarkable, with negative physical signs and laboratory findings.

II. METHODS OF TREATMENT

(I) Electro-Acupuncture with Magnesium Sulfate Administration Group (for short, it is called the "acupuncture group" below)

(1) Patient's position: Lying flat.

(2) Point selecting: Main acupuncture points: Riyue (right), Qimen (right). 6 cm needles inserted obliquely with an inclining angle of 30°.

Additional points. For cases with severe epigastric pain and with a distended gallbladder, point Danshu (right) and the mid-point of the line linking Juque and Fuai (right) should be used. The needle of 6 cm in length travels in the direction of the central part of the distended gallbladder and reaches underneath the external oblique muscle. Apparatus G6805 was connected to the needles inserted into the Riyue and Qimen points. Electric current of alternating sparse and dense waves was given. The intensity of the electric current was adjusted to be within the utmost endurance of the patient. Emergency cases were acupunctured, once immediately after admission, and thereafter the same treatment was given in the morning every day.

(3) After withdrawing the needles, 50 % $MgSO_4$ 40 ml was administered orally. Patients experiencing toxic shock, dehydration, acidosis, and so on, were treated separately. But acupuncture might be continued at the same time.

(4) After acupuncture, stools were collected after each excretion and stones were examined by the cleansing method for excreted stones.

(5) A course of treatment lasts 10 days. The patient may take a 5–7 day rest between two courses of treatment.

(II) Magnesium Sulfate Group

During the acute onset, 50 % $MgSO_4$ 40 ml was administered orally upon admission. Then 50 % $MgSO_4$ 40 ml was administered daily at 9 a.m. Except for the acupuncture, its treatment was the same as that of the acupuncture group in all other respects.

III. CLINICAL DATA

(I) General Data

1. **Acupuncture Group.** 522 cases, male 208 cases, female 314 cases. Male:female is equal to 1:1.5. The oldest, 76 years old; the youngest, 16 years old, the average age 51 years.

2. **Magnesium Sulfate Group.** 74 cases, male 30 cases, female 44 cases. Male:female is equal to 1:1.46. The oldest, 77 years old, the youngest, 23 years old, the average age, 48 years.

(II) Clinical Results

The curative effects of the two groups are compared, and given in Table 1.

The comparison shows that in the curative effect of the acute onset type, there is a significant difference between the "acupuncture group" and the control group ($P<0.01$)

The stone-excretion rate in the former is much higher than that in the latter. Since the rate of stone-excretion is highest in the acute onset type of the acupuncture group, the curative effect in the same type of the control group is also selected for comparison.

Time of stone-excretion (counted to the time when the stones were first recovered). Within 8 days stones were excreted by more than 95% of the cases of both groups.

Acupuncture group: 522 cases, stones excreted by 409 cases, rate of stone-excre-

Table 1. Curative effects of acupuncture group and magnesium sulfate group

Group	Type	Number of Cases	Number of Cases (Stones Excreted)	Rate of Stone-Excretion (%)
Acupuncture	Stable	100	35	35.0
	Acute onset	410	368	89.7
	Shock	12	6	50.0
Total		522	409	78.4
Magnesium sulfate	Stable	1	–	
	Acute onset	73	20	27.4
	Shock	–	–	
Total		74	20	27.2

tion, 78.4%. Stones not excreted but symptoms and signs disappeared, 97 cases, 18.2% of the total. Thus the total rate of effectiveness was 96.6%. There were 16 cases that failed to respond to acupuncture treatment and they were transferred to surgical treatment. Rate of surgical operation, 3.1%. Deaths, 6 cases; death rate, 1.2%. In this group, the total number of stones larger than 1.0 cm in diameter excreted by the 409 cases was 379, with the largest one among them measuring 4.5×3.5×3.5 cm (muddy and sandy stones as well as stones smaller than 1.0 cm were not included). The maximum total weight of excreted stones of a single case was 41 grams.

Magnesium sulfate group: 74 cases, stones excreted by 20 cases, rate of stone-excretion, 27.2%. Stones not recovered but symptoms and signs disappeared, 33 cases. Total rate of effectiveness, 72.6%. After a course of treatment by $MgSO_4$ administration, no stones recovered but subjective symptoms alleviated, 21 cases, making up 27.5%. Later on, these 21 cases were transferred to acupuncture treatment. 6 cases among them excreted stones, and consequently, symptoms and signs disappeared, and were cured. The remaining 15 cases who did not excrete stones, but their symptoms and signs disappeared. In this group of 21 cases, 16 pieces of stones larger than 1.0 cm in diameter were excreted, with the largest one measuring 2.0×1.8×1.8 cm. The maximum total weight of stones excreted in a single case amounted to 4 grams.

IV. A TYPICAL CASE

Liu--, male, 52 years old, No. of admission 138292. Admitted at 9:30 p.m. on July 5, 1976.

History: Recurrent right epigastric pain accompanied by chill, fever, jaundice, nausea, and vomiting for 12 years. There were 6–7 onsets every year, often induced by getting angry, catching cold, or by taking greasy food. Had been treated many times in his native place but without any lessening of the number of recurrences; the present onset started 4 days ago.

Physical examination: Body temperature 38.6°C, blood pressure 100/70 mm Hg. Acute suffering of pain shown, jaundiced sclera. Systolic blowing murmur of the 2nd degree was ausculated at the cardiac apex. The abdomen was flat. There was tenderness and guarding in the right epigastric area, and a distended gallbladder about 8 cm in diameter was palpated.

Laboratory data: Total number of WBC, 15,000/mm^3, neutrophil granulocytes, 94%; lymphocytes, 6 %; icterus index, 40 units: Van den Bergh test, direct reaction (+++); thymol turbidity, 4 units; cephalin cholesterol flocculation test (–); serum glutamic-pyruvic transaminase, 24 units. Diagnosis: Choledocholithiasis and cholecystitis.

After admission, fluid replacement proceeded and gentamicin was infused intravenously. Prednisone was administered orally. Meanwhile Riyue Qimen, and Danshu were acupunctured. Electric stimulation lasted 90 minutes, with alternating sparse and dense electric waves. The distended gallbladder was examined by palpation after the needles were withdrawn. It became more distinct. 50% $MgSO_4$ 40 ml was administered immediately after the acupuncture. Four hrs later, that is to say, at 2 a.m. on July 7, the gallbladder shrank somewhat, the pain alleviated, body temperature dropped to 36°C. At 7 a.m. of the same day, the above mentioned points were acupunctured once more; the stimulative parameters were the same as before. After withdrawing the needles, 50% $MgSO_4$ 40 ml was also

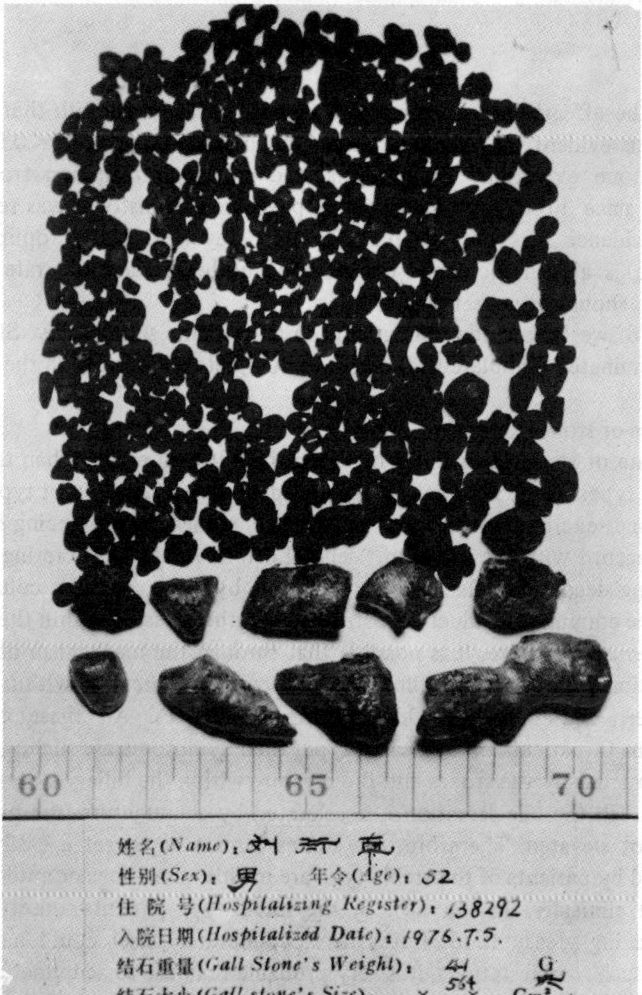
60
65
70
姓名(Name):
性别(Sex): 男 年令(Age): 52
住院号(Hospitalizing Register): 138292
入院日期(Hospitalized Date): 1976.7.5.
结石重量(Gall Stone's Weight): 41 G
结石大小(Gall stone's Size): 564 × × Cm

administered. At 10 a.m. the gallbladder could not be palpated entirely; the patient felt extremely comfortable. At 3 p.m. on July 8, 23 stones totaling 5 grams were recovered from the stools. The largest one among them measured 2.5×1.7×1.7 cm, and another one measured 1.5×1.0×1.0 cm. The remaining 21 pieces were small columnar stones less than 1.0 cm in diameter. From then on the patient was acupunctured once every day. On each day, stones of different dimensions were recovered. Stone-excretion lasted for 10 days. Total number of stones excreted amounted to 564 pieces, totaling in weight 41 grams. Jaundice disappeared completely on the 4th day. Laboratory examination: icterus index, 7 units; Van den Bergh test, (–). The patient returned to normal in all respects and was discharged from the hospital on the 12th day. He was called upon in September 1978 and had not experienced right epigastric pain for two years. The patient returned to normal physical labor soon after discharge from the hospital.

V. DISCUSSION

1. When the effectiveness of the $MgSO_4$ group is compared with that of the acupuncture group, it is evident that acupuncture is much more effective ($P<0.001$). But how is spontaneous stone excretion? Kameta analyzed clinical information from the past and indicated that since 1706, spontaneous disappearance of gallstones was reported time and again. The incidence was only about 1%[10]. Carey held similar opinions[11]. In our country, there is a high incidence of choledocholithiasis, and the rate of spontaneous stone-excretion should have been higher.

Since 1978, we have made radiography in 61 patients successively. Stones in 23 cases were found eliminated completely, the rate of complete elimination in the short term being 37.7%.

2. Features of stone-excretion

(1) The rate of stone-excretion is higher in the acute onset type than those in the stable and the shock types in the acupuncture group; patients of acute onset type amount to 410 cases, with stones excreted in 368 cases, the rate of stone-excretion being 89.7 % (see Table 1). This is in accord with the result of "general offensive" stone-excreting therapy and the "stone-excreting decoction" therapy[7, 8] reported by others in our country. During the acute onset, the common bile duct is obstructed and the pressure within the biliary system is increased. After acupuncture, it is possible that through the mechanism of neural elements the bile secretion increases, the gallbladder contracts, the pressure within the bile duct increases further, and then the Oddi's sphincter relaxes. All these changes promote stone-excretion. In patients of the stable type, their symptoms are slight– the bile duct has not been obstructed by the stones and the pressure within the biliary system is not elevated. Thus, even though the bile secretion is accelerated by acupuncture, the pressure within the bile duct is not elevated. Therefore, the stones cannot be excreted easily. Moreover, the stones excreted by patients of the stable type are mostly small ones or muddy-sandy like. We have observed clinically that in 50% of the stable type patients, onset could have been induced by taking greasy food. But after acupuncture, onset could hardly be induced. According to such manifestations, it is very probable that due to acupuncture treatment, the daily secretion of bile is increased; the remaining infection of the bile duct is alleviated by the rinsing effect. Furthermore, acupuncture has an anti-inflammatory effect in itself. Therefore, even though greasy food is taken, the onset would not be induced.

As to the patients of the shock type, it would be prudent to treat them cautiously. Owing to the severe infection and dehydration of varyingdegrees, the effect of acupuncture is influenced. Therefore, in the treatment of these patients, the shock should be corrected promptly and a surgical operation should be prepared while acupuncture is administered. A part of the patients were alleviated at once whether stones were excreted or not. In this group, there were 12 patients of the shock type. After acupuncture, 6 cases excreted stones and were cured clinically.

(2) Signs of stone-excretion. Before larger stones were excreted, the patient could feel the right epigastric colic pain increase. The body temperature elevated. Most of the distended gallbladders, whose dimensions could not be palpated distinctly before acupuncture, could be palpated distinctly after acupuncture. Gallbladers which were

palpated before acupuncture became tough after acupuncture. All of these indicate that after acupuncture, the pressure within the biliary system is increased. When pain disappears suddenly, it is very probable that the stones have been excreted into the intestinal tract. The Research Group of Acute Abdomen (Zunyi Medical College) which uses the "general offensive" therapy for cholelithiasis observed that similar phenomena mentioned above appeared when stones were excreted, and "stone-excretion phenomenon" was designated[9]. In this study, the above signs of stone-excretion appeared in 250 (61.1 %) of the 409 cases who excreted stones. Whether it was a sign of stone-excretion or impaction of stones which would aggravate the patients' condition often could not be determined easily. Especially when the stones had not been verified by biliary radiography and endoscopy, the discrimination was more difficult. Therefore, there were erroneous clinical judgements occasionally. For example, Wang--, female, 34 years old, No. of admission 140734, was admitted because of recurrent epigastric colic, chills and fever, and jaundice, for 4 days. Body temperature 38.5°C, blood pressure 100/70 mm Hg. jaundiced sclera. Obviously distended gallbladder, tenderness. After admission, fluid replacement and antibiotic drip infusion were given. Although the colic was alleviated after acupuncture, the gallbladder still could be palpated. The same treatment was repeated on the following day. When the needles were withdrawn, the gallbladder became tough evidently, with distinct border palpated. But there was no sudden relief of pain. On the third day, body temperature was 39°C, jaundice deepened, and the gallbladder was still distended. Acupuncture continued; pain became severe on the 4th day morning and the patient was restless. Blood pressure 90/60 mm Hg, pulse rate 110/min. Stricture of the lower parts of the common bile duct was suspected. After consultation of doctors, the needles were withdrawn immediately and a surgical operation was decided upon. During the operation, it became clear that the gallbladder was distended slightly. There was grass green bile in the enlarged common bile duct; no stones were seen.

Nevertheless, a stone about 1.0 cm in diameter was palpated in the third part of the duodenum. On the third day after the operation, a stone of 1.0×0.8×0.8 cm dimensions was recovered in the stools by the cleansing method.

The origin of this erroneous diagnosis is due to a lack of attention to all the changes of the patient at every stage. Even when surgical treatment is decided upon and the patient is already on the operating tble, one more inspection of the patient is necessary. Looking back on this patient after the operation, we found that the sudden obvious relief of abdominal pain occurred on the way from the ward to the operating room. Therefore, it was possible that at that moment the stone was excreted into the intestinal tract. From this it is clear that patients should be watched closely to avoid misdiagnosis.

(3) Relation between stone-excretion and course of disease (Table 2).

There is a very remarkable relation between the course of disease and the rate of stone-excretion ($P<0.01$) (see Table 3). The longer the course of disease, the lower the rate of stone-excretion. It is quite possible that along with the prolongation of the course of disease, the morphological and functional changes of the bile duct become more prominent. As the function of the gallbladder is more impaired, so the stone-excretion is inpaired.

(4) Effect of biliary operation on acupuncture stone-excretion.

After simple choledocholithotomy, stones could also be excreted after acupuncture when patients were suffering from cholelithiasis once again. After both

Table 2. Relation between stone-excretion and course of disease

Course of Disease (Years)	Number of Cases	Number of Cases (Excreting Stones)	Rate of Stone-Excretion (%)
<1	51	46	90.2
1–	112	99	88.4
3–	83	71	85.5
5–	107	80	74.7
10–	109	76	69.8
>20	60	37	61.6
Total	522	409	78.4

Table 3. Effect of surgical operation on acupuncture stone-excretion

Operation Performed	Number of Cases	Number of Cases (Excreting Stones)	Rate of Stone-Excretion (%)
Choledocholithotomy and cholecystectomy	14	6	42.9
Choledocholithotomy	182	142	78.1
Not operated	326	261	80.1
Total	522	409	78.4

choledocholithotomy and cholecystectomy, stone-excretion might be influenced to a certain degree (see Table 3).

The difference of the rates of stone-excretion between the choledocholithotomy group and the nonoperation group is not remarkable ($P<0.05$), and the stone-excretion rates of both the above groups are higher than those of the choledocholithotomy-plus-cholecystectomy group ($P<0.01$). Therefore, in the process of stone-excretion, a definite of the gallbladder, which still possesses some functions, is considered.

3. Analysis of the causes of the failure of acupuncture in stone excretion. We observed 25 cases which failed to excrete stones after acupuncture and were transferred to surgical treatment. The causes are roughly the following:

(1) Severe infection of the bile duct. In 9 cases, the walls of the common bile duct and the gallbladder were oedematous and thickened. There was empyema in the bile duct. Probably owing to the above metioned pathological changes, the function of the common bile duct and the gallbladder were impaired, even totally lost. The reactivity to stress lowered. The sphincter relaxed incompletely or could not relax at all. Thus, although the stone was not large, it was not easy to expel the stone.

(2) Peripheral fibrosis or stenosis of the lower portion of the common bile duct. 7 cases belong to these changes. Owing to the stone remaining in the ampulla portion of the common duct for a long period of time, chronic inflammation took place, and at last, scar formation developed at the lower part of the common bile duct; its periphery and its function of contractive-relaxant motility was lost. Therefore, these patients could hardly excrete their stones by acupuncture treatment.

(3) Diverticulum of the bile duct accompanied with lithiasis. In this study, two such

cases failed to excrete stones and were transferred to surgical treatment. During the operation, a dumbbellshaped stone was discovered. The stone in the diverticulum linked up with the stone in the common duct. Under such circumstances, undoubtedly the stone could not be excreted.

(4) Giant stone. In one case, the size of the stone in the common bile duct was 4.0×3.5×3.5 cm. The patient had been treated by acupuncture but no stones were recovered. Probably this might be due to the lowered reactivity to stress or to the various degrees of fibrosis of the ampulla and its periphery. But giant stone's are not incapable of being expelled absolutely, as we had encountered a recovered stone which was as large as 4.5×3.5×3.5 cm. Stones of excessive dimensions cannot be excreted easily.

(5) Unknown, 6 cases.

4. Problem of transferring to surgical operation. To excrete stones by acupuncture method is effective, but it does not rule out the possibility that a surgical operation is needed for a few patients:

(1) In some patients of the stable type, if recurrent onsets continued over a long period of time, symptoms disappeared but stones were not excreted after each acupuncture treatment. To these patients, radiography should be carried out in time in order to make a clear diagnosis as early as possible and to determine whether cholelithiasis and complications are present or not. If there is any one of the causes hindering the excretion of a stone, patients should not be observed and treated by acupuncture for long but surgery should be considered.

(2) Treating patients of the shock type is fairly difficult, but the shock induced by infection of the biliary tract takes place and develops slowly. Now, it is known that the increase of the pressure within the pancreatic duct, the countercurrent of the bile, ischemia, purulent toxin, etc., may result in a release of a large quantity of pancreatic lysosome and a production of myocardial depression factor (M. D. F.), which is involved in the onset of an acute cardiovascular disorder. It is practically proved that, even though microorganisms, pathogenic factors and so forth exist in the biliary tract, infection may not occur provided the bile passes through easily and smoothly. However, if the bile flow is retarded, owing to functional or morphological causes, a series of pathological changes will take place. Traditional Chinese theory holds that, to the six "Fu (viscerae)", opening and descending are natural. "While pain exists, Qi (air) is obstructed; while Qi is obstructed, pain exists." It appears that obstruction is the cause in most circumstances. In short, the basic contradiction lies in the free flowing or the obstruction of the bile. Therefore, while prompt correction of shock goes on, we must get rid of the obstruction at the same time; otherwise, the shock can hardly be corrected.

In view of the above mentioned causes and on the basis of our clinical practice of several years and the experiences of other districts, we recognized that patients of the shock type should be transferred to surgical operation rapidly if one of the following conditions is present.

(1) Development of toxic shock, systolic pressure below 80 mm Hg, pulse rate over 120/min, patients' conditions not improved after 6–8 hrs of active rescue.

(2) Shock patients accompanied with omen of renal failure, conditions not improved under quick expanding of the blood volume.

(3) Doubtful perforation of the gallbladder and the bile duct.

(4) When accumulation of pus in the gallbladder is considered.

VI. SUMMARY

1. The therapeutic effect of 522 cases with cholelithiasis treated by electroacupuncture of right Riyue and Qimen points as the main method with oral administration of 50 % magnesium sulfate is recommended. Stone-excretion occurred in 409 cases. Rate of stone-excretion is 78.4 %. Meanwhile the effectiveness is compared with that of a group to which only 50% magnesium sulfate is administered. The remarkable effect of the acupuncture of Riyue and Qimen is confirmed.

2. Features of stone-excretion are discussed, causes of failure of stone-excretion by acupuncture treatment are analyzed, and the proper time for transferring to surgical operation is suggested.

REFERENCES

[1] 龟田治南等：最新医学，30(60)：914，1975。

[2] 川岛震一：胆石症　内科的治疗一历史展望、胆石症、常冈键二编集、南汇堂，297 页，1974。

[3] 岩村键一郎：最新医学，30(6)：965，1975。

[4] 震井文隆：«实用针灸病理学»，高等针灸学院出版部，第一版 50 页，1927。

[5] 张子文等：中医杂志 (7)：27，1959。

[6] 胆石症分型及诊断标准：全国第一次中西医结合治疗胆系疾病经验交流会资料，1977。

[7] 贺瑞麟等：肝、胆管结石病的中西医结合"总攻"排石疗法，中国科学，2：206，1974。

[8] 青岛市立医院，胆石症，山东人民出版社，1973。

[9] 遵义医学院急腹症研究组：中西结合治疗肝、胆管结石病，全国第一次中西医结合治疗胆系疾病经验交流会资料，1977。

[10] 龟田治南等：最新医学，27(6)：1113，1972。

[11] J.B. Carey: *Modern TreatMent* 5(3); 493, 1968

CLINICAL OBSERVATION OF EFFECT OF ACUPUNCTURE ON ANGINA PECTORIS

Liu Fuzai, Li Jinglin, Liu Guizhi
(Beijing Tong Ren Hospital)

Wang Yizhong, Chi Huichang, Gao Benqi
(Beijing Second Hospital)

Mèng Jinghi, Liu Ruiting, Xu Huiren
(Institute of Acupuncture & Moxibustion, Academy of Traditional Chinese Medicine)

Since 1975, 621 patients with coronary heart disease have been treated with acupuncture. Part of these patients were studied with EKG, ultrasonic cardiography and rheoencephalography. Among them, dynamic changes in the left ventricular reserve in 123 cases, and those of 35 cases serving as self-controls were studied by synchronous recording of EKG, phonocardiogram (PCG), carotid pulse tracing (CPT) and apexcardiogram (ACG) before and after acupuncture in order to obtain objective data for studying the mechanism of the therapeutic effect of acupuncture in coronary heart disease.

I. METHODS

1. Points.

(1) Main points. Shanzhong point punctured with the needle tip directed subcutaneously for 2.5–2.8 cun toward Jiuwei point; Neiguan and Zusanli points.

(2) Supplementary points. According to the differential typing of traditional Chinese medicine, points Quchi, Waiguan, Zhongwan, Tongli, Shenmen, Jianshi, Rugen, Ximen, Xinshu, Jueyinshu, were selected (Fig. 1).

2. Manipulation. points were stimulated moderately, mainly with the "bu" (re-enforcing) method, the needle being retained for 20 minutes.

3. Needle sensation. Sinking, heavy and warm sensations were all obtained with points of the upper limbs. When Shanzhong point got "Deqi", there was usually an" Ah-effect".

4. Therapeutic course. Points were punctured once every other day. Each therapeutic course consisted of 10 treatments. Generally, each patient received 3 courses with intervals of 3–7 days.

5. All other treatments and drugs were suspended except that patients with hypertension might take hypotensive and sedative drugs.

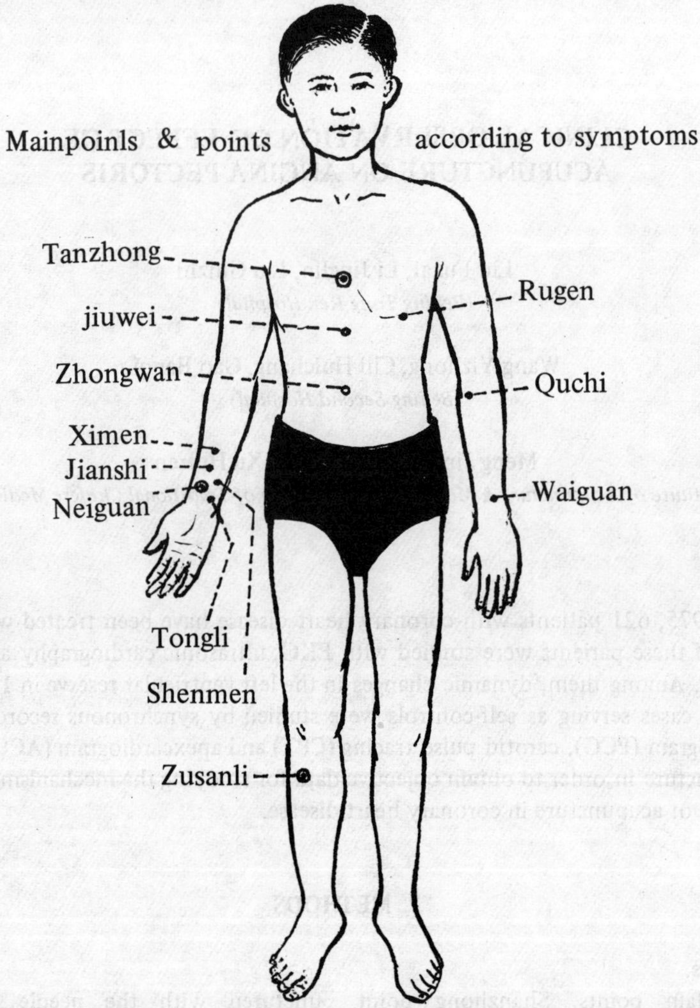

Fig. 1 Main Points and supplementary points.

6. Generally, the amount of physical activity remained just the same as before.

II. THERAPEUTIC EFFECT

1. Effect on angina pectoris.

(1) Effective rate. Total effective rate 89.2%, marked effective rate 47.8%.

(2) Time of appearance of therapeutic effect. Totally, there were 558 cases with therapeutic effect, and 85.8% of them appeared before the end of the 2nd course.

2. Discontinuation or reduction of nitroglycerine after acupuncture.

419 cases had oral nitroglycerine before the acupuncture therapy. It was gradually discontinued in 254 cases and reduced in 138 cases after therapy. The total rate of discontinuation and reduction was 93.6%.

3. Effect on the EKG. Among the 578 cases with abnormal EKG, 119 cases (20.6%) had a marked beneficial effect and another 189 cases (32.6%) were also improved. The total effective rate was 53.2%.

4. Correlation between the effect on ECC and that on the symptoms of angina pectoris.

In 578 cases, the effect on the symptoms of angina pectoris was mostly in paralel with that on the EKG changes, but in a part of the cases it was not.

5. Acupuncture effect upon the ECG of the patients with coronary heart disease under electrooscillography.

Since Nov. 1975, we had monitored the acupuncture effect on the ECG under electrooscillography in 100 patients with coronary heart disease. During acupuncture, the ECG was markedly improved 1–20 minutes after the start of treatment in 32 cases: S–T segments showed various degrees of improvement, changes in the T–waves being especially remarkable, turning from negative to positive.

After acupuncture, both the S–T segment and T–wave became normal in 23 cases, T–wave improved in 5 cases and S–T segment improved in 4 cases.

Case presentation. Case 1, patient Chen, female, technician, had suffered from coronary heart disease with angina pectoris for 1 year. She had precordial pain 1–2 times every day, each time lasting a few minutes. In addition, she often had dyspnea and tightness. Before acupuncture, her EKG TV_4 and TV_5 were inverted, and TV_6 flat, but the $TV_{4,\ 5,\ 6}$ all turned to positive 5 minutes after acupuncture, which was maintained for at least 2 hours. However, these T–wave changes only lasted a few hours, and then became inverted and flat again. When the acupuncture was repeated, they turned to positive again immediately. After nearly one course of treatment, these T–waves could be kept positive rather steadily, remaining so after two years and ten months. Nearly all her symptoms disappeared (see EKG 1,2,3.).

Case 2, patient Yi, male, mechanic, had suffered from hypertension for 4 years. The highest blood pressure reached 200/120 mmHg. He had had coronary heart disease for one year and had relatively severe precordial pain, 4–5 attacks every day, each lasting for a few

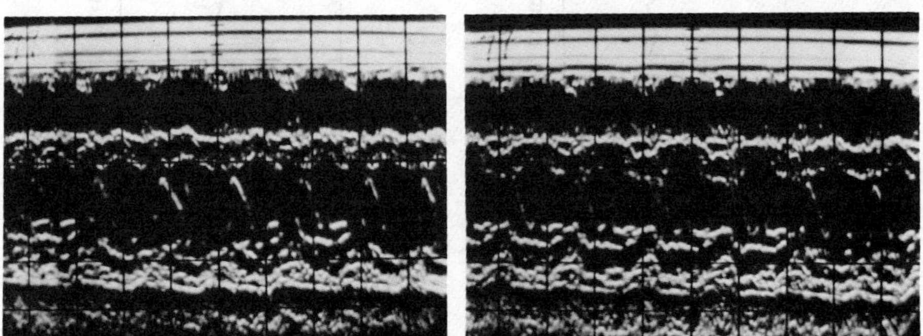

pre acup. **post acup.**

Fig. 2 Before acupuncture and after acupuncture.

EKG. 1

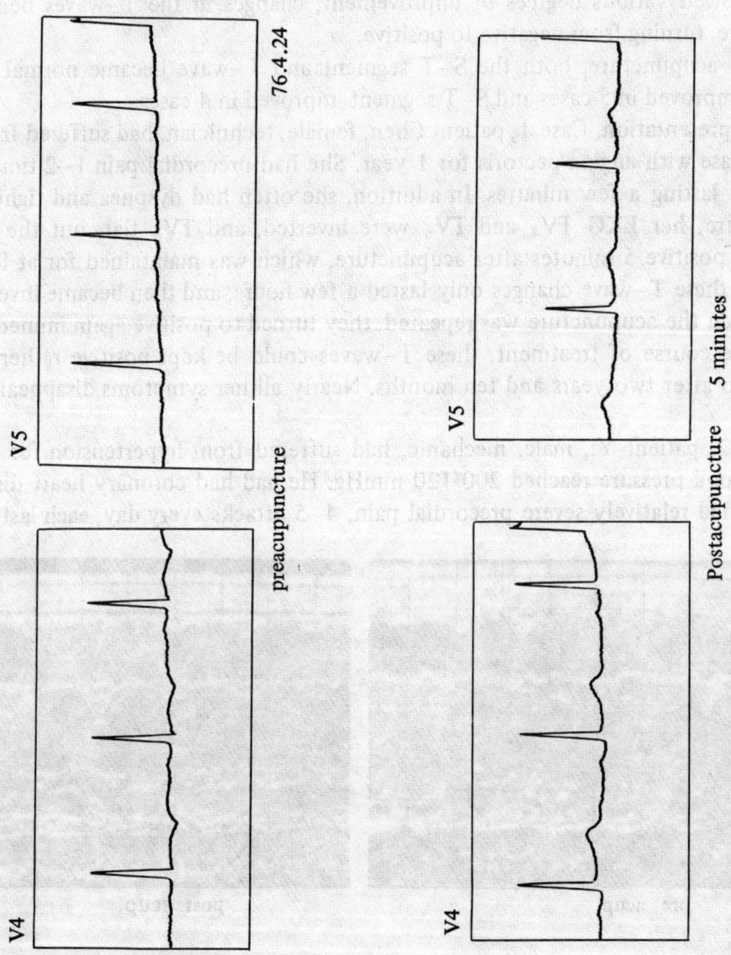

V4
V5
V6
preacupuncture
76.4.24
V4
V5
V6
Postacupuncture
5 minutes

EKG. 2

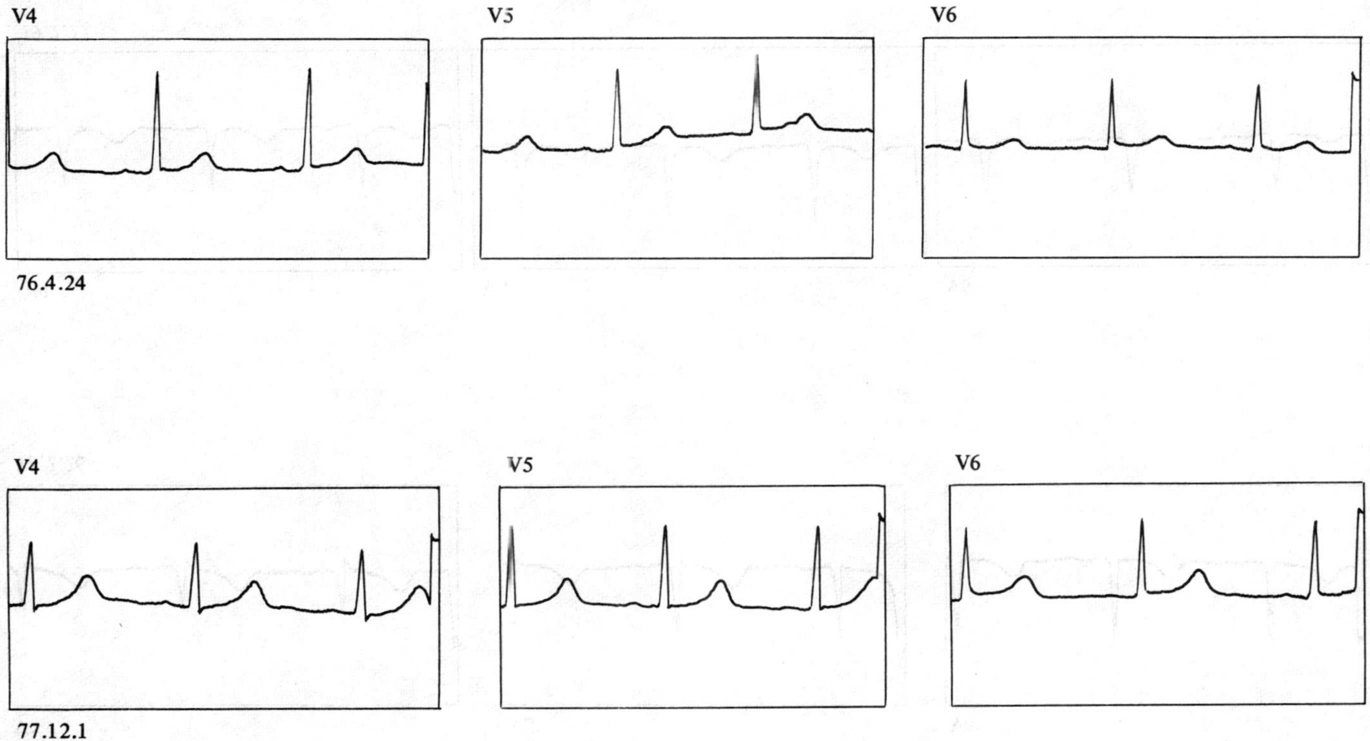

EKG. 3

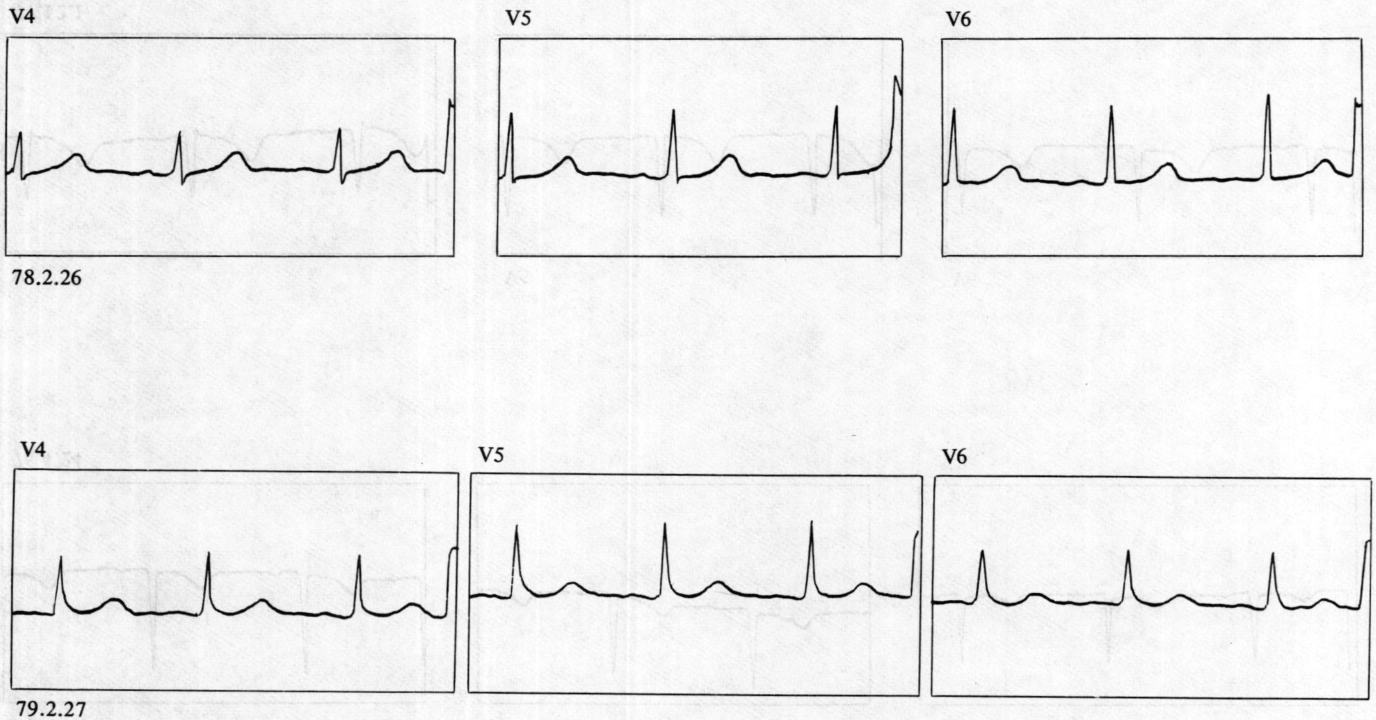

minutes. Before acupuncture therapy, the EKG TV_4 was inverted; TV_5 and TV_6 were biphasic. Five minutes after acupuncture, $TV_{4,5,6}$ all turned to positive and remained so for two hours. After 3 courses of treatment, symptoms became much better, precordial pain becoming milder and appearing only 1–3 times per day. Two years and two months later, the T–wave remained positive and precordial pain occurred only occasionally while attending to his full day's work (see EKG 4 and 5).

6. Effect on the left ventricular reserve in patients of coronary heart disease as evaluated by echocardiography (Fig. 2).

We studied the amplitude changes of the waves of the left posterior ventricular wall and the cardiac output before and after acupuncture in 100 cases of coronary heart disease and 40 normal persons as control. Defined points were punctured in both groups. Undefined points were selected and punctured in another 25 cases of coronary heart disease. Results are shown as follows:

(1) Variations in the pulsating amplitude (mm) of the posterior ventricular wall (see Table 1).

(2) Variations in cardiac output.

1) Stroke volume (Table 2).

2) Cardiac output (l/min) (Table 3).

3) Cardiac index (l/min/m) (Table 4).

Table 1.

	No. of Cases	Before Acu.		After Acu.		P Value
		Mean	Standard deviation	Mean	Standard deviation	
Defined points for CHD	100	6.84	±1.4305	8.78	±1.572	<0.001
Normal control	40	9.89	±1.920	9.98	±1.880	>0.05
Undefined points for CHD	25	7.22	±1.049	7.24	±1.180	>0.05

(2) Variations in cardiac output:
1) Stroke volume (Table 2)

(2) Variations in cardiac output:
1) Stroke volume (Table 2)

Table 2.

	No. of Cases	Before Acu.		After Acu.		P Value
		Mean	Standard deviation	Mean	Standard deviation	
Defined points for CHD	100	65.59	17.63	81.72	20.91	<0.001
Normal control	40	88.61	18.06	88.75	15.17	>0.05
Undefined points for CHD	25	63.91	28.06	64.24	27.63	>0.05

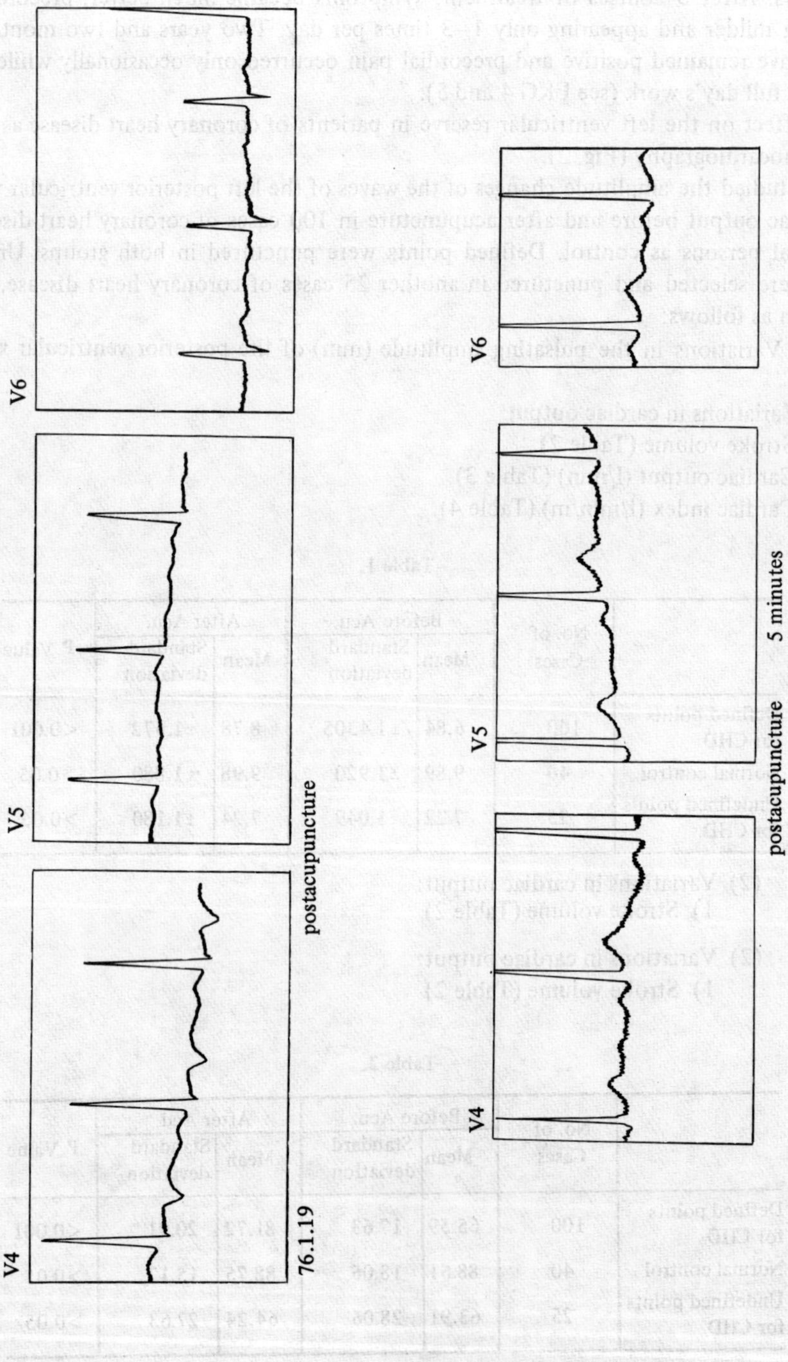
EKG. 4
V4
V5
V6
76.1.19
postacupuncture
V4
V5
V6
postacupuncture
5 minutes

EKG.5

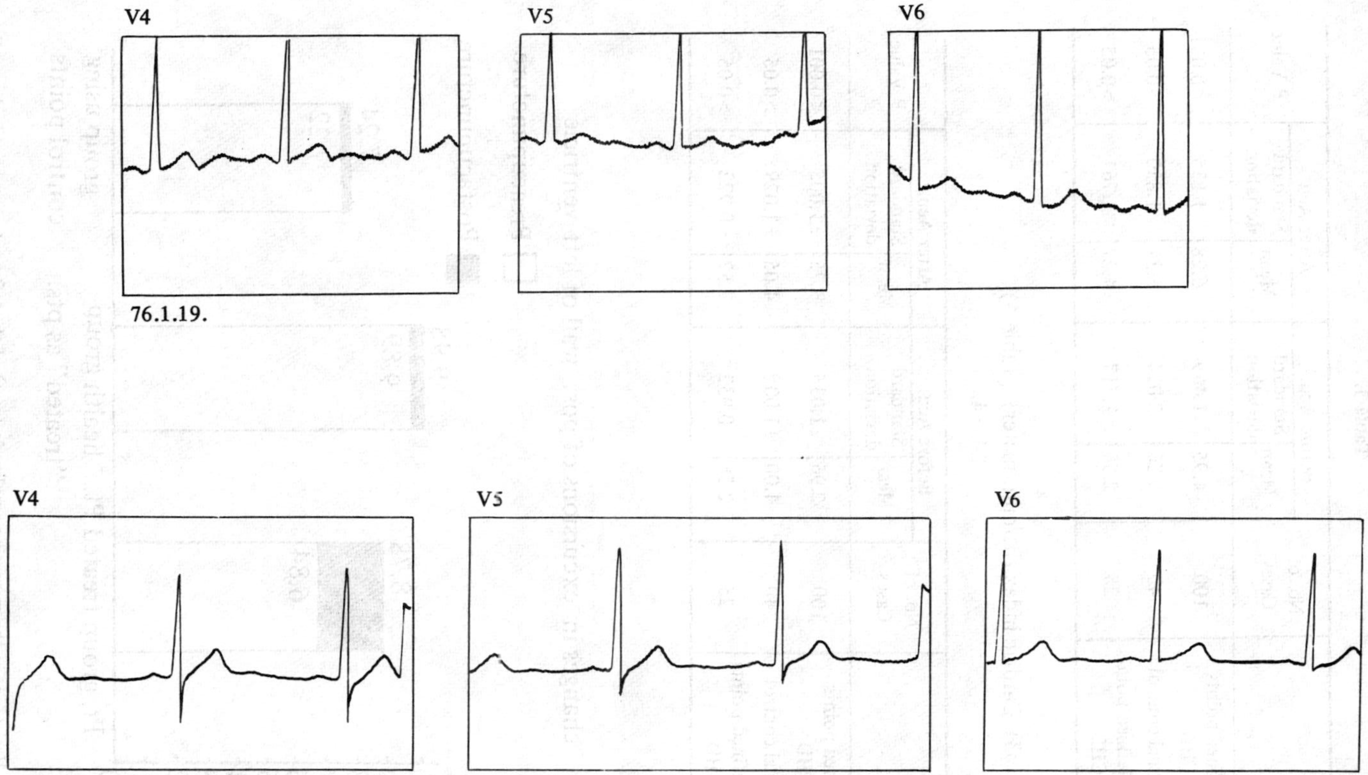

76.1.19.

78.3.30

2) Cardiac output (lit/min.) (Table 3)

Table 3.

	No. of Cases	Before Acu.		After Acu.		P Value
		Mean	Standard deviation	Mean	Standard deviation	
Defined points for CHD	100	4.95	1.469	6.28	1.835	<0.001
Normal control	40	6.26	2.024	6.34	1.830	>0.05
Undefined points for CHD	25	2.56	1.517	4.27	1.761	>0.05

3) Cardiac index (lit/min./meter) (Table 4)

Table 4.

	No. of Cases	Before Acu.		After Acu.		P Value
		Mean	Standard deviation	Mean	Standard deviation	
Defined points for CHD	100	2.96	±1.035	3.75	±1.005	<0.001
Normal control	40	4.00	±1.008	4.05	±1.029	>0.05
Undefined points for CHD	25	2.56	0.932	2.57	±0.922	>0.05

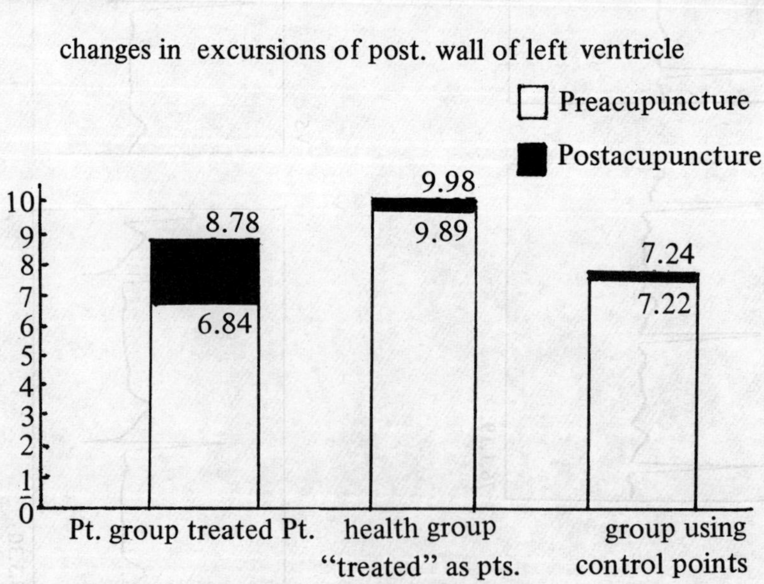

Fig. 3 Variations in the puesating amplitude (mm) of the left posterior ventricular wall.

As we can see from the above results:

1) There was no significant difference ($P>0.05$) in the normal group between the pre- and post-acupuncture pulsating amplitude of the posterior ventricular wall and stroke volume, while these figures were markedly increased in the coronary heart disease group after the defined points were punctured; the difference between pre- and post-acupuncture was significant ($P<0.001$). It was suggested that acupuncture might improve the left ventricular function of the patient with coronary heart disease.

2) When the points which were not defined were punctured in patients with CHD, there were no significant differences in the pulsating amplitude of the left ventricular wall and the cardiac output between pre- and post-acupuncture ($P>0.05$). However, the acupuncture results in patients with CHD were markedly different between the defined point group and the undefined point group ($P<0.001$). It was suggested that these defined points might have specificity in treating such a disease.

7. Effect of acupuncture on rheoencephalogram in patients with coronary heart disease (Figs. 4, 5).

Fifty patients with coronary heart disease and 20 normal controls were acupunctured at the above mentioned points. Twenty patients with coronary heary disease were acupunctured at random (undefined) points. The average ages of these three groups were 57, 55.6 and 56, respectively. Rheoencephalograms were obtained before and after acupuncture using a rheoencephalograph machine of Model XLJ 73, and the results are shown in Tables 5 and 6.

The above results indicated that:

(1) After needling the group of defined points for coronary heart disease, the in-flow time α was shortened, the wave amplitude H and the rapid in-flow segment H′ were both increased, and there was improvement in the shape of the wave. The diferences observed were highly significant ($P<0.001$). There was no remarkable difference in the parameters before and after acupuncture in the normal persons except for the considerably prolonged α ($P^{<0.05}_{>0.02}$). This could be due to nervous tension because they had never received acupuncture before, resulting in increased tone of the blood vessels and increased resistance to flow.

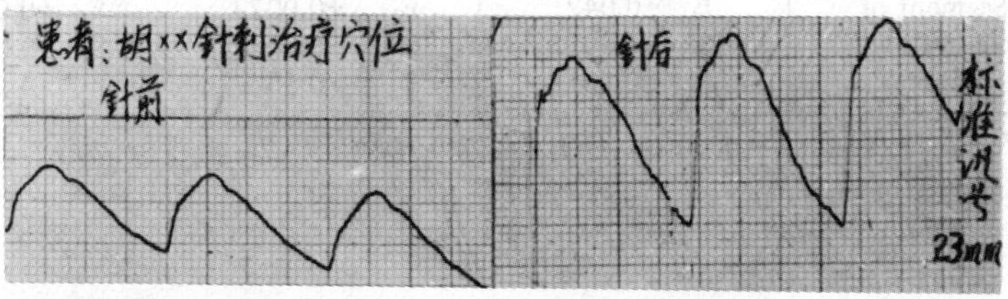

before acupuncture after acupuncture

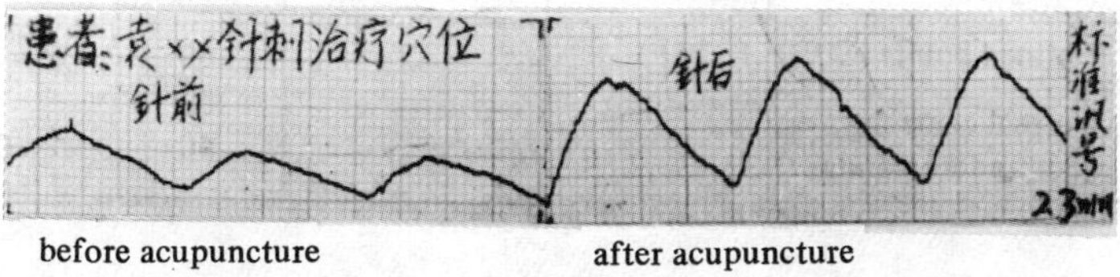

before acupuncture after acupuncture

defind points

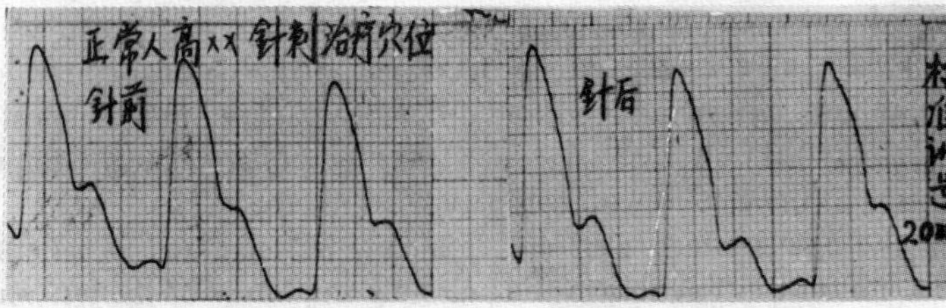

before acupuncture after acupuncture

undefind points

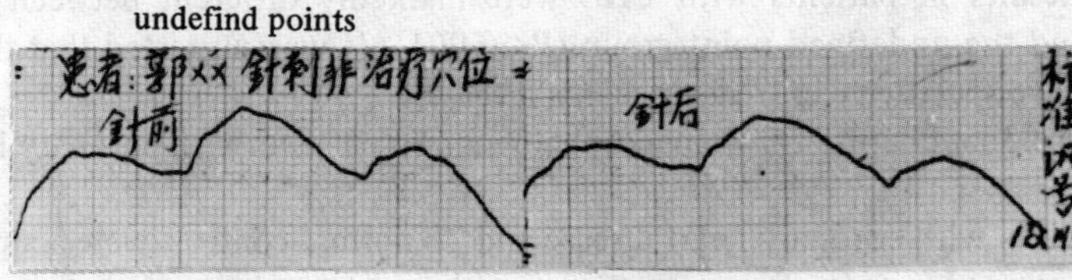

before acupuncture after acupuncture

Table 5.

Index	Defined Points (CHD)	Normal Control	Random Points (CHD)
Flow-in time (second)	E −0.029 S$\bar{x}$ ±0.004 P <0.001	E +0.007 S$\bar{x}$ ±0.0033 P <0.05 >0.02	E +0.0035 S$\bar{x}$ ±0.0028 P >0.20
Amplitude H (ohm)	E +0.044 S$\bar{x}$ ±0.0069 P <0.001	E −0.0075 S$\bar{x}$ ±0.0074 P >0.30	E −0.0023 S$\bar{x}$ ±0.0033 P >0.50
Segment of rapid in-flow H′ (ohm)	E +0.042 S$\bar{x}$ ±0.0055 P <0.001	E +0.0027 S$\bar{x}$ ±0.0086 P >0.50	E +0.0009 S$\bar{x}$ ±0.0027 P >0.50

Effect: + increase; − decrease. S$\bar{x}$: standard error.

Table 6. Effect on the shape of wave

Group	Improved	Unchanged	Total	P Value
Defined points (CHD)	15	35	50	$\chi^2 = 12.44$
Normal control and random points	0	40	40	P<0.001

However, the difference was significant when compared with the effect in the coronary patients acupunctured at the defined points ($P<0.001$). These results showed that acupuncture could improve not only the coronary circulation and the function of the left ventricle but also the circulation in the brain.

(2) No significant difference was observed before and after acupuncture in patients with coronary heart disease needled at random points ($P>0.2$). Highly significant differences were noted when compared with the group treated by needling the group of defined points for coronary heart disease ($P<0.001$). Therefore, these acupuncture points could be highly specific for treating the disease.

8. Effect of acupuncturing Neiguan on the systolic time interval in angina pectoris patients.

We have observed the acupunctural effect of point Neiguan on the systolic time intervals of 123 cases of angina pectoris with a control group of 35 cases of angina pectoris during bed-rest and another control group of 30 normal subjects.

After acupuncture was applied for 2 minutes and for 15 minutes, the heart rate was much slower and the electromechanical systole (QA2), mechanical systole (MS), ejection time (ET), isovolumetric relaxation period (IRP) and slow filling period (SF) were evidently prolonged. The preejection period (PEP)' isovolumetric contraction time (ICT), and the rapid filling period (RF) were shortened. The ratio PEP/ET was reduced while ET/ICT was increased. A-wave percentage of the apexcardiogram was significantly reduced. All these changes were statistically significant (see Table 7).

After the patients with angina pectoris had rested for 2 minutes and 15 minutes, most of the parameters did not show any significant change except lowering of the heart rate and prolongation of QA2, MS, and SF, which were related to the heart rate (Table 8).

In normal subjects the various parameters of the functional status of the heart did not change after acupuncture was applied continuously to both Neiguan for 2 minutes (Table 9).

Table 7. Effect on parameters of systolic time intervals and A-wave % in 123 angina pectoris patients

Item	Before Acup.	Mean ± Standard Error		P Value	
		Comparison before and during acup.	Comparison before and after acup.	Comparison before and during acup.	Comparison before and after acup.
HR	69.12	0.49 ± 0.30	2.18 ± 0.30	>0.1	<0.001
QA2	399.63	−3.09 ± 1.50	−6.09 ± 1.14	<0.05	<0.001
MS	345.04	−3.98 ± 1.09	−4.94 ± 0.81	<0.001	<0.001
PEP	110.06	5.63 ± 0.92	5.07 ± 1.71	<0.001	<0.001
ET	290.55	−8.08 ± 0.85	−10.45 ± 0.84	<0.01	<0.001
ICT	54.24	4.46 ± 0.94	5.75 ± 1.08	<0.001	<0.001
IRP	125.67	−1.16 ± 1.18	−5.17 ± 1.23	>0.3	<0.001
RF	76.59	2.02 ± 1.07	0.90 ± 1.04	=0.05	>0.5
SF	242.86	−18.61 ± 3.82	18.80 ± 3.90	<0.001	<0.001
PEP/ET	0.381	0.029 ± 0.004	0.029 ± 0.0045	<0.001	<0.001
ET/ICT	5.83	−0.74 ± 0.16	−1.05 ± 0.20	<0.001	<0.001
A-wave %	15.8	1.65 ± 0.72	2.78 ± 0.87	<0.05	<0.001

Table 8. Rest control analysis of effect on parameters of systolic time intervals and A-wave % in 35 angina pectoris patients

Item	Before Acup.	Mean ± Standard Error		P Value	
		Comparison before and during acup.	Comparison before and after acup.	Comparison before and during acup.	Comparison before and after acup.
HR	70.06	0.83 ± 0.46	2.23 ± 0.72	>0.1	<0.01
QA2	396.59	−1.11 ± 1.02	−3.69 ± 1.21	>0.3	<0.05
MS	345.51	−0.17 ± 1.36	−4.31 ± 1.49	>0.8	<0.05
PEP	112.31	−0.17 ± 1.70	0.26 ± 1.80	>0.5	>0.4
ET	289.54	0.175 ± 0.81	−2.83 ± 1.55	>0.7	>0.1
ICT	55.40	−0.34 ± 1.48	−0.77 ± 1.88	>0.7	>0.6
IRP	123.77	−0.40 ± 1.46	−4.43 ± 2.53	>0.7	>0.1
RF	73.11	−0.51 ± 1.84	−1.37 ± 3.01	>0.8	>0.6
SF	234.11	−8.14 ± 4.52	−27.14 ± 7.15	>0.1	<0.05
PEP/ET	0.391	0.034 ± 0.04	0.017 ± 0.007	>0.3	>0.7
ET/ICT	5.74	0.02 ± 0.18	0.16 ± 0.27	>0.8	>0.5
A-wave %	16.7	2.07 ± 2.58	1.21 ± 2.59	>0.4	>0.5
Δ ET	313.46	1.63 ± 1.09	3.37 ± 1.68	>0.1	⩽0.05

Table 9. Effect of acupuncture on parameters of systolic time intervals and A-wave % in normal adults

Item	Mean ± Standard Error		P Value
	Before acup.	After acup.	
HR	65.23 ± 1.17	65.40 ± 1.21	>0.5
QA2	335.83 ± 3.89	338.93 ± 3.00	>0.5
MS	92.30 ± 2.94	92.13 ± 2.74	>0.5
PEP	294.87 ± 2.74	294.93 ± 2.13	>0.8
ET	385.63 ± 3.30	387.83 ± 3.73	>0.5
ICT	41.97 ± 2.54	43.75 ± 2.74	>0.1
IRP	113.43 ± 2.60	112.80 ± 2.84	>0.5
RF	78.30 ± 3.40	79.23 ± 4.43	>0.5
SF	312.03 ± 16.33	310.40 ± 17.38	>0.7
PEP/ET	0.33 ± 0.02	0.31 ± 0.01	>0.3
ET/ICT	8.31 ± 0.94	8.54 ± 1.20	>0.4
A-wave %	7.0 ± 0.1	7.0 ± 0.1	>0.8

The preejection period in angina pectoris patients was apparently longer than in the normal subjects. After acupuncture, PEP of the patients was obviously shortened. After treatment by histogram with the electron computer, it showed that these were continuous changing processes, which implied that acupuncture improved the function of the heart to a certain extent.

In angina pectoris patients, ET was evidently shortened, ICT was evidently prolonged and ET/ICT was reduced. After acupuncture, ET was evidently prolonged, ICT was evidently shortented and ET/ICT was increased. It was implied that acupuncture promoted contractility of the myocardium. PEP, ICT, ET, PEP/ET and ET/ICT showed pathological changes in coronary heart disease patients, but all these parameters seemed to return to the normal ranges after adjustment by acupuncture. It was suggested that acupuncture improved the cardiac function.

The A-wave percentage of the angina pectoris patients was evidently higher than that of the normal person. After acupuncture A-wave % became significantly lower. It was suggested that acupuncture might improve the adaptability of the myocardium, decreasing the end diastolic pressure. Through the observation of the control group of the angina pectoris patients resting in bed, the results showed that the acupunctural effect mentioned above was not the effect of rest. The various parameters of the cardiac function of the normal persons were not affected by acupuncture either.

In summary, needling Neiguan probably resulted in an increase in the contractility of the myocardium, a prolongation of the ejection time, a lowering of the end diastolic pressure, and an improvement in the adaptability of the left ventricle.

EFFECTS OF ACUPUNCTURE ON EXPERIMENTAL ACUTE MYOCARDIAL INFARCTION

Yang Youmi, Liu Ruiting, Meng Jingbi,
Li Lianda*, Gao Xiuzi**, Wang Pingping
(Institute of Acupuncture and Moxibustion, Academy of Traditional Chinese Medicine)

In recent years, acupuncture has been applied to the treatment of coronary heart disease and angina pectoris caused by acute myocardial infarction with satisfactory results[1, 2]. To date, however no experimental observations on the effect of acupuncture on myocardial infarction has been reported. The present experiment studied the effects of acupuncture on the early stage acute myocardial ischemic injury and the size of infarction by means of epicardial ECG and morphological technique.

I. METHODS

Studies were carried out in 28 normal dogs weighing 13.9 kg on the average. They were divided into two groups: the acupuncture group and the control group. Dogs were anesthetized with intravenous pentothal sodium (25 mg/kg), and respiration was maintained with an electric respirator (Model SC-2). The heart was exposed through a left thoracotomy in the fourth intercostal space and suspended in a pericardial cradle. The root of the third branch of the left anterior descending coronary artery was isolated, used as the site of ligation. Then "the fixed multipoint" epicardial electrodes were fixed on the surface of the heart and connected with the RM-86 multipurpose polygraph ($V_1 - V_3$) through the waver[3].

Epicardial ECG of 30 points were recorded 10 times in order by switching the waver. Bilateral "Neiguan" were stimulated with SEN-3101 stimulator, pulse duration 5 ms, interval 100 ms, output at isolator 6 V.

During the experiment, epicardial ECG of 30 points were first, recorded as controls before ligation. Next the branch of anterior descending coronary artery was ligated for 20 minutes, and then the ligation was released slowly. Both "Neiguan" areas were given the electro-acupuncture five minutes before the release, and the stimulation lasted for 20 minutes. Epicardial ECG was recorded in the same way 15 minutes during ligation, stopping electro-acupuncture, and 15 minutes after the termination of electro-acupuncture,

*Xi Yuan Hospital, Beijing.
**The Second Hospital, Beijing.

respectively. The second ligation was made at the same place 30 minutes after the release. Beginning from the 16th minute after the second ligation, the animals were given electro-acupuncture five times, each time lasting for 10 minutes with an interval of 30 minutes. The hearts of the animals were removed 3.5 hours after coronary ligation, and histological preparations were made. The recording method, procedure and histological preparation were the same in the control group, except the electro-acupuncture. We referred to the reports of Maroko[4], Braunwald[5] *et al.*, using the number of S-T segment elevation exceeding 2 mV (N-ST) as the index of the extent of myocardial ischemic injury area. While Σ-ST, the sum of the S-T elevations from all 30 recording points represented the severity of the myocardial ischemic injury. In our observation the N-ST, Σ-ST values at the 15th minute during ligation were used as the standard for the effects of acupuncture on acute myocardial ischemic injury.

II. MORPHOLOGICAL INDEX

1. Nitro-blue tetrazolium (N-BT) stain[6]. The hearts of animals were removed. The left ventricle was dissected from the heart, weighed and cut transversely into two equal sections on the superior ligation site, and cut transversely into four equal sections from the ligation site to cardiac tip, then weighed, respectively. The sections of left ventricle were stained in N-BT solution. Normal myocardium was stained into blue color, while the necrotic myocardium was unstained. Thus, the range of infarction was clearly shown (Figs. 1, 2). The percentage of the infarcted zone in the total area and the percentage of the infarcted mass in the total weight of ventricular myocardium were then calculated respectively.

2. The patho-histological stain. The specimen of infarct was sectioned from the tissue of the infarction area in the third section of left ventriculum stained by N-BT stain. The specimen of the control was sectioned from the tissue of normal area. The different extent and range of myocardial necrosis could be demonstrated by the acid-fuchsinmethyl-green staining method[7]. Hematoxylin-eosin staining method was also used for comparison. The sever-

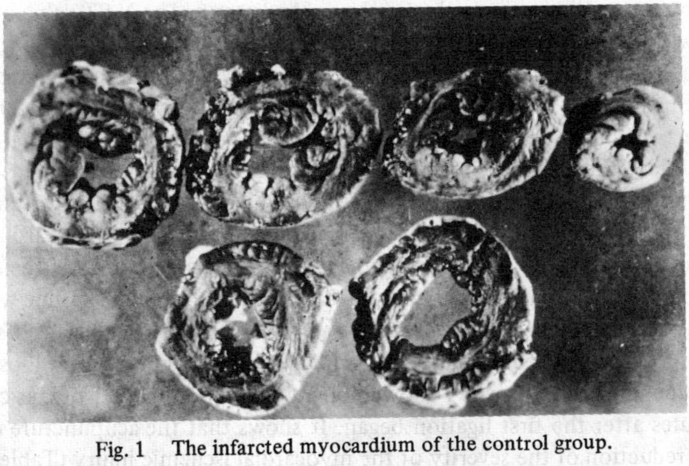

Fig. 1 The infarcted myocardium of the control group.

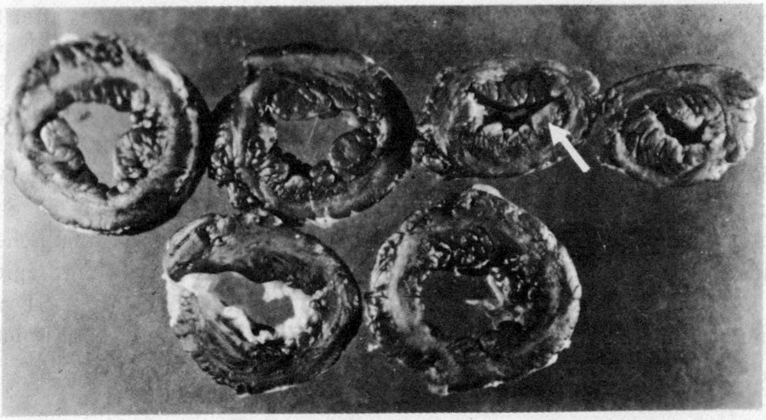

Fig. 2 The infarcted myocardium of the acupuncture group.

ity of myocardial lesions could be divided into three degrees: normal myocardium, the nuclei and myofibrils are clearly seen; moderate necrosis, the nuclei were pyknotic, the myofibrils disappeared and there were scattered or small areas of necrotic muscular cells; severe necrosis, the nuclei were pyknotic or in debris, the myofibrils dissolved and there were large areas of necrotic muscular cells.

III. RESULTS

1. Comparison of the extent and severity of acute myocardial ischemic injury.

(1) Comparison of N-ST and Σ-ST of the 15th minute during the loosening of the ligation.

Table 1 shows that there was no statistical difference in the extent of myocardial ischemic injury of the two groups, when they had been ligated for 15 minutes for the first time. It shows that the extent of myocardial ischemic injury in the acupuncture group before acupuncture was the same as that in the control group. The N-ST value of the acupuncture group was reduced considerably in the 15 minutes after loosening began in the ligation, and the change was great and of statistical significance. But the N-ST value of the control group remained at a higher level. There was a marked difference between the acupuncture and the control groups. The results mentioned above demonstrate that the extent of acute myocardial ischemic injury may be reduced by acupuncture.

There was no statistical difference between the Σ-ST values of the two groups 15 minutes after the first ligation started. It shows that the severity of the myocardial ischemic injury in the acupuncture group before acupuncture was the same as that of the control group. After loosening the ligation for 15 minutes, the control group's Σ-ST value was statistically significant, as compared with that 15 minutes after the first ligation began. It shows that the severity of myocardial ischemic injury may rapidly recover by itself after loosening the ligation. The acupuncture group's Σ-ST showed obvious variation in statistics, as compared with that 15 minutes after the first ligation began. It shows that the acupuncture may markedly promote the reduction of the severity of the myocardial ischemic injury (Table 2).

Table 1. Comparison of N-ST at the 15th minute during the first ligation and that at the 15th minute during the loosening

Group	15th Minute During the First Ligation M ± SE	15th Minute During the Loosening M ± SE	t	p
Control (12 dogs)	15.08 ± 1.15	12.58 ± 1.56	1.28	> 0.2
Acupuncture (16 dogs)	13.43 ± 1.35	7.81 ± 1.44	2.83	< 0.01

Table 2. Comparison of Σ-ST at the 15th minute during the first ligation and that at the 15th minute during the loosening

Group	15th Minute During the First Ligation M ± SE	15th Minute During the Loosening M ± SE	t	p
Control (12 dogs)	73.88 ± 12.77	40.63 ± 7.53	2.24	< 0.05
Acupuncture (16 dogs)	57.59 ± 7.75	24.78 ± 4.58	3.64	< 0.01

Table 3. Comparison of the N-ST values between the two ligations 15 minutes after they started

Group	15 Minutes After the First Ligation Began M ± SE	15 Minutes After the Second Ligation Began M. diff. ± SE	t	p
Control (12 dogs)	15.08 ± 1.15	1.08 ± 0.90	1.20	> 0.2
Acupuncture (16 dogs)	13.43 ± 1.35	2.94 ± 1.13	2.60	< 0.05

(2) Comparison of the extent and severity of myocardial ischemic injury between the two ligations 15 minutes after they started.

Tables 3, 4 show that there was no statistical significance of N-ST and Σ-ST values of the control group during two ligations of 15 minutes each. They also show that the effects of two ligations on the acute myocardial ischemic injury were the same and could be repeated. When the acupuncture group was ligated for 15 minutes once again the values of Σ-ST and N-ST were reduced markedly as compared with those of the first time. The difference shows marked significance in statistics. These results show that acupuncture could reduce the severity of ischemic injury and provide some protection to the myocardium, thus raising the defensive ability against the myocardial ischemic injury.

Table 4. Comparison of Σ-ST between the two ligations 15 minutes after they started

Group	15 Minutes After the First Ligation Began M ± SE	15 Minutes After the Second Ligation Began M. diff. ± SE	t	p
Control (12 dogs)	73.88 ± 12.77	2.33 ± 8.35	0.28	> 0.7
Acupuncture (16 dogs)	57.59 ± 7.75	15.96 ± 5.93	2.69	< 0.05

(3) Comparison of the range and extent of myocardial infarction and necrosis.

(i) Comparison of the percentages of the infarct area. (Table 5).

The percentage of infarct area of the acupuncture group is significantly smaller than that of the control group.

(ii) Comparison of the percentages of the infarcted mass in weight of the left ventricular myocardium (Table 6).

Table 5. Percentages of infarct area

Group	No. of Animals	Percentage of Infarct Area (%) M ± SE	t	p
Control	9	18.09 ± 2.69	3.44	< 0.01
Acupuncture	11	8.40 ± 1.30		

Table 6. Percentages of the infarcted mass in weight of the left ventriculum

Group	No. of Animals	Weight of Infarcted Mass (%) M ± SE	t	p
Control	9	11.33 ± 1.08	5.33	< 0.001
Acupuncture	11	4.62 ± 0.72		

Table 7. The incidence rates of various extents of myocardial necrosis

Group	No of Animals	No of Animals With Various Extents of Necrosis		Percentage (%)		χ^2	p
		Moderate	Severe	Moderate	Severe		
Control	7	2	5	28.57	71.43	3.233	≈ 0.05
Acupuncture	8	6	2	75.00	25.00		

The percentage of the infarcted mass in weight of the left ventricular myocardium is decreased significantly in the acupuncture group as compared with that of control group.

(iii) Comparison of the extent of myocardial necrosis (Table 7).

The severity of myocardial necrosis of animals with acupuncture is less than that of the animals without it.

IV. DISCUSSION

In the ischemic zone of acute myocardial infarction, oxygen deficiency would bring about irreversible necrosis of the myocardium. The increased severity of myocardial necrosis would influence prognosis directly, so the main object in the treatment of myocardial infarction is to reduce the size of the infarct zone.

The present results preliminarily show that acupuncture could significantly reduce the extent and severity of myocardial ischemic injury, promote recovery of injured myocardium and raise the defensive function of myocardium against injury. Morphological observations also show that acupuncture could reduce the size of myocardial infarction and the extent of myocardial necrosis. This indicates that in treatment of acute myocardial infarction by integrating traditional Chinese medicine with western medicine, the addition of acupuncture treatment is conducive to the enhancement of the therapeutic effect.

The effect of acupuncture is probably due to its regulating of the coronary blood flow, increasing of the supply of oxygen and as a result improving of the anoxic condition of the ischemic and marginal zones of myocardial infarction. Therefore, the amount of myocardial ischemic necrosis and the size of infarction are reduced.

Libby et al[8]. have reported that intravenously administered hydrocortisone could reduce and prevent myocardial ischemic necrosis and reduce the size of myocardial infarction. Braunwald et al.[9] and Barzilal, D. et al.[10] demonstrated that hydrocortisone could significantly reduce the size of myocardial infarction and the severity of myocardial ischemic injury. Vyden et al.[11] observed that after methylprednisolone was intravenously given to dogs with acute experimental myocardial infarction, blood flow in the anterior descending branch of the left coronary artery significantly increased and arteriovenous oxygen difference across the coronary circulation was decreased markedly. They claimed that methylprednisolone improved the oxygen balance of myocardium by increasing the coronary arterial blood flow. It is due to the increase of coronary blood flow that corticosteroid could reduce and prevent myocardial ischemic necrosis. Therefore, the effect of acupuncture against myocardial infarction may relate to the activation of function of suprarenal cortex and improvement of the anoxic condition of myocardium.

V. SUMMARY

The present study preliminarily demonstrates:

(1) Acupuncture could reduce the extent and size of myocardial ischemic injury.

(2) Acupuncture could reduce the size of myocardial infarction and the severity of myocardial necrosis.

REFERENCES

[1] 北京市冠心病协作组：全国针灸针麻学术讨论会论文摘要(一)，1979。

[2] 中医研究院西苑医院内科心血管组：中西医结合防治研究心血管病资料(1)，1977。

[3] 中医研究院西苑医院基础研究室药理组：新医药学杂志，(11)：52，1978。

[4] Maroko, P. R.: *Circulation*, 43: 67, 1971.

[5] Braunwald, E. *et al.*: *Circulation*, 54: 529, 1976.

[6] Shatney, C. H. *et al.*: *Amer. J. Cardiol.*, 37(4): 572, 1976.

[7] 中医研究院西苑医院：活血化瘀冠心II号方药及有关资料汇编(二)，1977。

[8] Libby, P. *et al.*: *J. Clinical. Invest.*, 52: 599, 1973.

[9] Braunwald, E. *et al.*: *Amer. J. Cardiol.*, 37(4): 550, 1976.

[10] Barzilal, D. *et al.*: *Chest*, 61: 488, 1972.

[11] Vyden, J. K. *et al.*: *Amer. J. Cardiol.*, 34(6): 677, 1974.

STUDY OF EFFECT OF ACUPUNCTURE ON BLOOD PRESSURE REGULATORY SYSTEM

(From the Control Theory Point of View)

Huang Bingxian, Pan Hua
(Institute of Automation, Academia Sinica)

Xiang Manjun, Wu Yulan
(Beijing Institute of Tuberculosis)

Yang Minggan, Yu Zhanjiu
(Hebei Academy of Medicine)

It has been demostrated[1, 2] that acupuncture exerts bidirectional control over abnormal blood pressure. However, the data now available are not enough to provide a quantitative evaluation of the effect, nor can they answer definitely what changes take place in the blood pressure regulatory system under acupuncture. In this paper is reported the effect of acupuncture on the blood pressure regulatory system in dogs studied experimentally by the system dynamic characteristics method used in control theory.

The work is divided into two parts:

I. EFFECT OF ACUPUNCTURE ON THE DYNAMIC CHARACTERISTICS OF THE CLOSED LOOP SYSTEM OF BLOOD PRESSURE

The so called "closed loop" is to keep an animal's regulatory system in normal physiological condition, because blood pressure is usually maintained steadily by a "closed loop" feedback system.

(I) Methods

Twenty-seven mongrel dogs weighing 10 to 15kg were anesthetized with nembutal (20mg/kg). One femoral artery and one femoral vein was exposed and cannulated. An endotracheal tube was inserted. Under artificial respiration, the animals were kept awake and immobilized with flaxedil (4mg/kg). The dynamic blood pressure response to a 5 sec arrest of artificial respiration was recorded[3]. Before acupuncture the response to a 5 sec arrest of artificial respiration of dogs was observed every 5–10 minutes interval. After the response became stable, acupuncture was introduced. After 20 minutes electro-acupuncture, the responses to the transient disturbance were recorded, and then we stopped the electro-acupuncture. Post-acupuncture responses of dynamic blood pressure were then observed many times.

The electrical stimulation was bidirectional sharp impulses with voltage 6–9 volts and frequency 20 Hz.

Acupuncture stimulation is on the "Neiguan" point (except 4 cases on "Renzhong", "Chengziang" points). In seven animals the blood gas P_{CO_2}, P_{O_2}, and the pH values were measured.

Similar experiments were performed on 6 dogs with hemorrhagic hypertension (90–100mmHg).

(II) Results and analysis

The dynamic blood pressure responses to a 5 sec arrest of artificial respiration are shown in Fig.1.

It shows that blood pressure deviates from normal value by the transient disturbance, and then deviation dies out under the action of the blood pressure regulatory system.

This dynamic process can reflect the performance of this regulatory system.

For quantitative evaluation, we chose three indices: (1) maximum amplitude of blood pressure (P); (2) time duration of oscillation of blood pressure (T); (3) number of oscillatory cycles (N), serving as the parameters for evaluating the dynamic characteristics of the system, as shown in Fig. 2.

Maximum amplitude of response P was in 20–40mmHg; time of osillatory T was in 20–90 sec; N was from 3/4 to 2 cycles. There are significant differences between individuals.

For each animal the first transient response was chosen as reference and compared with the responses of repeated disturbance at 20 minutes intervals without acupuncture. From the results of 42 repeated disturbances in 27 animals, P values were increased in 25 cases and reduced in 17 cases; only 9 cases were reduced over 15%. T increased in 30 cases and reduced in 12 cases; only 5 cases were reduced over 25%. It was shown that under our experimental conditions, the blood pressure response to 5 sec arrest of artificial respiration remained stable relatively.

Under acupuncture, P, T, N values showing the dynamic blood pressure responses to dis-

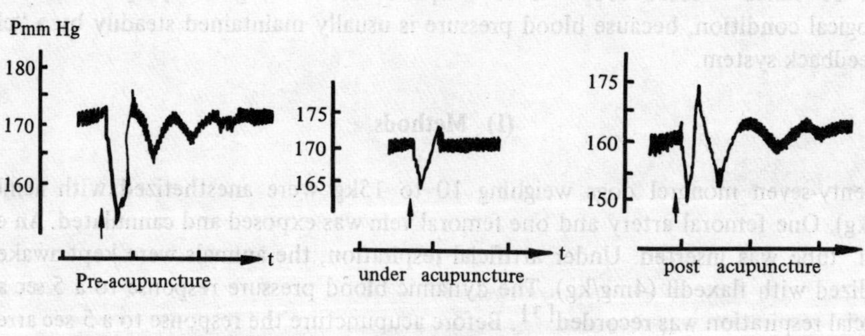

Fig. 1 Dynamic blood pressure responses.

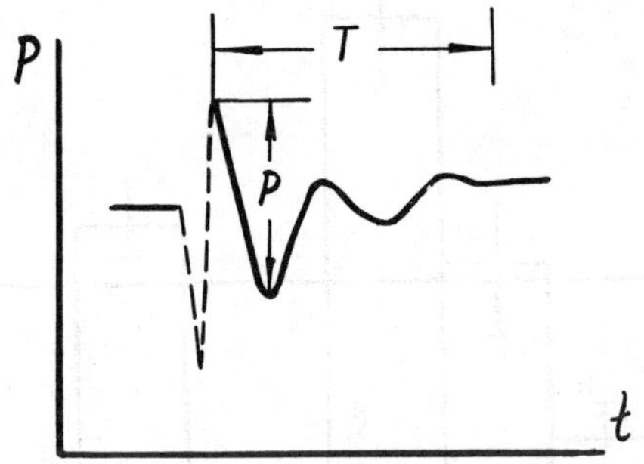

Fig. 2 Dynamic indices.

turbance in most cases were decreased compared with the pre-acupuncture values. The effect of acupuncture can be observed 10 minutes after insertion and it usually reached the maximum value about 30 minutes after the stimulation. The aftereffect of acupuncture can continue for 10 to 20 minutes.

In order to reduce the influence of respiratory activity, P, T, N values were calculated from the average response curves. For pre-acupuncture control, average response from 3 or more stimulations was taken.

To rule out spontaneous variation, we claimed improvement only when P decreased over 15% and T decreased over 25%.

Among the 30 experiments under acupuncture, there were 10 with all three indices improved (excellent), 11 with two indices improved (good) and 5 with only one index improved (poor), and 4 with no improvement at all (failed). About 70% of the experiments were excellent or good. It was shown that under acupuncture the dynamic characteristics of the blood pressure regulatory system were improved in most animals.

The indices P, T values were processed by statistics for different acupuncture effects. In cases of excellent effect P reduced to 63±6.36%, T to 48±6.6% of control value ($P<0.001$). The results are shown in Fig. 3. This showed that acupuncture speeded up the response of the system.

To evaluate the system stability, the frequency characteristic curve transformed from time domain curve was used. By Mihailov's criterion, the shortest distance from origin to the reverse frequency characteristic curve was considered as the index of stability. In the 30 experiments, there were 16 with improved index of stability. 21 cases with good to excellent effect, the average index of stability increased more than onefold.

In 6 dogs with hemorrhagic hypotension, the maximal amplitude of pressure response to distubance was less than those of normal pressure, but the duration of oscillation in dogs with hypotension was significantly longer than those of normal pressure (up to 4 minutes). Good to excellent effects were obtained in all six animals. On the average P, T values were reduced to 56% and 45.6% of those of pre-acupuncture control, respectively. Therefore the effect of acupuncture under hypotension is more prominent than that under normal pressure.

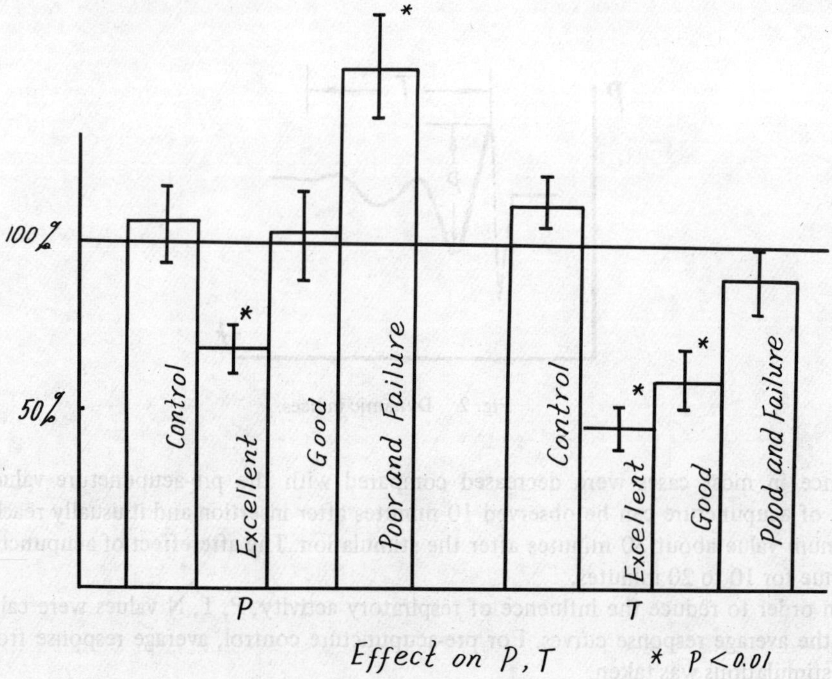

Fig. 3 Effect on P, T value.

Table 1. Acupuncture Effect Under he Morrhagic Hypotension

Number	P		T		N		
	Under/Pre acup. %	Post/Pre acup. %	Under/Pre acup. %	Post/Pre acup. %	Pre acup.	Under acup.	Post acup.
S1	73	–	14	–	3 ¼	1 ¼	–
S2	60	60	43	81	2 ¼	1 ¼	1 3/4
S3	68	88	34	144	2 ¼	3/4	2 3/4
S4	45	87	60	77	3 ¼	1/4	3 ¼
S5	41	70	43	83	2 ¼	1 ¼	2 3/4
S6	62	–	86	–	2 3/4	2 ¼	–
Average	56	76	45.6	95			

II. EFFECT OF ACUPUNCTURE ON THE OPEN-LOOP FREQUENCY CHARACTERISTIC OF CAROTID SINUS BARORECEPTOR FEEDBACK LOOP

Based on the result of part one, the purpose of this experiment was carried out to evaluate quantitatively the role of carotid sinus baroreceptor feedback loop in acupuncture effect on the blood pressure regulatory system, and to explore the pathway of acupuncture effect on this system.

(I) Method

By applying the frequency characteristic method in control theory, the carotid sinus baroreceptor was stimulated artificially by a changeable sine wave pressure (input), and the systemic arterial blood pressure serving as output was observed. Using the amplitude ratio of input to output and the phase lag relation, we obtained the open-loop frequency characteristic which was used in analyzing the system dynamic characteristic.

The experiment was carried out on 13 dogs weighing 8 to 15kg.

The carotid sinus of dogs anesthetised with nembutal were isolated and the femoral artery cannulated for measuring systemic blood pressure. To establish an open-loop circuit a membraneous blind sac was introduced through the common carotid artery to the level of carotid sinus[6]. The carotid sinus was through a T tube linked with an artificial sine wave pressure system[7], as shown in Fig. 4.

The frequencies of baroreceptor input signal were controlled by the motor speed. Baroreceptor was stimulated by sine pressure signals with constant amplitude (50–80mmHg peak to peak) of various frequencies (0.01–0.1cycle/sec). Both the sinusal and systemic pressures were recorded simultaneously with an X-Y recorder through pressure transducers and amplifier.

Carotid sinus feedback loop was "open" only unilaterally. The counterlateral blood flow was blocked temporally during observations.

The average pressure of carotid sinus was regulated by the position of the mercury bottle. The best operating point were determined by depressor reflex. The point of acupuncture stimulation and parameters and other conditions were the same as in part one.

(II) Results and analysis

The orignial records were a series of sine curves with different frequencies as shown in Fig. 5. Calculating the amplitude ratio of input to output and the phase lag for different frequencies from the curve, we obtained the amplitude-frequency characteristic and phase - frequency characteristic curves respectively. It is shown in Fig. 6. The frequency bandwidths which reflect the speeds of responses were calculated.

In the 4 cases of control set with no acupuncture, at 20 minutes interval the bandwidths were within 99.8–108% of the first record, change of phase lags were within–6°–+ 12° of the first record. In showed that before acupuncture the open-loop frequency characteristic was rather stable.

In 8 cases out of 10 acupuncture experiments, the frequency bandwidths were increased from 118 to 191% under acupuncture (average 153.8%). In 7 cases with phase record, phase lags were all decreased by an average of 36.5°. Twenty minutes after acupuncture was stopped, there was recovery to some extent. This showed that acupuncture improved the open-loop frequency characteristic which increased the frequency bandwidth and decreased the phase lag. In other words acupuncture speeded up the response and increased the stability of the system.

In order to obtain quantitative evaluation and to explore the pathway of acupuncture effect, we took 5 cases with prominent acupuncture effect and used the typical second order

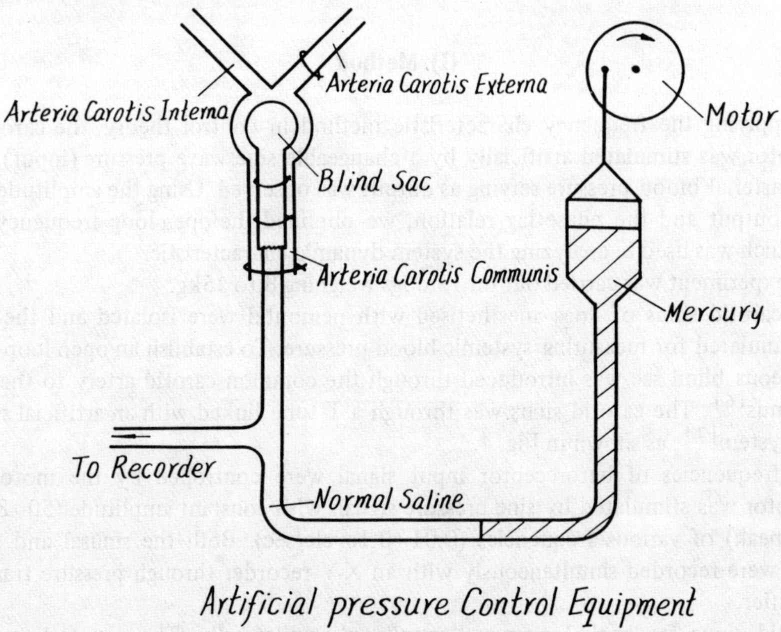

Fig. 4 Artificial pressure control equipment.

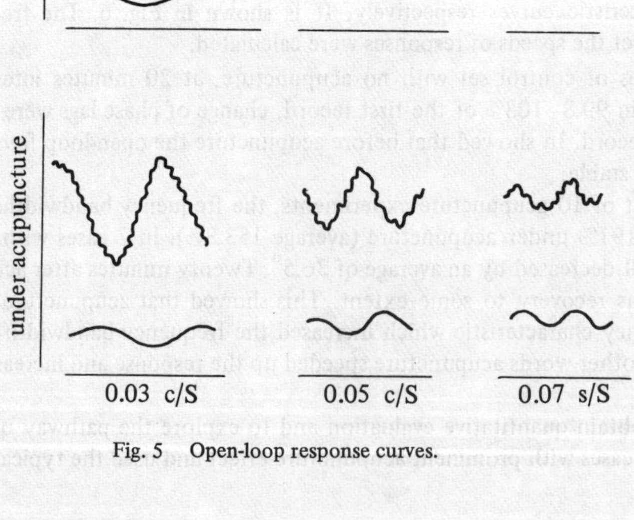

Fig. 5 Open-loop response curves.

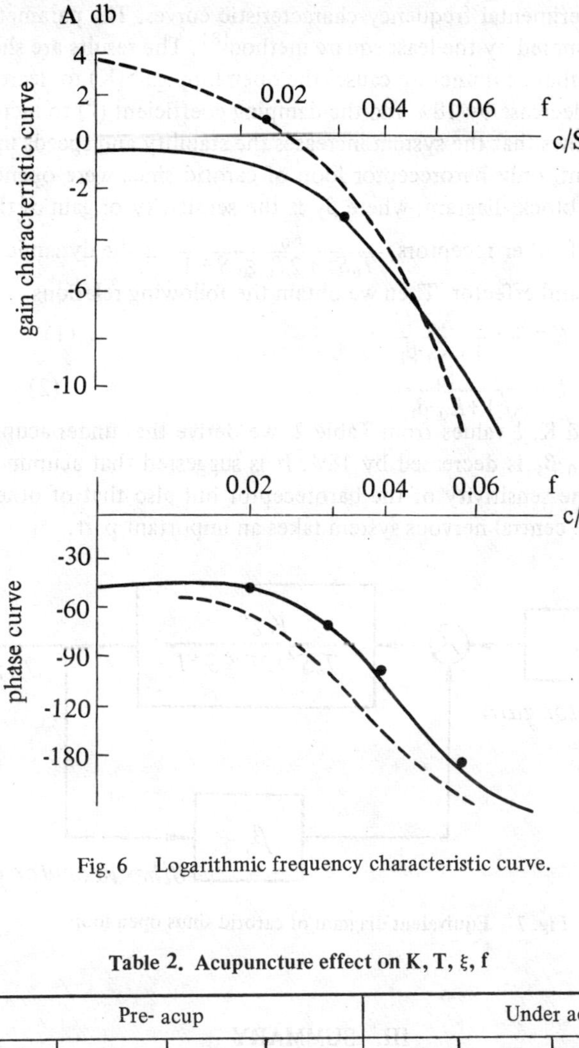

Fig. 6 Logarithmic frequency characteristic curve.

Table 2. Acupuncture effect on K, T, ξ, f

Number	Pre- acup				Under acup.			
	K	T	ξ	Δf	K	T	ξ	Δf
16	1.3973	6.5118	0.5245	0.1490	1.1523	5.1207	0.7398	0.1550
17	1.1260	5.0880	0.2790	0.1500	1.2500	4.9800	0.3310	0.1700
10–1	0.7172	3.3360	0.3630	0.1436	0.2998	2.7310	0.3030	0.3020
10–2	0.8020	2.4200	0.4230	0.2093	0.4750	1.7830	0.4000	0.5078
7	1.0646	4.6972	0.4542	0.2034	0.5264	3.3359	0.3902	0.2670
Average	1.007	4.412	0.409	0.171	0.741	3.595	0.433	0.280

$$G = \frac{K}{T^2 S^2 + 2\xi T S + 1}$$

system to fit the experimental frequency characteristic curves. The parameters of the open-loop system were estimated by the least square method[8]. The results are shown in Table 2.

The table shows that acupuncture causes the open-loop gain(K) to decrease by 26%, the time constant (T) to decrease by 18% and the damping coefficient (ζ) to increase by 5.9% on the average. It also shows that the system increases the stability and speeds up the response.

In our experiment, only baroreceptor loop of carotid sinus were opened. Fig. 7 is the equivalent open-loop block diagram, where β_2 is the sensitivity or gain of the baroreceptor, β_1 is the sensitivity of other receptors, $\frac{k_0}{T_0S^2+2T_0\,\xi_0\,S+1}$ is the dynamic characteristic of cardiovascular center and effector. Then we obtain the following relations

$$K=\beta_2\cdot\frac{K_0}{1+K_0\cdot\beta_1} \quad (1)$$

$$\xi=\frac{\xi_0}{\sqrt{1+K_0\cdot\beta_1}} \quad (2)$$

From (1), (2) and K, ξ values from Table 2, we derive that under acupuncture β_2/β_1 is decreased by 13%, $K_0\cdot\beta_1$ is decreased by 18%. It is suggested that acupuncture effects are manifold; not only the sensitivity of the baroreceptor but also that of other loops may be effected. Probably the central nervous system takes an important part.

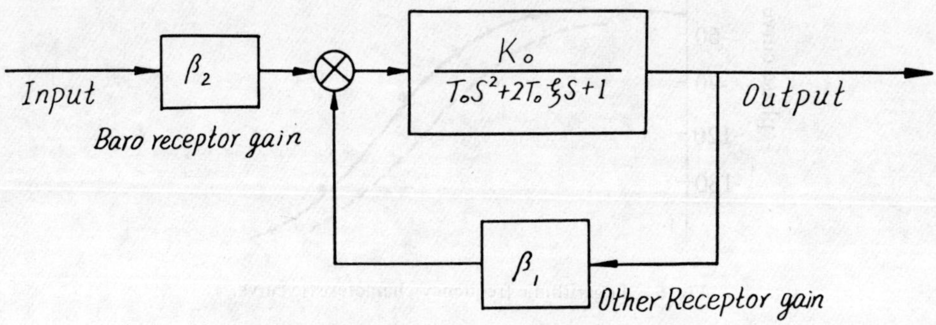

Fig. 7 Equivalent diagram of carotid sinus open-loop.

III. SUMMARY

The results were summarized as follows:

1. This paper gives some quantitative evaluations of the effect of acupuncture on the blood pressure regulatory system.

2. Under acupuncture, the dynamic characteristics were improved on most animals. Acupuncture can increase the anti-disturbance ability of the blood pressure regulatory system, stabilize the system and speed up the response.

3. The effect of acupuncture for cases of hypotension is more prominent than that for cases of normal pressure.

4. The effects of acupuncture are probably realized by changing many of the parameters of the system. The sensitivity of baroreceptor has been changed during electro-acupuncture. It is presumed that other loops may also be affected and that, probably, the central

nervous system takes an important part.

5. The phenomenon that during operation under acupuncture anesthesia the blood pressure remains rather steady can be partly accounted for by the speediness of the responses of carotid sinus to pressure change which is so increased by acupuncture that any minute vibration caused by external stimulation may be corrected immediately. On the other hand, since the gain and the time constant are decreased and the damping coefficient increased, the oscilation of blood pressure dies out rapidly.

REFERENCES

[1] 西安医学院，针麻基础理论研究协作组：针刺麻醉资料综述，人民卫生出版社，76 页，1973。

[2] 安徽医学院生理教研组：中华医学杂志，**53**：97，1973。

[3] Race, D.: *Circul. Res.*, **18**:525, 1966.

[4] 李振裕等译：自动控制系统实验计算法，上海科学技术出版社，16 页，1964。

[5] 刘 豹：自动调节理论基础，上海科学技术出版社，145 页，1963。

[6] Shen, T. C. R. *et al.*: *Science*, **128**: 784, 1938.

[7] 畠山一平：計測と制御，2:2，1963。

[8] Sims, J. B.: *Computer and Biomedical Research*, **5**:121, 1964.

[9] Sagawa, K. *et al.*: *Trans ASME series* G., **95**:339, 1973.

[10] 柯 志：自然科学争鸣 (1)：65，1976。

ANALYSIS OF THERAPEUTIC EFFECT OF ACUPUNCTURE IN 66 CASES OF GASTROPTOSIS

Gastroptosis Treatment Group, Radiological Department,
Institute of Acupuncture and Moxibustion and
Academy of Traditional Chinese Medicine

Based on the principle of "taking tenderness as the acupuncture point" of traditional Chinese medicine, 66 cases of gastroptosis were treated with acupuncture. They were all puncture (from roentgenographys), the tonicity of gastric muscle and the immediate effect of traditional Chinese medicine. The tonicity of gastric musculature and the immediate effect of acupuncture were studied in some patients in order to investigate the mechanism of the therapeutic effect of acupuncture and were evaluated by barium meal examination.

I. TREATMENT METHOD

Patients were asked to lie in a supine position during treatment. A 30–32 gauge filiform needle of 6–7 "cun" long was used and inserted subcutaneously into the reaction spot (tenderness or nodes) below the xyphoid process down to the reaction spot beside the umbilicus. If there were no tenderness spot or nodes, the needle should be inserted at about 2 cm below the xyphoid process down to the "Mang-shu" point beside the umbilicus.

When the patients had a feeling of soreness, distention at the apex of the needle or a feeling of tightness in lower abdomen or especially in the whole stomach, the doctor could provoke needling sensation at any time by manipulating the handle of the needle with fingers. The needle should be kept fixed at the point by the umbilicus for 40 minutes and then withdrawn. Treatment was performed once a week, 6 treatments as a course.

II. CRITERION OF DIAGNOSIS

In addition to some common symptoms of indigestion, X-ray examination was the main basis of diagnosis. As shown in Fig. 1, the angular notch of a normal stomach should be kept above the line between the iliac crests line (I.C. line), and the lower border of stomach should be below that line not more than 6 cm; otherwise it should be diagnosed as gastroptosis.

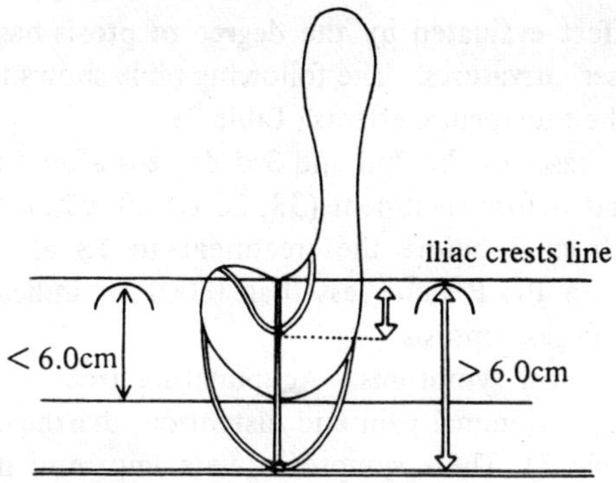

Fig.1 Criterion of diagnosis.

III. MEASURING METHOD OF GASTROPTOSIS

According to the roentgenographs the ascending or descending distances of the greater and lesser curvatures before and after the treatment are the criterion of the therapeutic effect (Fig. 2).

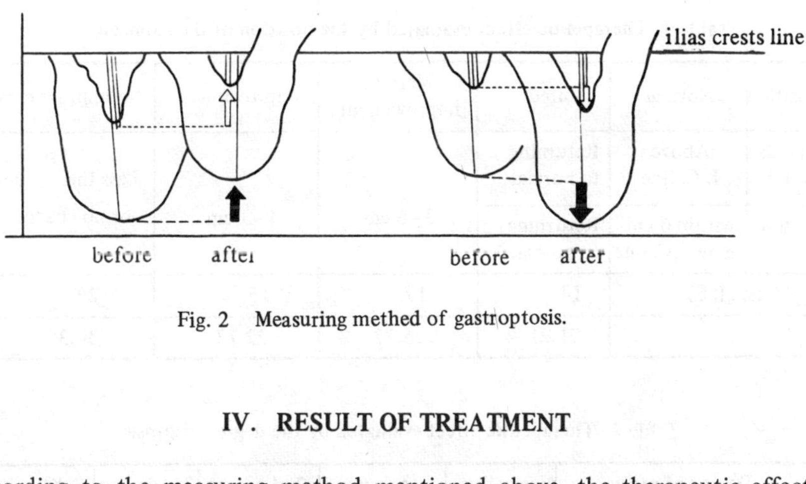

Fig. 2 Measuring methed of gastroptosis.

IV. RESULT OF TREATMENT

According to the measuring method mentioned above, the therapeutic effects were analyzed in several aspects of clinical symptoms in 66 cases of gastroptosis.

1. Therapeutic effect evaluated by the location of stomach based on the level of the greater and lesser curvatures (Table 1).

Among the 66 cases of gastroptosis, 14 cases were cured (21.21%) whose angular notch and the fundus were restored to normal; 17 patients had marked improvement (25.77%) whose angular notch and fundus elevated 3–6 cm; 15 cases improved (22.72%) whose notch and fundus ascended 1–3 cm; while 20 patients (30.30%) failed because their angular notch and fundus lifted less than 1 cm or no change. Therefore, the total effective rate was 69.70% (46 cases) and the percentage of cured and marked improvement reached 46.98% (31 cases).

2. Therapeutic effect evaluated by the degree of ptosis based on ptosis degree of the gastric greater and lesser curvatures. The following table shows the criterion for judging the degrees of ptosis and the therapeutic effects (Table 2).

As the number of cases of the 2nd and 3rd degrees after the treatment (24, 13 cases) was much less than that before treatment (33, 26 cases), while the number of cases of the 1st degree increased from 7 before the treatment to 18 after treatment, and 11 cases restored to normal, with the P value less than 0.001, it indicates that acupuncture may prominently improve the gastroptosis.

3. Relief of the clinical symptoms. Acupuncture treatment can relieve such clinical symptoms as: anorexia, abdominal pain and distention, diarrhea, belching, heavy feeling of the stomach, etc. (Table 3). These symptoms were improved in varying degrees (43.4%–75.8%) and the effective rate was approximately in conformity with that of the X-ray findings: 69.70%.

4. Long term therapeutic effect. 14 Cases with good short term effect were followed up for 4–8 months after the termination of treatment in order to observe the long term acupuncture effect. 9 cases of them were cured and 5 markedly improved in their short term effect. Roentgenologic examinations were made before the treatment, and immediately after treatment in the follow-up period.

As shown in Fig. 3, although both the lesser and greater curvatures of the long term effect group descended somewhat as compared with that of the short-term effect group

Table 1. Therapeutic effect evaluated by the position of the stomach

Position	Normal	Cured	Marked improvement	Improvement	No improvement
Angular notch	Above I. C. line	Returning to normal	3–6 cm	1–3 cm	Less then 1 cm or no change
Fundus	within 6 cm below I.C. line	Returning to normal			
Cases (66)		14	17	15	20
%		21.21	25.77	22.72	30.30

Table 2. Therapeutic effect evaluated by the degree of ptosis

Degree of ptosis		Normality	1st degree	2nd degree	3rd degree	X²	P
Criteria (cm)	Angular notch-I. C. line	Above I.C.line	Within 1.5	1.6–4.5	>4.6	21.6	<0.001
	Fundus→notch→I.C.line	Within 6.0cm	6–7.5	7.6–10	>10.1		
Therapeutic effect cases(%)	Before acup.	0	7 (10.6)	33 (50.00)	26 (39.40)		
	After acup.	11 (16.67)	18 (27.27)	24 (36.36)	13 (19.70)		

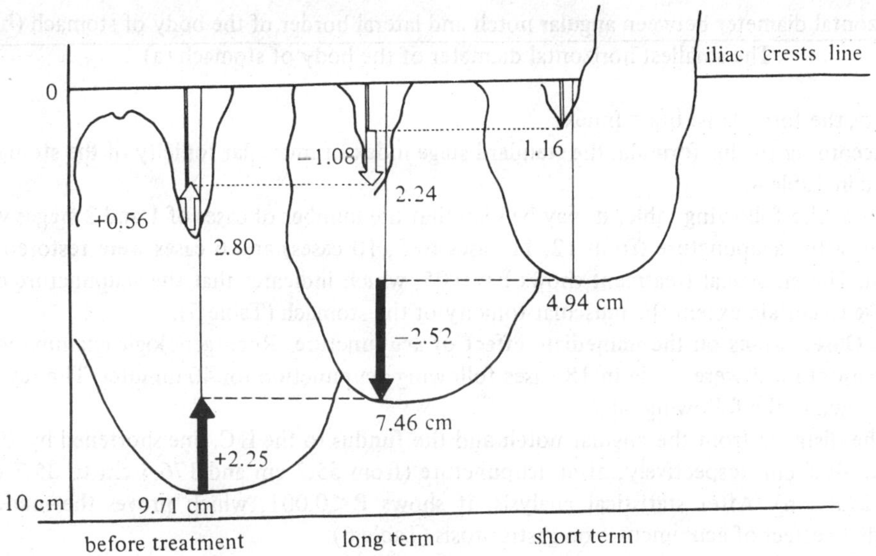

Fig. 3 Comparition of therapeutic effect.

Table 3. Relief of clinical symptoms

Symptom	Anorexia	Abdominal Pain	Abdominal distention	Diarrhea	Belching	Heavy feeling
Positive rate/case	29/46	27/44	23/53	25/33	30/49	24/45
%	63.0	61.4	43.4	75.8	61.2	53.3

(lesser curvature lowered by 1.08 cm, while the greater curvature lowered by 2.52 cm) on average, they were still kept higher than those before the treatment (lesser curvature kept 0.56 cm higher and greater curvature 2.25 cm higher). It implies that the therapeutic effect of acupuncture on gastropyosis may be maintained somehow in a long period.

V. INVESTIGATION OF THE UNDERLYING MECHANISM

In order to further elucidate the mechanism by which gastroptosis was cured by acupuncture (from roentgenographs), the tonicity of gastric muscle and the immediate effect of acupuncture were investigated through X-ray photographs.

1. Measuring method of the tonicity of the gastric muscle and its result. We measured the values of horizontal diameter between the angular notch and the lateral border, as well as the smallest horizontal diameter of the body of stomach in 35 out of 66 cases before and after treatment. The following formula was adopted for calculation of the index on the roentgenographs.

$$\frac{\text{Horizontal diameter between angular notch and lateral border of the body of stomach (b)}}{\text{The smallest horizontal diameter of the body of stomach (a)}}$$

= Index

In short, the formula is: b/a = Index

According to this formula, the standard stage index of muscular tonicity of the stomach is listed in Table 4.

From the following table, it may be seen that the number of cases of 1 and 2 stages was reduced after acupuncture (from 12, 11 cases to 5, 10 cases) and 6 cases were restored to normal. The statistical treatment shows $P \approx 0.05$, which indicates that the acupuncture can improve to certain extent the muscular tonicity of the stomach (Table 5).

2. Observations on the immediate effect of acupuncture. Roentgenologic examinations with barium meal were made in 18 cases following acupuncture for 40 minutes. The results were shown in the following table.

The distance from the angular notch and the fundus to the I. C. line shortened by 20.0 cm and 46.6 cm, respectively, after acupuncture (from 55.7 cm and 176.4 cm to 35.7 cm and 129.8 cm). After statistical analysis, it shows $P<0.001$, which proves the marked immediate effect of acupuncture on gastroptosis (Table 6).

Table 4. Standard stage index for gastric tonicity

Stage	1	2	3	4
Standard index (b/a)	1.6–2.0	2.1–2.5	2.6–3.0	>3.1

Table 5. Results of gastric tonicity determination

Comparison	Case	Stages of muscular tonicity of stomach					Stage percentage (%)					X^2	P
		Normal	1	2	3	4	Normal	1	2	3	4		
Before acup.	35	0	12	11	5	7	0	34.29	31.43	11.28	20.00	0.093	≈0.05
After acup.	35	6	5	10	6	8	17.14	14.29	28.57	17.14	22.86		

Table 6. Results of immediate effect

Position		Angular notch–I.C. line				Fundus–I.C. line			
Comparison	Case	Total value	Mean ± standard deviation	t	P	Total value	Mean ± standard deviation	t	P
Before acup.	18	55.7	3.09±0.38	4.115	<0.001	176.4	9.80±0.44	4.62	<0.001
After acup.	18	35.7	1.98±0.36			129.8	7.21±0.06		
Ascending value		20.0	1.11±0.02			46.6	2.59±0.38		

VI. SUMMARY

This paper has summarized the therapeutic effects of 66 cases of gastroptosis treated with acupuncture according to roentgenographs. The effective rate reaches 69.70%. It is noteworthy that before the acupuncture treatment all these 66 cases were resistent to prolonged combined treatment of physiotherapy and drug therapy from both western and traditional Chinese medicine. Therefore the value of acupunture in the treatment of gastroptosis is to be especially emphasized.

Although the long-term effect is not as good as the short term one, it at least can make some improvement. It had been proved in practice that acupuncture can elevate the angular notch and the fundus of the stomach, so as to reduce the degree of ptosis, especially to raise the muscular tonicity of the stomach. All those throw light in the future for the advancement of acupunctural therapeutic effect on gastroptosis.

CLINICAL OBSERVATION OF ACUPUNCTURE TREATMENT OF ACUTE PERFORATION OF PEPTIC ULCER

Zhuang Ding, Wang Yuanchao, Yang Xiuzhen
(Institute of Acupuncture and Moxibustion, Academy of Traditional Chinese Medicine)

Tian Zaishan, Liu Yingyun, Yuan Heping, Li Donghua
(Institute of Acute Abdominal Diseases, Tianjin)

Acute perforation of gastroduodenal ulcer, one of the serious complications of peptic ulcer, is a common acute abdominal disease. The nonoperative treatment by integrating traditional Chinese and western medicine of this complication may not only obtain good immediate results but also satisfactory long-term results[1, 2].

In the nonoperative therapy of acute perforation of peptic ulcer, acupuncture is employed as the chief means in the acute stage to facilitate the circulation of *vitality* and *blood*, and to relieve the severe pain, so as to enhance body resistance and to promote the sealing of the perforation. This will prepare the patient for herbal medication in the second stage.

In the present study the therapeutic effect was evaluated by recording the pneumographic curves and the EMG of rectus abdominis as objective indices of the changes and development of certain symtoms and the disease during the course of acupuncture treatment of acute perforation of peptic ulcer.

I. PATIENTS AND OBSERVATION METHODS

Forty-one patients (36 males, 5 females, at ages ranging from 20-73) of acute perforation of peptic ulcer admitted as emergency cases were studied. Precise diagnosis was made of all the cases. They all had the positive symptoms of the illness and these symptoms were further confirmed by roentgenography and abdominal paracentesis, etc.

Measures of treatment: Mainly by acupuncture, combined with gastrointestinal decompression, fasting, fowler's position, intravenous infusion, but generally without any analgesics or antibiotics.

The most frequently used acupuncture points were Zusanli (st. 36) or the adjacent tender points (bilateral), Zhongwan (Ren 12), Liangmen (St. 21) (bilateral), Tianshu (St. 25) (bilateral), and in case of severe nausea and vomiting, Neiguan (p. 6) (bilateral). After needle response had been produced, strong stimulation by hand manipulation was applied to enhance the needling sensation then the needle was connected with pulse current.

Electroacupuncture is applied for one hour with a frequency of 80/sec and an intensity tolerable to the patient. The interval between 2 needlings was 4 hours. The apparatus used was Bei-hang Model 57–6.

Method of electromyographic study: Two acupuncture needles of 1.5 cm in length were inserted into the rectus abdominis muscles at the maximal rigid points as recording electrodes. The electrodes, 0.5–1.0 cm apart, were fastened to the skin with adhesive tapes to ensure immobillization throughout the course of observation. The EMG of rectus abdominis, amplified by the type RB-5 Bio-electric amplifer (time constant 0.01 sec, high cut at "OFF", sensitivity 100 μV/cm) was recorded by RMG-5104 cassette tape recorder, and simultaneously monitored by cathode-ray oscilloscope and also recorded by the ink-writing RM-25 Polygraph for reference. Recording of the EMG of rectus abdominis for 1 minute should be made for every patient prior to treatment and at the end of the first trial of electroacupuncture treatment, and then every hour afterwards. The tape recordings were processed by the TQ–19(A) processor after the observations.

Method of pneumographic study: Tracings were made with the H3–327 ink-writing recorder, by means of carbonaceous transducer transmitted by Wheatstone bridge. The thoracic and abdominal respiration belts were placed paralled to the nipples and 1 cm above the umbilicus and fastened with nylon clips to ensure good immobilization throughout the course of observation. Synchronized tracings of both thoracic and abdominal pneumographic curves were recorded for 2 minutes prior to treatment and at the end of the first trial of the electroacupuncture. The speed of the tracing papers was 1mm/sec.

II. RESULTS

(I) Clinical Therapeutic Results

Criteria of therapeutic results

Good results: Obvious relief of severe abdominal pain after 1–2 trials of acupuncture, localization of tenderness, softening of abdomen, disappearance of board-like rigidity, reappearance of peristaltic sound, bowel movement, or passage of stool. These suggest the sealing up of the perforation and that herbal medicine can be administered with safety.

Poor result: No obvious alleviation of the symptoms after a few trials of acupuncture or recurrence of the symptoms and signs after brief relief. Operation is thus indicated.

26 of the cases had good results (63.4%) and 15 had poor results (36.6%).

(II) Physiological Investigation

1. Pneumographic curve. Marked restriction of respiratory movement caused by severe pain was observed in patients after perforation took place. In 31 cases, the pneumographic curve recorded before treatment showed increased respiration frequency and diminished amplitude, especially in abdominal respiration, and even temporary suspension of breath. In the majority of cases, improvements in both thoracic and abdominal respiratory movements as evidenced by obvious increase of respiratory amplitude were seen after the first trial of electroacupuncture. Such changes were found statistically significant in the good result

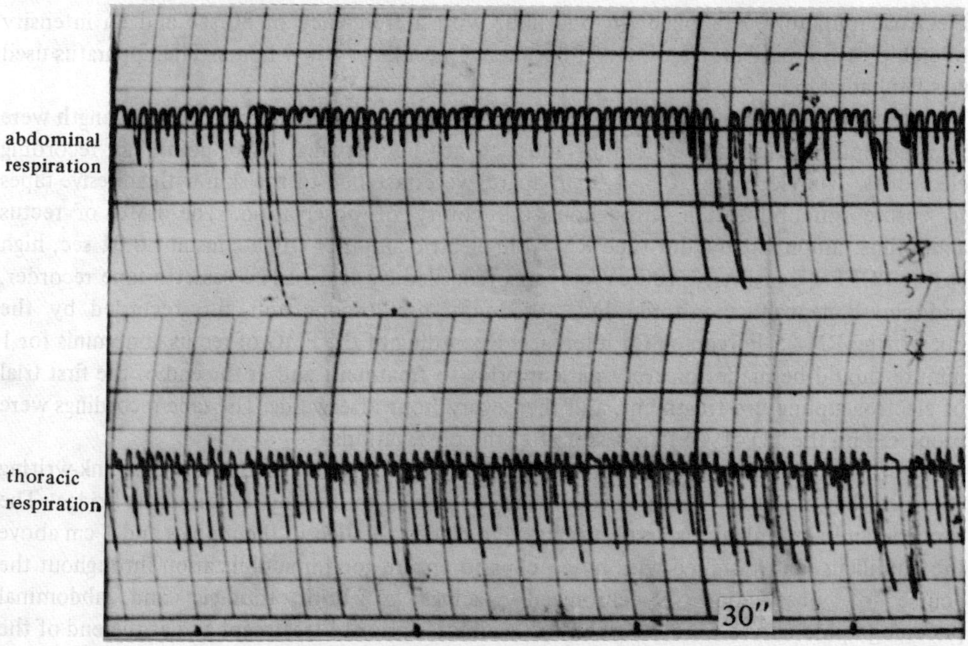

Fig. 1 Respiratory movement curve (prior the treatment).
Patient Yu (good result group)

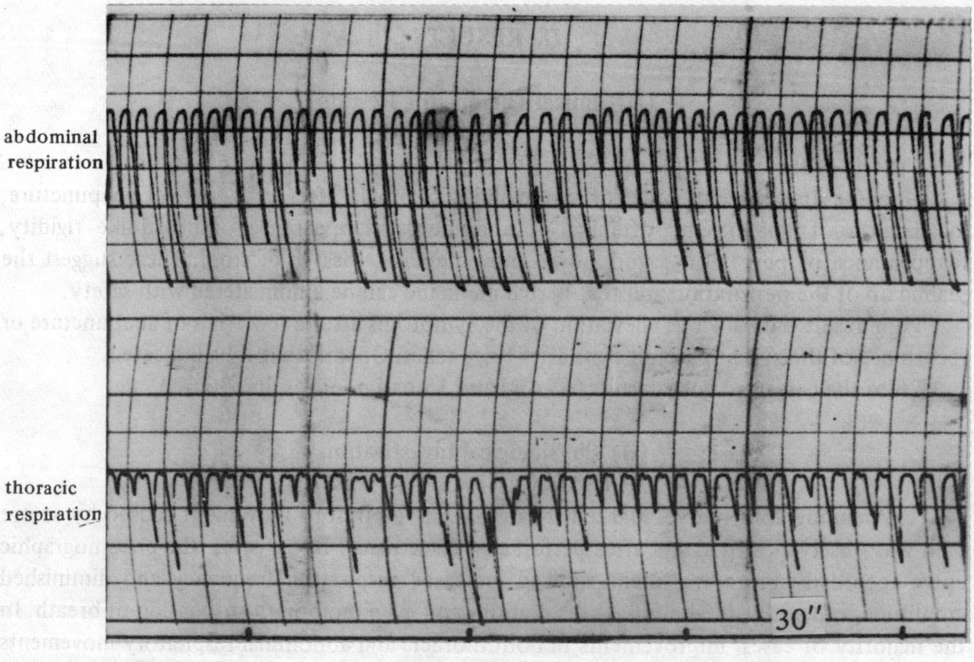

Fig 2 Respiratory movement curve (at the end of the 1st trial of electro-acupuncture).
Patient Yu (good result group)

group, but not in the poor result group (Table 1). Slight decrease in frequency was seen in 20 cases (64.2%) after the first trial of electroacupuncture, but this was not statistically significant.

Figure 1 and 2 demonstrate the pneumographic curves before and after electroacupuncture in a patient of the good result group.

Table 1. Amplitude variation of pneumographic curve before and after electroacupuncture

Group	Case	Modes of respiration	Pretreatment (mm)	Post-acupuncture (mm)	Difference (mm)	t	P
Good result	23	thoracic	10.24 ± 0.89	11.85 ± 1.08	1.89 ± 0.81	2.3259	<0.05
		abdominal	5.51 ± 0.58	7.91 ± 0.98	2.37 ± 1.04	2.2907	<0.05
Poor result	8	thoracic	10.72 ± 0.73	14.00 ± 5.02	3.28 ± 1.00	3.2679	<0.05
		abdominal	6.57 ± 1.36	6.75 ± 2.85	1.18 ± 1.19	0.1502	>0.5

In this group, most patients had their severe pain rapidly relieved during the first trial of electroacupuncture and many of them showed signs of sedation and sleepiness 15–20 min after electroacupuncture started. Meanwhile, increase of abdominal respiratory amplitude corresponds roughly with the amelioration of pain felt by the patients.

Figure 3 and 4 show the pneumographic curves before and after electroacupuncture in a patient of the poor result group. Pain was reduced slightly but not completely supressed, and

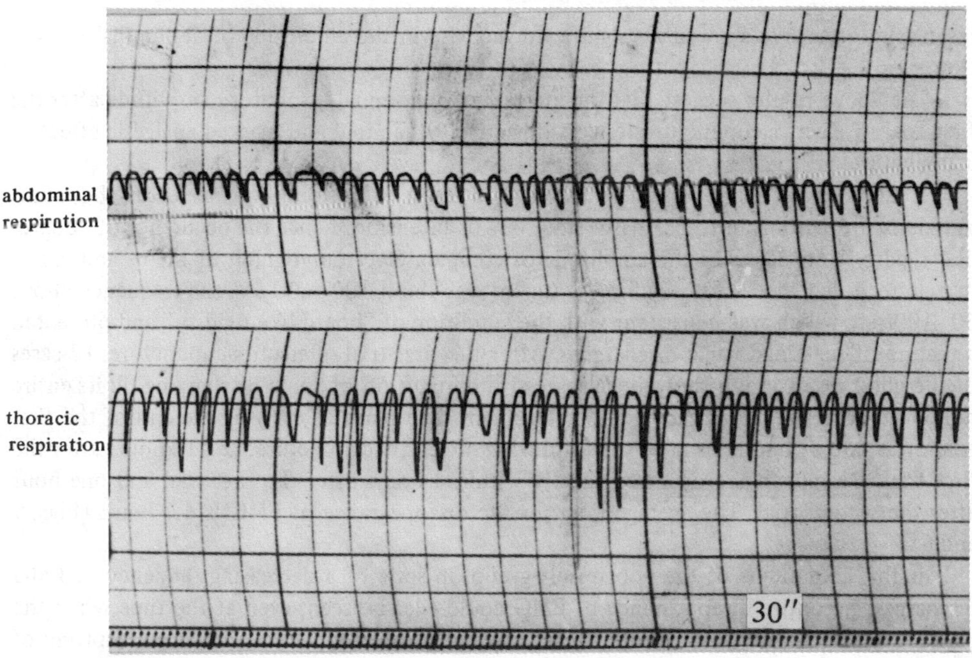

Fig. 3 Respiratory movement curve (prior to treatment). Patient Qi (poor result group)

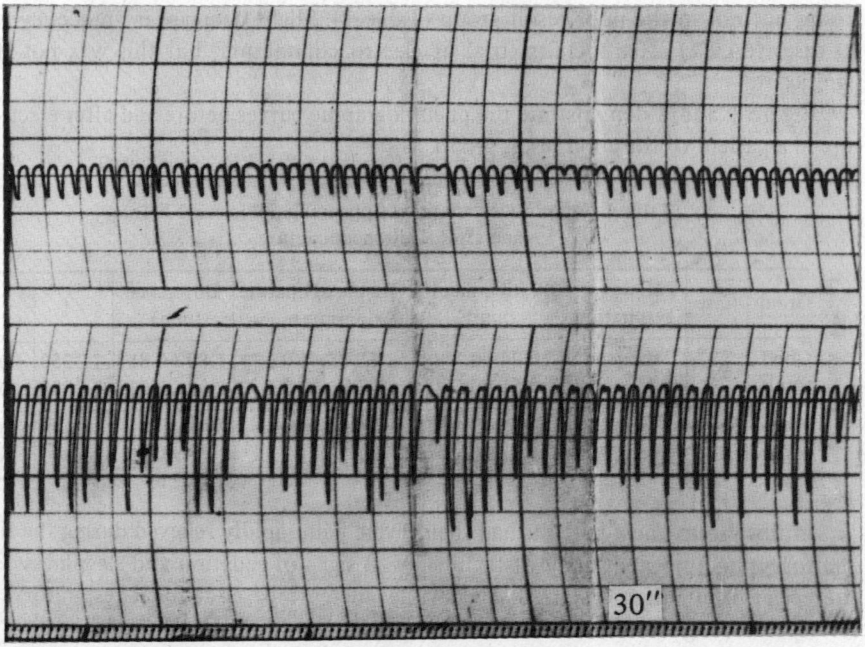

Fig. 4 Respiratory movement curve (at the end of the 1st trial of electroacupuncture).
Patient Qi (poor result group)

his respiratory curve showed no significant increase in the amplitude of abdominal respiration.

The above results suggest that the increase of abdominal respiratory amplitude after the first trial of electroacupuncture reflects objectively the rapid and marked analgesic effect of acupuncture.

2. EMG of rectus abdominis muscle. As a result of perforation, the rectus abdominis muscle is thrown into a tonic spasm state out of intension, hence the occurence of "board-like rigidity". In 30 cases the amplitude of complex electromyograph of rectus abdominis muscle recorded successfully before treatment was about 100–600 μV, the frequency about 50–100/sec, which was consistent with the condition of "board-like rigidity" and presented a picture of sustained tonic discharging. After the first trial of electroacupuncture, 17 cases of the good result group showed a progressive diminution of tonic discharging till its entire disappearance. The disappearence of EMG might take place as early as the end of the first trial or as late as one hour after the third trial of electroacupuncture, i.e., 10 hours after the first trial. Disappearance occurred mostly within 4 hours after the first trial and one hour after the second trial. The average time for the disappearance of EMG is 4.7 hours (Figs. 5 and 6).

In the 13 patients of the poor result group, in spite of a decreasing tendency of EMG discharges, no entire disappearance of EMG could ever be seen; even at the time when the patients were transferred to be operated on, some of them were still showing symptoms of recurrence (Figs. 7 and 8). In one case EMG discharges persisted for 37 hours after the first trial of electroacupuncture.

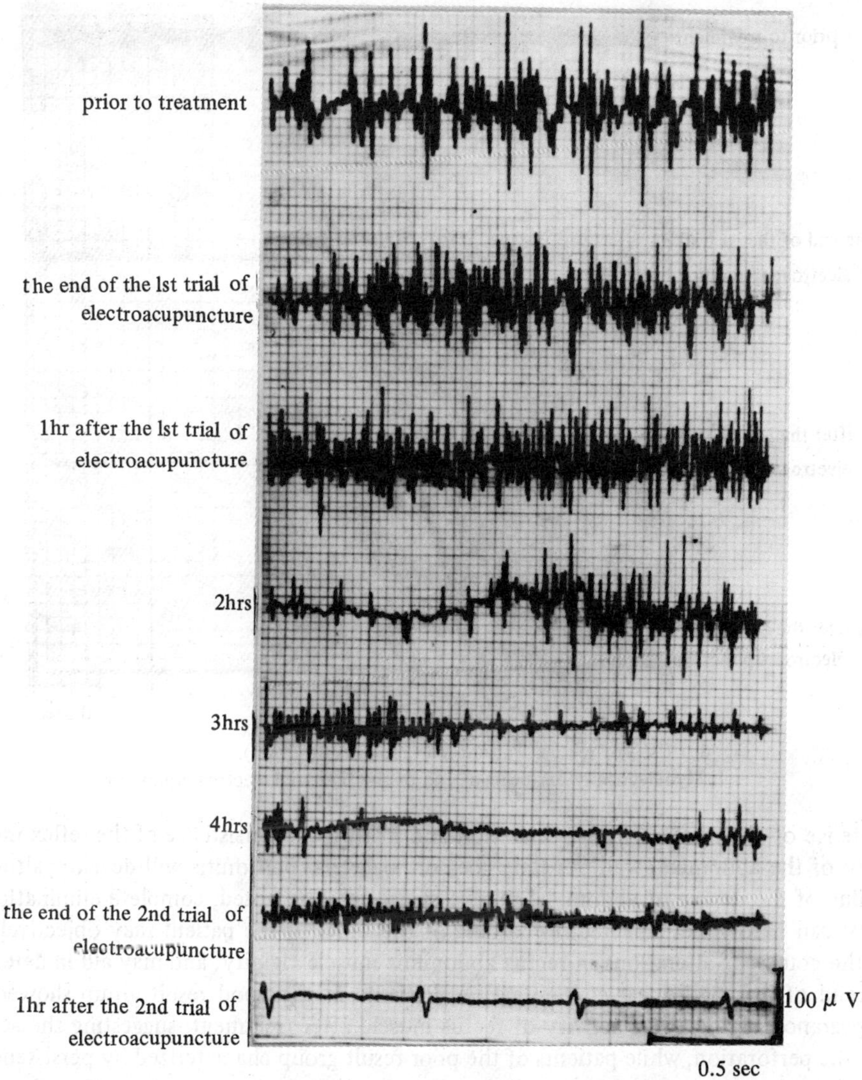

Fig. 5 EMG of rectus Patient Song (good result group). Myoelectricity disapears 1 hr after the 2nd trial of electroacupuncture.

EMG of rectus may reflect the degree of rectus abdominis muscle spasm. When perforation occurs, spillage of gastroduodenal contents in the peritoneal cavity causes chemical peritonitis, and marked peritoneal irritation by chemicals leads to rectus muscle spasm reflex. When the perforation is sealed after proper treatment the gastroduodenal contents will no longer spill out, and the loaked chemicals will gradually be diluted, neutralized and finally absorbed. Peritoneal irritation produced by the leaked chemicals will then become weaker and weaker and finally disappears, and rectus abdominis muscle spasm will be relieved accordingly and will finally disappear. On the contrary, should the perforation fail to seal, continuous spillage of the contents of the digestive tract would unavoidably cause the

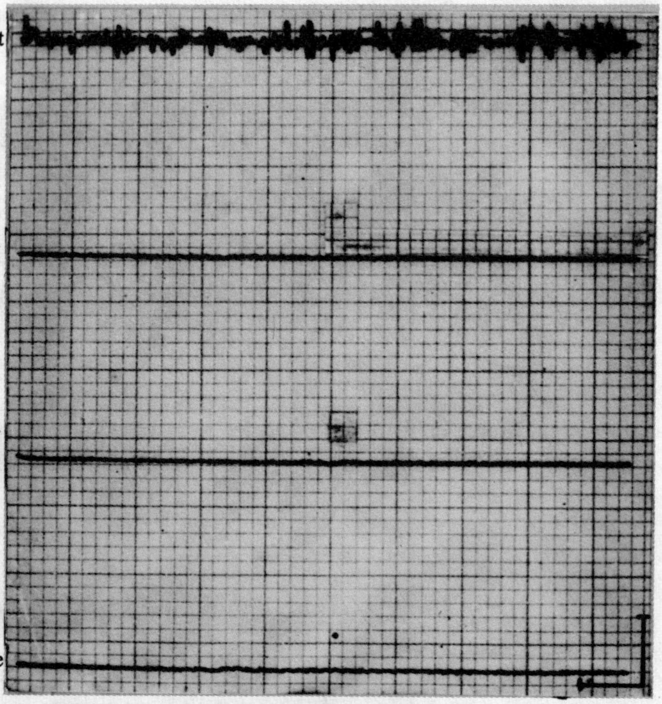

Fig. 6 EMG of rectus, Patient Yu (good result group). Myoelectricity disapears at end of the first trial electroacupuncture.

persistence of chemical peritoneal irritation and in turn the persistence of the reflex muscle rigidity of the abdominal wall. As time goes on, bacterial peritonitis will develop; although lessening of the degree of abdominal muscle spasm may be noted, complete elimination of rigidity can hardly be expected. Recording of the EMG of the patient may objectively reflect the course of alterations in rectus abdominis muscle rigidity, and may aid in detecting the trend of intraperitoneal contamination. Patients in the good result group showed the disappearance of the tonic activity of rectus muscle after treatment, suggesting the sealing up of the perforation, while patients of the poor result group characterized by persistence of rectus myoelectricity showed no sealing of perforation during operation. Therefore, the rectus myoelectricity may be considered as an indication of weather the perforation has been sealed up or not. This will decide whether the patient should be continuously treated nonoperatively or not.

(III) Relation of Needling Sensation to Therapeutic Result

In the present 41 cases, when the Zusanli point or its adjacent tender points were acupunctured, 22 out of 41 patients (53.6%) felt a needling sensation coursing towards the lesion; but for most of them, this sensation only reached beyond the knee joint, and rarely reached the lesion. The other 19 patients had only local needling sensation or felt it merely radiated to the foot. When the abdominal points were needled, 25 patients (60.9%) felt their

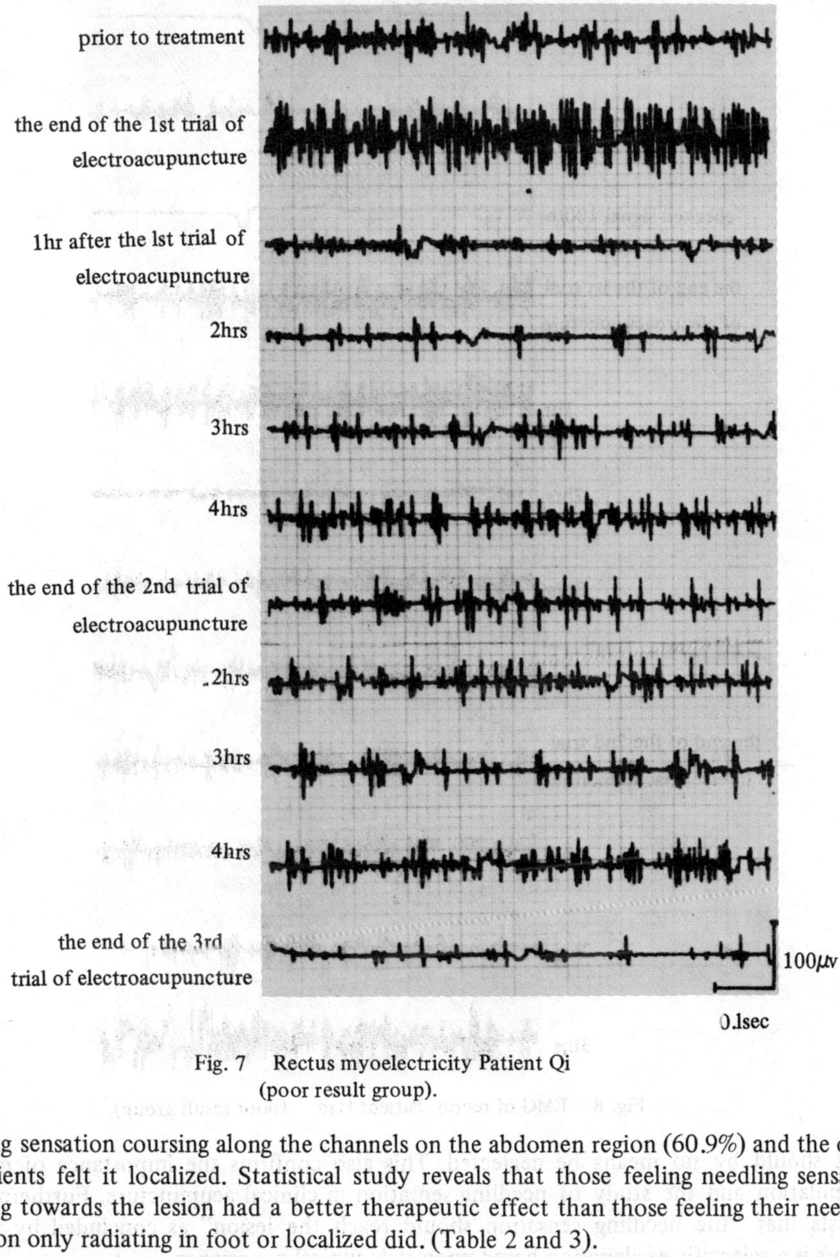

Fig. 7 Rectus myoelectricity Patient Qi (poor result group).

needling sensation coursing along the channels on the abdomen region (60.9%) and the other 16 patients felt it localized. Statistical study reveals that those feeling needling sensation coursing towards the lesion had a better therapeutic effect than those feeling their needling sensation only radiating in foot or localized did. (Table 2 and 3).

The "needling sensation" mentioned here denotes the sensation the patient felt and told about on the first trial of acupuncture during which the patient did not know why he was asked about his sensation of the needling; nor did the doctor know what the result would be; thus the acupuncture trial met to a certain degree the requirement of the "double-blind test". The above observation indicates that the relationship between the needling sensation, as to whether it is coursing towards the lesion or not, and the therapeutic

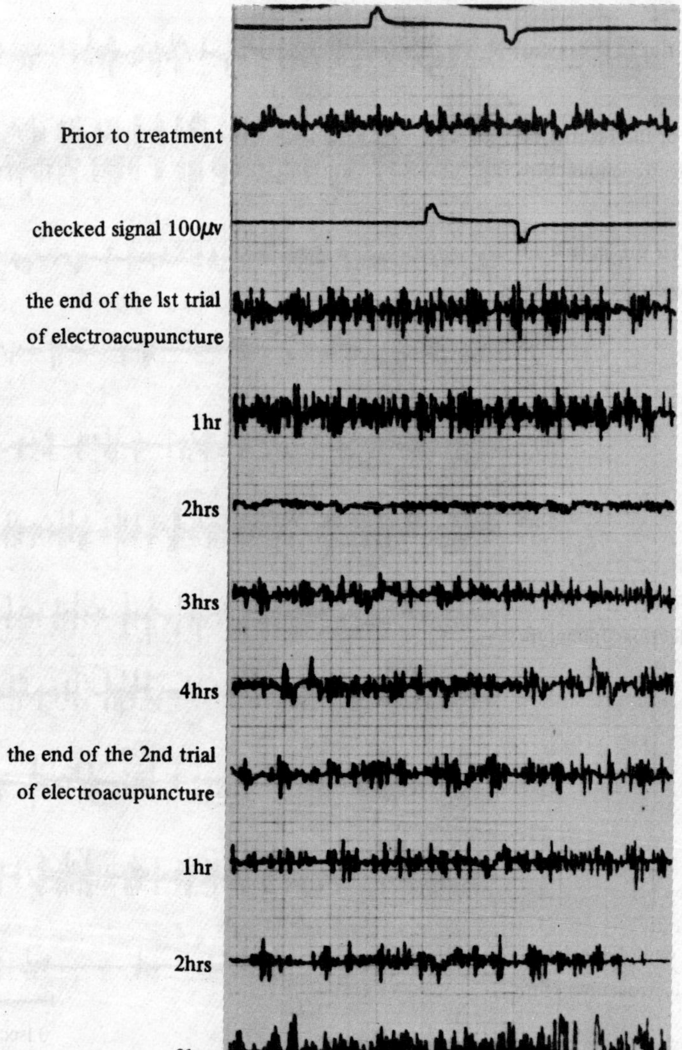

Fig. 8 EMG of rectus. Patient Han (poor result group).

result should by no means be neglected. This also confirms the importance of needling manipulation and the study of needling sensation in clinical acupuncture. Furthermore, it suggests that "the needling sensation should reach the lesion" as concluded by ancient doctors is a scientific explanation based upon rich clinical experience.

III. COMMENTS

1. More than 10,000 cases of acute perforation of peptic ulcer have been treated nonoperatively by integrating traditional Chinese and western medicines with satisfactory

Table 2. Relationship between the needling sensation on needling Zusanli point and the therapeutic result

Needling sensation	Case	Good result	poor result	% Good result	% poor result
Coursing towards the lesion	22	18	4	81.82	18.18
Localized or radiated in the foot	19	8	11	42.11	57.98
Total	41	26	15		

$X^2 = 6.9290$ $P<0.001$

Table 3. Relationship between the needling sensation on needling abdominal points and the therapeutic result

Needling sensation	Case	Good result	poor result	% Good result	% poor result
Coursing on the abdomen	25	19	6	76.00	24.00
Localized	16	7	9	43.75	56.25
Total	41	26	15		

$X^2 = 4.3716$ $P<0.05$

clinical results. 60–70% of the patients were free from the pains of operation. As a matter of fact, in this nonoperative treatment, in order to improve the therapeutic effect and to avoid any misjudgment, it is important to emphasize the importance of close observation during the first stage of treatment. The key points for improving the result of the first stage are: correct judgment of the indications for nonoperative treatment, close watch of the patients reactions during this stage of treatment, prompt decision of surgical intervention if indicated, and appropriate judgment of transferring to the second stage of treatment. Through the experiences obtained in the 41 cases under observation and investigation in the first stage treatment, we have preliminarily devised and developed some means for close watching, and found some objective criteria in evaluating the immediate effect of treatment during the acute stage and in determining the follow-up treatment in the second stage, i.e., operative or nonoperative. The criteria of rectus myoelectricity and pneumographic curve are applicable in monitoring the ulcer perforation patients in the acute stage. Judgment of the trend of the disease and the decision on the subsequent treatment (surgical intervention or continuous nonoperative treatment) based on certain objective criteria may avoid misjudgments that are entirely based on personal experience. Further clinical research on the nonoperative treatment by integrating acupuncture treatment with traditional Chinese and western medicines and efforts in the establishment of a monitoring system for patients of acute abdominal diseases will certainly raise the therapeutic levels of the treatment of such diseases and contribute to the popularization of nonoperating treatment.

2. Combined methods are generally adopted in the acute stage of treatment of acute perforation of peptic ulcer. Besides acupuncture, other methods are adopted too. For example, effective gastrointestinal decompression which by prompt suction of gastric contents will keep the stomach empty or even in a state of negative intraluminal pressure, reduce distention and promote retraction of the gastric wall, and as a result, minimize the leak of digestive contents into the peritoneal cavity. These effects are beneficial to reducing pains and promoting the sealing up of the perforation. The therapeutic effect should be attributed to the combined treatment. However, the role of acupuncture should by no means be belittled. Research data in regard with clinical acupuncture and acupuncture anesthesia and the underlying mechanism reveal that acupuncture may raise the pain threshold and the pain tolerance threshold, and adjust the secretory and motor functions of the gastrointestinal tract[3]. Acupuncture may also have an anti-inflammatory effect and accelerate the absorption of peritoneal exudate[4]. Moreover, acupuncture may promote the plugging, wrapping and adhesion of omental flap toward the perforation[4]. These acupuncture effects are of value in the treatment of ulcer perforation. We have observed the therapeutic effect on two patients of acupuncture treatment alone during the first trial of acupuncture (without gastrointestinal decompression). In the course of electroacupuncture treatment, the two patients were rapidly relieved of their pains, and put into a calm sleep state. At the end of acupuncture treatment the abdominal respiratory movement curve markedly improved with the increase of amplitude, and peristalsis began to recover. The fact that acupuncture, without G–I decompression, may also induce marked alleviation of symptoms signifies the important therapeutic action of acupuncture. Therefore, in the acute stage of treatment of acute perforation of peptic ulcer, the beneficial action of acupuncture is beyond question.

3. When perforation occurs, abdominal muscles contract reflexively to show board-like rigidity, restricting respiratory movements. In addition, because of severe pain the patient tries to restrain his respiration to a minimum, so the amplitude of abdominal respiration markdly decreases with increase of its frequency. At the end of the first trial of electroacupuncture, the patient talked of obvious relief of pain, in parallel with the improvement of the respiratory movement curve. However, at this moment EMG discharges of the rectus may not be reduced immediately, and may even be increased in some patients (Fig. 5). This fact indicates that when the patient talked of relief of pain, probably the peritoneal irritating effect of intra-abdominal chemical irritants is still not diminished accordingly, i.e., the defensive myotonic reflex at the level of the spinal cord induced by peritoneal stimulation is not suppressed. This suggests that relief of pain sensation may not be the result of diminution of pain stimulus. Experimental study in regard to the mechanism of acupuncture analgesia reveals that during acupuncture, a series of reactions are aroused in the central nervous system, such as the mobilization of intracerebral analgesic structures, release of morphine-like substances[5], alteration of neurotransmitters[6], convergences and interactions of pain signals and acupuncture signals at different levels in the center[7]. All these reactions may raise the pain threshold and the pain tolerance threshold. It seems that the analgesic effect of acupuncture in patients with acute perforation of peptic ulcer is the result of the rise of the pain and the pain tolerance thresholds. The rectus myotonic reflex elicited by peritoneal irritation can be completed at the level of the spinal cord;

and the changes in the degree of this reflex are not necessarily parallel to the relief of pain as felt by the patient. Therefore, the analgesic effect of acupuncture in the patient is likely to have been realized at higher supraspinal centers. Furthermore, the increase of abdominal respiratory amplitude may also be the consequence of pain relief.

IV. SUMMARY

1. This is a report on observation of the course of treatment in the acute stage of 41 cases of acute perforation of peptic ulcer.

2. Rectus EMG activity and pneumographic curve, reflecting certain pathological processes in the first stage, may be taken as an objective criterion for clinical monitoring in the acute stage, for the evaluation of the therapeutic effect and decision on continuing non-operative treatment or surgical intervention.

3. The relationship between needling sensation and therapeutic effect has been noted. Patients feeling a needling sensation coursing towards the lesion gained a much better result than those feeling only a local needling sensation or one coursing in the opposite direction of the lesion.

4. The role of acupuncture in the treatment of ulcer perforation is discussed.

Acknowledgments

The authors are indebted to Professor Wu Xianzhong for his valuable direction. We also thank the staff members of the Department of Surgery, Nankai Hospital, Tianjin, for their indefatigable efforts in supporting the work.

REFERENCES

[1] 天津市南开医院：中华医学杂志 54 (2): 66，1974。

[2] 天津市南开医院、天津市中西医结合急腹症研究所：中华医学杂志 57 (11): 655，1979。

[3] 上海第二医学院等：全国针灸针麻学术讨论会论文摘要(一)，第 236 页，1979。

[4] 黄观清等：全国针灸针麻学术讨论会论文摘要(一)，第 44 页，1979。

[5] 张安中等：全国针灸针麻学术讨论会论文摘要(一)，第 22 页，1979。

[6] 韩济生等：全国针灸针麻学术讨论会论文摘要(一)，第 22 页，1979。

[7] 张香桐：中国科学 4: 465，1978。

EFFECT OF NEEDLING "ZUSANLI" ON GASTROINTESTINAL FUNCTION AND ANALYSIS OF ITS AFFERENT PATHWAY

Zhuang Ding, Gao Huihe, Yang Xiuzhen,
Wang Yuanchao, Zai Shixing
(Institute of Acupuncture and Moxibustion, Academy of Traditional Chinese Medicine)

Lin Yinli, Wang Wensu, Chen Xiaomei,
Li Zhonghua, Shen Mingbao, Yu Lili
(Shanghai Second Medical College)

Jiang Songlin, Yu Bin, Li Fenglian,
Jin Guilian
(Heilongjiang College of Traditional Chinese Medicine)

Gong Qihua, Ouyang Zirong, Fan Li
(Shanghai Institute of Traditional Chinese Medicine)

Hua Xingbang, Zhang Wanwen, Qiu Yongchao,
Gong Yanhua, Zhu Lingying
(Jiangsu Institute of Traditional Chinese Medicine)

"Zusanli" is one of the commonly used points of acupuncture in clinical practice. Its significant curative effect on gastrointestinal diseases was even recognized by the ancients and there is the saying: "For abdominal diseases, leave the needle in the Sanli." In modern times, there have been many reports confirming the close relationship between the "Zusanli" point and the gastrointestinal tract.

This paper deals with the effect of needling the "Zusanli" point on gastrointestinal function and the investigation results of its relative point specificity and its possible afferent pathway.

I. THE EFFECT OF NEEDLING THE "ZUSANLI" POINT ON GASTROINTESTINAL FUNCTION AND ITS RELATIVE SPECIFICITY

(I) The effect of needling the "Zusanli" point on gastric potential (EGG) and gastric secretion.

The experiment was carried out on 7 dogs of both sexes, weighing 7.6–11 kg. They were operated on under sterile conditions. A pair of platinum electrodes of 0.5 mm in diameter was implanted in the muscular layer near the great curvature about 3–4 cm from the pylorus. The wire was passed from the peritoneal cavity and led subcutaneously to the cervical region from where it could be connected with the outside. Gastrostomy was performed at the lower end of stomach body. The experiment began after the animal had entirely recovered following 2–3 weeks' rest. Hyperactivity of stomach was produced by continuous intravenous infusion of pentagastrin (0.5–1 μg/Kg/hr). EGG was recorded by a polygraph with the time constant of 0.3 sec. Under such circumstance, the EGG pattern was characterized by an acceleration of basic rhythm as an increase of the number and amplitude of action potentials. Meanwhile, gastric juice was collected through the gastric fistula for determination of gastric acidity and cAMP content by means of the modified titration method and the saturation analysis method respectively. After pentagastrin infusion for 1 hour, the gastric acidity gradually rose to a peak and remained stable at this high level during the entire course of needling. The experiment was divided into 3 groups: electroacupuncture of the "Zusanli" point of the Stomach Channel, electroacupuncture of the "Heyang" point of the Urinay Bladder Channels and the control group without needling.

Our results demonstrate that under the influence of pentagastrin the excitability of the stomach was raised. Needling of "Zusanli" point under such background caused an inhibition and a lowering of the basic rhythm which decreased by 0.24 times/min ($P<0.05$) following 5 minutes of acupuncture and by 0.29 times/min ($P<0.01$) following 25 minutes of acupuncture. This effect declined gradually following withdrawal of the needle and would disappear complely 1 hr. after withdrawal of the needle. No marked effect was observed either on needling of "Heyang" point or in the control group. Gastric secretion was determined once every 15 minutes and 10 samples were collected in the whole course of experiment (4 samples before, 2 during, and 4 after needling). It was found that gastric acidity was decreased by needling of "Zusanli" point. The acidity measured 15 minutes following needling (5th sample) was significantly lower than that of control before needling

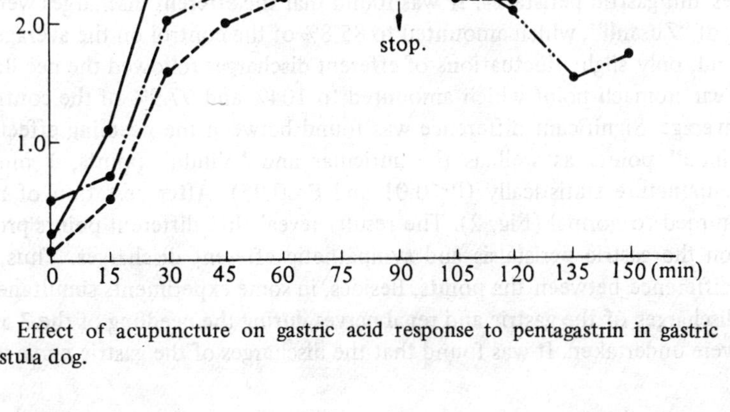

Fig. 1 Effect of acupuncture on gastric acid response to pentagastrin in gastric fistula dog.

(4th sample) ($P<0.05$) (Fig. 1). A lowering of cAMP content was observed simultaneously which paralleled with the declining tendency of gastric acidity, but its variation was not significant statistically. An aftereffect was manifested so that the depression of cAMP content did not pass away until 1 hour after needling. No evident change of gastric acidity was observed following needling of "Heyang" point, while the cAMP content was raised rather than decreased after acupuncture.

The results mentioned above demonstrate that needling of "Zusanli" point may depress the excitability of stomach smooth muscle as well as the gastric acidity under the hyperactive state of stomach produced by pentagastrin, but no marked or different effect is observed by needling of "Heyang" point. It seems that different points produce different effects under needling, so a special needling effect does exist for every point.

(II) The effects on gastric motility and the efferent discharges of the sympathetic nerve produced by needling certain points in the rabbits

67 rabbits weighing 2–3 kg were operated on under light ether anesthesia. The gastric branch and renal branch of the postganglionic fibers of the sympathetic nerve were dissected and the spontaneous discharges of them were recorded by a platinum electrode of 0.3 mm in diameter. A balloon was inserted into the stomach to record the gastric motility by pressure transducer. All animals were paralyzed by Flaxedil and artificial respiration was maintained. During experiment the nerve discharges and the gastric peristalsis were recorded intermittently before needling, 1 minute following needling and 2 minutes after cessation of needling. This sequence of experiment was repeated at intervals of 15–20 minutes. The points selected were "Zusanli" of the stomach Channel, "Yindu" of the Kidney Channel and the point of stomach on the ear. Electroacupuncture was applied by means of a G6805 stimulator, using an interrupted pulse at a frequency of 26 c/min and an intensity of 6–8 volts.

The results revealed that the gastric peristalsis was strengthened by needling of "Zusanli" point (increased by 0.8 c/min of the average), depressed by needling of "Yindu" point (reduced by 0.6 c/min) and slightly depressed by auricular acupuncture. The effect on the efferent discharges of the gastric nerve by needling was evaluated quantitatively by integrating the pulse numbers. A reciprocal interrelationship existed bytween the efferent fischarges and gastric peristalsis. It was found that the efferent discharges were decreased by needling of "Zusanli", which amounted to 85.8% of the control on the average. On the other other hand, only slight fluctuations of efferent discharges followed the needling of "Yindu" and the ear stomach point which amounted to 104% and 97.9% of the control respectively on the average. Significant difference was found between the needling effects of "Zusanli" and "Yindu" points as well as the auricular and "Yindu" points, 1 minute following electroacupuncture statistically ($P<0.01$ and $P<0.05$). After cessation of needling, all of them returned to normal (Fig. 2). The results reveal that different points produce different effects on the gastric peristalsis and sympathetic efferent discharges. Thus, there exists a certain difference between the points. Besides, in some experiments simultaneous recordings of the discharges of the gastric and renal nerves during the needling of the 3 aforementioned points were undertaken. It was found that the discharges of the gastric nerve were decreased,

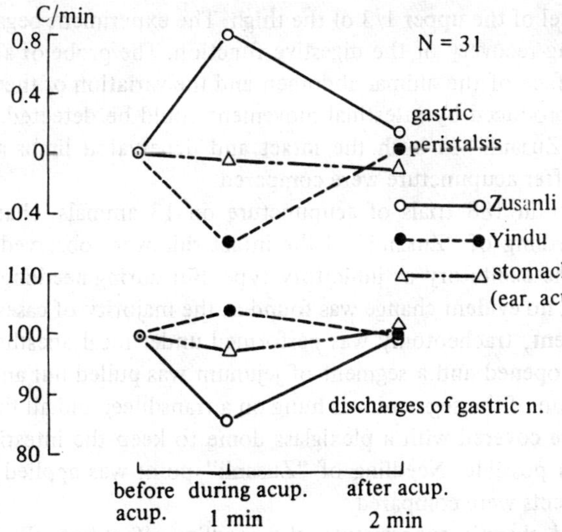

Fig. 2 Effects on gastric peristalsis and discharges of gastric n. by acupuncture of various points.

while that of the renal nerve was increased by needling of "Zusanli" point ($P<0.01$ in comparison with the control before needling; $P<0.05$ in comparison with the other nerve). On the other hand, the discharges of both nerves were increased by needling of "Yindu" point ($P<0.01$ in comparison with the control before needling; $P>0.5$ in comparison with the other nerve). No evident change in the discharges of both nerves was onserved in needling of ear points. Similar results were obtained in experiments on cats.

These results show that the gastric motility and the discharges of the gastric nerve may either be modified by either needling of "Zusanli" of "Yindu", but the patterns of modification are different. Though both discharges of the gastric and the renal nerves are affected by needling of the "Zusanli" point, the effects are different. It is thus suggested that the needling effects of "Zusanli" point is relatively specific, which is an evidence in support of the opinion of the relative specificity of the various points regarding various ponding visceral organs.

II. ANALYSIS OF THE INFLUENCE OF THE AFFERENT PATHWAY ON THE NEEDLING EFFECT OF "ZUSANLI" ON INTESTINAL MOTILITY

(I) The effect of denervation on needling effects in rabbits bothe acute and chronic experiments were performed in 40 rabbits

In chronic experiment sterile surgical operations were undertaken under pentobarbital narcosis. Median incision was made in the ipigastric region and a segment of jejunum 2–3 cm long was fixed beneath the muscular layer of the abdominal wall. A piece of magnet 3 mm in diameter was sutured into this segment. Then the sciatic nerve and femoral nerve of one side were severed at the level of the upper 1/3 of the thigh. The experiment began one week after the operation following recovery of the digestive function. The probe of a Hall Gauss meter was placed on the surface of the animal abdomen and the variation of the magnetic field of the piece of magnet produced by intestinal movement could be detected. Electroacupuncture was applied to "Zusanli" in both the intact and denervated limbs and the intestinal motilities before and after acupuncture were compared.

It was found that in 188 trials of acupuncture on 13 animals, changes in intestinal motility following needling of "Zusanli" of the intact side were observed in a majority of cases which were of the excitatory or inhibitory type. But during needling of the "Zusanli" of the denervated side, no evident change was found in the majority of cases (see table 1).

In acute experiment, tracheotomy was performed under local anesthesia and then the abdominal cavity was opened and a segment of jejunum was pulled out and fixed on a glass rod. The middle portion of the segment was hung on a transducer and all the wound and the intestinal segment were covered with a plexiglass dome to keep the intestinal segment in as normal a condition as possible. Needling of "Zusanli" point was applied before and after denervation and its effects were compared.

Both in acute and chronic experiments, the needling effect entirely disappeared after the severance of the sciatic nerve in majority animals. The difference in the needling effects of "Zusanli" before and after denervation was very significant statistically.

Table 1. Comparison between the effects of acupuncturing the intact and denervated "Zusanli" points

Groups	No. of cases				Percentage(%)			
	Marked	Not marked	No effect	Total	Marked	Not marked	No effect	Total
Needling of intact "Zusanli"	8	3	2	13	61.54	23.08	15.38	100
Needling of denervated "Zusanli"	2	3	8	13	15.38	23.08	61.54	100
Total	10	6	10	26	–	–	–	

Statistical analysis $X^2 = 7.194$ $P<0.05$

Note: Marked: Amplitude variation $\geqslant \pm 20\%$

Not marked: Amplitude variation $\geqslant \pm 10\%$

No effect: Amplitude variation $< \pm 10\%$

(II) The role of the vascular wall in needling effect

The experiments were performed on rabbits. Under urethane narcosis the sciatic nerve, femoral nerve, femur bone and all the muscles of one limb were severed, and the femoral artery and vein were left intact. Two segments of the femoral artery and vein, each 5 cm long, were dissected and the cotton threads wound around the vascular wall were used as an electrode to record the electric activity of the vascular wall. The intestinal peristalsis was recorded from the exposed segment of the intestine by means of photoelectric technique.

The effects on intestinal motility by needling the "Zusanli" of both the intact and the severed linbs and by traction of the isolated femoral artery were compared.

It was found that needling of "Zusanli" of the isolated limb in which only the femoral artery and vein were left intact still initiated intestinal movement. Similar effect was also observed during traction of the femoral artery. After block of the femoral arterial wall with 0.6 mm lidocaine, the effect persisted in half of the experiments, which was greatly attenuated following high concentration lidocaine (0.1% and 2%) block as well as painting the arterial wall with phenol. Cutting both the femoral artery and vein and recanalizing them with plastic tubes gave negative results, which was just the same as that of the blank experiment (Table 2). Simultaneous recording of the electrical activity of the arterial wall revealed that during manual needling, the amplitude of the electrical activity was often depressed, and would recover after cessation of needling. Thus, in the needling effect of "Zusanli" on intestinal motility, the vascular smooth muscle and the perivascular vegetative nerve element may have been implicated in the afferentation of the impulses.

Table 2. Analysis of affent pathway

Groups	Effect	No effect	Total
Needling intact "Zusanli"	27* (64.28%)	15 (35.72%)	42 (100%)
After cutting sciatic N., femoral N., femur bone and all the muscles of the limb, needling "Zusanli"	25 (56.81%)	19 (44.19%)	44 (100%)
During traction of femoral artery	24 (64.8%)	13 (35.2%)	37 (100%)
After block of the femoral a. wall with 0.6 mL lidocaine, needling "Zusanli"	9 (45%)	11 (55%)	20 (100%)
After block of the femoral a. wall with 0.1% lidocaine, needling "Zusanli"	9 (34.61%)	17 (65.39%)	26 (100%)
After block of the femoral a. wall with 2% lidocaine, needling "Zusanli"	9 (39.13%)	14 (60.87%)	23 (100%)
After painting the a. wall with phenol, needling "Zusanli"	4 (36.36%)	7 (63.64%)	11 (100%)
After cutting both femoral a. and v., needling "Zusanli"	8 (28.57%)	20 (71.43%)	28 (100%)
Control	28 (28.28%)	71 (71.72%)	99 (100%)

* No. of cases (percentage)

III. DISCUSSION

1. Numerous clinical and experimental studies have proved the effect of "Zusanli" on gastrointestinal function, which is also confirmed by our study. From the results mentioned above, needling of "Zusanli" in animals produces an evident influence on EGG, gastric secretion, and gastric motility as well as the efferent discharges of the gastric branch of the splanchnic nerve. Such effect is relatively specific in comparison with that induced by needling other unrelated cntrol points. But the difference is not clearcut, as needling of other points may also initiate certain more or less attenuated alterations in the gastrointestinal tract, indicating that various points may exhibit similar needling effect. Besides its effect on gastrointestinal activity, "Zusanli" may cause definite changes in the efferent discharges of the renal branch of the sympathetic nerve. On the other hand, by needling "Yindu" of the "Kidey Channel", variation in the efferent discharges may be observed accordingly not only in the renal branch but also in the gastric branch of the sympathetic nerve. These discharges present a different picture from those initiated by needling "Zusanli". Thus, acupuncture of a given point may initiate different responses in different branches of the sympathetic nerve. It is shown by numerous data[1–7] that the sympathetic control of visceral function is differentiated from that of peripheral vasomotor activity. Therefore, the different needling effects from various points are probably correlated with the segmental and central differentiation of the vegetative nervous activity. This may be considered to be the material basis of point specificity.

Besides, point specificity may also be associated with the functional state of the body. According to some reports[8], needling effect is closely related with the functional state of the organism as well as the background activity of the receptors. Our study also supports this opinion, as needling of "Zusanli" produces a suppressive action on the over-activated stomach by pentagastrin, while in a normal stomach a strengthening of gastric motility may be observed under similar circumstances. Moreover, the needling effect of "Zusanli" on intestinal motility may either be excitatory or inhibitory, depending on the functional state of the body. Thus, the needling effect of a given acupuncture point is not constant but variable. The point specificity manifests itself only under certain conditions. The linkage between acupuncture points and various visceral organs is not simple a direct relationship between two corresponding sites, but rather a morphological and functional complex which may be considered to be the basis of the readjusting mechanism of acupuncture.

2. The fact that needling of superficial body points may initiate functional changes in corresponding internal organs has been systematically described by the channel theory in ancient Chinese medical literature. Our responsibility tody is how to elucidate the mechanism of such actions with modern scientific knowledge and techniques.

Since the beginning of this century extensive studies have been made in regard with the somato-visceral sympathetic reflex[9,10], which is considered to be the basis of certain clinical therapies. It is obvious that in the needling effect on visceral functions the somato-visceral reflexes is one of its physiological bases. Profound study of somato-visceral reflex may produce more evidence for better understanding of the essence of the traditional channel theory.

As to the afferent pathway for the needling effect of "Zusanli" on gastrointestinal activites, the majority of authors propose the somatic nerves as the main route[11, 12]. In our experimentation the needling effects are greatly suppressed after severance of the sciatic and femoral nerves, indicating that the somatic nerves actually play the chief role in the propagation of needling effect. However, the study of vascular wall mentioned above presents evidence to show that the vegetative nerves on the vascular wall as well as the smooth muscle may have a part in the afferent propagation of needling effect. Therefore, it is assumed that the pathway carrying the needling effect is: needling activates certain structures of the acupuncture point, including various receptors, nerve endings and the perivascular neural elements, the excitation of which passes mainly along the somatic nerves, involving also the vascular smooth muscle and perivascular vegetative nerves. After reaching the CNS, inpulses are integrated there and then by way of the vegetative nerve system they regulate the visceral functions reflexively. As a matter of fact, the sympathetic efferent fiber is one of the important stations involved, as the efferent discharges and gastric motility are modified accordingly under the influence of acupuncture in our experiments. As to the general features of the linkage between the body surface and the visceral organs, further studies are needed.

IV. SUMMARY

1. This paper reports on the needling effect of "Zusanli" on gastrointestinal functions. The results reveal that needling of "Zusanli" may inhibit the hyperactivity of the stomach initiated by pentagastrin, both in secretion and motility, while in a normal stomach a potentiation of gastric motility is usually observed under such circumstances. The spontaneous efferent discharges of the gastric and renal branches of the sympathetic nerve are modified accordingly under the influence of acupuncture, in which a relative point specificity is noted.

2. The afferent pathway carrying the needling effect of "Zusanli" on gastrointestinal tract involves mainly the somatic nerves, but the smooth muscle on the arterial wall and the perivascular vegetative nerves may also have a part in it.

3. A tentative hypothesis for point specificity and pathway of needling effect is suggested and discussed.

REFERENCES

[1] 张锡钧、陈尚恭：生理学进展第 163 页，上海科技出版社，1963。

[2] 马如纯：生理学报 **29**; 172, 1966.

[3] Iriki, M. *et al.*: *Jap. J. Physiol.*, **22**: 585, 1972.

[4] DeLius, W. *et al.*: *Acta Physiol. Scand.*, **84**: 177, 1972.

[5] Capa B, H.K.: C C C P **45**: 65, 1959.

[6] Simon, E. *et al.*: In, *Central Rhythmic and Regulation, Circulation, Respiration, Extraphyramidal. Motor System*, edited by Umbach W. *et al.*, Hippokrates Verlag, Stuttgart, pp. 220–227, 1974.

[7] Riedel, W. *et al.*: *ibid.*, pp. 228.

[8] 西安医学院针麻理论研究组：针刺对机体的调整作用(参考资料)。

[9] Mountcastle, V. R.: *Medical Physiology,* Vol. 1. pp. 801–802, Mosby. st. Louis, 1974.

[10] Sato, A. and Schmidt, R.F.: *Physiol. Rev.,* **53**: 916, 1973.

[11] 郭协勋 等：全国中医经络针灸学术座谈会资料选编 PP：286—294，人民卫生出版社，1959。

[12] 南京第一医学院生理教研组：全国中西医结合研究工作经验交流会议资料选编，1961。

INVESTIGATION OF MECHANISM OF ACUPUNCTURE TREATMENT OF PERFORATED PEPTIC ULCER

Huang Guanqing, Tang Meilai, Wang Kaizhi, Liu Shihua
(Surgical Department, The Provincial People's Hospital of Hunan)

The combined treatment by traditional Chinese and western medicine of acute perforation of peptic ulcer is usually carried out in three stages, as formulated by the Tianjin Institute of Acute Abdomen and the Institute of Acupuncture and Moxibustion, Academy of Traditional Chinese Medicine, Beijing. Electro-acupuncture is one of the important means of treatment during the first stage. The clinical application of this means often quickly brings the treatment of acute perforation and the diffuse peritonitis it induces into the second stage, during which the abdomen becomes softer, the borborygmus audible and the bowel begins moving.

In order to investigate the mechanism of the curative effect of acupuncture by which it enhances the closure of peptic perforation, animal experiments were carried out as follows.

I. METHOD

Observation of the effect of electro-acupuncture on the anatomical relationship between the omentum and the site of artificial perforation of the stomach in the experiment animals.

Twenty-four rabbits, each weighting 2–3 kg., were equally divided into two groups: the experimental and the control. All rabbits underwent fasting before experimentation. Hairs were shaved and skin sterilized before operation. Under local infiltration with procaine, the abdomen was laid open by a median incision. A stab was made with a No. 2 scalpel into the anterior wall of the stomach 4–5 cm from the pylorus, making an artificial perforation of 0.6 × 0.6 cm in size. Gastric contents were seen spilling. Then the abdomon was closed and dressed. Parenteral fluid was given for one day under fasting after the operation. In the experimental group, bilateral Zusanli points on both legs were electrically acupunctured 4–6 times, each lasting for 15–20 minutes with an interval of 1to 2 hours. The electro-acupuncture apparatus used is Shanghai G6805. The needles are made of silver, 2.5–3 cm. long; electric current: 3–3.5 mA; and frequency: 120–250 per min. Nothing was done to the rabbits of the control group except the paranteral fluid administration under fasting. All animals were killed 17–24 hours after operation, their abdomens were again opened and examined for the relative positions of the gastric wound and the omentum.

Result. In the acupuncture group, the omentum was found closely affixed to the gastric wound in ten of the twelve rabbits and free in the remaining two. In the control group, only four out of twelve showed such adhesion and the remaining eight showed no adhesion at all. This figure is statistically significant as seen in Table 1.

Table 1.

	Total no. of animals	Relationship between the gastric wound and the omentun	
		Affixed	Free
Acupuncture group	12	10	2
Control group	12	4	8

$X^2 = 6.1704 \quad P < 0.01$

II. METHOD

Observation of the movement of the omentum toward the artificial gastric perforation through scanning the labelling ^{131}I.

Thirty rabbits, each weighing 3–2.5 kg, were equally divided into two groups. The preoperative and operative procedures as well as the acupuncture treatment in the two groups were the same as those in the above experiment. Sixty samples of isotope ^{131}I, 30–60 microcuries each (equivalent to about 6 mg in weight) were sealed in 60 tiny and air-tight plastic tubes, 5 mm long and 0.15 mm in diameter. Two of them were surgically fixed in each animal, one just above the gastric wound and the other at the lowermost edge of the omentum. All animals were scanned immediately after operation. Scanning was repeated at the 1st, 2nd, 3rd, 5th and 7th hour after electro-acupuncture with a total of six readings for each animal.

Result. A glance at the scanning maps of isotope ^{131}I would find a difference between the two groups. In the treated animals, the omentum moved toward the gastric wound in 9 of the 15 animals. But, in the control group, the omenta of only two out of the 15 rabbits showed such movement and very little movement was noted in the other 13. The statistical significance is also apparent, as shown below (Table 2).

Table 2.

	Total No. of animals	No. of animals with marked omental movement	No. of animals without marked omental movement
Acupuncture group	15	9	6
Control group	15	2	13
	$X^2 = 7.032$	$P < 0.01$	

Note: Marked omental movement means gradual and apparent shortening of the distance between the two samples of isotope ^{131}I scanning of the gastric wound and the omentum. Some of them even overlapped or joined each other finally (See Figs. 1,2).

Figs. 1 and 2 show the relative positions in a series of scanning maps of the isotopes at different times.

From the above observations, it may be concluded that electro-acupuncture can accelerate the omental movement toward the artificial gastric perforation in animals. This action probably is one of the most important factors in healing and closing of peptic ulcers in the early stage.

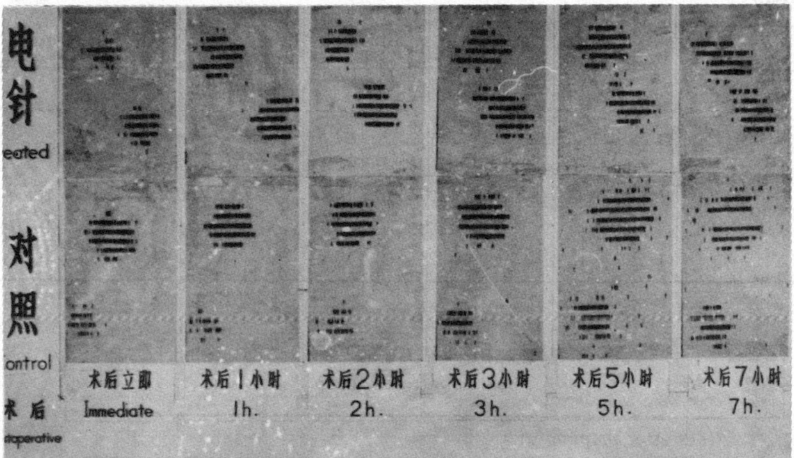

图例：大网膜与穿孔部位相对位置I^{131}同位素标记扫描图
Illustrative Case: Scanning of Relative Positions of Omentum and Perforation Marked by I^{131}

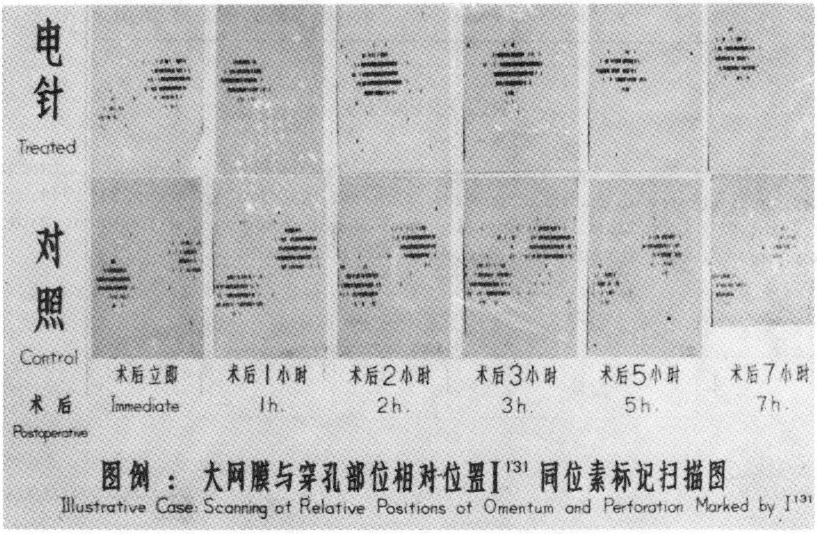

图例：大网膜与穿孔部位相对位置I^{131}同位素标记扫描图
Illustrative Case: Scanning of Relative Positions of Omentum and Perforation Marked by I^{131}

Table 3. Average distances between the two maps (the maps of the omentum and the gastric wound) in acupuncture and control animals

Table 3–1.

	Hour after acupuncture	Average distance ±standard error in cm	Compared with distance before acupuncture T	P
Acupuncture group	0	2.92		
	1	1.51 ± 0.2073	6.7773	< 0.01
	2	1.39 ± 0.3012	5.0680	< 0.01
	3	1.14 ± 0.2054	7.1086	< 0.01
	5	2.10 ± 0.1941	9.5419	< 0.01
	7	0.82 ± 0.1491	10.7551	< 0.01
Control group	0	4.11		
	1	4.02 ± 0.1860	0.5015	> 0.50
	2	4.06 ± 0.1450	0.3218	> 0.50
	3	3.94 ± 0.2142	0.6791	> 0.50
	5	3.80 ± 0.2143	1.4629	> 0.10
	7	3.35 ± 0.4725	1.5660	> 0.10

Table 3–2. Comparison of T and P between treated and controled group

Hour after acupuncture	T	P
1	5.3814	< 0.01
2	4.7066	< 0.01
3	5.4640	< 0.01
5	7.8789	< 0.01
7	9.8333	< 0.01

REFERENCES

[1] The Institute of Science and Technology, Shansi: Treatment of experimental artificial gastric perforation in rabbits with electric acupuncture, *Materials of Medical Science.* p. 21, 1974.

[2] The Institute of Traditional Chinese Medicine, Shansi: Experimental treatment with electric acupuncture in gastric perforation in rabbits, *Materials of Science.* p. 12, 1972.

OBSERVATION OF THE EFFECTS OF ACUPUNCTURE THERAPY ON VESICLE AND ANAL INCONTINENCE CAUSED BY CONGENITAL SPINA BIFIDA OVER THE LUMBOSACRAL REGION

Research Group on Vesical and Anal Incontinence, First Hospital, Bethune Medical College

Vesicle and anal incontinence caused by congenital spina bifida over the lumbosacral region is a very painful disease. Its principal manifestations are vesicle and anal incontinence, impairment or loss of sensation in the perineal region with saddle-shaped distribution and various extent of anomalies of lower extremities. It is generally recognized that such a disease is due to congenital myelospinal nerve dysplasia and/or secondary degeneration, and that it is irreversible. Hence, urinary diversion is usually performed or an electronic stimulator is to be mounted on the bladder[1,2]. Up to now, it remains a refractory disease still to be dealt with. Since 1970, 500 cases have been treated with acupuncture therapy in our hospital and the results are encouraging.

I. MATERIAL

All the patients included in this report were over 7 years old, and the diagnoses of their illness were verified by systematic physical examination, plus X-ray film, and so all cases of vesical and anal incontinence caused by factors other than congenital spina bifida were excluded.

Of the 500 patients, 326 were male and 174 female; 331 aged 7 to 15 years, 93 aged 15–20, 70 aged 20–40, and 6 over 40.

On the basis of whether a mass protruded from the spina bifida or not, they were divided into two types. There were 358 cases with mass protrusion and 142 cases without. So the former formed the dominant type and the latter was of the occult type. Vesicle and anal inconence frequently occurred after birth in the dominant type, but gradually manifested itself during the growing period in the form of the occult type as late as at age of 54.

Anal and vesical incontinence persisted in 302 cases (60.4%), who had undergone either meningomyelorrhaphy or spinaneurolysis operation half a year to ten years before the present admission.

II. THERAPEUTIC METHOD

According to the various principal symptoms and signs in different patients, different groups of points of acupuncture were selected.

1. Selection of the points (see Table 1).

Table 1. Selection of points

Main symptoms	Points selected
Unconscious dribbling of urine	Zhongji, Henggu, Sanyinjiao
Enuresis	Jiaji points over the lumbosacral segment
Dysurea	Changqiang, Huiyin, Zhibian
Anal incontinence	Changqiang, Huiyin Points around anus

The points in each group may be used continuously, alternatively or simultaneously.

2. Manipulation. Generally, needles of size 26–28 gauge were used. Insert the needle quickly with a sudden flick of the finger, and advance it with moderate strength to a depth of 1.5–2.0 cun. When the root of urethra or anus has a sense of contracting, desire to excrete or prolapse, it means the effect of needling is on, technically called "Deqi". After "Deqi", moxibustion should be applied for the first group of points and electrostimulation (Stimulator Model G 6805, made in Shanghai) with intermittent waves at intensity tolerable to the patient for the remaining groups of points. The needle is retained for 30 minutes.

3. Course of treatment. Treatment is given once a day for 10 consecutive days as a therapeutic course and, after an interval of 3–5 days, another course of treatment begins if necessory. Desire to make water mostly appeared during the first course of treatment. Generally speaking, 5–6 courses of treatment were required.

4. Things worthy of note during acupuncture therapy. All of the 80 cases who had mass protrusion (meningomyelocele) or who had spina bifida occulta with doubtful therapeutic effect or who failed to respond to acupuncture therapy due to bombardment of the protruded mass were all operated on by meningomyelorrhaphy or spinoneurolysis. Nevertheless, the postoperative incontinence should still be treated by acupuncture. During the course of acupuncture therapy, attention should be paid to the functional exercise of urination and defecation, training the patients to know the desire to void, and treating the complication of urinary infection with antibiotics and herb drugs in time. All of these measures served to consolidate and promote certain acupuncture therapeutic effects.

III. THERAPEUTIC RESULTS

1. Criteria of therapeutic effects. According to the changes of the main clinical symptoms and signs, residual urine and uroflow rate, etc., the therapeutic effects were determined and divided into three groups:

(1) Excellent: Dribbling of urine basically stopped with stable sense for urination which could be controlled for more than two hours during the day, and enuresis at night ceased, and defecation could be controlled basically. The residual urine was reduced to zero or less than half the volume before treatment, and the uroflow rate was markedly improved.

(2) Improved: Sense of urination restored with only occasional dribbling of urine. Urination could be controlled for more than one hour during the day time, and enuresis only occurred occasionally at night. Anal incontinence ensued as liquid stool appeared. Residual urine was less than pre-therapy and the uroflow rate was slightly ameliorated.

(3) Ineffective: There was no significant change after the acupuncture therapy. Among them were those with whom the treatment was effective but the effectiveness did not last.

2. Analysis of the therapeutic results. After the acupuncture therapy, judged from the above criteria, the results are as follows:

Excellent in 97 cases (19.4%), improved in 327 cases (65.4%), and ineffective in 76 cases (15.2%).

Analysis and comparison of the main symptoms and special findings before and after acupuncture are presented below:

(1) Clinical symptoms: The clinical symptoms were improved after the therapy (see Table 2).

(2) EMG: Electromyograph of external urethral and anal sphincteric muscles had been recorded since 1973. The differences between the patient and the normal control groups are as follows:

(a) At rest. Fibrillation potentials were found in both sphincteric muscles of the patients, but none in the normal control group.

(b) During contraction. All the subjects in the normal control group showed increasing of the electric activity with the formation of an interferential type in most of them, while in most of the patients no electric activity was observed. Even though a few of them had some scanty electric activity, they could never attain the interferential type.

Table 2. Improvement of symptoms after acupuncture therapy

Symptoms \ Cases	Before therapy	After therapy	Improved cases (%)
No sense of urination	455	81	374 (82.0)
Dribbling of urine	472	98	374 (79.2)
Enuresis	478	114	364 (75.0)
Anal incontinence	433	60	373 (90.9)

(c) The duration of motor unit potentials in both urethral and anal sphincteric muscles of the patients was remarkably prolonged in comparison with that of the subjects in the normal control group.

The above changes indicated that the EMG of both sphincter muscles of the patients were abnormal, and corresponded to the EMG patterns of muscular atrophy due to lower motor neuron lesions.

Comparison of the EMG patterns before and after treatment shows that therapeutic results would be poor when EMG had no reaction both before and after treatment, while it would be better when EMG had some reaction even before treatment.

3. Measurement of the residual urine and uroflow rate[3]. Since 1974, in order to get objective evidence to judge therapeutic effects, the residual urine volumes of 240 patients were measured before and after complete treatment with the SSL–31 A–2 type of sonolayergraph made in Japan (the anterior and posterior diameters of the fluid level in the

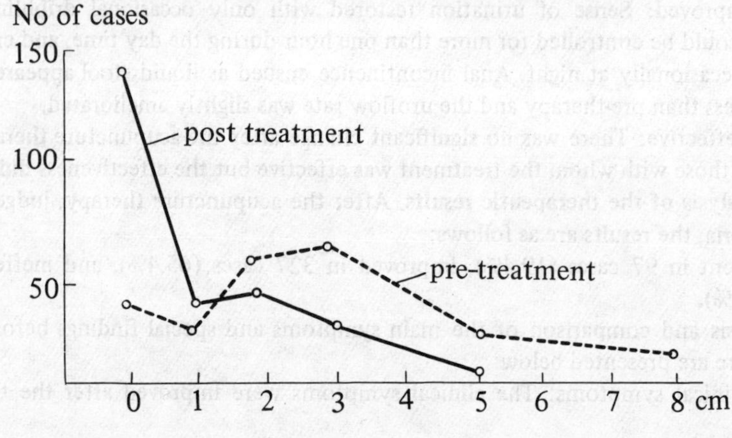

Fig. 1 Comparative diagram of residual urine columes of 240 patients pre- and post-treatment.

bladder was expressed in centimeters). At the same time the uroflow rates were calculated from the recorded curves made with the Mingograph 34 type uroflowmeter made in Sweden. From the recorded curves the mean maximum urinating rate (F, ml/sec.), the mean maximum urine volume (V, ml.) and the urinating time (S, sec.) could be calculated. The results obtained with the two medical instruments are given in Fig. 1 and Table 3, respectively.

It is demonstrated in Fig. 1 that the number of cases in which residual urine completely disappeared after acupuncture therapy was remarkably increased, while in the rest of them it also more or less decreased.

It can be seen in Table 3 that the patients' maximum urinating rates and volumes were all increased after treatment and the residual urine volumes were decreased, with $P<0.01$. It is suggested that the functions of urination and evacuation of the bladder were all improved under acupuncture therapy. The urinating time was slightly shortened in the adult group, but $P>0.05$, so the decrease has no statistical significance. In the children group, the urinating time was prolonged which was compatible with its clinical changes, because the patients could only expel a small amount of urine each time, or only dribble before

Table 3. Comparison between the residual urine volumes and the uroflow rates before and after acupuncture therapy in 240 patients

Items measured	Children group 167 cases		Adult group 73 cases	
	Increased values	P-value	Increased values	P-value
Max. urinating rate (ml/sec)	5.7 ± 0.51	< 0.01	5.2 ± 0.93	< 0.01
Urination volume (ml)	66.0 ± 6.2	< 0.01	58.0 ± 10.5	< 0.01
Urinating time (sec)	4.4 ± 1.87	< 0.05	−0.8 ± 1.54	> 0.05
Residual urine volume (cm)	−1.4 ± 0.11	< 0.01	−1.7 ± 0.21	< 0.01

acupuncture therapy, but after therapy, urinating volume each time was increased; therefore the urinating time was prolonged. It means that the patients still passed urine with difficulty after treatment.

4. Follow-up studies. 234 cases with improvement at discharge were followed up for 1–9 years. Those cases in which the therapeutic results at discharge were maintained stable were considered as "effect persisted", those that were not as "effect decreased", and those that disappeared completely or regressed to the pretreatment state, as "effect vanished".

The follow-up results are shown in Table 4.

Table 4. Follow-up studies

Remote effect	Effect persisted	Effect decreased	Effect vanished
Cases	91	70	67
%	38.9	29.8	28.9

Six patients (2.4%) died during this period because of severe urinary tract infection and uremia.

IV. DISCUSSION AND SUMMARY

The incidence of vesicle and anal incontinence caused by congenital spina bifida remains obscure, but the incidence of spina bifida is not rare. According to foreign reports, there might be one dominant type in 5,000–10,000 newborns and one occult type in 2–4 newborns[4]. Among the 3,003 persons surveyed in the forest region of Dashitou and the mine area of Liaoyuan in Jilin province from 1975–1976 there was one belonging to the dominant type and 1,019 (34%) of the occult type. Therefore, it is inferred that vesicle and anal incontinence caused by spina bifida would not be too rare. It is known that the vesical and rectal dysfunction, loss of sensation of urination, dribbling of urine, residual urine, anal incontinence and loss of sensation at the saddle area over the perinium are caused by congenital degeneration of spinal nerve. All of these manifestations should be considered as impairment of spinal nerve function. In addition, it was proved by the EMG patterns of urethral and anal external sphincters[5].

It was recognized that such neuro-lesions could not recover spontaneously, so that spinoneurolysis or urinary diversion was often performed. According to foreign reports, in order to control urination artificially, an electronic stimulator had been mounted to the detrusor urinae or muscles at the pelvic floor. All of these measures are not aimed at the recovery of urination function in the patients themselves.

According to the theory of traditional Chinese medicine, kidney is the source of heredity, kidney controls water circulation and water metabolism within the organism, and kidney controls bone and marrow production; and according to the theories about that both "Ren" and "Du" channels are originated from "Baozhong" (after birth) and come out from the perineum, etc., it is considered that this kind of disease is originated from an inherent shortage of vital energy in the kidney and from the fire decline in the "Mingmen", so they cannot warm up the urinary bladder, and as a result, both urination and defecation are interrupted. Therefore, acupuncture therapy was suggested to treat the disease and the points along the kidney, urinary bladder, "Ren" and "Du" Channels were selected. It has been proved in practice that the short-term acupuncture therapeutic effective rate for the disease was 84.8%. The long-term therapeutic effect as follow up investigation for 1–9 years show there are 38.9% patients who kept the level of therapeutic effect at discharge. Their sense for urination, dribbling of urine and ability to control urination improved or recovered to various degrees. The decreased residual urine volume, increased uroflow rate and urinating volume of urine discharged each time after acupuncture therapy indicated that such a treatment was effective, and the results obtained were mainly due to the recovery of the discharging power and the function of urination of the bladder. Besides, the function of defecation was improved too. Before the treatment, the patients could not feel the urge for defecation and the stool turned into dried hard balls that were not evacuated consciously and sometimes dropped out from the rectum spontaneously. After therapy, patients obtained the sense for defecation, the stool balls changed into soft strips and could be evacuated voluntarily. All of these changes indicated that the function of defecation and the peristalsis of the intestine were restored.

It can be seen that acupuncture based upon the theories of Chinese traditional medicine has positive therapeutic effects on this disease, either in function of urination or in defecation. Everybody knows that the function of degenerated spinal nerves can hardly be restored by acupuncture therapy, but, the above concrete therapeutic results are facts and as such must have a material basis. We infer that the incompletely degenerated nerves and their related Channels may have developed a certain ability of adaptation and compensation following acupuncture therapy. As a result, the function of urination and defecation is improved. Although the underlying mechanism is not yet clear, the acupuncture treatment is simple and easy to practice, with satisfactory therapeutic effect, painless and therefore highly appreciated by the patients. Especially the treatment can promote the recovery of physiological functions which can hardly be achieved through other therapeutic means. 302 cases (60.4%) of the patients had undergone meningomyelorrhaphy and/or spinoneurolysis before admission without being completely cured. Vesicle and anal incontinence was completely stopped by acupuncture. However, patients of the dominant type, i.e., with spinal protrusion mass had frequent relapse of symptoms due to compression of the protrusion mass during therapy, so operation was again called for. Acupuncture and operation should be coordinated and complementary to each other so as to raise the therapeutic effect.

As this is a congenital disease, many of the patients never felt the desire to void and never urinated actively. Therefore during the treatment, attention should be paid to train them how to urinate by themselves. On the other hand, the disease is a rather complex one and is frequently complicated by urinary infection and even chronic renal dysfunction. Since 1975, 98 (46.5%) out of 211 cases have been found to have urinary infection, BUN increased in 62 of 336 cases, and PSP tests were below normal limits in 54 (30.7%) of 176 cases, but the PSP data were often distorted by the dysfunction of urination and residual urine, and were not completely reliable. We had tried to make PSP test by catheterism, but this was given up because it often caused urinary infection. Urinary infection should be controlled promptly with drugs. All of these factors would exert certain effects on the elevation and consolidation of the therapeutic effect of acupuncture.

In light of our experiences, children below 6 years old of age should not be admitted for such acupuncture treatment, because they would not cooperate in it.

As to the mechanism by which this disease is cured by acupuncture, further investigation is required.

REFERENCES

[1] Merrill, D.C.: *J. Urol.*, **112**: 823, 1974.

[2] Merrill, D.C.: *J. Urol.*, **113**: 335, 1975.

[3] Iwatsubo, E. *et al.*; *J. Urol.*,**114**: 871, 1975.

[4] Badell-Ribera, *A. et al.*: *Arch. Phys. Med.*,**45**: 443, 1964.

[5] Dept. of New Traditional Medicine and Dept. of Physiology, Jirin Medical College: *J. Jilin Medical College*, **2**: 93, 1975.

THE INDUCTION OF LABOR BY ELECTROACUPUNCTURE STIMULATION — ANALYSIS OF 771 CASES

Zhu Renlie, Gao Xiuhui, Zhou Yulian, Yu Jin
(Hospital of Obstetrics & Gynecology, Shanghai First Medical College)

In obstetrics, when pregnancy is complicated by medical and surgical diseases, postmaturity, fetoplacental dysfunction or toxaemia etc., prompt termination of pregnancy is often indicated. As the mechanism of the initiation of labor is still not clearly understood, obstetricians are still looking for a simple, effective and safe method for starting labor. Electroacupuncture, a combination of modern technique and traditional Chinese medicine, is now a new method for induction of labor in obstetrics.

I. MATERIAL AND METHODS

Between January 1977 and October 1978 labor was induced by electroacupuncture in 771 pregnant women for postmaturity and premature rupture of membranes. 604 were primiparas (78.43%), and 167, multiparas (21.66%). The duration of gestation ranged between 37–44 weeks. In another 118 cases, labor was induced by intravenous pitocin drip as a control for comparison.

Preinductional preparations. In cases not in labor but with prematurely ruptured membranes, electroacupuncture was employed shortly after rupture without additive preparation. The cases with intact membranes were divided into two groups: 216 cases admitted in 1977 were given enemas before induction; 157 cases treated in 1978 were given enemas first, then stripped of membranes.

Urinary pergnandiol and blood cortisol were determined from urine 12 hours before induction and 6 hrs after acupuncture.

Acupuncture points and stimulation parameters. The points were "Hegu" on the hand and "Sanyinjiao" on the ipsilateral lower leg. The electrostimulator was connected to the needle after the needling sensation was felt, and the intensity of stimulation regulated to the patient's tolerance. Two types of electroacupuncture apparatus were used, one, a DF–1 model with a frequency of 300 cycles per second, producing alternate biphastic square waves of 3 msec wave length; the range of output is 5–15 volts. The other was a BT–701 model with frequency of 120 cycles per second, producing monophasic sharp peaked waves; the wave length was 0.5 msec and the output about 6 V.

Our criterion for success of induction in cases with ruptured membranes is labor commencing within 24 hrs after acupuncture. In cases with intact membranes, the limit of commencement of labor is extended to 48 hrs. The same criterion is applied to the control group.

II. RESULTS

In the present study, labor was induced by electroacupuncture in 771 cases; 556 cases were successful (72.11%), 215 cases failed (27.89%). Of the 118 cases induced by pitocin drip, 83 cases were successful (70.34%), 35 cases failed (29.66%). There is no significant difference in success rates of the two groups.($P > 0.05$).

Some of the results of induction by different methods in the literature are as listed below (Table 1).

The results of electroacupuncture induction in relation to the condition of the membranes, ruptured or not are shown in Table 2, and the relation of results to parity in Table 3.

The above tables reveal a higher success rate in cases with ruptured membranes than in those with membranes intact ($P < 0.01$). There is no statistical difference between parities ($P > 0.05$).

Comparison of results of different types of electrostimution. Among 424 cases using the square wave stimulation for induction, a success rate of 69.34% was obtained, and for 347 cases using sharp wave stimulation the success rate obtained was 75.5%. There was no significant difference statistically ($P > 0.05$).

Effects of preinductional procedures. Stripping of membranes was not used in 1977. In 1978, membranes were stripped before induction (Table 4). There is no statistical difference between the two groups.

The results of induction by electroacupuncture in relation to pelvic scoring. Pelvic scoring represents an estimation of the conditions of the cervix and the presenting part of the fetus before induction. The criteria of pelvic scoring were as follows (Table 5).

In the present study, pelvic scoring was adopted in 222 cases (Table 6).

The relationship between pelvic scoring and the results of induction may be more accurately reflected after ruling out other factors such as multiparity, ruptured membranes, etc. 133 cases were chosen according to these conditions (Table 7).

From the above two tables, it may be seen that the rates of success rise with the increases in scoring. To draw an arbitrary line between score number 6 and 7 there exists a significantly higher success rates in the latter group (7 or more) ($P < 0.01$). This shows the important role of the cervical status in relationship to the success of induction. The riper the cervix, the higher the success rate.

Changes of pregnandiol pre- and post-induction of labor by electroacupuncture. Progesterone is one of the main hormones for maintenance of pregnancy and its level rapidly drops before the initiation of labor. Cortisol at a certain level is considered to be the "trigger" of the initiation of labor.

The values of pregnandiol and cortisol before and after electroacupuncture induction were evaluated in a limited number of cases (Tables 8, 9).

The mean cortisol level in the successful group was higher than that in the unsuccessful group. The preinductional mean values of pregnandiol were higher than the postinductional values in both groups.

Table 1. Results of induction by various methods

Authors	Year	Cases	Methods of induction	Success rate	Complications
Tsuei[3]	1977	47	Electroacupuncture	78%	None
Spellacy[6]	1973	115 107	$PGF_2\alpha$ Pitocin	74.5% 66.4%	Phlebitis, Hypertonisity of contraction
Anderson[9]	1972	46 27	$PGF_2\alpha$ Pitocin	79.6% 85.2%	Hypertonisity of contraction
Karim[6]	1971	100	$PGF_2\alpha$ Pitocin	67% 56%	Hypertonisity of contraction
Peterson[7]	1965	Primiparous 63 Hultiparous 260	Spartein	51% 65%	None
Yip[8]	1973	57	PGE_2 (oral)	80%	None
Present study		771 118	Electroacupuncture Pitocin	72.11% 70.34%	None

Table 2. Results of groups with ruptured and with intact membranes

Membranes	Wave type	No. of success	%	No. of failure	%	Total: No. of cases	Total: Success rate	P
Ruptured	Square	169	76.47	52	23.53	221	80%	< 0.01
	Sharp	149	84.12	28	15.88	177		
Intact	Square	125	61.58	78	38.42	203	63.8%	
	Sharp	113	66.47	57	33.53	170		
		556	72.11	215	27.89	771		

Table 3. Comparison of the results between parities

Parities	Membranes	No. of success	%	No. of failure	%	Total: No. of cases	Total: Success rate	P
Primiparas	Ruptured	258	79.95	73	22.05	604	70.86%	> 0.05
	Intact	170	62.27	103	37.73			
Multiparas	Ruptured	60	89.55	7	10.45	167	76.64%	
	Intact	68	68.00	32	32.00			
		556	72.11	215	27.89	771		

Table 4. Comparison of results of membranes stripped and not stripped

Membranes	No. of cases	No. of success	%	No. of failure	%	P
Stripped	216	132	61.11	84	38.89	> 0.05
Not stripped	157	109	69.42	48	30.58	

Table 5. Pelvic scoring

Score	0	1	2	3
Cervical dilation (cm)	0	1–2		
Effacement (%)	0–30	40–50	60–70	80
Consistency	firm	medium	soft	
Position	post.	mid.	ant.	
Station	–3	–2	–1~0	+1~+2
Birth weight	>4000	3500~	3000~	< 3000
Total				

Table 6. Pelvic scores and success rate

Scores	2	3	4	5	6	7	8	9	10	11	12	Total
Success	4	9	16	25	27	22	25	28	17	3	1	177
Failure	1	2	9	12	12	4	2	2	1	0	0	45
Fractional success rate	81/117 = 69.2%					96/105 = 91.4%						
P	< 0.01											

Table 7. Pelvic scores and success rate (ruling out nonpelvic factors)

Scores	2	3	4	5	6	7	8	9	10	11	12	Total
Success	3	3	6	10	12	13	14	18	10	2	1	92
Failure	1	2	9	9	12	3	2	2	1	0	0	41
Fractional success rate	34/67 = 50.7%					58/66 = 87.9%						
P	< 0.01											

Table 8. Plasma cortisol levels (Radioimmunoassay)

Success					Failure				
Parity	Weeks	Birth Weight	Preinduction μg/100ml	Postinduction μg/100ml	Parity	Weeks	Birth Weight	Preinduction μg/100ml	postinduction μg/100ml
G_2P_0	42	3320	55	18	G_1P_0	41	3400	28	14
G_1P_0	42	3300	9.5	14.5	G_1P_0	42	4080	14.5	14.5
G_1P_0	42	3600	26.5	3.6	G_1P_0	42	3400	55	18
G_2P_0	42	3800	50	35	G_1P_0	42	3700	13.5	38
G_3P_1	42	3650	35	55	G_1P_0	42	3300	39.6	17
G_1P_0	42	3580	15	19	G_1P_0	43	4100	74	70
G_1P_0	43	3350	75	112					
G_1P_0	42	3400	54	105					
G_1P_0	42	3150	60	66					
G_1P_0	42	3150	47	22.5					
Mean values			42.7	45.0				37.4	28.6

Table 9. Urinary pregnandiol level (Gas chromatography)

Success					Failure				
Parity	Weeks	Birth Weight	Preinduction mg/12hrs	Postinduction mg/12hrs	Parity	Weeks	Birth Weight	Preinduction mg/12hrs	Postinduction 12hrs
G_2P_1	42	3320	33.75	27.8	G_1P_0	41	3400	22.43	10.21
G_1P_0	42	3300	15.04	13.94	G_1P_0	42	3020	15.2	14.28
G_2P_0	42	3800	11.83	14.18	G_1P_0	42	4280	25.91	8.98
G_1P_0	42	3150	20.2	4.46	G_1P_0	42	3400	16.93	20.81
					G_1P_0	43	4100	25.54	15.44
Mean values			20.3	15.1				21.2	13.94

The status of the newborn. Two pairs of twins were among the 556 cases of successfully induced labor, making the total of infants 558. The birth weights of 22 infants were ⩾ 4000 g; 528 infants, 2501–3999 g; and 8 infants ⩽ 2500 g. There was one stillbirth due to rupture of a blood vessel of a velamentous placenta, and a neonatal death due to prolapse of the cord. The remaining infants were born alive and well. This indicates that induction by this method produces no deleterious effect on the infant.

III. DISCUSSION

The use of electroacupuncture to induce labor is a new method in obstetric practice. The results presented in this study, and from the literature, indicate that its effectiveness is comparable to induction by pitocin drip. Moreover, there were neither side effects such as nausea, vomitting or phlebitis as those occurring in prostaglandin induction, nor hypertonic uterine contractions as those sometimes occurring with pitocin drips. We consider it to be a simple, safe and effective method for induction of labor.

The main factors affecting the results of this method are rupture of the membranes and ripeness of the cervix. If membranes are not ruptured, softening and ripeness of the cervix is the main factor to be considered before induction. Any method of induction is unlikely to succeed with an unloosened, unsoftened cervix, as seen by a significantly higher success rate with pelvic scores of 7 or more in comparison to scores of 6 or less in our data. Turnbull *et al.*[4] showed when the level of blood estradiol rises, the cervix becomes softened and relaxed, and the same result can be obtained by an intravenous drip of 17β-estradiol. According to Gustavii[5], decidual lysosomes might be of significance in the initiation of labor. Lysosomal phospholipase A_2 is released into the cytoplasm which triggers increased prostaglandin synthesis. These effects are said to be induced by altered levels of sex steroids, namely a rise in estrogen and the decline of progesterone. Thus one may consider injecting estradiol first when attempting to induce labor in a pregnant woman with a stiff cervix.

Results show no statistical difference between cases with stripped membranes and those without, indicating that it was electroacupuncture, but not stripping of membranes that was responsible for the success of induction.

The exact mechanism of electroacupuncture induction of labor has not yet been clearly understood. Relevant investigations[3] show that there is a definite relationship between acupuncture and the autonomic nervous system. Acupuncture of the "Renzhong" point results in a sympathomimetic reaction of the cardiovascular system. Administration of propranolol prior to acupuncture of "Renzhong", inhibits the sympathomimetic effect. Stimulation of the "Zusanli" point results in a parasympathomimetic-like reaction of the cardiovascular system.

Stimulation of "Sanyinjiao" produces effects within the area of the L4 dermatone, in which the point is located. Uterine activity is controlled by the sympathetic nerve system. The stimulation of acupuncture of "Sanyinjiao" possiblly passes through the pelvic plexus which receives preganglionic fibers from T5 to L4, and alters the physiologic function of the uterus, causing it to contract. The effect of acupuncture on "Hegu" is believed[3] to be mediated through the central nervous system, but this has not yet been fully confirmed.

Based upon observations of the uterine contractions among our cases, we found two types of uterine response; one, the uterus responds by contraction only under continuous needle stimulation, but the contraction ceased as soon as the needles withdrawn; in the other, uterine contractions continue until delivery despite cessation of needle stimulation. It is assumed that in the former, needle stimulatory effect is probably effected through transmission via the nervous system, and in the latter it is probably not only neural, but also hormonal[1]:

In regard to the hormonal factor in the initiation of labor views differed formerly. It was believed that during pregnancy the gradual rise of progesterone inhibits nervous transmission and activities of the uterine musculature, thus maintaining pregnancy. Prior to delivery, the level of progesterone rapidly falls and the uterine musculature is released from the inhibition and labor ensues. This view is mainly based on animal experiments. There is dispute in regard to events in the human being, because the level of progesterone does not invariably fall before the onset of labor; moreover, injection of progesterone does not delay the natural course of labor[2].

In a few determinations made by us, the mean preinductional level of pregnandiol is higher than that 6 hrs after acupuncture in both successful and unsuccessful groups. However, among the cases classified as failures, labor commenced within 72 hrs. These results seem to be compatible with the concept of the relationship between the decline of progesterone level and the initiation of labor.

Recently, it is said[2] that the fetus is involved in the initiation of labor. When the fetus matures, its pituitary releases a large amount of ACTH, which promotes increased production of fetal cortisol, acting on the placenta and causing a release of more estrogen and a diminished production of progesterone. Meanwhile, the synthesis of prostaglandin in the decidua also increases. The rising estrogen then acts on the maternal pituitary causing release of pitocin. Under such conditions, the uterus begins to contract regularly. Thus, it is considered[5] that cortisol acts as a trigger in the initiation of labor. Our few cortisol determinations show that the preinductional levels of cortisol among successfully induced cases are higher than those of the failed ones. This, it seems, is compatible with the above viewpoint; however no conclusions can be drawn yet because of the limited number of cases.

SUMMARY

1. The labor of 771 pregnant women between 37–44 weeks of gestation was induced by electroacupuncture with a success rate of 72.11%, similar to the success rate of 70.34% of intravenous pitocin drip induction.

2. The main factors affecting the results of electroacupuncture induction are prelabor pelvic scoring and whether the membranes are ruptured or not. The higher the score, the greater the chance for success, and a higher success rate occurs in cases with ruptured membranes.

3. The relationship of progesterone and cortisol to initiation of labor was observed, but no conclusion can be drawn due to the limited number of cases.

4. The mechanism of electroacupuncture induction of labor is discussed, although it is not yet clearly understood.

REFERENCES

[1] 浙江大学:«针刺与内脏器官功能的关系»。1972 年参加全国针麻会议资料。
[2] 朱岩平:«国外避孕研究进展» 43～80 页,上海避孕药领导小组办事处编印 1977。
[3] Tsuei, J. J.: *Obstet. & Gynecol.*, **50**:479, 1977.

[4] Turnbull, A.C. *et al.*: *Lancet*, **1**:101, 1974.
[5] Gustavii, B.: *Brit. J. Obstet. & Gynecol.*, **82**:117, 1975.
[6] Spellacy, W.N. *et al.*: *Obstet. & Gynecol.*, **41**(1):14, 1973.
[7] Peterson, W.F.: *Obstet. & Gynecol.*, **26**:408, 1965.
[8] Yip, S.K.: *Brit. J. Obstet. & Gynecol.*, **80**:442, 1973.
[9] Anderson, G.G. *et al.*: *Am. J. Obstet. & Gynecol.*, **112**:382, 1972.

ACUPUNCTURE TREATMENT OF PERIPHERAL FACIAL PARALYSIS

Yang Zhaomin
(*Nanjing College of Traditional Chinese Medicine*)

Wang Juming, Hu Ningqi
(*The Research Institute of Traditional Chinese Medicine of Jiangsu Province*)

Clinically, facial paralyses are classified into two categories, namely the central and the peripheral facial nerve paralyses. The main manifestation is disturbance of the movement of the mimetic muscles on one side, resulting in a state of paralysis, which is known as facial paralysis. It is a frequent disorder in neurology. We have separately applied body and auricular acupuncture to treat 46 cases of peripheral facial paralysis. Satisfactory results have been obtained. We have also used electromyogram to observe EMG changes of facial muscles in some cases before and after needling. The results show that acupuncture exerts an obvious influence on EMG changes.

I. CLINICAL DATA

(I) Cases for Observation

Cases of simple peripheral facial paralysis with typical symptoms and signs, such as difficulty in frowning and shutting eyes and deviation of the mouth, are mainly selected. Acupuncture therapy was applied to those cases, the majority of which had been treated with Chinese and Western drugs or physical therapy without obvious improvement. During acupuncture treatment, other therapies were stopped.

(II) General Data

A total of 46 cases were studied in this group. Among them 21 cases were male and 25 female. The youngest was 14 years old, the eldest 61. 40 cases were in the age between 21 to 50. Up to the moment of acupuncture treatment, the shortest history of the disease was 3 days, the longest 22 years, while 38 cases had been ill for 8 to 25 days. There were 4 other cases who were old sufferers of the disease.

(III) Etiology

Cause of disease: 6 cases were caused by otitis media and cervical lymphadenitis, 2 cases were due to traumatic injuries, 2 cases of herptic paralysis, while the other 36 cases were due to exposure to cold or causes still unknown, but all fell victim to the illnesses suddenly.

(IV) The Site of Paralysis

20 cases were left sided, 24 cases right sided and in 2 cases the paralysis was initially on the right side and then shifted to the left.

(V) Previous Treatments

27 cases had been treated with western drugs, such as hormone, vitamins, oryzanol and dibazol, 15 cases with Chinese drugs. acupuncture physiotherapy and massage, and 4 cases with application of eel's blood or ointment on the affected side.

(VI) EMG Findings Before Treatment

The results suggested that the facial muscles (i.e., orbicularis oculi muscle) of 14 cases were completely denervated, 28 cases partially denervated and 4 cases with irritability lowered.

II. METHODS OF OBSERVATION

(I) Methods of Treatment

46 cases were divided into two groups, namely 25 cases treated by body acupuncture and 21 cases by auricular acupuncture. Points Hegu, Dicang, Jiache and Zhanzhu were mainly selected for body acupuncture with Yifeng, Sibai, Quanliao, Yangbai, Chengjiang, Yingxiang and Waiguan as auxillary points. 4 to 5 points were selected each time and points on the affected side were punctured and medium stimulation was given to local points while the medium and strong stimulation to distal points. The needle was retained for 30 minutes and treatment was given once every other day. Electric needling or plum-blossom needling was added for some cases. Points of Mouth, Cheek and Liver were chiefly selected for ear acupuncture with Eye, Spleen, Ear-Shenmen and Forehead as auxillary points. 3–4 points were selected for every treatment. The affected side was punctured. The needle was retained for 30 minutes. Treatment was given once every other day and electric needling was also added for some cases. Seven treatments were considered as one course of treatment for both groups. Therapeutic effect was assessed after the completion of 3 successive courses.

(II) Criteria of Therapeutic Effects

Recovery: Disappearance of clinical manifestations, recovery of functions, normal appearance, no sequelae and follow-up EMG basically normal.

Marked result: Remarkable alleviation of symptoms and signs, fundamental recovery of functions, weakness of muscle tone, slight dropping of the angle of the mouth or eyelids and improvement in follow-up EMG.

Improvement: Partial improvement of symptoms and signs, incomplete shutting of the eye, obvious deviation of the mouth while speaking and showing teeth and slight improvement in follow-up EMG.

Failure: No improvements in symptoms and signs as well as in follow-up EMG.

(III) Examination of EMG

The EMG activities in the facial muscles both on the affected and the healthy side were measured before and after treatment and the immediate EMG changes after auricular needling were also recorded.

Stimulating electrode: A pair of acupuncture needles, 1–2 cm apart, were inserted along the pathway of temporozygomaticoorbital branch of the facial nerve anterior to the ear lobe.

Parameters of stimulus: The duration was 0.1 ms, frequency 0.5 c/s, intensity 20 to 130 V.

Recording electrode: The concentric bipolar electrode was inserted into the lower orbicularis oculi muscle. EMG activities under resting and weak to strong contractive condition were displayed in oscillograph and recorded by camera. Before treatment they were measured in all the 46 cases, among which follow-up study was taken in 12 cases so as to observe EMG changes before and after acupuncture. Besides, in 8 cases, during EMG examination, ear points of Mouth, Cheek, Liver and Ear-Shenmen were punctured with a needle retained for 30 minutes. After withdrawing the needle, EMG was recorded again so as to observe immediate effect on EMG by auricular acupuncture.

III. RESULTS OF OBSERVATION

(I) Clinical Therapeutic Effects

Of the 46 cases, 30 cases were cured (65%), 9 cases markedly improved (20%), 4 cases improved (9%) and 3 cases failed (6%). Total effective rate was 94%. The following tables show the relationships between therapeutic effects and acupuncture group, etiology, course of disease, and times of treatments as well as nerve degeneration.

From Table 1 we may find that both body and ear acupuncture are rather efective in treating facial paralysis. Although there exists a difference in cure rates and marked effective rates between these two groups, the total effective rates are about the same. Statistically there is no significant difference. Therefore, all the numbers in the following tables are calculated from the two groups as a whole.

From Table 2 we can see that there is certain correlation between therapeutic effect and etiology. Better results are obtained in cases caused by exposure to cold. Among 2 cases due to traumatic injuries, 1 case due to injury in the retroauricular region was cured after 9 treatments; while another case due to operation on mastoid process with a history of 10 years failed after several dozen trials of acupuncture.

From Table 3 we may find that the shorter the history of the disease, the better the therapeutic effects. This is identical with the data reported elsewhere.

From Table 4 we may see that the therapeutic effect is closely related to the times of treatments. Highest cure rate was obtained following 14–20 trials of acupuncture.

Table 1. Relationship between therapeutic effect and acupuncture group

Grouping	Total cases	Recovery	Marked effect	Improved	Failed
Body-acup.	25	18	3	2	2
Ear-acup.	21	12	6	2	1

Table 2. Relationship between therapeutic effect and etiology

Classification of etiology	Total cases	Recovery	Marked effect	Improved	Failed
Exposure to Cold or Idiopathic	36	25	7	3	1
Otitis Media or Cervical	6	4	1		1
Lymphadentitis Herpes	2		1	1	
Trauma	2	1			1

Table 3. Relationship between therapeutic effect and course of disease

History of disease	Total cases	Recovery	Marked effect	Improved	Failed
1–10 Days	17	14	2	1	1
11–20 Days	13	10	3		
21–30 Days	8	4	2	1	1
31–40 Days	4	2		1	1
Above 1 Year	4		2	1	1

Table 4. Relationship between therapeutic effect and times of treatment

Times of treatment	Total cases	Recovery	Marked effect	Improved	Failed
1–7	2	1			1
7–14	13	8	3	1	1
14–21	18	15	2	1	
21–28	7	4	2	1	
Above 28–35	6	2	2	1	1

We can see from Table 5 that the therapeutic effect is directly related to the degrees of nerve degeneration. After treatment, those cases with decrease of irritability and partial denervation are rapidly cured and the therapeutic effect is satisfactory, while those with complete denervation are cured very slowly and the therapeutic effect is poor.

(II) EMG Changes

The results of follow-up EMG of 12 cases before and after treatment, as well as the immediate effect on EMG in 8 cases by auricular needling, indicate that acupuncture exerts obvious effects on EMG, EMG changes of 12 cases before and after treatment are mainly shown as follows:

1. Evoked potential. Comparing with that of the healthy side before treatment, among 12 cases the latent period of 9 cases was prolonged, the duration in 4 cases shortened, the amplitude in 7 cases decreased and electric silence occurred in 4 cases (i.e., no reaction to stimulation). After treatment, the latent period in 4 cases was restored to normal, the duration in 7 cases prolonged, the amplitude in 7 cases increased and the evoked potential reappeared in 3 cases presenting electric silence before treatment (see Table 6).

Table 5. Relationship between therapeutic effect and nerve degeneration

Classification of nerve degeneration	Total cases	Recovery	Marked effect	Improved	Failed
Complete Degeneration	14	7	4	1	2
Partial Degeneration	28	19	5	3	1
Decrease of nervous Irritability	4	4			

Table 6. Changes of induced EMG potential in 12 cases pre- and post- treatment

	Latent period		Reflex potential		Duration		Voltage	
	Prolonged	Normal	Disappeared	Prolonged	Prolonged	Shortened	Increased	Decreased
Pre* treatment	9		4	2	5	4	2	7
Post** treatment	5	4	2	2	7	2	7	2

*No reaction to stimulation in 3 Cases.

**Appearance of action potential in 3 cases.

2. EMG during strong contraction. Comparing with that of the healthy side before treatment, the peak value of EMG potential was lowered and frequency decreased in 10 cases, simple pattern in 9 cases, intermediate pattern in 1 case and electric silence in another two cases. After treatment the peak value of EMG potential in 4 cases was restored to normal; the peak value of EMG Potential in 6 cases as well as the frequency of 4 cases improved; the number of occurence of simple pattern decreased from 9 to 3 cases, while the number of intermediate pattern increased to 2 and the number of interference pattern increased to 5. EMG potential reappeared in 2 cases originally with electric silence (see Table 7).

The results of EMG changes in 8 cases treated by ear acupuncture show that immediately after 30 minutes' auricular needling the amplitude and frequency of EMG in 6 cases during voluntary contraction was increased and no change occurred in 2 cases, indicating that acupuncture can produce immediate regulatory functions.

Table 7. EMG changes of 12 cases during strong contraction pre- and post- treatment

	Voltage			Pattern			Frequency		
	Normal	Improved	Decreased	Simple	Intermediate	Interference	Improved	Decreased	Normal
Before* Treatment			10	9	1			10	
After** Treatment	4	6		3	2	5	4	1	5

*Electric silence appeared in 2 cases.
**EMG potential appeared in 2 cases.

(III) Case Example

Wang, 28 years old, male, electrician, complained that 12 days ago there appeared dropping and discomfort in his left cheek, deviation of the mouth to the right, incomplete shutting of the left eye and distension and pain in the retro-auricular region. When the attack occurred, he went to the factory clinic to receive Vit. B1 and B12 injection, without obvious result. So he asked for acupuncture treatment.

Physical examination: The shutting of the eye, frowning, whistling and showing teeth on the left side were significantly inhibited, the naso-labial groove disappeared and there was a grain-like abscess on the left inferior palpebral margin without other abnormal changes.

EMG report: It was found that the latent period of evoked potential on the affected side and H-reflex had prolonged, duration shortened, voltage lowered, scanty diphasic potential appeared during voluntary contraction and simple pattern emerged during forceful contraction and peak-value of voltage markedly decreased, indicating that the left facial nerves was denervated partially.

Treatment: After 3 auricular acupuncture treatments, the eye could shut, the deviated mouth became normal but still deviated, while showing teeth and muscle tone improved. After ten treatments the symptoms had disappeared, functions were restored and appearance became normal, which can be considered as clinical cure.

Follow-up EMG: The latent period of evoked potential on the left side and H-reflex were slightly shortened, duration slightly prolonged, intermediate pattern appeared during voluntary contraction, interference pattern emerged during forceful contraction, peak-value of voltage increased and frequency enhanced, indicating that the left facial paralysis had fundamentally been cured.

IV. DISCUSSION

To treat nerve paralysis, acupuncture can regulate the circulation of qi and blood and set free the channels and collaterals so as to restore the functions of nerves and muscles. In peripheral facial paralysis, because of the lesions of peripheral facial nerve, the mimetic muscles are thus denervated, resulting in difficulty in frowning, shutting of the eye and whistling. Some cases of peripheral facial paralysis may recover spontaneously. However, it may develop into an old and untreatable case due to delay of treatment. EMG examination may not only afford an objective index for clinical diagnosis and treatment, but also provide evidence for judging the prognosis of the disease, so that the risk of blind expectation of spontaneous recovery or improper treatment may be avoided.

Viewed from the results mentioned above, it is assumed that the shortening of latency of the evoked muscle potential following acupuncture treatment may be considered to be an elevation of excitability of facial nerve and restoration of nerve conduction, while prolongation of duration and increase of amplitude of the evoked response indicate that nerve regeneration and formation of collateral branches may occur under the influence of acupuncture, which increases the amount of muscle fibers innervated, thus giving rise to an increase of spatial and temporal dispersion of the muscle potential. Evidence of reinnervation of muscle fibers is also shown by the EMG patterns during voluntary contraction following acupuncture, i.e., the electrical silence no longer exists and the simple pattern is shifted to intermediate or interference pattern. Whether such beneficial actions of acupuncture are local reactions arised from needling or mediated reflexively by way of the corresponding brain stem centers requires further study.

V. SUMMARY

This paper reports the clinical significance of acupuncture therapy for peripheral facial paralysis. Definite therapeutic effect of body and auricular acupuncture on this disease is confirmed. A follow-up EMG study presents some evidence for better understanding of the mechanism by which the facial paralysis can be cured by acupuncture. It suggests that acupuncture has the effect of adjusting the function of the nervous system.

ACUPUNCTURE OF "XIANGYANG" POINT IN TREATMENT OF CENTRAL SEROUS CHORIORETINOPATHY

ANALYSIS OF 600 CASES*

Department of Ophthalmology, First Hospital Zhejiang Medical College

Central serous chorioretinopathy, a common ocular disease first described by Von Grafe in 1866, has been well-documented in this country and abroad. The early embarrassment of the central vision and the protracted clinical course have markedly threatened sufferers. Various remedies have been prescribed throughout the world and some improvement, though far from satisfactory, has been achieved. However, the lengthy therapy and high cost prevented their general acceptance by the vast majority of patients.

Since we began to treat this malady with needling Xiangyang point in 1970, encouraging results have been attained with a cure and improvement rate up to 97.66%. Our practice and follow-up study lasting for 7 years reveals that acupuncture in the treatment of serous central chorioretinopathy not only is effective, but also significantly shortens the conventional therapeutic course, providing a simple, safe and almost painless procedure, which demands low cost and least equipment and thus has been well accepted by most people.

I. POINT SELECTED FOR NEEDLING AND ITS APPLICATION

(I) Selection of Acupuncture Point

"Xiangyang" is a point at the intersection of the level line through hyoid with anterior border the sternocleidomastoid muscle, opposite the medical aspect of the lower jaw (see following Fig. 1).

(II) Procedure

The patient lies supine, with the shoulders slightly elevated on a pillow support and the anterior aspect of the neck fully exposed by extending the head a little downward. The skin is sterilized as routine. The operator holds the needle with his right hand and pierces abruptly through the skin keeping the shaft of the needle at an angle of 75 degrees with the skin surface and avoiding the blood vessels. Then insert the needle gradually, inward and upward to a depth of about 3cm until the sense of "deqi" (needle sensation, i.e. soreness, distension, and numbness over the periauricular and temporal regions) is felt. Twist the needle and retain therein for 15–20 minutes.

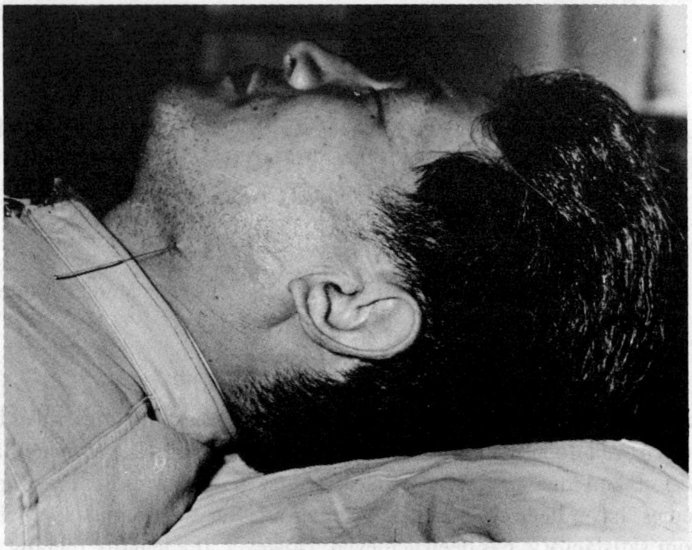

(III) Regimen of Therapy

Needle once daily the Xiangyang point on the diseased side, while in cases of bilateral involvement the Xiangyang points on both sides. Each therapeutic course last for 10 days and then starts on the second course if necessary after an interval of 2–5 days.

II. CASE ANALYSIS

Over a period of 7 years in the OPD of ophthalmology more than 1000 patients with central serous chorioretinopathy have been treated by acupuncture. 600 cases (624 diseased eyes) receiving more than one therapeutic course and comparatively well-documented were analyzed.

(I) Sex

There were 527 male (87.83%) and 73 female (12.17%) patients in a ratio of 7:1.

(II) The Side Affected

There were 576 cases with unilateral involvement (96%) and 24 bilaterally involved (4%) in a ratio of 24:1. In the cases of unilateral involvement, right eye affection counted 304 (50.66%), and left 272 (45.34%). More common was unilateral involvement.

---

* Compiled by Ye Lingmei

(III) Age

10–20 years of age, 1 case (0.16%); 21–30, 61 cases (10.16%); 31–40, 290 (48.34%); 41–50, 236 (36.34%); 51–60, 12 (2%). The majority of patients fell into the age group of 31–50 (87.68%).

(IV) Occupation

Workers, 335 cases, (55.83%) counted more than one half of the patients; cadres, 130 cases (21.67%); peasants, 40 cases (6.67%); miscellaneous, 38 cases (6.33%); school teachers, 32 cases (5.34%); medical personnel, 14 cases (2.33%) and truck driver, 11 (1.83%). Workers and cadres constitute the great majority of the patients.

III. CLINICAL RESULTS

(I) Criteria in Assessing Results

1. Cured: Distant vision more than 1.0 (International Vision Test Chart under Artificial Light), absence of subjective symptoms, resolution of inflammation and presence of central light reflection at the macular region.

2. Improved: Visual acuity improved, subjective symptom absent or markedly alleviated and inflammation at the macular region significantly lessened.

3. Failed: Neither visual acuity nor macular inflammation improved.

(II) Clinical Results

Of the 600 cases so treated, 277 (46.16%) were cured, 309 (51.5%) improved, and 14 (2.34%) failed. The percentage of the cured and improved is 97.66%.

(III) CORRELATION BETWEEN THE CLINICAL RESULTS AND PRIMARY OR RECURRENT ATTACK

Of 519 cases of primary attack, 243 (46.82%) were cured, 265 (51.05%) improved, and 11 (2.13%) failed, while of 81 cases of recurrent attack, 33 (40.74%) were cured, 45 (55.56%) improved, and 3 (3.7%) failed. It appears that acupuncture produces better responses in primary cases. However, there is no significant difference statistically.

(IV) Correlation of Therapeutic Courses with Clinical Results (Table 1) .

Treated for 1–4 courses, the majority (95–97%) of cases would be cured or improved. Persistent acupuncture would result in further improvement in those who failed. No adverse effect was ever found.

In the 14 cases that failed (9 underwent 2 and 5 underwent 4 courses), no further acupuncture treatment could be continued for one or another reason and from the table it can be seen they would be cured or improved if treatment were continued, as none failed with 5 or more courses.

(V) History of Disease Versus Clinical Results

Favorable results were obtained in cases suffering the disease less than 6 months (Table 2). It seems that the shorter the history, the better the results would be. However, so few were the patients who had suffered the illness for more than 6 months that no conclusion can be drawn without further investigation.

Table 1. Therapeutic Courses and Clinical Results

No. of Courses	Clinical Results			
	Cured & Improved		Failed	
	cases	%	cases	%
1–2	183	95.31	9	4.67
3–4	200	97.56	5	2.44
5–6	131	100.0	– –	– –
7–8	46	100.0	– –	– –
9–10	19	100.0	– –	– –
11–12	7	100.0	– –	– –

Table 2. History of Disease versus Clinical Results

Duration	No. of Cured or Improved (%)	No. of Failed (%)
less than 1 mon.	315(97.53)	8(2.74)
1–3 mon.	193(98.97)	2(1.03)
3–6 mon.	53(98.15)	1(1.85)
6–12 mon.	13(92.86)	1(7.14)
over 12 mon.	12(85.72)	2(14.28)

IV. ILLUSTRATIVE CASES

Case I. Wang, a 40 year old, male carpenter, complained of blurring of vision, seeing black spots and distorted image with his right eye for more than 2 months. Some remedies (such as vit. B_1, dibazol, etc.) made it better. He had never had this eye trouble before.

On examination distant vision O.D. 0.5, near vision 3/30 cm. (Jaeger's Test Chart). Nothing particular found in externac examination. Ophthalmoscope examination: disc margin sharply defined, central light reflection at macular region doubtful with marked edema and abundant yellowish-white spotty exudate. Diagnosis: central serous chorioretinopathy O.D. (cause unknown).

Progress note: examination carried out at the end of the 1st therapeutic course revealed: distant vision (O.D.). improved to 0.9, central light reflection brighter but remained diffuse, edema markedly reduced, more red in color but no hemorrhage, majority of the spotty exudation resolved.

After the 2nd course of acupuncture: distant vision O.D. 1.2, near vision 1/30cm, central light reflection much brighter than before, edema mild, exudation scanty.

At the end of the 3rd course of acupuncture: distant vision O.D. 1.2, near vision 1/30cm, central light reflection excellent, edema and exudation completely resolved.

Case II. Xin, male, 42 years old, a school teacher, complained of blurring of vision for 2 weeks. No improvement following treatment received elsewhere; no previous history of the complaint.

On examination: distant vision O.D. 0.4, near vision 4/30cm. Nothing peculiar found in external examination. Optic disc well defined, loss of central light reflection at the macular region, more red in colour but no hemorrhage, plenty of yellowish white exudative spots, edema marked.

Diagnosis: serous central chorioretinopathy O.D. (cause unknown).

Progress note: after the 1st course of acupuncture, distant vision improved to 0.6, no central light reflection at macular region, retinal color fainter, edema and exudation reduced.

After the 2nd course of therapy: distant vision O.D. 1.0, central light reflection indistinct at the macular region, exudation and edema greatly resolved. As the 3rd course of needling was completed, distant vision O.D. 1.5, notmuch change except edema became mild.

After the 4th course: distant vision O.D. 1.5, near vision 1/30cm., central light reflection excellent, edema and exudation entirely absorbed.

V. CONCLUSIONS AND COMMENTS

1. Assessment of clinical results. A lot of remedies, both western and traditional Chineses ones, have been tried. It is reported in the literature that some patients recovered spontaneously, but there were cases refractory to any form of therapy. In general, cost is treatment. No steroid was ever prescribed and only occasionally was some vitamin B_1 given. In all the 600 cases we have treated, 586 were cured or improved, for a rate of 97.66% and only 14 or 2.34% failed. 397 of 383 cases (95–97%) after 1–4 therapeutic courses were cured or improved. All 177 cases that underwent 5–8 therapeutic courses were cured or improved.

From our clinical experience of over 7 years, we found acupuncture treatment of this disease has a high response rate. As a rule, 1–4 therapeutic courses will suffice to attain a cure or improvement of it. Continued acupuncture treatment would either cure or improve those that failed to respond to the first 4 courses.

2. The role of acupuncture Xiangyang point. It has been well documented in traditional Chinese medical literature that "Jinglao" (channel) is the pathway for circulating "Qixie" (air-blood) throughout the human body. "Jingqi" (humour-air) of "Zangfu" (viscerae) flows

cephalicly along the pathway and expresses itself in both eyes. And thus viscerae correlate with both eyes closely.

Whether "Jinglao" is closely connected with the nervous system or not is still controversial, but we would like to present a few facts: (1) "Jinglao" is not the small vessels, because once small vessels were pierced through, the patients would experience no "needling sensation" ("deqi"), but only a very painful sensation would be felt. (2) "Jinglao" is intimately related with the nervous system. Occasionally we had to needle through various kinds of scars at the site of Xiangyang point, and "Deqi" could hardly be felt or not at all, as scars are made up mainly of connective tissues which are devoid of nerve endings.

We postulate that the unique distribution of cervical nerve plexus and sympathetic chains would account for the favorable response in needling Xiangyang point. By the aid of current fluorescin angiography, permeability changes of choricapillaris have been demonstrated in this malady. Mild stimulation from needling may regulate the malfunctioned cervical sympathetic plexus, decrease the permeability of choriocapillaris and promote the resolution of edema and exudation.

However, further investigation is still needed for elucidating the nature of "Jinglao". For the time being we would like to assume that "Jinglao" is closely correlated with the nervous system.

OBSERVATION OF SENSORINEURAL DEAFNESS TREATED WITH ACUPUNCTURE

Audiological Research Group, Bethune Medical College and
Deaf-mutism Research group, Unit 81112, PLA

It has been reported by many medical workers in our country that they have achieved definite therapeutic effects with acupuncture in a part of sensorineural deafness and deaf-mutism. To study the mechanism of this therapeutic effect of acupuncture, observations were carried out both experimentally and clinically.

I. PATHOLOGICAL STUDY OF THE INNER EAR[1]

To find out whether acupuncture can influence the pathological process of the inner ear, 70 guinea pigs were subjected to 128dB white noise for ten hours. Auditory threshold shift can be observed. On the next day 35 animals received acupuncture at "Tinggong" (32 remained because 3 animals died accidentally during the experiment). The other 35 animals without acupuncture were served as controls. Excluding 7 animals that died or the cochlea being broken, the group consisted of 28 animals. Animals were sacrificed 8 weeks later and the whole cochlear surface preparation from the left ear of each animal was dissected and examined[2]. The whole cochlea was shown in Fig. 1, the prepared Corti's organ in Fig. 2.

White noise stimulation caused damage of some hair cells in the cochlea. Fig. 3 showed the surface preparation of the 1st turn (near the basal part) of guinea pig's cochlea under phase-contrast microscope. The noise-induced damage in this turn is very slight and damaged hair cell can not be found in this area. Fig. 4 showed the third turn; in this preparation the damage is very serious, the majority of the hair cells had been damaged and only two cells are normal in this part.

The damaged hair cell population was counted. The mean damage value and range of hair cells at each mm of the organ of Corti was first calculated for both groups. The arithmetic damage values were substituted by logarithms. Then, the mean damage curves were plotted logarithmically with the mean damage value of each mm for both groups. Both curves were compared in turn.

It can be seen in Fig. 5 that the damage curve of the control group is highest at the third turn, then falls gradually at the second turn, and the amount of the damage is very small and nearly normal at the first turn. The mean damage curve of the acupuncture group is essentially the same as the control group at the 3rd and 1st turn. But the curve for the acupuncture group is significantly lower than that of the control group and the ranges do not overlap at 8–14mm in the second turn. It means that the damage in the acupuncture

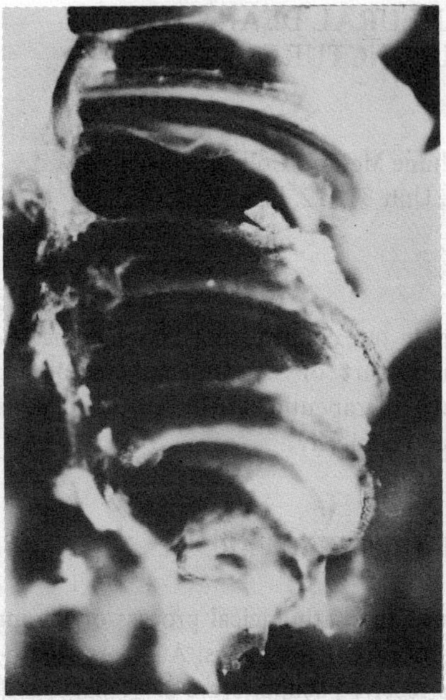

Fig. 1 The whole cochlea.

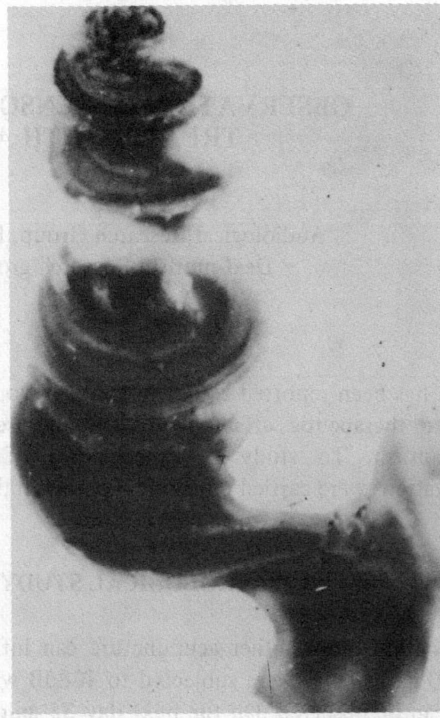

Fig. 2 The organ of Corti.

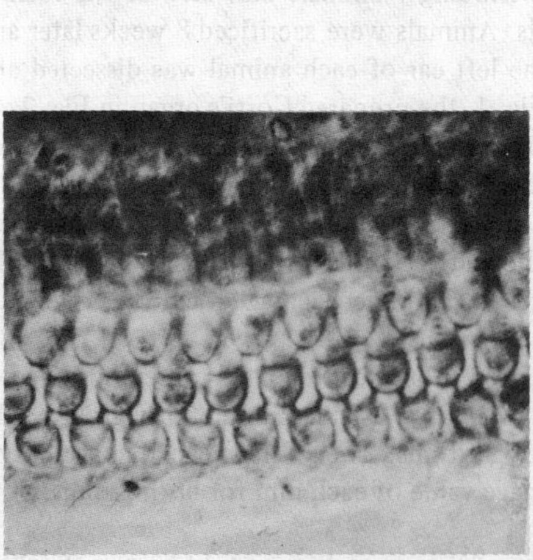

Fig. 3 Surface preparation of the 1st turn.

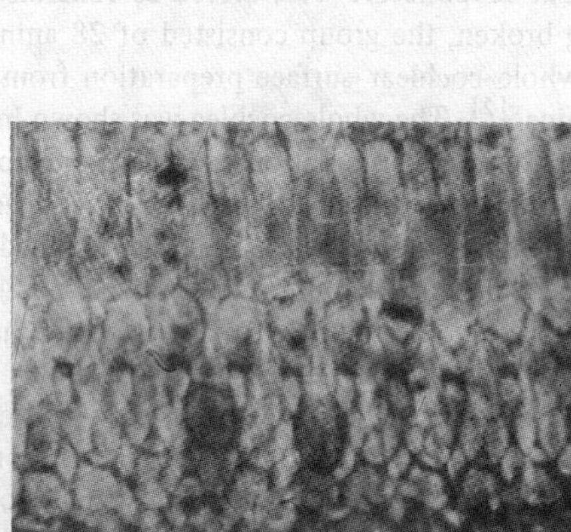

Fig. 4 Surface preparation of the 3rd turn.

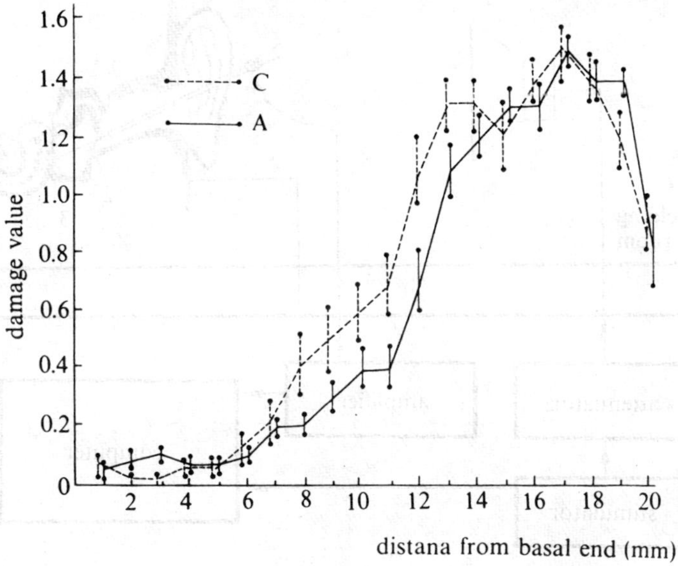

Fig. 5 Comparison of mean damage curve of acupuncture group with control group.
C: Control group A: Acupuncture group

group is less than in the control group only in this part. It is possible that the second turn was just in a reversible stage of damage process. The necrosis of the hair cells might be prevented by acupuncture which can improve the microcirculation of the cochlea and the nutrition for hair cells. At the third turn the failure of acupuncture for repairment may be related to the serious damage and necrosis of the hair cells.

II. PHYSIOLOGICAL STUDY OF HEARING

To explain whether acupuncture can raise the function of the inner ear, the effect of electro-acupuncture at the "Tinggong" point and the promontory area upon the cochlear potentials (i.e., electrocochleogram, EochG) was observed in sensorineural deafness of various types[3, 4]. The transtympanic technique was used. After disinfection and local anesthesia of eardrum, the specially-made promontory needle was penetrated through the eardrum and to the promontory area; the potential was carried in this needle, then conveyed into the amplifier and treated with the averaging computer.

The 90 dB click generated from the stimulator served as a sound stimulation for audiometry (Fig. 6).

Under the stimulation of 90 dB click, the range of fluctuation of the amplitude (from peak to trough) of cochlear potentials was observed in 60 ears (53 deaf patients), and the upper limit of 95% individuals treated statistically was found to be 28.44%. Therefore, the fluctuations of the amplitudes of cochlear potentials over a value of 29% in either direction in comparison with the amplitudes before electro-acupuncture stimulation would be

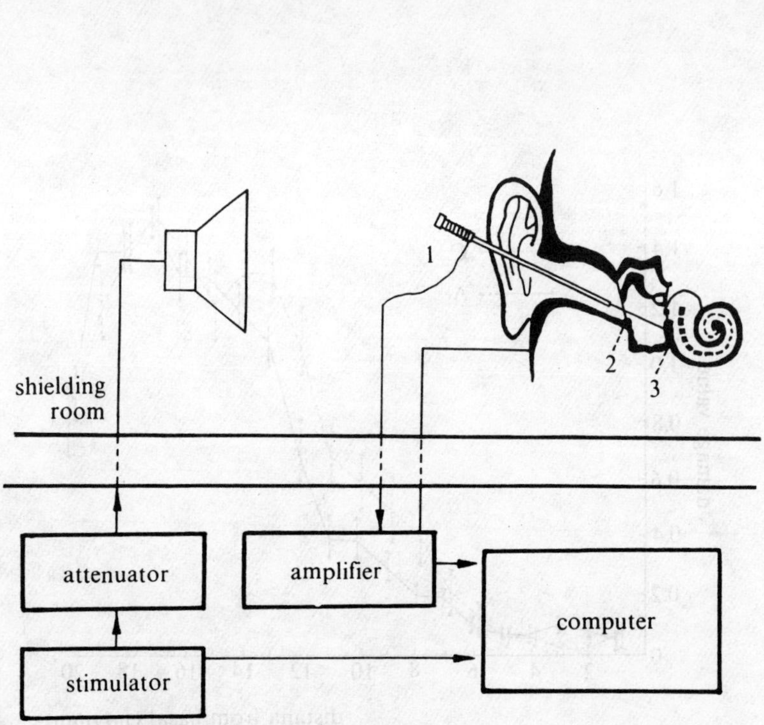

Fig. 6 Experimental equipments.
1: Promontory needle 2: Ear drum 3: Promontory area

considered to be significant. The results after five minutes electro-acupuncture stimulation were shown in the following table (Table 1).

It can be seen from Table 1 that the cochlear potentials were raised with the application of electro-acupuncture to either "Tinggong" or the promontory area in some of the patients (about 20%). As we know, an increase in the amplitude of cochlear potentials would be a reflection of the promotion of cochlear hair cell function. This might partly account for the therapeutic effect of electro-acupuncture at "Tinggong" point or the promontory area. The experimental records were shown in Figs. 7 and 8. Fig. 7 showed the results of stimulating "Tinggong", while Fig. 8 showed the results of stimulating the promontory area.

The amplitude of cochlear potentials was increased in both cases after stimulation as compared with control.

The therapeutic effects of the electro-acupuncture at the promontory area in relation to changes in cochlear potentials in 42 ears were analyzed. It was found that 7 of the 8 ears with increase of cochlear potentials were therapeutically effective and only one ineffective.

Table 1. The influence of stimulation with electro-acupuncture upon the cochlear potentials

Site of stimulation	Change of Potential			Total
	Increase	Decrease	No change	
"Tinggong"	11 (18.3%)	2 (3.3%)	47 (78.4%)	60 ears (53 Cases)
Promontory	11 (20.7%)	1 (1.9%)	41 (77.4%)	53 ears (41 Cases)

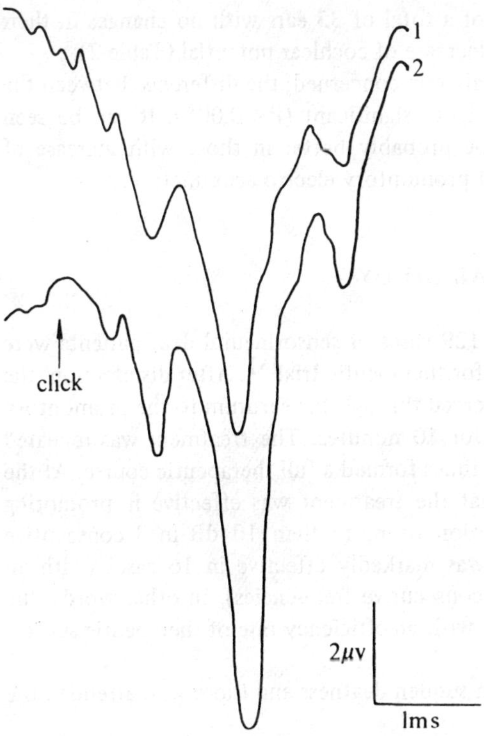

Fig. 7 The recorde of stimulating "Ting gong".
1. Before stimulation
2. After stdmulation

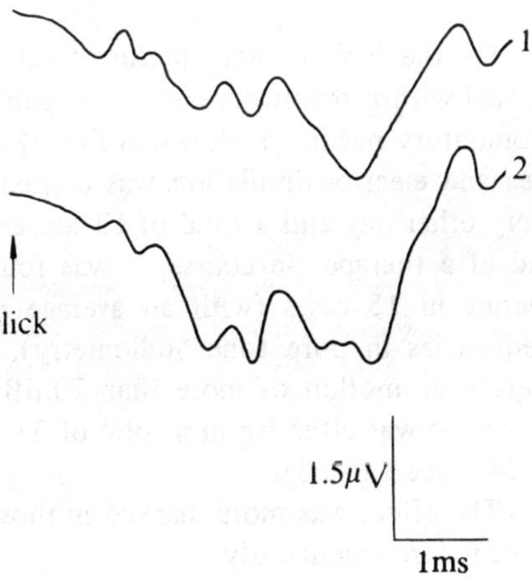

Fig. 8 The recorde of stimulating promontory.

Table 2. Relationship between therapeutic effects and the increase of cochlear potentials

Group	Increase	Decrease	No change	Total
Effective	7		6	13
Ineffective	1	1	27	29

Table 3. Therapeutic effect of the sensorineural deafness with promontory electro-acupuncture

Therapeutic effect	Markedly effective	Effective	Ineffective	Total
Number of cases	16	15	98	129
%	24		76	100

There was no therapeutic effect at all in 27 of a total of 33 ears with no changes in their cochlear potentials and also in the one with a decrease of cochlear potential (Table 2).

As far as the increase of cochlear potentials was concerned, the difference between the two groups (effective and ineffective) was highly significant ($P<0.005$). It can be seen therefore that the therapeutic effect would be probably better in those with increase of cochlear potentials following the application of promontory electro-acupuncture.

III. CLINICAL STUDY

On the basis of acupuncture treatment, 129 cases of sensorineural deaf patients were treated with promontory electro-acupuncture for therapeutic trial[5]. After disinfection, the promontory needle (as shown in Fig. 6) was pierced through the eardrum to the promontory area and electro-stimulation was carried out for 10 minutes. The treatment was repeated every other day and a total of 10 consecutive times formed a full therapeutic course. At the end of a therapeutic course, it was found that the treatment was effective in promoting hearing in 15 cases (with an average promotion of more than 10 dB in 3 consecutive frequencies in pure tone audiometry), and was markedly effective in 16 cases (with an average promotion of more than 20 dB in 3 consecutive frequencies). In other words, the treatment was effective in a total of 31 cases, with an efficiency rate of therapeutic success of 24% (see Table 3).

The effect was more marked in those with sudden deafness and those who attended the clinic for treatment early.

The relations between therapeutic effects and etiology were shown in Table 4.

Table 4. Relationship between the therapeutic effect and etiology

Etiology	Effective	Ineffective	Total
Traumatic	2	10	12
Noise-induced	3	16	19
Sudden deafness	6	2	8
Virus-induced	4	20	24
Toxication by streptomycin	3	10	13
Sequelae of encephalitis	0	5	5
Familial progressive deafness	2	3	5
Meniere's disease	0	4	4
Cause unknown	9	13	22
Congenital deaf-mute	1	2	3
Others	1	13	14
Total	31	98	129

The standard of therapeutic effect was deduced on the basis of investigation upon the fluctuated range of auditory threshold of deaf-mute students[6]. Comparing 250,310 fluctuation values obtained by the examination of 2400 ear-times in 182 deafmute students of two deaf-mute schools, it was found statistically that the effect was less than 5% with an average promotion of 10 dB in 3 consecutive frequencies, 15 dB in two consecutive frequencies and 20 dB in one frequency (Table 5)

As we know, according to the statistical principle, it isn't belonging to the natural fluctuation if the pro bability of one thing is less than 5%. Therefore it is reasonable that the hearing promotion which is more than 10 dB in 3 consecutive frequencies on the average was considered as effective.

Besides pure tone audiometry, the speech audiometry was also carried out in some of the patients treated with promontory electro-acupuncture[7]. It was found that there were improvements of more than 5 dB in speech reception threshold (SRT) in 17 of the 20 ears whose pure tone audiometry were found to be effective, and in the ineffective group there was only one ear. Statistically, the differences between effective and ineffective groups with standard of improvement of 5 dB in SRT were highly significant ($P<0.005$). There was promotion of 10% in maximum discrimination score (PBmax) in 17 of the 21 ears that belonged to the effective group of pure tone audiometry, and only one ear to the ineffective group (Table 6). The differences between the effective and the ineffective groups with the standard of promotion of 10% in PBmax were also highly significant (P<0.005).

Therefore in speech audiometry the hearing promotion can be found also in those patients whose hearing promotion was determined to be effective in pure tone audiometry, and prediction of the therapeutic effect by combining the indices of pure tone (hearing promotion of more than 10 dB in 3 consecutive frequencies on average), SRT (im provement more than 5 dB) and PBmax (promotion more than 10%) would prove to be more accurate and reliable.

Table 5. Fluctuation of auditory threshold of deaf-mutism

Consecutive frequencies	Fluctuation (dB)	Probability (%)
1	20	3.11
2	15	0.7
3	10	0.9

Table 6. Comparison between the results of pure tone audiometry and speech audiometry

Group (Pure tone audiometry)	Improvement of SRT		Increase of PBmax	
	>5 dB	<5 dB	>10%	<10%
Effective group	17	3	17	4
Ineffective group	1	19	1	19

IV. SUMMARY

This paper reported observations on the mechanism of the therapeutic effect of acupuncture concerning sensorineural deafness both experimentally and clinically.

It is possible that in a stage of reversibility the necrosis of the damaged hair cells was prevented by the application of acupuncture.

The amplitude of cochlear potentials of some patients (about 20% ears) suffering from sensorineural deafness showed increase with the application of electro-acupuncture to nigher "Tinggong" or promontory area.

Hearing promotion was observed in 24% patients suffering from various sensorineural deafness and treated with promontory electro-acupuncture therapy.

From the experimental results cited above and clinical observations, we considered that there was theoretical basis of acupuncture therapy in treating sensorineural deafness. However, to understand the mechanism of acupuncture in the treatment of sensorineural deafness as a whole, much research work in this field has to be done.

REFERENCES

[1] 戴树宏 王春阳：吉林医大参加全国耳鼻喉科学术会议论文汇编，第 41 页，1978。

[2] 戴树宏等：同上 第 37 页。

[3] 姬柏春等：吉林医大学报 (3)：8，1978。

[4] 同上：同上 (2)：19，1977。

[5] 王金远等：同上 (2)：27，1977。

[6] 佘蕴山等：白求恩医科大学学报 (3)：24，1979。

[7] 孙云章等：同上 (3)：20，1979。

PART IV
CLINICAL RESEARCH ON ACUPUNCTURE ANESTHESIA

ACUPUNCTURE ANESTHESIA IN NEUROSURGERY

National Cooperative Group of Acupuncture Anesthesia for Neurosurgery*

From November 1965 to December 1978, according to incomplete statistics, at 21 units of neurosurgery in this country, 7,469 successfol craniocerebral operations were performed under acupuncture anesthesia. Beginning from March 1975, the 21 units mentioned above were organized into coordination groups to carry out further researches on this subject. Before the end of December 1978, 4,466 craniocerebral operations under acupuncture anesthesia had been accomplished in accordance with the research plan of the coordination group, including 1,865 cases (41.8%) of the anterior cranial fossa, 1,594 (35.7%), the temporo–parieto-occipital region and 1,007 (22.5%), the posterior cranial fossa. The success rate of acupuncture anesthesia in these cases was over 90%, and the satisfactory rate (grade I,II rate) was 76.6%. This illustrats that acupuncture anesthesia is safe, effective, simple and economical. Although some defects still exist in acupuncture anesthesia at present, it has, nevertheless, become one of the common methods of anesthesia in craniocerebral operations. This article presents the basic experiences in the application of acupuncture anesthesia in craniocerebral operations and reports some results of our studies of the action of the nervous system in acupuncture analgesia.

I. METHODS OF ACUPUNCTURE ANESTHESIA IN CRANIOCEREBRAL OPERATIONS

(I) Selection of cases and preoperative management

1. Indications for craniocerebral operation under acupuncture anesthesia:

(a) General conditions: All of the patients were volvnteers, over 18 years of age, and had clear consciousness. Those with obvious mental disturbances and/or intellectual defects were excluded.

(b) Site of the lesion: In 2,837 out of the 4,466 cases, lesions were mainly situated in the cerebral hemisphere, 622 in the sellar region, 566 at the cerebellopontine angle and 441 in the cerebellum.

(c) The nature of the lesion: Indications for craniocerebral operation under acupuncture anesthesia were chiefly tumors of various types as illustrated in Table1.

* Compiled by Chen Gongbai, Din Yuji, Li Qingbin, Gao Yuhua, Yin Shida, Chen Huahai Luo Qizhong Ma Lie.

Table 1. Pathological classification of diseases indicating craniocerebral operation under acupuncture anesthesia

Nature of the disease	No. of Cases
Glioma	1,058
Meningioma	393
Pituitary tumor	521
Craniopharyngioma	101
Cerebral abscess	101
Intracranial hematoma	232
Vascular malformation and aneurysm	57
Neurofibroma	364
Trigeminal neuralgia	292
Vasoanastomosis (cerebral thrombosis)	12
Torkildsen's operation (hydrocephalus)	58
Scalp and skull disorders	792
Other disorders	485
Total	4,466

Table 2. Selection of points for craniocerebral operation under acupuncture anesthesia and adjustment of stimulus parameters

Site of operation	Selection of points and polarity (+) or (–)	Frequency of stimuli
Anterior cranial fossa	Quanliao point (–), with indifferent electrode set at ear-lobe (+)	500–1000/min.
	Ear needling: through Naogan to Pizhixia (–), through Shenmen to Shen (–), Jiaogan (+), Waifei (+)	500–1000/min.
	Jinmen (–), Taichong (+)	120–200/min.
Temporo-parieto-occipital region	Body needling: Jinmen (–), Taichong (+), through Fengchi to Anmian$_2$ (+), through Shangxing to Conghui (–)	200–400/min.
	Ear needling: through Naogan to Zhennie (–), Waifei (+), through Jiaogan to Taiyang (–), through Shenmen to Shen (+)	500–1000/min.
Posterior cranial fossa	Ear needling: through Naogan to Pizhixia (–), through Shenmen to Shen (–), Jiaogan (+), Waifei (+)	500–1000/min.
	Body needling: through Dazhui to Yamen (–), through Houding to Naohu (+) Zulinqi (–) Yifeng (+)	1000–2000/min. 200–400/min.

2. The Craniocerebral operation under acupuncture anesthesia was relatively contraindicated when the patient was in coma, deaf, dumb, or incooperative owing to mental disturbances; when their lesions were too deep or extensive; or when artificial hypothermia and hypotension were required during the surgery.

Areoperative interview with the patient should be properly carried out to gain the patient's cooperation. Test needlings might be given to determine the patient's adaptability to acupuncture.

(II) Selection of points and adjustment of stimulus parameters

On the basis of past experience, we had, since 1975, set up a number of standards concerning the selection of acupuncture points and stimulus parameters. They were classified as one of 7 groups according to the site of operation (Table 2). Through out the clinical practice of the past four years, theresuits in the 4,466 cases of the 7 groups, were quite similar and stable. The acupuncture points were all selected on the same side as the lesions were located. The stimuli were all derived from the electro-acupuncture apparatus. 20–30 minutes of induction for the acupuncture anesthesia was considered to be most suitable.

(III) Preoperative administration of drugs and choice of proper adjuvants during operation

Premedications were used routinely for craniotomy. Sodium phenobarbital 0.1 gram i.m. and atropine 0.5 mg or scopolamine 0.3 mg subcutaneously were given one hour before operation. For those with history of epilepsy, those whose tumors were situated in the central region, those with mild mental disturbances (e. g. tendency to develop exhilaration or excitement), and those who were quite nervous, the dosage of sodium phenobarbital was doubled (up to 0.2 gm). In addition 5 ml of 5% dilantin were given intramuscularly at the same time.

To enhance the analgesic effect, intramuscular injection or slow intravenous drip of pethidin hydrochloride (dolantin), 1 mg/Kg was given 15 minutes before operation. If the operation exceeded 2 hours, one half of the above dosage was administered again. Haloperidol, a better sedative and antiemetic, administered by intravenous drip 15 minutes before incision or intramuscularly 30 minutes before, would usually enhance the analgesic effect of acupuncture. In addition, haloperidol could control the cranial hypotension and reduce the reactions from the meninges or diaphragma sellae. For those patients in whom an inadequate effect of acupuncture anesthesia was expected, procaine 0.1% less than 150 ml was sometimes infiltrated under the scalp as an additional adjuvant.

(IV) Problems existing in craniocerebral operation under acupuncture anesthesia and their countermeasures

(a) Incomplete analgesia over the scalp: Whenever a patient complained of pain to some degree during cutting or suturing of the skin, especially the latter, additional needles at paraincisional points were applied with relatively high frequency (40,000–60,000/min.). The intensity and frequency of the stimuli at each point should be adjusted from time to time throughout the course of the operation, the intensity being appropriately increased when the incision and sutures were made. For those patients whose preoperative evaluation of the effect of acupuncture anesthesia was poor, adjuvants should as a rule be used more liberally.

(b) Reactions from the meninges and diaphragma sellae to the stimuli: These were frequently noted in operations of the anterior cranial fossa. Mild reactions were nausea and perspiration, and severe reactions included vomiting, profuse perspiration and restlessness, which occasionally hindered the operative procedures. Surgical manipulations under acupuncture anesthesia should be as gentle as possible so as to avoid stimulating the structures at the base of the cranium. The patient's apprehensions must be eliminated by a thorough explaination of the procedure in order to obtain his full cooperation. Whenever an ill reaction did occur, patients were instructed to take deep breaths. Before opening the bone flap, an intravenous drip of 0.25 mg of atropine or haloperidol could reduce the incidence of these reactions. When the reaction was mild, needling the points Neiguan, Taichong etc. was helpful, and when it was severe, intramascular injection of metoclopramidum (maxolon) was given.

(c) Intracranial hypotensive reactions: After a large amount of cerebrospinal fluid had been drained away, intracranial pressure fluctuated abruptly or violently. This would give rise to nausea and vomiting. To control such reactions, the same measures mentioned above for managing reactions from the meninges and diaphragma sellae to stimuli were taken. In patients with signs of high intracranial pressure, intracranial decompression was carried out before operation so as to avoid too abrupt or violent fluctuations of intracranial pressure after craniotomy. During operations, drainage of cerebrospinal fluid was slow and intermittent so that the declining of intracranial pressure might be rendered gradually and steadily.

II. "TRIPLE COUNTERING EFFECT" OF ACUPUNCTURE ANESTHESIA

(I) Anti-pain or analgesia

Patients receiving craniotomies were divided at random into two groups, of 50 patients each. In the control group, acupuncture was not given, procaine 0.1% was injected under the scalp over the operation field, and at the same time, dolantin 1 mg/kg was administered by intravenous drip. In the case of only one patient was the operation carried through to the end while all the others required additional adjuvants including local or even general anesthesia. In the other group receiving acupuncture anesthesia, procaine 0.1% local infilbration was as a rule omitted but dolantin intravenous drip was given routinely. Success was achieved in 46 cases, and 68% of them had results of Grade I or II. This definitely proved that acupuncture had analgesic effects.

Since 1975, we have set up criteria for evaluating the effects of acupuncture anesthesia with a four-graded classification being generally accepted (see Table 3).

According to these criteria for the effect of acupuncture anesthesia, in the 4,466 cases, 1,855 cases (41.5%) belonged to Grade I, 1,566 cases (35.1%) to Grade II, 696 cases (15.6%) to Grade III and 349 cases (7.8%) to Grade IV. The 4,117 cases (92.2%) with Grades I, II and III put together were considered successful, while the 3,421 cases (76.6%) with Grades I and II, being satisfactory.

Of the 4,466 cases, 64.3% were male and 35.7% female. As to the age (overall range 10–81 years), 75% were aged 21–50, 14.3% 51–60, 6.9% below 20 and 3.6% over 60.

Table 3. Criteria adopted nationwide for evaluating the effects of acupuncture anesthesia in craniocerebral operations

Grade	The patient's manifestations and proceeding of the operation	Dosage of pethidin hydrochloride (Dolantin) within 2 hrs.	Dosage of procaine
I	Quiet without pain. Operation smooth.	1 mg/Kg (or less)	none
II	Relatively quiet with occasional complaining or expression of pain. Operation not affected.	1.5mg/Kg (or less)	none
III	Marked pain, abated after additional adjuvants. Operation barely finished.	2 mg/Kg (or less)	procaine 0.5%<10ml,
IV	Marked pain, no improvement even after adjuvants. Acupuncture anesthesia was changed to another kind of anesthesia	over 2 mg/Kg	procaine 0.5%>10ml.

By occupation, 32.2% were workers, 28.9% peasants, 17.7% cadres and 21.2% other vocations. Statistics showed that difference in sex, age and occupation did not have significant influence on the effect of acupuncture anesthesia. The following factors, however, are considered to be influential.

(a) Prescription of acupuncture points: Our experience revealed that if acupuncture points were selected on the basis of Xun jing qu xue (selecting the acupuncture points along the main meridians), while paring attention to the distribution of the more relevant nerve segments so as to select acupuncture points identical with or close to the nerve segment related to the operative field, analgesic effects were much enhanced. We had the experience of performing frontal craniotomy in 40 patients and non-frontal craniotomy in another 40 patients under acupuncture anesthesia induced by needling the same point quanliao. Since this point is closely related to the nerve segment supplying the frontal region, the analgesic effects were Grades I and II in 83.7% cases of the frontal craniotomies and in only 57.1% of the non-frontal group. The difference between the two groups ($P< 0.05$ by χ^2 test) was significant.

(b) The frequency and intensity of stimulus: The frequency and intensity of the stimulus was not determived blindly but had to be decided in accordance with the location of the acupuncture points, the physical condition of patients and their tolerance for acupuncture, and the various procedures of the operation. Stimulation with constant frequency and intensity for a long time tends to develop adaptability, thus reducing the analgesic effect. Therefore, the intensity of stimulus should be frequently adjusted during the operative procedures. For example, it was intensified when the skin was incised or sutured. In general, stimuli of high frequency were used for the points over the ear and proximal segments, and those of low frequency for the points of remote segments.

(c) Individual variations: Preoperative evaluation of the effect of acupuncture anesthesia was carried out in a number of patients. The essentials of this evaluation consisted of determining various indexes before and after acupuncture. To assess the acupuncture analgesic effect, a comparison of these indexes measured preoperatively with the actual efficacy of acupuncture anesthesia was made after operation and their similarities calculated statistically (Table 4). With the exception of galvanic skin response, the other six indexes were highly significant for predicting the effect of acupuncture anesthesia. It showed the existence of individul variation.

Preoperative evaluation was shown to be of some help in selecting suitable patients thus ensuring a better effect of the acupuncture anesthesia.

(d) Site of operation: The effect of acupuncture anesthesia was Grades I and II in 83.9% of the operations over the anterior cranial fossa, 81.7% over the posterior cranial fossa,and only 74.1% over the temporo-parieto-occipital region. The relatively poor effect of the latter group might be attributed to the thick temporal muscles over this area.

Table 4. Predetermination of individual variation

Item	No. of Cases	Coincidence	χ^2 test
Pain threshold	69	69.57%	$P<0.05$
Pain tolerance threshold	69	76.81%	$P<0.05$
Heart rate	69	75.36%	$P<0.05$
Blood vessel volume (Plethysmogram)	69	84.05%	$P<0.05$
Skin temperature	47	72.30%	$P<0.05$
Galvanic skin response	71	50.00%	$P>0.05$
Pain reaction to venous puncture	64	80.00%	$P<0.05$

(II) Anti-shock

Acupuncture anesthesia not only left the physiologic functions of the body almost undisturbed, but also rendered the blood pressure, pulse rate and respiration stable during the operation. A comparison between the two groups of 50 patients each, who underwent surgical removal of tumors over the sellar region, was made, with operations of one group performed under acupuncture anesthesia and the other under drug anesthesia. In the group of acupuncture anesthesia only one patient's blood pressure dropped over 20mm Hg during the operation, while in the group of drug anesthesia there were 32 such cases. In the group of acupuncture anesthesia only 9 patients' pulse rate increase exceeded 20/min., while in the group of drug anesthesia there were 29 such cases (Fig. 1). In addition, the two groups of 20patients each, which had the resection of acoustic neurinoma investigated, had the operations in one group performed under general anesthesia and that in the other group under acupuncture anesthesia. The former group had 7 patients whose blood pressure fluctuated more than 40mm Hg, while in the latter group there was none. In the group of general anesthesia 9 patients had bradypnea and 2 had apnea during the operation, while in the group of acupuncture anesthesia only 2 had the former and none had the latter. In addition,

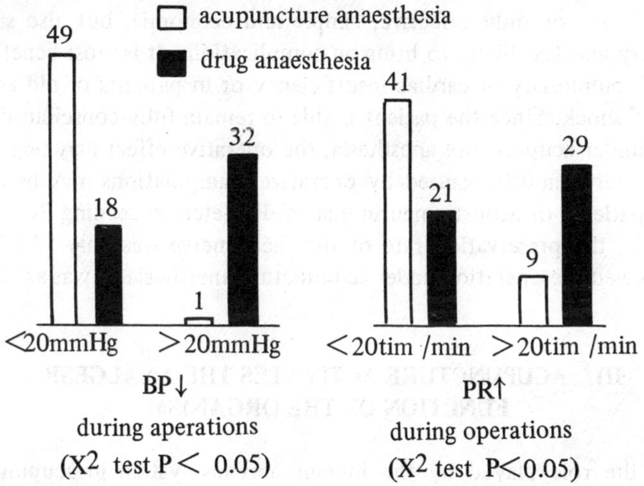

Fig. 1 Comparison between acupuncture and drug anaesthesia about BP, pulse rate during operation, patients with pituitary tumor, each 50 cases.

in the group of general anesthesia, 4 patients had the functions of the brain stem and/or cranial nerves impaired after the operation, while in the group of acupuncture anesthesia none showed impairment.

(III) Anti-infection

Experiments proved that needling the points Hegu and Zusanli induced leucocytosis and increase the phagocytic power of leucocytes. This indicated that acupuncture had a definite anti-infection effect. Comparing the incidence of postoperative pneumonia in 644 patients of acoustic neurinoma resected under general and acupuncture anesthesia, we found that among the 333 patients who received the operation under general anesthesia, 35 (10.5%) had postoperative pulmonary complication, while in the 311 patients under acupuncture anesthesia there were only 9 (2.8%). Statistically, the difference was significant (Fig. 2).

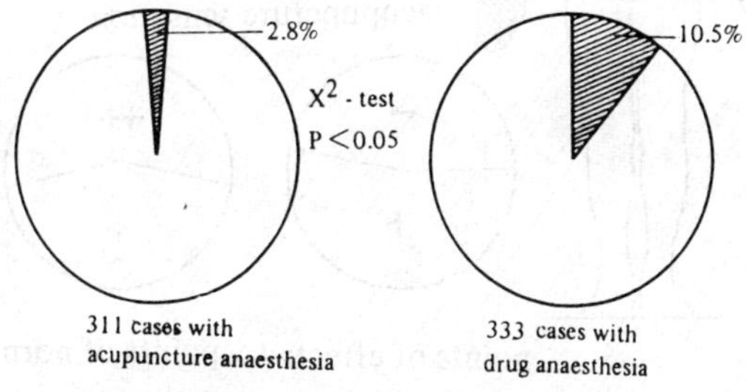

Fig. 2 % of postoperative complicated pneumonia in patients with acoustic neuroma.

As acupuncture anesthesia has the above-mentioned anti-pain, anti-shock and anti-infection effects, it is not only effective, simple and economic, but also safer capable of hastening recovery and less likely to bring on complications. It is most beneficial in patients of hepatic, renal, pulmonary or cardiac insufficiency or in patients of old age, poor health, or in the state of shock. Since the patient is able to remain fully conscious during an operation performed under acupuncture anesthesia, the operative effect may be assessed quickly, and unnecessary nerve injuries caused by operative manipulations may be minimized. For example, in 22 patients of acoustic neurinoma of diameters exceeding 3 cm resected under general anesthesia, the preservation rate of the facial nerve was only 54.5%, while in 137 patients that received the operation under acupuncture anesthesia, it was as high as 80.3%.

III. ACUPUNCTURE ACTIVATES THE ANALGESIC FUNCTION OF THE ORGANISM

Studies on the role played by the human nervous system in acupuncture analgesia were conducted in the neurological clinic with care being taken not to produce any untoward effects on the course and treatment of the disease. Preliminary observations in the following three areas aspects were made:

(I) The spinal afferent pathway for needling sensations

Supposing that "De qi" (i. e. the sensations of soreness, distension, numbness and heaviness induced by needling an acupuncture point) and myoelectro-activity at the point

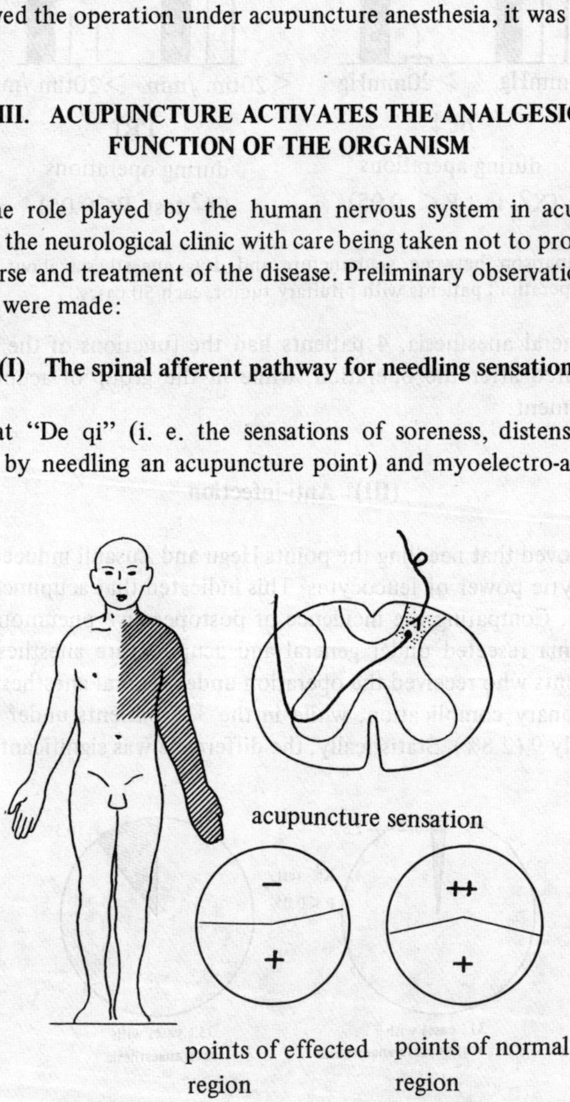

Fig. 3 Lesion of superficial sensory tract (syringomyelia) 40 cases.

represent the needling sensations, and the rise in the pain threshold and pain tolerance threshold after needling together with the cortical inhibition of the somatosensory evoked potential could represent acupuncture effects in 101 cases with various spinal diseases, the affected areas were needled with the normal area as a control to compare the effects. Cases of complete transverse section of the spinal cord gave no acupuncture sensations or effects at all below the sectioned level which indicated that acupuncture sensation depended upon the impulses ascending from the spinal tracts to the brain. When the spinal pathway of the motor impulse or of deep sensation was impaired, needling the points over the affected area evoked acupuncture sensations and effects, which illustrated that acupuncture sensations were independent of the tracts for spinal motor impulses or those for deep sensations.

In 40 cases of syringomyelia, whose dorsal horn or anterior commissure was impaired so that the spinal sensory pathway (the superficial sensations of pain and temperature passing through the ventrolateral bundle of the spinal cord) was destroyed, needling the points over the affected area could only produce feeble or even negative acupuncture sensations (Fig. 3). Accordingly, the acupuncture effect either rémarkably decreased or completely disappeared. Inhibition of the evoked cerebral potential was insignificant and therefore the rise in the pain threshold was indefinite.

These results illustrated that the ventrolateral bundle was the spinal afferent pathway for the acupuncture sensations.

(II) The role of the caudate nucleus in acupuncture analgesia

21 patients of late stage cancer with severe pain were treated with electric stimulation through retained electrodes on the dorsal side of the head of the caudate applied by stereo-orientational operation. The stimulation could abate pain, raise the pain and pain tolerance thresholds, lower the skin electricity response and reduce the respiratory as well as the finger-vessel volume reactions. The analgesic effect produced by stimulating the caudate nucleus was similar to that of acupuncture needling. Both were capable of relieving pain and inducing sedation; both had a latent period and after effects; and neither had any marked seg mental distribution. Evoked electropotential could be recorded from the caudate nucleus when electrical stimulation of the needling points was given. This electropotential appeared as a complex wave comprising several positive and negative elements. The latent period of the peak potential of the predominant element was P100–180 msec and N148–332 msec (Fig. 4). Electric stimulation at either the acupuncture needling points or the dorsal side of the head of the caudate nucleus had an inhibiting effect upon the latent elements of somatosensory evoked potential of the cerebral cortex and upon that of the thalamic central nucleus (see Figs. 5 and 6). These results indicated that the caudate nucleus nuinght plays an important role in acupuncture analgesia.

(III) Relationship between endorphin in the cerebrospinal fluid and acupuncture analgesia

In 8 patients that underwent ventriculostomy, 6–8ml of cerebrospinal fluid was collected before and after needling the acupuncture points. (The cerebrospinal fluid dropped

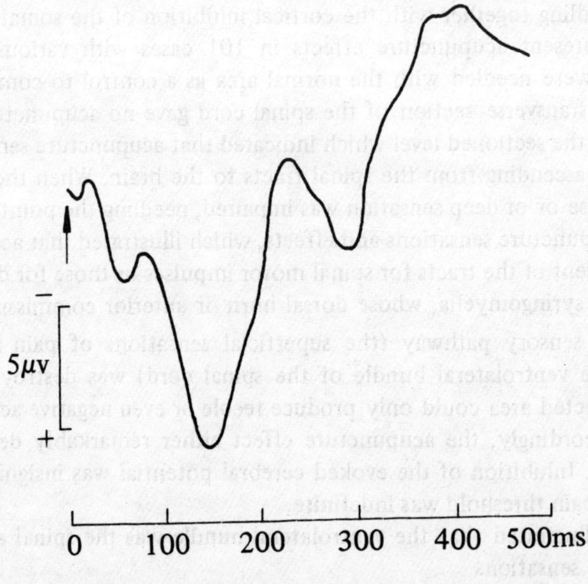

Fig. 4 Ep. from head of caudate, unipolar En-50 stimulating points Ho-Ku, Nei-Kuan.

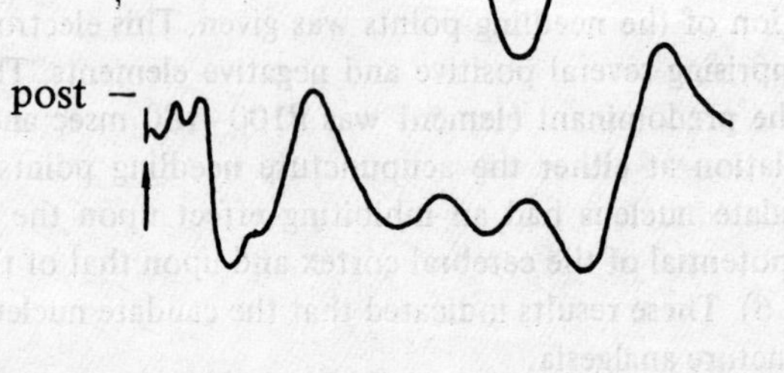

Fig. 5 Effects of caudate stimulation on SEP stim. R. median nerve on Wrist Lead. L. CPR-Al. En-50.

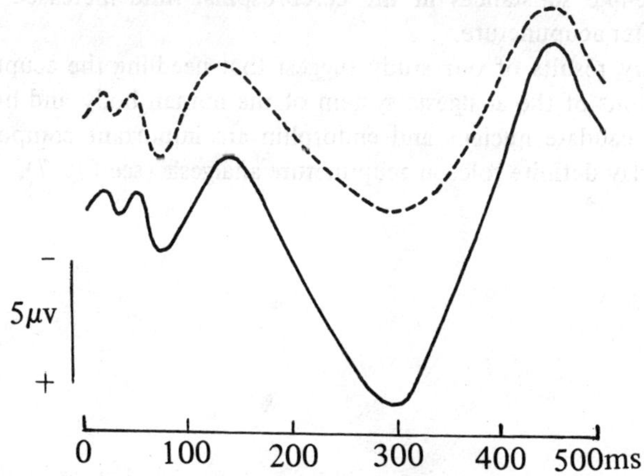

Fig. 6 Effects of caudate Stim. on EPs from C.M. of thalamus. pre-stim. — post-stim, ...

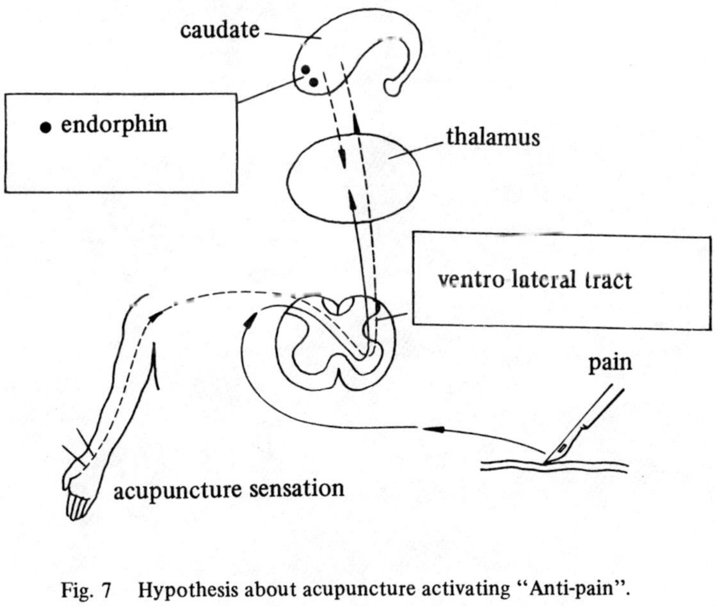

Fig. 7 Hypothesis about acupuncture activating "Anti-pain".

directly into a scaled centrifuge tube refrigerated by dry ice.) Hypothermic ultra-filtration with CXA-10 ultra-filtration membrane (cross-passing molecular weight 10,000) was carried out and 5 ml of ultra-filtered cerebrospinal fluid was taken, dried in hypothermic vacuum and subjected to chromatography on Sephadex G-10 molecular sieve. The final solution was collected in separate tubes and was assayed by radioreceptor analysis. It was found that the level of morphine-like substances in the cerebrospinal fluid increased markedly (average increase 36.6%) after acupuncture.

These preliminary results of our study suggest that needling the acupuncture points can activate the functions of the analgesic system of the human body and hence produce analgesic effects. The caudate nucleus and endorphin are important components of the analgesic system and play definite roles in acupuncture analgesia (see Fig. 7).

LARYNGECTOMY UNDER ACUPUNCTURE ANESTHESIA
(REPORT OF 430 CASES)

Huang Henian

(ENT Department, EENT Hospital, Shanghai First Medical College, Shanghai)

Four hundred and thirty cases of advanced carcinoma of the larynx unsuitable for radiotherapy had been treated by total laryngectomy under acupuncture anesthesia from June, 1970 to December, 1978. Favorable anesthetic results were observed in 73.5% of these cases. As the results of acupuncture anesthesia were quite satisfactory, we persistently used this kind of anesthesia all through that period.

The present paper sums up our clinical experience in the above-mentioned 430 patients, evaluates the results of the acupuncture anesthesia using combinations of ear points, body points and points around the incision, and discusses the "three barriers". i.e. incomplete analgesia, reaction to traction of the larynx and irritative cough which we met with during the laryngectomy under acupuncture anesthesia, as well as the solution to these difficulties.

I. MATERIALS AND METHODS

(I) Selection of Patients

Laryngectomy has been one of the effective methods in treating carcinoma of the larynx. We used to routinely perform this operation under general anesthesia, but some cases were done under local anesthesia as well. From June, 1970 onwards, we selected patients who were emotionally stable and willing to receive the acupuncture anesthesia, and whose lesions were localized. We treated them with laryngectomy under acupuncture anesthesia. The effect of the acupuncture anesthesia was very good. Generally postoperative reactions were mild. Tracheal secretion was reduced, and so there was not much coughing. Wounds heales fast. Therefore in this operation acupuncture anesthesia was obviously superior to general anesthesia. The method was also welcomed by the patients. Later, we also selected cases in which more tissue was involved in the disease process, such as those in which the lesions were beyond the laryngeal cavity and even involved the base of the tongue, the periform sinus, the thyroid, and muscles of the anterior neck, or those cases that had been treated by radiotherapy preoperatively and had adhesions. Satisfactory results were also observed in such cases. Since then, we have gradually used acupuncture anesthesia as our first choice in laryngectomy instead of general anesthesia. Among the 430 patients of laryngectomy under acupuncture anesthesia, the oldest was 83 years of age, and the youngest was 21.

(II) The Method of Acupuncture Anesthesia

1. The selection of the points. At the beginning, the body points hoku, nei-guan, and chih-kou were tried. Later, we changed the body points to the ear points 'lung', 'shenmen', 'sympathetic', 'neck', 'pingchuan', 'adrenal', and 'pharyngolarynx'. Since 1974, points fu-tu, tien-ting and chi-she have been added, which are on the two sides of the neck.

2. The technical procedure of the acupuncture anesthesia. At first, we continuously twisted the needles which were inserted in the points by hand. Since this was laborious, we connected the needles to an electric stimulor. Generally, an induction time of 20–30 minutes was needed.

The frequencies for the ear needles and body needles were 2–3 Hz, and for the needles around the skin incision they were 8–16 Hz. The intensity of the stimulation was adjusted according to the tolerance of the patient.

3. Supplementary medication. We gave the patients luminal 0.1g orally two hours before operation, and phethidine 75 mg intramuscularly half an hour before operation.

(III) Classification of the Effect of the Acupuncture Anesthesia and Its Recording

The whole procedure of the operation was divided into ten steps in the following order:

Incision of the skin, dissection of muscles of the anterior neck, resection of the hyoid bone, dissection of the thyroid gland, suturing of the artificial skin fistula, resection of the trachea, dissection and removal of the laryngeal body, suturing of the mucous membranes of the pharyngolarynx, and suturing of the skin.

According to the degree of the pain shown by the response of the patients during the operation, four grades were observed: no pain, slight pain, moderate pain and severe pain. At the same time, attention was paid to the expressions of the patients, such as knitting of the eyebrows, tenseness in the extremities and sweating. All these manifestations were recorded. After the operation, we performed a follow up examination and completed the records.

The four-graded classification of the results of the anesthesia: Grade one (Excellent). The patient had no apparent pain, the operation was carried out smoothly without adding any local anesthesia.

Grade two (Good). The patient suffered from slight pain occasionally, but the operation was still successful, without adding local anesthesia.

Grade three (Fair). The patient complained of pain. 1% procaine not exceeding 5c.c. or pethidine (less than 75 mg) was required, and the operation could be performed through to the end.

Grade four (Poor). The patient complained of severe pain. The operation couldn't be carried out and general or local anesthesia had to be substituted for acupuncture anesthesia.

(IV) The Clinical Effect of the Acupuncture Anesthesia

In our 430 cases, the Excellent and Good rate totalled 73.5%. According to the four-graded classification, the result of the acupuncture anesthesia is shown in the following table.

Table The results of the classification of the 430 cases of laryngectomy under acupuncture anesthesia

Grade	I Excellent	II Good	III Fair	IV Poor
No. of cases	174	142	66	48
Percentage	40.5	33	15.3	11.2

II. DISCUSSION

Laryngectomy under acupuncture anesthesia is quite safe and convenient. But the operation is rather extensive. It is necessary to dissect all the muscles of the anterior neck, section the isthmus of the thyroid, free the larynx, section the trachea and repair the esophagus. Nearly every important structure of the neck is involved. Under such circumstances, the duration of the operation is usually long, taking 3–4 hours in general, and this makes the operation difficult to be performed under acupuncture anesthesia. In our experience, laryngectomy is a typical surgical procedure for studying the acupuncture anesthesia of the neck. Thus, it is of great clinical significance to carry out meticulous research in dealing with the "three barriers".

Through our clinical practice in the past eight years, we have found that the "three barriers" in laryngectomy under acupuncture anesthesia are incomplete analgesia, reaction to the traction of the larynx, and irritatant cough. The causes of the "three barriers" and their interrelations as well as the solution to these problems are summarized as follows:

(I) Searching for Effective Points

The selection of the points is extremely important in producting the effect of the acupuncture anesthesia. Incomplete analgesia appears to be a matter of the utmost importance. If incomplete analgesia occurs during the incision of the skin or dissection of the muscles of the neck, the operation will be rather difficult. Finally, the acupuncture anesthesia has to come to an end if an irritative cough, suffocation or bleeding make it hard for the patient to endure. Finding various effective points and using them in appropriate combinations so that the patient feels no, or only slight, pain in the early stages of the operation and so that he keeps mentally relaxed and cooperative, are the keys to the smooth performance of the operation under acupuncture anesthesia.

Back in 1970 when we performed laryngectomy under acupuncture anesthesia for the first time, we used the body points-hoko, nei-guan, chih-kou, chih-ze, and chu-chih. Later, we changed to the ear points 'lung', 'shenmen proceeding on to sympathetic', 'neck proceeding on to pingchuan', and 'adrenal proceeding on to pharyngolarynx'. However, in practising this, we found neither of the methods was very successful. Then we tried combining the ear points with body points on the left. Since then, the Excellent and Good rate has been raised from 53% to over 70%. But there were still some patients complaining of pain around the skin incision at the beginning of the operation so they could not endure any further steps of the operation and general anesthesia had to be used.

Since 1974, the points fu-tu, tien-ting and chi-she on both sides of the skin incision have been added. Two fine long needles have been used to penetrate the three points over a distance of about 3–4 cm on either side. This method greatly alleviated the pain around the skin incision. However, there arose the disadvantage that the patient had to tolerate too many needles. To remedy this short-coming, the ear points have been reselected. We used a combination of the ear points 'lung', 'shemen proceeding on to sympathic', the body points he-gu and lie-que, and the points around the skin incision fu-tu, tien-ting and qi-she. We would like to recommend this method of acupuncture anesthesia. It consists of eight points in three different groups. By using these points, the acupuncture anesthesia seems to have become more effective.

(II) Improving the Surgical Procedure

In our experience, the "three barriers" are related not only to the acupuncture anesthesia itself, but also to the technique of the surgery. We have found that the tractional reaction and irritative cough during the dissection and resection of the larynx or the trachea are mainly due to the surgical procedure which is suitable for the patient under general anesthesia, but not for the patient who is conscious under acupuncture anesthesia. The heavy irritation makes it hard for the patient to endure the operation. This is the usual cause of failure. Now, we have improved the surgical procedure in dissecting and sectioning the larynx and the trachea as described below.

1. Rapid section of the hyoid bone and relaxation of the structure of the upper part of the neck. When induction of the acupuncture anesthesia is complete, a midline incision is made from the level above the hyoid bone to just below the level of the middle of the suprasternal notch. Next the sternohyoid muscles, sternothyroid muscles and their tendons which are attached to the upper and lower margins of the hyoid bone are dissected. The hyoid bone is sectioned with a pair of scissors as quickly as possible. In this way, the structures of the upper part of the neck are relaxed and the traction reduced.

2. Section of the isthmus of the thyroid gland, exposure of the trachea and prevention of suffocation. Before freeing and dissecting the larynx, we section and ligate the isthmus of the thyroid. Subsequently, the thyroid is dissected from the trachea, so that the upper end of the trachea can be exposed. This makes it convenient to do a tracheotomy when it is necessary to release dyspnea and prevent suffocation.

3. Suturing the severed end of the trachea quickly to prevent the blood from flowing into the respiratory tract, which will produce an irritaant cough. After the upper portion of the trachea has been dissected from the esophagus, we proceed to cut the greater horn of the hyoid bone with a pair of scissors, dissect the constrictor pharyngeal muscles, prepare the rounded artificial orifice in the skin, cut the upper part of the trachea at safe distance from the growth, and suture the severed end of the trachea to the skin orifice just made. Coughing often occurs during the cutting of the trachea because of blood flowing into the trachea, and because of over-manipulation by the surgeon. Severe coughing often makes the patients unable to restrain themselves. Therefore, it is important to pay attention to the hemostasis, see that suction be at hand all the time, suture the artificial tracheal orifice as fast as possible, and manipulate carefully during the operation, in order to avoid unnecessary irritation to the mucous membrane of the trachea.

4. Dissection of the larynx from below to relax the traction. As soon as we finish suturing the severed end of the trachea, the laryngeal body is dissected from below moving in an upward direction The periform sinus is pushed upward, the pharyngolaryngeal cavity is entered from the posterior margin of the arytenoids, and finally the laryngeal body is removed below the hyoid bone. Then the mucous membrane is sutured to the esophagus. At this point, we usually ask the patient to swallow so as to see immediately if there is any leakage to be repaired.

5. Keeping the airway open by means of the inner tube of the tracheal cannula If the lesions are extensive and the patient is already tracheotomized, we withdraw the outer tube when the plate of the outer tube interferes with the surgical field. Instead, a no. '6' inner tube is used. With this, the airway is maintained and the operation can be carried on smoothly.

III. SUMMARY

The present paper sums up 430 cases of laryngectomy under acupuncture anesthesia in the past eight years. The "three barriers", namely, incomplete analgesia, irritaant cough, and reaction to the traction of the larynx, have also been discussed. A combination of ear points, body points and points around the skin incision, in other words, an acupuncture anesthesia method which uses a total of eight points has been recommended. In order to enhance the effect of the acupuncture anesthesia, five main surgical technical improvements have been suggested. The Excellent and Good Rate in the 430 cases of laryngectomy under acupuncture anesthesia was 73.5%.

ACUPUNCTURE ANESTHESIA IN 1,965 CASES OF MAXILLARY SINUSOTOMY

National Cooperative Group of Acupuncture
Anesthesia for Radical Sinusotomy*

From March to December 1975, 1,965 radical maxillary sinusotomies were done under electroacupuncture anesthesia. There were 909 male and 611 female patients with ages ranging from 12 to 72 years, the majority being from 20 to 40. The occupation of the patients included 462 workers, 489 peasants, 175 cadres, 165 students, and 188 others. Most of the patients suffered from chronic maxillary sinusitis. As for their attitude toward acupuncture anesthesia, 26 patients asked for it of their own accord, 1072 patients showed full agreement, 137 patients consented after explanation, and 151 patients were not informed beforehand.

I. METHODS OF ACUPUNCTURE ANESTHESIA

In the majority of the patients, the acupuncture anesthesia apparatus used was of the G–6805 type. The patients were divided into two groups according to the acupuncture points used: In the first group, there were 1,149 patients in whom the adjacent points Quanliao and Sibai were adopted, and in the second group there were 816 patients in whom the distant points Hegu and Zhigou were selected, all being on the homolateral side of the affected sinus. The parameters of the electrical stimulation were 1,000–10,000 times per minute for the adjacent points, and 100–500 times per minute for the distant points. The pulse wave of stimulation was continuous. The induction time was generally 15–30 minutes, the shortest being 10 minutes, and the longest more than 60 minutes. The preoperative medication and supplemental drugs were as follows:

1. Phenobarbital 0.1 gm. given 30 minutes before operation,
2. Demerol 1 mg. per kilo 30 minutes before operation,
3. Phenobarbital and demerol in combination,
4. No supplemental drug at all.

II. ANALYSES OF THE EFFECT OF ACUPUNCTURE ANESTHESIA

(I) Criteria of grading the anesthetic effect

Grade 1: The operation was performed smoothly without the patient's feeling any pain.

* Compiled by the Departments of Otolaryngology and Anesthesiology, Bethune University of Medicine.

Table 1.

Group	No. of Cases	Grade 1		Grade 2		Grade 3		Grade 4		Good analgesic effect (Grade 1+2)		Success (Grade 1+2+3)	
		Cases	%	Cases	%	Cases	%	Cases	%	Cases	%	Cases	%
Quanliao & Sibai	1149	681	59.77	326	28.37	114	9.92	28	2.44	1007	87.64	1121	97.56
Hegu & Zhigou	316	450	55.14	255	31.25	86	10.54	25	3.06	705	86.40	791	96.94
Total	1965	1131	57.56	581	29.56	200	10.18	53	2.70	1712	87.12	1912	97.30

Table 2.

Occupation	No. of cases	Grade 1 and 2 analgesic effect		Success (Grade 1+2+3)	
		Cases	%	Cases	%
Workers	462	405	87.66	451	97.62
Peasants	489	427	87.32	481	98.36
Cadres	175	155	88.57	172	98.36
Students	165	126	76.36	158	95.75
Miscellaneous	188	167	88.82	184	97.87

There was no need for any supplemental drug, so not more than 1 mg. per kilo of demerol was used.

Grade 2: There was slight pain which did not influence the operation. The dose of demerol was within 1.5 mg. per kilo. A small amount of topical anesthetics was applied onto the sinus mucosa.

Grade 3: The pain was relatively marked, and the operation could be carried on only by the aid of supplemental drugs. The dosage of demerol was within 2 mg. per kilo, or less than 5 ml of 0.5% procaine was used locally.

Grade 4: The pain was so marked that the operation could not be carried on without changing to local anesthesia. The dosage of demerol was more than 2 mg. per kilo, and more than 5 ml of 0.5% procaine had to be used.

(II) Relation between various factors and the effect of acupuncture anesthesia

1. Relation between the points used and the effect of acupuncture anesthesia. The above Table 1 shows that the effect of analgesia was satisfactory in both groups. Grades 1 and 2 showing good analgesic effect was 87.64% for the adjacent points group and 86.4% for the distant points group. Thère is no significant difference between the two groups statistically ($P>0.05$).

2. Relation between sex and the effect. Comparison between Grades 1 plus 2 analgesic effect in the male and female groups shows no significant difference statistically ($P>0.05$).

3. Relation between age and the effect. Acupuncture anesthesia was less satisfactory in the group of young people below 20 years of age, as compared with its use in older groups ($P<0.05$).

4. Relation between occupation and the effect. It is evident from Table 2 that acupuncture anesthesia was less satisfactory in the student group ($P<0.05$).

5. Relation between patient mood and the effect. The figures in Table 3 shows that the patient mood did bear some relation to the anesthetic effect. Patients experiencing nervous tension had poorer results as compared with those who were in a quiet state ($P<0.05$).

6. Relation between acupuncture sensation and the effect. From Table 4 we can see that the transmission of the acupuncture sensation of a patient seemed to bear some rela-

Table 3.

Mood	No. of cases	Grade 1 and 2 analgesic effect		Success (Grade 1+2+3)	
		Cases	%	Cases	%
Quiet	775	708	91.59	758	98.06
Nervous	458	356	77.73	441	96.28

Table 4.

Acupuncture sensation	No. of cases	Grade 1 and 2 Analgesi ceffect		Success (Grade 1+2+3)	
		Cases	%	Cases	%
Propagated	314	284	90.44	306	97.45
Local	361	507	85.04	348	96.40
Poor	53	40	75.46	49	92.45

Table 5.

Operation time (minutes)	No. of cases	Good analgesic effect (Grade 1+2)		Success (Grade 1+2+3)	
		Cases	%	Cases	%
30 or less	386	356	92.22	383	99.22
31–60	674	952	87.83	666	98.81
over 60	360	287	79.72	335	93.06

tionship to the efficacy of acupuncture anesthesia, namely, the more intense the sensation of transmission, the better the effect of acupuncture anesthesia.

7. Relation between supplemental drugs and the effect. It is interesting that patients without any supplemental drug had better analgesic effect than those who received demerol and phenobarbital in combination before the operation. Therefore, the use of supplemental drugs is not a prerequisite to acupuncture anesthesia.

8. Relation between induction period and the effect. The optimal duration of induction was within 15 minutes. Prolonged induction did not produce any of the good effects of acupuncture anesthesia.

9. Relation between duration of the operation and the effect. It is clear from Table 5 that better results of acupuncture anesthesia were obtained when the operation was completed within 30 minutes.

III. DISCUSSION

It is our experience that maxillary sinusotomy under electroacupuncture anesthesia possesses the following advantages over local anesthesia:

1. There is less postoperative edema over the cheek of the operated side owing to the anti-inflammatory action of acupuncture: hence a more rapid convalescence.
2. There is persistent analgesia postoperatively so that most patients had only slight pain after operation. Out of the 1,965 patients who had their maxillary sinuses operated on under acupuncture anesthesia only 125 patients (6.18%) asked for analgesic drug postoperatively. This is less often than those who lave had local anesthesia.

As the analgesic effect of electroacupuncture anesthesia is not perfect, the operative manipulations should be steady, exact, gentle, and brisk to avoid unnecessary and inadvertent stimulus as much as possible. The following modifications are recommended:

1. Adrenalinized normal saline is injected in the labiogingival fold on the side of the operation to avoid excessive bleeding during operation.
2. A curved incision is made down to the bone in the labiogingival fold with a sharp knife, and retractors are gently placed.
3. The anterior wall of the maxillary sinus is opened with a drill instead of a chisel and hammer.
4. The counter opening at the inferior meatus is made while the sinus is packed with adrenalinized gauze and before the pathological mucous membrane of the sinus is removed.
5. At the end of the operation, the sinus may be packed with gelfoam, arubber balloon, or vaselin gauze strips to avoid pain on withdrawal.

As successful analgesic effects of electroacupuncture anesthesia for maxillary sinusotomy are obtained in only about 86% of cases, there still remains the problem of obtaining a complete analgesia. This requires further investigation.

CLINICAL ANALYSIS AND PRELIMINARY EXPERIMENTAL OBSERVATIONS OF 1,802 CASES OF ORO-MAXILLO-FACIAL OPERATIONS UNDER ACUPUNCTURE ANESTHESIA

Qiu Weiliu*, Lin Guochu*, Yuan Wenhua*, Liu Shixun*,
Ha Qi*, Fan Baohua*, Chen Shaodong**, Liu Yugui**,
Shen Jiannan***, Ma Guizhen*** Lü Juying***

(Ninth People's Hospital, Shanghai Second Medical College)

From May 1966 to November 1977 we performed 1,802 oro-maxillo-facial operations using acupuncture anesthesia (Selecting distal points according to the course of the channels and retaining the needles after 'Deqi', i. e. the normal needling reaction). Partial data were reported in 1973[1]. This paper offers an analysis of the factors which influence the analgesic effect of acupuncture anesthesia, and a preliminary discussion of the mechanism of our method.

I. MATERIALS AND METHODS

1. Patients. Of a total of 1,802 cases, 1,072 were male and 775 were female. Ages ranged from 13 to 88 years, and 88.6% of the cases involued persons over twenty.

2. Disease and operative regions. There were about 45 kinds of diseases in the 1,802 cases. Since many operations were not done by standard procedures, we divide our cases into nine groups according to anatomic regions:

(1) Parotid region: included mixed tumor, carcinoma, cyst of the parotid, etc. Superficial parotidectomy and total parotidectomy make up 90.4% of the total cases of this region.

(2) Submaxillary region: included mixed tumor, chronic inflammation of submaxillary gland, hemangioma, etc. Dissection of the submaxillary triangle and excision of the maxillary gland make up 77.8% of the total cases of this region.

(3) Labio-buccal region: included lip cleft and carcinoma, hemangioma and defects of this region. Repair of clefts and excision of cancer plus reconstruction with flaps account for 73% of the total cases of this region.

(4) Cervical region: These were chiefly metastatic carcinomas. Unilateral neck dissection alone and combined with resection of the primary lesion were the main operations.

* Department of Oro-Maxillo-Facial Surgery
** Department of Traditional Chinese Medicine
*** Department of Anesthesiology

(5) Palatal region: including mixed tumor, cleft palate, etc. Excision of mixed tumors amounts to 76% of the total cases of this region.

(6) Mandibular region: including ameloblastoma, ossifying fibroma, cysts, etc. Unilateral partial or total mandibulectomies make up 27.9% of these cases, and removal of cysts and cleaning up of lesions of osteomyelitis make up 39.8% of the total respectively.

(7) Temporo-Mandibular joint region: including ankylosis and hypertrophy of the condyle: arthroplasty and condylectomy make up 74.1% and 20.9% of the total respectively.

(8) Maxillary region: including ameloblastoma, ossifying fibroma, etc. The operation which was performed, was chiefly resectioning (subtotal or total) of the maxilla.

(9) Others.

3. Point prescription. Points used in our series were selected according to the Jing-Luo theory, namely, selecting distal acupuncture points according to the course of the channels. We chiefly used points distal to the elbow or knee joint, and only in 23 cases were local points (the fifth cranial nerve) used for a control.

4. Mode of stimulation. The needles were inserted by hand at the prescribed points. It is essential that the patient has a feeling of soreness, distention, heaviness and numbness, and the anesthetist have a feeling of "Deqi".

The modes of stimulation in the present study were of four types.

A. Continuous manipulation: During both the induction and the operation, lifting-thrusting and rotating of the needles were used (180–200 revolutions per min.)

B. Continuous manipulation was used only for half an hour prior to operation in the induction period. The condition was the same as above but when the operation began, the manipulation was stopped but the needles were retained.

C. Continuous pulsating electric current stimulation: The electric instrument G6805 made in Shanghai was used (frequency 400 Hz; wave length 800 μs; intensity 0–30 v).

D. Retention of the needles after 'Deqi': After inserting the needles and obtaining 'Deqi', no manipulation or electric stimulation was used. But the anesthetist nust check from time to time whether the feeling of 'Deqi' still remains during the operation. If the feeling of 'Deqi' no longer exists, then he ought to correct it immediately until 'Deqi' is regained.

Dolantin 50 mg and Phenergan 50 mg i.m. were routinely used half an hour prior to operation. If necessary, Dolantin 25 mg i. v. was added during the operation.

II. ANALYSIS OF THE ANALGESIC EFFECTS AND THE FACTORS AFFECTING ANALGESIC EFFECTS OF ACUPUNCTURE ANESTHESIA

(I) The analgesic effects were graded in four classes

Grade I (excellent): Blood pressure and pulse were stable; the patient did not complain of pain, or had only slight pain in certain steps of the operation. These comprised 44.2% of the total (797 cases).

Grade II (good): Blood pressure and pulse were stable; the patient had slight pain, and 1% procaine below 10 ml was needed. These comprised 29.46% of the total (531 cases).

Grade III (fair): Blood pressure and pulse were fairly stable; the patient had considerable pain, and adjuvant druge such as Dolantin or Fentanyl were administered intravenously more than twice. In some cases over 10 c.c. of 1% procaine was needed. Such cases amounted to 18.75% of the total (338 cases).

Grade IV (poor): Blood pressure and pulse were unstable. The patient could not endure the operation, and some conventional anesthesia had to be substituted. In some cases over 20ml of 1% procaine was needed. 7.55% of the total (136 cases) belonged to this group.

According to this standard; the success rate (I+II+III) was 92.43% (1666/1802), the excellent plus good rate (I+II) was 73.68% (1328/1802), and the failure rate (IV) was 7.5% (136/1802).

(II) Analysis of factors affecting the analgesic effect of acupuncture anesthesia

1. Analgesic effect and sex. In neither the success rate nor the excellent plus good rate was there any significant difference between the male and female cases ($P>0.05$).

2. Analgesic effect and age. As table 1 shows, the success rate and excellent plus good rate of the 20–29 and 40–49 year old groups are higher than that of the group below 20 years ($P<0.05$ and 0.01), and the 40–49 old year group is still higher than the 20–29, year old group ($P<0.05$).

Table 1. The analgesic effect and age

Age group	No. of successes (I+II+III)	Success rate %	No. of excellents and goods (I+II)	Excellent plus good rate %	No. of failures (IV)	Failure rate %
< 20	171	87.69	127	65.12	24	12.30
20—	743	91.72	593	73.20	67	8.27
40—	428	90.48	284	60.04	45	4.51

3. Analgesic effect and mode of stimulation. The success rate at the 0.05 level, is not statistically different among the 4 groups of different modes of stimulation. We also compared the effect of different modes of stimulation in operations of the parotid (659 cases) and submaxillary (361 cases) regions. The results showed that neither the success rate nor the excellent plus good rate were significantly different in the two groups ($P>0.05$).

4. Analgesic effect and the anesthetist and surgery personnel. Before 1975, the anesthetists and surgical team were relatively stable (fixed team), but after 1975, there was no fixed personnel for the team (nonfixed team). Table 2 shows that the success and excellent plus good rates of the fixed team were significantly higher than those of the nonfixed team ($P<0.01$ and $P<0.05$ respectively).

5. Analgesic effect and point prescription. An example of this categort is the point prescription for operations of the parotid region. We have tested the efficacy of six point

Table 2. The analgesic effect and the organization of the anesthetist and surgical team

Group	No. of successes (I+II+III)	Success rate %	No. of excellents (I+II)	Excellent plus good rate %	No. of failures (IV)	Failure rate %
Fixed team	1,045	94.22	837	75.47	64	5.77
Nonfixed team	621	89.61	491	70.85	72	10.38

Table 3. The analgesic effects and operative regions

Operative region	No. of successes (I+II+III)	Success rate %	No. of excellents and goods (I+II)	Excellent plus good rate %	No. of failures (IV)	Failure rate %
Parotid	613	93.01	464	70.40	46	6.98
Submaxillary	342	94.73	289	80.05	19	5.26
Labiobuccal	171	91.93	156	83.67	15	8.06
Cervical	12	92.30	10	76.92	1	7.69
Palatal	105	98.13	92	85.98	2	1.86
Mandibular	215	88.47	162	65.58	28	11.52
T. M. J.	56	90.32	37	59.67	6	9.67
Maxilla	36	85.72	28	66.66	6	14.28
Others	107	89.16	90	75.00	13	10.28
Total	1,666	92.45	1,328	73.69	136	7.54

Table 4. The analgesic effect and duration of operation*

Duration (hr.)	No. of successes (I+II+III)	Success rate %	No. of excellents and goods (I+II)	Excellent plus good rate %	No. of failures (IV)	Failure rate
<2	524	87.77	441	73.86	73	12.22
2–	599	92.01	437	67.12	52	7.98
4–	101	97.11	62	59.61	3	2.88

* 451 cases were excluded since the duration was not recorded

prescriptions* for simplifing the prescription. We found that their success rate and excellent plus good rate were not significantly different ($P>0.05$). The sixth point prescription has been widely used in other oro-maxillo-facial operations.

6. Analgesic effect and region of operation. Table 3 shows there were significant statistical differences among the various operative regions ($P<0.01$). The success rate of the parotid, submaxillary, palatal or labial region was higher than that of the mandibular region ($P<0.01$). The excellent plus good rate of the submaxillary, parotid, palatal and labial region was also higher. In comparing the soft tissue operations with the bone structure operations, it was shown that the success and excellent plus good rates were both higher in the soft tissue operations than in the bone structure operations ($P<0.01$ in both cases).

7. Analgesic effect and the duration of operation. Table 4 shows there were no statistical differences in the success rate of the different groups based on operation duration ($P>0.05$). But the excellent plus good rate of the group in which operations lasted less than 2 hours was the highest ($P<0.05$ and 0.01).

III. DISCUSSION

1. It is generally considered that 'Deqi' is the key to success of acupuncture anesthesia. Most clinics have adopted the electric pulse stimulation method. However, our data show that once 'Deqi' is achieved, the mere retention of needles without using any electric pulse stimulation or manipulation can provide a sufficient amount of stimulation for an oro-maxillo-facial operation.

We carried out[1] an experiment in which convergent light was focused on a rabbit nose for a pain test. The pain reaction time was 24.4 seconds in the acupunctured and needle retaining group as compared to 13 seconds in the non-acupunctured group. The nearly 90% prolongation of pain reaction time is statistically significant ($P<0.05$). This clearly demoustrates the prolonged analgesic effect of simple needle retention after 'Deqi'. This result parallels the clinical analgesic effect of acupuncture. Furthermore, it seems to show more precisely what the role of acupuncture in anesthesia is by excluding the cooperating analgesic effect of electric stimulation.

The method of retaining the needles is simple and convenient, and it requires no special instruments.

2. Clinical and experimental studies in our series were based on theories of the traditional Chinese medicine:

A. Since "the head is the converging site of the 'Yang' channels", we mainly used the Yang channels.

---

* 1. Waiguan Huizong Houxi Sanjian Wangu Hegu Foot-Linqi Yangfu Gongsun Neiting Taichong Xiangu

2. Hegu Huizong Waiguan Houxi Wenliu Zhizheng Taichong Yangfu Foot-Linqi Gongsun Xiangu Fenglong Xingjian

3. Hegu Xiangu Taichong

4. Sanjian Houxi Hegu Wangu Huizong Neiguan

5. Fenglong Yangfu Foot-Fuyang Taichong Xiangu Xiaxi

6. Fenglong Taichong Gongsun

B. "In order to kill pain, intercrossing channels are selected"; so the points used were usually intercrossed and intersected.

C. "Lower points should be selected for upper ailments"; so we usually used the points on the extremities, especially on the lower extremities, whereby the anesthetist is kept out of the way. This is very important in oro-maxillo-facial operations.

More than 10 years' practice has shown us that although the entire system of the Jing-Luo is still unclear, the Jing-Luo phenomenon is an objective reality.

The Jing -Luo phenomenon manifested itself in the following observations:

A. In 1779 out of the 1802 cases, we selected distal points according to course of channels, with a success rate of 92%, and with an excellent or good rate of 73%. This shows that distal points along the course of the channels are effective.

B. As we reported previously[2], a patient with fibrous temporo-mandibular ankylosis was prepared for arthoplasty, and after acupuncture was given [points selected were Fenlong, Yangfu, Taichong, Gongsun etc.], his mouth immediately opened from the original 2mm to 35mm, making the operation unnccessary. This case demonstrates the typical phenomenon of propagation through Jing-Luo from the lower extremities to the head and facial region.

C. Utilizing Na^{125} I isotopic scanning in the propagation study of Jing-Luo, 4 positives were obtained in 58 cases.

Method: Na^{125} I was injected in the Neiguan point of the "pericardial" channel, and was measored at points Ximen, Quze and Tianquan, which are "pericardial" channel points, were at 40 sec. intervals. It was also measned at the control points on the ulnar and radial sides of the pericardial channel. The figures obtained show a higher uptake of Na^{125} I at the pericardial channel points than at the controls in a typical case (Figs. 1–3).

3. In oro-maxillo-facial operations we found the following advantages to vsing acupuncture anesthesia:

A. As compared with general anesthesia, acupuncture anesthesia is safe, produces fewer functional disorders and promotes an early recovery. In our series no anesthetic accident occurred, little postoperative care was needed, and the period of hospitalization was relatively short, reducing the patients' expenses.

B. Acupuncture anesthesia can be used in patients who show allergic reactions to local anesthetics, and in the resectioning of malignant tumors which is unsuitable for local infiltration anesthesia.

C. Special interest is paid to plastic operations where tissue deformity caused by local infiltration anesthesia can be avoided.

However, at present, acupuncture anesthesia still can not be applied to some oro-maxillo-facial operations such as 1) complex operations, 2) protracted operations, or 3) extensive operations.

Owing to incomplete analgesia and the uncomfortable reaction to stretching, acupuncture anesthesia has not been accepted by all patients and surgeons. It is necessary to continue the study to clarify its mechanism and improve its method. We feel that acupuncture anesthesia is soitable for medium-sized operations such as parotidectomy, excision of submaxillary gland, temporomandibular arthoplasty and bucco-labial operations. It can also be used in unilateral radical neck dissection in selected cases.

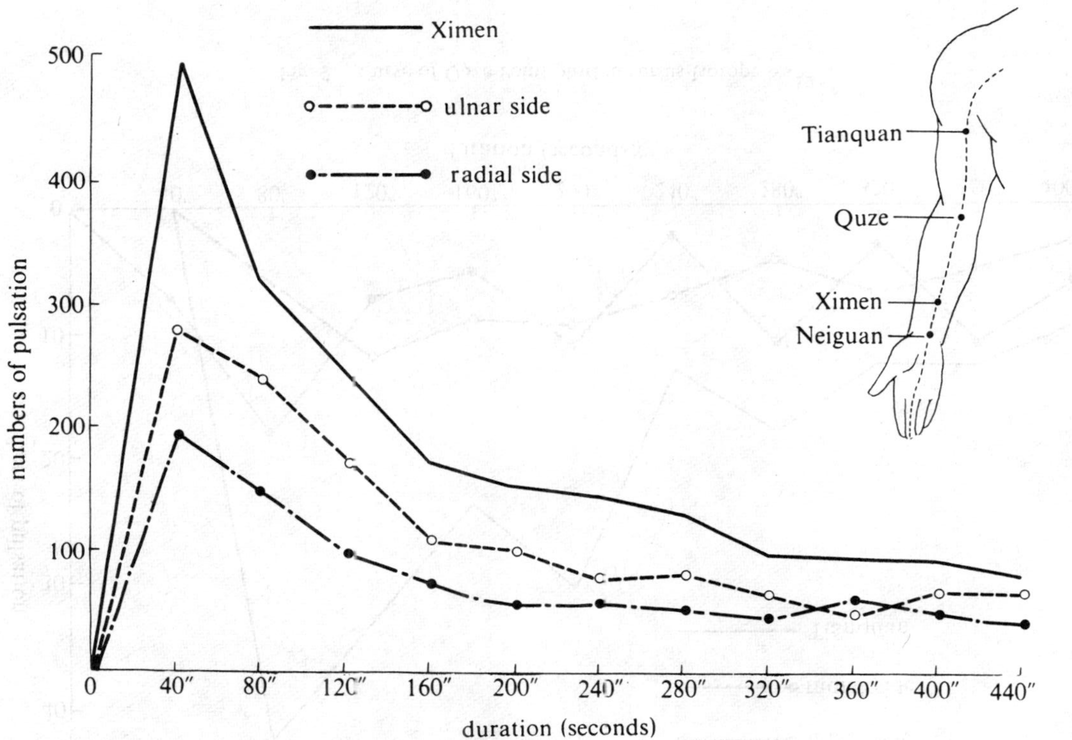

Fig. 1 Curve of Ximen point plotted versus Isotope Na^{125}.

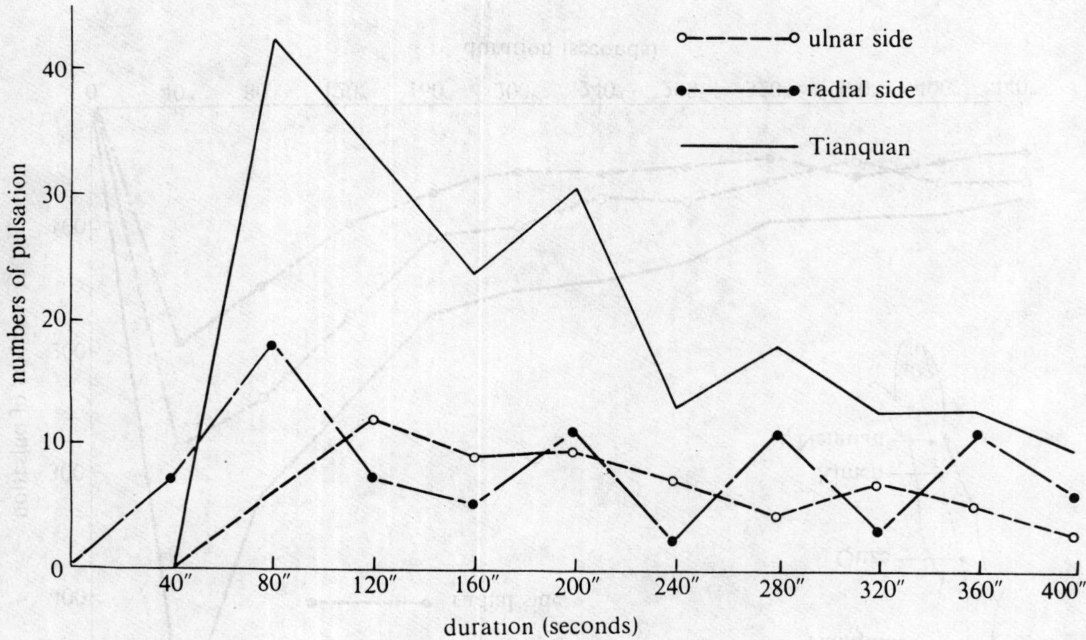

Fig. 2. Curve of Quze Point plotted versus Isotope Na^{125}.

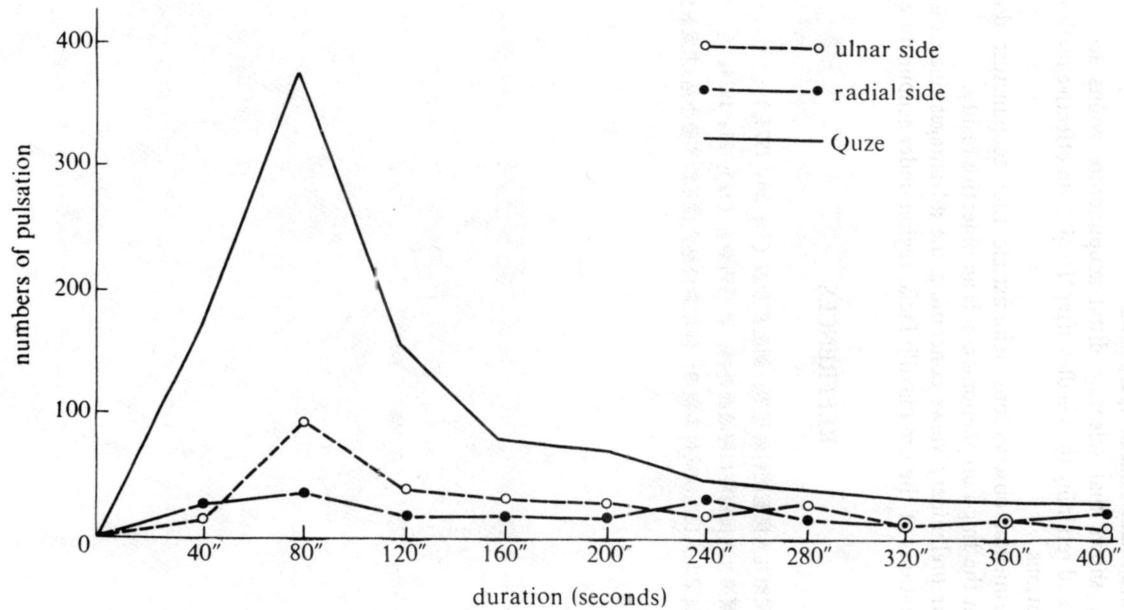

Fig. 3 Curve of Tianquen Point versus Isotope Na^{125}

IV. SUMMARY

We have discussed the effectiveness of acupuncture anesthesia and the factors affecting it in 1,802 cases of oro-maxillo-facial operations.

The present study shows that selecting distal acupuncture points according to the course of the channels and retaining the needles after 'Deqi' is an effective method for use in oro-maxillo-facial operations.

Clinical and experimental observations demonstrale that acupuncture does have an analgesic effect and that the Jing-Luo phenomenon is an objective reality.

We have given our preliminary views concerning the advantages, indications and existing problems in operations of the oro-maxillo-facial region under acupuncture anesthesia.

REFERENCES

[1] 上海第二医学院附属第九人民医院针麻组等：新医药杂志（3）：20，1973。

[2] 上海第二医学院附属第九人民医院口腔颌面外科：新医药杂志（12）：21，1974。

[3] 上海第二医学院附属第九人民医院同位素室等：同位素经络穴位示踪实验小结，未发表资料，1977。

SUMMARY OF 9,375 CASES OF THYROIDECTOMY UNDER ACUPUNCTURE ANESTHESIA

National Cooperative Group for Acupuncture Anesthesia
in Thyroidectomy

Before 1975 acupuncture anesthesia (A.A.) was used in 8,171 cases of different types of thyroid operations, with a successful rate of 95.4% and an excellent plus good rate of 84.8%. But for the hyperthyroidism cases the excellent plus good rate was only 74.2%. In order to find out what inherent rules govern A.A. in hyperthyroidism operations, we performed another 1,204 cases in 1976 and found that the excellent plus good rate was raised to 82.6%. The following is a summary of these 2 groups (9,375 cases).

I. CLINICAL DATA

(I) General

1. Sex: Male 2,339 cases; female 6,246 cases; M:F=1:2.7.
2. Age: Youngest 8 yrs; oldest 82; yrs; under 20, 538 cases; above 60, 151 cases; 21–40, 6,160 cases; 41–60, 2,326 cases.
3. Occupation: Workers 2,312; peasants 4,744; cadres 1,477; students 222; others 619.
4. Disease: Thyroid adenoma 3,882; cysts 1,843; nodular struma 856; hyperthyroidism 1,514; others 187.

(II) Methods of A.A.

1. Point prescription: 1st group: Hegu-Neiguan (both sides); 2nd group: neck Futu (both sides); 3rd group: ear points (Shengmen, Lung, Neck & sympathetic).
2. Frequency of stimulation: G–6805 type A.A. apparatus was used for most of the patients, using continuous waves. The frequency for the 1st group was 120–400 c./min., and for the 2nd & 3rd groups, 2,400–5,00 c./min. The intensity of stimulation was gradually increased to the maximum that the patient could tolerate.
3. Induction period: Usually 20–30 minutes.
4. Preoperative medication: Sod. luminal 0.1–0.2 gm. Certain patients might need valium, chlorpromazine, droperidol, scopolamine hydrobromide, etc. There were

Compiled by Chen Shude

384 patients receiving no preoperative drugs at all.

5. Adjuvant drugs: Dolantin 1mg./Kg body wt. iv. may be administered 15 min. prior to operation and another 25 mg may be be added 2hrs. later or if the result are not satisfactory. For some hyperthyroidism patients sedatives such as valium or droperidol may be administered. No adjuvants were given in 402 cases.

(III) Analysis of effect of A.A.

1. General results:

(1) Among the 8,171 cases of ordinary thyroid operations, the excellent plus good rate was 84.8% and the success rate was 95.4%.

(2) In the 1,204 cases of hyperthyroidism the excellent plus good rate was 83.7%, and the success rate was 95.2%.

2. Effect of A.A. in the 3 groups by points:

(1) In the 8,171 cases of ordinary thyroid operations the excellent plus good rate in the 3 groups was 85.5%, 83.8% and 85.7% respectively. No statistically significant difference was found among them (χ^2 equals 4.62, $p>0.05$); but the failure rate of the Futu group was higher than the other 2 groups showing a very significant difference statistically (χ^2 equals 14.15, $p<0.01$)(Table 1).

Table 1. Effect of A.A. in the 3 groups

Points	No. of pts.	Grades I & II		Grade III		Grade IV	
		No.	%	No.	%	No.	%
Hegu-Neiguan	3,175	2,714	85.5	336	10.9	125	3.9
Futu	3,221	2,699	83.8	339	10.6	183	5.4
Ear points	1,775	1,520	85.7	187	10.6	68	3.7
χ^2	-	$p>0.05$		-		$p<0.01$	

Table 2. Points used in hyperthyroidism operations and the effect of A.A.

Points	No. of pts.	Grades I & II		Grade III		Grade IV	
		No.	%	No.	%	No.	%
Hegu-Neiguan	423	375	84.3	42	11.4	18	4.2
Futu	73	54	73.9	12	16.4	7	9.5
Ear points	57	51	89.4	6	10.5	0	0
Taichong, Xiangu	137	102	74.4	28	20.3	7	5.1
χ^2	-	$p<0.01$		-		$p<0.01$	

(2) 1,204 cases of operations under A.A. on hyperthyroidism:
4 groups with atotal of 696 cases having different point prescriptions with complete records, and containing more than 50 cases each were compared. We found that the results were better in the Hegu-Neiguan & ear points group and worse in the Taichong and Futu groups. Statistically the difference was very significant (χ^2 equals 12.1, $p<0.01$) (Table 2).

3. The type of operation and the effect of A.A.: The effect of A.A. was less satisfactory in complicated operations, especially those with severe traumatization. So the results in thyroid adenoma or cyst extirpations were usually better than in Partial and total thyroidectomies. There was a very significant difference ($p<0.01$)(Table 3).
4. Duration of operation and the effect of A.A.: The longer the duration, the less satisfactory the effect of A.A. were meaning the excellent plus good rate would drop and failure rate would raise. Statistically there was a very significant difference ($p<0.01$) (Table 4).

Table 3. Types of operations and results of A.A.

Operations	No. of pts	Grades I & II		Grade III	Grade IV	
		No.	%		No.	%
Excision of thyroid adenoma	2,396	2,137	89.1	198	61	2.5
Thyroid cyst extirpation	1.092	975	89.2	92	25	2.2
Subtotal thyroidectomy	1.975	1,596	80.8	271	108	5.4
Total thyroidectomy	414	343	82.8	50	21	5.0
Others	144	107	74.3	18	19	13.1
χ^2	-	$p<0.01$		-	$p<0.01$	

Table 4. Duration of operation and effect of A.A.

Duration of operation	No. of pts.	Grades I & II		Grade III		Grade IV	
		No.	%	No.	%	No.	%
<1 hr.	1,346	1,255	93.2	70		21	1.5
1 to 2 hrs.	2,282	1,966	86.1	241		75	3.2
2 to 4 hrs.	1,514	1,189	78.5	224		101	6.6
>4 hrs.	234	161	68.7	50		23	9.8
χ^2	-	$p<0.01$		-		$p<0.01$	

(IV) Blood pressure and pulse rate during A.A.

Owing to the regulatory action of A.A., the patients' circulatory function was unusually stable.

1. Change in blood pressure: In 145 out of 179 cases (81%) the blood pressure was stable (fluctuation < 20 mm Hg), and in the remaining 34 cases (19%) the fluctuation was above 20 mmHg.
2. Change in pulse rate: The pulse was stable (fluctuation < 20/min.) in 173 out of 193 cases (89.63%) and markedly fluctuated (>20/min.) in 20 cases (10.27%).

(V) Preoperative estimation of A.A. effect

1. Needling endurance test: Of the 871 cases receiving such tests, we found that in 664 cases the needling endurance test conformed well to the A.A. effect (positive, 76.23%) and negative in 204 cases (23.77%). Studying 433 cases from the above group we found that in 337 cases forecasted as Grades I and II, had such results. The conformation rate was 93.77%. But comparing 96 cases forecasted as Grades III and IV with their actual results of A.A., the conformation rate was only 56.2% (54 cases). Therefore further studies are necessary in order that better estimation of the effect of A.A. can be made.
2. Pain threshold estimation: We did preoperative K^+ iontophoresis tests in 195 cases and found that the pain threshold and the pain tolerance threshold were both increased in patients with 9000 A.A. effects.

II. DISCUSSION

(1) Selection of points. The following 3 groups of points were selected according to the clinical experience of certain hospitals in the country: 1, Hegu-Neiguan according to the Channal theory; 2, neck-Futu in view of stimulation of the related nerves and 3, ear points. The excellent plus good rates were 85.5%, 83.8% and 85.7% respectively, with no significant difference statistically (χ^2 equals 4.62, p>0.05). But the Futu group showed a marked failure rate compared to the other 2 groups (χ^2 equals 14.5, p<0.01). Since 1976 we have selected 22 groups of points such as Taichong-Xiangu, Taichong, Hegu-Zusanli, Hegu-Zhigou and points of scalp needling, nasal needling, etc. Their excellent plus good rates were quite similar to those of the 3 groups mentioned above. But because they were mostly reported by only one hospital and since the number of patients were not enough for analysis (over 100 cases in only 10 groups), they need further study. From the clinical study of more than 10 thousand cases, we would recommend these 3 groups of points for clinical use, because the effect was quite steady and reliable. We found also that each group had its own characteristics. When the Hegu-Neiguan were needled with intensive electrostimulation the patient would usually feel a soreness and distention in the hand and also a weakness of the thumb when grasping for several postoperative days. In operations on large thyroid tumors acupuncturing the Futu point, would inevitably interfere with the operation field. If the nee-

dle is placed in too deep there is a chance of injuring the vagus and/or the phrenic nerve thus influencing the respiratory and cardiac function. In a deep ear point acupuncture there is a chance of producing auricular chondritis or even causing auricle atrophy. So selecting the ideal points is of prime importance for best clinical results.

(2) Individual difference and the A.A. effect: In order to assess the individual differences, preoperative evaluations were performed by methods such as type-differentiation according to principles of traditional Chinese medicine, propagation of sensation along the channels (P S C), needle manipulation test of the pain threshold and pain tolerance threshold, plethysmogram, temperature and galvanic skin reflex etc. None of these methods helped very much except the manual pain threshold and pain tolerance threshold tests which not only were easy to perform but afforded a rather high conformation rate in the preoperative estimation of A.A. effect during thyroid operations. From observations on a large number of patients we found that the excellent plus good rate was high in mentally stable and quiet patients especially in those who requested this anesthesia. Otherwise the result were so good unless the patient was completely persuaded and well informed before operation so that their worries and misunderstandings were eliminated.

(3) Subsidiary medication: 402 cases of our thyroid operations under A.A. did well without any subsidiary medication. With some patients however, small amounts of drugs may be necessary in order to eliminate pain, lessen their worries and enhance the effect of A.A.. It is also important not to administer an excess of drugs because this might produce untoward effects such as a semi-comatous condition or even excitement, which would of course interfere with the operation. The condition of patients with respiratory obstruction may be worsened on such occasions.

(4) Modification of operative technique: From our experience we found that the effect of A.A. was closely related to the type of disease, the mode of operation and the duration of the operation. For instance, the results of A.A. in hyperthyroidism operations or in partial and total thyroidectomies were usually worse than those in thyroid adenoma or cyst extirpations. The longer the duration of the operation, the lower the excellent plus good rate. In operations of less than 1 hr's duration, the excellent-good rate was 93.2%, but in operations longer than 4 hrs it dropped to 68.7%. So it is necessary to modify the operative technique both to minimize trauma and to shorten the period of operation. In other words, in all thyroid operations under A.A., steady, accurate, fast and light surgical manipulation is essential for an ideal result to be obtained.

(5) Hyperthyroidism operation under A.A.: The handling of hyperthyroidism patients is rather complicated because of their specific physiopathological characteristics. One should pay special attention not only to the operation but also to the pre- and post-operative care. Drug anesthesia was routinely used in the past. But it has been found that acupuncture anesthesia is much better than both epidural or general anesthesia because of its effectiveness, reliability and lower frequency of complications. In our 1,204 cases, we found that the successful and excellent plus good rates was 95.2% and 82.6% respectively. We believe that A.A. produces a reliable effect in both hyperthyroidism and other thyroid operations. In hyperthyroidism operations we consider good pre-operative preparation and a certain amount of adjuvant drugs to be essential. The pre-operative requirements for such patients include a very stable mental state, a gain in body weight, B.M.R. below +20% and a pulse rate under 100/min. In our group, postoperative crises happened in 3 patients, whose B.M.R.

was fairly high before the operation. The beta-receptor inhibitory drugs like inderal and practolol are all useful for lowering the pulse rate before the operation and keeping it stable during the operation.

(6) Indications and complications: As the results of thyroid operations under A.A. are quite steady with high success and excellent plus good rates, we recommend this anesthesia for all sorts of thyroid operations except in the case of persons who firmly refuse it. In cases in which the effect of A.A. was relatively poor, the blood pressure rose and the pulse rate increased. Thus, for the severe types of hyperthyroidism cases, especially those with unfavorable sings preoperatively (e.g. having ill-controlled B.M.R., recent attacks of thyroid crisis, auricular fibrillation and/or heart failure etc.,) one must see to it that they be treated satisfactorily before operation. Complications during operation are usually produced by improper body posture, rough manipulation of the thyroid tissue, and pressure deviation of the trachea which causes difficulty in breathing. Some patients may have headaches caused by: (a) long hyperextension of neck, (b) heavy traction during dissection of the upper pole of the thyroid, (c) functional change in autonomous nerves due to clamping of thyroid vessels, (d) immobilization of the neck due to post-operative pain. Postoperative headaches, in most cases, can be prevented by careful manipulation.

III. SUMMARY

(1) We have summed up our experierce from 9,375 cases of thyroid operations (including 1,204 cases of hyperthyroidism) under acupuncture anesthesia, which we would recommend as the anesthesia of the first choice to be used in all kinds of thyroid operations because it is simple, effective and reliable.

(2) The following aspects have been discussed in some detail: (a) selection of points, (b) individual differences in behaviour toward A.A., (c) subsidiary medication, (d) modification of operative technique, (e) hyperthyroidism operation under A.A., (f) indications and complications.

(3) A.A. can be used in all thyroid operations except when the patients are incooperative.

(4) In some patients the analgestic effect of A.A. is not complete, so certain analgesic or adjuvant drugs should be given. Further studies are needed to made the anesthesia more effective.

OPERATIVE TREATMENT OF HYPERTHYROIDISM UNDER ACUPUNCTURE ANESTHESIA

Zhu Yu, Yang Baoheng, Wang Xiuhua,
Luo Laikui, Zhuang Liding
(Department of Surgery, Capital Hospital, Chinese Academy of Medical Sciences, Beijing)

The choice of anesthesia for the surgical treatment of hyperthyroidism is usually a complicated problem which challenges many surgeons. Local anesthesia is sometimes not satisfactory for huge goiters, and cervical epidural block with its high technical requirement and an anesthetic level difficult to control, is known for its high incidence of complications, such as respiratory inhibition, disagreeable sensation sequential to the puncture and nerve injuries. General anesthesia with endotracheal intubation will apparently cause more of a burden to the patient, and in carrying out the operation with the patient in an unconscious state, it is not uncommon to find neglect of a recurrent laryngeal nerve injury. Also the incidence of postoperative thyroid crisis and other complications is high in cases of severe hyperthyroidism. Therefore, there is not yet am ideal anesthetic procedure for thyroid surgery.

The introduction of acupuncture anesthesia into clinical use opened up new vistas in the area of anesthesia for operative treatment of hyperthyroidism. Based on our own practice, acupuncture anesthesia used in subtotal thyroidectomy for hyperthyroidism distinguishes itself by its stability in effect, safety and simplicity in use, and low incidence of complication. Our results are presented as follows.

I. CLINICAL DATA

A total of 276 cases of hyperthyroidism were operated on under acupuncture anesthesia in our hospital from Jan. 1972 to Dec. 19, 1977. Of these, 37 were male and 239 were female, trovs having a ratio of 1:6.5. The ages of the male patients ranged from 13 to 54, with an average of 38; the ages of the female patients varied widely from 14 to 67, with an average of 34. Of the 276 cases of hyperthyroidism, 253 belonged to the diffuse type and 23 were nodular (not including the adenomas of the thyroid with hyperfunction); the ratio between the two was 11:1.

Antithyroid drugs such as tabazole and thiouracil were given to most of the patients in this group of hyperthyroidism in the out-patient-department until the symptoms were controlled. For about one week prior to admission, iodine preparation (Lugol's solution) was administrated when the condition of the patient was considered fit for operation. There was also a small number of patients treated first in the medical ward and then transferred to the surgical department. The standard of preoperative evaluation was generally identical to that adopted previously with drug anesthesia. Details of the criteria chiefly consisted of subsidence of the subjective symptoms, mental stability, increase of body weight and both pulse rate and the BMR being brought down to normal limits.

Acupuncture anesthesia was carried out by electric needling and the patients were divided into groups at random with different acupuncture point prescriptions using Futu, Hegu, Neiguan, Zusanli, and auricular needling. Frequency of the electric needling was 500–600 for Hegu, Neiguan and Zusanli; and 5,000–6,000 for Futu and the auricular needling. Maintenance medication during the operation and the evaluation of the anesthetic effect were both based upon nationally adopted standards. There was only one failure in the case of a 14 year old child who refused to cooperate during the operation, which was then carried out under intravenous anesthesia. The rest of the 276 cases were operated upon under acupuncture anesthesia. Effect of acupuncture anesthesia: Grade I: 129 cases (46.7%), Grade II: 121 cases (43.8%), Grade III: 25 cases (9.1%), and Grade IV: one case (0.4%). The rate of success was 99.6% and the effect was satisfactory in 89.5%. Compared with the 762 cases of thyroid operations of various kinds done in the same period under acupuncture anesthesia in our hospital, no significant difference was seen in the anesthetic effect (Table 1).

Table 1. Effect of acupuncture anesthesia for hyperthyroidism operation

	Cases	Effect				Rate of	Satisfactory
		GR.I	GR.II	GR.III	GR.IV	success	
Thyroid operation of various kinds	762	391	294	69	8	98.9	89.9
Hyperthyroidism	276	129	121	25	1	99.6	90.5

II. DISCUSSION

1. The theoretical basis for the selection of acupuncture points Hegu and Neiguan: Evaluation of the effect of acupuncture anesthesia among groups of patients given different point prescriptions was done during these periods by comparatively fixed observers (including the personnal engaged in anesthesia and the operation team). The results are summarized in Table 2.

Based on the above results of observations, one is very easily impressed with the fact that, irrespective of the kind of thyroid operation and the choice of the acupuncture point prescription, the rate of success and satisfactory effect were uniformly high, being 92% and 85% respectively. The best results were seen among the cases with bilateral Futu points, and those with bilateral auricular needling ranked second. The effects among the cases with Hegu and Neiguan points was also fine. Only the Zusanli group seemed unsatisfactory. Although a relative specificity among the different point selections seemed to exist after a

Table 2. Anesthetic effect of acupuncture at different points

Points	Frequency (time/min)	Cases	Effect GR.I	GR.II	GR.III	GR.IV	Rate of success (%)	Exellent plus good rate (%)
Futu (bilat)	5000–6000	79	46	31	2	0	100.0	97.4
Hegu+Neiguan (bilat)	500–600	546	298	180	63	5	99.1	87.5
Auricular points	5000–6000	22	12	8	2	0	100.0	90.9
Hegu+Neiguan+Auricular		18	8	8	2	0	100.0	88.9
Zusanli (bilat)	500–600	27	15	8	2	2	92.6	85.6

general survey of the clinical data, the results were of no statistical significance (P>0.05). A synergistic effect was not produced by adding Hegu and Neiguan points to auricular needling.

In our own clinical practice, it was realized that acupuncture at the Futu point distinguished itself by its superficial analgesic effect over the neck, especially when a high frequency electric needling (5,000–6,000 times/min.) was adopted. This gave the patient a sense of numbness during skin incision. But this point is situated just within the operative field, interfering with the sterile technique. Furthermore, oozing from the wound was more profuse. For this reason we became reluctant to select this point and our preference was shifted to the points Hegu and Neiguan.

The selection of the points Hegu and Neiguan finds its sound theoretical basis in the classics of Traditional Chinese Medicine. As recorded in Zhen Jiu Da Quan (Compendium of Acupuncture and Moxibustion), Hegu is the point of origin on the Large Intestine channel of Hand-Yangming, "The 12 Channels and the 15 Collaterals are passages of 'Blood' and 'Qi' (vital engery) distributed in the human body"; ...... "Channels are the main trunks, while the Collaterals are their branches. Derangement of 'Blood' and 'Qi' (vital engery) results in diseases ......" Therefore, as stated in Canon of Medicine, when the disease process starts from Yang (positive factor), it will stay within the Channels. Consequently pathology originating in the face and neck will transmit downward to Yang-Ming. For this reason the Hegu point on the Hand-Yangming channel is used for treatment of diseases over the face and the neck regions, and the effect is especially good for analgesic purposes. Neiguan is a point on the Pericardium Channel of Hand-Jueyin. As stated in Tong Ren Yu Xue Zhen Jiu Tu Jing (Illustrated manual of the points for acupuncture and moxibustion as found on the red copper figure) "The channel of Hand-Jueyin commences from the chest, where it connects with its pertaining organ, the Pericardium. Then it descends through the diaphragm into the abdomen, linking up the upper, middle and lower portions of the body cavity (Sanjial). That is why very often the patient feels hot in the palm...... palpitation and flushing...... and the disease mainly manifests itself in cardiodynia and heat in the palms." The above passage points out the functional correlation between the cardiovascular and sympathetic systems and the Pericardium Channel of Hand Jueyin. Hence needling of the point Neiguan on this channel is very often used for sedation and to check vomiting. With the selection of Hegu and Neiguan points, acupuncture anesthesia brings about sedation and analgesia for surgical treatment of hyperthyroidism. At present, these two pairs of acupuncture points are routinely used for thyroid surgery in our hospital.

2. Advantages of acupuncture anesthesia for surgical treatment of hyperthyroidism.

According to our own clinical observations, acupuncture anesthesia, in addition to its simple procedure, gives rise to a more stable effect with a steady cardiac rate, and a speedier postoperative convalescence with fewer complications than the drog anesthesia previously osed. (Table 3).

Comparative data of three groups of hyperthyroidism treated operatively are shown in table 3. The first group consisted of 101 cases, operated on during the period 1961–1966, all with drug anesthesia. Of these, 75 were performed under intravenous anesthesia, three under ether, 11 with cervical epidural block, nine with intravenous anesthesia combined with epidural block, two with cervical plexus block and one under local infiltration. The second and third groups included 220 cases with complete history records treated during the period 1972–1974. The 103 cases in the second group were specially assigned as research cases to a cooperative research group consisting of fined personuel of Surgcon, acap uncture auesthesirt, and rearchworkers of the Institute of Base Meehcal Sciences. in 1972–1974. The 117 cases in the third group were treated in 1975–1977 when acupuncture anesthesia was already an accepted procedure, and so the patients were managed by the regular unselected personnel. The results of the above two groups of patients were essentially the same except that there were three cases of wound infection and two cases of postoperative hemorrhage requiring reoperation in the third group.

As is clearly shown in table 3, surgical treatment of hyperthyroidism under acupuncture anesthesia, in contrast to those done under drug anesthesia, causes insignificant changes in pulse rate during and after the operation, low incidence of thyroid crisis and vocal cord paralysis, low wound infection rate, few complications and no mortalities. These facts demonstrate the superiority of acupuncture anesthesia over the other methods. Of course, this does not mean that all cases of hyperthyroidism should be operated upon invariably under acupuncture anesthesia, since the analgesic effect can sometimes be un-satisfactory.

Conditions influencing the result of the operative treatment are multiple. Besides the selection of anesthesia, the pre-operative preparations, skill and cooperation of the operation team, appropriate post-operative care and individual differences on the part of the patients are all factors of consideration. The occurrence of Post-operative complications in thyroid surgery is closely related to the nature of the lesion, to the surgeon's knowledge of possible complications and his proper management of the patient. In thyroid operations perforred abroad mostly under general anesthesia, and with progressive surgical technique, in competent hands, the operative mortality has approached zero and the incidence of vocal cord paralysis, tetany and other complications has become low. Foelowing the introduction of β–blockers such as propranolol into the pre-operative preparation for hyperthyroidism, the incidence of thyroid crisis has also decreased remarkably. Propranolol was used in a small number of cases in this group.

The highest preoperative average pulse rate in cases of either the drug or the acupuncture group was around 80/min. As shown in table 3 and Fig.2 the pulse rate was remarkably

Table 3. Data analysis of acupuncture and drug anesthesia for hyperthyroidism

Date	Anesthesia method	No. of cases	Highest mean pulse rate* time/min			Thyroid crisis	Vocal cord paralysis	Wound healing**	Complication
			Day before operation	During operation	3 days after operation				
1961–1966	Drug	101	81	113	121	Crisis 2 precrisis 15	5 all unilateral	A:91 B: 5 C: 5	Re-operation for hemorrhage 3 Pneumonia 5 Hypocalcemia (transient) 5 Tracheotomy 2 Death from trachea collapse 1
1972–1974	Acupuncture	103	80	87	109		1 unilateral transient	A:101 B: 2 C: 0	Hypocalcemia (transient) 7
1975–1977	Acupuncture	117	82	88	102		1 unilateral transient	A:112 B: 2 C:3	Re-operation for hemorrahage 2 Hypocalcemia (transient) 3

* Average of the highest pulse rate of all patients.

** A—Primary healing;
B—healing with minor defect;
C—wound infection.

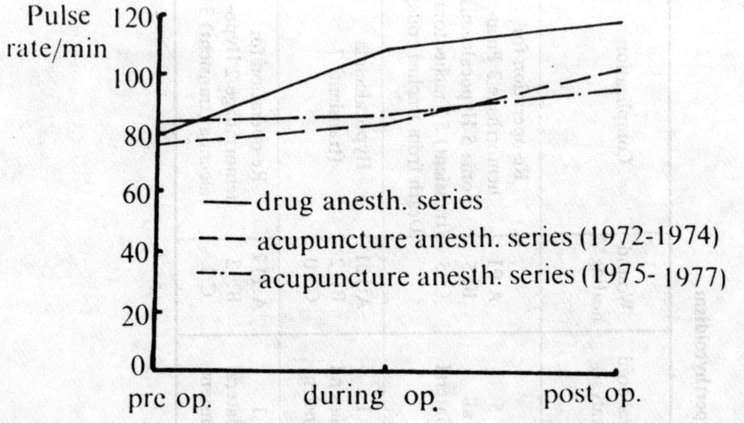

Fig. 1 Relationship between anesthetic method and pulse rate in patients with hyperthyroidism underwent operation

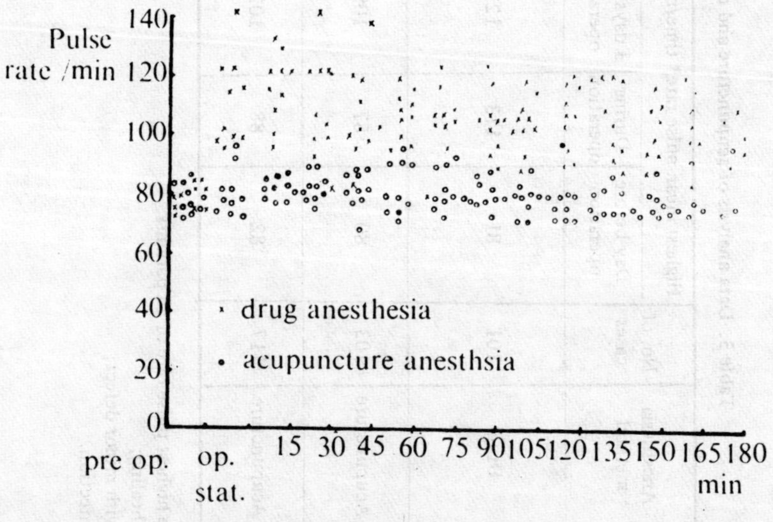

Fig. 2 Pulse rute changes during subtotal thyroidectomy for hyperthyroidism with different anesthetic method

increased during and after the operation in the cases of the drug anesthesia group. Two cases of thyroid crisis and 15 cases of pre-thyroid crisis occurred in the 101 cases of the drug anesthesia group, while none occurred in the 220 cases of the acupuncture group. The wound infection rate was also higher in the drug anesthesia group. After reviewing the records of the hyperthyroidism cases operated on under acupuncture anesthesia and selected at random, it was found that in about 1/4 of the cases the highest pulse rate during operation was the same as or a bit slower than that before operation. In the case of a 14 year old child whose highest pulse rate was 84/min on the day before operation, the anesthesia was changed from acupuncture to intraveneous because of his lack of cooperation during surgery. His pulse rate increased to 100/min following the administration of intravenous anesthesia. On the second postoperative day his pulse rate was still 144/min. Ten cases each from the drug and acupuncture anesthesia groups were selected at random and the changes of their pulse rate during the operation were analysed (none of the acupuncture anesthesia cases received β–blocker preoperatively). It was observed that, although the pre-operative pulse rate was around 80/min., In both groups, following the induction of anesthesia and commencement of the operation, aremarkable increase in the pulse rate was observed in the drug anesthesia group. In this group the polse rate rose to 100–120 for the most part, with some as high as 144/min., and an average of 110/min. In contrast, no remarkable change of the pulse rate was seen in the acupuncture anesthesia group during the operation. It was steady at the rate of 80/min. throughout the operation (Figs. 2,3). These facts suggest that there is a close relationship between the selection of the anesthesia and the change of pulse rate during and after the operation for hyperthyroidism and the frequency of occurrence of thyroid crisis and wound infection. The data also show that acupuncture anesthesia for hyperthyroidism operation, in addition to its analgesic effect, is accompanied by a possible potentiality for regulating different physiological functions, including those of the cardiovascular, endocrine and immune systems. This conforms to the concept of regulating the "blood" and "qi" or "Yin" and "Yang", a well-known function of the acupuncture and moxibustion therapy. Naturally the research into the material base of these regulating functions, the pathways of their transmission, and their internal correlations will pave the way for understanding the mechanisms of acupuncture anesthesia.

3. A few remarks on the surgical procedure for hyperthyroidism under acupuncture anesthesia.

The operation is performed on conscious patients under acupuncture anesthesia, which as currently practiced still has some unsolved problems, these include incomplete analgesia and inadequate muscular relaxation, despite the well known fact that the effect of acupuncture anesthesia is generally satisfactory in thyroid surgery. Therefore the surgeon must follows the principles of certainty, accuracy, gentleness, and nimbleness during the operation. For the practical details of operative treatment of hyperthyroidism, we propose the following:

Certainty: The operation should not be carried out in a hurry and with disorder. Operations upon a hyperfunctioning thyroid are usually accompanied by a large amount of hemorrhaging for the gland is congested and the capsule is friable. Therefore every step must be carried out with careful consideration. Bleeders are to be controlled by light pressure with the finger or with a gauze sponge, and ligation sutures applied after the source of bleeding is clearly identified. Avoid blind clamping in haste which will not only increase bleeding, but also

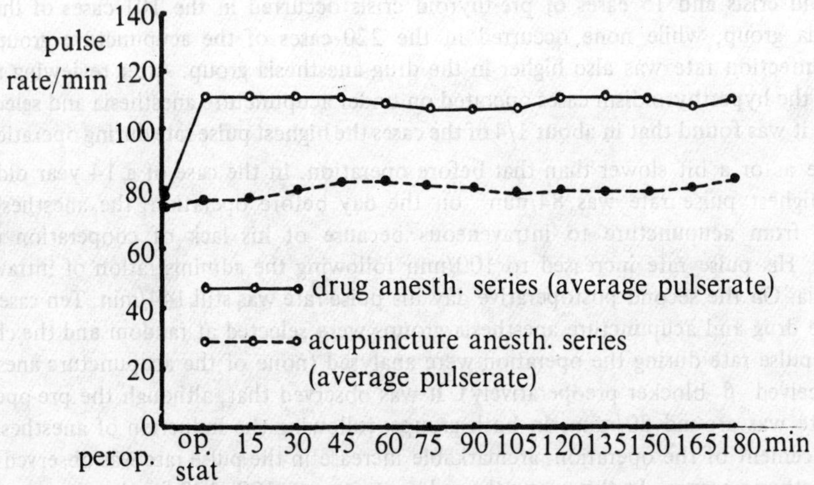

Fig. 3 The comparison of the average pulse rate curves using different anesthetic method.

cause more tissue injury. After the thyroid is excised, the wound should be carefully examined for active bleeders. Appropriate drainage material should be placed to prevent postoperative fluid collection.

Accuracy: The manipulation must be precise. Surgeons are familiar with the anatomy of the thyroid and its anatomical relations with the adjacent organs. The main blood vessels of the gland must be accurately identified and ligated. The surgeon may hold the posterior thyroidal capsule to control the bleeding and the amount of gland removal during the final step of excision. Manipulation adjacent to the posterior aspects of the gland is better accompanied by simultaneous oral communication with the patient. This will help detect the function of phonation from time to time, in order to avoid recurrent laryngeal nerve injury.

Gentleness: This requires a skillful and delicate technique. Unnecessary traction upon the tissue should be avoided under acupuncture anesthesia. For the purpose of adequate exposure, we usually transected the ribbon muscles higher than usual above the level of the skin incision. This will prevent forcible traction at the time of the handling of the upper pole. Infiltration with small amounts of local anesthetic may be given to abolish the painful sensation in a small number of cases with unsatisfactory analgesic effect.

Nimbleness: So long as a successful operative technique is insured,shortening the operation time will,to a certain extent,improve the effectiveness of acupuncture anesthesia. Dissection and hemostasis are the most time-comsuming parts of an operative procedure for hyperthyroidism. In competent hands with strict basic training, the operation should be carried out with skill and nimbleness. Time can be saved by accurate cooperation and tacit understanding within the surgical team. Sharp instruments should be used for skin incision and suture.

Certainty, accuracy, gentleness, and nimbleness should be viewed as an integral whole. Accuracy is the primary requirement and follows from veteran experience. Only with experience can the dissection and manipulation be done with certainty. Gentleness and nimbleness are only possible when the manipulation is precise. Therefore, among the four requirements accuracy is of top importance. These facts are familiar to all surgeons engaged in acupuncture anesthesia.

III. SUMMARY

1. The effect of acupuncture anesthesia is satisfactory for operative treatment of hyperthyroidism. In this group of 276 cases, the rate of success was 99.6%, and the rate of satisfactory result was 90.5%.

2. The general characteristics and the relative specificities of the different point prescriptions used for thyroid operations are discussed by analyzing the anesthesic effect of the groups operated upon with different acupuncture points. The selection of Hegu and Neiguan points for analgesia and sedation is explained according to theories set forth in the Chinese traditional medical literature.

3. A comparison is made between hyperthyroidism cases operated under acupuncture anesthesia and drug anesthesia performed in different periods of time. In the acupuncture group, the changes in pulse rate during and after the operation were slight, the incidence of thyroid crisis and wound infection were low, and complications were few. These facts bring forth the possibility of a potential effect of regulating different physiological functions, including cardio-vascular, endocrine and immune systems in addition to the analgesic effect of acupuncture anesthesia.

4. The special features of the operative procedure for hyperthyroidism are discussed and comments are made upon the practical application of the principles of certainty, accuracy, gentleness and nimbleness.

REFERENCES

[1] 北京医学院第一附属医院麻醉科：中华外科杂志 15：159，1977。

[2] 张双全：中华外科杂志 13：969，1965。

[3] 张肇祥等：中华外科杂志 5：283，1957。

[4] Freemzln G. C. : *Surg Clin Nor Amer* **50**:409, 1970.

[5] Beahro O.H. *et al* : *J Clin Endocrinol metab* **16**:1450, 1956.

[6] Beahrs O.H., Sakulsky S.B. : *Arch Surg* **96**: 512, 1968.

[7] Mackin J.F. *et al* : *New Eng J Med* **291**:1396, 1974.

[8] Lee T.C. *et al: Ann Surg* **177**:643, 1973.

CLINICAL STUDIES OF ACUPUNCTURE ANESTHESIA FOR LUNG RESECTION

Department of Acupuncture Anesthesia,
Beijing Tuberculosis Research Institute

Studies of acupuncture anesthesia (AA) started in 1965 in our research institute. Up to 1978 a total of 1,048 cases of lung resection were performed under AA. The success rate was 97.2% with Grades I and II results in 78.1%. Based on clinical data, factors affecting the efficacy of AA, especially the selection of acupuncture points and the individual variation in the efficacy of AA, were analyzed. Preliminary studies and observations were made on the regulatory functions of acupuncture.

I. GENERAL CLINICAL DATA

Of the 1,048 cases receiving AA in this series, 750 were males and 298 were females. 238 cases were under 25 years of age, 725 cases were aged 26–49 years and 85 cases were over 50 years old. There were 544 manual workers and 504 mental workers. Statistical analysis showed that sex, age and occupation had nothing to do with the efficacy of AA.

The diseases included pulmonary tuberculosis (856 cases), pulmonary abscess (107 cases) and lung cancer (85 cases). The types of operation included lobectomy (820 cases), segment or wedge resection (180 cases) and pneumonectomy or combined resection (48 cases).

Table 1. Relationship between kind of disease, type of operation and efficacy of AA

Kinds of Disease & Types of Operation	No. of Cases	Efficacy of AA I	II	III	IV	Rate of Excellent & Good Results
Kinds of Disease:						
Lung T.B.	856	228	405	207	16	73.9%
Lung abscess	107	23	41	36	7	59.8%
Lung cancer	85	13	35	31	6	56.5%
Total	1,048	264	481	274	29	71.7%
Types of operation:						
Lobectomies	820	197	385	214	24	71.0%
Segmenectomies or wedge resections	180	60	78	41	1	76.7%
Pneumonectomies or combined resections	48	7	18	19	4	52.1%
Total	1,048	264	481	274	29	71.1%

Table 1 shows the relationships between the efficacy of AA and types of disease and operation.

II. THE EFFECTIVENESS OF AA AND SELECTION OF POINTS

When we started to doalung resection under AA, points were selected on each Channel according to the principle of selecting points along the Channels. Altogether 40 points were selected on the 12 Channels. It was discovered from practice that so many points were not readily accepted by the patients, and furthermore, primary points could not be differentiated from secondary ones and some points might interfere with one another, thus lessening the clinical effect. After trying more than 80 combinations of points, the number of points were gradually reduced from 40 to 32, 16, and 12. Lung resections were successfully carried out under AA using points on one upper limb or lower limb or only at point Sanyangluo.

(I) Comparison of efficacy of AA between multiple points and Sanyangluo

In this series, lung resections were carried out under AA using multiple points in 234 patients, among whom 175 cases showed Grades I and II results, amounting to 74.8%. Out of 133 patients undergoing lung resection under AA using Sanyangluo alone, 114 cases showed Grades I and II results, amounting to 85.7%. The analgesic effect produced by the single point Sanyangluo was significantly better than that of multiple points ($P<0.01$).

(II) Comparison of effect produced by points on the upper limb and the lower limb

In this series the points Yangfu, Jinmen, etc., on the lower limb were used in 30 cases; 15 showed Grades I and II results, amounting to 50%, which was significantly lower than those of the Sanyangluo group (85.7%) ($P<0.02$).

The results indicate that the points have relative specificity.

III. THE EFFECT OF INDIVIDUAL VARIATION ON THE EFFECTIVENESS OF AA

(I) The mental types and the efficacy of AA anesthesia

Clinically the patients were divided into mental types: (1) excitable type: emotionally irritable, active, talkative and quick in response; (2) depressed type: dull, apathetic, reticent, quiet and slow in response; (3) balanced type: calm, unruffled, restrained, and thoughtful with a responsiveness between the excitable and depressed types.

Clinical observation showed that 81 out of 144 patients of the excitable type had Grades I and II results, amounting to 56.3%; among 275 patients of the balanced type, 203 showed Grades I and II results, amounting to 73.8%. The efficacy of AA was significantly better in the balanced than in the excitable type patients. In 36 cases of the depressed type, Grades I and II results were obtained in 26 cases, amounting to 72.2%.

(II) The patient's attitude toward acupuncture and emotional state and the efficacy of AA

In 174 patients who had confidence in AA and were cooperative, the rate of Grades I and II results was 74.1% (129/174); in 72 patients who lacked confidence and understanding, the rate of Grades I and II results was 52.8% (38/72) ($P<0.001$). The rate of Grades I and II results was 88.6% (62/70) in 70 patients who were emotionally stable and calm when entering the operating room. 31 apprehensive patients showed Grades I and II results in 41.9% (13/31) ($P<0.0015$). This indicates that there is a positive correlation between the efficacy of AA and the patient's emotional state and attitude toward acupuncture.

(III) Skin sensitivity and the efficacy of AA

106 patients were tested for: (1) sensitivity to electric stimulation (start to feel it) at point Sanyangluo; (2) threshold of response to electric stimulation at point Sanyangluo (fingers begin to twitch); (3) sensitivity to electric stimulation at the site of operation; (4) pain threshold at the site of operation. The results showed that in 68 insensitive patients the rate of Grades I and II results was 93.6% (63/68); while in 38 relatively sensitive patients it was 57.9% (22/38) ($P<0.0015$), indicating a positive correlation between skin sensitivity and the efficacy of AA.

(IV) The patient's tolerance to needling

Clinical observation of 158 patients operated upon under AA showed that the rate of Grades I and II results for 116 patients with good needling tolerance (could stand strong stimulation) was 78.4% (91/116), and for the 42 patients with poor needling tolerance (could not stand strong stimulation) was 52.4% (22/42) ($P<0.0015$), indicating that the efficacy of AA was intimately related to the patient's tolerance to needling.

(V) The efficacy of AA and the preoperative examination of physiologic parameters

Respiration, finger-plethysmogram and galvanic skin reflex were used for preoperative prediction and postoperative evaluation of effectiveness of AA in 473 cases. The corresponding rate was 80%. The results showed that the efficacy of AA was better in patients in resting and quiet conditions with little changes in respiration, pulse wave and galvanic skin reflex during insertion of needle and induction; otherwise the effect was poor (Table 2).

(VI) Relationship between the preoperative "abdominal breathing exercise" and the respiration during operation

In order to alleviate the patient's feeling of suffocation after thoracotomy and mediastinal flutter produced by open pneumothorax, patients were asked to relax their glottis and

Table 2. Relationship between efficacy of AA and respiration, pulse, galvanic skin reflex during insertion of needle

Physiologic Parameters	Efficacy of AA				χ^2
	Good	Medium	Poor	Total	
Amplitude of G.S.R. (millivolts)					
< 1.0	36(37.50)	30(31.25)	30(31.25)	96(100.00)	
1.1–3.0	55(26.96)	61(29.90)	88(43.14)	204(100.00)	15.211
> 3.1	10(13.16)	24(31.58)	42(55.26)	76(100.00)	
Total	101	115	160	376	
Respiratory response*					
(–)	29(29.29)	23(23.23)	47(47.47)	99(100.00)	
(+)	31(21.38)	64(44.14)	50(34.48)	145(100.00)	16.465
(++)	10(13.89)	24(33.33)	38(52.78)	72(100.00)	
Total	70	111	135	316	
Change in pulse amplitude(%)					
< 20	3(10.00)	8(26.67)	19(63.33)	30(100.00)	
21–50	56(27.32)	60(29.27)	89(43.41)	205(100.00)	7.170
over 50	41(27.70)	49(33.11)	58(39.19)	148(100.00)	
Total	100	117	166	383	

N.B. For convenience of analysis, good (grade I and better part of grade II), poor (grade III and worse part of grade II), medium means grade II.

* (–) means no response, (+) means increase or decrease of frequency, change of amplitude 1–2 times/min, (++) means hold of breathing or change of respiration for 2 cycles.

do abdominal breathing slowly, smoothly and naturally before the operation. The criteria of evaluation were as follows:

(1) abdominal breathing: the results were evaluated as "Good" when the breathing was natural and with a frequency less than 10 times/min.

(2) respiration during operation: Good—when the respiration was fairly smooth with a frequency of 15–20 times/min. Moderate—not very smooth with frequency of 21–30 times/min. Poor—when the patient felt suffocation with a respiratory frequency over 31 times/min.

Observation of 87 patients with good preoperative abdominal breathing exercise showed that the distribution of good, moderate and poor respiration during operation were 33 cases (37.9%), 50 cases (59.5%) and 4 cases (4.6%), respectively. Of the 13 patients with poor preoperative abdominal breathing, none showed good respiration during operation, while 4 patients had moderate respiration (30.8%) and 9 patients had poor respiration (69.2%). The differences were statistically significant between the two groups ($P<0.001$).

In order to evaluate the effect of respiration objectively, blood gas analysis was performed in 26 patients under AA with endotracheal intubation and 16 patients under general anesthesia. The results indicated that in patients operated upon under AA the blood gas values could be kept at normal levels after thoracotomy, but there was slight retention of CO_2. The operation could be carried out smoothly and uneventfully with oxygen administration and through the regulatory mechanisms of the body. The blood gas values returned to normal 4 hours after operation.

IV. REGULATORY AND ANALGESIC EFFECT OF ACUPUNCTURE

(I) Elevation of pain tolerance of the body after needling

Point Sanyangluo was needled with hand manipulation in 21 normal subjects. Before and after induction, electric stimulation was applied over the chest with 4 different intensities and they were asked to report 5 different feelings: no stimulation, touch, slight pain, pain and severe pain. The results showed that after needling, the incidence of severe pain was reduced on an average by 67.8%; the incidence of severe pain and pain was reduced on an average of 38.6% ($P<0.001$). Thus, needling significantly raised the body's pain tolerance.

(II) The changes in blood histamine and endorphin levels after needling

Experiments were performed on the above mentioned 21 normal subjects. They were divided into two groups—acupuncture group and control group (some of them took part in both groups). The effect of needling on blood histamine level (acupuncture group–19 subjects, control group–10 subjects) and blood endorphin level (acupuncture group –17 subjects, control group–11 subjects) was observed. The results showed that in the control group when pain stimulations were given the blood histamine level increased far above that of the acupuncture group ($P<0.05$), while in the acupuncture group group the blood endorphin level was markedly higher ($P<0.01$). The acupuncture group was further divided into two groups —groups with good and poor effects, according to whether the decrease of the incidence of severe pain was over or under 75%. The effect of acupuncture on blood histamine and endorphin levels was observed. The results showed that in the group with good effects fewer cases had a histamine increase, but cases with an increase in endorphin were markedly more (as compared with the group with poor effect, P values were less than 0.05 and 0.01, respectively). This indicates that acupuncture can regulate blood histamine and endorphin levels which are intimately related to its analgesic effect.

Observation of 45 patients undergoing lung resection under AA revealed that 8 out of 36 cases with Grades I and II results showed an increase in histamine, accounting for 22.2%, while 6 out 9 cases of Grades III and IV showed increased histamine level, accounting for 66.7%. The difference was significant ($P<0.01$).

(III) Blood pressure changes during operation under AA

Observation of similar types of lung resection performed under AA and general anesthesia was made on 500 cases each. It was discovered that the systolic pressure dropped to below 90mmHg after induction in 73 patients receiving general anesthesia, accounting for 14%, while only 12 patients receiving AA developed hypotension.

In order to further prove the regulatory effect of acupuncture, induced hemorrhagic shock was brought about in 37 rabbits (body weight 2.5–3 kg) under AA (13 rabbits),

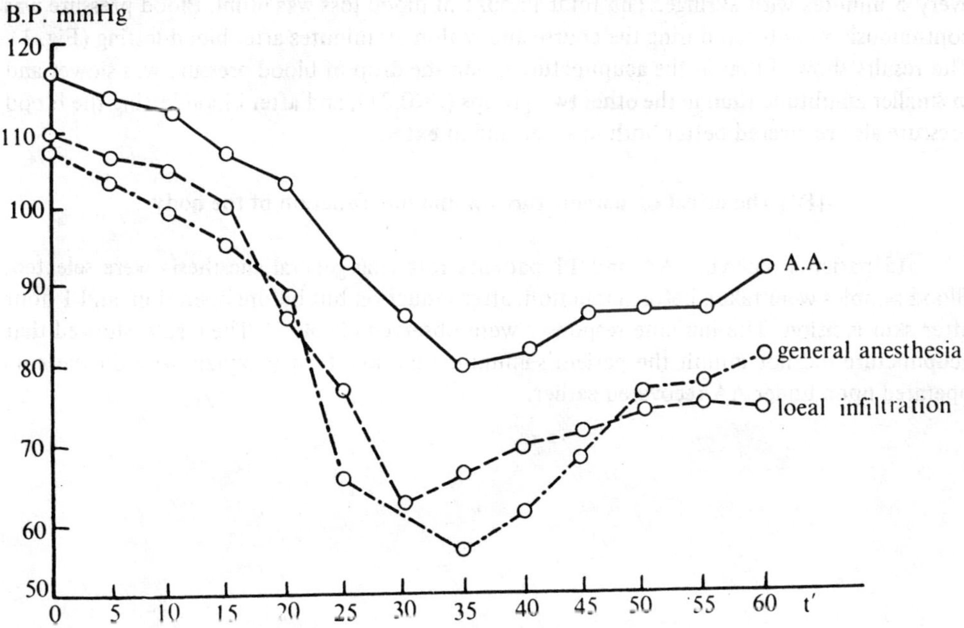

Fig. 1 Blood Pressure Changes.

Table 3. Observation of immunologic index before, during and after AA and general anesthesia (means ± S.E.)

Observation Index	15 Cases of AA			11 Cases of General Anesthesia		
	Before needling	Needling	During operation	Before anesth.	During anesth.	During operation
No. of W.B.C.	7,047 ±405.8	6,900 ±304.5	9,590 ±877.5	9,186 ±960	7,064 ±644	9,676 ±1497
Phagocytic capability*	24.3 ±5.0	23.1 ±1.5	20.4 ±1.3	25.5 ±1.9	19.6 ±2.4	17.6 ±2.4
Phagocytic index	0.703 ±0.066	0.667 ±0.114	0.727 ±0.095	0.849 ±0.107	0.651 ±0.118	0.609 ±0.192
Lymphocytic cell transformation	56.3 ±4.8	53.7 ±5.2	50.0 ±4.5	46.5 ±4.8	39.2 ±4.6	36.6 ±4.6
Rosette formation	39.6 ±9.8	43.9 ±3.0	43.2 ±3.7	40.4 ±8.8	42.9 ±6.2	39.7 ±6.4

* Phagocytosis of B. subtilis by neutrophils.

general anesthesia (14 rabbits) and local anesthesia (10 rabbits). 10ml of blood were drawn every 5 minutes with syringe. The total amount of blood loss was 60ml. Blood pressure was continuously monitored during the course and within 30 minutes after blood-letting (Fig. 1). The results showed that in the acupuncture group the drop of blood pressure was slower and in smaller amplitude than in the other two groups ($P<0.01$), and after blood-letting the blood pressure also recovered better both in speed and in extent.

(IV) The effect of acupuncture on immune function of the body

15 patients receiving AA and 11 patients receiving general anesthesia were selected. Blood samples were taken before induction, after induction but before operation, and 1 hour after skin incision. The immune responses were observed (Table 3). The results showed that acupuncture did not inhibit the patient's immune function. It may explain why the patients operated upon under AA recovered earlier.

CLINICAL STUDY OF 1,067 CASES OF PULMONARY RESECTION UNDER ACUPUNCTURE ANESTHESIA

Shanghai First Tuberculosis Hospital and Shanghai Institute of Acupuncture and Moxibustion

Starting from June 1960, inspired by a paper on 13 cases of pulmonary resection under acupuncture anesthesia reported by Liuzhou City Tuberculosis Hospital, Guangxi Province, up to November 1978, we performed 1,067 pulmonary resections under acupun cture anesthesia in cooperation with the Shanghai Research Institute of Acupuncture and Moxibustion. The effective rate was 96.1% (1,025 cases), Grades I and II combined rate was 82.4% (879 cases), and Grade IV (failure) was 3.9% (42 cases).

I. METHODS

(I) Preoperative Preparation

1. In order to win cooperation of the patient, a full explanation of the operative procedure of pulmonary resection should be given to him, including all the possible reactions that might occur during the operation. The patient should be trained to exercise deep and slow abdominal respiration ("Qi Gong") with the purpose that he would be able to respire 5–6 times per minute for more than 1 hour.

2. Prior to operation the patient should be needled several times in order to find out his tolerance and adaptability toward the acupuncture stimulation (the "needling test").

3. We examined the pain tolerance threshold and some physiological indices pre- and post-acupuncturally to estimate the effectiveness of the acupuncture analgesia.

4. Preoperative medication. At the night before operation and in the morning of the day of the operation, doses of amytal 0.1 g were given, and atropine 0.5 mg was injected hypodermically before the operation.

(II) The method of Acupuncture Anesthesia

1. Selection of acupuncture points.

We have studied more than 20 prescriptions of acupuncture points; the biggest used 87 needles and the simplest used only one needle. We present here 3 typical prescriptions for illustration:

(1) 20 pairs of acupuncture points. The points were selected according to the theory of

traditional Chinese medicine that points be chosen along the Channels and in accordance with differentiation by the patient's symptoms and signs. This prescription consists of 20 pairs of points along the Channels which are intercepted by or near the incision in relation to the "Lung " or "Heart" Channels which can control the functional changes in the cardiopulmonary system during the operation.

(2) 7 pairs of points. According to the experimental results of our hospital in cooperation with the Shanghai First Medical College, these points were chosen as being most effective in producing analgesia of the thoracic region.

(3) Using only a few points or one single needle. Points were used which induced a strong " Deqi" sensation, or produced a strong radiating sensation toward the operation field, such as "Binao" on the side of operation. We also chose the points of "Head needling" which refer to the chest region, such as the "Chest region" point on the scalp.

2. The technique of acupuncture stimulation.

(1) The locations of the selected points were accurately determined by eliciting the "Deqi" sensation. The depth of the needle was determined individually, generally between 1–3cm. The insertion was done swiftly and accurately, followed by rotating the needle to and fro slowly with lifting and thrusting movements to produce a feeling of soreness, distension and heaviness, or that of "Deqi".

(2) The preoperative induction period was about 30 minutes generally. It was prolonged when more points were selected.

(3) Method of hand maneuver. The stimulation was performed by lifting, thrusting and rotating movements. The frequency of up and down movement was maintained at 100–200 times per minute, the range of rotation between 90–360 degrees and that of lifting and thrusting less than 10mm. The hand maneuver should be smooth and even, keeping the tip of the needle in line with its shaft. It was adjusted as needed by the operative procedure and according to the response of the patient, so that he could tolerate. Electric needling or electric needling combined with hand maneuver was also used.

3. Adjuvant drugs. Adjuvant drugs were administrated in small or moderate amounts according to the preoperative estimation of the effectiveness of acupuncture anesthesia and the patient's response to the skin incision.

Small amount:
0.5% procaine 10ml, intercostal block,
Dolantin 50–100mg,
or 0.25% procaine 10ml, local infiltration.

Moderate amount:
0.5% procaine 10ml, intercostal block,
Dolantin 101–200mg,
or 0.25% procaine 30ml, Local infiltration.

4. The effectiveness of acupuncture anesthesia was divided into 4 grades, based on the pain response, grade of mediastinal flutter, and whether of not adjuvant drugs were used (See Table 1).

(III) Management During Operation

1. Nursing care.
2. Using adjuvant drugs when incomplete analgesia appeared.

Table 1. Acupuncture anesthesia technique for lung resection

Steps of Operation	Points	Adjuvant Drug, if Necessary
1. Incision of skin	Kongzui, Shenmen	Dolantin 50 mg i.v. drip
2. Incision of extracostal muscles	Kongzui, Shenmen	
3. Incision and separation of periost	Hegu, Sanyangluo directed toward Ximen	0.5% procaine 10 ml, intercostal block
4. Incision of parietal pleura and propping the chest open	" "	O_2 Mask
5. Dissection of adhesions	" "	
6. Check of bleeding	Sanyangluo directed toward Ximen	Dolantin 50 mg i.v. drip
7. Management of pulmonary arteries	" "	0.5% procaine infiltration or Dolantin 50 mg i.v. drip
8. Management of pulmonary veins	Sanyangluo directed toward Ximen	
9. Management of bronchi	" "	
10. Management of interlobar fissure	" "	Marked assisted respiration to inflate lung
11. Division and suturing up of bronchial stump	" "	
12. Irrigation of pleural cavity and insertion of drainage	Hegu, Sanyangluo directed toward Ximen	
13. Applying stitches in chest wall and tying the stitches	" "	
14. Suturing up extracostal muscles	Kongzui, Shenmen	
15. Suturing up skin and subcutaneous tissue		

3. Management of open pneumothorax and tracheabronchial secretion.

(1) During the state of open pneumothorax, the patient was asked to make deep and slow abdominal respiration, oxygen was supplied by nasal tube or mask, or assisted respiration performed for inflation of the lung by mask if necessary.

(2) When irritative cough occurred during management of bronchial tree or lung the patient was asked to respire with the mouth open or 0.25% procain used to infiltrate the hilus pulmonis.

(3) For patients with massive secretion or low pulmonary function intratracheal intubation was used.

II. ANALYSIS OF DATA

1. General. There were 1,067 cases of pulmonary resection under acupuncture anesthesia including 799 male cases (74.9%), and 268 female cases (25.1%). The youngest was 10 years of age, and the oldest 68 years of age. Most were 21–50 years of age. Tuberculosis, 841 cases (78.8%); lung tumor, 131 cases (12.3%); and miscellaneous, 90 cases (8.4%). The results were: grade I without adjuvant drugs 140 cases (13.1%), grade II 739 cases (69.3%), grade III 146 cases (13.7%) and failure 42 cases (3.9%). There were no significant differences between the sex, age, and occupation groups.

In the group younger than 20 the rate of Grade IV (12.8%) was greater than that of the other groups.

The rate of Grades I plus II among cases taking the 20 pairs of points prescription was 85.5%, those with pairs of points 75.7%, and with one single point 81.6%. The rate of Grades I plus II in the hand maneuver group was 84%, and in the electric stimulation group, 77.7%. The rate of Grades I plus II among cases whose induction period was less than 30 minutes was 80%, and in those longer than 30 minutes 86%. The pain tolerance threshold before and after acupuncture was tested with a pair of toothed forceps equipped with a pressure indicator which recorded the force that the patient could no longer tolerate. The result showed a significant individual variation among the patients. The pain tolerance threshold of those patients of Grades I and II was mostly higher (51.7%–69.8%) than those of the Grades III and IV groups. There was a significant difference between pain tolerance thresholds before and after acupuncture anesthesia ($P<0.01$).

2. Laboratory examination. We examined physiological and biochemical indices of some patients before acupuncture, during induction and during operation. The results were as follows.

(1) Pain threshold and pain tolerance threshold increased in different degrees after acupuncture. During the operation blood pressure, pulse rate, temperature, white cell count, 17–hydroxycorticosterone in the urine and 11–dehydrocorticosterone in the blood were elevated.

(2) VMA concentration in urine decreased.

(3) There were no changes in bleeding time, coagulation time, blood cholesterase, electroencephalogram, and electrocardiogram. Temperature, pressure, taste sensations and two point discrimination were all present. In the data of gas analysis there can be found acidosis of various degrees in the acupuncture anesthesia group, in the group of general anesthesia with tracheal intubation, as well as in the group of acupuncture anesthesia with tracheal intubation, but in the latter it was the slightest.

3. Preoperative estimation of effectiveness of acupuncture anesthesia by the changes in pain tolerance threshold and skin temperature was carried out in 197 cases. The rate of accuracy was 78.2%.

III. DISCUSSION

The well known analgesic effect of acupuncture was proved by clinical practice of pulmonary resection under acupuncture anesthesia. The effective rate amounted to 96.1%, including 13.1% (140 cases) in which no adjuvant drugs were used at all, so that acupuncture anesthesia is an established method combining the traditional Chinese and western medicines. But the problems of incomplete analgesia and control of mediastinal flutter should be further studied.

1. Factors influencing the effectiveness of acupuncture anesthesia.

(1) The pain tolerance threshold goes parallel with the effectiveness of acupuncture anesthesia.

(2) There was an individual difference in the effectiveness of acupuncture anesthesia, the influencing factors being such as the cooperation between patient and surgeon, the degree of adhesion of the pulmonary lesion, the skill with which the operation was done and the duration of operation.

2. The factors which influence the effectiveness are very complicated, and the anesthesia is the result of regulation by acupuncture of anti-pain function in the organism, so that the patients receiving acupuncture anesthesia should be selected. The surgical manipulations should be carried out steadily, precisely, lightly and nimbly. We had 28 cases with low pulmonary function and massive secretion undergoing pulmonary resections smoothly under acupuncture anesthesia.

IV. CONCLUSION

1. The present paper analyses 1,067 cases of pulmonary resection under acupuncture anesthesia with an effective rate of 96.1%.

2. The effectiveness was related to the pain tolerance threshold.

3. Preoperative evaluation is helpful in selecting the cases and guiding the use of adjuvant drugs.

4. In cases of low pulmonary and liver functions it is preferable to choose acupuncture anesthesia.

REFERENCES

[1] 上海第一结核病院：中华医学杂志(2)：80，1973。

[2] 上海第一结核病院：上海市针刺麻醉资料汇编(第一册)，第 16 页，1974。

[3] 上海第一医学院生理教研组等：针刺麻醉理论研究资料选编。

[4] 上海市针麻机制研究组临床生理小组：针刺应用于肺切除临床生理资料初步小结(内部资料)，1966。

[5] 上海市第一结核病院等：针麻肺切除术 45 例血液气体分析(内部资料)，1977。

[6] 上海第一医学院生理教研组等：针刺麻醉理论研究所资料选编，第 45 页，上海人民出版社，1973。

[7] 上海市针麻效果预测协作组：上海市针麻资料选编(第一册)，第 128 页，1974。

[8] 上海第一医学院生理教研组等：针刺麻醉时皮肤电反射的研究(内部资料)，1972。
[9] 上海市第一结核病院等：针麻时痛觉变化及其与针麻效果关系的观察(内部资料)，1972。
[10] 上海市第一结核病院等：针麻时皮肤温度变化的初步观察(摘要)(内部资料)，1972。

CLINICAL OBSERVATION OF ACUPUNCTURE ANESTHESIA FOR OPEN HEART OPERATIONS UNDER EXTRACORPOREAL CIRCULATION WITH RELATED PHYSIOLOGICAL AND BIOCHEMICAL CHANGES–A REPORT OF 230 CASES

Third People's Hospital of Shanghai Second Medical College and Acupuncture Research Laboratory of Shanghai Second Medical College

We initiated the first open heart operation under acupuncture anesthesia with success in April 1972. Up to August 1978 we had performed a total of 230 cases of open heart operations under acupuncture anesthesia. This is a report of the clinical results with particular emphasis on the analysis of ECG, EEG, breathing tracing and volume, plethysmography, galvanic skin response, myography and also arterial pH $PaCO_2$ and other items of blood gas analysis, through which we attempt to find some guide for our clinical practice and gain information for the research of the principles of acupuncture anesthesia.

I. CLINICAL RESULTS

1. General materials. In this series, 125 patients were males and 105 were females. The age ranged from 10 to 48. The intracardiac lesions and corresponding operations are listed in Table 1, with ventricular septal defect in preponderance.

2. Method and result of acupuncture anesthesia. Preoperative preparation: abdominal respiration training was carried out for one to two weeks before operation in all cases.

Method of acupuncture anesthesia. Needles were inserted 15 minutes before operation and twirled manually. When needling sensation was felt the needle was connected to an electric stimulator with a current of 3–4 Hz in frequency. The intensity of stimulation was then regulated according to surgical procedures but was never beyond the endurance of the patient.

Prescription of needling points. In accordance with the principles of selection of points along the course of Channels, 10 groups of acupuncture points were selected consecutively (Table 2).

Since various factors may influence the effect of acupuncture anesthesia there was no apparent difference in effect among these groups.

Supplementary medication. Phenobarbital 2mg/kg was administered intravenously 15 minutes prior to operation. During the operation an additional dose of pethidine 0.5mg/kg was given when indicated. If necessary, fentanyl and haloperidol were administered in order to enhance the analgesic effect. Local infiltration of 1:200,000 adrenaline saline solution was made along the incision line in order to reduce bleeding and 0.25% xylocaine solution 40ml was used for local infiltration in case the analgesic effect was not satisfactory.

Table 1. Diagnosis and surgical method

Diagnosis and Operation	No. of Cases
Ventricular septal defect (closure by simple suture or with a patch)	112
Tetralogy of Fallot (infundibulectomy and repair of V.S.D.)	29
Atrial septal defect (ostium secundum) (closure by simple suture)	40
Rupture of aneurysm of aortic sinus of valsalva (repair of the defect)	17
Triology of Fallot (pulmonary valvulotomy)	10
Rheumatic mitral stenosis (removal of left atrial blood clot and mitral commissurotomy)	11
Partial A-V communis (closure with a patch and suturing of mitral valve cleft)	6
Right ventricular stenosis (infundibulectomy)	4
Rheumatic mitral insufficiency (mitral prosthetic valve replacement)	1
Total	230

Effect of acupuncture anesthesia. According to the nationwide adopted standard, the effect of acupuncture anesthesia was graded as excellent (Grade I) in 42 cases (18.3%), good (Grade II) in 117 cases (50.9%), fair (Grade III) in 52 cases (22.7%) and poor (Grade IV) in 19 cases (8.2%) with a favorable effect rate of 69.2%, and an effective rate of 91.8%.

Surgical technique. The median sternotomy approach was adopted in all cases. After opening into the pericardial sac, the ascending aorta was cannulated with an arterial catheter (in the early days femoral arteries were cannulated for perfusion). The superior vena cava and the inferior vena cava were cannulated via the right auricular appendage and the right atrial wall, respectively. In the early stage we performed single or intermittent cross-clamping of the aorta to induce anoxic cardioplegia or additional topical application with ice slush for local hypothermia. Later, from 1976 on, in order to bring about even cooling of the full thickness of the myocardium to ensure its protection, for complicated intracardiac lesions we began to employ coronary perfusion under pressure through the root of the aorta with 4°C Ringer's solution 200–300ml. After the intracardiac operation had been finished, the aortic clamp was released.

Heart beat resumed after electric defibrillation and cardio-pulmonary bypass were terminated. The wound was then closed in layers after careful hemostasis.

3. Perfusion time over 60 minutes was found in 72 cases, over 100 minutes in 15 cases, the longest one being 132 minutes. For all cases except 6, the ascending aorta was occluded, the occlusion time being 6–80 minutes (See Table 3).

4. There were 11 operative mortalities and the causes of death were not related to acupuncture anesthesia.

Table 2. Ten groups of acupuncture points and respective no. of cases

Group	No. of Cases	Ear Points	Limb Points
1	4	left ear: 'chest' point 'neck' point, ping-chuan 'subcortex' point, 'kidney' point, 'lung' point,	left Nei-Kuan Wai-kuan; San-yung-lu Chieh-men Pi-nao Chien-yu
2	11	left ear: "	bilateral Nei-kuan Wai kuan Ho-ku Kung-sun
3	4	both ears: 'kidney' point Ping chuan 'subcortex' point	bilater al Fu-tu paraincisional subcutaneous electrical needles
4	7	"	bilateral Fu-tu; Leih-chueh
5	28	left ear: 'chest', neck, 'kidney' 'lung' points	bilateral Ho-ku; Nei-kuan
6	77	"	bilateral Nei-kuan; Leih-chueh
7	28		bilateral Nei-kuan; leih-chueh Kung-sun; Chao-hai
8	25	left ear: 'kidney', 'lung' points	bilateral Nei-kuan; Leih-chueh; Kung-sun Chao-hai
9	44		bilateral Nei-kuan; Lieh-chueh Yunmen
10	2	"	special points of low electrical resistance in the upper extremities

Table 3. Aortic occlusion time and cardiac resuscitation

Aortic Occlusion Time (min)	No. of Cases	Heart not Arrested	Spontaneous Resuscitation	Electric Defibrillation
5–10	43	16	13	14
11–20	76	9	29	38
21–30	43	1	5	37
31–40*	26	–	4	22
41–50** or longer	36	1	5	30
Total	224	27	56	141

* Aorta clamped twice in 5 cases.
** Aorta clamped twice in 4 cases;
Aorta clamped 3 times in 2 cases.

II. ANALYSIS OF PHYSIOLOGICAL AND BIOCHEMICAL DATA

During the entire operative course the electro-encephalogram and five other parameters were continuously monitored with a R–M 85 polygraph. Tracings were recorded at different surgical steps such as skin incision, sternum splitting, etc. Blood pH, $PaCO_2$ and other biochemical parameters were determined before and after sternotomy, during cardiopulmonary bypass, at termination of bypass and three hours after operation.

The result of the analysis is presented as follows:

1. Electroencephalogram. Thirty cases were analysed. There was a predominance of α rhythm with sporadic β rhythm. In some cases during cardiopulmonary bypass there was sporadic or transient θ or δ rhythm. When slowing of the EEG wave appeared, a number of patients were found asleep. Transient loss of consciousness was observed in 3 patients, while EEG still showed a predominance of α rhythm; yet soon after the termination of cardiopulmonary bypass, the patients regained consciousness, and EEG returned gradually to normal status.

2. ECG. In a group of 32 cases with complete data, ECG was essentially normal, only a few patients having atrial and ventricular premature beats or ventricular tachycardia. Arrhythmia appeared mainly during cardiopulmonary bypass, when all the patients had ventricular fibrillation and temporary cardiac arrest after occlusion of the ascending aorta. 30 patients resumed heartbeat after a single electric shock, 4 patients needed it twice, and in two patients even 4 and 7 shocks were necessary. After the termination of cardiopulmonary bypass 19 patients were in sinus rhythm, 12 were in supraventricular tachycardia and 1 had a nodal rhythm.

3. Tracings of plethysmography, galvanic skin response electromyography and respiratory spirometry. An analysis of the corresponding parameters before and after the operation was carried out during the various steps of the surgical procedure, which is summerized in Table 4.

(1) Plethysmography may reflect the status of the peripheral circulation, and its amplitude diminishes when pain is present. During cardiopulmonary bypass, plethysmographic waves disappeared and they returned slowly after the resumption of the heartbeat and termination of perfusion.

(2) Galvanic skin response. It is a complicated process of reaction and may be influenced by emotional changes and thinking activities as well as by pain. It appeared at any maneuver on the patient's body surface such as skin disinfection, skin incision, etc., but subsided or even disappeared after the chest had been opened.

(3) Electromyogram response was present throughout the entire course of the operation, and to a certain extent its occurrence might indicate existence of pain and discomfort. Thus, electromyography response could be useful as a means of evaluating the effect of acupuncture anesthesia.

(4) Respiratory spirometric wave. During the operation the common changes in respiratory spirometric waves were the occurrence of acceleration and breath-holding, reflecting the presence of pain; but these changes might be influenced by a number of factors. During cardiopulmonary bypass they might also show whether spontaneous respiration

Table 4. Changes of physiological parameters in groups of different grades

Surgical Procedure / Index / Grade of Anesthetic Effect	Skin Incision					Sternotomy					Cardiopulmonary Bypass					Skin Suturing				
	Heart rate	Plethys-mography	Galvanic skin response	EMG	Respi-ration	Heart rate	Plethys-mography	Galvanic skin response	EMG	Respi-ration	Heart rate	Plethys-mography	Galvanic skin response	EMG	Respi-ration	Heart rate	Plethys-mography	Galvanic skin response	EMG	Respi-ration
I	0.75	2.89	0.97	241	0.53	0.78	2.8	1.11	197	0.68				164		0.55	2.52	0.14	298	0.74
II	1.55	1.82	1.52	561	0.88	1.32	3.5	0.55	365	1.2				251		0.33	2.23	0.91	431	0.51
III	0.47	2.4	1.25	311	0.73	1.17	4.65	0.05	138	0.99				381		0.27	1.23	0.20	589	0.80

Note:

1. Changes in heart rate and respiration designate difference in No. of times at 6'' intervals.
2. Plethysmography is the average amplitude in mm of all the plethysmographic waves in 6''.
3. Galvanic skin response is calculated according to the area similar to a cycle of sinus wave.
4. EMG is calculated according to the bipeak wave in μv.

had occurred. In a series of 40 cases, spontaneous respiration ceased temporarily in 24, and became intermittent in 16 with slowing and lengthening of the intervals. Spontaneous respiratory waves recovered one to two minutes after termination of cardiopulmonary bypass.

(5) Determination of ventilatory volume. In 35 cases, minute expiratory volume was measured by means of a wet-type spirometer; the result is shown in Table 5. In another 8 cases, a photoelectric rotatory spirometer was used for measurement which is summerized in Table 6. These results showed that there was no significant change in the ventilatory volume during the preoperative and postoperative periods or at the end of the operation.

(6) Blood pH changes. In 49 operative cases, pH value, buffer base, standard bicarbonate, and base excess were determined successively after opening of the chest, 30 minutes after the institution of perfusion, after termination of perfusion and three hours after the operation. Metabolic acidosis of mild degree in the preperfusion period was observed, but it recovered to normal after termination of cardiopulmonary bypass; in the meantime, $PaCO_2$ remained normal throughout the entire course.

Table 5. Observation on ventilatory volume in 36 cases

Surgical Procedure	Total Expiratory Volume l/min
Preoperative	5.24
Induction of acupuncture anesthesia	5.39
After skin incision	6.50
After sternotomy	5.50
After institution of cardiopulmonary bypass	5.20
Termination of operation	5.50

Table 6. Respiration rate and ventilatory volume in 8 cases

Surgical Procedure	Expiratory Volume l/min	Respiration Rate l/min	Total Volume l/min
Induction of acupuncture anesthesia	0.36	15.6	5.38
After skin incision	0.37	18.8	7.34
After sternotomy	0.36	18.1	6.70
After cardiopulmonary bypass	0.35	19.0	6.54
Termination of operation	0.40	20.0	8.00

III. DISCUSSION

(I) Physiological Changes

1. Central Nervous System. One of the main differences between acupuncture anesthesia and conventional general anesthesia is that in the former case, for instance, open heart surgery under acupuncture anesthesia, the patient remains conscious and therefore can cooperate, while in the latter case he is unconscious. The electroencephalogram in this series showed a pattern of predominant α rhythm with intermingled β waves. Even when the patient fell asleep during cardiopulmonary bypass, only a slight increase of θ or δ waves was found. The basal activity was closely related to the mean arterial pressure, perfusion rate and perfusion blood oxygenation during cardiopulmonary bypass. In order to keep the patient fully conscious, it is necessary to keep (1) the PaO_2 in the oxygenator above 100mmHg and blood oxygen saturation above 95%; (2) the flow rate above 60–80 kg/min; (3) the mean arterial pressure above 50mmHg, during perfusion. Besides, it is also related to temperature, medication and surgical maneuver. When hypothermia was adopted in combination with acupuncture anesthesia, the patient became dull and even began to lose consciousness as he was cooled down to 33°C, and meanwhile, diminished EEG amplitude was observed. In one patient a temporary superior caval catheter occlusion due to improper maneuver brought about unconsciousness. Sometimes in order to stop spontaneous respiration a small dose of muscle relaxant would be required, and then the patient would not be able to answer the anesthetist's inquiries after the administration, yet his EEG remained normal. Therefore, closely watching the mental status and EEG monitoring during perfusion would help to reveal whether anoxia is present, and meanwhile they might also serve as a guide to judging whether the perfusion being performed fulfilled the physiological demand or not.

2. Circulatory System. During cardiac operations, especially open heart operations, the occurrence of arrhythmia is not infrequent. An analysis of ECG recorded continuously during the operation showed that not a single case of serious arrhythmia had ever occurred before perfusion, which was apparently different from what was observed in general anesthesia. Acupuncture anesthesia has less cardiac depressing effect than general anesthesia and may also be exempt from sideeffects induced by endotracheal intubation and hypothermia. During perfusion following occlusion of the ascending aorta and local application of ice-chips for hypothermic cardioplegia, ventricular fibrillation and cardiac arrest occurred, similar to those that happened under general anesthesia. However, after releasing the aorta clamp and electric defibrillation no serious arrhythmia was observed with the exception of ventricular tachycardia in four cases.

At the termination of cardiopulminary bypass and completion of the operation, normal cardiac rhythm was resumed in a part of the cases and supraventricular rhythm occurred in some other cases. The cause of the tachyarrhythmia is believed to be related to various factors, such as hemodynamic changes, hemodilution, hypovolemia, prolonged operation time, emotional state of the patient and incomplete analgesia. Fluctuation of arterial blood pressure is also less marked in acupuncture anesthesia patients. Comparing 60 cases under general anesthesia with 155 cases under acupuncture anesthesia, a drop of blood pressure was present in 19 cases (31.7%) of the general anesthesia group before perfusion and 34 cases (56.7%) after it, requiring the administration of vasopressor, while in the acupuncture group there were only 11 cases (7.1%) before perfusion and 43 cases (27.7%) after it ($P<0.01$). With the introduction of many new anesthetics and ever-improving anesthetic techniques, the margin of safety for drug-induced anesthesia has been greatly increased; but on the other hand, ill effects in various degrees upon the circulatory function still exist in most anesthetics and their improper handling may affect the function of the circulatory system or even provoke serious complications. Since only small doses of sedatives and narcotics are used as supplementary medication for acupuncture anesthesia, the ill effects of such drugs on circulatory functions will be thus reduced. According to the literature and clinical practice it is suggested that acupuncture may also possess the ability to regulate body functions besides its analgesic effect. An article in the medical literature reported that an instant effect had been observed in coronary heart patients upon needling Neiguan points. The resultant changes were manifested in the preejection period (PEP) and a dozen other parameters, all showing improved myocardial functions. Therefore, the fact that the influence on blood pressure and cardiac rhythm during open heart operation under acupuncture anesthesia is very slight may be explained by the regulating effect on the cardiac performance of needling Neiguan and other points. Our experience in regard to this aspect in the present study is only preliminary and further research is needed.

3. Respiration. For the majority of cases of this series endotracheal intubation was not employed. There was no marked difference in the ventilatory and tidal volumes determined preoperatively, after sternotomy and after completion of the operation. There was a slight increase in respiration rate during skin incision and after sternotomy. In our early practice patients complained of sensations of oppression and heaviness over the anterior chest when the sternum was split. Later on patients were trained to practice a respiration exercise, which was to perform abdominal respiration at a rate of 10 per min, with a sandbag weighing 5–10kg placed over the precordium and epigastrium. After sternotomy, oxygen was supplied through a nasal tube and the patient was asked to start abdominal respiration immediately. The aforementioned sensations of oppression and heaviness would soon diminish. In case the pleural cavity should be opened by accident with subsequent lung collapse, mediastinal flutter and respiratory embarrassment, a catheter should be inserted promptly through the anterior chest wall and connected to an underwater drainage. The opening in the pleura should then be closed either by suturing or by packing with gauze in order to facilitate re-expansion of the lung. In 18 cases with perforated pleura, the central venous pH was determined with a mean value of 7.308, and an average $PaCO_2$ of 49.9mmHg, showing the presence of respiratory acidosis.

In two cases, bilateral perforation of the pleura occurred before perfusion, and in one of them the arterial blood pH was found to be 7.32 and $PaCO_2$ of 28mmHg, which may be considered as the result of compensation contributed by abdominal respiration. Thus the proper performance of abdominal respiration is important. Nevertheless, the prevention of perforation of the pleura is far more important. From the anatomical point of view, as the reflection of pleura on the right side extends toward the midline just behind the lower part of the sternum, it is liable to be torn by the sternum saw during sternotomy. However, at the level of the manubrium the reflection of the pleura on neither side is so close to the midline, so we prefer to perform sternotomy by pulling the sternum saw from the suprasternal notch down to the xiphid, so that tearing of the pleura may be avoided.

In this series respiratory complications in the postoperative period were much less than those under general anesthesia. 155 cases of intracardiac operations under acupuncture were compared with 60 contemporary cases under general anesthesia. There were only 5 cases with respiratory complications in the former group. Among these, 2 were intubated during the operation and one case was intubated before the operation. So, besides these 3, only 2 of the 152 non-intubation cases had respiratory complications. In general, there was no cough and expectoration during the postoperative period. In the general anesthesia group, however, 14 cases had respiratory complications, including 9 cases of pulmonary infection, 3 cases of various degrees of aphonia, one case of atelectasis and one case of pleuritis, and besides, cough and expectoration occurred more frequently. This suggests that acupuncture anesthesia without endotracheal intubation may reduce postoperative respiratory complications. However, for cyanotic cases with severe hypoxia and cardiac function under Grade II an oxygen mask should be applied or a tracheal tube should be inserted preoperatively to insure respiratory tract patency and to provide a sufficient supply of oxygen.

(II) Objective Evaluation and Improvement of the Effect of Acupuncture Anesthesia

While observing the physiological changes in open heart operations under acupuncture anesthesia, we also paid attention to the changes in heart rate, plethysmography, galvanic skin response, electromyography, and spirometry during each operative maneuver to evaluate the anesthesic effect (See Table 4). We found that there were a number of factors which could influence these physiological parameters, such as various kinds of electric field interference, movement of the patient's body and limbs, surgical manipulations and drugs administered during the operation, etc. After analyzing the above mentioned parameters we found that there was no parallelism between the changes in those parameters and the grading of the effect of acupuncture anesthesia. Nevertheless, we came to the conclusion that changes in plethysmography and other physiological parameters may serve as objective indices of pain, but they should not be regarded as quantitative indices for the reflection of pain.

Acupuncture anesthesia in this series showed an effective rate of 91.8% and an excellent plus good rate of 69.2%.

Further research is thus needed to enhance the analgesic effect and reduce the patient's uncomfortable feelings during the operation. The prescriptions of needling points had been revised ten times, yet no marked improvement had been obtained. Therefore, besides the selection of acupuncture points, we should also consider such items as the selection of cases, preoperative preparation, supplementary medication and improvement of surgical technique in order to improve the effect of acupuncture anesthesia. In this series most of the patients graded as poor were children under 14 years of age. Furthermore, complicated lesions and a prolonged operation also brought ill effects. Hence we believe that, at present, acupuncture anesthesia for open heart operations under extracorporeal circulation should be limited to patients over 14 years of age who are willing to cooperate, with a definite diagnosis of either congenital or acquired cardiac lesions which are not very complicated. Of course, with improvement of techniques the indication for acupuncture anesthesia may be extended gradually. For the present we wish to emphasize the following points: (1) Abdominal breathing training with a respiratory rate of 10/min should be carried out for one or two weeks before the operation, and explanation to the patient to eliminate worries about the operation should be given. (2) Local infiltration of 0.25% xylocaine and saline solution subcutaneously along the incision line should be done to reduce pain and lessen oozing of blood so as to eliminate the necessity of using electric coagulation. (3) Haloperidol 2.5–5.0 mg should be given intravenously just before needling, and a dose of pethidine 1mg/kg given 15 minutes before the operation, an additional dose of fentanyl (0.1 mg) intravenously before sawing the sternum and another dose of pethidine 0.5 mg/kg if necessary after the operation has been going on for 2–3 hours. (4) All the manipulations must be done lightly and swiftly, including the insertion of urethral catheter and the monitoring of arterial and venous pressures. (5) Operative technique and the heart–lung machine should be improved to ensure sufficient oxygen supply, such as shifting of the arterial perfusion cannula from the femoral artery to the ascending aorta so as to eliminate numbness and discomfort in the lower extremities, and the adoption of the bubbling oxygenator instead of using the rotating disc. Through clinical application of the above mentioned steps the effect of acupuncture anesthesia has been gradually improved, but our aim has not yet been fulfilled, and endeavors for further improvement remain to be made.

REFERENCES

[1] 上海第二医学院附属第三人民医院，中华外科杂志，4：197，1978。

[2] 上海第二医学院针麻研究室、上海第二医学院附属第三人民医院针麻组：针刺麻醉临床和原理研究资料选编，27页，1977。

[3] 上海第二医学院附属第三人民医院：第九届外科学会论文选编，1978。

[4] 中医研究院经络研究所：针刺对冠心病心绞痛病人左心功能状态的影响，中西医结合防治研究心血管病资料，1977。

ACUPUNCTURE ANESTHESIA IN MITRAL COMMISSUROTOMY FOR SEVERE MITRAL STENOSIS

Shanghai Chest Hospital

One hundred consecutive patients of severe mitral stenosis who were operated upon with closed commissurotomies under acupuncture anesthesia from Feb. 1972 to Dec. 1975 were studied. These amounted to 19.17% of all closed commissurotomies during the same period in this hospital. The anesthesia was successful in 89% of the cases, among which 70% were classified as Grades I and II. No one died of the anesthesia. In this paper two problems are discussed:

1. Is it safe to perform commissurotomy for severe mitral stenosis under acupuncture anesthesia?
2. How is the respiration properly managed during thoracotomy under acupuncture anesthesia?

PART I

(I) Methods

1. Criteria of severe mitral stenosis (Table 1).

Some patients had a history of hemiplegia caused by thrombosis; some were cases of restenosis and had to be operated on for the second time; and some suffered from acute left heart failure and received urgent operations. Cases whose cardiopulmonary functions were greatly impaired or who had multiple valvular disease were not included in this series.

2. The points and methods of acupuncture anesthesia (Table 2).

Electric needling was done with an electric stimulator (G 6805); frequency was 140–180/min.

The intensity of the stimulation was determined by the tolerance of the patient, being increased when the muscular twitches weekened. Induction time lasted for at least 20 minutes; all points were stimulated simultaneously.

3. Respiratory management. Respiration was assisted by intubation in 88 cases; respiration assisted with masks in 12 cases.

4. Premedication and supplementary medication. Phenobarbital 0.1 and scopolamine 0.15mg intramuscularly given were one hour before operation. In 92% of the cases, morphine 0.1–0.2 mg/kg was administered intravenously before intubation. In eleven cases, ketamin 0.5–2 mg/kg was added to overcome the incomplete analgesia with the acupunc-

Table 1.

Heart Function[3] Diameter of mitral orifice* Cardiothoracic ratio Pulmonary hypertention by X-ray[1]	III or IV < 0.7 cm > 60% +	III or IV < 0.5 cm < 60% +	III or IV > 0.7 cm >70% +
Number of cases	86	10	4

Table 2.

Points Used	No. of Cases
1. Hegu, Neiguan, Sanyangluo, Zhourong	56
2. Hegu, Neiguan, Zhigou	9
3. Hegu, Neiguan, gongsun, Yangfu, Zhigou, Ximen, Xiangu, Taixi	13
4. Ear-Acupuncture (Shenmen, "sympathetic", "lung", "spleen", "kidney") and Scalp-acupuncture ("thoracic" region)	22

ture. These cases were classified as failure of the acupuncture anesthesia.

5. The effect of acupuncture anesthesia was appraised according to the nationally adopted standards.

(II) Clinical Data and Analysis

1. General data.

Male:42 cases, female:58 cases. Age 18 to 50.

Among these 100 cases, 50 had had cardiac symptoms for more than 10 years, 47 had a history of heart failure and the smallest diameter of mitral orifice found at the operation was 0.4 cm. The highest cardiothoracic ratio was 90%. 31% of the cases had Grade IV cardiac function. In 62% of the cases the EKG. revealed atrial fibrillation before operation. The diameter of the mitral orifice was less than 0.5 cm in 55 cases; the cardiothoracic ratio was above 70% in 30 cases; 31 cases belong to Grade IV of cardiac function. The data as mentioned above indicate that even in cases of severe mitral stenosis, acupuncture anesthesia is not contraindicated.

2. Comparison between the 100 severe cases and 123 mild and moderate cases[2] (Table 3).

The rates of Grades I and II were similar in both groups (P>0.05), while the failure rate of the severe cases was much higher than that of the mild and moderate cases (P<0.01). The causes of failure were:

(1) The supplementary medication exceeded the routine dosage for fear of development of pulmonary edema from tachycardia.

(2) Since pain is bad for severe heart cases, ketamin was administered whenever incomplete analgesia became obvious.

Table 3.

Severity of the Disease	No. of Cases	Efficacy of Acupuncture Anesthesia			
		I	II	III	IV
Severe M.S.	100	9	61	19	11
		70% (I–II)			
Mild to moderate M.S.	123	37	51	34	1
		71.5% (I–II)			

Table 4.

Groups of Points	No. of Cases	Efficacy of a.a.				Successful Rate of Grades	
		I	II	III	IV	rate %	I-II
I	56	3	30	16	7	76.6	51.6
II	9	1	7	1		100	88.8
III	13	2	11			100	100
IV	22	3	13	2	4	81.8	72.7

(3) Therelationship between the points used and the efficacy of acupuncture anesthesia (Table 4).

Although the rate of Grades I and II was apparently higher than that in groups of II and III, further proof is needed because the cases were too few. Comparing group I with IV, the difference has no statistical significance ($P>0.05$).

(4) The changes in PaO_2 and acid-base value of the arterial blood. Acid-base values were determined in 21 cases before and during operation. PaO_2 and SaO_2 were determined in 19 cases simultaneously. In order to exclude the influence of mitral stenosis, specimens were taken during the operation before and after commissurotomy. O2 was given by intubation in all the cases determined.

(5) The changes in PaO_2 in the arterial blood. Before operation. 8 cases of the 19 inhaled O_2 with mask, and this average PaO_2 value was 208 mmHg, while in the other 11 with no inhalation of O_2, the PaO_2 was less than 85 mmHg.

During the operation, average PaO_2 values were 224 mmHg both before and after dilation of the valve. The above facts show that when an operation for severe M.S. is performed under acupuncture anesthesia. 1) O_2 given with a mask before the operation can increase PaO_2 effectively, and 2) A higher level of PaO_2 maintained by intubation during the operation is not only of benefit to the maintenance of the cardiac function, but also useful in preventing arrhythmia.

(6) Changes in the acid-base index. pH, $PaCO_2$, B.B., S.B., B.E., and pH either before or after dilation of the valve were all ranged within normal limits. Comparing with the average values before the operation, there was no significant difference.

In severe M.S., the acid-base index can be kept within the normal range during thoracotomy under acupuncture anesthesia. This fact may illustrate that under AA the regulating mechanisms of the body are at work and that the safety for severe patients is increased with effective respiratory management (Table 5).

(7) Changes in blood pressure and heart rate.

Blood pressure.

The systolic pressure was kept above 80mmHg throughout in 70 cases, below 80 mmHg in 30 cases; among these, automatic return to normal range occurred in 14 cases, and in the other 16 cases with the help of inotropic agents.

Heart rate.

Before commissurotomy, heart rate was under 100/min in 60 cases, and over 100/min in 40 cases; 31 of these returned to normal after commissurotomy (77.5%).

These illustrate that the blood pressure and heart rate in most cases were kept stable during the operation. Most cases recovered from tachycardia after commissurotomy, which suggests that the diameter of the orifice has influence on tachycardia, while no appreciable relation was found between intubation and tachycardia ($P > 0.05$).

Table 5.

Index / Period	PaO_2 (mmHg)	SaO_2 (%)	pH	$PaCO_2$ (mmHg)	BB (mEq/L)	BE (mEq/L)	SB (mEq/L)
Before operation	208 (with O_2)	99.7					
	85 (with air)	96.6	7.42	36.6	51.5	−0.2	23.8
Before commissurotomy	224	99	7.37	39.1	49.9	−1.1	21.9
After commissurotomy	224	99	7.39	37.1	47.8	−0.76	22
Normal range	93–103	96	7.35–7.45	35–45	45–50	±3.0	21–25

all are average values.

(III) Discussion

Safety of acupuncture anesthesia in severe M .S.

Patients with a small mitral orifice, large heart, poor function, and low out-put, accompanied by pulmonary hypertension and cardiogenic cirrhosis, cannot tolerate general anesthesia very well[4]. Formerly, sodium pentothol was used for induction,so myocardial contractivity was decreased and peripheral vasodilation occured. With the deepening of the anesthesia, severe hypotension and arrhythmia would appear in some cases. According to the statistics for 3,245 cases of closed commissurotomy under general anesthesia, 0.4% died in the inductive stage. Through the practice of operating on severe M.S., we have realized that one of the prominent advantages of acupuncture anesthesia is stable circulation, which may be related to the following facts:

(1) The cardiac function suffers no depression due to anesthetics.

(2) The patient is kept in a fully conscious condition so that the normal organic regulative functions can be maintained. It has been proved that the severity of disease is not a contraindication to acupuncture anesthesia. 70% of the cases had results of Grades I and II

and not a single case died of the anesthesia. Therefore, it is indeed a safe method of anesthesia for closed commissurotomy, especially in the severe cases.

PART II

Thoracotomy under general anesthesia needs tracheal intubation, but under acupuncture anesthesia, in some cases thoracotomy was performed without intubation, oxygen, or strict respiratory management. But what about safety? This must be answered through careful study. Blood gas analysis in 74 cases and oxygen consumption measurements in 9 cases were done during acupuncture anesthesia for mitral commissurotomy. Arterial blood specimens were taken before the operation, before commissurotomy and before closing the thorax. The clinical effects of the respiratory management ,were studied among the following three groups:

spontaneous respiration with oxygen;
assisting respiration with 100% oxygen by means of mask;
assisting respiration with 100% oxygen by means of intubation.

(I) Data and Analysis

(1) Irrespective of the size of stenosis, the PaO_2 would be higher than 155 mmHg if oxygen was given before the operation; it was lower than 85 mmHg if no oxygen was given ($P<0.01$).

Table 6.

Orifice (cm)	> 0.7								
Respiratory management (No. of cases)	Spontaneous respiration (12)			Assisted resp. with mask (10)			Assisted resp. with intubation (20)		
Stage	B.O.	B.C.	B.T.	B.O.	B.C.	B.T.	B.O.	B.C.	B.T.
PaO_2 (mmHg)	103.75 ±26.31	203.16 ±104.40	181.50 ±95.50	108.40 ±68.48	257.10 ±114.10	219.00 ±116.10	100.85 ±62.45	243.10 ±121.20	267.80 ±126.50
SaO_2 %	97.53	98.40	98.11	96.25	99.40	98.60	94.92	97.97	99.03
pH	7.41 ±0.01	7.36 ±0.06	7.34 ±0.07	7.40 ±0.29	7.30 ±0.26	7.29 ±0.10	7.38 ±0.26	7.35 ±0.15	7.37 ±0.07
$PaCO_2$ (mmHg)	39.04 ±3.97	42.58 ±8.82	44.80 ±9.63	38.31 ±5.62	50.65 ±18.7	48.44 ±14.78	38.51 ±5.83	41.57 ±11.00	36.90 ±10.38
BE (mEq/L)	+0.96 ±2.44	−1.65 ±2.68	−2.67 ±2.97	−0.24 ±1.90	−4.09 ±2.15	−5.51 ±1.56	−1.74 ±2.78	−2.89 ±2.59	−3.82 ±2.35

B.O.–Before operation; B.C.–Before commissurotomy; B.T.– Before closing thorax.

Table 6. (Continue)

Orifice (cm)	< 0.7								
Respiratory management (No. of cases)	Spontaneous respiration (5)			Assisted resp. with mask (7)			Assisted resp. with intubation (20)		
Stage	B.O.	B.C.	B.T.	B.O.	B.C.	B.T.	B.O.	B.C.	B.T.
PaO_2 (mmHg)	86.02 ±18.38	197.00 ±180.60	193.60 ±164.30	168.86 ±155.00	225.71 ±100.80	226.85 ±127.30	126.20 ±87.15	217.35 ±99.20	198.15 ±80.12
SaO_2 %	95.70	94.62	95.40	97.42	98.66	98.92	96.78	98.57	98.29
pH	7.42 ±0.20	7.35 ±0.05	7.31 ±0.05	7.43 ±0.22	7.33 ±0.07	7.33 ±0.02	7.41 ±0.05	7.37 ±0.01	7.39 ±0.08
$PaCO_2$ (mmHg)	31.10 ±4.02	34.54 ±6.73	36.12 ±7.30	34.57 ±1.14	43.09 ±10.49	43.85 ±12.60	38.60 ±9.18	39.09 ±10.34	37.63 ±9.66
BE (mEq/L)	−2.90 ±3.73	−5.76 ±5.99	−6.10 ±4.51	+0.19 ±2.74	−3.54 ±3.12	−3.96 ±2.66	−0.36 ±3.68	−2.39 ±3.45	−2.22 ±4.25

(2) PaO_2 and $PaCO_2$ remained in the normal ranges for the three groups. The BE value, however, reached – 6.1 mEq/L in cases with the mitral orifice diameter under 0.7 cm in the spontaneous respiratory group, whereas it was – 2.22 mEq/L in the intubation group (Table 6).

(3) The gas analysis before commissurotomy and before closing the thorax showed that the metabolic index in the intubation group was stable in cases whose orifice was under 0.7 cm, while in the spontaneous respiration group, the BE value dropped from – 5.76 to – 6.10, and pH from 7.35 to 7.31. This shows that the metabolic acidosis was gradually increased owing to the lengthening of the operation.

(4) The degree of pulmonary collapse in 68 patients was recorded when the blood specimen was taken. The results can be divided into three groups: the PaO_2 was the highest (265.75) when the lung was in full expansion, median (208.38) when it was completely collapsed, and the lowest (106.60) when it was partially collapsed.

Most cases with full expansion of the lung belonged to the intubation group (77.5%), and the other two groups belonged mostly to the non-intubation cases (89.28%) ($P<0.01$). It means that intubation contributes to expansion of lung and increase of PaO_2.

5. Before the thorax was closed the oxygen consumption value in the mask group was 472.80 ml, which is similar to the value before the operation, while in the spontaneous respiration group, it was as high as 918.75 ml ($P<0.05$).

(II) Conclusion

(1) The average value of blood gas analysis was normal in the intubation group, while in the other two groups, metabolic acidosis occurred though their PaO_2 and $PaCO_2$ were

kept normal. Acidosis was more marked in those whose mitral orifice was under 0.7 cm. In the spontaneous respiration group, the oxygen consumption value just before closing the thorax was twice that before operation. The increment of acidosis and oxygen consumption may be related to augmented activity of respiratory muscles.

(2) Results of blood gas analysis were obviously affected by whether oxygen was given, the means of supplying the oxygen, the severity of disease and the degree of pulmonary collapse. Therefore, it was suggested that respiration be strictly controlled during thoracotomy under acupuncture anesthesia, including the supply of oxygen before the operation. For those cases whose orifice was under 0.7cm we should lay stress on the necessity of intubation, the assisted or controlled respiration and the maintainance of complete expansion of the lung during operation.

(3) Assisting respiration with a mask could reduce oxygen consumption, and it is a useful method when patients appear to be in dyspnea during thoracotomy.

* The diameter of the mitral orifice was judged by feeling with the finger during the operation; its accuracy was only relative. Therefore, the affirmation of severe M.S. was based on the four criteria.

REFERENCES

[1] 刘玉清等：中华放射学杂志，6(1)、11，1958。
[2] 上海胸科医院：针刺麻醉资料汇编，第 23 页，1974。
[3] 胡旭东等：中华外科杂志，10(2)，86，1962。
[4] Leroy, D.V.: *Cardiac Surgery*, 23(3), 1971, p. 94.

REGULATORY FUNCTION OF ACUPUNCTURE IN SUBTOTAL GASTRECTOMY UNDER ACUPUNCTURE ANESTHESIA

Zhou Shu, Lou Ailin, Zhou Lü, Luo Qingdao*, Zhou Longwu,
Zheng Chaoqiang, Cui Suying, Cheng Lanying,
Chen Yuzhen, Xu Rongkun,
Zheng Xiaozhao
(Department of Theoretical Study of Acupuncture Anesthesia, Institute of Basic Medical Sciences, Chinese Academy of Medical Sciences)

By regulatory function of acupuncture, we mean the effect of needling which, after a certain period of induction, enables major operations to be done without intolerable pain and obvious physiological disturbances. As a rule, the more fully developed the regulatory function by acupuncture, the better the anesthetic effect. But what is the mechanism of such regulatory function; how could it be fully developed; how is it related with the relief of pain; and how does it overcome the sensation of visceral traction? All these problems could be solved only by extensive clinical and experimental investigation.

In our work, the physiological functions of 294 patients during subtotal gastrectomy under acupuncture anesthesia were carefully observed and recorded, and the changes were correlated with the anesthetic effect. Our findings may be grouped under the following three topics.

I. THE IMPORTANCE OF THE PROPER SELECTION OF ACUPOINTS FOR BRINGING THE REGULATORY FUNCTION INTO FULL PLAY

It is necessary to select the proper acupoints in accordance with the actual condition of the patients during the operation. In subtotal gastrectomy if the anesthetic effect is poor, the patient would often complain of pain, nausea, palpitation, uneasiness, sweating, cold limb, etc. (Table 1).

The pulse is tense, tight, rapid, fine, feeble or knotted (Table 2). According to the theory of Chinese traditional medicine, these symptoms may be grouped into three categories, viz., 1. stasis of vital energy and stagnation of blood, characterized mainly by pain; 2. belching from the stomach characterized by nausea and vomiting; 3. disturbances of the heart vitality, characterized by palpitation, uneasiness and sweating. The therapy taken is directed : 1. to activate and promote blood circulation to combat pain; 2. to modulate the

* Anhui College of Traditional Chinese Medicine.

Table 1. Symptoms of Grades II, III subtotal gastrectomy under acupuncture anesthesia (50 Cases)

Symptoms	Pain	Nausea	Vomiting	Palpitation	Uneasiness	Unwillingness to Talk	Limb Coldness	Sweating		
								Light	moderate	heavy
No. of Cases	50	28	15	26	40	42	34	5	30	15
%	100	56	30	52	80	84	68	10	60	30

Table 2. Pulse conditions of Grades II, III subtotal gastrectomy under acupuncture anesthesia (50 Cases)

Pulse Condition	Tense & Rapid	Tense & Tight	Tense & Fine	Fine & Rapid	Fine & Weak	Hasty	Intermittent	Knotted
No. of Cases	50	25	48	39	28	6	12	4
%	100	50	96	78	56	12	24	8

Table 3. Symptoms, diagnosis, principles of therapy and acupoints in subtotal gastrectomy

Process of Operation	Main Symptoms	Differential Diagnosis	Principles of Therapy	Acupoints
Incision & suture of skin	Pain	Stasis of vital energy and blood	To activate the blood circulation	Renzhong Chengjiang
Incision & suture of peritoneum	Palpitation, restlessness, sweating coldness of limbs	Disturbances of heart vitality	To relieve uneasiness of heart & mind	Neiguan Xinshu
Clamping of omentum & gastric arteries Pulling out & cutting off the stomach Anastomosis of stomach & intestine	Nausea and vomiting	Belching of stomach	To modulate the gastrointestinal function	Zusanli Pishu

gastrointestinal function to overcome the visceral traction sensations; 3. to tranquilize the mind to relieve uneasiness and prevent sweating and palpitation. The acupoints are Renzhong and Chengjiang in combating pain, Zusanli and Pishu to overcome the gastrointestinal disturbances caused by traction, and Neiguan and Xinshu to eliminate uneasiness and to prevent sweating (Table 3).

The apparatus for acupuncture anesthesia in our series is Bei-hang Type 57–6 with succesive wave 6000 cycles per minute for points on limbs and 12,000 for those on hips and back.

During the operations, not all of the three groups of symptoms appeared. In some patients pain was the main one, while in others nausea and vomiting, and in still others uneasiness, palpitation and sweating. The intensity of the electrical stimulation of various acupoints was regulated from time to time in accordance with the clinical manifestations of the patients during the operation.

In order to ensure the anesthetic effect of the acupuncture, the patients should do deep breathing excercises (Qigong) 3–5 days before the operation. In doing so, the patient is asked to lie on his back with a sand bag weighing 2–3kg on his abdomen and then breath deeply and slowly with the rate of 5–6/min for a duration of two or more hours.

The effect of acupuncture anesthesia is graded into four categories, namely, excellent (I), good (II), poor (III) and fail (IV). In our series, the abovе mentioned acupoints were used in 151 cases of subtotal gastrectomy and the anesthetic effect was Grade I– 128 cases (84.7%), Grade II– 20 (13.3%), Grade III– 3 (2%). In a comparable group of 143 cases in which other combinations of acupoints were used, 57 cases belonged to Grade I (39.8%), 64 to Grade II (47.5%) and 13 to Grade III (12.5%). Thus the acupoints correctly selected in accordance with the condition of the patients during operations have resulted in better regulatory function. In subtotal gastrectomy a small amount of 0.5% procaine (not more than 5 ml in total) is given as local infiltration when the peritoneum is incised and sutured, and when the gastric arteries are clamped. 10 mg of scopolamine is injected just before the operation and 50 mg of dolantin when the stomach is under traction.

II. THE RELATION BETWEEN THE CHANGES OF CARDIOVASCULAR FUNCTION, ITS REGULATORY FACTORS AND THE EFFECT OF ACUPUNCTURE ANESTHESIA

(I) The Changes of Cardiovascular Function and Acupuncture Anesthetic Effect

Long clinical practice demonstrated that acupuncture can regulate the cardiovasoular function so as to enable the individual to combat shock better, and this function goes in parallel with the relief of pain. In this paper, some indexes such as blood pressure, heart rate, stroke volume, cardiac output and total peripheral resistance were measured for observing the state of cardiovascular function. The relation between the change of cardiovascular function and acupuncture anesthetic effect was investigated in 100 cases of subtotal gastrectomies.

Type XYT–2 autosphygmomanometer made in China was used for serial measurement of blood pressure before acupuncture, after induction and during the operation. After the patients were placed on the operation table and rested for 10 minutes, blood pressure was measured three times at half minute intervals, and the average value was used as control. During the operation, blood pressure was measured in every main operative step when it was expected to change; if the step was long, it was measured every 10 minutes.

Simultaneously, Type SZR–1 2–channels impedance plethysmograph and LM–6B polygraph were used to observe the heart rate, the stroke volume, the cardiac output and the total peripheral resistance[1]. The impedance plethysmography which recently has gained world wide acceptance is a simple and atraumatic method for measuring the stroke volume, and the data obtained by this method are as reliable as that by Fick's method, dye dilution method, electromagnetic flowmeter and isotope dilution method, etc.[2,3]. In our own study, comparison was made between the impedance plethysmography and Fick's method with 28 patients who were examined with cardiac catheterization. The relative coefficiency was significant (γ=0.805, $P<0.01$)[4]. The lead of extremities with four electrodes method was used because it was more convenient and equally stable as the thoracic lead. The heart rate and the total peripheral resistance were separately calculated from the intervals of the impedance plethysmogram and the slope of its decline (Ω/sec.).

1. The control value before acupuncture. The differences of blood pressure, heart rate, stroke volume, cardiac output and total peripheral resistance among Grades I, II and III cases, were not statistically significant. The results show that the levels of cardiovascular activity of the patients with eventually different acupuncture anesthetic effects were more or less the same before acupuncture (Table 4).

2. Changes during induction and operation. Blood pressure: The systolic pressure showed a tendency to rise in Grades I, II and III cases after induction. It went up further in different degrees during the process from abdominal incision to the cut-off of the stomach. It increased 20–30mmHg in Grade I cases and 30–40mmHg in Grades II and III cases. The differences of the systolic pressure between Grades I and III cases were statistically significant ($P<0.01$) during some procedures such as abdominal incision, the division of the right gastroepiploic artery, the right gastric artery and the left gastric artery, and the division of the stomach. The systolic pressure gradually returned to the control level in Grade I cases in the later part of operation, but still maintained a level higher than the control throughout the operation in Grade III cases. The diastolic pressure was almost stable in Grade I cases, but fluctuated considerably in Grade III cases (Fig. 1).

Heart rate: Though the heart rate obviously increased in all cases during the operation, the increase was less in Grade I cases as compared with that in Grade III. Starting from the procedure of gastrointestinal anastomosis, it gradually returned to the preoperative level in Grade I, but not in Grade III, cases (Table 5).

Stroke volume: Though not statistically significant, the stroke volume 15 minutes after induction showed a tendency to increase in Grade I cases and a tendency to decrease in Grade III cases, compared with the control values. During the operation, up to the time of division of the stomach, the stroke volume in Grade I cases decreased less than that in Grade III ($P<0.05$). Starting from the procedure of gastrointestinal anastomosis, it returned to the preoperative level in Grade I cases, but remained at a lower level in Grade III cases (the different value between Grades I and III, $P<0.01$). Thus it can be seen that the stroke volume in Grade I cases was more or less stable in the course of the operation except in the early period but in Grade II and especially in Grade III, it decreased throughout the operation (starting from anastomosis, the different value between Grades II and III, $P<0.01$) (Table 6).

Cardiac output: During induction and operation, the cardiac output in Grade I cases was definitely increased ($P<0.01$ or 0.05), and it did not return to the pre-acupuncture level until the abdomen was closed. However, the cardiac output in Grade III cases did not have any distinct increase, but in fact showed on the contrary some decrease, starting from the procedure of gastrointestinal anastomosis ($P<0.05$).

Table 4. States of cardiovascular function before acupuncture in different grades

Grade	S.V. (c.c.)	H.R. (time/min.)	C.O. (L./min.)	T.P.R. (Ω/sec.)	B.P. (mm Hg.)
I (58 Cases)	102.07 ±2.78	70.33 ±1.46	7.07 ±0.18	0.08 ±0.07	117.94/73.57 ±1.56/1.33
II (30 Cases)	95.00 ±4.11	71.77 ±1.59	6.69 ±0.24	0.77 ±0.11	120.20/78.23 ±2.13/2.06
III (12 Cases)	96.58 ±7.63	71.25 ±2.39	6.98 ±0.63	0.84 ±0.13	126.33/81.33 ±6.24/2.75

Table 5. Changes in heart rate during subtotal gastrectomy under acupuncture anesthesia

Grade	No. of Cases	Operative Procedures: 15 min. after induction	Abdominal incision	Subtotal gastric resection	Anastomosis between stomach and intestine	Abdominal closure
I	58	** △△ 2.8±0.93	** △△ 20.3±1.95	** △△ 15.1±1.98	△△ 2.0±2.69	△△ 2.4±1.54
II	30	** △ 4.6±1.05	** 34.6±3.40	** 26.3±2.34	** 9.7±1.88	** 11.6±2.37
III	12	** 9.2±2.17	** 31.9±2.08	** 30.1±3.32	** 17.1±3.50	** 18.5±3.57

** Different value between operatioe procedure and pre-acupuncture intra-grade, P<0.01.

△ Different value between Grades II and III, P<0.05.

△△ Different value between Grades I and III, P<0.01.

Table 6. Changes in stroke volume during subtotal gastrectomy under acupuncture anesthesia

Grade	No. of Cases	Operative Procedures: 15 min. after induction	Abdominal incision	Subtotal gastric resection	Anastomosis between stomach and intestine	Abdominal closure
I	58	1.38±1.05	** 15.29±2.16	** △ 9.58±2.63	△△ 0.88±2.21	0.19±2.15
II	30	0.67±1.63	** 21.69±2.98	** 15.50±2.81	** △△ 6.62±2.17	10.63±2.96
III	12	-2.18±1.70	-24.83±3.38	-23.67±3.69	-19.67±4.76	-23.08±3.97

** Different value between operative procedure and pre-acupuncture intra-grade, P<0.01.

△ Different value between Grades I and II P<0.05.

△△ Different value between Grades III or II and III, P<0.01.

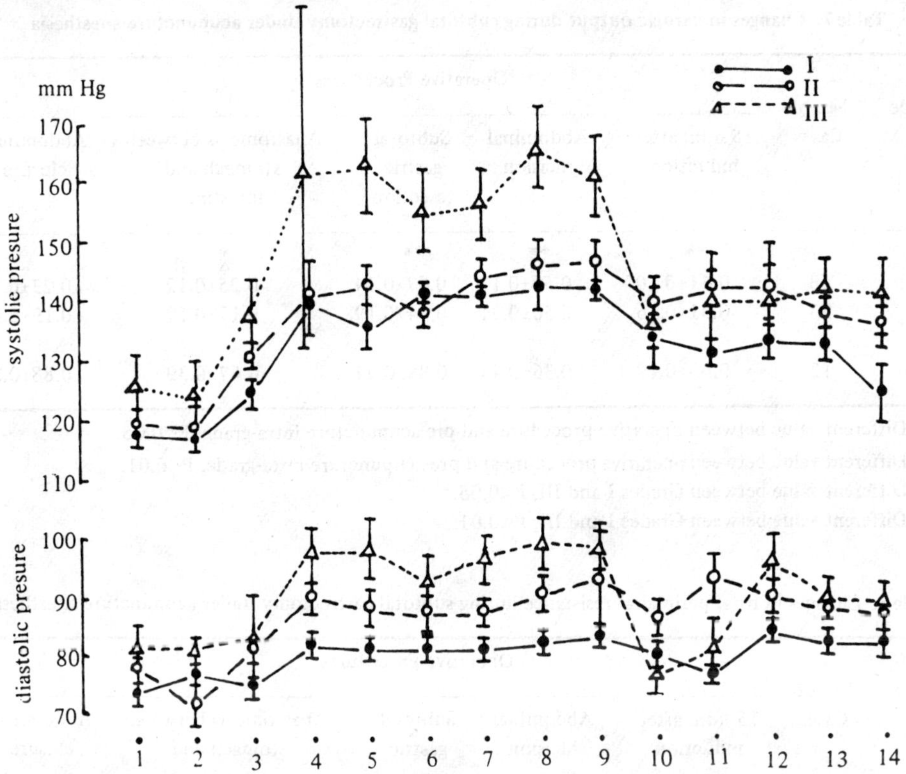

Fig.1 Changes in blood pressure during subtotal gastrectomy under acupuncture anesthesia

1. before acupuncture; 2. during needling; 3. 15 minutes after induction; 4. skin incision; 5. peritoneal incision; 6. division of right gastroepiploic artery; 7. division of right gastric artery; 8. division of left gastric artery; 9. subtotal gastric resection; 10. gastrointestinal anastomosis 10 minutes; 11. gastrointestinal anastomosis 30'; 12. gastrointestinal anastomosis 50'; 13. peritoneal closure; 14. skin closure.

It is necessary to point out that 500–700cc of 5% glucose –0.9% saline was routinely given intravenously starting 1–2 minutes before acupuncture in all subtotal gastrectomy patients, and this might affect the cardiac output, but the differences between the Grade I and Grade III cases seemed significant. Evidently, circulation of patients with excellent anesthetic effect was much better than that of patients with poor anesthetic effect (Table 7).

Total peripheral resistance: Though the changes of the values of the total peripheral resistance 15 minutes after induction in comparison with the control value were not significant in all cases. It showed a tendency to decline in Grade I and Grade II, and a tendency to increase in Grade III. During the operation, the peripheral resistance went up in different degrees in all cases (0.05–0.01), but much less in Grade I than in Grade III cases (Table 8).

Table 7. Changes in cardiac output during subtotal gastrectomy under acupuncture anesthesia

Grade	No. of Cases	Operative Procedures: 15 min. after induction	Abdominal incision	Subtotal gastric resection	Anastomosis between stomach and intestine	Abdominal closure
I	58	** 0.41±0.10	** 0.59±0.12	** 0.67±0.14	* △ 0.25±0.12	△△ 0.23±0.13
II	30	0.31±0.16	0.56±0.21	0.54±0.19	0.17±0.17	0.19±0.21
III	12	0.03±0.19	0.36±0.44	0.88±0.24	0.67±0.39	* 0.88±0.39

* Different value between operative procedure and pre-acupuncture intra-grade, $P<0.05$.

** Different value between operative procedure and pre-acupuncture intra-grade, $P<0.01$.

△ Different value between Grades I and III; $P<0.05$.

△△ Different value between Grades I and III, $P<0.01$.

Table 8. Changes in total peripheral resistance during subtotal gastrectomy under acupuncture anesthesia

Grade	No. of Cases	Operative Procedures: 15 min. after induction	Abdominal incision	Subtotal gastric resection	Anastomosis between stomach and intestine	Abdominal closure
I	58	0.019±0.015	** 0.117±0.026	△ ** 0.082± 0.021	△ 0.018 ±0.023	△ ** 0.077±0.016
II	30	* 0.056±0.022	** 0.121±0.036	* 0.111±0.046	** 0.116±0.037	** 0.135±0.031
III	12	0.074±0.069	** 0.232±0.064	* 0.270±0.081	* 0.278±0.105	** 0.245±0.072

*** △ Same as Table 7.

The above findings showed that in Grade I cases, after induction the total peripheral resistance was either unchanged or slightly decreased, so that heart blood backflow and the stroke volume were not affected, and even somewhat increased. In addition to the simultaneous moderate increase in the heart rate, the cardiac output volume showed a significant increase. It was expected that these changes would be advantageous to the patients for combating the operative trauma, as it had been found that the effect of acupuncture anesthesia was closely related to the state of circulation. If during induction, and especially during the later part of the operation, the circulation is not in a good state marked by the increase of pulse rate and peripheral resistance, as well as decrease of stroke volume, then the effect of acupuncture anesthesia is regarded as poor.

(II) The Change of Plasma Dopamine-β-Hyroxylase (DβH) Activity and Prostaglandin E (PGE)

In Operations Under Acupuncture Anesthesia. Cardiovascular function is closely related to the autonomic nervous system. When the sympathetic nerve is in an excitative state, DβH (an enzyme for synthesis of norepinephrine) in plasma is released from the peripheral sympathetic nerve terminals together with noradrenaline (NA), and may have some correlation with the activity of the peripheral noradrenergic neurons. It has been known that the release of NA may induce the synthesis and release of PGE on the membrane of locally effected cells[5,6,7]. PGE plays a negative feedback role in reducing the adrenergic neurotransmitter release. In our work the changes in plasma DβH and PGE were determined simultaneously.

1. **The changes of plasma DβH activity.** Three samples of plasma DβH taken before induction, after induction and during operation on 50 patients of subtotal gastrectomy under acupuncture anesthesia[8] were examined by the T. Negatsu method. In cases of Grade I, the plasma DβH activity after induction was decreased significantly as compared with that before acupuncture, and the lower activity of the enzyme was kept unaltered during operation. But in cases of Grades II and III, no significant changes were observed (Table 9).

Table 9. The relationship between the plasma DβH activity and the effectiveness of acupuncture anesthesia on the patients in subtotal gastrectomy

Grade		DβH Activity nmole/10μl Plasma/hr 37°C		
		Before acupuncture	After induction	During operation
		*	**	***
I	38	46.96±1.7	43.72±1.95 P<0.01	43.45±2.06 P<0.00
II	8	37.56±2.08	40.22±3.27 NS	40.19±3.32 NS
III	4	30.87±1.14	33.27±1.27	36.60±1.43

* S.E.M.
** After induction / before induction
*** During operation / before operation

2. **The changes of plasma PGE level.** The plasma PGE levels of 40 cases subjected to subtotal gastrectomy under acupuncture anesthesia were determined by extraction, thin layer chromatography and bioassay[9,10,11]. In cases of Grade I, the average level of plasma PGE after induction was apparently higher than that before acupuncture and even higher during the operation. In cases of Grade II, the plasma PGE level was unchanged during the operation. In cases of Grade III, the PGE level was actually reduced or showed no change before and after the operation (Table 10).

Parallel determinations of the plasma PGE levels and DβH activities at various intervals were carried out in 37 patients undergoing gastrectomy under acupuncture anesthesia. There was a negative relation between the PGE and DβH levels in 94% of cases (Table 11).

Table 10. The relationship between the plasma PGE level* and the effectiveness of acupuncture anesthesia in 40 cases of subtotal gastrectomy

Grade	Before Acupuncture	After Induction	During Operation	After Operation
I	0.62±0.19 (n=28)	** 1.4±0.28 (n=28)	*** 1.78±0.30 (n=28)	** 1.50±0.31 (n=18)
II	1.23±0.40 (n=8)	1.31±0.57 (n=8)	1.40±0.65 (n=8)	—
III	0.35±0.20 (n=4)	0.15±0.10 (n=4)	0.32±0.28 (n=3)	0.69±0.13 (n=3)

* Unit ng/ml±S.E.
** Compare with before acupuncture $P<0.01$
*** Compare with before acupuncture $P<0.001$

Table 11. The correlation between the variations of PGE levels and DβH activities of 37 patients undergoing gastrectomy under acupuncture anesthesia

Grade	After Induction Variation of PGE / of DβH	Relevance Coefficient	During Operation Variation of PGE / of DβH	Relevance Coefficient
I	+0.78 / -2.17, n=26		+1.11 / -3.71, n=25	
II	-0.17 / +5.10, n=7	-0.194 P<0.3	-0.09 / +2.51, n=7	-0.489 P<0.01
III	-0.20 / +2.85, n=4		-0.14 / +6.12, n=3	

Analysis of the correlation between the variation of the two assays mentioned above and the effectiveness of acupuncture anesthesia showed that decreased activity of DβH and increased level of PGE were observed after induction in cases of Grade I but entirely different results were obtained at the same interval in cases of Grade III.

According to the results mentioned above and the clinical changes in cardiovascular functions, we assume that the important role of acupuncture anesthesia consists of modulating the sympathetic nerve activity and rendering it relatively stable or less active. Due to the stimulation by surgical trauma at the beginning of the operation, the sympathetic nerve is excited temporarily. When the modulating function of acupuncture anesthesia is exerted further, DβH, and PGE are quickly modulated to a new synchronous level of homeostasis, i.e., the PGE level is higher than that after induction; DβH activity is decreased. At the same time, the cardiovascular function is regulated to a higher level of homeostasis than that before acupuncture. When the regulatory function of acupuncture anesthesia is not satisfactory, the sympathetic activity after induction and during the operation would be apparently excited, the cardiovascular functions would be in an unstable state, the DβH levels would be increased and the PGE unchanged. It seems probable that DβH and PGE may be two important factors in cardiovascular homeostasis. Our results indicate that some cases are contrary to the above rule of variation. This shows that there may be some other substances taking part in regulating the function of acupuncture anesthesia. Among these, the parasympathetic nerve activity and the metabolic changes of cholinergic neurotransmitters might also play some important roles. Later reports show that PGF, the counterpart of PGE, is found to be connected with the parasympathetic nerve activity. Therefore, in what state is the parasympathetic activity throughout the course of acupuncture anesthesia? What changes of the humoral factors are related to parasympathetic activities? What is the correlation between these factors and those mentioned above? All these problems are worthy to be studied further.

III. THE RELATION BETWEEN THE CHANGES IN THE PLASMA KININ SYSTEM AND THE EFFECT OF ACUPUNCTURE ANESTHESIA

1. Relation between the pain-producing activity of blood in the traumatic area and the effect of acupuncture anesthesia.

It is usually believed that some chemical pain-producing substances are locally liberated from damaged tissue cells and platelets, such as BK (bradykinin), 5–HT (serotonin), histamine, etc.[12, 13]. In order to find out whether the liberation of these pain-producing chemical factors was influenced by acupuncture anesthesia, a blister test was performed.

1–2 drops of a tinctura containing 0.2% cautharidin was spread on the skin of the flexor surface of the left forearm of one undergoing the test and a blister with a diameter of about 1 cm was formed. The next day the epidermis of the blister was cut off and its base exposed. Then a plastic ring was clasped tightly on to the traumatic surface to form a small cup. Sterile Lock's solution was dropped into the cup, and the blister base was bathed completely in the solution. During the experiment, the bathing fluid was removed and the standard pain-producing solution (8 mN KC1, 0.5 ml) was dropped into the cup for 1½ minutes. The pain sensation was recorded by a mechanical device [14]. If there was no response to 8 mN KCl, then 16, 32, 48 mN KCl were used.

A blood sample was collected from the traumatic area along the incision wound and it was centrifuged and the plasma was used for experiment. The plasma was placed in the cup to be in contact with the base of the blister for 2 min, and the intensity, property and latency of the sensation were determined. The pain intensity was classified into four grades: none, slight (as the pain response induced by less than 4 mN KCl), marked (as the pain response induced by 4 mN KCl), and severe (as the pain resoponse induced by 8 mN KCl).

In 10 out of 12 Grade I cases there was no pain response to the wound blood, while in

7 out of 9 Grades II and III cases marked or severe pain responses were observed. This showed that the amount of pain-producing substances in the blood was definitely influenced by the effect of acupuncture anesthesia.

The latent period of the pain-producing response to the wound blood was compared with that of KCl. Among 33 experiments with KCl, the latent period of pain response was under 20 seconds in 70%, while among 17 experiments with blood sample, it was above 21 seconds in 70%. Thus the pain response induced by the blood of patients under acupuncture anesthesia had a longer latent period than that by KCl. Besides, the pain produced by wound blood lasted much longer. The longest duration was over 30 minutes (Fig. 2) (Table 12). As to the character of the pain, the wound blood gave a burning or sometimes paroxysmal sensation, while pain induced by KCl had a pinching sensation. Thus, the painproduced by wound blood had the same characteristics as that by bradykinin[14].

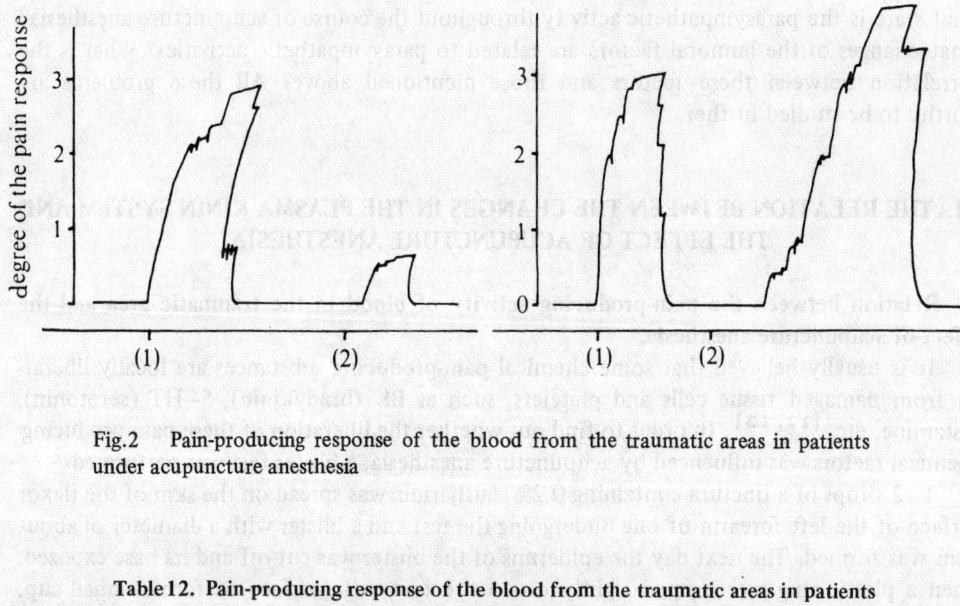

Fig.2 Pain-producing response of the blood from the traumatic areas in patients under acupuncture anesthesia

Table 12. Pain-producing response of the blood from the traumatic areas in patients under acupuncture anesthesia

Grade	Pain-producing Response				
	No	Mild	Marked	Severe	Sum
1	4	6	2	0	12
2	0	2	3	3	8
3	0	0	0	1	1
Sum	4	8	5	4	21

2. The relation between the changes of the plasma kinin system and effect of acupuncture anesthesia. The favorable influence of acupuncture anesthesia was evidenced by the fact that in Grade I patients, there was little pain reaction to wound blood. Our next problem is to find out if it is related to the plasma bradykinin system, so the changes of plasma kininase, bradykinin and kininogen have been studied.

Bradykinin is an intense pain-producing substance. During surgical manipulation a lot of bradykinin may be liberated, but it is very soon inactivated by kininase. We measured both the activity of kininase and the content of bradykinin in patients of subtotal gastrectomy under acupuncture anesthesia.

Kininase activity was determined by the improved method of Watanabe and Greenbaum[15,16]. Bradykinin was extracted by Bracklehurst Lonhija's method[17,18] and determined by biological assay with rat uterine preparation[19–22]. The contraction of the uterine preparation, either caused by the test sample or the standard bradykinin was turned into an electrical signal through a displacement transducer. The signal was then sent to a discrimination error meter and registered by electronic potential recorder. Ratio of equal efficiency was used to identify the bradykinin content of the test sample and then to calculate the kininase activity.

The change in plasma kininase has been observed in 38 cases. In 15 Grade I patients, kininase activity was increased by 8% after induction and during operation; in Grade II cases, there was no significant change, while in Grade III cases there was a decrease of 24% during operation (Table 13).

The amount of bradykinin in the blood taken before acupuncture and during the operation was compared in 24 cases. The results showed that bradykinin decreased by 63% during the operation in Grade I cases, while in Grade III cases, it increased three fold. As the number of Grade III cases was small, supplementary experiments were done on 15 dogs. Amputation of the limb of dogs was carried out without any anesthesia. The content of plasma bradykinin during the operation was elevated markedly. In the blood from the traumatic area, the content of kinin during the operation was about 9 times that of the preoperative figure. Shortly after the operation, bradykinin from the femoral vein of the operative side was about 3.7 times, and that from general circulation 3.3 times (Table 14).

During an operation or other traumatic process under the action of kallikrein, kininogen is transformed to bradykinin. Bradykinin is easily destroyed in plasma, but kininogen is more stable, so the change in kininogen can be used to reflect the level of plasma bradykinin.

The content of plasma kininogen was determined with Diniz-Habermann's method[23] in 49 cases of subtotal gastrectomy under acupuncture anesthesia. It was shown that the plasma kininogen did not change in Grade I cases and had a tendency to decrease in Grade II cases. In Grade III cases it decreased markedly after induction, and remained so during the operation (Table 15).

The plasma kinin system consists of various factors influencing not only the formation but also the destruction of bradykinin. All these factors are controlled by complex enzymatic systems and kept in the dynamic balance. Bradykinin is formed from the decomposition of kininogen under the action of the kinin formation enzymekallikrein. Under normal physiological conditions, kallikrein exists in an inactive state, and is activated by platelet XII factor. The tissue damage leads to a situation in which XII factor and a series of enzymes are

Table 13. The changes of plasma kiniase activity in patients of subtotal fastrectomy under acupuncture anesthesia

Grade	No. of Cases	Inactivition Rate of Bradykinin		
		Before acupuncture	After acupuncture	During operation
1	15	73.8±4.48	80.26±4.53 P<0.05	79.53±4.06 P<0.05
2	15	74.2±5.37	76.57±4.06 P<0.05	69.60±5.074 P<0.05
3	8	70.0±6.28	76.47±4.06 P<0.05	53.5±8.57 P<0.01

Table 14. The change in bradykinin content in the blood of amputated dogs

Place for collecting blood	Time for Collecting Blood	Content of Kinin in Blood (μg/ml)		
		No. of Cases	Average Value	P Value
Anterior limb vein	Before operation	15	0.03±0.01	
Traumatic area	During operation	12	0.30±0.08	<0.01
Femoral vein of operative side	After operation	13	0.14±0.04	<0.05
Anterior limb vein	After operation	14	0.13±0.05	<0.05

Table 15. The changes of plasma kininogen content in patients of subtotal gastrectomy under acupuncture anesthesia

Grade	No. of Cases	Before Acupuncture	After Acupuncture	During Operation
I	14	10.53±1.41	-0.7 NS.	-0.02 NS.
II	17	10.99±5.18	-0.91 NS.	-0.80 0.05<P<0.1
III	18	12.88±7.44	-2.75 P<0.05	-2.47 0.05<P<0.1

activated and bradykinin is formed. Bradykinin can be released locally from the operated traumatic area and is destructed by kininase as soon as it is formed. Our results indicated that acupuncture may increase the kininase activity, and as a result the bradykinin concentration was reduced. Particularly, kininase activity began to increase quickly after acupuncture induction, indicating that acupuncture can activate hydrolytic enzymes to counteract the great kinin production from the traumatic area and maintain bradykinin at a low level, so that the pain sensation and physiological disturbances were decreased. As the change of bradykinin in blood from the traumatic area and from the vein of the amputated dog was so similar to that of the subtotal gastrectomy patients under acupuncture anesthesia, it can be concluded that the determination of plasma bradykinin level in patients under acupuncture anesthesia might reflect the change of bradykinin in blood from the traumatic areas. We consider that the changes of the kinin system mentioned above represent one aspect of the regulatory function of acupuncture.

IV. CONCLUDING REMARKS

Acupuncture has a diversified effect on the regulation of bodily functions. On the basis of the regulatory function of acupuncture, the ability of the organism to tolerate operative trauma is elevated. This report indicates that selecting acupoints in accordance with the condition of manifestations during the operation seems to make fuller development of the regulatory function of acupuncture. The acupuncture can stabilize the sympathetic nervous system, promote cardiovascular function, and decrease the formation of the pain-producing substance, bradykinin. All of these may be a part of the factors which make the operation capable of being done without intolerable sensation and physiological disturbances.

This report would not have been possible without the assistance of all members of the Research Group of Acupuncture Anesthesia, Chinese Academy of Medical Sciences, especially the assistance of Dr. Zhu Yu, Zhong Shouxian, Yao Shuqing, Tong Yongsheng.

The authors also wish to thank Prof. Huang Jiasi, Director of Chinese Academy of Medical Sciences, and Dr. Guo Fuzhi, Director of Institute of Basic Medical Sciences, Chinese Academy of Medical Sciences, for their advice and support.

REFERENCES

[1] 魏金河等：针刺麻醉资料汇编，中国医学科学院，307 页，1979。
[2] Save J: *Ann. N. Y. Acad. Sci.* **170**:577, 1970.
[3] Lababidi A *et al*: *Pediatrics,* **47**:879, 1971.
[4] 魏金河等：针刺麻醉资料汇编，中国医学科学院，317 页，1979。
[5] Geffen L: *Life Science,* **14**: 1593, 1974.
[6] Brody M J *et al*: *Fed Proc* **33**:48, 1974.
[7] Hedqvist, P.: *Ann. Rev. Pharmacol. Toxicol.,* **17**:259, 1977.
[8] Nagatsu, T. *et al*: *Clinical Chemistry,* **18**:980, 1972.
[9] William, G. V.: *Nature,* **223**:336, 1974.

[10] Green, K. *et al*: *J. Lipid. Res.*, **5**:117, 1964.
[11] Coceani, F. *et al*: *Can. J. Physiol. Pharmacol.*, **44**:933 1966.
[12] Lim, R. K. S.: *Anesthesiology*, **28**:107, 1968.
[13] Keele, C. A. *et al*: *Substances Producing Pain and Itch*, **Edward Armold, London, 1964.**
[14] Keele, C. A.: *Ann. Rev. Med.*, **21**:67, 1970.
[15] Watanabe, N.: *Tohoku J. Exp. Med.*, **92**:63, 1967.
[16] Brackleburst, W. E. *et al*: *Brit. J. Pharmac. Chem.*, **27**:256, 1966.
[17] Brackleburst, W. E. *et al*: *Brit. J. Pharmac. Chem.*, **27**:256, 1966.
[18] Lonhija, A. *et al*: *Biochem. Pharmac.*, **21**:1151, 1972.
[19] Brackleburst, W. E. *et al*; *J. Physiol.*, **191**:417, 1969.
[20] Horton, E. W.: *Brit. J. Pharmac. Chem.*, 14125, 1959.
[21] Trautschold, J.: *Advances in Exp. Med. and Biol.*, **Vol. 8.** Bradykinin and Re*lated Kinines*, P. 55, 1970.

CLINICAL EVALUATION OF ACUPUNCTURE ANESTHESIA IN SUBTOTAL GASTRECTOMY AND A STUDY OF TYPE-CLASSIFICATION BASED ON DIFFERENTIATION OF SYNDROME IN TRADITIONAL CHINESE MEDICINE

Zhang Guangzheng, Ye Qiang, Xiang Limin, Wu Chuande,
Zhu Meimei, Gu Yanqing, Xue Lunxian
(Shuguang Hospital, Shanghai College of Traditional Chinese Medicine)

Zhou Shaoci, Weng Enqi, Dai Yongzhen
(Department of Biology, Shanghai Normal University)

Mao Liang, Yang Zhen, Zhang Meili, Ke Xuefan
(Faculty of Basic Medical Science, Shanghai College of Traditional Chinese Medicine)

The relaxation of abdominal muscles is rather highly demanded in abdominal operations. In order to discover the rules of acupuncture anesthesia applied to abdominal surgery, since October 1964, we have evaluated the effectiveness of acupuncture anesthesia by studying the observational records of surgeons' findings of the tenseness and relaxation of the abdominal wall, the patients' complaints and expressions, blood pressure, pulse rate, perspiration, nausea, vomiting, bulging of the viscera, and the amount of adjuvant drugs used mainly during subtotal gastrectomy in accordance with the national unified standard 4-grade criteria[1].

Altogether the records of 1,100 cases performed were examined and it was found that 1,055 cases were basically successful, covering 95.9% of the total, out of which 184 cases belonged to Grade I (16.7%), 493 cases to Grade II (44.8%), 378 cases to Grade III (34.4%) and 45 cases to Grade IV (4.1%). Seeing that the effectiveness of acupuncture anesthesia was affected by personal differences, we began from 1974 to investigate the relationship between the type-classification based on differentiation of syndrome according to traditional Chinese medical lore and the effect of acupuncture anesthesia. We found that the effect in patients of the "Yang-deficient" type was better than that in patients of the "Yin-deficient" type. This discovery provided a clue for studying the principles of acupuncture anesthesia by combining traditional Chinese medical art with western medicine.

I. METHODS

1. Subjects. Patients with gastric or duodenal ulcers willing to undergo operations under acupuncture anesthesia were selected for experiment and observation, excluding those with complicated foci, overanxiety, excessive fatness of abdominal wall or serious hypertension.

2. Points. Thirty-one groups of point-prescriptions had been adopted successively. According to the characteristics of the combinations, the points prescribed could be divided into six groups:

(1) Group of multiple points: 15–22 pairs of points along the four extremities were selected;

(2) Group of lower limb points: 5–8 pairs of points were selected;

(3) Group of upper-limb points: 2–3 pairs of points were selected;

(4) Group of auricular points;

(5) Group of Zusanli and Shangjuxu points;

(6) Group of Zusanli, Shangjuxu and other 1–2 pairs of points.

3. Methods of Stimulation.

(1) Manual manipulation: Rotating angle: 180–360°; amplitude of lifting and thrusting: 3–10mm; frequency: 180–220 times/min.

(2) Mechanical manipulation: Parameters same as those in manual manipulation.

(3) Electro-stimulation: Model-G-6805 and Beihang-576 electro-stimulators all made in China were chiefly used. Output: Double phase spiked wave impulse. Unloaded peak value: 0–50 v. Frequency: remote points 180–220 times/min, adjacent points 200–300 times/sec.

(4) Inductive duration: About 20 minutes. During certain procedures such as gastro-enterostomy, if surgical stimulation was slight, the needles were retained in sites without other stimulation.

(5) Adjuvants: Dolantin 50mg and Scopola mine 0.3mg administered intramuscularly if required. For 10% of the cases, no drugs were required; only a few of the cases required scopolamine 0.3mg administered intramuscularly and fentany10.1mg intaueuously.

II. ANALYSIS OF DATA

Of 1,100 cases of subtotal gastrectomy under acupuncture anesthesia, chronic gastric ulcers, duodenal ulcers and duplicated or multiple ulcers amounted to 971, ulcers complicated with pyloric stenosis and repairs of gastric perforation amounted to 46; gastric cancer and other gastric surgery amounted to 83. According to statistical data, the effect of acupuncture anesthesia, in respect to patients' sex, age, particular disease and surgical method manifested no significant difference.

(I) The Relationship Between the Combination of Points and the Effect of Acupuncture Anesthesia

Any one of the selected 31 groups of point prescription was able to enhance the patients pain threshold to various degrees, and to resist the functional disorders induced by surgical trauma. The efficacy rate of even the least effective group also reached 62.5%. The effect of acupuncture anesthesia of Zusanli and Shangjuxu group was the best. Its effective rate and rate of excellent result were higher than those of the multiple-point group used in the early stage as well as the groups other than Zusanli and Shangjuxu in the same stage (Table 1).

Table 1. Comparision of the effect of acupuncture anesthesia among the Zusanli-Shangquxu points, multiple points and points other than Zusanli and Shangjuxu

1	2	3	4	5	6	7
Group	Point-prescription	Cases	Grade I-II Cases %	Grade III Cases %	Grade IV Cases %	T-test
1	Zusanli and Shangjuxu	179	126 70.4	50 27.9	3 1.7	Group 1 & 2 Rate of excellent effect t=3.63 P<0.01
2	Multiple-points 15–22 pairs	57	25 43.9	22 38.6	10 17.5	Group 1 & 3 Rate of excellent effect t=3.00 P<0.01
3	Non Zusanli and Shangjuxu	68	34 50.0	28 41.2	6 8.8	

(II) The Relationship Between the Methods of Stimulation and the Effect of Acupuncture Anesthesia

From 1967–1970, 179 operations of subtotal gastrectomy under acupuncture anesthesia were performed. We compared the anesthesia effect of manual manipulation with that of mechanical manipulation under the same conditions of applying Zusanli and Shangjuxu points regularly and keeping fixed stimulating frequency and intensity and found the difference was significant ($P<0.05$). The anesthetic effect of mechanical manipulation was better than that of manual manipulation.

From 1972–1974, by applying the point on the right side ear-radix in addition to the same Zusanli and Shangjuxu points, 130 operations were performed. Comparing the anesthetic effect of mechanical manipulation with that of the electro-stimulator (Model G6805 or BT 701) we found the anesthetic effect of the former was also much better than that of the latter.

(III) The Relationship Between Some Personal Peculiarities of the Patients and the Effect of Acupuncture Anesthesia

1. Tolerance of needling means the intensity of acupuncture manipulation which the patients can endure. If the patient could endure the stimulation for ten minutes at sensitive points, such as Hegu, Neiguan, Zusanli, etc. by puncturing, twisting, lifting and thrusting, his tolerability is good, while the patient of poor tolerability could only endure gentle twist-

ing, lifting and thrusting (the amplitude smaller than 2mm). Therefore, the better the tolerability, the higher the rate of excellent effect ($P<0.05$) (Table 2). This revealed that the effectivenese of acupuncture anesthesia was realized through "needling sensation". Patients of good tolerability could endure stronger "needling sensation", and therefore the analgesic effect of the points could be exploited more fully.

Table 2. The relationship among the tolerance, mental condition and focus of the patient and the effect of acupuncture anesthesia

Groups	Cases	Grade I-II Cases	%	Grade III Cases	%	Grade IV Cases	%	T-test Rate of Excellent Effect
Tolerable	132	103	78	29	22	0	/	t=2.13
intolerable	104	68	65.4	35	33.7	1	0.9	P<0.05
Sufficient mental preparedness	225	172	76.4	52	23.1	1	0.5	t=2.56
Insufficient mental preparedness	51	30	58.8	19	37.3	2	3.9	P<0.05
1st Grade foci	82	66	80.6	16	19.3	0	/	t=2.41
3rd Grade foci	113	70	61.8	36	31.8	7	6.4	P<0.05

2. Personal Emotions or Mental State also Affect the Effect of Acupuncture Anesthesia.

According to mental preparedness for acupuncture anesthesia, patients were divided into two groups: the sufficiently prepared group and the insufficiently prepared group on the day before gastrectomy. In the former group are patients who were actively enthusiastic, willing and fearless about the operation under acupuncture anesthesia, while in the latter group were patients who were worried about or afraid of the operation under acupuncture anesthesia. Comparison of the effect of acupuncture anesthesia with the patients, mental preparedness showed the effect of acupuncture anesthesia in psychologically well prepared patients was better (Table 2).

3. Whether the nature of the ulcer focus is complicated or not and the indicated operation is easy or difficult affect the effectiveness of acupuncture anesthesia significantly. For convenience of analyzing, different ulcer foci are arbitrarily divided into three classes:

1st class—Simple ulcers in the duodenal bulb or in the lesser curvature of the stomach, with no adhesions, easily excised, duodenal stump easily closed or gastroduodenostomy performed easily by routine practice.

2nd class — duodenal ulcers with deformed bulb, with adhesion, but could be excised, stump closed and gastrojejunostomy performed by routine practice; gastric ulcers (or penetrating ones) with close adhesion at lesser curvature, but could be separated and gastrojejunostomy performed.

3rd class — Seriously deformed duodenal bulb in ulcers with extensive and dense adhesion could not be excised casily so that anterior exclusion gastrectomy might be performed; extensive adhesion due to previous repair of perforation or bile duct surgery; high located ulcers in the lesser curvature, close adhesion to retroperitoneal tissues or mesentery due to previous perforation, more difficult to be excised.

From 1968–1971, 195 operations of gastrectomy under acupuncture anesthesia were performed. We compared the effect of acupuncture anesthesia in 1st class foci with that of the 3rd class foci under similar preoperative medication (Table 2). It showed that the anesthetic effect of the 3rd class was significantly lower than that of the 1st class. There were seven failures during which acupuncture anesthesia had to be given up. As to 1st class foci, the rate of excellent effect was high and no failure was recorded. All these show that physiological peculiarity, mental state, complicacy of the focus and the personal response of each patient to external stimuli affect much the effectiveness of acupuncture anesthesia.

(IV) The Electromyographic Scanning of Rectus Abdominalis in Operations Under Acupuncture Anesthesia

In order to ascertain objectively the effect of acupuncture anesthesia, observations of 16 surgical procedures in subtotal gastrectomy under acupuncture anesthesia were carried out through electromyographic scanning of the rectus abdominalis. The results of an analysis of 72 cases, in which both the clinical data and electromyographic findings were complete, are as follows: The Grade I effect of acupuncture anesthesia, 11 cases; Grade II, 37 cases; and Grade III, 24 cases. Their mean value of electromyointegram area was $196.8 mm^2$, $443.9 mm^2$ and $661.5 mm^2$, respectively. Fig. 1 shows that the curves of variations of electromyographic discharge of 16 gastrectomy procedures in Grades I, II, and III were basically identical. The discharge amount was large during the exploration of the abdomen, detachment of the duodenum and recheck, while the amount was much small during the incision and gastrojejunostomy. For evaluating the effect of anesthesia during the incision and the exploration separately, we compared it with the amount of electromyographic discharge during these two procedures. The comparison showed that the relationship between the discharge amount and the effect of acupuncture anesthesia in a single surgical procedure was inversely proportional.

Moreover, in contrast, observations of 12 gastrectomy cases under epidural anesthesia show that in only 2 cases a small amount of electromyographic discharge was accompanied, by the patients suffering from nausea and vomiting induced by the traction of internal organs. Another two cases with slight reaction on visceral traction had no electromyographic discharge. Electromyographic discharge of short duration took place in one case only when the patient complained of pain. In the rest of the cases, there was no electromyographic discharge throughout the entire operation.

All the above indicates that there exists a close relationship between the amount of electromyographic discharge and the effect of acupuncture anesthesia. This relationship is reflected objectively in the degree of pain, the tenseness of the muscles and the reaction on visceral traction in the different surgical stages. It suggests that at present the effect of acupuncture anesthesia is still not as good and sure as that of epidural anesthesia.

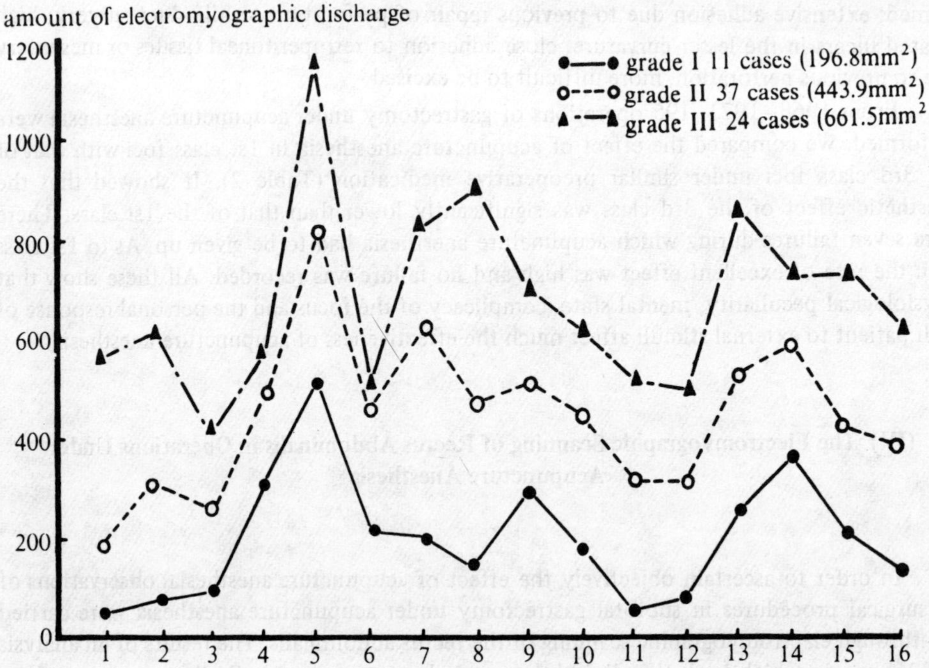

Fig. 1 Relationship between the Electromyographic Discharge of Rectus Abdominatis and Effect of Acupuncture Anesthesia.

1. Incision of skin
2. Incision of muscles
3. Hemostasis
4. Insicion of peritoneum
5. Exploration
6. Ligation of vessels on Greater Curature
7. Detachment of the duodenum
8. Incision and suturing of the duodenum
9. Ligation of the left gastric artery
10. Resection of stomach
11. Gastro-enterostomy (backwall)
12. Gastro-enterostomy (Frontwall)
13. Recheck
14. Suturing of peritoneum
15. Suturing of muscles
16. Suturing of skin

(V) Analysis of the Disappearance of the Inhibition of the Intestinal Peristalsis After Operation Under Acupuncture Anesthesia

Between 1969 and 1970, the duration from the end of operation till the first conscious flatus in patients under acupuncture anesthesia (62 cases) and in patients under epidural anesthesia (20 cases) were recorded in order to compare the difference of duration between these two anesthetic methods in the inhibition of intestinal peristalsis. As a result, the patients under acupuncture anesthesia recovered flatus sooner after operation than those under epidural anesthesia. According to statistical data (P<0.01), acupuncture anesthesia is beneficial for the recovery of the alimentary motor function.

(VI) The Relationship Between the Type-classification Based on the Differentiation of Syndrome in Traditional Chinese Medicine and the Effect of Acupuncture Anesthesia

The individual differences between patients affect the effect of acupuncture anesthesia. From 1974, according to traditional Chinese medical lore[2], 116 cases were divided into three types — the Yang-deficient type, the Yin-deficient type and the atypical type. According to the principle of "double blind method" we tested the preoperative physiological and biochemical indues of the patients simultaneously. Then a statistical analysis was made of the type classification, the effect of acupuncture anesthesia, and the physiological and biochemical indices (the experimental conditions were relatively regular).

Of 116 cases, the rate of excellent effect in the Yang-deficient type patients was 83.3%, in the Yin-deficient type patients 39.1%, and in the atypical type patients 57.6%. These results suggest that the effect of acupuncture anesthesia in patients of the Yang-deficient type was better than that in patients of the Yin-deficient type (Table 3).

1. The relationship between the digital pulse wave, type classification according to traditional chinese medical lore and the effect of acupuncture anesthesia.

Table 3. Relationship between type-classification and effect of acupuncture anesthesia

Type Classifaction	Cases	Grade I Cases	%	Grade II Cases	%	Grade III Cases	%	Grade IV Cases	%	X^2 Test
Yang-deficient type	60	18	30	32	53.3	10	16.7	0	0	
Yin-deficient type	23	1	4.3	8	34.8	12	52.2	2	8.7	P<0.005
Neutral	33	2	6.1	17	51.5	12	36.4	2	6.1	
TOTAL	116	21		57		34		4		

The fluctuation of the digital pulse wave was recorded by a pulse wave transducer, and the variations of the digital pulse wave were observed after twenty minutes' inductive period and during needle-retention. Analysis of the effect of acupuncture anesthesia with the variation of the digital pulse wave showed that in the patients with amplified broad amplitude, the effect of acupuncture anesthesia rated Grade I or II in the majority, and in the patients with diminished narrow amplitude, the effect of acupuncture anesthesia rated Grade III or IV in the majority. After the analysis of 53 type-classified cases, it was discovered that in 29 cases of broad wave amplitude, the Yang-deficient type patients covered 69%; in 24 cases of narrow wave amplitude, the Yang-deficient type patients covered 33% (Table 4). This indicated that in those Yang-deficient patients whose digital pulse wave became broad after induction, the effect of acupuncture anesthesia was better in the majority; in patients of the Yin-deficient type or atypical type, whose digital pulse wave became narrow after

Table 4. Relationship among variation of digital pulse wave after induction, type classification and the effect of acupuncture anesthesia

Digital pulse wave	Cases	Yang-deficient type Cases	%	Yin- deficient atypical tapes Cases	%	Cases	Grade I+II Cases	%	Grade III+IV Cases	%
Amplitude dilated	29	20	69	9	31	32	29	91	3	9
Amplitude contracted	24	8	33	16	67	24	4	17	20	83
TOTAL	53	X^2=5.337		P<0.05		56	X^2=28.01		P<0.005	

induction, the effect of acupuncture anesthesia was also worse in the majority.

Under the same experimental conditions, when a fixed amount of pain stimulation was given, generally speaking, the amplitude of the digital pulse wave would become narrower. When the reaction of digital pulse wave after pain stimulation was compared with the effect of acupuncture anesthesia, it was discovered that when the digital pulse wave varied ⩽20%, the effect of acupuncture anesthesia rated Grade I or II in the majority; and when the digital pulse wave varied ⩾40%, the effect of acupuncture anesthesia rated Grade III or IV in the majority.

Analysis of 49 type-classified cases out of 116 showed the pain reaction in the Yang-deficient type patients was less than that in the Yin-deficient type ones. This result shows clearly that there is a definite close relationship between the extent of pain reaction, the type-classification and the effect of acupuncture anesthesia (Table 5).

2. The relationship between the saliva contents of potassium and sodium and the type-classification according to traditional chinese medical lore.

Before acupuncture, the saliva sodium content of the Yang-deficient patients was high and the potassium content was low. After acupuncture induction, the potassium content increased with a long lasting duration (still lower than that of the Yin-deficient patients), but the sodium content decreased markedly. In the case of the Yin-deficient patients the saliva content was just the reverse. After acupuncture induction, though the potassium con-

Table 5. Relationship among pain induced variation of digital pulse wave, type classification and effect of acupuncture anesthesia

Percentage of contraction Amplitude	Cases	Yang-deficient type Cases	%	Yin-deficient atypical types Cases	%	Cases	Grade I+II Cases	%	Grade III+IV Cases	%
⩽20%	17	13	76.5	4	23.5	19	14	74	5	26
21–39%	18	9	50	9	50	18	9	50	9	50
⩾40%	14	4	29	10	71	14	4	29	10	71
TOTAL	49	X^2=7.179		P<0.05		51	X^2=6.68		P<0.05	

tent increased too, the lasting duration was shorter. The sodium content showed no significant change. This result might suggest that the adrenal cortical function of the Yang-deficient patients was originally low, and that after acupuncture induction, the function was strengthened and prolonged. The improvement of the cortical function induced by acupuncture in the Yin-deficient patients would not last long[2].

3. The relationship between the pulse rate, blood pressure, body temperature and type-classification based on traditional chinese medical lore.

In the entire observation before, during and after operation, it was found that the average body temperature of the Yang-deficient patients was lower than that of the Yin-deficient ones before operation, and the lasting duration of absorption fever was also shorter. During the operation the changes in the blood pressure and pulse rate in the Yang-deficient patients were smaller than those in the Yin-deficient ones. In the course of exploration, ligating the vessels of the greater curvature, detachment of the duodenum, and ligation of left gastric arteries, a comparison between two types of patients was carried out, and there were marked differences between the two.

III. DISCUSSION

(I) A Number of Factors That Influence the Effect of Acupuncture Anesthesia

1. Points for acupuncture anesthesia have their relative peculiarities. Practice proved that puncturing of different points produces different degrees of analgesic effect. In a subtotal gastrectomy with median incision, the analgesic effect of points Zusanli and Shangjuxu is relatively peculiar.

Both of the two points are distributed along the Stomach Channel of Foot-Yang-Ming. According to the principle that "the site where the channel passes by is the site where major treatment should be applied", it is most appropriate to select points along the Stomach Channel in gastrectomy. Ancient and modern literature and experimental and research findings concerning the point Zusanli are very voluminous. It is recorded in the "Treatise on Acupuncture and Moxibustion" that "when the gastric gas goes the wrong way, bitter juice would come up and be vomited; so for patients suffering from vomiting bile, the point Zusanli should be selected to cure it". It is also said in "Lingshu" that visceral disorders should be treated by points of conjugation. The stomach conjugates Zusanli and the large intestine Shangjuxu. According to the summation of ancient literatures, the points Zusanli and Shangjuxu are points of conjugation. They have the function of regulating the spleen and the Stomach, dissolving intestinal stasis, and improving vitality and blood circulation within the channels, and are important points in treating visceral disorders within the abdominal cavity.

The effective pathway of point Zusanli was observed in experiments. By puncturing the Zusanli point of a rabbit peristalsis of the intestine would be improved. If the sciatic and femoral nerves are severed and the artery is coated with saturated carbolic acid, then this reaction would disappear[3]. It shows that the function of acupuncture depends upon the conduction of the nerves. Discharge evoked by pain from the midbrain reticular formation of guinea pig was recorded by microelectrode technique. Such discharge would probably be inhibited if Zusanli points were punctured. In general, the inhibitory effect on inductive potential evoked by pain stimulation on the abdomen was more evident than that on the extremities[4]. This might probably be the reason why the points Zusanli and Shangjuxu could exert better anesthetic effect in subtotal gastrectomy.

2. Different stimulant methods produce different anesthetic effects. Whether or not the analgesic effect could be produced was determined first by the "needling sensation". According to acupuncture analgesic experiments on man, there would be no sensation of soreness, distension, heaviness, etc. during acupuncture, as soon as the points were infiltrated with local analgesics, nor would there be any more elevation of the pain threshold. The rate of effect in Grades I and II of mechanical manipulation was higher than that of manual manipulation. The reason why the anesthetic effect of mechanical manipulation was better than that of manual manipulation was that the mechanical manipulation after getting excellent needling sesation, fixed the needling direction and depth, kept an even and rhythmical stimulation, to maintain an excellent needling sensation and exert a better analgesic effect of the points. Stimulation produced by the electrostimulator was a kind of electric stimulus which possessed a sensation of numbness. Such sensation was quite different from that of the mechanical manipulation. But owing to the simplicity of the electrostimulator, it is still much used clinically.

3. The intensity of surgical stimulation is related to the effect of acupuncture anesthesia to a certain extent. When all other conditions are similar, the larger the surgical stimulation is, the worse the anesthetic effect would be and vice versa. The intensity of surgical stimulation is, however, affected by the seriousness of diseased the focus. In the cases of complicated foci and long surgical duration, the stimulation of surgical trauma would be stronger. So it is quite reasonable to ask the surgeon to perform operations steadily, exactly, gently, and quickly. Constantly improving the surgical technique could not only avoid unnecessary surgical stimulation but also facilitate the anesthesic effect.

For many years, we had met a number of patients who had no evident pain reaction and complaints during operations under acupuncture anesthesia. The reasons were analyzed as follows: most of them had good tolerability for needling, so they were able to accept stronger needling manipulation. They were emotionally stable, and accepted willingly operations under acupuncture anesthesia. Most of them were thin and tall men, their abdominal walls were thin, loose and soft, their stomachs were low, or of gastroptosis, and their ulcer foci were simple and no extensive exploration was required. The fact that individual variation affects anesthetic effect suggests to us that forecasting the effect of acupuncture anesthesia is important for enhancing the effect itself.

(II) Clinical Evaluation

The most frequently used anesthetic method in subtotal gastrectomy is epidural anesthesia, which in comparison with acupuncture anesthesia has its own advantages and disadvantages. The advantages of acupuncture anesthesia are: simple and convenient in method, simple in equipment, no anesthetic side reactions and no other fatal accidents. During the operation, the blood pressure is stable with a slight elevation; after operation, the patients could recover their physical activities quickly and their peristalsis would resume function and begin flatus soon. All these are beneficial to postoperative recovery and nursing. But the disadvantages of incomplete analgesic effect, tension of abdominal muscles and reaction due to visceral traction which, to a certain extent, affect the surgical operation still exist.

According to the analysis of electromyography of rectus abdominalis[5], a certain amount of myoelectric discharge was observed in every step of operation under acupuncture anesthesia. Under epidural anesthesia, only a small amount of myoelectric discharge could be observed when the patients complained of serious visceral dragging pain. These objective reflections showed the anesthetic effect of epidural was better than that of acupuncture. In acupuncture anesthesia, the correlation between the myoelectric discharge and surgical procedures, and between the surgeon's feeling on operation and patients' complaint was corresponding. For example, the patients suffered most during the course of exploration and the detachment of the duodenum due to visceral dragging pain; surgeons met difficulty in operation due to deep seated ulcers, extensive adhesion and foci with thick scar; the patients complained most, and the myoelectric discharge was greatest. During the course of incision and gastro-anterostomy, the patients generally complained of nothing due to the easiness of surgical manipulation; then the myoelectric discharge was least. This suggested to us that in abdominal operations, the method of acupuncture anesthesia and surgical technique should be both appropriately improved, and adjuvant drugs should appropriately be administered according to the different amount of stimulation in various surgical procedures. This is also the key to enhance the effect of acupuncture anesthesia.

Regarding the improvement of surgical technique, we considered that in subtotal gastrectomy, upper abdominal median incision is better than paramedian incision or transrectus incision, because the stimulation caused by this incision is small, the viscera are less liable to be cut, cutting and closing the abdominal cavity is simpler and more covenient. Since we lessened the length of the incision from 15–20 cm to 8–10 cm, and managed to take out the stomach segmently out of the incision for operation, painful stimulation could be reduced greatly. The whole operation should be performed steadily, exactly, gently, quickly and flexibly. Blunt dissection or pulling of the viscera should strictly be avoided. In drawing the stomach, a steady pulling force should be kept, so as to reduce the stimulation of visceral traction. The patients were then instructed to breathe deeply and slowly in order to relax their abdominal muscles and reduce the morbidity of nausea and vomiting. In the ligation of left/right gastric artery, because of the distribution of abundant nerves around, a small amount of anesthetics was advised to be infiltrated locally, so as to reduce the reaction of visceral traction and to facilitate smooth performance of the surgery.

(III) The Relationship Between the Type-classification Based on Traditional Chinese Medical Lore and the Effect of Acupuncture Anesthesia

The relationship between the two discussed above, shows that the anesthetic effect in the Yang-deficient patients is better than that in the Yin-deficient patients. The reasons follow:

1. From the point of physiology. The syndrome of both Yang-deficiency and Yin-deficiency is physiologically correlated with disorders of the autonomic nerves. The digital pulse wave is a sensitive index of vasomotion, which reflects the sympathetic tension of the vessels. The amplitude of digital pulse wave of the patients of the Yang-deficient type, under a definite amount of painful stimulation, does not contract much; but after acupuncture induction, the amplitude would become dilated. It probably indicates that the sympathetic tension in the Yang-deficient patient is regulated approriately after acupuncture. This is one of the factors that make the anesthetic effect in the Yang-deficient patients superior to that in the Yin-deficient patients. Therefore, the blood pressure and pulse rate of the Yang-deficient patients do not vary much during the operation, and the post-operation variation is slight too[6].

2. From the point of biochemistry. The potassium and sodium contents in the saliva of the patients are affected by the autonomic nerves and adrenal cortical hormone. After acupuncture induction, the rise of the potassium and the fall of the sodium contents in the saliva of Yang-deficient patients were marked and they lasted for a quite long while. This shows acupuncture regulates the function of autonomic nerves and adrenal cortex, so that the anti-stress function of the organism against surgical trauma is enhanced. As to the patients of Yin-deficiency, after acupuncture only the potassium content in their saliva varied and lasted a relatively short while. This might be another factor that causes different anesthetic effects between Yang-deficient and Yin-deficient patients.

3. From the point of channel theory in traditional chinese medicine. Clinical experiments showed Zusanli and Shangjuxu are more appropriate points to patients of the Yang-deficient type. As to Yin-deficient patients, these are contradictory to the principle of "applying treatment according to the differentiation of syndrome". This might be one of the reasons why the anesthetic effect in Yin-deficient patients was worse, even though a similar pointprescription was made.

The above investigation findings show that at present, the same point-prescription used clinically on different patients in operation under acupuncture anesthesia do not conform to the principle of applying treatment according to the differentiation of syndrome in traditional Chinese medicine. This demands us to analyze further the rule of clinical acupuncture anesthesia, which will be beneficial to improving the effect of acupuncture anesthesia and promoting the theoretical research of acupuncture anesthesia.

REFERENCES

[1] The Acupuncture Anesthesia Cooperative Group of Shuguang Hospital, Shanghai College of Chinese Traditional Medicine: *National Medical Journal of China,* **55** (10): 703, 1975.

[2] The Acupuncture Anesthesia Cooperative Group of Shuguang Hospital, Shanghai College of Traditional Chinese Medicine: *Selected Papers on Clinical and Fundamental Study of Acupuncture Anesthesia,* Shanghai People's Publishing House, No 3, No.15, p.307, 1977.

[3] Physiology Department of Shanghai College of Traditional Chinese Medicine: *Journal of Traditional Chinese Medicine,* **11.** 1, 1964.

[4] Shanghai College of Traditional Chinese Medicine et al.: *National Medical Journal of China,* **53**: 136, 1973.

[5] Shanghai Normal University et al.: *Selected Papers on Clinical and Fundamental Study of Acupuncture Anesthesia,* Shanghai People's Publishing House, p.53, 1973.

[6] The Acupuncture Anesthesia Cooperative Group of Shuguang Hospital, Shanghai College of Traditional Chinese Medicine: *Papers on Shanghai Annual Meeting of Traditional Chinese Medicine,* 1977, p.43, 1978.

OBSERVATION OF VISCERAL DRAGGING-PAIN-REACTION DURING SUBTOTAL GASTRECTOMY

Chen Peixi, Pan Wenzheng, Zhang Ming,
Weng Jiwei, Feng Jianjiang
(Physiological Research Section of Acupuncture Anesthesia, Zhongshan Medical College)

A complex reaction of visceral dragging pain often occurred during subtotal gastrectomy and influenced the smooth proceeding of the operation. Neither acupuncture anesthesia nor epidural anesthesia could inhibit such reaction completely. Recently, much basic and clinical research of the inhibitory effect of acupuncture on visceral dragging pain was made, and some data and findings have been gained[1–6, 11–14]. We have observed the changes of finger plethysmogram, blood pressure and heart rate of 197 cases of subtotal gastrectomy and analyzed the occurrence and expression of visceral dragging-pain-reaction, as well as how it was influenced by electro-acupuncture, in order to understand the rule of the inhibitory effect by acupuncture on visceral-dragging-pain and to improve the effect of acupuncture anesthesia to provide some basis for further investigation of the mechanism of acupuncture anesthesia.

I. METHODS

The changes of the plethysmogram, blood pressure and heart rate were continuously observed with a 4-guides recorder during operation; at the same time, nausea, vomiting and other patient's subjective feeling were recorded. The finger plethysmogram was observed with a photo-electric transducer which was fixed at the tip of the finger and recorded after amplification. The unit of its wave amplitude was milivolt. The blood pressure was examined intermittently by indirect method. A little air sac for depression, connected with a pressor transducer was bound onto the root of the finger, and the pulsation of the finger tip was demonstrated by photoelectric plethysmography. During each measurement, the pressure within the air sac increased gradually from zero upward; thus the wall of the finger blood vessel was pressed. While the pulse wave of the finger tip began to disappear, the pressure within the sac representing the systolic pressure was recorded on paper through the transducer and amplifier. The height of the curve expressed the value of blood pressure. The measurement was taken every 30 seconds. Before and after the main steps of operations we also measured the brachial arterial pressure by auscultation and pulse rate at the same time for comparison. Heart rate was recorded through a tachometer triggered by ECG signal. The amplitude of the heart rate curve expressed the duration of the cardiac cycle; the higher curve showed the longer cycle period, i.e., slower heart rate.

Grouping of electro-acupuncture: (1) Control group: Jiuwei, bilateral Zhangmen (with the frequency of 500 Hz), bilateral Qimai (50 Hz), bilateral Geshu (50 Hz); (2) Strengthened Backshu group: Bilateral Geshu (50 Hz), Danshu, (100 Hz), and others same as control group; (3) Ear-radix stimulating group: Aq. dist. 10ml injected into the left ear-root, and right Neiguan, Jiuwei, Shuifen and bilateral Zhangmen, Weishen, and Danshu, electro-acupunctured; (4) Ear-radix Blocking group: 0.5% procaine 10ml injected into the left ear-root, and others same as group (3).

After operation, the efficacy of acupuncture anesthesia was divided into four grades on the basis of the patient's reaction and according to the national standards.

II. RESULTS AND DISCUSSION

1. Manifestations of the Visceral Dragging-Pain-Reaction. Manifestations of the visceral dragging-pain-reaction were analyzed by the following changes of the physiological indices during operation.

(1) Changes in the amplitude of the plethysmogram during operation.

The whole course of operation was divided into 25 successive steps for convenience sake to analyze the changes on the wave amplitude. The control value (0) was the amplitude taken before skin incision. The changes of amplitude in various steps were counted separately, and they were called change values (+means increase, -means decrease). Table 1 shows the mean values and standard errors of the change values in various steps of a group of 42 cases under acupuncture anesthesia, and Figure 1 was plotted from these values.

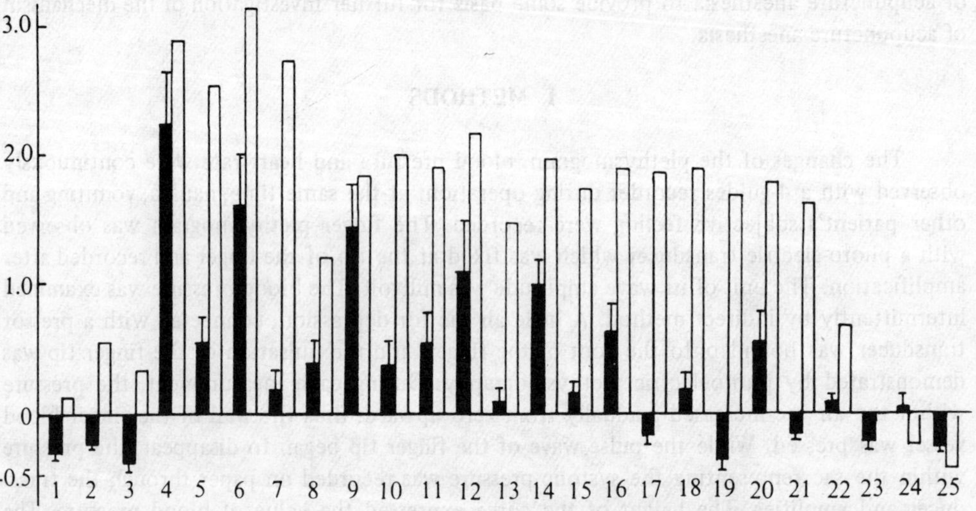

Fig. 1 The changes of amplitude values of plethysmogram wave during subtotal gastrectomy (mean values ± standare errors). The number under the column shows the step of operation, same as Table 1.
The solid columns indicate the values of 42 Cases under acupunture anesthesia, the hollow columns indicate 50 cases under epidura anesthesia.

Table 1. The changes of amplitude value of plethysmogram wave during subtotal gastrectomy under acupuncture anesthesia

Steps of operation	Change value of wave amplitude	
Before skin incision	0	
1. Incision of skin	-0.3±0.04	...
2. Incision of peritoneum	-0.19±0.06	..
3. Ascertainment	-0.39±0.06	...
4. Freeing greater curvature	2.34±0.44	...
5. Dragging A. gastroepiploica dext.	0.58±0.24	.
6. Ligating A.g.e.d.	1.71±0.47	..
7. Freeing pylorus	0.19±0.17	
8. Dragging A. gastrica dext.	0.42±0.24	
9. Ligating A.g.d.	1.50±0.35	...
10. Dragging gastric wall	0.39±0.22	
11. Cutting pylorus	0.55±0.26	
12. Closure of duodenal stump	1.17±0.40	..
13. Dragging A. gastrica. sin.	0.12±0.13	
14. Ligating A.g.s.	1.05±0.22	...
15. Dragging gastric wall	0.10±0.15	
16. Incision of ant.gastric wall	0.69±0.23	.
17. Dragging gastric wall	-0.16±0.10	
18. Incision of post. gastric wall	0.23±0.15	
19. Dragging jejunum	-0.35±0.10	..
20. Suture of post. gastric wall	0.62±0.24	.
21. Resection of stomach	-0.10±0.99	
22. Suture of ant. gastric wall	0.12±0.08	
23. Testing anastomosis	-0.18±0.12	
24. Closure of peritoneum	0.07±0.14	
25. Suture of skin	-0.23±0.07	..

· P<0.05 ·· P<0.01 ··· P<0.001

From Fig. 1 we found that the amplitude decreased during the opening of the abdomen (including the incision of the skin, muscle and peritoneum and the ascertainment). During the separation of the greater curvature (omentum), the amplitude increased gradually; the maximum increase could be several times the control value, and after that it would decrease gradually. In the later period of gastro-intestinal anastomosis, the value approached that before operation or somewhat below that. It is necessary to point out that in the 7th, 8th, 10th, 11th, 13th, 15th, 17th, 19th, 21th, and 23th steps, the amplitude dropped suddenly for a short while, and then climbed up to a higher level. All such manipulations strongly stimulated the wall of the stomach, the intestine and the blood vessels.

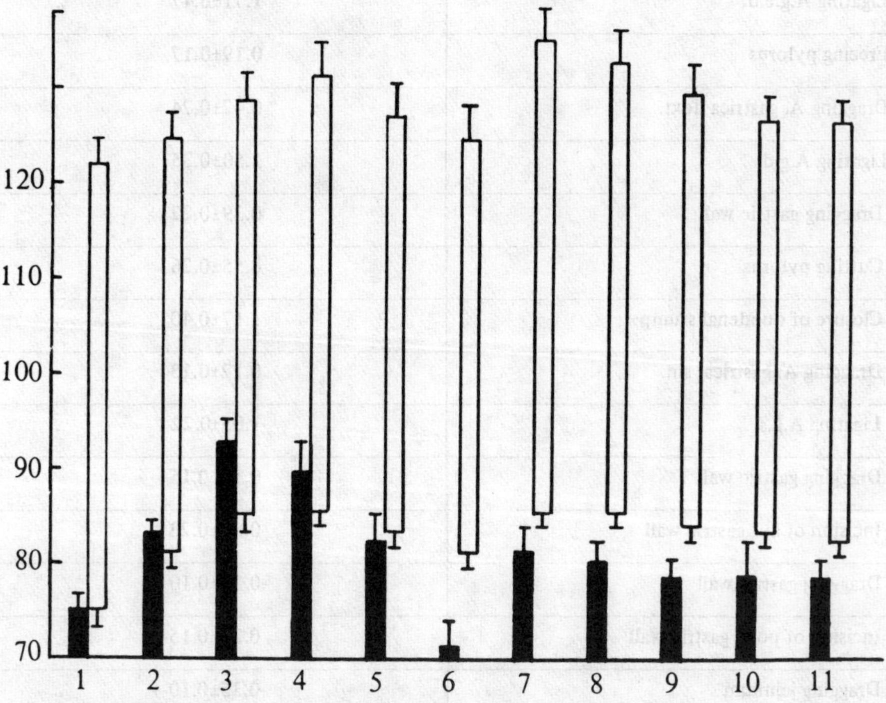

Fig. 2 The changes in the heart rate and the blood pressure during subtotal gastrectomy under acupuncture anaesthesia. (mean values ± standard errors) The solid column shows the heart rate (beats/min.). The upper end of the hollow column shows the systolic pressure, the lower end, diastolic pressrue (mm Hg). The numbers under the columns were the steps of operation: 1. Before induction. 2. During induction. 3. Incision of the skin. 4. Incision of the peritoneum. 5. Ascertainment. 6. Separation of the greater curvature. 7. Separation of the lesser curvature. 8. Handling of the duodenal stump. 9. Gastrointestinal anastomosis. 10. Suture of the peritoneum. 11. Suture of the skin.

We also compared the amplitude values before (1 minute) and after various steps and analyzed the number of those patients who had increasing amplitudes and those who had decreasing ones (changes over 10%). We found that most patients' amplitude values increased during the separation of the greater curvature; 86 of 145 cases showed increasing effect (86/145), while 7 cases showed decreasing effect. On the contrary, most of the patients showed decreasing effect during separation of the posterior wall of the pylorus; 67 of 130 cases showed decrease in amplitude, while 14 cases showed increase in it. Many patients showed the decreasing effect during the dragging of the wall of the jejunum (42/50) and of the gastric arteries (53/122).

(2) The change in the heart rate during operation.

Different degrees of changes in the heart rate occurred in the various steps of the operation. Fig. 2 shows the mean values of the heart rate in 10 steps of the operation of 50 patients. The heart rate increased during the induction period, and further increased during the incision of the skin and the peritoneum. But it decreased during the ascertainment and became the slowest during the separating of the greater curvature (omentum); it was either on the same level before induction or below that. But the heart rate went up again while the lesser curvature was being separated and the duodenal stump closed. During the period of gastro-intestinal anastomosis the heart rate changed slightly, and it returned to the level before operation after the closure of the abdomen.

Comparison of the changes in the heart rate before and after the various steps showed that there were two kinds of reaction, i.e., increasing reaction and decreasing reaction. The decreasing reaction mostly occurred during the separation of the omentum on the greater curvature, and out of 127 cases 42 cases decreased while in 4 cases the rate increased. Increasing reaction mainly appeared during dragging the gastro-intestinal wall and the gastric arteries. Out of 64 cases 47 cases increased, while 4 cases decreased.

(3) The changes in blood pressure during operation.

Different changes in blood pressure were induced in different steps of the operation. Fig.2 shows the average changes in blood pressure in 10 steps of the operation of 50 patients. In this figure we found that the blood pressure increased during induction, and further increased while skin and peritoneum were incised, but decreased during freeing the greater curvature and then increased again during freeing the lesser curvature, and recovered gradually during gastro-intestinal anastomosis, and returned to the preoperation level while the skin was sutured. The changes on the diastolic pressure were similar to those in the systolic one.

Comparing the changes in blood pressure before and after various steps of operation, we found that the pressor reaction mainly occurred at the step of dragging the left gastric artery. Out of 85 patients, the blood pressure of 62 cases increased, and the depressor reaction occurred mainly during freeing the greater curvature.

Fig. 3 shows the changes in three physiological indices of one case of subtotal gastrectomy under acupuncture anesthesia. During the step of freeing the greater curvature (omentum), the amplitude of the plethysmogram increased gradually; at the same time the blood pressure decreased and the heart rate became lower. The maximum amplitude was 5 times over that before operation. While the pyloric portion was being separated, the amplitude began to diminish gradually and after the abdomen was closed, it returned to the preoperation level. Several times when the gastric wall was dragged, the amplitude diminished

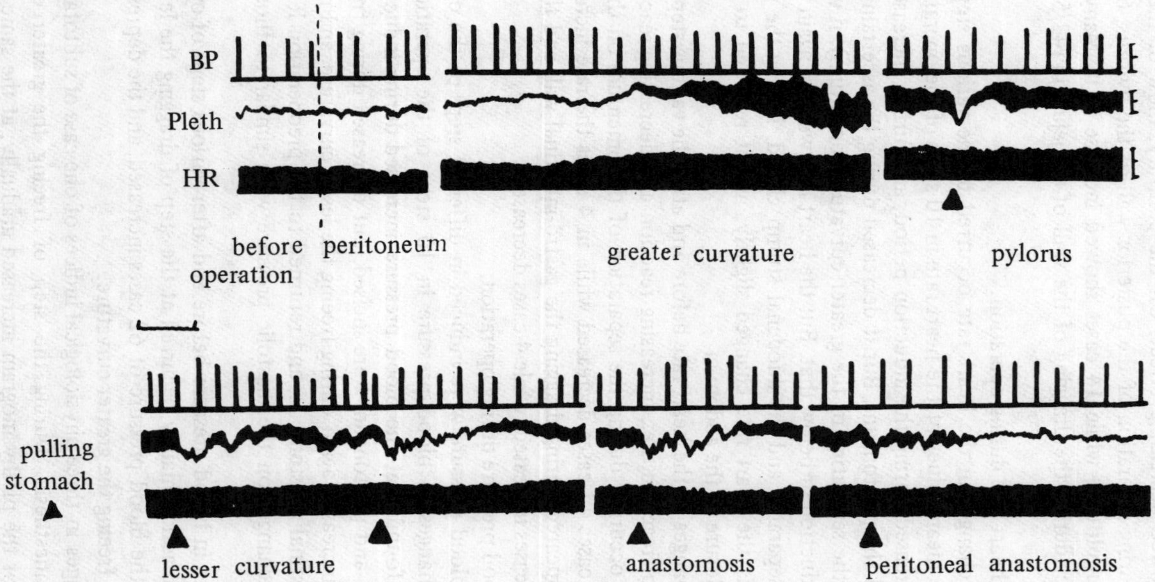

Fig. 3 Changes in 3 indices of one case during subtotal gastrectomy.

BP=blood pressure, Pleth=plethysmogram, HR=heart rate, ▲indicate pulling stomach

Time scale ; BP scale, 100, 50 mmHg; Pleth. scale, mV; HR scale, 50, 80 beats/min quickly and markedly, and at the same time both blood pressure and heart rate increased (Fig. 3).

(4) Nausea and vomiting during operation.

Out of 180 patients of subtotal gastrectomy under acupuncture anesthesia, nausea occurred in 72 cases for 150 times; it occurred mainly during the step of separation of the omentum of the greater curvature, and then during the step of handling the duodenal stump, 20 cases vomitted for 28 times; it occurred mainly during manipulating the duodenal stump (10 times) and freeing the greater curvature (5 times). Most patients also felt fullness of the chest during these periods.

According to the changes mentioned above, different manipulations induced different characters of stimulation, and stimulation at different locations induced different visceral dragging-pain-reactions. These are very complicated processes. As to the characters of stimulation, there are mechanical stimulation, including dragging, pressing, cutting, clamping, ligating, and sticking, etc. Strongest reactions are induced by dragging, clamping and ligating. As to the location stimulated, strongest reactions are caused by manipulating the peritoneum, dragging the lesser curvature, and ligating the gastric arteries. Meanwhile all the physiological indices observed showed changes of various degrees in the finger tip pulse wave, heart rate and blood pressure, and dragging pain, fullness of the chest nausea were felt by the patients; even vomiting, hiccuping and swallowing might occur.

From the changes mentioned above, the reaction of visceral dragging-pain could be divided into two types, i.e., the sympathetic exciting reaction and the sympathetic inhibiting reaction. In the sympathetic exciting reaction, the plethysmogram and the pulse wave decreased, but the blood pressure and the heart rate increased. The durations of these reactions were short; the patients felt pain, which was mainly due to visceral pain reaction. In the sympathetic inhibiting reaction, these four physiological indexes were opposite to those of the exciting reaction. The duration was also longer. The patients felt nauseous and vomited. That was mainly due to the visceral dragging reaction. During gastrectomy, these two types of reactions often occurred together; however the sympathetic exciting reaction might happen in some steps of operation, while the sympathetic inhibiting reaction appeared in some other ones.

Some of these results coincided with what were reported previously by other investigators[1-7]. Similar reactions occurred during operations for other abdominal organs. Dividing these complex visceral dragging-pain-reactions into visceral dragging reaction and visceral pain reaction might be of practical significance for further clarifying the characters and mechanisms of these reactions so as to eliminate them more completely.

2. The Occurrence of Visceral Dragging Pain. (1) The visceral pain reaction. Figs. 1 and 3 show significant amplitude decreasing reaction of the plethysmogram during dragging of the gastric wall, especially during freeing the wall of the pyloric portion. Dragging the wall of the jejunum and that of the gastric blood vessels also induced significant amplitude decreasing effects. The amplitudes of 28 cases out of 47 patients decreased during dragging the wall of jejunum, but those of 5 cases increased. The amplitudes of 24 cases out of 44 patients decreased during dragging the wall of the left gastric artery, but those of 7 cases increased. The upper curve in Fig. 4 shows the marked sympathetic exciting reaction due to dragging the gastric wall two times successively, i.e., plethysmogram waves decreased, blood pressure and heart rate increased, and the patient felt severe pain. This suggests that the

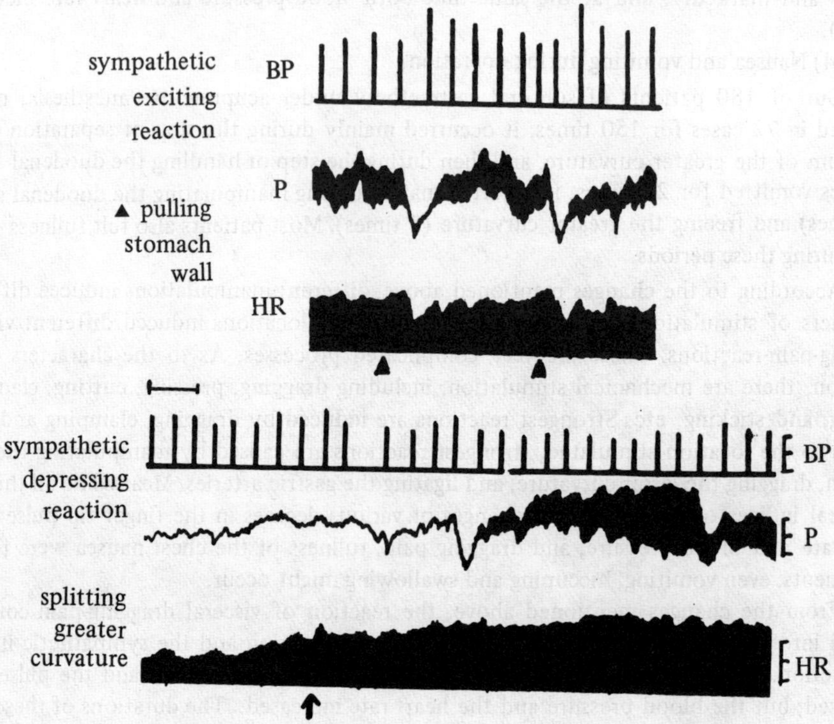

Fig. 4 Sympathetic exciting reaction (upper) and sympathetic inhibiting reaction (lower)
▲ indicate dragging of gastric wall, ↑ indicates freeing of greater curvature.

visceral pain reaction may be caused by the stimulation given to the receptors within the gastric wall, the intestinal wall and the blood vessel wall.

Under epidural anesthesia, $T_4 - T_{10}$ blocked, the sympathetic exciting reaction was obviously reduced (Fig. 1), and only 4 of 17 patients felt pain (23.5%). While under acupuncture anesthesia, 115 of 180 cases felt pain (63.9%). The difference is very significant ($P<0.01$). The greater splanchnic nerve enters the spinal cord at T_{4-10}, and so it suggests that the greater splanchnic nerve might be the main afferent pathway of visceral pain reaction.

(2) The visceral dragging reaction. From Figs. 1 and 3 we can see that during separating the greater curvature most of the patients have an obvious increase reaction of the pulse amplitude, and many of them felt nauseous. The lower curve of Fig. 4 shows the sympathetic inhibiting reaction during separation of the greater curvature, i.e., the amplitude increased but both the blood pressure and heart rate diminished; the patients felt fullness in the chest and nauseous. Nausea and vomiting occurred more frequently during the step of handling the duodenal stump. It suggests that the visceral dragging reaction might be due to the stimulation of the receptors of the tissues surrounding the stomach and the intestine.

Under epidural anesthesia, the amplitude increasing reaction of the plethysmogram could not be reduced, and patients appeared nauseous and vomited more frequently. Out of 17 patients 16 cases (94.1%) appeared nauseous, 12 cases (70.6%) had vomiting. But out of 180 patients under acupuncture anesthesia, only 72 cases (40%) were nauseous; 20 cases (11.1%) had vomiting. The difference is very significant ($P<0.01$). It shows that the visceral dragging reaction could not be inhibited by epidural anesthesia. It suggests that the greater splanchnic nerve is not the main afferent path of this reaction and the afferent impulses might pass through the vagus or other nerves.

The abdominal visceral mechanoreceptors might be divided into slowly adapting and rapidly adapting receptors. These receptors exist in the gastro-intestinal wall, mesenterium and omentum[15]. The receptors which induce visceral pain reaction belonged to slow adaptation, and the receptors which induce visceral dragging reaction may either belong to slow adaptation or relate to fast adaptation. According to the papers published before, the afferent fibers of upper abdominal visceral pain exist in the greater splanchnic nerve, while the afferent fibers which induce nausea and vomiting exist in the vagus nerve[8–13]. It has practical significance to determine the receptors and afferent paths of these two kinds of reactions, because it will be benificial to the study for eliminating the visceral dragging-pain-reaction.

3. The Effect of Acupuncture on Visceral Dragging-Pain-Reaction. (1) The effect of Back-shu point on the visceral pain reaction. Out of 22 patients of control group, 13 cases (59.1%) experienced strong visceral pain reaction, while of strengthened Back-shu group, out of 29 patients only 9 cases (31.9%) reacted strongly. The difference is statistically significant ($P<0.05$). It showed that the electro-acupuncture at Back-shu points could inhibit the visceral pain reaction.

(2) The effect of ear-radix points on the visceral dragging reaction.

In 70 patients of ear-radix blocked group, 15 cases (21.4%) vomited; while in the 38 patients of ear-radix stimulated group, only one case (2.6%) vomited. The difference is very significant ($P<0.01$). It showed that the ear-radix points could inhibit the visceral dragging reaction.

During subtotal gastrectomy under acupuncture anesthesia we observed that acupuncture could inhibit the visceral dragging reaction to some degree, especially nausea and vomiting reactions. Nausea and vomiting reactions were fewer under acupuncture anesthesia than epidural anesthesia. But the inhibitory effect of acupuncture on visceral pain reaction showed individual difference, some were obviously inhibited and some lesser. So, this difference might have some connection with the electro-acupuncture points selected. In the strengthened Back-shu group, we found that more Back-shu points and higher electric frequency made the visceral pain reaction weakened and the ratio of good result elevated. It suggests that Back-shu point could inhibit visceral pain. The segment at which the Dushu and Danshu enter the spinal cord corresponds to that of the greater splanchnic nerve, so it conforms to the conception that the points related to the spinal segment strengthened the inhibition effect[14]. The ear-radix points are close to the entrance of the vagus nerve into medulla oblongata. Therefore, we consider that the appropriate coordination of the Back-shu points with the ear-radix points might further inhibit the visceral dragging-pain-reaction and enhance the effectiveness of acupuncture anesthesia.

From the facts mentioned above we believe that during subtotal gastrectomy, gastrointestinal dragging manipulation induces complex visceral dragging-pain-reaction, which may be divided into visceral pain reaction and visceral dragging reaction. The visceral pain reaction is expressed in the form of sympathetic exciting reaction, and induced mainly by the mechanical stimulation of the receptors of the gastro-intestinal wall or the walls of gastric vessels, whose afferent impulses enter the spinal cord through the greater splanchnic nerve; Back-shu points could inhibit this reaction. The visceral dragging reaction expressed in the form of sympathetic inhibiting reaction is induced mainly by the mechanical stimulation of the receptors of the peri-gastrointestinal tissues (omentum, etc.) whose afferent impulses enter the medullar oblongata perhaps through the vagus nerve, and the ear-radix points could inhibit this reaction (Fig. 5).

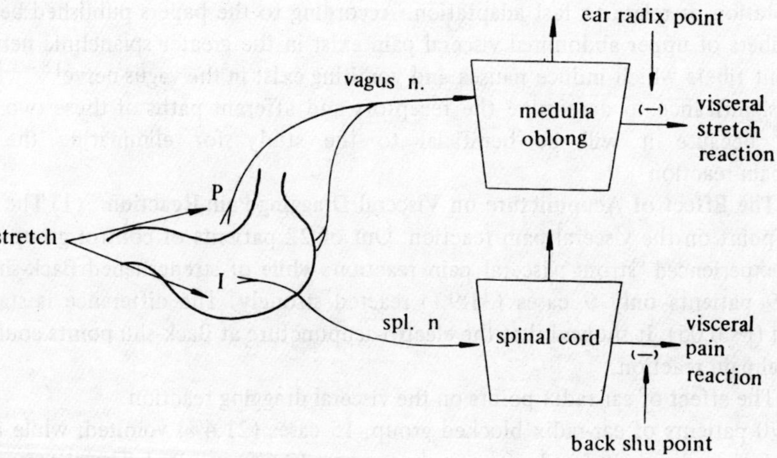

Fig. 5 Diagram of visceral dragging pain reaction.
P=perigastrointestinal tissue
I=gastrointestinal wall

III. SUMMARY

During subtotal gastrectomy (under acupuncture anesthesia or epidural anesthesia), the changes in several physiological indices were recorded in order to study the rule of the inhibitory effect of acupuncture on the visceral dragging-pain-reaction. We found that the visceral dragging-pain-reaction consists of two kinds of reactions, i.e., visceral pain reaction and visceral dragging reaction. The visceral pain reaction is shown in the diminishing of the plethysmograth, raising of the blood pressure and increasing of the heart rate; these belong to the sympathetic exciting reaction. At the same time the patients often complained of pain. The visceral dragging reaction is shown in the increase of the plethysmogram, the diminishing of heart rate and blood pressure; these belong to the sympathetic inhibiting reaction. At the same time the patients often feel fullness of the chest accompanied by nausea and vomiting. These two types of reactions often interlapped in the course of gastrectomy, but during some steps there was marked sympathetic exciting reaction, and during others there was marked sympathetic inhibiting reaction.

The visceral pain reaction occurred mainly during dragging the walls of the stomach, and the intestine or blood vessels, which diminished markedly under epidural anesthesia, and could be inhibited by stimulation of the Back-shu points. The visceral dragging reaction occurred mainly during separating the omentum around the greater curvature; it did not diminish under epidural anesthesia, but the stimulation of the ear-radix points could inhibit it.

REFERENCES

[1] 广州部队针麻协作组：中华医学杂志（4)：256，1975。

[2] 上海中医学院曙光医院：中华医学杂志（10)：703，1975。

[3] 北京医学院第三附属医院针麻研究组：全国针麻研究资料选编，第60页，上海人民出版社，1977。

[4] 中医研究院针灸经络研究所生理组等：中医药研究参考（7)：21，1974。

[5] 中医研究院针灸经络研究所生理组：中医药研究参考（6)：10，1974。

[6] 上海市第一人民医院：针刺麻醉原理的探讨，第367页，人民卫生出版社，1974。

[7] Folkow, B. *et al*: *Ann, Surg.*, **156**:905, 1962.

[8] Moore, R. M. and Galveston, M. D.: *Surgery*, **3**:534–555, 1938.

[9] Herin, C. and Mark, W. J. : *Am. J. Physiol.*, **144**:720–723, 1945.

[10] Ray, B. C. and Neill, G. L.: *Ann Surg*, **126**: 709–724, 1947.

[11] 山东医学院针麻原理研究组：全国针麻研究资料选编，第250页，上海人民出版社，1977。

[12] 杜焕基等：新医药学杂志 4：25，1975。

[13] 重庆医学院针麻原理研究组 针刺麻醉，第87页，1976。

[14] 吴建屏等：科学通报 **5**：238，1973。

[15] Leek, B. F.: Handbook of Sensory Physiology V. III/I Enteroceptors, 114–156, Springer-Verlag. N. Y., 1972.

PREOPERATIVE COMPREHENSIVE FORECAST OF THE EFFECTIVENESS OF ACUPUNCTURE ANESTHESIA IN SUBTOTAL GASTRECTOMY FOR PEPTIC ULCER*

Acupuncture Anesthesia Coordinating Group for Gastrectomy, Beijing Medical College

Acupuncture anesthesia is a new anesthetic method different from current anesthesia methods. How to further improve the effect of acupuncture anesthesia–which depends upon the regulatory function of the human body and the physiological characteristcis of each individual–is an urgent task of clinical importance to medical workers. Therefore, to find out a sure method that will enable the doctor to choose the kind of anesthesia suitable for each patient will enhance the effect of acupuncture anesthesia. We call this "preoperative forecast of acupuncture anesthesia".

As the functional status of the human body is influenced by many complicated factors, it is necessary to use amulti-index method, which can complement each other, instead of the single index one in order to get more objective and precise forecasts.

This article is a report on how since 1976, the effect of acupuncture anesthesia was forecasted in 51 cases of subtotal gastrectomy by three norms of different physiological meanings, which were analyzed with multivariable statistical analyzing method and the preliminary results obtained.

I. METHOD

In the 3 days before operation, the basic pain tolerance threshold at the incision area of the upper abdominal wall was measured with 57–9A potassium iontophoresis dolorimeter, while the patient was lying in a quiet laboratory. Then Shangjuxu point on the right side of the lower leg was needled, and the changes in the pain tolerance threshold were observed at the 10th, 20th and 30th minute after acupuncture At the 31st minute after needling, the needle was drawn out, and at the 40th minute the threshold was measured once more. During these measurements, the basic curve of vasomotority of the finger vessels was observed by photoelectric plethysmography of the finger with Galileo E8c polygraph. The curve which fluctuated within a 0–7mm range belongs to Type A, while that beyond the 0–7mm range belongs to Type B.

After operation these data were analyzed with reference to the anesthetic records of the effect of acupuncture anesthesia and skin analgesic effect. The classification of the effect

*Compiled by Wang Youliang.

of acupuncture anesthesia was done according to the national unified standards of four grades, but in this article we combine them into two main grades, the good group (Grades I and II) and the poor group (Grades III and IV). The clinical condition under which the investigation was carried out was basically stable.

Through preoperative measurements and actual clinical effects, we found out the corresponding relations and their possibilities between each norm and the effect of acupuncture anesthesia or skin analgesic effect. Then the value of various possibilities was converted into an index by multivariable statistical analyzing method (likelihood method). A forecast chart of the efficacy of acupuncture anesthesia was tabulated from these indices calculated from various possibilities. The value of each index is the sum of the logarithms of its possibilities plus one, and then multiplied by 10. It ranged from −10 to +10.

The multivariable statistical analyzing method is a comprehensive forecast method which can make the forecast digitalized, and more systematic and scientific. It is a useful and scientific tool for the forecast of the effect of acupuncture anesthesia.

II. RESULTS

1. Basic Pain Tolerance Threshold.

41 cases were analyzed from complete data and anesthetic records.

In the good effect group (Grades I or II) of acupuncture anesthesia, there were 13/25 cases whose basic pain tolerance threshold was more than 3.5 mV (52%) and 8/23 cases less than 3.5 mV (34.8%); in the bad effect group (Grades III or IV) of acupuncture anesthesia, there were 10/18 cases whose basic pain tolerance threshold was more than 3.5 mV(55.5%) and 8/18 cases less than 3.5 mV (44.4%).

In the good effect group of skin analysis, there were 17/23 cases whose basic pain tolerance threshold was more than 3.5 mV (73.9%) and 6/23 cases less than 3.5 mV (26.1%); in the bad effect group of skin analgesia there were 8/18 cases whose basic pain tolerance threshold was more than 3.5 mV (44.4%) and 10/18 cases less than 3.5 mV (55.5%).

2. Changes in Pain Tolerance Threshold After Acupuncture.

The values of pain tolerance threshold measured after needling were divided into two groups. Increasing group means that all the four values measured after needling increased, while decreasing group means that one or more than one of the values decreased.

In the good effect group of acupuncture anesthesia 12/26 cases belonged to the increasing group (60%) and 8/20 cases to the decreasing group (40%); in the bad effect group of acupuncture anesthesia, 8/16 cases belonged to the increasing group (50%) and 8/16 cases to the decreasing group (50%).

In the good effect group of skin analgesia, 15/19 cases belonged to the increasing group (78.9%) and 4/19 cases to the decreasing group (21.1%); in the bad effect group of skin analgesia, 5/17 cases belonged to the increasing group (29.4%) and 12/17 eases to the decreasing group (70.6%).

3. The Patterns of the Curves of the Finger Plethysmograph of the Finger Were Divided Into Type A and Type B, as Mentioned Above.

In the good effect group of acupuncture anesthesia, 13/17 cases were Type A (76.5%) and 4/17 cases Type B (23.5%); in the bad effect group of acupuncture anesthesia, 8/13 cases were Type A (61.5%) and 5/13 cases Type B (38.5%). In the good effect group of skin analgesia, 15/16 cases were Type A (93.8%) and 1/16 cases Type B (6.3%); in the bad effect group of skin analgesia, 6/14 cases were Type A (42.9%) and 8/14 cases Type B (57.1%).

A forecast chart of the efficacies of acupuncture anesthesia and skin analgesia is drawn with the above data (see the table below).

Table1 Forecast chart of acupuncture anesthesia effectiveness in subtotal gastrectomy

		Effectiveness of acupuncture anesthesia		Effectiveness of acupuncture anesthesia on skin incision	
		Good (I, II)	Bad (III, IV)	Good (I, II)	Bad (III, IV)
Basal pain tolerance	>3.5 mA	8	7	9	6
threshold	>3.5 mA	5	6	4	7
Rate of change of pain tolerance		8	7	9	5
threshold after acupuncture		6	7	3	8
Pulse wave curve	A	9	8	10	6
	B	4	6	-2	8

According to the values of the norm measured preoperatively, add up the corresponding indices of each column longitudinally, and compare the sums of each pair respectively; the greater one indicates which grade the efficacy of acupuncture anesthesia or skin analgesia belongs to. For example, if a patient's basic pain tolerance threshold was 3.5 mV, the pain tolerance threshold after needling belonged to the increasing type, and the pattern of the curve of the plethysmograph was Type A, we find out the corresponding indices and add up them longitudinally as follows:

Table2	Acupuncture anesthesia effect		Skin analgesia effect	
	8	7	9	6
	8	7	9	5
+)	9	8	10	6
	25	22	28	17

As 25>22, so the forecast of the effect of acupuncture anesthesia is of the good grade, and as 28>17, that of skin analgesia effect is also of the good grade.

The rate of correct forecasts of acupuncture anesthesia is 67% and that of skin analgesia 80%.

III. DISCUSSION

1. The three norms selected for forecasting should neither be closely related, nor have the same physiological meanings, but they must be closely interrelated to the effect of acupuncture anesthesia. Of the three norms which we chose, the basic pain tolerance threshold reflects the patient's basic pain endurance. The rate of change of the pain tolerance threshold after needling reflects the dynamic change in the pain endurance of the patient under prolonged acupuncture. Actually the patient's regulatory response to acupuncture, and the basic curve of the plethysmograph of the finger reflect more or less the function of the autonomic nervous system. By correlating the above three norms with the effect of acupuncture by the multivariable analyzing method, the degree of accuracy of the forecast of each norm can be enhanced. This is the chief feature of the present method, which should be further tested through clinical practice.

2. These factors influencing the efficacy of acupuncture anesthesia are rather complicated. The true rate of the present forecast method is not satisfactory yet. This may be due to the fact that many factors such as the seriousness of the disease, the psychological factors of the patients, etc., have not been included in our consideration. These factors should be studied in order to improve the degree of accuracy of forecast.

3. It is possible to forecast the effect of acupuncture anesthesia for subtotal gastrectomy by multiple indices which are analyzed by the likelihood method.

4. The forecast chart drawn up by this method is convenient, scientific and can be popularized in clinical practice.

CLINICAL ANALYSIS OF 1,000 CASES OF CESAREAN SECTION UNDER ACUPUNCTURE ANESTHESIA

The Research Group of Acupuncture Anesthesia for Cesarean
Section, Beijing Obstetrics and Gynecology Hospital

Acupuncture anesthesia has been widely used as an anesthetic method for cesarean section in hospitals all over China. During the operation the patient's blood pressure and pulse are stable, blood loss is less and the effectiveness of the anesthesia is rather steady. An analysis of a thousand cases of cesarean section done under acupuncture anesthesia from 1966 to 1978 by this hospital is given below.

I. METHOD OF ACUPUNCTURE ANESTHESIA

1. **Prescription of the Acupuncture Points.** Seven different prescriptions of acupuncture points have been used since we started cesarean sections under acupuncture anesthesia. Through actual practice, Sanyinjiao (Sp. 6), "external anesthesia" point and para-incisional needle are finally chosen as the basic prescription. In recent years according to the principle of 'bian-zheng' (symptom identification) method of Chinese traditional medicine, another two prescriptions are used selectively. They are: (1) Sanyinjiao, Taichong (Liv. 3) and Xiajuxu (St. 39); (2) Sanyinjiao, Neiguan (P.6) and Zusanli (St. 36).

2. **Method of Stimulation.** Kind of Stimulation: Electric pulse stimulation is used.

Frequency of Stimulation: For the points on the legs 2 Hz are used, and 800 Hz for para-incisional needles.

Table 1. Standards of grading the effectiveness

Grade	1	2	3	4
Anesthetic effect	Excellent	Good	Moderate	Poor
Dose of pethidine used (mg)	Within 50	Within 50	50–100	Over 100
0.5% Procaine used (ml)	Within 5 ml	Within 10 ml	With 20 ml	Over 20 ml
Effect on operation	Carried on smoothly	Carried on smoothly	Can be carried on	Have to change anesthesia
Pain sensation	Generally free from pain	May have slight pain	Carried on more pain	Anesthesia marked pain

Intensity of Stimulation: To be adjusted in accordance with patient's tolerance.

Length of Time of Induction: 15 to 30 minutes.

3. **Supplementary Medication.** Pethidine 50 mg is given intravenously 10 minutes before operation or after delivery of the baby. Two ml of 1% dicaine is applied locally to the peritoneum. For skin incision 5 ml of 0.5% of procaine may be used for supplementation and 20 ml may be used for the excision of old abdominal scar.

4. **Standards of Grading the Effectiveness.** The effectiveness of acupuncture anesthesia is divided into four grades according to the subjective feeling of the patient, the pain response, use of adjuvant drugs and its effect on the operation (Table 1).

II. CLINICAL DATA

1. **Indication for Operation.** The indications for cesarean section in this series of cases are shown in Table 2.

Other indications such as elderly primipara, overterm, premature rupture of membranes, history of laceration of cervix, etc., made a total of 151 cases, accounting for 15.1%.

2. **Effectiveness.** For the 1,000 cases under study, the rate of success is 98.4% and the rate of Grades 1 and 2 is 75.8% (Table 3).

Table 2. Indications for cesarean section

Indication	No. of Cases	%
Contracted pelvis	522	52.2
Pregnancy after cesarean section	137	13.7
Fetal distress	79	7.9
Abnormal presentation	50	5.0
Precious baby	36	3.6
Antepartum hemorrhage	25	2.5

Table 3. Effectiveness of acupuncture anesthesia

	Total	Grade			
		1	2	3	4
No. of cases	1000	290	468	226	16
Percentage	100.0	29.0	46.8	22.6	1.6
Rate of success (%)			98.4		
Rate of Grades 1 & 2 (%)		75.8			

3. **Observation of Clinical Conditions and Physiological Parameters.** Excluding the cases with complications which might affect the blood pressure and the amount of bleeding, such as toxemia of pregnancy, anemia, antepartum hemorrhage, twins, etc., the remaining 664 cases were analysed and in 51 cases the physiological parameters were observed (Fig. 1).

(1) Blood pressure. In the various steps of the operation, the changes in blood pressure were not marked (Fig. 1). During the whole course of operation the changes in systolic and diastolic pressures within 20 mm Hg were 67.6% and 85.7%, respectively. When the baby is being delivered, the physiological disturbance in circulation is the greatest. At this moment the blood pressure changes within 20 mm Hg were 82.9% and 90.5% for systolic and diastolic pressures, respectively (Tables 4 & 5).

(2) Pulse and plethysmogram. Clinical observation shows the average range of changes in pulse rate throughout the course of operation and during delivery of the baby were 15.4/min and 12.1/min, respectively (Table 6). The finger plethysmogram records also show the stability of the pulse rate. Between various operative steps the difference of pulse rate on the average was only 4.3/min. After the operation started, there was a decrease in the wave amplitude. During the delivery of the baby the amplitude was 2.1 mm less than that after induction on the average, and it rapidly recovered when the uterus was sutured. While the wave amplitude decreased, the blood pressure, pulse rate, respiration rate and skin galvanic potential were relatively stable (Fig. 1).

(3) Respiration. It was also stable. The difference of respiration rate between various operative steps was 3.3/min on the average (Fig. 1).

(4) Skin galvanic potential: It was stable and the greatest amplitude was only 1.5 mv (Fig. 1).

Table 4. Change in blood pressure during the course of operation

Pressure	No. of Cases	Range of Change mmHg						Average Value	Unknown	
		20		21–30		30				
		Cases	P.C.*	Cases	P.C.	Cases	P.C.		Cases	P.C.
Systolic pressure	664	449	67.6	11	16.6	73	11.0	21.6	32	4.8
Diastolic pressure	664	569	85.7	49	7.4	14	2.1	15.5	32	4.8

*P.C.=Per cent

Table 5. Change in blood pressure during delivery of baby

	No. of Cases	Range of Change mmHg						Average Value	Unknown	
		⩽ 20		21–30		> 30				
		Cases	P.C.*	Cases	P.C.	Cases	P.C.		Cases	P.C.
Systolic pressure	664	551	83.0	52	7.8	27	4.1	14.2	34	5.1
Diastolic pressure	664	601	90.5	21	3.2	5	0.7	9.2	37	5.6

* P.C.=Per cent

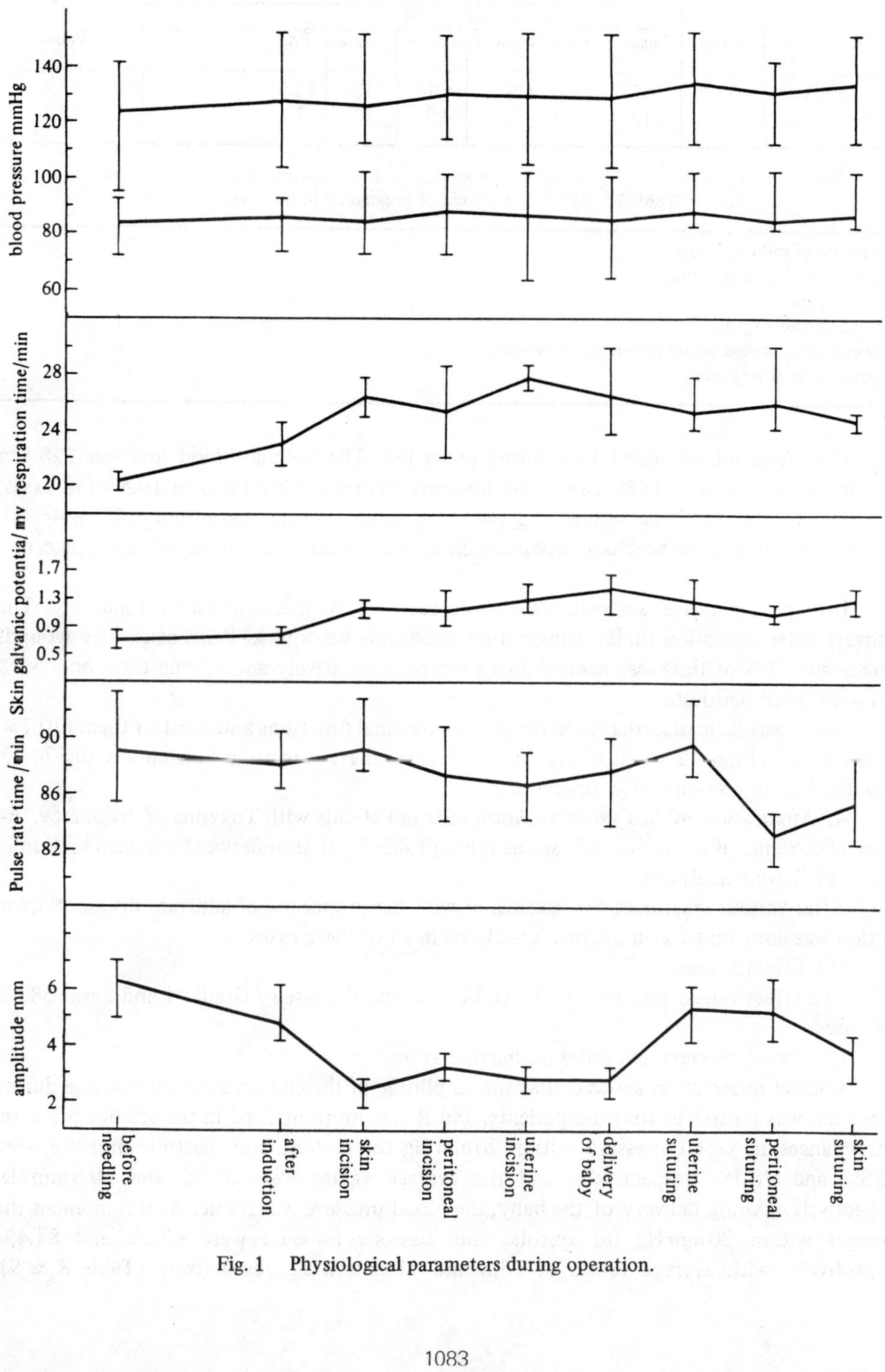

Fig. 1 Physiological parameters during operation.

Table 6. Change in pulse rate during operation

	No. of Cases	Range of Change (time/min.) ≤ 20 Cases	P.C.	21–30 Cases	P.C.	> 30 Cases	P.C.	Average Value
During operation	373	265	71.0	60	16.1	48	12.9	15.4
During delivery	373	313	83.9	33	8.9	27	7.2	12.1

Table 7. Types of toxemia of pregnancy in 64 cases

Light type of mild toxemia	37
Severe type of mild toxemia	6
Pre-eclampsia	4
Antepartum eclampsia	1
Toxemia complicated with chronic hypertension	6
Hypertension during labor	10

(5) Amount of blood loss during operation. The average blood loss was 278.8 ± 5.19ml. In 66.1% cases (439 cases) the loss was less than 300ml and in 10.8% (72 cases) over 500ml. As to the cause of bleeding, poor uterine contraction was responsible for 44.4%; the rest were due to hemorrhage from uterine sinuses, wound laceration, adherent placenta, etc.

(6) Postoperative analgesic effect and recovery of gastro-intestinal functions. The recovery after operation under acupuncture anesthesia was quick. Pains caused by wounds were slight. 50% of the cases needed analgesics postoperatively and among them only 5.2% had to be given pethidine.

There was little disturbance in the gastro-intestinal functions and most of them (70.7%) passed flatus within 12 to 48 hours. In 82.8% cases there was no gas distention and 74.8% took food 12 to 48 hours after operation.

4. Application of Acupuncture Anesthesia in Patients with Toxemia of Pregnancy. 64 cases of toxemia of pregnancy of various types (Table 7) that underwent cesarean section in 1976–1977 were analyzed.

After various treatment for toxemia or with the proper use of adjuvant drugs, cesarean section was done under acupuncture anesthesia in all of these cases.

(1) Effectiveness.

The effectiveness rate was 98.4% (63 cases) and the rate of Grades 1 and 2 was 68.8% (44 cases).

(2) Blood pressure and pulse during operation.

Clinical observation showed that the amplitude of the change in blood pressure during operation was greater in toxemic patients, and it was more marked in the systolic pressure. The changes in blood pressure within 20mm Hg for systolic and diastolic pressure were 32.8% and 78.1%, respectively, and the average values were 36.25 and 20.8mm Hg, respectively. During delivery of the baby, the blood pressure was stable. At this moment the changes within 20mm Hg for systolic and diastolic pressure were 67.2% and 84.4%, respectively, with average values of 18.6 and 11.26mm Hg, respectively (Table 8 & 9).

Table 8. **Changes in blood pressure of toxemic patients during operation**

Time	Blood Pressure	No. of Cases	Range of change (mmHg)						Average Value (mmHg)
			$\leqslant 20$		21–30		> 30		
			Cases	P.C.*	Cases	P.C.	Cases	P.C.	
During course of operation	Systolic	64	21	32.8	17	26.6	26	40.6	36.25±2.1
	diastolic	64	50	78.1	9	14.1	5	7.8	20.8±1.57
During delivery of baby	Systolic	64	43	67.2	13	20.3	8	12.5	18.6±1.96
	diastolic	64	54	84.4	5	7.8	5	7.8	11.26±1.45

* P.C.=Per cent

Table 9. **Changes in pulse rate of toxemic patients during operation**

	No. of Cases	Range of Change (time/min)						Average Value
		$\leqslant 20$		21–30		> 30		
		Cases	P.C.*	Cases	P.C.	Cases	P.C.*	
During course of operation	64	46	71.9	7	10.9	11	17.2	22.5±1.77
During delivery of baby	64	52	81.3	4	6.3	8	12.5	9.23±1.16

* P.C. =Per cent

The range of change in pulse rate during the couring the course of operation was 22.5 beats/min and during delivery of baby, 9.23 beats/min.

(3) During operation, the average blood loss was 267.98 ± 21.94 ml. There was 68.8% with blood loss over 300 ml and 14% over 500 ml. In comparison with the group without complications, there was no significant difference ($P>0.05$).

(4) Complications: With the exception of one case of postural shock, the course of operation was smooth and without any complication due to the anesthesia. There were five cases of asphyxia neonatorum. Two of them had intrauterine asphyxia, and the other three were due to cord around the neck, abruptio placentae and the internal version transverse lie of the baby. It is evident that acupuncture anesthesia can be used equally effectively with toxemic patients as with is nontoxemic patients.

5. **Comparison of Acupuncture Anesthesia and Epidural Anesthesia for Cesarean Section**

237 cases of cesarean section of similar conditions done under epidural anesthesia by the same group of doctors since 1966 have been analyzed for comparison with acupuncture anesthesia.

(1) Blood Pressure Changes: Throughout the operation the changes in systolic and diastolic pressures were evident in epidural anesthesia group. Changes in systolic pressure within 20 mm Hg in acupuncture anesthesia and epidural anesthesia were 71% and 51% respectively ($P<0.05$). Those for diastolic pressure were 90% and 78.1% respectively ($P<0.01$). The differences are significant, but during the delivery of the baby, they are not significant (Tables 10 and 11). This shows that under acupuncture anesthesia the patient was not affected by physiological disturbance. It could deep the blood pressure stable even dur-

Table 10. **Comparison of blood pressure changes during operation between acupuncture and epidural anesthesia**

Blood Pressure	Anesthesia	No. of Cases	Range of Change (mm Hg) ≤ 20 Cases	P.C.	21–30 Cases	P.C.	> 30 Cases	P.C.	Average Value (mm Hg)	P
Systolic	Acupuncture	632*	449*	71.0	110	17.4	73	11.6	21.6	<0.01
	epidural	237	123	51.9	54	22.8	60	25.3	26.7	
Diastolic	Acupuncture	632*	569	90.0	49	7.8	14	2.2	15.5	<0.01
	epidural	237	185	78.1	34	14.3	18	7.6	17.4	

* 32 cases without data are excluded.

Table 11. **Comparison of blood pressure changes during delivery of baby between acupuncture and epidural anesthesia**

Blood Pressure	Anesthesia	No. of Cases	Range of Change (mm Hg) ≤ 20 Cases	P.C.	21–30 Cases	P.C.	> 30 Cases	P.C.	Average Value (mm Hg)	P
Systolic	Acupuncture	630*	551	87.5	52	8.2	27	4.3	14.2	>0.05
	epidural	237	200	84.4	23	9.7	14	5.9	11.6	
Diastolic	Acupuncture	627**	601	95.8	21	3.4	5	0.8	9.2	>0.05
	epidural	237	224	94.5	10	4.2	3	1.3	9.3	

* 34 cases without data are excluded.
** 37 cases without data are excluded.

ing the moment of comparative strong operative interference.

(2) Blood Loss during Operation: The average blood loss for acupuncture and epidural anesthesia were 278.8±5.19 ml and 390±37.19 ml respectively, P<0.05 and the difference is significant. The blood losses under 300 ml in acupuncture and epidural anesthesia groups were 66.1% (439 cases) and 32.9% (78 cases) respectively, and above 500 ml 10.8% (72 cases) and 29.9% (71 cases) respectively, P<0.01, and the difference is very significant. More blood was lost under epidural anesthesia.

(3) Use of Postoperative Analgesics: Postoperative analgesics used in acupuncture and epidural anesthesia groups were 50% (500 cases) and 62.9% (149 cases) respectively, P<0.01. The need for pethidine occurred in 5.2% and 27.5% cases respectively. The difference between the two groups is very significant, P<0.01.

(4) Complications: The incidences of postural shock, anesthesia accident, and postpartum hemorrhage in the two groups of anesthesia were compared and the rates of all these were higher in the group of epidural anesthesia. One accident of punctural trauma occurred in epidural anesthesia, but none in acupuncture anesthesia. Postural shock occurred in 1.3% and 6.75% cases in the acupuncture and epidural groups respectively, and the postpartum hemorrhage rates were 10.8% and 29.9% respectively.

Erom comparison it is evident that the main advantages of acpuncture anesthesia are safety, effectiveness, no anesthesia accident, fewer postural shocks, fewer postpartum hemorrhage cases and stable blood pressure and pulse throughout the course of operation.

6. Factors Affecting the Effectiveness of Acupuncture Anesthesia.

(1) Obstetrical factors. Whether the cesarean section is primary or secondary, a planned one or an emergent one will influence the effectiveness of acupuncture anesthesia. The difference is especially marked in Grade 1 cases. In primipara, first and planned cesarean section the rate of Grade 1 was high (Table 12).

(2) Type and duration of operation. Among the various types of operations, the effectiveness in simple lower segment cesarean section was the best, with 31.1% of Grade1, while in cesarean section with sterilization it was only 22.8%. P<0.05 and the difference is significant. There is a close relationship between effectiveness and duration of operation. The combined rate of Grades 1 and 2 decreased as the duration of operation increased. There were 172 cases with durations of operation within 30 min and the combined rate was 84.9%, while in 82 cases with duration of operation over 90 minutes, the combined rate was 53.7%. P<0.001 and the difference was very significant (Table 13).

(3) Mental State and Effectiveness. There is a close relationship between mental states and effectiveness of acupuncture anesthesia. The rate of Grade 1 in calm patients was higher than in patients with tension, and the number of Grades 3 and 4 cases was less in the former, P<0.001 (Table 14).

Table 12. Relationship between parity, time and nature of operation and effectiveness of acupuncture anesthesia

Factors		No. of Cases	Grade I Cases	Grade I P.C.	Grade II Cases	Grade II P.C.	Grades 1 & 2 Combined Cases	Grades 1 & 2 Combined P.C.
Parity	Primipara	542	181	33.4	236	43.5	417	76.9
	multipara	458	109	23.8	232	50.7	341	74.5
Time	First time	471	215	32.0	302	45.0	517	77.0
	repeated	329	75	22.8	166	50.5	241	73.3
Nature of operation	Planned	744	246	33.1	327	43.9	573	77.0
	emergency	256	44	17.2	141	55.1	185	72.3

P<0.01

Table 13. Effectiveness and duration of operation

Duration of Operation (min)	No. of Cases	Grade 1 Cases	Grade 1 P.C.	Grade 2 Cases	Grade 2 P.C.	Grade 3 Cases	Grade 3 P.C.	Grade 4 Cases	Grade 4 P.C.	Rate of Success (%)	Combined Rate of Grades 1 & 2 (%)
⩽ 30	172	93	54.7	52	30.2	26	15.1			100.0	84.9
31–60	471	142	30.2	231	49.0	95	20.2	3	0.6	99.4	79.2
61–90	250	34	13.6	136	54.4	73	29.2	7	2.8	97.2	68.0
> 90	82	9	11.0	35	42.7	32	39.0	6	7.3	92.7	53.7
Unknown	25	11	44.0	14	56.0					100.0	100.0

For groups ⩽ 30 min and 31–60 min,P> 0.05.
For group ⩽ 30 min and > 90 min,P < 0.001.

Table 14. Effectiveness and mental state

Mental State	No. of Cases	Grade 1 Cases	Grade 1 P.C.	Grade 2 Cases	Grade 2 P.C.	Grade 3 Cases	Grade 3 P.C.	Grade 4 Cases	Grade 4 P.C.	Rate of Success (%)	Combined Rate of Grades 1 & 2 (%)
Calm	273	117	42.9	114	41.8	41	15.0	1	0.3	99.7	84.7
Tense	272	66	24.3	128	47.0	66	24.3	12	4.4	95.6	71.3
P		<0.001				<0.001					

III. DISCUSSION

1. As a result of the physiological and pathological changes during pregnancy and labor, there is an increase of total blood volume, augmented circulatory function, changes in endocrinological functions, establishment of placental circulation, pressure of the gravid uterus on the vena cava, disturbances in the vasodilation function, etc. These make it not easy to maintain the hemodynamic stability. It is also not easy to adapt to these rapid and severe changes, which increase the complexity of obstetric anesthesia. The choice of obstetric anesthesia. aside from its effectiveness, also demands the maintenance of hemodynamic stability during the course of anesthesia, so as to safeguard the health of the mother and the child. In recent years acupuncture anesthesia has been used clinically as an anesthetic method. Its advantages are that it is safe, simple, easy to manage, with definite analgesic effect and good regulatory effect. It can satisfy the requirements of operation, keeping the physiological functions stable during the operation with little changes in blood pressure and pulse and with less loss of blood. There are none of the untoward reactions common to drug anesthesia, no accident and no associated complications. Postoperative recovery is also smooth and rapid.

Toxemia of pregnancy is a common complication in obstetreics. Owing to pathological changes, the vascular regulatory function is disturbed. Therefore, the chances of obstetric shock and postpartum hemorrhage are greater and this increases the incidence of sudden drop of blood pressure or massive hemorrhage during cesarean section. Under such circumstances the conduct of anesthesia is a rather complicated matter. In obstetrics, it is stressed clinically to avoid giving any stimulation to the patient. At present, the problem of incomplete abatement of pain in acupuncture anesthesia has not been solved yet. Whether its use in a toxemic patient would give rise to any complications is of great concern. Through many Years'clinical practice, we realized that the analgesic and regulatory effect of acupuncture anesthesia not only can meet the requirements of cesarean section upon a toxemic patient, but there would also be less blood loss during operation, relatively stable blood pressure and pulse rate even during the delivery of the baby, and no complications. According to the conditions of different types of toxemic patients, it is better to take all possible measures to give proper preoperation treatment, including adjuvant medication such as the use of a mixture of phenergan and pethidine or a mixture of chlorpromazine, and a small amount of local anesthesia for skin incision. From these we think acupuncture anesthesia is a fairly good anesthetic method suitable for cesarean section not only for normal patients but also for toxemic ones; basically there is no contraindication. Nevertheless, there are still the problems of incomplete abatement of pain and insufficient muscular relaxation. It cannot meet the requirement of operation in cases of a deeply engaged head or extensive abdominal adhesions. Therefore, for such patients and nervous patients, epidural anesthesia is still preferred. On the other hand, for patients constitutionally allergic or hypersensitive to anesthetic drugs, or with deformity in the spinal column or contraindication for epidural puncture, acupuncture anesthesia should be taken.

2. The obstetrical factors affect the effectiveness of acupuncture anesthesia to different extents. The close relationship between duration of operation and effectiveness is especially important. The rate of Grades 1 and 2 effectiveness decreases as the duration of the operation increases. This indicates that improvement of operation skill and shortening of the duration of the operation would help raise the effectiveness. Through clinical practice in recent years some improvement has been made in operation technique and procedure on the basic principle of steadiness, precision, lightness, nimbleness, and quickness.

(1) The mid-line incision below the umbilicus was used and lower segment cesarean section was done. The site and length of abdominal incision was determined according to the station and size of the fetal head so as to make an incision of the adequate length at the right place. A proper incision with easy exposure will lessen or abolish the use of tractors.

(2) No pad was used in the abdominal cavity.

(3) The exploration is made with definite purpose. Before delivering the baby, the operator's fingers should be inserted gently into the abdominal cavity on the lower uterine segment to find out the position and station of the fetal head and the position of the uterus in order to decide the site and length of the uterine incision. Later on, before closure of the peritoneum the adnexa on both sides were examined.

(4) The fetal head is to be delivered during the intervals between the uterine contractions with the close cooperation between the operator and the assistant. The direction of the force used must be appropriate. For high floating head, after sucking out the amniotic fluid, the fetal head descends. The assistant fixed the fundus of the uterus per abdomen with his hand and the operator inserted his hand into the uterine cavity and brought the fetal head to the uterine incision. Then the assistant pressed on the fundus of the uterus and the fetal head was delivered. If the fetal head was deeply engaged, the operator firstly delivered the head to the uterine incision and pushed it outward. Then the assistant pressed on the fundus, so as to deliver the head.

(5) The myometrium of the uterus is sutured in two layers. The first layer is sutured with two to three stitches of interrupted continuous sutures and continuous mattress suture is used for the second layer. In this way the wound would be regular. It is good for hemostasis and would also shorten the time of suturing.

(6) The process of suturing must also be skillfully arranged so as to finish all the manipulations at one time on one side and then go to the other side, in order to lessen the to-and-fro traction of the uterus and to reduce the sense of traction.

(7) Oxytocics are given intrauterinely and intravenously after the fetal head was delivered. This will shorten the time of separation of the placenta and reduce the necessity of manual removal of it.

(8) The close cooperation between the operator, the assistants and the instrument nurse together with the improvements mentioned above would shorten the duration of

the operation and thus improve the effectiveness of acupuncture anesthesia. No complication has been found due to this improved procedure. There were 60 cases of repeated cesarean section and 15% showed light adhesions on omentum and peritoneal reflexion which were easily separated; none was found with serious adhesions that interfered with operation.

IV. CONCLUSION

1. 1000 cases of cesarean section under acupuncture anesthesia were studied. The rate of successes is 98.4% and the rate of Grades 1 and 2 successes is 75.8%. The clinical effects and conditions during and after operation were analyzed. Similar cases of cesarean section under epidural anesthesia during the same period were taken for comparison.

2. Acupuncture anesthesia is a fairly good anesthetic method for cesarean section. It can be used with patients with toxemia of pregnancy, anemia and other complications. Its advantages are stability of blood pressure and pulse during operation, less blood loss, rapid recovery after operation, safety, simplicity, and no complication or anesthesia accident.

3. Improvements on operative procedure in cesarean section made in those years of this study and their relationship with effectiveness are presented in the paper.

REFERENCES

[1] 北京结核病研究所：北京结核病研究所针麻资料汇编(内部资料)，1976。

[2] 北京结核病研究所：北京结核病研究所针麻资料汇编(内部资料)，1976。

[3] 北京妇产医院：中华医学杂志，4：260，1975。

[4] 上海中医学院曙光医院等：针刺麻醉临床和原理研究资料选编(上海)，1978。

[5] 中国科学院心理研究所王振盛等：全国针灸针麻学术讨论会论文摘要(一)，1970。

[6] 上海实用麻醉学编写组：实用麻醉学(第一版)，528 页，上海科学技术出版社，1978。

[7] 谢荣：麻醉学(第二版)，467 页，人民卫生出版社，1963。

INVESTIGATION OF ELECTRO-NEEDLING OF JIZHONG POINT IN ABDOMINAL TOTAL HYSTERECTOMY

Xu Zhengyi*, Xue Biru*, He Shufang** , Zheng Zehui**

We have reported previously that electro-needling of Jizhong and Yaoshu on the Dumai Channel for acupuncture anesthesia gave satisfactory results in abdominal total hysterectomy (ref. Chinese Medical Journal (11):6, 1978). From January 1975 to December 1977, 674 cases of total hysterectomy were performed with the same points group to observe further their efficacy. The effective rate was 83.1%.

Previous clinical experience showed the penetration of the needle at these points must reach a definite depth in order to obtain a good anesthetic effect. Specifically the point of the needle must reach the epidural space, and short of this, it would fail to produce the characteristic subjective sensation in the patient, whereas beyond this, there is the danger of injuring the spinal cord. Formerly the depth of needle puncture was determined by the hand feeling of the acupuncturist and the subjective sensation of the patient. Obviously some objective criteria would be much more desirable in order to put acupuncture anesthesia in this operation on a scientific basis and make it more reliable.

In order to locate accurately the acupuncture points, roentgenographic examination of the epidural space was performed with part of the patients to determine the relative positions of the needle point and the epidural space with the purpose of establishing some bases for improving the anesthetic effect.

I. METHOD

Combination of acupuncture points selected (Fig.1).

1. Jizhong (between the11th and 12th thoracic vertebrae);
2. Yaoshu (the needle penetrating into the sacral hiatus);
3. Ciliao (bilateral, the needle going into the posterior sacral foramen).

The technique of introducing the acupuncture needles, the method of electro-needling, and the adjunct medication used are essentially the same as reported in the past.

Roentgenographic location of the depth of the acupuncture needle.

In order to ascertain the proper depth of needle insertion at Jizhong point, roentgenographic examination was done with 7 patients with 60% Conray injected into the epidural

* The International Peace Maternity & Child Health Hospital, Shanghai.
** Shanghai Institute of Physiology, Academia Sinica, Shanghai.

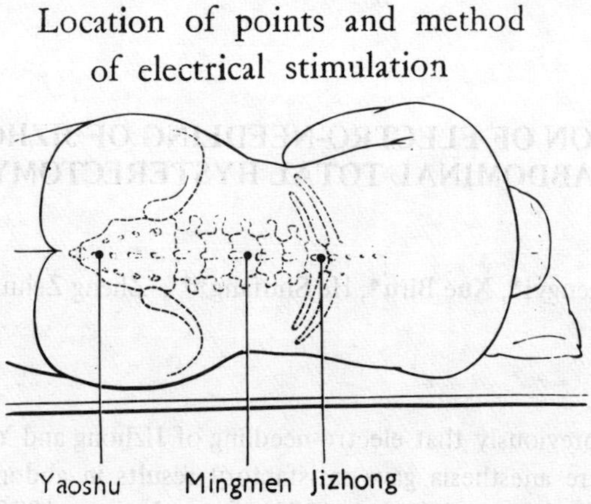

Fig. 1 Location of points and method of electrical stimulation.

space as contrast medium. The patient lay sidewise, an epidural puncture was made between the Th_{12} and L_1, and an acupuncture of Jizhong point was followed. 2 ml of the contrast medium were injected within one minute through the catheter into the epidural space. Immediately films of the A. P. and lateral views of the thoracic and lumbar spines were taken.

Observations on the change of impedance.

Observations were made on 11 cases of abdominal tubal sterilization. Insulated (with the exception of the tip) fine needle was slowly inserted at Jizhong point. At every 3 mm depth of insertion, the change in impedance was measured and the hand-feeling of the acupuncturist as well as the subjective feeling of the patient in response to electric pulsation from a stimulator was noted.

Method of the measurement of impedance.

An audio-voltage of 500 Hz was produced by an XDI signal generator and through a high resistance, a constant current was obtained, which was passed into the body via the fine needle. The indifferent electrode was a 2X3 cm silver foil placed on the skin of one of the lower extremities. As the current was constant, the frequency voltage from the needle to the indifferent electrode was directly proportional to the impedance. The ratio could be adjusted by means of a standard resistance.

Changes in the impedance during the entry of the needle were observed in 4 dogs. Needles were left in various places with different impedance levels to fix the positions for anatomical identification. Four dogs each weighing about 10 kg were anesthetized by sodium pentothal given intravenously at a dose of 25 mg per kg body weight. The apparatus used and the method of investigation were all the same as those used and adopted clinically. At the end of the experiment, the acupuncture needles were left in situ. The whole length of the lumbar spine was resected and fixed in 10% formalin for 24 hours. Afterwards the exact positions of the needles point were determined by dissection.

Observation of the histological changes in the spinal cord after long period of electric stimulation.

The dorsal sides of the 1st, 4th or 5th lumbar vertebrae of 6 cats were exposed aseptically. With a dental drill small holes were made in the vertebral laminae at the basal portion of the spinous processes of the vertebrae. #32 stainless steel wires with bent tips were then implanted inside the holes. Epidural electric needling was simulated. The indifferent electrodes used were silver chips about 1 square centimeter large. While the cats were in a state of deep anesthesia, the intensity of the electric stimulation was gradually increased to the point when tremor, but not tonic contraction, of the muscles of the lower extremity appeared. The electric stimulation was continued for 3 hours. Afterwards the animals were kept alive for a week. The exact site of the buried electrode was carefully located when the segment of the spinal cord together with the adjacent dura mater under the point of stimulation was dissected out. A segment of normal spinal cord was taken for control. The specimens were fixed simultaneously in Carnoy's solution for 3 hours, dehydrated with 95% absolute alcohol, made transparent by chloroform, and embedded in wax for slicing transverse sections each 10μ thick, and finally stained with cresyl violet.

II. RESULTS

1. Analysis of Results of Acupuncture Anesthesia. A total of 674 abdominal total hysterectomies were done using Jizhong and Yaoshu as the principle points for stimulation in acupuncture anesthesia. The effective rate was 83.1% (560 cases); Grade I and Grade II success rates were 35.8% (228 cases) and 33.8% (221 cases), respectively, while 16.9% (114 cases) failed. Of the 114 failures, 33.3% were due to pain, 32.2% to bulging of the intestinal loops so that the intestine could not be replaced, 12.3% to tenseness of the abdominal muscles and 17.6% to adhesions which interfered with exposure of the operative field.

2. Factors Affecting the Effectiveness of Acupuncture Anesthesia. Among the various factors which may influence the effectiveness of acupuncture anesthesia are the tolerance to needling and the threshold of pain tolerance ($P<0.01$). Grade I success rate was higher in patients who were calm. Other factors such as period of induction, amount of stimulation, duration of operation, age and occupation of the patients do not influence the effect of acupuncture anesthesia directly ($P>0.05$).

3. Comparison Between Postoperative States of Acupuncture Anesthesia and Epidural Anesthesia. In 1977, 30 cases of abdominal total hysterectomy chosen at random were operated on under acupuncture anesthesia, using the Jizhong point group, and 15 cases of the same operation were done under epidural anesthesia and the results were compared. In the acupuncture group, recuperation was more rapid, complications fewer and the pain of the abdominal incision was mild; the postoperation complaining of wound pain began on the average after 10.5 hrs. But in the epidural group this complaint began on the average only after 3 hrs. 56.7% of the patients in the former group did not need postoperative analgesics, whereas 86.7% of the patients in the epidural group had to take pethidine to alleviate pain ($P<0.01$).

4. Roentgenographic Location of the Depth of Needle at Jizhong Point. Lateral films of 6 of the 7 cases studied showed that the anterior and posterior outlines of the contrast medium column were sharp and distinct. Its anterior side and the advancing portion of the medium were clearly marked out by a boundary line. Because the needle at Jizhong point is only one vertebra away from the epidural catheter and the amount of Conray used is small, the lateral portion and anterior border of the epidural space contained only a very small amount of the contrast medium. Therefore the tip of the needle and the low density contrast medium did not overlap to interfere with the location of the acupuncture needle.

The AP widths of the contrast medium column were 0.3–0.5cm. In 6 of the 7 cases, the tips of the needles overlapped with the medium (Fig. 2) but they did not go beyond their range. The anesthetic effect of these cases was Grade I or II. In one case, the puncture was so shallow that the needle tip was still 0.1 cm away from the posterior limit of the contrast medium, showing the peneration was not deep enough, and the anesthetic effect was of Grade III (Fig. 3).

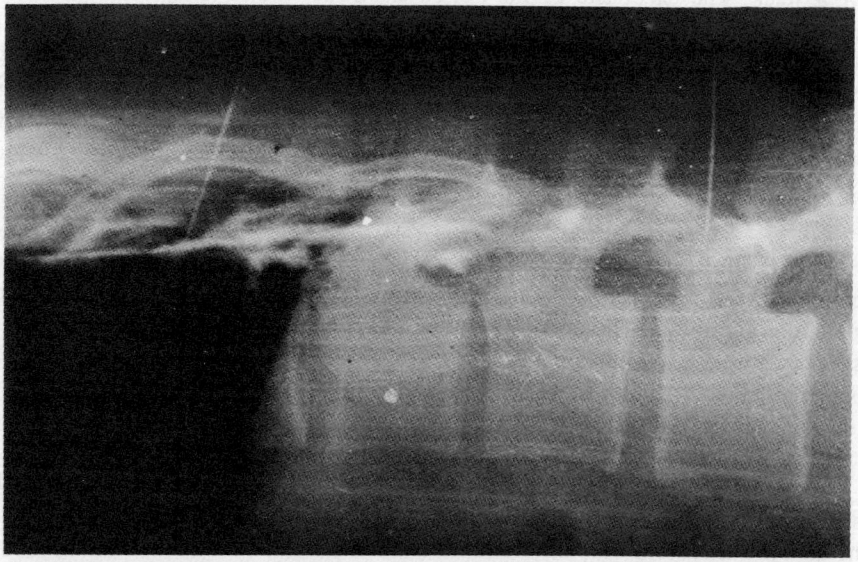

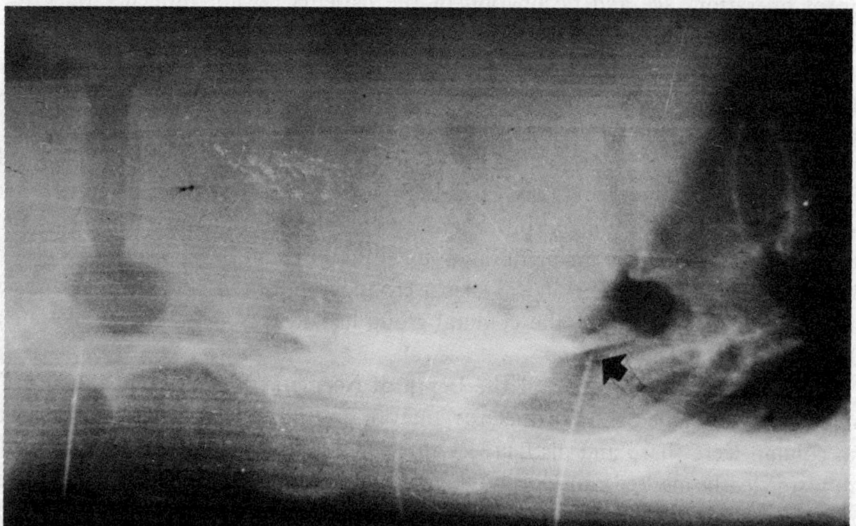

Fig. 3

5. Changes in Impedance During the Course of Needle Insertion. In 8 of our pateints, the needle was inserted intermittently, each time not exceeding 1–2 mm. There were slight variations in the impedance (1–4kΩ) in the superficial tissues within 3 cm beneath skin surface. Stimulation at these points produced a sensation of heaviness and distension in the back and tightness of the chest with contraction of local muscles. Only when the point of the needle reached a depth of around 3 cm, the hand feeling of the anesthetist became dense and tough and there was a marked increase in impedance ranging from 10 to 40kΩ. With deeper insertion of the needle, the impedance dropped suddenly to a low level, lower than that obtained in the superficial layer, although the dense and tough hand feeling remained. The needle should be left here for induction of acupuncture anesthesia. By electric stimulation at this level, i.e., of dense and tough hand feeling and low impedance, the subjective sensations reported were slight tremor and numbness of the gluteal region, perineum and the deep structures of both lower extremities, as well as undulating wind blowing sensation, "ants crawling" sensation on the skin, and shifting and sliding down sensation of the lower extremities.

Observations on the changes in the impedance and hand feeling of 23 points at various segments of the lumbar spine in 4 dogs show that the changes in impedance agree in the main with those of our previous clinical observations (Fig. 4). Anatomic dissection proved when dense and tough hand feeling is obtained, the tip of the needle was outside the yellow ligament; when the impedance suddenly decreased, but the hand feeling was still dense and tough, the needle had just pierced the yellow ligament and was on the dorsal layer of the dura mater; when a piercing through feeling was obtained, the point of the needle was 1–2mm inside the epidural space, and sometimes the point of the needle was closely attached to the dura mater. When the lower extremities of the experimental animal suddenly contracted, anatomic dissection showed that the needle had pierced into the ventral aspect of the spinal cord.

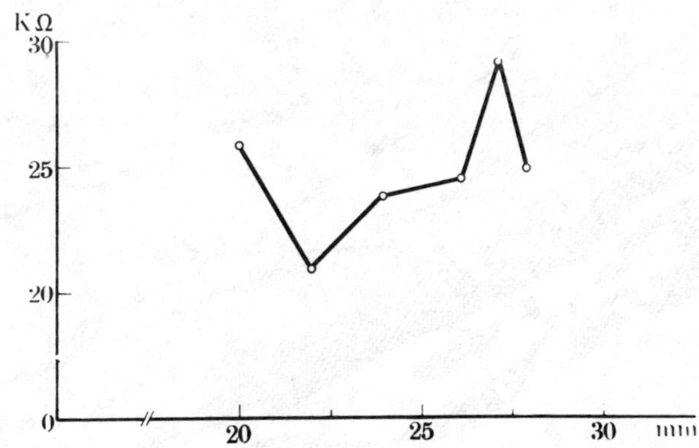

Fig. 4 The change of impedance in needling into lumbar vertebral interspace in dogs.

6. Histological Changes in the Spinal Cord After Long Period of Electric Stimulation. It was noted that with an electric current less than 23 mA (10–23 mA), no histological changes were observed in the nerve tissue of the spinal cord, but only mild swelling was observed in areas of the dura mater directly under the point of stimulation. When the current was increased to 23 mA, the connective tissue became darkly stained with coagulative necrosis of tissue fibers, and there was also a tendency for the cells to coagulate, and swelling of the connective tissues was more extensive, extending from the dorsal to the lateral aspect of the dura (Figs. 5 & 6).

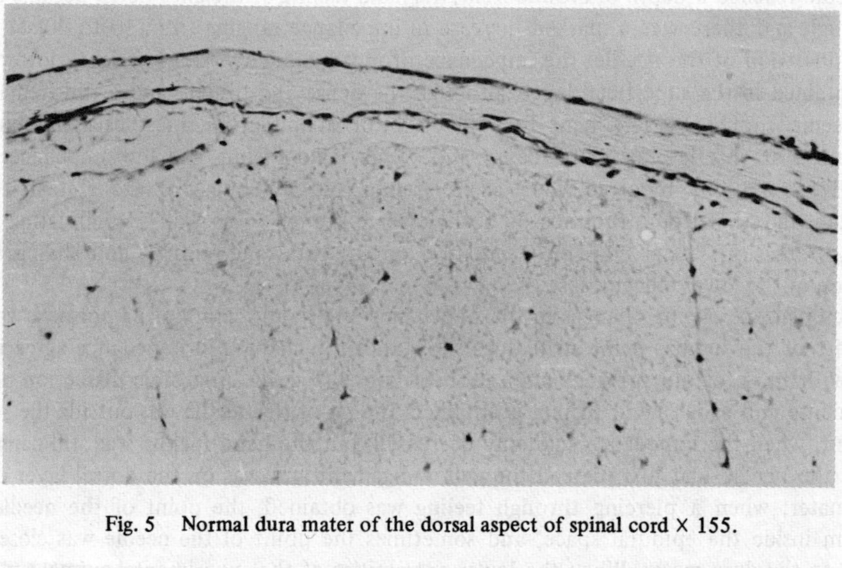

Fig. 5 Normal dura mater of the dorsal aspect of spinal cord × 155.

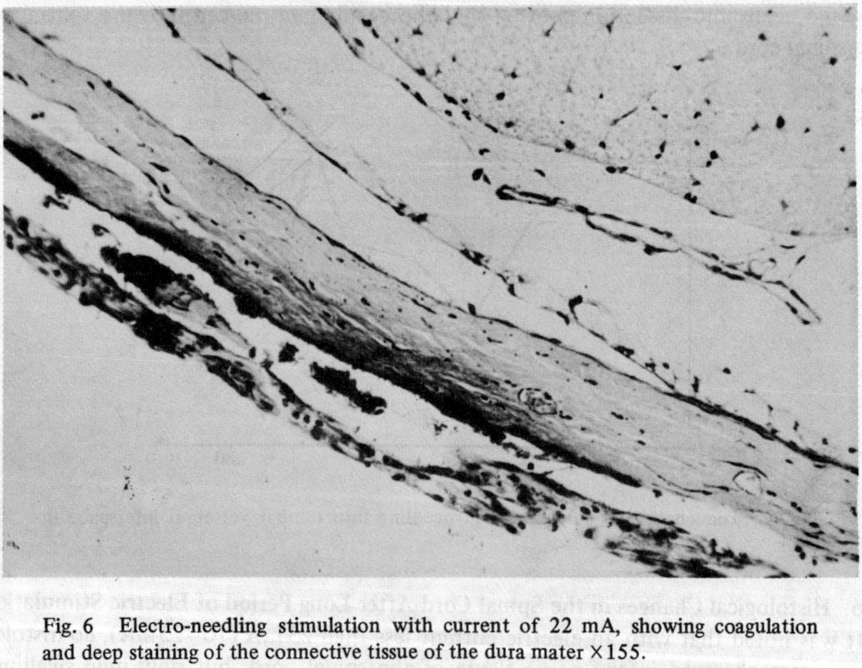

Fig. 6 Electro-needling stimulation with current of 22 mA, showing coagulation and deep staining of the connective tissue of the dura mater ×155.

When the stimulating current was over 32 mA (32–54 mA), in addition to the changes in the dura mentioned above, swelling of some nerve fibers in the superficial portion of the lateral fasciculus of the cord under the point of stimulation was also observed. The changes involved the myelin sheath as well as the axons (Fig. 7).

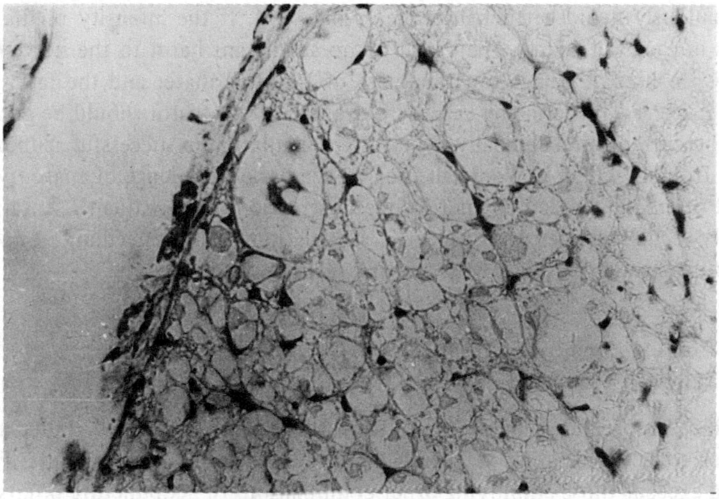

Fig. 7 Electro-needling stimulation with current of 54 mA, showing edema of the superficial fibers of the lateral fasciculus ×27.

III. DISCUSSION

On the effectiveness of Jizhong point.

674 cases of abdominal total hysterectomy using Jizhong and Yaoshu as the principal points for acupuncture anesthesia were analyzed. Compared with the results of the same operation using Mingmen and Yaoshu, the results were more satisfactory as evidenced by better relaxation of abdominal muscles and great reduction of adjunct drugs used. This shows that the key to the increase of the effectiveness of acupun cture anesthesia lies in the selection of the right acupuncture points, the proper technique for introducing the needles and the producing of the desired acupuncture sensations in response to electro-needling. Jizhong point lies between the 11th and 12th thoracic vertebrae, under which there is the spinal cord. The tip of the needle is in the epidural space. The subjective sensations and the sustained analgesic effect produced by electric stimulation at this point probably come from the excitation of the spinal cord. Up to now, the reaction of visceral traction after acupuncture of Jizhong points remains to be solved. At present we are looking for new adjuvant acupuncture points to enhance the anesthetic effect of Jizhong point. At the same time, measures are taken to prevent the displacement of the tip of the needle during operation.

The results of X-ray studies show that to secure good anesthetic effect, the point of the needle must reach the epidural space. This means that the hand feeling of the acupuncturist and the subjective sensation of the patient at that depth of puncture are specific, and they could be relied upon as clinical criteria for the depth of acupuncture.

In animal experiments, when the stimulating current reached a certain intensity, the dura mater was the first to show reactive changes. We are of the opinion that the dura with its surrounding fatty tissues and the cerebral spinal fluid afford great protection to the spinal cord. Nevertheless, the point for acupuncture must be carefully determined and the needle should meticulously avoid getting into the spinal cord. If the intensity of the stimulating current does not exceed 23 mA, there will be no significant harm to the nerve fibers of the cord. Besides, in human beings the thickness of the dura mater and the fatty tissue layer surrounding it exceed those in the cat; therefore, the safety factor should be greater in man. At present the current used clinically for electric stimulation in successful acupuncture anesthesia varies from 10–15 mA. We deem that with a basic knowledge of anatomy, after a definite period of training, aided by meticulous observation of the patient's sensation induced by a carefully regulated intensity of electric stimulation, electric needling of Jizhong point for acupuncture anesthesia should be a safe and satisfactory procedure.

IV. SUMMARY

1. 674 cases of abdominal total hysterectomy were performed under acupuncture anesthesia using electro-needling of Jizhong and Yaoshu as the primary points. The effective rate obtained exceeds those employing other combinations of acupuncture points.

2. Clinical and experimental studies prove that satisfactory results of acupuncture anesthesia can be achieved only when the point of the needle is in the epidural space. The proper depth of needle penetration is determined by integrating the hand feeling of the acupuncturist, the subjective sensations of the patient induced by electro-needling, changes in the impedance along the trajectory of the needling and roentgenographic methods.

3. Basing on the results of animal experiments, we conclude that the 10–15 mA intensity of the stimulating current used clinically is effective and safe for abdominal total hysterectomy.

CLINICAL STUDY OF ABDOMINAL TUBOLIGATION UNDER ACUPUNCTURE ANESTHESIA

National Cooperative Group of Acupuncture Anesthesia
for Abdominal Tuboligation

A program for investigating acupuncture anesthesia for abdominal tuboligation was launched and carried out by research workers and clinicians of the provinces, municipalities and autonomous regions of Shanghai, Jiangsu, Fujian, Shandong, Anhui, Jiangxi, Zhejiang, Shanxi, Heilonjiang, Henan, Hubei, Hunan, Guangxi, Sichuan, Yunnan, Ningxia, Guangdong, and Gansu. From 1975 to 1977 operations were performed on 23,554 patients with a rate of success of 97.9% and a rate of excellent-good result of 85.8% (Table 1).

I. CHOICE OF POINTS

Clinical observation and comparison were made of five groups of different acupuncture points. The result was that in the body acupuncture group (6,290 cases) the rate of success was 97.6%, and the rate of excellent-good results was 85.5%; in the lip acupuncture group (8,412 cases) the rate of success was 97.9%, and the rate of excellent-good results 85.2%; in the ear acupuncture group (6,136 cases) the rate of success was 97.8%, and the rate of excellent-good results 85.2%. The above three groups all obtained satisfactory effectiveness. There was no remarkable difference between the three groups statistically ($P>0.05$) in the rate of success and in the rate of excellent-good results (Table 2).

Having collected the clinical data of 9,097 cases from Ningxia, Henan, Jiangxi and Yunnan, we made an analysis of the analgesic effects of acupuncture on six manipulations. The result was that during skin incision, skin suture, peritoneum incision, and peritoneum suture, the analgesic effect was better in the lip acupuncture group; during fetching tubes, the analgesic effect in the body acupuncture group was better (Table 3). This shows that the points have both general analgesic effect and relative specificity. Thus, search and selection of specific points for specific analgesic effect is an important task in the future.

In April 1976 in the National Symposium of Acupuncture Anesthesia for Abdominal Tuboligation, another two groups of acupuncture points were chosen in addition to the above three groups. The first group consists of Renzhong, Chengjiang and Cijiao; the second group – ear acupuncture of Point Shenmen penetrated towards Point Uterus, Point Brain penetrated towards Point Lung and paraincisional acupuncture. The data of 2,716 cases from clinical observation for a year by 9 medical units in Shanghai, Jiangsu, Ningxia, Guangxi, Shandong, etc., show that in the Renzhong, Chengjiang and Ciliao group, the rate of success was

Table 1. Rate of success of acupuncture anesthesia

Year	No. of Cases	Effects of Acupuncture Anesthesia								Rate of Excel-lent-good Effect		Rate of Success	
		Grade I		Grade II		Grade III		Grade IV					
		No.of Cases	%	No.of Cases	%	No. of Cases	%	No. of Cases	%	No. of Cases	%	No. of Cases	%
1975	3573	1843	51.2	1252	35.5	385	10.6	93	2.7	3095	86.7	3480	97.3
1976	16702	8601	51.5	5553	33.2	2183	12.6	365	2.7	14154	84.7	16337	97.3
1977	3294	1802	54.9	1163	35.5	271	8.3	43	13.3	2965	90.4	3236	98.7
Total	23554	12246	51.9	7968	33.9	2839	12.1	501	2.1	20214	85.8	23053	97.9

Table 2. Statistics of effects of acupuncture anesthesia

Point Px	No. of Cases	Effects of Acupuncture Anesthesia								Rate of Excel-lent-good Effect		Rate of Success	
		Grade I		Grade II		Grade III		Grade IV					
		No.of Cases	%	No.of Cases	%	No. of Cases	%	No. of Cases	%	No. of Cases	%	No. of Cases	%
Sanyinjiao, Cijiao	6290	3172	50.4	2209	35.1	757	12.1	152	2.4	5381	85.5	6138	97.6
Renzhong, Changjiang	8412	4472	53.2	2703	32.0	1064	12.7	173	2.1	7175	85.2	8239	97.9
Ear point	6136	3205	52.2	2027	33.0	768	12.6	136	2.2	5232	85.2	6000	97.8
Renzhong, Changjiang, Cijiao	1430	772	54.0	535	37.4	95	6.6	28	2.0	1307	91.4	1402	98.0
Ear point near the incision	1286	625	48.6	494	38.4	155	12.1	12	0.9	1119	87.0	1274	99.1
Total	23554	12246	51.9	7968	33.9	2839	12.1	501	2.1	20214	85.8	23053	97.9

Table 3. Comparison of the responses appearing during the process of operation of the three groups of acupuncture points

Process of operation	Renzhong, Chengjiang (3422)								Sanyinjiao, Cijiao (2846)								Ear Point (2829)								P Value "-"
	–		+		++		+++		–		+		++		+++		–		+		++		+++		
	No. of Cases	%	No. of Cases	%	No. of Cases	%	No. of Cases	%	No. of Cases	%	No. of Cases	%	No. of Cases	%	No. of Cases	%	No. of Cases	%	No. of Cases	%	No. of Cases	%	No. of Cases	%	
Skin incision	2482	72.5	864	24.9	71	2.4	5	0.2	1854	65.2	899	31.5	86	3.1	7	0.2	1929	68.2	839	29.6	57	2.1	4	0.1	P<0.01
Peritoneum incision	2536	74.1	758	22.2	124	3.6	4	0.1	1885	66.2	845	29.8	110	3.8	6	0.2	1912	67.5	806	28.5	98	3.5	13	0.5	P<0.01
Probe	1524	44.5	1448	42.5	411	11.9	39	1.1	1329	46.7	1236	43.4	251	8.8	30	1.1	1194	42.3	1331	47.0	270	9.5	34	1.2	P<0.01
Tube tying	2720	79.4	574	16.9	122	3.5	6	0.2	2198	77.3	568	19.9	78	2.7	2	0.1	2172	76.8	550	19.4	96	3.4	11	0.4	P>0.05
Peritoneum suture	2758	80.6	573	16.8	87	2.5	4	0.1	2161	75.9	627	22.1	54	1.9	4	0.1	2249	79.5	524	18.5	50	1.8	6	0.2	P<0.01
Skin suture	2462	71.6	854	25.1	98	2.8	8	0.2	1723	67.5	830	19.2	85	3.0	8	0.3	2032	71.8	733	25.9	56	2.0	8	0.3	P<0.01

Notes "–" means quiet, without sign of pain,
"+" means occasional painful feeling,
"++" means marked painful feeling, and
"+++" means intense painful feeling.

Table 4. The relationship between duration of induction and the effect of acupuncture anesthesia

Duration of induction (min)	No. of Cases	Effect of acupuncture anesthesia								Success		Excellent-good	
		Grade I		Grade II		Grade III		Grade IV					
		No. of Cases	%	No. of Cases	%	No. of Cases	%	No.of Cases	%	No. of Cases	%	No. of Cases	%
5–	584	382	65.4	170	29.1	32	5.5			584	100	552	94.5
10–	607	351	57.8	197	32.5	55	9.1	4	0.6	603	99.4	548	90.3
15–	1459	735	50.4	504	34.5	192	10.9	28	1.9	1431	98.1	1239	84.9
20–	2113	1073	50.7	769	36.4	232	10.9	39	1.9	2074	98.1	1842	87.1
Total	4763	2541	53.3	1640	34.5	511	10.7	71	1.5	4692	98.5	4181	87.8

Note: The above data are of studies made in 1975–1976.

98.0%, and the rate of excellent-good results 91.4%; in the ear and paraincisional acupuncture group, the rate of success was 99.4%, and the rate of excellent-good results 87.0% (Table 2). This indicates that these two groups have better effect of acupuncture anesthesia. A remarkable difference was noted between the rate of excellent-good results in these two groups and that of the previous three groups (the body, lip and ear acupuncture groups) ($P<0.01$), i.e., the effectiveness in the Renzhong, Chenjiang and Ciliao group was the best and that in ear acupuncture and paraincisional group was better.

II. STIMULATION PARAMETERS

Practice in acupuncture anesthesia has demonstrated that suitable stimulation parameters are an important factor in stimulating the body to produce analgesia. The clinical observation of 16,702 cases showed that a certain degree of effectiveness was obtained with the wave types and frequencies designed in the National Symposium (Model G6805 acupuncture stimulator, continuous waves at various frequencies: ear needling: 1,500–3,000 cycles/min; lip needling: 300/min; body needling: Saninjiao 160–200 cycles/min; Ciliao 4,000 cycles/min). Comparison was made in Heilongjiang between the conventional electric waves of Model G6805 acupuncture stimulator and the sonoelectric waves of a self-made acupuncture apparatus. In 469 cases with conventional electric waves the rate of excellent-good results was 83.2%; while in 531 cases with sonoelectric waves the rate of excellent-good results was 93.9%. It is found that the conventional acupuncture stimulator provides regular waves, to which the body is easy to develop adaptation, resulting in a decreased effect at a longer period. The sonoelectric waves are irregular, and the body could hardly adapt to it. Hence the effect may be steady even in prolonged operating time.

The effects of different durations of induction were observed (in Fujian, Guangxi, Zhejiang, Anhui, etc.) in 4,763 patients, who were divided into four groups. Group I: in 584 cases, the duration of induction was 5–9 min with 94.5% of the rate of excellent-good results; Group II: the duration of induction was 10–14 min and in 607 cases the rate of excellent-good results was 90.3%; Group III: the duration of induction was 15–19 min and in 1,459 cases the rate of excellent-good results was 84.9%; Group IV: the duration of induction was more than 20 min and in 2,113 cases the rate of excellent-good results was 87.1%. The average of excellent-good rate of the four groups was 87.8% (Table 4). From these figures we can see that all the various durations of induction could have good effectiveness of acupuncture anesthesia, and comparison of the rates of excellent-good results between the four groups shows their similarity, i.e., no more effectiveness of acupuncture anesthesia in tuboligation could be obtained by further prolonging the induction time longer that 5–10 min. For checking this conclusion, in 1976, further clinical observation of 1,799 patients for abdominal tuboligation in Jiangsu, Jiangxi, Anhui, Guangdong, Guangsi, Shanxi, Hunan, Hubei and other provinces was carried out in two groups. For the first group the duration of inducation was 4–6 min and in 974 cases the rate of excellent-good results was 89.1%, and for the second group the duration of induction was 14–16 min and the rate of excellent-good results of 825 cases was 81.4% (Table 5). These results support the above preliminary conclusion that 5–10 min was the most optimal induction duration for tuboligation.

Table 5. The relationship between duration of induction and the effect of acupuncture anesthesia

Duration of induction	No. of Cases	Effect of acupuncture anesthesia								Success		Excellent-good	
		Grade I		Grade II		Grade III		Grade IV					
		No. of Cases	%	No. of Cases	%	No. of Cases	%	No.of Cases	%	No. of Cases	%	No. of Cases	%
4'–6'	974	539	55.3	329	33.8	98	10.1	8	0.8	966	99.2	868	89.1
14'–16'	825	370	44.8	302	36.3	142	17.3	11	1.3	814	98.7	672	81.4
Total	1799	909	50.5	631	35.1	240	13.3	19	1.1	1780	98.9	1540	85.6

Rate of excellent-good P<0.01 (Note: data from studies 1976–1977)

III. SUPPLEMENTARY MEDICATION

Proper supplementary medication is one of the measures to enhance the effect of acupuncture anesthesia. The data from 931 patients in Shanghai in 1975 indicated that in the first group of 403 cases given dolantin (50 mg) before operation, the rate of excellent-good results was 68.9%; in the second group of 423 cases not given dolantin before operation, the rate of excellent-good results was 82.9%; in the third group including patients forecasted as Grades I and II (result of preoperative test) without dolantin and those forecasted as Grade III with dolantin (50 mg) before operation, the rate of excellent-good results was 86.8%. In order to further investigate the relationship between dolantin and acupuncture effect, observation and analysis of 728 cases were made in Shanghai and Jiangsu. The results were for the first group (with supplementary medication) of 240 cases, and the rate of excellent-good results was 93.3%; for the second group of 241 cases, without supplementary medication, the rate of excellent-good results was 84.6%; for the third group of 247 cases with supplementary medication selectively the rate of excellent-good results was 88.1% (Table 6). So, in order to enhance the acupuncture effect, it is necessary to give an adequate dose of dolantin selectively to those who were under nervous tension and had a lower pain threshold.

Table 6. The relationship between supplementary medication and the effect of acupuncture anesthesia

State of medication	No. of Cases	Effect of acupuncture anesthesia								Success		Excel-lent-good	
		Grade I		Grade II		Grade III		Grade IV					
		No. of Cases	%	No. of Cases	%	No. of Cases	%	No. of Cases	%	No. of Cases	%	No. of Cases	%
Group with Drug	240	127	52.9	97	40.4	15	6.3	1	0.4	239	99.6	224	93.3
Group without Drug	241	81	33.6	123	51.0	34	14.2	3	1.2	238	98.8	204	84.6
Group with selected drug	247	80	32.4	133	53.8	33	13.4	1	0.4	246	99.6	213	86.2
Total	7328	288	39.6	353	48.5	82	11.2	5	0.7	723	99.3	641	88.1

Rate of excellent-good, P<0.01.

IV. METHODS FOR FETCHING THE TUBES

At present, although methods for fetching the tubes are rather numerous, the matter that counts in all of them is the degree they are mastered. In Jiangsu and Shanghai tubes were fetched with a hook to reduce stimulations and overcome the difficulties in performing operations on patients with a posteriorly deviated uterus. According to reports from various provinces, the number of patients with a posteriorly deviated uterus is quite large, so it is advisable that the hook fetching method should be popularized.

V. PREOPERATIVE ESTIMATION OF EFFECT OF ACUPUNCTURE ANESTHESIA

Determination of pain threshold by potassium ionophoresis or spring pressure is considered an important method for finding out individual pain endurance and predicting the effectiveness of acupuncture anesthesia. But these methods could hardly be popularized in rural areas. In 1975, a decision was made that in preoperative estimation for abdominal tuboligation, the measurement of pain tolerance of manual needling should be applied to all patients. Point of needling is Hegu in the right hand. Estimation of pain tolerance of needling is divided into three grades: Grade I–tolerance of those who could endure heavy whirling; Grade II–tolerance of those who could not endure heavy whirling, but who could endure middle stimulation; Grade III–tolerance of those who are very sensitive even to inserting or light whirling. In Shanghai, Sichuan, Gansu and other places clinical observations of the tolerance of manual needling of 4,284 cases were made. The results were as follows: 1,769 cases belonged to Grade I needling tolerance. There were 1,275 cases with Grade I acupuncture anesthesia representing 72.6%; while of 2,091 cases of Grade II tolerance, only 832 cases had Grade I acupuncture anesthesia, representing 39.8%; and of 423 cases of Grade III tolerance, only 119 cases had Grade I acupuncture anesthesia, representing 28.1%. The results indicate that measurement of manual needling has a high coincidence rate with the effectiveness of acupuncture anesthesia. This is a simple valuable method that should be popularized.

Practice has proved that abdominal tuboligation under acupuncture anesthesia had many abvantages such as safety, simplicity, effectiveness and rapid recovery after operation. It is therefore a reliable and effective method of anesthesia for abdominal tuboligation.

AN ANALYSIS OF DIFFERENT METHODS OF ANESTHESIA FOR PROSTATECTOMY

Zhuang Xinliang, Qu Guilian Chen Shoulin, Zhang Lingdi
(Shanghai First People's Hospital)

Prostatesctomy is a comparatively difficult operation in urological surgery. This is not only due to the difficulty in surgical manipulation but also due to the important fact that the patients undergoing such operation belong mostly to the old age group often with cardiovascular diseases or certain functional impairment of other important organs. The anesthetic management used for the prostatectomy, therefore, bears characteristics for the aged either during the operation or pre- or post-operatively. Formerly, the anesthetic methods for prostatectomy were usually general or epidural. Since 1966 we began to use acupuncture anesthesia for the prostatectomy with satisfactory results, and it has been adopted as the most commonly used method up to now. This report presents analysis of 300 cases of prostatectomy performed under different methods of anaesthesia including 150 cases of acupuncture, 100 cases of continuous epidural and 50 cases of general anesthesia.

I. THE EFFECTIVENESS OF ACUPUNCTURE ANESTHESIA OF 150 CASES OF PROSTATECTOMY

1. Selection of Acupuncture Points and Effectiveness of Acupuncture Anesthesia. The acupuncture points were selected according to the principle of selecting points along the course of meridian combined with that along the course of nerve. The basic points used were Ciliao (bilateral), Yaoshu and para-incisional needlings (bilateral) or Wushu (bilateral), Weidao (bilateral). Some supplemental points were also added. According to the different supplementary points selected the whole series was divided into three groups: Group I was Mingmen, Group II Jizhong, and Group III Mingmen and Zusanli (bilateral), Sanyinjiao (bilateral). The anesthetic effects of the three groups are listed in Table 1.

Table 1. Anesthetic effects of acupuncture anesthesia of 150 cases of prostatectomy

Grade of effectiveness		I		II		III IV		I	II
Group	No. Cases	No. Cases	%	No. Cases	%	No. Cases	%	No. Cases	%
I	45	12	26.7	20	44.4	13	28.9	32	71.1
II	30	14	46.7	12	40.0	4	13.3	26	86.7
III	75	14	18.7	47	62.6	14	18.7	61	81.3
Total	150	40	26.7	79	52.6	31	20.7	119	79.3

The percentages of Grade I plus Grade II cases in all the three groups add up to above 70%. The anaesthetic effect of Group II was the best, that of group III the next best, and that of Group I the least.

The Procedure of Anesthetic Manipulation. The parameters of the electric needling, the premedication, supplementary drugs and the criteria of grade evaluation were similar to those described in the previous paper[1].

II. COMPARISON OF ACUPUNCTURE AND MEDICINAL ANESTHESIA

The clinical data of 300 cases of prostatectomy under different methods of anesthesia are compared. The data compared include the patient's condition before operation, the blood pressure changes and use of hypertensors during the anesthesia, post-operative complications and the use of analgesics within 24 hours after operation.

1. Pre-operative Condition of the Patients. Tables 2 and 3 show the average age of the prostatectomy patients and the incidence of electrocardiogram abnormalities before operation.

Table 2. Ages of patients undergoing prostatectomy

Method of Anesthesia	No. Cases	Age		
		Average	Range	
Acupuncture	150	69.4	54	88
Epidural	100	66.5	52	79
General	50	55.2	45	85
Total	300	66.0	45	88

Table 3. Pre-operative electrocardiogram abnormalities

Method of anesthesia	No. Cases	1*	2	3	4	5	6	Total No. Cases	Total %
Acupuncture	150	16	2	10	14	12	1	55	36.6
Epidural	100	5	0	8	7	2	0	22	22.0
General	50	1	1	6	0	6	0	14	28.0
Total	300	22	3	24	21	20	1	91	30.3

* 1. Bundle block 2. Auricular fibrillation 3. Other abnormal rhythms 4. High tension of left heart 5. Chronic cardiac ischemia 6. Old myocardial infarction

The average age and the incidence of pre-operative electrocardiogram abnormalities are both greater in the acupuncture group than in either of the other two anesthetic groups.

2. Blood pressure Changes and Use of Hypertensors during Anesthesia. The amplitudes of blood pressure fluctuations during prostatectomy, which refers to the maximal value of elevation or depression of mean blood pressure during operation, under three different anesthetic methods are analyzed in Table 4.

Under acupuncture anesthesia, 75% of patients showed an elevation of the mean arterial

Table 4. Mean arterial pressure changes during three types of anesthesia

Method of anesthesia	No. Cases	Elevation or Depression	Amplitude fluctuation (mm Hg)	No. Cases	%	Total No. Cases	Total %
Acupuncture	150	Elevation	>20	54	36.0	113	75.2
			6–20	59	39.3		
		No change	±–5	31	20.7	31	20.7
		Depression	>20	1	0.7	6	4.0
			6–20	5	3.3		
Epidural anesthesia	100	Elevation	>20	0	0	4	4.0
			6–20	4	4.0		
		No change	±–5	22	22.0	22	22.0
		Depression	>20	29	29.0	74	74.0
			6–20	45	45.0		
General anesthesia	50	Elevation	>20	14	28.0	19	38.0
			6–20	5	10.0		
		No change	±–5	9	18.0	9	18.0
		Depression	>20	12	24.0	22	44.0
			6–20	10	20.0		

blood pressure with the amplitude of fluctuation exceeding 20mmHg in 36% of the cases; for the patients under epidural anesthesia, the finding is to the contrary, i.e., about 75% of them showed a fall of the mean arterial blood pressure, in which 29% of the cases exceeded 20 mm. For those patients under general anesthesia, the rate of either elevation or depression of the mean arterial blood pressure is about 40%; the range of elevation and depression exceeding 20mmHg are 28% and 24% respectively. The rate of using hypertensors and other measures to combat hypotension during anesthesia are shown in Table 5. The percentage of cases requiring the use of hypertensors is lowest in the acupuncture anesthesia group (6%), comparatively high in the general anesthesia one (18%) and the highest in the continuous epidural anesthesia one (55%).

3. Post-operative Condition. The rate of using analgesics within 24 hours after operation is 22.0% (33 cases) for the acupuncture anesthesia group, 66.0% (66 cases) for the epidural anesthesia group, and 40% (20 cases) for the general anesthesia group. Table 6 shows

Table 5. Uses of hypertensors in three types of anesthesia for prostatectomies

Method of anesthesia	No. Cases	50% Glucose solution	Ephedrini hydrochloridum	Phenylephrine	Vasoxyl	Norepinephrine	Atropini Sulfas	Total No. Cases	Total %
Acupuncture	150	7	1	0	0	0	1	9	6.0
Epidural	100	14	20	1	2	5	13	55	55.0
General	50	4	3	0	0	1	1	9	18.0
Total	300	25	24	1	2	6	15	73	24.3

Table 6. Post-prostatectomy complications using different anesthetic methods

Method of anesthesia	No. Cases	1*	2	3	4	5	Total No. Cases	Total %
Acupuncture	150	2	2	3	4	4	15	10.0
Epidural	100	6	0	5	3	1	15	15.0
General	50	6	1	1	1	1	10	20.0
Total	300	14	3	9	8	6	40	13.3

* 1. Pulmonary infection 2. Bed-sores 3. Urinary infection 4. Secondary infection 5. Transitory urinary incontinence.

the post-operative complications, the rate of which is lowest in the acupuncture anesthesia group (10.0%), next lowest in the continuous epidural anesthesia group and the highest in the general anesthesia group (20.0%). Among the post-operative complications, pulmonary infection occupies the most prominent position. The infection was seen in 14 of a total of 300 cases, but in 6 of 50 cases of general anesthesia, in only 2 of 150 cases of acupuncture anesthesia, and in only 2 of 150 cases of acupuncture anesthesia.

III. HEMODYNAMIC CHANGE BEFORE AND AFTER ACUPUNCTURE AND EPIDURAL ANESTHESIA

In 9 patients a preliminary investigation on hemodynamic changes produced by acupuncture and epidural anesthesia during prostatectomy was made by means of recording the plethysmogram, the first derivative thoracic impedance cardiogram and cardiophonogram with an 8-channel polygraph before and after the induction of these two types of anesthesia. The values of stroke volumes, cardiac output, cardiac index and the ventricular ejection time calculated from the impedance cardiogram, cardiophonogram and electrocardiogram are shown in Table 7.

During the epidural anesthesia the amplitude of the plethysmographic wave was increased while the stroke volume, cardiac output and the cardiac index were reduced and the ventricular ejection time was shortened. Whereas after the induction of acupuncture anesthesia, the change of most hemodynamic indices were in the reverse direction, except for the ventricular ejection time which was also shortened. Thus, the amplitude of plethysmographic waves was reduced, while the stroke volume, cardiac output and cardiac index were all increased after induction. However, the frequency of the plethysmographic wave was not significantly changed in both cases.

IV. DISCUSSION

It has been shown in this study that epidural anesthesia exerts a comparatively greater influence on hemodynamics as manifested by an increase of the amplitude of the digital plethysmogram, a decrease of stroke volume, a diminution of cardiac index, a shortening of the time of ventricular blood ejection and also a fall of mean arterial blood pressure. All

Table 7. Hemodynamic changes before and after acupuncture and epidural anesthesia

Method of anesthesia / Indices	Epidural anesthesia n=4		Acupuncture anesthsia n=5	
	Before anesth.	After anesth.	Before induction	After induction
Frequency of plethysmographic wave (Beats/min)	67.0	68.3	78.0	78.0
Amplitude of plethysmographic wave (mm)	8.25	13.6	8.2	7.4
Stroke volume (ml)	98.6	68.7	90.7	97.9
Cardiac output (L)	6.6	4.7	6.6	7.5
Cardiac indices (L/min/M²)	3.8	2.4	3.95	4.27
Ventricular ejection time (sec)	0.35	0.31	0.32	0.29

these suggest that such kind of anesthesia causes peripheral vascular dilatation within the blocked area, which leads to the reduction of venous return to the heart, and which in turn exerts an inhibitory effect on the myocardium. As a consequence the compensatory action of the circulatory function is weakened. Therefore, during the epidural anesthesia the incidence of hypotension is high, especially in aged patients and those already suffering from circulatory decompensation.

In 100 cases of epidural anesthesia for prostatectomy, there are 74% patients showing a fall mean arterial blood pressure over 5 mmHg, among whom 29.0% cases showed a fall exceeding 20mmHg. 55% of the epidural anesthesia patients needed hypertensors, for which 50% glucose or ephedrine hydrochloride was usually used. 8% of the patients, however, required the use of ordinary hypertensors many times, or even more potent ones, such as noradrenalin, phenylephrine, or even the use of more than two types of hypertensors to combat the vascular hypotension.

The influence of general anesthesia on hemodynamics varies with the method of anesthesia used, the variety of the anesthetics and the depth of anesthesia attained. Tracheal intubation under light anesthesia is liable to induce hypertension, while, deep general anesthesia has an inhibitory effect on the cardiovascular function. Sudden marked blood pressure changes are most likely to happen during the induction period of anesthesia.

In contrast to the other two types of anesthesia, acupuncture anesthesia after its induction causes slight decrease of the amplitude of the digital plethysmogram, an increase of cardiac output, stroke volume and cardiac index, and an elevation of arterial blood pressure. These suggest that the acupuncture anesthesia gives a difinite stimulating effect on the cardiovascular function, which explains the lowest incidence of vascular hypotension during the operation under acupuncture anesthesia. In 150 cases of prostatectomies under acupuncture anesthesia about 75% of the patients showed an elevation of blood pressure, and only 6% of them needed the use of hypertensors. Elevation of blood pressure under acupuncture anesthesia does not need any special treatment and was followed by no adverse effect. However, in severely hypertensive patients originally treated with hypotensor drugs, such medications are generally not discontinued before operation under acupuncture anesthesia, thus the amplitude of blood pressure elevation produced by acupuncture during operation is minimized.

Acupuncture gives a relatively good anesthesia effect for prostatectomy with a Grade I+II rate above 70%. Furthermore, acupuncture anesthesia exerts only slight influence on hemodynamics, and its postoperative complications are less frequent than in either epidural or general anesthesia. Hence, for the aged patients undergoing prostatectomy it seems advisable to use acupuncture as an anesthetic method. Since adopting acupuncture anesthesia for prostatectomy in our hospital, the indication for the operation has been somewhat extended, and the average age of the patient undergoing the operation elevated. A few patients with impaired cardiopulmonary function, for whom we had had some apprehension for the safety of the operation, smoothly underwent prostatectomies under acupuncture anesthesia. Acupuncture anesthesia for prostatectomy as for many other operations has also its disadvantages, such as incomplete analgesia and insufficient muscular relaxation with the result of poor exposure in a few obese patients. These defects would be overcome by improving the anesthetic method.

REFERENCE

[1] 上海市第一人民医院：中华医学杂志 **57** (2): 97。1977。

CLINICAL EXPERIENCE IN ACUPUNCTURE ANESTHESIA FOR CERVICAL SPINE OPERATION THROUGH ANTERIOR APPROACH

Wang Kuan, Ma Lihua

(Acupuncture Anesthesia Group, The Third Teaching Hospital, Beijing Medical College)

Dong Fangchun, Zhang Tancheng

(Department of Orthopedics, The Third Teaching Hospital, Beijing Medical College)

In the past, general anesthesia was routinely used in operations performed by anterior approach for resection of cervical disc and interbody grafting at the Third Teaching Hospital of the Beijing Medical College.

In September 1970, acupuncture anesthesia was first used for this operation with success. Since then, up to May 1978, 255 such operations were performed under acupuncture anesthesia. In the clinical practice in this series of operations, the effect of acupuncture anesthesia has been progressively improved from an excellent to good rate of 69.9% in 1974 to 92.7% in 1977. At present, acupuncture anesthesia is routine for this kind of operation at this hospital.

I. CLINICAL DATA

1. Selection of cases. All the patients who were indicated for this operation were considered suitable for acupuncture anesthesia. This series of cases consists of 239 cases of various types of cervical spondylosis, 9 cases of fracture dislocations of the cervical spine, 6 cases of subluxation of the cervical spine and 1 case of congenital deformity of the cervical spine.

2. Sex and Age. Males, 200; females, 50. The youngest was 19 years old and the eldest 74, with an average of 48.

3. Occupation. Workers, 119; cadres, 64; peasants, 22; medical workers, 17; and others, 41.

4. Range for operation. See Table 1.

5. Duration of operation. Ranged from 1 hour 15 minutes to 5 hours 45 minutes with an average of 2 hours and 20 minutes.

II. METHOD AND EFFECT OF ACUPUNCTURE ANESTHESIA

1. Preoperative Preparations. Besides the usual preoperative preparations, the patient was taught to lie on his back with a pillow between the shoulder blades to extend his neck

Table 1. Range for operation

No. of discs removed	I	II	III	IV	V	Total
No. of cases	29	59	119	42	6	255
Percentage	11.4	23.1	46.7	16.7	2.3	100

Table 2. Prescription and effect of a.a.

Grading of effect / No. of cases / Prescription	I	II	III	IV	Total	Grades I and II rate %
Bilateral futu right Hegu and Waiguan	85	102	23	1	211	88.6
Bilateral Fuyang and Feiyang	12	10	7	0	29	75.9
Others	0	10	5	0	15	66.7
Total	97	122	35	I	255	85.9

and to push his trachea sidewise to the left. These procedures would adapt the patient himself to the requirement of the operation.

The doctor should allay the patient's anxiety by explaining the procedure of the acupuncture anesthesia and the sensations in the main steps of the operation, such as skin incision, traction of the trachea and bone chiselling, etc., so that the patient would be able to cooperate actively. In order to make out the patient's reaction and tolerance to acupuncture, trial needling should be made before the operation.

2. Selection of Points. Bilateral Futu, right Hegu and Waiguan used in most cases, and in a number of cases, bilateral Fuyang and Feiyang were used for comparison. In a small number of cases, ear and body points were used in combination.

3. Method of Stimulation. The inserted needles were connected with a weak electric current to achieve effective continuous stimulation. The current flowing from the electric acupuncture apparatus is in the form of biphasic pulse waves. Frequency for Futu points is 100Hz, and for points on appendages 2–4Hz. Intensity was adjusted to the level that the patient was able to tolerate. During operation, the acupuncture sensation was maintained.

4. Induction time. 20–30 minutes.

5. Adjuvants.

The pre-medication: Scopolamine 0.3mg, Dolantin 1mg/kg, Sodium luminal 0.2g or Haloperidol 5mg were used when indicated.

During operation: If the patient felt some discomfort or pain, 0.5% procaine might be infiltrated locally or Dolantin injected intravenously when necessary.

6. Prescription and Effect. See Table 2.

III. DISCUSSION

1. On Specificity of Acupuncture Points. There is still considerable controversy on the question of the specificity of the acupuncture points. From June 1976 to September 1977, two groups of cases were chosen for comparison. In one group of 32 cases, local and near points along the Channel were selected (Futu, Hegu and Waiguan), while in the other group of 29 cases, distal points along the Channel were chosen (Fuyang and Feiyang). Comparative observations were made on the acupuncture anesthesia effects between these two groups. The results are shown in Table 3.

Table 3. Effect comparison between 2 groups

Grading of effect / No. of cases / Prescription	I	II	III	IV	Total	Grades I and II rate %
Bilateral Futu right Hegu and Waiguan	20	11	1	0	32	96.9
Bilateral Fuyang and Feiyang	12	10	7	0	29	75.9

Note: Statistically, $X^2=5.89$, $P<0.025$.

Observations on the main steps of operation such as skin incision and bone chiselling showed the analgesic effect of the group with points Futu, Hegu and Waiguan was better than that with points Fuyang and Feiyang (statistically $P<0.05$)

It is evident that needling has analgesic effect in general, but different points used in the same sort of operation may produce different effects. Experimental studies on needling certain points on the body of a normal person revealed that different points gave influence remarkably differently on the pain threshold of the same site of the body. From the data mentioned above, it is clear that every acupuncture point has its own specificeffect of analgesia.

Chinese traditional medicine believes that the Channels distributed in the body are different pathways with different functions. In traditional Chinese medicine there is a saying: "Where the Jing Mai Channel pathways traverse where is the place amenable to treatment." The results of this series of cases showed that the group of Hegu-Waiguan-Futu produce better effects. This also explains that every point has its relative specificity.

2. Characteristris of Acupuncture Anesthesia in Anterior Cervical Intervertebral Operation.

(1) Recognition of the effect of acupuncture anestheisa.

In 255 operations under acupuncture anesthesia, discpuncture was carried out during operation in order to determine the site to be operated upon. There was no pain felt at puncturing the disc. In 22 cases, discographs were taken with liquid iodine contrast medium in order to find out the pathological changes of the nucleus pulposus and except that there was one case who felt shoulder pain, and another case who had distension sensation in the back of the neck, all the rest had no significant pain reaction. For comparison, Wang Dao Xin reported 5 cases of cervical discograph with liquid contrast medium under local anesthesia. The patient would have distension pain in the back of the neck when the nucleus pulposus is normal, and radiating pain in the arm when the nucleus pulposus is ruptured or degenerated. Under acupuncture anesthesia, above 80% of cases had no pain sensation at the time of removal of the disc.

In order to confirm the analgesic effect of acupuncture anesthesia, 10 operations were carried out under local anesthesia as control with the same pre-operative medication as those under acupuncture anesthesia. The amount of 1% procaine used under local anesthesia was 23ml on the average, while under acupuncture anesthesia (40 cases) it was 6.2ml on the average, or 3/4 less than the former.

(2) Safety and less physiological disturbance.

In this series of 255 cases, there were patients with various concomitant diseases, and they stood the operation well under acupuncture anesthesia. Since acupuncture helps to regulate the normal body functions, under acupuncture anesthesia there is very little fluctuation of blood pressure and pulse rate, and the respiration rate is much more steady. In this group of 255 cases, 22 cases had hypertension, 18 cases with systolic pressure 160–180 mmHg, 8 cases over 180 mmHg; 8 cases had coronary disease, 1 case had remote cardic infarct and carditis, and one had diabetes. They all stood the operation well.

Cervical spondylosis is often found in middle-aged or aged people. Some of them might also have concomitant diseases in other systems of the body, especially the cardiovascular system; with such patients it is more safe to operate under acupuncture anesthesia.

(3) Prevention for injuring the recurrent laryngeal nerve.

Since acupuncture anesthesia exists with the patient mentally alert and has the advantage of the patient being able to cooperate actively during the operation, injury of this nerve can be easily avoided. Under local anesthesia, the tissue was infiltrated with drug solution and the operation field became unclear. In addition to this fact, the nerve might be also infiltrated and became interrupted chemically, so that it could not be differentiated from true nerve injury.

As to the nerve injury in anterior cervical vertebral operation, Wu Zu-Yao reported 8 cases operated under cervical plexus block and local anesthesia with one case having recurrent laryngeal nerve injury and one case being complicated with Horner's Syndrome. In the past, of 78 cases of anterior cervical vertebral operations performed at our hospital (70 of which were done under general anesthesia, 6 under epidural anesthesia and 2 under cervical plexus block and local anesthesia), 3 cases were found to have their recurrent laryngeal nerve injured. In 225 cases operated on under acupuncture anesthesia, only 2 cases were found to have their nerve being under traction, and this was discovered in time and nerve injury was avoided during operation.

(4) Rapid postoperative recovery, less complication and less nursing care.

Generally, the patient could take food on the very day of operation, need no fluid infusion, could do arm and leg excerises, and could turn unaided in bed. Incision pain is slight. About one half of the patients do not require any analgesics. No bedsores. Recently, a plaster neck collar was introduced for immobilization of the neck and when the patient returns to his ward, he would be able to sit up and get out of the bed the day after operation. Thus, possible complications were reduced to a minimum and nursing care became much simplified.

Although the effect of acupuncture anesthesia for this operation is comparatively good and stable, there still remains such problem as incomplete analgesia of which the theoretical basis must be further explored.

IV. SUMMARY

This article sums up the data of acupuncture anesthesia collected from 255 cases of anterior cervical intervertebral operation. The anesthesia effect is recognized as good and positive.

By comparison of the effects between two different acupuncture point groups, it was noticed that each acupuncture point has its relative specificity.

Observations on the postoperative course of the patient show that under acupuncture anesthesia there is a rapid postoperative recovery and a minimum of complications .

We are convinced that acupuncture anesthesia is an effective and reliable anesthesit method for anterior cervical vertebral operation.

REFERENCES

[1] 汪道新: 中华神经精神科杂志 **9** (4): 333，1965。

[2] 吴祖尧: 天津医学杂志骨科(副刊) **8** (3): 159，1964。

ACUPUNCTURE ANESTHESIA USING YEPING POINT FOR UPPER EXTREMITY OPERATIONS—A REPORT ON 72 CASES

Lei Yunshan, Li Baoxiang, Wang Dongsheng
(The People's Hospital of Southeastern District, Shanxi)

I. INTRODUCTION

The Yeping point applied by us in acupuncture anesthesia for upper extremity operations was derived from experience by Dr. Huo Zenglian, who used to treat pain and numbness in the arms with it for over 50 years with good results.

From May 1976 to Sept. 1978, we prescribed Point Yeping for acupuncture anesthesia for 90 cases of upper extremity operations, the data of 72 cases of which are complete, and the following is a report and analysis of the 72 cases based on them.

Location of the point. The patient to be acupunctured lies on his back with his affected arm abducted to 30 degrees. The Yeping point is located at the tip of the main plica axillaris anterior. If there are several main plica, select the deepest and broadest one that is parallel to the axis of the trunk (Fig. 1).

Pathe of needling to the Yeping point. The needle, having pierced through the skin and subcutaneous tissue, traverses the m. pectoralis major, the m. pectoralis minor, the axillary adipose tissue and then passes between the medial side of the neurovascular sheath of the brachial plexus and the n. thoracis longus to reach the loose tissue or into the m. subscapularis. The depth of the needle tip in the tissue is about 4.5cm (Figs. 2,3).

Manipulation of needling. Insert the needle perpendicularly into the Yeping point with the arm abducted to 30 degrees. Manipulate the penetrating needle to and fro, twist it back and forth to produce vigorous stimulation. Push the needle until a special needling feeling somewhat like tingling sensation, called Deqi, is brought about around the operation area or along the whole limb.

If an electric needling apparatus is used, penetrate another needle at a point about 0.5cm medial to the Yeping point for connection with the electrode. As to the electric apparatus the Beihang Model 57–6D or the Shanghai Model G6805 is preferred. The length of induction is 15–30 minutes at a frequency of 6000–12000 cycles per minute. The intensity of the stimulating current is adjusted to the tolerance of the patient. Turn on continuous wave during induction and loose-dense alternative wave during operation.

Preoperative medication. If necessary, 0.1–0.2g of phenobarbital and 0.3mg of scopolamine hydrobromide or 0.5mg of atropine sulphate may be given intramuscularly one hour prior to operation. If supplementary analgesic is required, a dose of demerol 1–1.5mg per kg of body weight is given half an hour preoperatively by intramuscular injection or 15

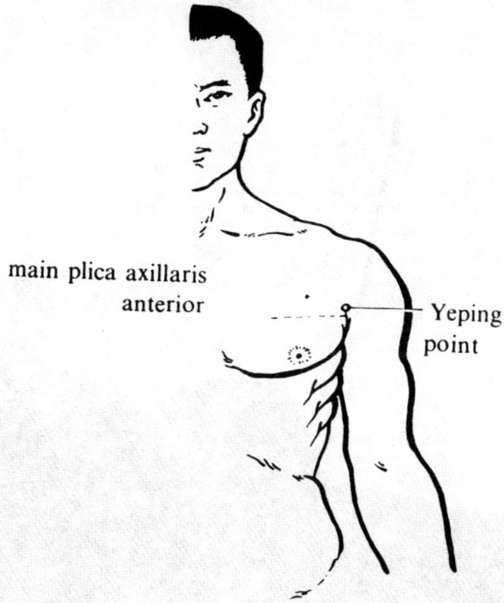

Fig. 1 The site of Yeping point.

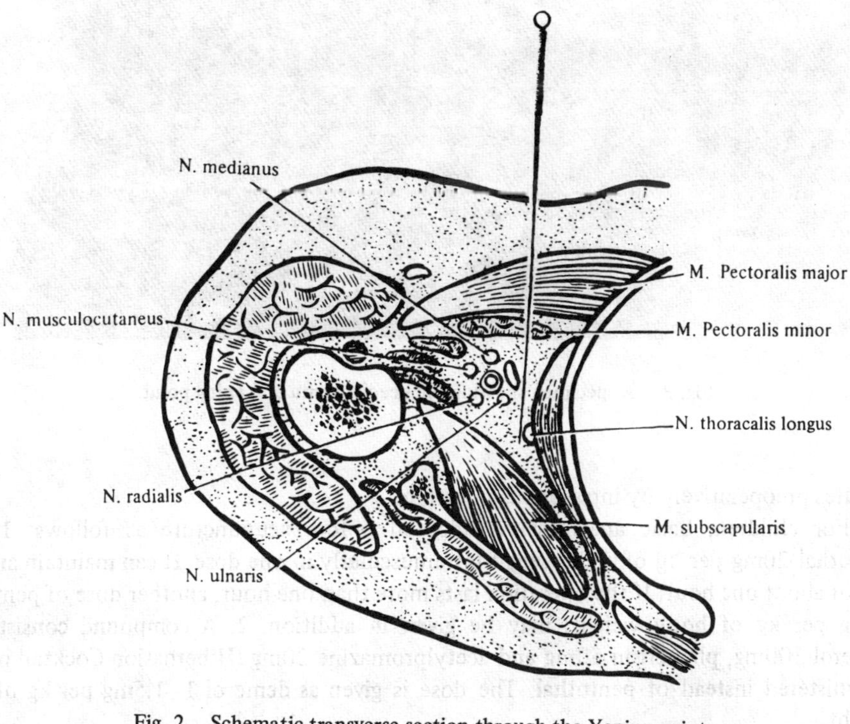

Fig. 2 Schematic transverse section through the Yeping point.

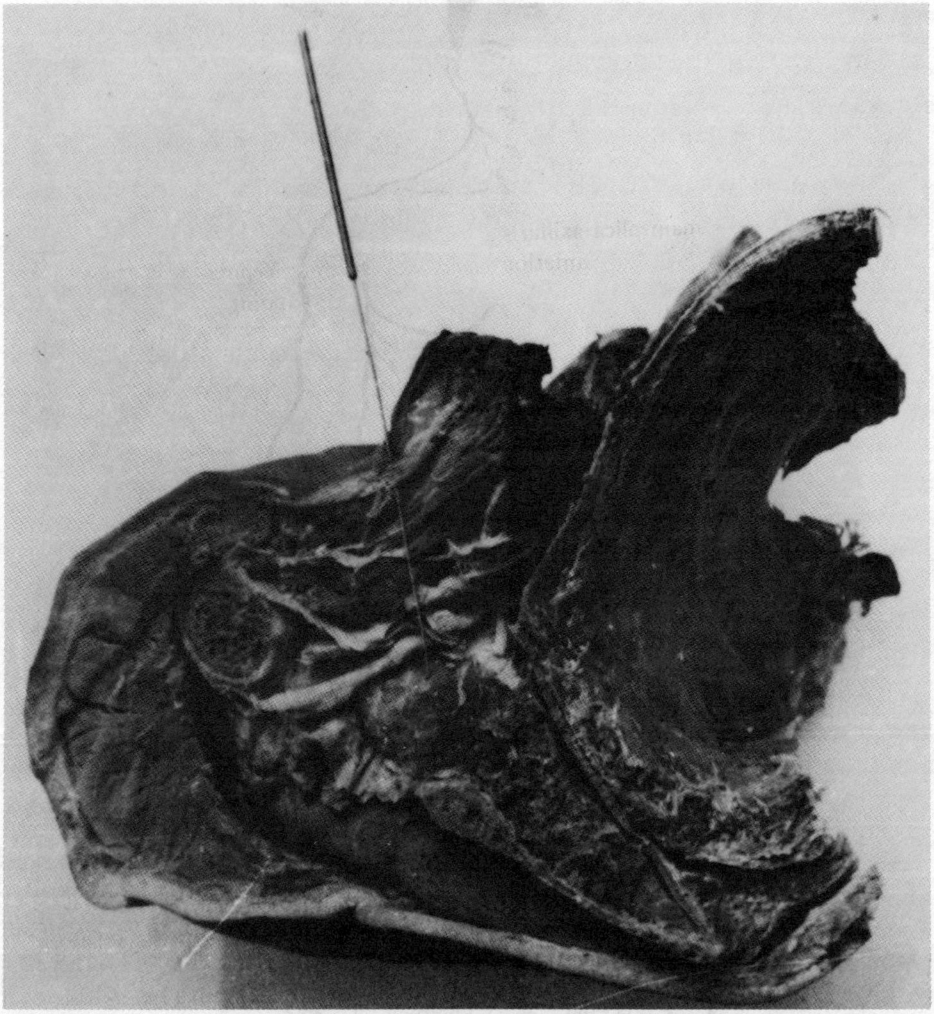

Fig. 3 A specimen showing the needle in situ at Yeping point.

minutes preoperatively by intravenous injection.

For children, basic anesthesia is adopted before acupuncture as follows: 1. Give pentothal 20mg per kg of body weight intramuscularly in one dose. It can maintain anesthesia for about one hour. If the operation lasts more than one hour, another dose of pentothal, 10mg per kg of body weight, may be given in addition. 2. A compound consisting of demerol 100mg, phenergan 50mg and acetylpromazine 20mg (Hibernation Cocktail no.4) is administered instead of pentothal. The dose is given as demerol 1–1.5mg per kg of body weight.

II. CLINICAL DATA

According to the four-grade score system suggested by the National Acupuncture Anesthesia Conference in Tianjin in 1976, the effects of acupuncture anesthesia via Yeping point in this series of 72 cases are: Grade 1(excellent effect) 46 cases, amounting to 63.89%; Grade 2 (good effect) 17 cases, amounting to 23.61%; Grade 3(fair effect) 6 cases, amounting to 8.33%; and Grade 4(poor effect) 3 cases, amounting to 4.16%. The rate of satisfaction (Grades 1,2) is 87.5%, and that of success is 95.83%.

Among the 72 cases, 49 cases are men, 23 cases, women. The eldest is 65 years old, the youngest, 2 years. There is no significant difference between the effects of anesthesia in the various age groups statistically.

25 of the 72 cases are emergencies; 22 cases(88.8%) give Grades 1 and 2 effects. The others are selective operations. 41 cases of them (87.2%) give Grades 1 and 2 effects. It was found that acupuncture anesthesia via Yeping point was especially effective in operations for the hand, the wrist and the forearm (Table 1).

Table 1. Effects of acupuncture anesthesia in operations for different parts of the upper extremity

	Effects				Total no. of cases	No. of cases of success (%)	No. of cases of Gr.1 effect(%)	No. of cases of Gr.1&2 eff.(%)
	Gr.1	Gr.2	Gr.3	Gr.4				
No. of cases	46	17	6	3	72	69 (95.83)	46 (63.88)	63 (87.50)
Hand, wrist	22	7		1	30	29 (96.67)	22 (73.33)	29 (96.66)
Forearm	16	8	2		27	26 (96.29)	16 (59.62)	24 (88.88)
Elbow	5	2	4	1	11	11 (100)	5 (45.45)	7 (63.63)
Upper arm	3			1	4	3 (75)	3 (75)	3 (75)

Statistically, there is no significant difference between the effects of anesthesia for operations for bones, muscles, or the mix of the two (Table 2).

The duration of operation under acupuncture anesthesia lasted 15 minutes to 2½ hours in this series of operations. The effectiveness of acupuncture anesthesia is not affected by the length of the operation in time. The shortest tourniquet tolerance time is 30 minutes and the longest, 1¼ hour. To apply the tourniquet only once would generally be enough for the completion of an entire operation, especially in the excellent or good cases.

In 70 cases of this series, 27 cases were given preoperative medication, 43 cases were not, and 33 cases were given preoperative supplementary analgesics, and 37 cases were not. There is no statistically significant difference between them so far as the effect of acupuncture anesthesia is concerned (Table 3).

Table 2. Effects of acupuncture anesthesia for different kinds of upper extremity operations

	Effects (Grade) 1	2	3	4	Total no. of cases	No. of cases of success (%)	No. of cases of Gr.1 effect (%)	No. of cases of Gr.1&2 eff. (%)
No. of cases	46	17	6	3	72	69 (95.83)	46 (63.88)	63 (87.50)
Ops. for Bones	21	9	2	2	34	32 (94.11)	21 (61.76)	30 (88.23)
Ops. for Tendons	19	3	1	1	24	23 (95.83)	19 (79.16)	22 (91.62)
Ops. for the Mix	3	2	1		6	6 (100)	3 (50)	5 (83.33)
Reduction of closed fracture	3	3	2		8	8 (100)	3 (37.50)	6 (75)

Table 3. Comparison of effects with or without preoperative medication

With or without preoperative medication	With medication	Without medication	With supplementary analgesic	Without supplementary analgesic
No. of cases	27	43	33	37
Grade 1 eff.	15	35	23	27
Grade 2 eff.	9	5	8	6
Grade 3 eff.	3	2	1	4
Grade 4 eff.	0	1	1	0
Rate of success (%)	100	97.67	96.96	100
Rate of Grade 1(%)	59.25	81.39	69.96	72.97
Rate of satisfaction (%)	88.88	93.02	93.93	89.18

III. DISCUSSION

1. Deqi (needling sensation) in relation to the effect of acupuncture anesthesia.

"Lingshujizhu", a traditional medicine work, states that"to reach the Qi should be the first object of the practitioner of acupuncture." "Lingshujiuzhenshieryuan" also emphasizes that "the xecret of acupuncture is that it can be effective only when the Qi is reached." All these tell us that we must try by all means in acupuncture to obtain or reach the Qi (Deqi), and set it in motion. During acupuncture anesthesia, we have to obtain the needling sensation in the region of operation. We once treated a patient whose ring finger was cut off by accident and the stump left had to be sterilized and sewn up. Though it was a minor operation, the anesthesic effect by acupuncture was poor, because the needling sensation reached the thumb and the index finger instead of the remnant of the lost finger.

2. The analgesic effect of the Yeping acupuncture point and the functional state of the body.

Clinical experience found that acupuncture point with strong needling sensation would also produce strong analgesic effect, and the effect of acupuncture anesthesia would also be good.

Needling of the Yeping acupuncture point produces strong needling sensation along the upper limb so that we attained a rate of 87.5% Grades 1 and 2 effects in upper extremity operations. This fact confirms the specificity of the Yeping point to that part of the body. But in individual cases, though needling sensation was remarkable, the effect of acupuncture anesthesia was unsatisfactory. Moreover, there were cases when the analgesic effect of the same acupuncture point was good for the first time, but poor for the next. The reason is probably connected with the state of the physical functions of the patient at the moment that prevented the same acupuncture point from producing the same analgesic effect.

In ancient Chinese acupuncture therapeutics, it is emphasized that "the cause of disease (pathogenecy) should be sought in the symptoms", and that "the restoration of the proper function of the Qi(vitality) should be realized through studying the cause of its malfunction." "To deplete when too full" and "to refill when too depleted" are two general principles of therapeutics. According to these principles, weak stimulation is applied to patients who were weak and had a weak pulse, and strong stimulation is applied to patients who are strong and had a strong pulse.

3. The relation between the propagation of needling sensation and the channels and collaterals and the nervous system.

The points from which the channels and collaterals originate and in which they end and the viscerae governed by them are described in detail in traditional Chinese medicine. However, the Yeping point is a discovery of an unknown acupuncturist among the people and therefore there is no mention of it in any ancient Chinese medical works. We have observed the propagation by needling the Yeping point. Of 69 cases, needling sensation reaching the entire length of the arm and the whole hand was reported in 39. It reached the upper arm and the elbow in 9 cases, the thumb and the index finger in 5, the thumb, index and middle fingers in 6, the thumb, index, middle and ring fingers in 5, the index, middle, ring, and little fingers in 3, and the thumb and index fingers and the elbow in 1. This propagation of the needling sensation has the same characteristics as those of the Shousanyin channels and collaterals. It is stated in the "Lingshujinmai", a traditional Chinese medical work, that Shousanyin has three channels that pass through the axilla down to the upper arm, the elbow, the forearm, and finally end at every finger tip. These are similar to the needling sensation passages of the Yeping point, which can thus be considered as the converging point of the Shousanyin channels. As the Yin and Yang channels are mutually the exterior and interior channels, therefore needling at the Yeping point may produce analgesia over the whole limb.

From observations on the cross section of the axillary fossa through Yeping point and in 3 cases of radical operations for breast cancer and 1 operation for disarticulation at the shoulder, it was found that the needle inserted through Yeping point lies about 0.5–1.5cm medially to the vagina neurovasorum.

From the facts mentioned above, we can conclude that the Yeping point has a close relation with the nervous system as well as with the channel system.

IV. SUMMARY

A report of 72 cases of acupuncture anesthesia at the Yeping point for upper extremity operations is made in this paper. The rate of satisfactory anesthetic effect of the Yeping point is 87.5%, and that of success, 95.83%. The location, topography and manipulation of acupuncture anesthesia via the Yeping point are defined. The needling sensation in relation to the effect of acupuncture anesthesia, the relative specificity of the acupuncture point and the functional condition of the patient, and the propagation of the needling sensation in relation to the channel line and the nervous system are discussed.

REFERENCES

[1] 山西省晋东南地区人民医院：针刺麻醉 **4**：13，1977。

[2] 张隐庵等(合注)：素问・灵枢。

[3] 上海第一医学院人体解剖教研组：针刺麻醉理论研究资料选编，上海人民出版社，第262页。

[4] 陕西中医学院：针刺麻醉资料综述，人民卫生出版社，第32页，1973。

[5] 西安医学院针麻基础理论研究协作组：针刺麻醉资料综述，人民卫生出版社，第98页，1973。

ON THE PROPOSED MECHANISM OF ANALGESIC EFFECT OF ACUPUNCTURE ANESTHESIA IN LATERAL MENISCECTOMY

Guo Bangfu, Yao Zhiyin, Zhang Qingcai, Shen Lei, Wang Liujiang

(The Institute of Traumatology and Orthopaedics, Shanghai Department of Traumatology and Orthopaedics of Rui Jin Hospital, Shanghai Second Medical College, Shanghai)

Lateral meniscectomy puts high demands on anesthesia. Orthopedic surgeons always believe that if a patient can tolerate the incision of the joint capsule, it shows that the anesthesia is effective. Clinical exprience of 504 cases of meniscectomy proves acupuncture anesthesia to be effective. Now acupuncture anesthesia is used as routine anesthesia in our department and is greatly welcomed both by the medical staff and the patients.

According to the theory of channel pathway, the operation field of lateral meniscectomy is in the vicinity of the Gall Bladder Channel of Foot-Shaoyang. The aterior portion belongs to the Stomach Channel of Foot-Yangming and the posterior portion belongs to the Urinary Bladder Channel of Foot-Taiyang. According to the dermatome, the operation field is in the vicinity of the lateral femoral cutaneous nerve, the anterior portion belongs to the femoral nerve and the posterior portion belongs to the sciatic nerve. Therefore, whether the acupuncture point is selected along the Meridan Channel or the nerve system, the channel and the nerve system coincide more or less with each other. Judged from their effectiveness of acupuncture anesthesia, they are definitely related with each other.

The following conceptions come from observations made during operations of lateral meniscectomy. Many efforts have been made to hypothesize its mechanism in the hope of throwing more light on the mechansim of acupuncture anesthesia in this operation.

I. THE REQUIREMENTS OF LATERAL MENISCECTOMY

Injury of lateral meniscus has the highest incidence rate in this country. From 1966 through September 1978, 504 meniscectomies have been performed, in which the ratio of lateral to medial was 3:1, which is just the reverse of that in foreign countries reported in the literature. This shows cartilage injuries in the Chinese have their special anatomical and developmental characteristics and mechanism of injury. Another noteworthy thing is that the incidence of discoid cartilage injuries has a much higher rate. All these raise the incidence rate of lateral injuries that call for meniscectomy.

The lateral meniscus is easier to be loosened than the medial one as it is not restricted by the lateral collateral ligament and its posterior horn is in close contact with the popliteus. Therefore, the lateral meniscus is more easily detached from the anterior and middle portions, while the detachment of the posterior horn requires strong traction. This is the reason why patients often complain of an uncomfortable traction sensation which is no less painful than the dragging sensation of the viscera. Therefore, not only should the pain of the skin and the capsule be overcome, but also the dragging sensation of the meniscus should be eliminated. In meniscectomy, though there is no muscle tension experienced, yet the ischemic pain will increase the uneasiness of the patient; when the operation is prolonged, it is also unbearable. A good acupuncture anesthesia should overcome these difficulties in order to carry on the operation smoothly.

II. THE POINT SELECTION FOR LATERAL APPROACH OF KNEE OPERATION

Six pairs of Points were used at the beginning. They are bilateral Zusanli, Yanglingchuan, Yinlingchuan, Fenglung, Juegu and Taichong. These Points produced good results irrespective of manual control or electro-stimulator. The shortcomings were too many Points used and the inconvenience in operation[1].

Since 1969, we have re-evaluated our Point selection. We selected Points on the Urinary Bladder and the Gall Bladder channels at the proximal end. It is laid down in ancient medical literature that "the important thing in acupuncture is that effectiveness can be obtained only when the 'Qi' is reached", and that "pain would be cured when the needle reaches the place of pain." Since September 1969 the Qihaishu, Dachangshu and Yinmen of the Urinary Bladder Channel, and the Fongshi of the Gall Bladder Channel have been chosen. Qihaishu and Dachangshu are in the vicinity of the intervertebral foramina of L_{3-4} and L_{4-5} respectively. These are the places from which the L_4 nerve roots emerge. The L_2 and L_3 roots form together the femoral nerve and the lateral femoral cutaneous nerve. The anterior branches of the latter are distributed in the anterior and lateral portions of the thigh down to the knee, and the nerve-endings are connected with the anterior cutaneous nerve branches of the femoral nerve, forming the patellar plexus. Therefore, the stimulation of the Qihaishu and Dachangshu will produce anesthetic effect in the anterior and lateral portions of the knee. Yinmen is in the area governed by the posterior femoral cutaneous nerve, and is originated in the $S_{1, 2}$, and $_3$, and distributed only in the posterior side of the thigh down to the posterior portion of the knee and the calf and connected with the sural nerve. With stimulation of these three Points on the Urinary Bladder Channel, anesthetic effect will be produced in the anterior, lateral and posterior sides of the knee. In addition, the effect in the lateral side will be further enhanced by stimulation of Fongshi of the Gall Bladder Channel at the nerve endings of the lateral femoral cutaneous nerve. Ten year's clinical experience shows the principle of Point selection along the Channel is correct. It proves that the Meridian Channels and the nervous systems have a close relationship.

III. THE RESULTS OF ACUPUNCTURE ANESTHESIA

Three hundred and eighty-five cases of lateral meniscectomy have been performed since September 1969. In the first stage, distal selection of points was adopted in 83 cases, and 28 cases graded excellent, i.e., complete analgesia or painlessness, 41 cases graded good with only slight painful sensation or uncomfortable feeling, but the operation was still carried on smoothly, 7 cases graded fair with incomplete analgesia, but the patient still could stand the operation and the cemaining 7 cases graded as failure, and operation was completed only with the addition of drug anesthesia. In the second stage, proximal selection of Points was adopted in 302 cases with the results of 188 cases graded as cxcellent, 93 cases as good, 20 cases as fair and one as fail (see table). Therefore, in comparing the results of these two stages, the latter is obviously superior to the former ($P<0.005$). On the other hand, the proximal needling will not interfere with the operation. The way of proximal Point selection not only supports the principle of Meridian Channel, but also coincides with the pathway of the nerve system. Consequently, the Meridian Channel and innervation have a very close relation. There is an analogy between these two.

Table Two different approaches of point selection for 385 cases of lateral meniscectomy with comparison of results ($P<0.05$)

Grading		Cases of distal selection	%	Cases of proximal selection	%
Acceptablc	I (Excellent)	28	33.7	188	62.2
	II (good)	41	49.4	93	30.7
	III (Fair)	7	8.45	20	6.7
Unacceptable	IV (Failure)	7	8.45	1	0.4
Total		83	100.0	302	100.0

IV. THE ANALGESIC FACTORS OF ACUPUNCTURE ANESTHESIA DURING MENISCECTOMY AND ITS POSSIBLE MECHANISM

From the final results of this long series of meniscectomy, it seems without doubt that the superiority of acupuncture anesthesia is confirmed. Not only does it produce the analgesic effect required, but also reduces the post-anesthetic complications almost to nil. Patients underwent operations smoothly and recovered and rapidly convalesced. However, the mechanism of acupuncture anesthesia is still being investigated by many authors. We propose to interpret the mechanism of the analgesic effect in terms of lateral meniscectomy.

(1) The Relationship between Points and Receptors. Anatomically, the Points are mostly in the vicinity of nerve trunks and their branches. In the organisms beneath the points are concentrated free nerve-endings. In some Points, muscle spindles are also heavily packed. According to experiments on animals, the mechanical stimulation of a fine needle can set multi-receptors of stretching, touching and pressure into action and also can activate the I, II, III and IV afferent fibers. The evoked potential can even last for more than ten minutes after removal of the needle. The deep receptor apparatus under a Point has a close

relationship with analgesia. It mainly depends upon the afferent activity of medium-sized fibers, i.e., A_δ of cutaneous nerve and III fibers[2].

It goes without saying that not all Points are along nerve trunks and their branches. Therefore, in such cases the action of a Point should be transmitted through receptors, producing a coding impulse that then, by way of the medium-sized fibers of the deep nerves, goes to the spinal cord. The impulse will go upwards through the lateral column to the reticular structure in the brain stem, and then is reflected to the hypothalamus, basal ganglion, finally to the non-specific thalamic-cortical system. The medial reticular structure projects the descending fibers to the spinal cord, and connects them with the different parts of the central system to integrate the messages of regulation of the pain. The recent advances in neurochemistry strongly confirm that the 5-HT and endorphin have analgesic effect and have action antagonistic to noradrenaline.

In our coordination of Points, we adopted the Points Qihaishu and Dachangshu that are innervated by the lumber plexus. Mechanical stimulation can increase the blood circulation in the nerve roots and spinal cord. The stimulation of these Points transmits impulses centripetally; at the same time, it also gives segmental analgesia with the integrated activity of posterior horn cells, thus establishing the analgesic effect.

(2) The Relationship between Channels and Nerves. The basic principle of acupuncture anesthesia is the theory of Meridian Channels. This theory was established by the vast amount of clinical experience of our ancestors and through further practice a complete system was evolved. It gives the idea of interrelationship between different parts of our body with mutual coordination and antagonism, mutual defense against and protection from external stress. So long as needling gives analgesic effect, it must have some relation with the nerve system, at least the analgesic effect can only be obtained through the pathway of the nerve system. In traditional medicine, the theory of Channels is used to intepret the analgesic action. Obviously, Channels and the nerve system must have a close relationship, and even common characters. By Channel, we mean there is a complex network lengthwise and crosswise, such as the twelve main and branch Channels, the eigtht specific Channels, the twelve subordinate Channels and numerous other small or tiny Channels. It is connected internally with the viscera, externally with the muscles and skin. They form a complete system of intercommunications in the body, to nourish and protect the streaming of the blood and the vital energy "Qi". It is pointed out in the ancient medical work "Ling Shu" that "as to the Channels and their branches, their function is to circulate the blood and the vital energy, balance and nourish the 'positive' and 'negative', nourish the muscles and bones and activate the joints." As we all know, the Channels running the whole body are the blood vessels, the lymphatics and the nerves. Therefore, in a broad sense Channels must be a conception including all these structures. Physiologically, the Channels also include the physiological phenomena of metabolism and endocrinal action. In short, for the time being we believe that the theory of Meridian Channel is a broad anatomical and physiological concept.

In lateral meniscectomy we chose the Urinary Bladder and Gall Bladder Channels. This accords with Meridian Channel Theory. Qihaishu and Dachangshu are in the paraspinal region. By stimulation, they could activate the lumbar plexus, they by way of the lateral femoral cutaneous nerve, down to the patellar plexus. Fongshi is also a Point which can have the stimulation passed directly to the lateral femoral cutaneous nerve. The stimulation on

Yinmen, by way of the posterior femoral cutaneous nerve, gives effect at the popliteal space. There fore, by stimulating these four Points the analgesic effect could be dispersed all over the anterior lateral and posterior regions. This further proves the close relationship between the Meridian Channels and the nerves.

(3) The Action of Acupuncture Anesthesia for Pain Alleviation. Pain is a kind of sensation sent to the brain as a message in order to alarm the higher center in the central nervous system to make an appropriate response. At the same time, it activates a series of protective responses. Therefore, the pain is a plain subjective manifestation of physiological activities, which will reflect·the degree of pain. It is possible to obtain the mechanism of analgesic effect of acupuncture anesthesia from the basis of physiological and biochemical changes.

Stimulation of Points will directly or indirectly stimulate receptor, or non-myelinated free nerve-endings. The damage of these tissues will liberate intrinsic factors, such as bradykinin, histamine, potassium ion, 5-HT, acetylcholine, etc. These chemical substances will act upon the nerve endings (or chemical receptors) producing the impulse of pain. This impulse is usually transmitted by A-fibers and C-fibers to the spinal cord. This activates the posterior horn deep cells. By way of the spino-thalamic tract, the sensory nuclei in the thalamus, the impulse is reflected to the sensory area of the cerebral cortex to fix the location of sensation[3].

From the above hypothesis, it seems that the analgesic action of the Meridian Channels and that of the nerves are identical. We believe that the Meridian Channels include the nerves, but they are not the same thing. In certain cases, the manifestation of the Meridian Channels can be mainly of the nerves, but in others it includes also the physiological action of other tissues. However, it is still a mystery if there is a real anatomical structure that has not yet been explored. Further research should be carried on with great effort.

V. SUMMARY

In reviewing the results of 385 cases of lateral meniscectomy under acupuncture anesthesia, we analyze the way of Point selection under the guidance of the Channel Theory and the relation between the Channels and the nerves, so as to explore the nature of the Channel. Our preliminary concept is that Channels represent in a broad sense various physiological functions, including the nerve system. It is incorrect to put an equal symbol between the two.

The conductive functions of the nerve can be accomplished by stimulating the Point to activate the nervous activities and to produce the antagonistic action towards the pain-producing factor and finally to reach the goal of the alleviation of pain. This might be the mechanism of the acupunctural analgesic effect.

As to the analgesic effect of acupuncture in meniscectomy, it might be the activation of the Point receptor, with the impulse transmitted to the brain to make the pain threshold of the operation field elevated. We are convinced that the Channel and the nerves have something in common.

REFERENCES

[1] 上海市伤骨科研究所等：针刺麻醉膝关节半月板摘除术 440 例临床小结，针刺麻醉 **4**：14，1977。

[2] 吴珏等：实用麻醉学，第 85 页，上海科技出版社，1978，上海。

[3] 江振裕，张清才等：针刺镇痛效应外周传入途径的分析，中国科学，2：157，1973。

RELATIONSHIP BETWEEN EFFECT OF ACUPUNCTURE ANALGESIA AND SYMPATHETIC FUNCTIONAL ACTIVITY

Cao Xiaoding, Mo Huanying, Su Qingfen
(Department of Physiology, Shanghai No. 1 Medical College)

Li Kaiqiao
(No. 1 Tuberculosis Hospital of Shanghai)

Li Shengchang, Xu Cixiong
(Huashan Hospital, Shanghai No. 1 Medical College)

Our preliminary observations on patients during pulmonectomy under acupuncture anaesthesia showed that there were no abnormal changes in EEG and ECG and no significant changes in knee jerk, tendon jerk, touch sensation and taste sensation[1]. Their changes in blood pressure, pulse rate and respiratory movements were less than those under general anesthesia[2]. However, there were marked changes in pain threshold, pain tolerance threshold, galvanic skin reflex, finger plethysmogram and skin temperature measured at the palm and fingers[3–5].

Clinical experience has shown that there are individual variations in the efficacy of acupuncture analgesia (AA) among different patients and normal subjects[6–8]. In order to devise a suitable method for selecting patients for operation under acupuncture anesthesia and to provide clinical material for studying the mechanism of acupuncture analgesia, we recorded in the present work the magnitude of changes of the pain sensibility and the warmth sensation and of certain autonomic nerve responses due to acupuncture of the patients before operation, and correlated these results with the efficacy of acupuncture analgesia afterwards during the operation .

I. METHODS AND RESULTS

1. Effect of Acupuncture on Pain Threshold and Pain Tolerance Threshold. The skin at the site of incision was pinched with a pair of tooth forceps equipped with a micrometer for measuring the force of pinch in grams. The force used to produce a just perceptible pain was recorded as the pain threshold. The pinching was then gradually strengthened up to the point when the pain was no more tolerable by the patient. This strength of pinching is called pain tolerance threshold. Next the effect of acupuncture was assessed. Bilateral twenty pairs of points or unilateral twenty points including "Hegu" and "Neiguan" were needled in different patients by hand maneuver for about one hour, after which the pain sensibility was tested again. These patients were later operated upon under acupuncture and the efficacy of analgesia was graded I, II, III and IV according to national unified standards, Grade I being the excellent analgesic group. It was found that in 109 cases of pulmonary operation, acupuncture significantly increased the pain threshold both in the "good analgesic effect group" (Grade I+II—55 cases) and the "poor analgesic effect group" (Grade III+IV —54 cases) ($P<0.001$); there was no correlation between the magnitude of changes of pain threshold and analgesia efficacy (Table 1).

The case of pain tolerance threshold, however, was different. Table 2 shows that 50% of patients with good analgesic effect during operation had a high pain tolerance threshold before acupuncture in the preliminary test, but the rate went up to 80.4% after one hour of acupuncture. On the other hand the rate of low pain tolerance threshold of the same good efficacy group was 16.1% before acupuncture and 0% after acupuncture. The result suggeste that first, acupuncture is able to elevate pain tolerance threshold and secondly, most patients with high pain tolerance threshold manifest a good analgesic effect.

Table 1. Changes of pain threshold during acupuncture in 109 cases of pulmonary operation

Efficacy	No. of cases	Pain threshold (grams)		
		Before acup.	Acup. for 1 hr.	T test
Good	55	266±19	438±20	$P<0.001$
Poor	54	200±16	360±19	$P<0.001$

Values represent the mean values±S.E.

Table 2. Correlation between changes of pain tolerance threshold during acupuncture and analgesic efficacy during operation

Pain tolerance threshold	Tested before acup.					Tested after acup.				
	Good efficacy		Poor efficacy		Total	Good efficacy		Poor efficacy		Total
	No. of cases	%	No. of cases	%		No. of cases	%	No. of cases	%	
800–1000gm	28	50	12	20.7	40	45	80.4	20	35.1	65
600–790gm	19	33.9	28	48.3	47	11	19.6	26	45.6	37
<600gm	9	16.1	18	31	27	0	0	11	19.3	11
Total	56	100	58	100	114	56	100	57	100	113
X^2	$P<0.01$					$P<0.001$				

2. **Effect of Acupuncture on Warmth Threshold.** The warmth threshold of the skin of the left hand (corresponding to "Hegu" point) and the forehead was tested before and during acupuncture in normal subjects and patients[9]. It was found that after 30 minute's acupuncture of the "Hegu" and "Neiguan" points, the warmth threshold of skin of the hand and the forehead rose significantly ($P<0.01$, $P<0.05$) (Table 3). In the control group no noticeable changes were found ($P>0.05$). However, in 36 patients it was found that the change of the warmth threshold did not correlate very well with the efficacy of acupuncture during operation, so it seems that warmth threshold is not suitable to be used as an index for the prediction of the efficacy of acupuncture analgesia.

Table 3. Changes of warmth threshold during electro-acupuncture

Group	No. of cases	Changes of warmth threshold (°C)	
		"Hegu" Point	Forehead
Acupuncture	44	+0.895±0.282**	+0.550±0.251*
Control	8	+0.275±0.125	−0.119±0.226

Values represent the mean values ±S.E. *$P<0.05$. **$P<0.01$

3. **Effect of Acupuncture on Skin Temperature.** Earlier work showed that the rectal temperature and the skin temperature of the forehead of the patients were relatively stable during operation under acupuncture anesthesia, but the skin temperature of the palm varied significantly[3]. Therefore, the latter was measured during acupuncture as a preliminary test in 47 patients scheduled for surgical operation and the result was correlated with the efficacy of acupuncture analgesia during operation. At a stabilized room temperature of 22°C, the skin temperature of the palmar surface of the distal phalanges of the index and ring fingers and the center of the palm contralateral to the acupuncture point were measured once every 10 minutes by a transistorized thermometer. As it reached a relatively stable level, Hegu and Neiguan points were needled. Then the skin temperature was measured again at the 5th, 20th and 30th minute during acupuncture and the 10th and 20th minute after the cessation of acupuncture.

As shown in Figs. 1, 3 patterns of changes in skin temperature were obtained. (1) The skin skin temperature rose gradually during acupuncture and kept on rising after acupuncture. All patients with such a curve had a good acupuncture analgesic effect during operation. (2) The skin temperature fell during acupuncture but rose up to or above the control level afterwards. Patients with such a curve also had a good effect. (3) The skin temperature fell during acupuncture and kept on falling after acupuncture. Such patients had a poor analgesic effect during the subsequent operation. In the control group without acupuncture no noticeable changes in skin temperature were found. The data show a correlation between changes of skin temperature and the efficacy of acupuncture analgesia.

4. **Effect of Acupuncture on Galvanic Skin Activity (GSA).** Observations were performed on 40 healthy persons in a quiet room at a temperature of 18–25°C. After a person had rested for 20–30 minutes, his GSA was recorded from the palmar surface of the distal phalange of the middle finger at intervals of 3 minutes[5]. A pinch with forceps, the

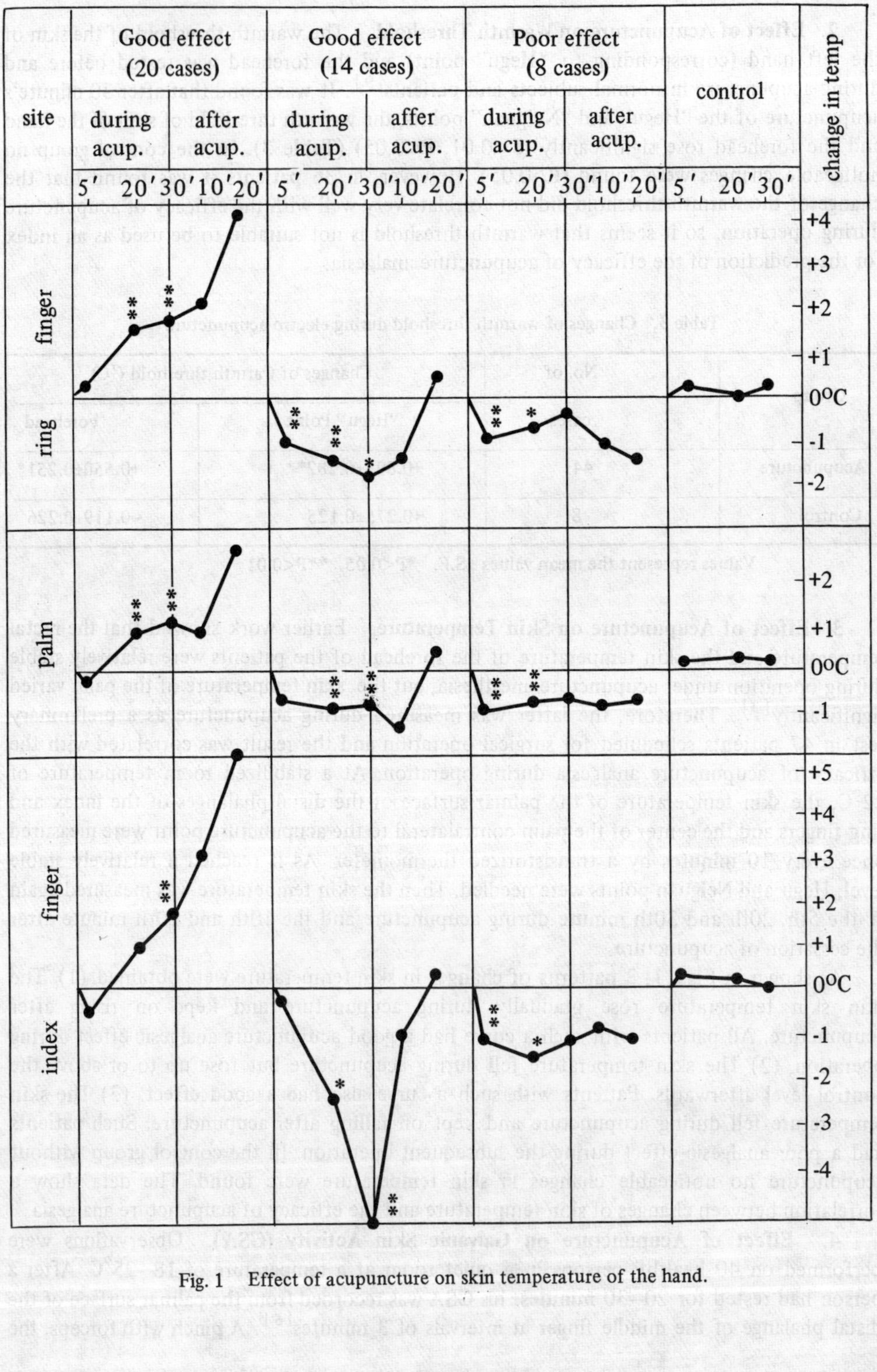

Fig. 1 Effect of acupuncture on skin temperature of the hand.

sound of a ring or a flash light were used as stimuli. As shown in Table 4, after 20 minute's acupuncture of Hegu, Huizong, Shenmai and Fenglong points, the GSA elicited by these 3 kinds of sensory stimuli were all greatly depressed ($P<0.001$). No significant changes were found in the control group without acupuncture ($P>0.05$). Thus a spontaneous decline of GSA could be ruled out. The results indicate that acupuncture could inhibit the GSA.

5. Effect of Acupuncture on Finger Plethysmogram. The finger plethysmograms of 20 persons kept in a quiet and relaxed state at a room temperature of 22–27°C[10] were recorded. Changes in pulse wave elicited by pain stimulation were tested before, during and after acupuncture. Observations were made once every 10 minutes. As shown in Table 5, a significant reduction in the amplitude and dicrotic index of the pulse wave, and the shortening of the left ventricular ejection time was elicited by pain stimulation ($P<0.005$). Thus these changes could be taken as pain responses.

As shown in Fig.2, before acupuncture a marked reduction in the amplitude of the pulse wave was observed following pain stimulation. During 20 minutes' acupuncture the reduction of waves due to pain stimulation was less than that before acupuncture. It means that the pain response was depressed during acupuncture. At the 30th minute after cessation of acupuncture, the amplitude of the pulse wave was markedly reduced again. The results from 20 persons revealed that acupuncture exerted an inhibitory effect on the pain response of

Table 4. Inhibitory effect of acupuncture on GSA elicited by pain, sound and light stimuli

Stimuli	No. of cases	Amplitude of GSA	
		Changes in amplitude (mV)	T Test
Pain	22	−2.00±0.31	P<0.001
Sound	21	−2.06±0.32	P<0.001
Light	22	−1.74±0.27	P<0.001
Control	18	+0.16±0.38	P>0.05

mean values ±S.E.

Table 5. Pain responses of pulse wave

	No. of cases	Control	During Pain stimulation	P Value
Amplitude (Ω)	20	0.482±0.019	0.333±0.029	<0.005
Dicrotic index	16	0.672±0.082	0.347±0.047	<0.005
Left ventricular Ejection Time(sec)	16	0.302±0.004	0.280±0.007	<0.005
Pulse rate (c/min)	20	66.03±1.712	66.11±1.988	>0.05

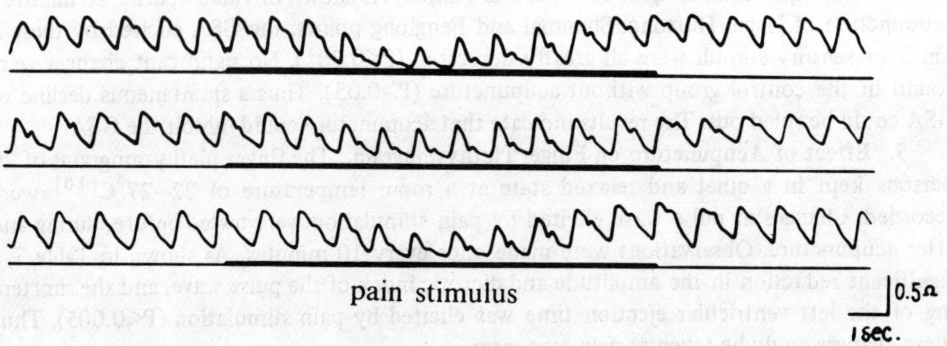

Fig. 2 Inhibitory effect of acupuncture on pain response of plethysmographic pulse wave.
The finger plethysmogram of a normal person — 10 second pain stimulation.
Acupuncture points: Hegu, Neiguan 10 c/sec, 18V.
Upper curve: Before acupuncture.
Middle curve: During 20 minutes acupuncture.
Lower curve: 30 minutes after cessation of acupuncture.

the plethysmographic pulse wave ($P<0.01$), but there was no noticeable effect on the pain response of the left ventricular ejection time ($P>0.05$) (Table 6).

6. Overall Observations on Effect of Acupuncture on Pain Response of Patients. At a stable room temperature of 22°C, observations were made on 42 patients before operation. The respiratory movement, the GSA and the finger plethysmogram were simultaneously recorded by a polygraph (RM-150)[11]. A pain stimulus was applied to the center of the forehead by placing on it a 350g calibrated spring rod dolorimeter for 30 seconds.

As shown in Fig. 3, the pain stimulation elicited a significant reduction in the amplitude of pulse wave, a significant augmentation in the GSA and significant changes in the respiratory movement ($P<0.001$). These alterations could be taken as pain responses. After needling Hegu and Neiguan points for 30 minutes the pain responses were depressed. Twenty minutes after cessation of acupuncture they tended to recover.

Table 6. Effect of acupuncture on pain response of pulse wave

	No. of cases	Percentage of pain response		
		Before acup.	During acup.	P Value
Amplitude	20	68.65±4.324	80.48±3.636	<0.01
Dicrotic index	16	54.95±4.602	65.04±4.920	<0.05
Left ventricular ejection time (sec)	16	92.13±2.745	93.47±2.832	>0.05

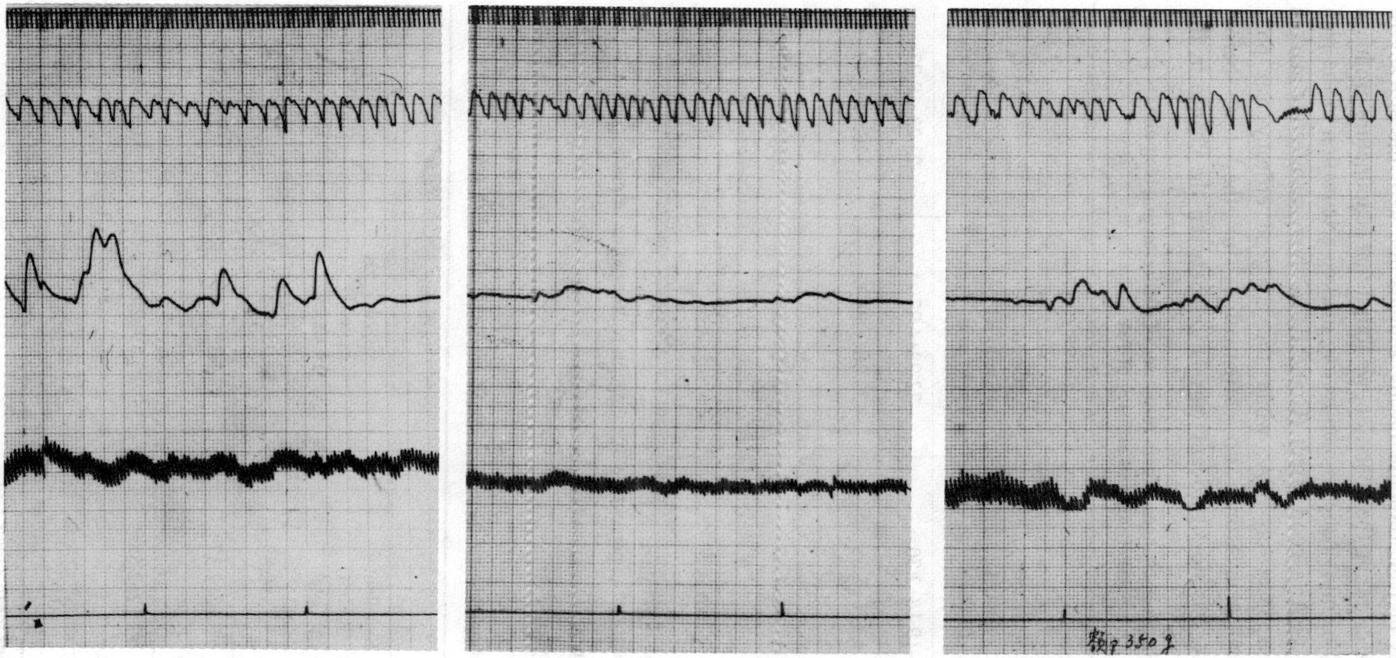

(a) before acup.

(b) during acup. (30min)

(c) after acup. (20min)

Fig. 3 A record from a patient with excellent analgesic effect.
From top to bottom; time(sec); respiratory movement (inspiration upward); GSA; plethysmographic pulse wave; and signal of the beginning and end 30 seconds' pain stimulation.
(a) Pain stimulation only.
(b) Pain stimulation given during 30 minutes' acupuncture.
(c) Pain stimulation given after cessation of 20 minutes acupuncture.

Comparing these changes in pain response during acupuncture with the efficacy of acupuncture analgesia afterwards during the operation, we found that acupuncture produced an excellent effect (Grade I) in most patients manifesting marked attenuation in the pain responses of pulse wave and GSA; a good effect (Grade II) in those manifesting marked attenuation only in pain responses of GSA; while the analgesic efficacy was poor (Grade III+IV) in those manifesting no attenuation in the test before operation (Tables 7,8). There was no significant correlation between the change in the

Table 7. Correlation between changes of pain responses of plethysmographic pulse wave amplitude and efficacy of AA

	Efficacy		
	Excellent (Grade I) 20 Cases	Good (Grade II) 14 Cases	Poor (Grade III+ IV) 8 Cases
Before acup. (%)	–19.18±2.70	–22.92±4.97	–23.23±10.07
During acup. (%) (30 min)	–7.26±3.68	–20.38±4.96	–26.10±5.79
After acup. (%) (20 min)	–17.98±4.87	–32.05±4.31	–20.78±2.47
P Value	<0.025	>0.05	>0.05

Values represent mean values ±S.E.
Numerals representing the percentage of change in pain response of pulse wave amplitude

$$= \frac{\text{Pain response values-control values}}{\text{Control values}}$$

Table 8. Correlation between pain responses of GSA and efficacy of AA

	Efficacy		
	Excellent (Grade I) 20 Cases	Good (Grade II) 14 Cases	Poor (Grade III+ IV) 8 Cases
Before acup. (mV)	15.15±2.88	23.05±4.51	8.33±2.73
During acup. (mV) (30 min)	8.17±2.37	14.30±2.90	9.95±1.71
After acup. (mV) (20 min)	12.12±2.53	17.59±2.83	10.72±3.67
P Value	<0.005	<0.01	>0.05

Values represent mean values ±S.E.
Numerals denote the Summation of the amplitudes (peak to peak) of GSA per minute.

patient's respiratory frequency and amplitude in response to pain stimulation with the analgesic effcacy during the operation.

II. DISCUSSION

1. Individual Variation in Efficacy of Acupuncture Analgesia. In the present paper it is stated that clinical observation found that acupuncture is able to elevate pain threshold, pain tolerance threshold, and attenuate changes of autonomic functions induced by pain stimulation, but there are marked individual variations. Most patients with high pain tolerance threshold before acupuncture or with raised pain tolerance threshold after acupuncture had a better analgesic effect during the operation and vice versa. The fact that pain tolerance threshold is a better index for forecasting analgesic efficacy rather than pain threshold shows that the patient's emotional status plays an important role in the efficacy of acupuncture analgesia.

It has also been found that acupuncture elevates not only the pain threshold but also the warmth threshold, and both changes are parallel[9]. Since the afferent pathway of "Deqi" sensation of acupuncture was closely related to that of the pain and the temperature sensation in the spinal cord[12], it suggests that the signals of acupuncture could simultaneously inhibit the signals of the pain and the warmth sensations in the central nervous system.

Eletrophysiological studies have revealed that the analgesic effect of acupuncture is essentially the result of interaction between the afferent impulses from the point of acupuncture and the afferent impulses from the source of pain at different levels of the paramedial ascending system. The paramedial ascending system is highly polysynaptic and most easily influenced by ascending or descending impulses. This may partly account for the existence of individual variation in the efficacy of acupuncture analgesia[13].

From clinical and experimental practice it is known that the development of acupuncture effect usually requires a 20–30 minute induction and its aftereffects may last for some time. This suggests the individual variation of acupuncture analgesia may also correlate with the level of some neurotransmitters in the brain.

2. Effect of Acupuncture on the Autonomic Nervous Functions. From the present investigation it is evident that during acupuncture the skin temperature of the palm and the fingers are markedly changed; the pain responses of GSA, the pain responses of the amplitude and dicrotic index of the plethysmographic pulse wave are significantly depressed. It has been reported that the final common pathway of galvanic skin reflex in the spinal cord is sympathetic cholinergic fibers and the GSA could be taken as a sensitive index to reflect the functional state of the sympathetic nervous system and the psychoemotional state of the patient[14]. The palm and the finger skin in man are known to contain abundant arteriovenous anastomoses innervated by the sympathetic vasoconstrictor nerve fibers alone; vasodilatation in these skin areas is chiefly due to the release of sympathetic vasoconstrictor tone[15]. Therefore the results suggest that acupuncture is able to inhibit the sympathetic functional activity.

It has also been observed in this paper that there exists a correlation between the inhibition of pain responses during acupuncture and analgesic effect, i.e., most patients with the elevation of skin temperature and marked attenuation in the pain responses of GSA and pulse wave during acupuncture manifest a good effect of acupuncture analgesia during operation. On the contrary, those manifesting drop of skin temperature and no attenuation in pain responses usually have a poor effect. The results further suggest that those patients with inhibition of the sympathetic functional activity by acupuncture have a good analgesic effect. It means that the efficacy of acupuncture analgesia is also related with the activity of the sympathetic nervous system.

III. SUMMARY

1. Acupuncture is able to elevate the pain and the warmth threshold and the pain tolerance threshold, but only the last one correlates well with the efficacy of acupuncture analgesia.

2. There exists individual variation in acupuncture analgesic effect. Patients with high pain tolerance threshold, rise of skin temperature, and inhibition of pain responses in finger plethysmogram and GSA during acupuncture may get a good effect.

3. Acupuncture is able to inhibit the functional activity of the sympathetic nervous system.

The authors wish to express their sincere gratitude to Prof. Xu Fengyan for his guidance. Cai Zeji, Lin Yinli and Ye Zhijun participated in padrt of this research.

REFERENCES

[1] 上海市针麻机制研究组临床生理小组：针刺麻醉应用于肺切除术临床生理资料初步小结。1966年全国针刺麻醉会议资料。

[2] 上海市第一结核病院等：针刺麻醉应用于肺切除术的临床应用。同上。

[3] 上海市第一结核病院等：针麻时皮肤温度变化的初步观察。针刺麻醉资料汇编（上海第一医学院）1972。

[4] 上海市第一结核病院等：针麻时痛觉变化及其与针麻效果关系的观察。同上。

[5] 上海第一医学院生理学教研组等：针刺麻醉时皮肤电反射的研究。同上。

[6] 上海市针麻机制研究组临床生理小组：用生理学方法探讨针刺镇痛的个体特异性的初步印象。1966年全国针刺麻醉会议资料。

[7] 上海第一医学院生理学教研组等：针刺麻醉资料汇编，第一册（上海） 109，1972。

[8] 上海第一医学院生理学教研组等：同上，119，1972。

[9] 上海第一医学院生理学教研组等：针刺麻醉资料汇编，第二册（上海） 1，1974。

[10] 上海第一医学院基础部针麻研究组：针刺麻醉（4）：41，1977。

[11] 上海第一医学院生理学教研组等：针麻效果术前预测中某些生理指标变化的观察。上海第一医学院医学科研资料，1977。

[12] 上海第一医学院生理学教研组等：中华医学杂志 （10）：619，1973。

[13] 上海第一医学院生理学教研组：痛和镇痛的生理学问题，针刺麻醉资料汇编（上海第一医学院） 1972。

[14] Wang GH: *Am. J. phys. Med.*, **36**:295, 1957; **(37)** 35, 1958.

[15] Bareroft H.: Physiol Rev. 40, Suppl (4):81,1960.

ON RELATIONSHIP OF INDIVIDUAL DIFFERENCE AND EFFECTIVENESS OF ACUPUNCTURE ANESTHESIA

Department of Acupuncture Anesthesia, Beijing
Institute of Tuberculosis

There are many factors that affect the efficacy of acupuncture anesthesia (AA), among which individual difference is an important one. Investigation of the relationship between individual variation and the efficacy of AA has been carried on through physiological characteristics such as mental state, cutaneous pain sensitivity, evoked and spontaneous cortical spike potentials, skin temperature, et al., in order to find some criteria for ascertaining patients suitable for AA and to clarify the underlying mechanism of AA. Since 1973 we have been studying different individual characteristics of different degrees of efficacy of AA with some physiological parameters and predicting the efficacy of AA by the results obtained. These results are presented in this articles.

I. METHOD

The patient indicated for lung resection under AA was examined 1 day to 1 week before operation. In the examination, polygraphic recordings of plethysmograph, galvanic skin reflex (GSR) and respiration were made. The patient was asked to lie quiet with eyes closed. Respiratory movement was taken by a mechanico-electric transducer fastened to the abdomen. Photoelectric plethysmograph was used to record the pulse wave of the index finger. The potential difference of the palm and the dorsum of the hand under acupuncture was taken by a 3.0X4.5cm. Ag-AgCl plate. After having the patient lie down for several minutes to adapt to the surroundings, the natural wave within three minutes was taken as the basal control. Then changes in the various indices were recorded by needling points Xiayifeng and Sanyanluo for 15 minutes with continuous electro-stimulation or twisting of the needle.

The efficacy of AA was judged by a clinician after the operation and the result was correlated with the preoperative examination. Because of the total number of Grade I and Grade III efficacy were too small for analysis, the upper part of Grade II and those in Grade I was listed as good effect, and the lower part of Grade II and those classified in Grade III was listed as poor effect. The middle part of Grade II remained as Grade II and was listed as medium.

In GSR the maximal amplitude was estimated, and percentage of activity which was calculated from "period of active GSR/ period of total observation" was measured in the basal 3 minutes and total 15 minutes of induction. The pulse wave was calculated by frequency and the height of wave amplitude, and the respiratory wave by frequency and wave amplitude.

II. RESULT

1. GSR. The spontaneous GSR appears infrequently in most patient during quiet rest control recording. When a needle was inserted, a conspicuous GSR was initiated and abolished gradually in the successive induction period. Both the maximal amplitude and percentage of activity showed great individual difference. Correlating GSR with efficacy of AA, it was found that the percentage of patients with high voltage of spontaneous GSR was higher in the poor efficacy group. As shown in Table 1, the patients giving GSR amplitude greater than 2mV. during quiet condition only accounted for 5% of the 99 cases of good efficacy group. But they reached 25.3% in the poor efficacy group.

Comparing the average amplitudes of GSR induced by insertion of the needle in different efficacy groups, it was found that there was statistically significant differences between them. It was 0.98, 1.8, and 2.7 mV in Grades I, II and III groups respectively.

In Table 2 the occurence of various amplitudes of GSR is correlated with the efficacy of AA. It was found that the percentage of patients with amplitude less than 1 mV was highest in the good efficacy group, while the percentage of patients with amplitude over 3mV was the highest in the poor efficacy group. This difference is also statistically significant.

During the induction period the percentage of patients with activity percentages over 20% was 18 out of 87(19.7%) in the good efficacy group, while it was 56 out of 151 (37.1%) in the poor efficacy group.

The results indicate that the individual difference in GSR, either spontaneous or induced is closely related with the efficacy of AA.

2. Plethysmograph. The patient whose plethysmograph wave was relatively stable during quiet rest condition gave good efficacy. The volume amplitude was reduced during needle insertion. The extent of reduction seemed related with the efficacy of AA (Table 4). Among 103 cases of different efficacy the "vol. amp. during insertion of needle/vol. amp. in rest condition"% averaged 58.9±5.4% in 22 cases of good efficacy group. It was only 41.4±5.4% in 23 cases of poor group ($t=2.33$, $P<0.025$). Pulse rate was increased in some patients during needle insertion, but it was not related with the efficacy of AA.

3 Respiration. The respiratory rate is related with the efficacy of AA. The respiratory rate was below 20 per minute in 15 out of 17 cases of Grade I patient, while in Grade III patients the rate might attain 25/min and even 30/min.

During insertion of needle the patient might hold his breath shortly or the respiration became accelerated or slowed down or irregular in rhythmicity. It is found that the patient who shows more remarkable changes in respiration would probably give poor efficacy (Table 6).

The efficacy of AA may be good in patients with less fluctuation in respiratory rhythm and pulse amplitude during induction period.

Summarizing the results obtained, it seems that efficacy of AA is closely related with: 1. functional activity of respiration and pulse in rest condition; 2. responsiveness of GSR,

Table 1. Efficacy of AA and maximal amplitude of GSR in quiet atmorphers

	Less than 0.9mV	1–2mV	Over 2.0mV	Total
Good	74(75%)	20(20%)	5(5)	99
Moderate	67(57%)	34(29%)	17(14%)	118
Poor	75(48%)	43(27%)	40(25%)	158
Total	216(58%)	97(26%)	62(16%)	375

X^2=25.875 P<0.005

Table 2. Efficacy of AA and amplitude of GSR induced by needle insertion

	<1.0mV	1.1–3.0mV	<3.1mV	Total
Good	36(36%)	55(54%)	10(10%)	101
Moderate	30(26%)	61(53%)	24(21%)	115
Poor	30(19%)	88(55%)	42(26%)	160
Total	96(26%)	204(54%)	76(20%)	376

X^2=18.80 P<0.005

Table 3. Efficacy of AA and GSR activity percentage during induction

	<20%	21–50%	50%	Total
Good	69(79%)	15(17%)	3(3.5%)	87
Moderate	76(75%)	17(17%)	8(8%)	101
Poor	95(63%)	32(21%)	24(16%)	151
Total	240(71%)	64(19)	35(10%)	339

X^2=12.35 P<0.025

Table 4. Efficacy of AA and changes in volume of plethysmograph during needle insertion

	<20%*	21–50%	<50%	Total
Good	3(3%)	56(56%)	41(41%)	100
Moderate	8(7%)	60(51.3%)	49(42%)	117
Poor	19(11%)	89(54%)	58(35%)	116

X^2=7.24 P $\ddot{<}$0.05

$$* \frac{\text{Amp. during needle insertion}}{\text{Amp. in quiet condition}}$$

Table 5. Efficacy of AA and respiratory rate in quiet atmosphere

	Less Than 20/min.	21–25/min.	Over 25/min.	Total
Grade I	15	2	0	17
II	32	16	0	48
III	11	5	3	19

X^2=15.4 P<0.001

Table 6. Efficacy of AA and respiratory changes during needle insertion

	–	+	++	Total
Good	29(42%)	31(44%)	10(14%)	70
Moderate	36(29%)	64(52%)	24(19%)	124
Poor	47(35%)	50(37%)	38(28%)	135
Total	112(34%)	145(44%)	72(22%)	329

X^2=9.85 P<0.05

Table 7. Method of grading of the records of the parameters according to response to needle insertion

	–	+	++	+++
Induced GSR	No reaction	0.1–0.9mV	1.0–3.0mV	<3.1mV
Amp. of plethy. during needle insertion / Amp. of plethys. in quietitude	≯100	51–500%	21–50%	<20%
Resp. response	No response	Change 1–2 times	Breath holding or change over 2 times	–

Table 8. Rate of correctness of prediction of efficacy of AA

Year	No. of Cases	No. of Correctness	Percentage of Correctness(%)
1973–1974	103	93	90
75	102	79	78
76	70	54	77
77	75	65	87
78	123	91	74
Total	473	382	81

respiration and amplitude of plethysmograph to insertion of needle; 3. activity of GSR, regularity of respiratory rhythm during induction period. The patient with good efficacy showed less fluctuation of respiration and pulse amplitude of plethysmograph, response to needle insertion was small, with less active GSR and amplitude of plethysmograph enlarged gradually in the course of continuous stimulation. On the contrary, the patient with poor efficacy showed marked fluctuation in GSR, respiration and plethysmograph, gave prominent responses to needle insertion and the 3 parameters remained unstable in the induction period.

4. Clinical application for prediction of efficacy of AA. When evaluated singly, the significance of the above 3 parameters was different in regard to their correlation with the efficacy of AA. The response of each parameter was different in different individual. Therefore for the purpose of clinical application to prediction of efficacy of AA, we used the above mentioned 3 parameters in combination since 1973. A scheme, based mainly on the magnitude of the response to insertion of the needle with reference to the recording taken during rest and induction period, is proposed(Table 7).

As shown in Table 7, if the summation of the patient's response to needle insertion reached 6^+ or over, the patient was predicted as to have poor efficacy. If it was less than 6, the patient was predicted as to have good efficacy. When the patient predicted as having good efficacy actually obtained Grade I or II efficacy, the prediction is said to be correct. Cases predicted as having poor efficacy is correct when Grade III or IV efficacy was obtained. The percentage of correctness of prediction was around 80% (Table 8).

III. DISCUSSION

The results of most analysis of clinical observations show that the efficacy of AA is related with the patient's mental status. The patient with mental calmness would probably gives good efficacy. It is a difficult problem to measure the mental state of a patient with objective means. Is it possible to find out some parameters related to the function of the central nervous system on the one hand and to the efficacy of AA on the other hand? The parameters used by us having long been adopted in studying the autonomic nervous activities in different physiologic and pathophysiologic conditions. Neurons controlling respiratory and vasomotor activities are concentrated in the reticular formation of the brain stem, and are connected extensively with the visceral afferent and efferent fibers. Their activities are influenced by neural and humoral factors. GSR, considered as a sensitive indicator of emotional status and sympathetic activity, is related to the nervous activity of various levels, especially the facilitative and inhibitory activities of the reticular formation. The facts observed by us seems to suggest that the activities of the neurons related to GSR, vasomotor and respiration perhaps take some part in the mechanism of AA. The question raised is whether the results obtained are valid for tuberculous patients and a chest clinic only. The proposed scheme and the method of examination have been applied to cesarean sections and craniotomies under AA and similar results and persentage of correctness have been obtained. Under AA the overall regulatory and integrative functions of the nervous system make respiration, vasomotor tone and GSR to be less affected, thus the effect of acupuncture may be achived more satisfactorly.

Furthermore, response to pain stimuli experimentally produced or appeared in operation is very similar to the reaction to needle insertion as indicated by the 3 parameters used. [2] Although the pain sensitivity was not estimated directly in our test, the degree of response to the insertion of needle may reflect the tolerance of pain to some certain extent. The patient with a strong response to needle insertion may also tolerate pain badly.

According to the theory of traditional Chinese medicine, effect of acupuncture is to clear the meridian channels for the proper circulation of the vital energy and blood. When the amplitude of the finger pulse wave was enlarged after acupuncture, respiration would become smooth and regular without spontaneous GSR potential and the effect of AA would mostly be good. Do these reflect the results of the improvement of the circulation of the vital energy and blood by acupuncture? This is a point worthy of special attention. Of course, vital energy and blood are not respiration and circulation simply, but they can at least explained partly by them. Our present work may serve as a beginning for the further exploration of the relationship between respiration and circulation and the proper function of the vital energy and blood.

Besides individual difference, there are a number of factors effecting the efficacy of AA, such as the clinical condition of the patient, the extent of surgical trauma, the dosage and the time of drugs used, et al. It is difficult to estimate all these factors previously and adequately, so they should all be taken into considearation in making preoperation prediction of the effectiveness of AA. All the 3 parameters used are nonspecific, particular attention must be paid to the environment under which the examination is carried out. The reliability of the examination can be raised by relieving the patient's nervousness by proper explanation and elimination of environmental interference.

REFERENCES

[1] 北京市结核病研究所针麻组：全国针刺麻醉研究资料选编，第5页，上海人民出版社，1977。

[2] 同上：针刺麻醉，第41页，1976年合订本。

COMPREHENSIVE PREOPERATION FORECAST OF EFFECTIVENESS OF ACUPUNCTURE ANESTHESIA AND SCREENING OF VARIATIONS

National Cooperative Group of Preoperation Forecast of Effectiveness of Acupuncture Anesthesia

Years' of experience in clinical practice proves that satisfactory result of acupuncture anesthesia (AA) depends on the selection of effective points and appropriate parameters of stimulation and the screening of the patients for ones suitable for AA by physiological, biochemical and psychological means. There are things that must be done for preoperation forecast of effectiveness of AA. As the basis of AA is the functional regulation of the various organs of the body by means of acupuncture, it is influenced by numerous complex factors. The results of studies show at present that no single physiological, biochemical or psychological index can reflect the functional state of the patient independently; in other words, it is hardly possible to forecast whether a patient is suitable or not for AA by a single index. It requires a study of all indices involved. The object of the present study is to select the indices by a multivariable statistical method, and sum them up in a mathematical formula for preoperation forecast. We call it "comprehensive forecast of the effectiveness of AA by multiple indices."

I. METHOD

On the basis of a careful study of experience of preoperation forecast of the effetiveness of AA from various regions of our country, from October to December in 1978, 566 operations of 8 kinds were performed under AA. The types of operation were: craniotomy, strabotomy, lung resection, subtotal gastrectomy, hysterectomy, caesarean section, appendectomy, and operation on the extremeties. The following parameters were selected:

1. Cutaneous pain theshold and pain tolerance threshold.
2. Finger plethysmogram.
3. Heart rate.
4. Cutaneous threshold of two-point discrimination and threshold of tactile sensation.
5. The change of the above parameters 15 minutes after needling.
6. Psychological indices.

Processing of information: Hu Shulan, Wang Sulin, Yao Jihua; Data processing: Sun Shanggong; Writing: Wang Youliang, Sun Shanggong.

The combination of the above indices makes 19 variables for forecasting statistical analysis which are listed in Table 1.

Instruments and measurement of the indices.

1. Pain and pain tolerance thresholds.

Instrument: 57–9DK$^+$-algometer (the inner diameter of electrode, 1.5mm, made by Haidian Factory of Electronic Instruments, Beijing).

Parameters: Large step, direct current; autostep rising current; step height 0.15mA and wave amplitude 0.6ms. The electrode is filled with KCl saturated solutions.

Measuring method: Place the electrode on the centre of the incision, and hold it against the skin. The measurement is done in the following way: Pain threshold — "When you begin to feel pain on the site of the electrode, please tell me so." Pain tolerance threshold —"When you feel you cannot stand the pain, please tell me so and remember the degree of pain, which will be a standard in the measurements following."

2. Finger plethysmogram.

Instrument: HB-2A polygraph.

Parameters: Paper rate 2.5 mm/sec, time constant 0.03, recording of respiratory waves synchronized for observing the effect of spontaneous respiratory waves.

Collecting data: Maximal amplitude at rest and minimal amplitude after needling (the norm of needling intensity is that when needling sensation appeared clearly. Plethysmogram is recorded for 10″ immediately after needling for 15′, take mean amplitude value and calculate the pulse rate. Spontaneous waves fall into two types: the uniform and the non-uniform (the type of plenty fluctuation in amplitude, deducting the effect of respiration and other factors, belongs to the non-uniform type).

3. Tactile sensation.

Instrument: Modified BY-7A electro-anaesthetizer. Method. Put the electrode on the right Neiguan point (incision) and the indifferent electrode on Zusanli (or in the vicinity of Sanyinjiao or Hegu). When the patient begins to have the sensation, read the datum; measure three times, and averaged the last two values.

Parameters: 220 Hz in frequency

4. Cutaneous threshold of two-point discrimination.

Instrument: Protracter (Modified)

Sites and method of measuring: Measure the Waiguan point of the left arm and the incision site. Two points along the direction of long axis of the upper extremities should be touch tested with equal force at the same time. During the measurement, let the patient feel one point first, then the distance between two points should be increased by 1–2mm every time until they feel two points. Conversely, the distance between two points may be shortened gradually until they become one point. The cutaneous threshold of two points discrimination is the mean value of the two values measured.

5. Psychological indices.

Under the condition of no suggestion, the patient is asked to answer two questions: (1) Do you wish to receive anesthesia operation? (2) Are you afraid of anesthesia operation? The patients who wish to receive it and are not afraid of it belong to one group, and those who do not want to receive it and are afraid of it belong to another group.

The room for making these forecasting measurements is kept quiet and at constant temperature. The patient is tested three days before operation. Medical workers conducting the test should explain the method to the patients according to instructions but they must not be suggestive. The patient is first asked to lie still; and then to lie another 5 minutes after he is already in a calm mood. The plethysmogram recorded at rest is used as a control.

The order of measurements is: threshold of tactile sensation, threshold of two-point discrimination, pain threshold and pain tolerance threshold. Then right Neiguan was tested. In abdominal operations, the Zusanli point; in operations on the head and the face the right Hegu point; in gynecological operations, the right Sanyinjiao is tested in addition; and in operations on the extremities and the chest, no extra point is added.

After needling the above points and the needling sensation gained, acupuncture needles are connected to Type 57-6 or G-6805 electro-anaesthetizer (in operations on the extremities and the chest, the indifferent electrode was put on the right Waiguan point) with 80–100Hz frequency. After induction for 15', the value changes after needling are measured.

The information is tabulated, divided into groups and processed statistically by computer.

II. TREATMENT OF DATA

The data of pain threshold, pain tolerance threshold and threshold of tactile sensation are converted into logarithm. The above norms are indicated by relative values in order to be compared with themselves for reflection of the changes before and after needling. Thus 19 forecast variables before operation are obtained in the first column of Table 1.

Signs used for the indices: in sex, male is represented by 0, while female represented by 1; uniform spontaneous pulse waves is represented by 0, while non-uniform spontaneous pulse waves represented by 1; and in psychological index, patients who wish to receive and are not afraid of AA are represented by 1, while patients who do not want to receive and are afraid of AA are represented by 0. Thus, the 19 variables in Table 1 become quantitative indices. Besides, due to incomplete recording of some indices or the limitation of storage capacity of our table computer, the variables considered in eight operations were not the same.

In our analysis, the efficacy of AA and the efficacy of cutaneous analgesia were considered as criterion variables. Grades I and II of efficacy of AA merged into Group 1 while Grades III and IV merged into Group 2 for analysis. Data of there two groups were processed by the Discriminant Analysis Method of multivariable statistics analysis. The cutaneous analgesic effects are expressed by –, +, ++ and +++ and these signs are used as subscripts of 0, 1, 2 and 3. The variables are screened by the multiple regression equation method. The results of our screened variables are shown in Table 1. The effect of the variables on the efficacy of AA is processed by the t-test formula of multiregression analysis. P vaues are divided into 5 grades, e.g., $P<0.01$, $P<0.05$, $P<0.10$, $P<0.15$ and $P\leqslant 0.15$; t or p values are the scales for measuring the importance of the variables.

All variables with t values greater than 1 are formed into the following forecasting formulas:

For craniotomy: $Yc=-59X_1-69X_2+70X_4+232.44X_7+94.96X_8-42.28X_{18}-241.$

If $Yc \leqslant 0$, the prediction result will belong to Group 1; if $Yc \geqslant 0$, the prediction result will belong to Group 2.

For strabotomy: $Ys=21.499X_3+67.735X_7+18.903X_8-26.295X_{10}-94.039X_{11}-0.359X_{13}-0.756X17+104.$

If $Ys<0$, the result of forecast will belong to Group 1; if $Y_s \geqslant 0$, the result will belong to Group 2.

For lung surgery (there are no Grades III and IV, so Grade I is considered as Group 1 and Grade II as Group 2):

$Y_L=16.214X_2-12.264X_4+4.604X_5-25.91X_11+4.22X_18+21.90$. If $Y_L<0$, the result of forecast will belong to Group 1; if $Y_L \geqslant 0$, the result will belong to Group 2.

For subtotal gastrectomy: $Y_{sg}=25.367X_1+19.651X_{10}-53.2$

If $Y_{sg} \geqslant 0$, the result of forecast will belong to Group 1; $Y_{sg}<0$, the result will belong to Group 2.

For hysterectomy: $Y_h=9.989X_9-19.45X_{16}-7.5$. If $Y_h \leqslant 0$, the result of forecast will belong to Group 1; if $Y_h>0$, the result will belong to Group 2.

For caesarean section: $Y_{cs}=61.4X_1-52X_4+53.49X_{10}-0.53X_{13}-149$. If $Y_{cs}<0$, the result will belong to Group 1; if $Y_{cs} \geqslant 0$, the result will belong to Group 2.

For appendectomy: $Yap=8.8052X_1+3.1304X_3-13.446X_4-13.27X_5-11.429X_6+1.8469X_8+1.7084X_9+31.412X_{11}-0.0865X_{13}+3.3732X_{14}-4.7563X_{15}-0.1858X_{17}+2.0648X_{18}-24.6$. If $Y_{ap}<0$; the result of forecast will belong to Group 1; if $Yap \geqslant 0$, the result will belong to Group 2.

For operation on extremeties: $Y_{oe}=-78.476X_2+30.365X_3+12.792X_9+109.04X_{10}-41.046X_{19}-140$. If $Y_{oe}<0$, the result of forecast will belong to Group 1; if $Y_{oe} \geqslant 0$, the result will belong to Group 2.

The tallying rates of the forecasts for all operations are shown in Table 2, among which the tallying rate of appendectomy is the highest (100%), that of craniotomy is the next highest and those of subtotal gastrectomy and hysterectomy are lowest.

The efficacy of cutaneous analgesia can also be shown by the following forecasting formulas (represented by U): $Uc=-55.02X_2+398.12X_7+1.04X_{13}-1.328X_{17}-24.88X_{18}-445$.

If $Uc<0$, the result of forecast will be good; if $Uc \geqslant 0$, the result will be poor.

$Ul=-13.314X_4+14.794X_7+1.733X_{15}-17$

If $Ul<0$, the result of forecast will be good; if $Ul \geqslant 0$, the result will be poor.

$Usg=62.774X_1+81.81X_2-96.11X_5+28.44X_{10}+24.31X_{16}+1.134X_{17}-162.$

If $Usg \geqslant 0$, the result of forecast will be good; if $Usg<0$, the result will be poor.

$U_h=33.91\ X_1-27.284\ X_9+51.16\ X_{10}+36.69\ X_{16}-101$. If $U_h \geqslant 0$, the result of forecast will be good; if $U_h<0$, the result will be poor.

$U_{cs}=31.55\ X_6+21.104\ X_{15}-1$. If $U_{cs} \geqslant 0$, the result of forecast will be good; if $U_{cs}<0$, the result will be poor.

$U_{ap}=5.293\ X_3+14.14\ X_5+8.576\ X_7-2.513\ X_8+0.1412\ X_{13}-2.786\ X_{14}-0.11\ X_{17}-3.302\ X_{18}-13.5$.

If $U_{ap} \leqslant 0$, the result of forecast will be good; if $U_{ap}>0$, the result will be poor.

$Uoe=157.08\ X_1+174.94\ X_2-55.33\ X_3+0.9494\ X_{12}-52.98\ X_{15}-30.702\ X_{18}+75.03\ X_{19}-230$.

If $U_{oe} \geqslant 0$, the result of forecast will be good; if $U_{oe}<0$, the result will be poor.

The tallying rates of the efficacy of cutaneous analgesia are shown in Table 3.

III. CONCLUSION

1. The effectiveness of acupuncture anesthesia (AA) can be forecasted more or less correctly before operation. In Table 2, the forecasts of some operations (such as appendectomy) coincide completely with the actual results. Though the rate of coincidence of subtotal gastrectomy forecast is low (0.662 and 0.611), it still has a statistical significance (X^2=6.47, P<0.02). There is no specific variable in Table 1, but it shows that if the appropriately selected variables are put together, it is possible to select the patient suitable to AA.

2. Different variables should be selected for forecasting the effectiveness of AA for operations of different locations; even for operations of the same location, the forecast of effectivenss of AA requires different variables from those for the efficacy of cutaneous analgesia. Table 1 shows that the variables selected for forecasting the overall effectivenss of AA and those for analgesic effect on the skin of the same operations are different, and the same is true with operations of different locations. Efforts should be made to find out more specific variables for particular operations in addition to the common variables selected for all operations (e.g., threshold of basic pain tolerance, etc.) in order to raise the accuracy of the forecast of effectivenss of AA Only a number of such variables are listed in Table 1; more new variables are searched for.

3. The effectiveness of AA is also influenced by psychological factors. In all the cases studied, data on such factors were complete in only four kinds of operations. If the effect of cutaneous analgesia is considered as a part of the overall effectiveness of AA, their effect in three out of the four kinds of operations listed in Table 1 is related with psychological factors. Psychological factors can exert some defenite influcnceon the effectiveness of AA.

4. Automatic analysis of the effectiveness of AA and the effect of cutaneous analgesia can be obtained by putting the program drawn up according to the forecast formula of the various operations into the computer.

IV. DISCUSSION

1. On the problem of how to raise the tallying rate of forecast of the effectiveness of AA.

There are generelly three factors that determine the accuracy of the forecast on the effectiveness of AA:

(1) The individuality of the patient;

(2) The conditions of the operation, especially the condition of the lesion, simple or complicated, and the skill of the surgeon;

(3) The reliability of the data on the various pain thresholds of the patient undergoing the operation, especially the objectivity of the final overall judgement.

The present paper is mainly concerned with the investigation of the functional state of the patient and the interrelation between the efficacy of needling and the effectiveness of AA under laboratory conditions. It does not include the status of the patient at the operation and the conditions of operation; the measurement of various psychological, physiological and biochemical indices should be done under the condition of the operation theater. According to past experience, preoperation talk to the patient to dispel his worries and increase his confidence in the effect of AA and the professional skill of the operation team will all contribute substantially to the success of AA. All of these should be considered in the preoperation forecast.

2. How to treat the variables not selected in Table 1.

From the mathematical viewpoint, there are generally 3 possibilities:

(1) The variable in question is significant for forecast, but it is not selected because it is an individual difference, the error in its measurement is large and there are not enough number of cases of it. That is to say the variable would be selected, and their t-value would be increased when the number of cases increases and the accuracy of its measuresuent is improved.

(2) Some variables closely relating to other variables selected were not selected. This could indicate that only their correlated part would be significant for forecast while their uncorrelated part would not.

(3) The variable is actually not signficant for forecasting the effectiveness of AA.

With the above reasons we could explain why certain indices (i.e., basic pain tolerance threshold X_1) are not selected in a number of operations. For instance, in case of strabotomy, the coefficient of correlation between X_1 and X_{17} is as great as 0.61 ($P<0.01$) and between X_1 and X_3 is as great as 0.23 ($P<0.05$), and X_3 and X_{13} have been selected, so X_1 might not be selected, and X_1 would meet with the same fate in lobectomy. Nevertheless, we cannot conclude that X_1 is not significant for forecasting the effectiveness of AA in strabotomy and lobectomy.

3. The common variables for effectiveness forecast in different kinds of operations.

Following the foregoing discussion, the variables with more "*" symbols in Table 1 could be taken as the common variables for forecast of the effectivenes of AA. There are 9 of them: the basic pain tolerance threshold, X_1; the tactile sensation threshold of Neiguan point before needling, X_{10}; the pulse rate at rest, X_{13}; psychological factors, X_{16}; Sex, X_{18}; age, X_{17}; the change in pain tolerance threshold after needling, X_2; the change in tactile sensation threshold at the site of incision after needling, X_4; and the change in pulse rate after needling, X_7.

These variables fall into 4 main categories:

(1) The sensitivity of cutaneous sensation (X_1 and X_{10});

(2) The functional state of the autonomic nervous system (X_{13});

(3) The efficacy of needling (X_2, X_4 and X_7);

(4) Psychic and other variations (X_{16}, X_{17} and X_{18}).

Further studies of the underlying rules and the materialistic basis of the above variables will throw more light on the nature of AA.

4. The following items should be considered in clinical application of the forecast formula:

(1) The conditions necessary for applying the formula. The forecast was made in the present study with assigned instruments and defined criteria 3 days before operation. The discrepancies between hospitals and especially the evaluation of the efficacy of AA should

be reduced to the minimum.

(2) The flexibility in the application of the formula. All the formulas mentioned above take the complex value Y=0 as a limit. But in practice, for ensuring the reliability of the forecast, the Y values of each kind of operation can be divided into 3 ranges: (i) the range indicating that the result would certainly belong to Group 1, (ii) the range indicating that the result would certainly belong to Group 2, (iii) the range that cannot predict the result with certainty. In cases of this range, other clinical data should be consulted in order to forecast their effectiveness.

According to the distribution of the Y-value of each operation, the 3 ranges of each Y-value are specified as follows:

Craniotomy: if $Y_c \leqslant -12$, effectivenesswould be Group 1; if $Yc \geqslant 40$; it would be Group2; if Yc lies between –12 and 40, other clinical data should be consulted.

Strabotomy: if $Ys < -17$, effectiveness would be Group 1; if $Ys \geqslant -17$, other clinical data should be consulted.

Caesarean section: if $Ycs \geqslant 10$, effectiveness would be Group 1; if $Ycs \leqslant -20$, it would be group 2; if Ycs-values lie between –20 and 10, other clinical data should be consulted.

Lung resection: if $Y_L \geqslant 3$, effectiveness would be Group 1; if $Y_L \leqslant -3$, it would be Group 2; if Y_L-values lies between –3 and 3, other clinical data should be consulted.

Appendectomy: if $Yap \geqslant 3$, effectiveness would be Group 1; if $Yap \leqslant -3$, it would be Group 2; if Yap lies between –3 and 3, other clinical data should be consulted.

Operation on extremities; if $Yoe \geqslant 15$, effectiveness would be Group 2; if $Yoe \leqslant -40$, it would be Group 1; and if Yoe lies between –40 and 15, other clinical data should be consulted.

Y-values of subtotal gastrectomy and hysterectomy overlap each other, and their ranges are difficult to determine. The forecast of cutaneous analgesic effect could be made in the same way as above, but it is still more difficult, because to a certain extent it is already included in the evaluation of the effectiveness of AA. So it will not be discussed here at length.

(3) The reliability and stability of the formulas. Theoretically, the formulas for forecast in each kind of operation stated above is generally reliable and stable if the number of cases is very large, as the cases reflect the actual objectivity. In the present study, the number of cases is not very large, and it is questionable whether they really represent the actual condition objectively. For instance, in craniotomy, a conclusion was reached from the forecast formula that females are more suitable for AA. than the males, but the reverse is true in other kinds of operations. This controversy leads to doubt about whether the cases selected in each kind of operation can objectively reflect the actual conditions. In order to improve the reliability and stability of the forecast formulas, we should, first of all, start with the further investigation of the effect of AA objectively and increase the number of cases to as many as possible, so the practical value of the formulas in the present study can be verified and modified.

Table 1. Screening of Forecast Variations of the A.A. and C.A. in Various Operation

Operation	Craniotomy				Strabotomy				Lung Resection			
No. of Cases	38				78				30			
Efficacy	A.A.		C.A.		A.A.		A.A.		C.A.		A.A.	
Name of Variables	t	p	t	p	t	p	t	p	t	p	t	p
x_1 lg Basic PTT	2.169	***	0.551		0.565		0.4045		0.2939		1.391	**
x_2 lg $\frac{\text{PTT After Needling}}{\text{Basic PTT}}$	1.151	*	1.078	*	0.327		1.2485	*	0.6279		0.633	
x_3 lg $\frac{\text{PT After Needling}}{\text{PT Before Needling}}$	0.366		0.349		1.475	**	0.9665		0.0729		0.166	
x_4 lg $\frac{\text{Incision TS After Needling}}{\text{Incision TS Before Needling}}$	1.455	**	0.230		0.434		1.4903	**	1.5313	**	0.480	
x_5 lg $\frac{\text{TTpD of Forearm After Needling}}{\text{TTpD of Forearm Before Needling}}$	0.362		0.034		0.182		1.1539	*	0.5074		0.312	
x_6 lg $\frac{\text{TTpD of Incision After Needling}}{\text{TTpD of Incision Before Needling}}$	0.015		0.823		0.279		0.4095		0.6493		0.169	
x_7 lg $\frac{\text{Heart Rate After Needling}}{\text{Heart Rate Before Needling}}$	1.362		1.629	**	1.107	*	0.2361		1.3544	**	0.602	
x_8 lg $\frac{\text{Wave Amplitude After Needling}}{\text{Wave Amplitude Before Needling}}$	2.612		0.529		1.366		0.7473		0.3305		0.064	

Subtotal Gastrectomy				Hysterectomy				Caesarean Section				Appendectomy				Operation on the Extremities			
100				99				71				39				77			
C.A.		A.A.		C.A.		A.A.		C.A.		A.A.		C.A.		A.A.		C.A.		C.A.	
t	p	t	p	t	p	t	p	t	p	t	p	t	p	t	p	t	p	t	p
2.789	****	0.188		1.765	***	2.315	***	0.546		2.255	***	0.234		0.619		2.676	****	0.946	
1.948	****	0.162		0.023		0.556		0.571		0.103		0.005		1.414	**	2.032	***	0.906	
0.185		0.058		0.494		0.068		0.587		1.203	*	1.901	***	1.081	*	1.130	*	0.860	
0.269		0.606		0.113		1.519	**	0.485		3.571	****	0.536							
1.421	**	0.185		0.064		0.124		0.121		2.882	****	2.258	***	0.088		0.148		0.229	
0.349		0.2001		0.358		0.500		1.023		3.629	****	0.170							
0.084		0.041		0.378		0.591		0.862		0.373		1.159	*	0.565		0.243		0.182	
0.035		0.702		0.175		0.885		0.970		1.200	*	1.397	**						

Table 1. Screening of Forecast Variations of the A.A. and C.A. in Various Operation

Operation	Craniotomy				Strabotomy				Lung Resection			
No. of Cases	38				78				30			
Efficacy	A.A.		C.A.		A.A.		A.A.		C.A.		A.A.	
Name of Variables	t	p	t	p	t	p	t	p	t	p	t	p
x_9 lg $\frac{\text{Wave Amplitude After 15' Incision}}{\text{Wave Amplitude at Rest}}$	0.560		0.965		0.570		0.0283		0.4590		0.784	
x_{10} lg "Neiguan" TS Before	0.066		0.290		2.090	**	0.1628		0.7897		1.182	*
x_{11} $\frac{\text{Pulse Rate After 15' Incision}}{\text{Pulse Rate at Rest}}$	0.428		0.780		1.584	**	1.008		0.5672			
x_{12} Pulse Rate After 15, Incision											0.112	
x_{13} Pulse Rate at Rest	0.283		1.223	*	1.057	*	0.7502		0.6396		0.478	
x_{14} Spontaneous Wave at Rest	0.363		0.595		0.2293		1.1197	*	0.5926		0.561	
x_{15} Spontaneous Wave After 15′ Incision	0.678		0.784		0.118		0.2842		1.3035		0.272	
x_{16} Psychological Factor											0.793	
x_{17} Age	0.173		1.083	*	1.449	**	0.1862		0.4382		0.069	
x_{18} Sex	1.924	***	1.407	**	0.493		1.4704	**	0.7206			
x_{19} Incision TS After Needling					0.460							

PTT— Pain Tolerance Threshold PT— Pain Threshold

Subtotal Gastrectomy				Hysterectomy				Caesarean Section				Appendectomy				Operation on the Extremities			
100				99				71				39				77			
C.A.		A.A.		C.A.		A.A.		C.A.		A.A.		C.A.		A.A.		C.A.		C.A.	
t	p	t	p	t	p	t	p	t	p	t	p	t	p	t	p	t	p	t	p
0.108		1.002		2.049	***	0.470		0.025		1.387	**	0.601		1.31	**	0.844		0.595	
1.314	**	0.071		1.902	***	1.503	**	0.693		0.337		0.072		3.057	****	0.646		0.664	
		0.002		0.078		0.364		0.128		2.569	****	0.167							
1.116	*													0.577		1.112	*	0.613	
0.810		0.235		0.325		1.079	*	0.804		1.521	****	1.639	**	1.064	*	0.612		1.069	
0.037		0.927		0.630		0.770		0.693		1.435	**	1.610	**	0.998		0.367		0.235	
0.738		0.734		0.221		0.802		1.574	**	2.633	****	0.961		0.134		1.544		0.583	
1.452	**	2.186	***	0.897		0.503								1.108	*	0.0054		0.800	
1.843	***	0.442		0.115		0.252		0.157		2.493	***	1.309	*	0.195		0.028		0.482	
										1.617	**	1.860	***	0.551		1.134	*	0.242	
														1.155	*	1.615	**	1.027	

TS— Tactile Sensation

TTpD— Threshold of Two-point Discrimination

Table 2. Rate of Agreement of the Forecast Efficacy of Anaesthesia in Various Operation

Name of Opesation	Craniotomy		Strabotomy		Lung Resection		Subtotal Gastrectomy		Hysterectomy		Caesarean Section		Appendectomy		Operation on the Extremities	
Group	Group 1	Group 2	Group 1	Group 2	Group 1	Group 2	Group 1	Group 2	Group 1	Group 2	Group 1	Group 2	Group 1	Group 2	Group 1	Group 2
No. of Cases	37	9	57	21	20	10	68	35	77	22	52	20	22	17	35	64
Rate of Agreement	0.838	1.00	0.702	0.810	0.850	0.800	0.662	0.600	0.611	0.720	0.750	0.900	1.00	1.00	0.886	0.50

Note: Here the number of cases is greater than that of Table 3 In the Operations of Lung resection, Group 1 is of Grade I, Group 2 is of Grade II (Here is no Grades III and IV)

Table 3. Rate of Agreement of Forecast Efficacy of Cutaneous Analgesis of Various Operation

Name of Opesation	Craniotomy		Lung Resection		Subtotal Gastrectomy		Hysterectomy		Caesarean Section		Appendectomy		Operation on the Extremities	
Group	Group 1	Group 2	Group 1	Group 2	Group 1	Group 2	Group 1	Group 2	Group 1	Group 2	Group 1	Group 2	Group 1	Group 2
No. of Cases	32	10	25	5	48	53	37	55	15	56	11	28	54	45
Rate of Agreement	0.906	0.700	0.680	0.600	0.813	0.623	0.568	0.673	0.600	0.572	0.818	0.964	0.778	0.556

EXPERIMENTAL STUDY OF SCREENING OF STIMULATION PARAMETERS OF ELECTRIC NEEDLING IN ACUPUNCTURE ANESTHESIA

Shi Minsheng, Zhang Jian, Cong Yinbin, Liu Runqi, Li Baoqin, Jia Zhiping
(Research Group of Acupuncture Anesthesia, Department of Surgery, Beijing Chaoyang Hospital)

In the clinical practice and theoretical study of acupuncture anesthesia, instead of manual needling, the acupuncture anesthesia apparatus is at present widely used as a means of stimulation to maintain the needle sensation at the point. In clinical practice, the selection of electric acupuncture parameters is generally considered to be closely connected with the effect of acupuncture anesthesia. Therefore, a reasonable control of the amount of stimulation is an importment condition for increasing the efficacy of acupuncture anesthesia, which makes it necessary to select the stimulation parameters of electric acupuncture so as to obtain the appropriate stimulation conditions for acupuncture anesthesia. For this reason, under the guidance of the Higher Mathematic Research Group and the Department of Biology of Beijing University, we have designed a set of animal experiments to observe the influence of several related main stimulation parameters of electric acupuncture on the effect of acupuncture anesthesia.

I. METHOD

1. Experimental subject. Adult grey-haired rabbits, regardless of kind and sex, weighing 2–3kg, are randomly assigned experimental numbers.

2. Pain Stimuli. The simulated acute traumatic process in surgical abdominal exploration is used as pain stimuli in the following way: Without any anesthetics, a paramedian incision of about 10 cm in length is made on the abdomen of the animal, and the whole process is carried out in five steps, namely, cutting of the skin, cutting of the muscle and the peritoneum, traction of the mensentery, sewing of the muscle and sewing of the skin.

The operation is performed by preassigned persons according to the prearranged procedure, so as to keep the condition for pain stimulation as stable as possible.

3. The determining and recording of behaviour responses to pain. An inflated rubber bag of 20 by 8 cm is put under the back of the animal lying fastened on the operation table, and the changes in the bag pressure produced by the struggle of the animal are recorded on paper by the blood pressure graphic device of the Galileo four-lead physiological recorder. The struggle reaction of the animal during the simulated operative process is quantitatively

calculated with the sum of the altitudes of wave amplitude.

During the experiment, in the closed system in which the blood pressure graphic device is connected to the bag on the operation table, a constant pressure of 50 mmHg. is maintained in order to keep the sensitivity of the graphic pen constant. The running rate of the recording paper is 2.5 mm/s.

4. Conditions for acupuncture anesthesia.

(1) Acupuncture points: Corresponding to the human bilateral "Zusanli" and "Sanyin-jiao".

(2) Acupuncture parameters: See orthogonal design of experiment project.

(3) Induction time: 20 minutes. In the initial 5 minutes of induction, the intensity of stimulation is gradually increased to the fixed electric current.

(4) The constant current quantitative acupuncture anesthesia apparatus made by ourselves is used for electric acupuncture. Its intensity of electric stimulation, wave amplitude and frequency are adjustable, and the range of different parameters can meet the requirement of the designed experiment, and the quantitative mesurements are shown in figures.

II. DESIGN AND RESULTS

In order to obtain in fewer experiments the main electric acupuncture parameters influencing the effect of acupuncture anesthesia our group used the mathmatical design of multiplefactor orthogonal tables to arrange groups. The factors and grades of the electric acupuncture stimulation parameters observed selectively are as follows.

Grade / Factor	1	2	3
1 Intensity	3mA	4mA	5mA
2 Ratio of loaded to unloaded	1%	10%	20%
3 Wave amplitude	1,000μs	250μs	2.5μs

Under the fixed wave amplititude and the ratio of loaded to unloaded the frequency is observed by mobile gradation, and out of the range of 10,000–100,000 Hz, 9 grades of 10, 20, 100, 200, 400, 800, 4,000, and 80,000 Hz are made.

Wave form of the electric acupuncture stimulation. Bidirectional rectangular wave.

As the experiment reguires, the selected orthogonal table $L_9^{(3^3)}$ is a 9-experiment project with 3 factors and 3 grades. For the quantitative analysis of the experiment design and results, see Table 1.

This table includes two items:

1. Experiment design. 1,2 3 show the three grades of the respective factors, and the figures in parentheses represent the parameters of the respective grades.

2 Responses. They are the struggle responses of the rabbit in the whole process of the experimental operation; the figures in the lower part of the table are calculations made

on the basis of these responses

It can be seen from Table 1 that when the simulated surgical abdominal exploration is made on the rabbit under acupuncture anesthesia the observation of the effect of such factors as stimulation intensity wave amplitude, frequency and the ratio of loaded to unloaded of electric acupuncture on the acupuncture anesthesia reveals:

(1) The polar differences between the 3 grades of each factor are not equal According to orthogonal analysis, it is believed that the difference between the total responses of the 3 grades of intensity is the biggest which is the main factor influencing the efficacy of acupuncture anesthesia.

(2) Among the intensity factors, the total response of the third grade is the smallest and among the nine combinations formed by each grade with a different grade of another factor, the best combination is the 5mA combination of the third grade. In the three combinations of 5mA (experiment nos. 3,6,9), all the struggle responses of the animal are

Table 1. Experiment Design — **Exp. Results**

Factor / Exp. No.	Intensity mA	Loaded: Unloaded %	Freq. (Hz)	Wave Amplitude μs	Struggle response mm
1	1(3mA)	1(1%)	(4000)	3	366
2	2(4mA)	1	(10)	1	447
3	3(5mA)	1	(40)	2	134.5
4	1	2(10%)	(400)	2	349
5	2	2	(40000)	3	538
6	3	2	(100)	1	376
7	1	3(20%)	(200)	1(1000)	518
8	2	3	(800)	2(250)	439
9	3	3	(80000)	3(2.5)	391.5
1 Sum of 3 struggle responses in grade 1	1233	947.5		1341	
2=Sum of 3 struggle responses in grade 2	1424	1263		922.5	
3=Sum of 3 struggle responses in grade 3	902	1348.5		1269.5	
Polar diff. R=maximum no, in 1,2, 3 minus minimum no.	522	401		418.5	

smaller.

(3) In the second grade of wave amplitude and the first grade of the ratio of loaded to unloaded, the response to pain is the least in the three grades of the factor. According to orthogonal analysis, wave amplitude 250 μs and the ratio of loaded to unloaded, 1% are better conditions.

(4) Frequency is a mobile grade under the condition of selected wave amplitude and the ratio of loaded to unloaded, and in our experiment its relation to the effect of acupuncture anesthesia is not obvious

To further prove the experiment results given in Table 1, under the better conditions of the three factors of intensity, wave amplitude and frequency, we arranged a set of densified experiments. The two grades of each of the three factors selected for densified observation are given in Table 2.

According to the requirement of experiment, the selection of orthogonal Table $L_4(2^3)$ is a four experiment program of 3 factors and 2 grades. The experiment design and the quantitative analysis of the results are given in Table 3. The explanation is the same as of Table 1.

Table 2.

Factor / Grade	Intensity	Wave Amplitude	Frequency
1	4.4mA	500μs	100Hz
2	5.4mA	250μs	50Hz

Table 3.

Experiment Design				Experiment Result
Factor / Exp. No.	Intensity mA	Wave Amplitude μs	Frequency Hz	Struggle response mm
1	1(4.4mA)	1	1(100)	354
2	2(5.4mA)	1(500μs)	2(50)	475
3	1	2(250)	2	227
4	2	2	1	161
1=Sum of 2 struggle responses in grade 1	581	829	575	
2=Sum of 2 struggle responses in grade 2	636	388	702	
Polar diff. R=maximum no. in 1,2, minus minimum no.	55	441	187	

It can be seen from Table 2:

1. The difference between two grades 4.4mA and 5.4mA of the intensity factor is very small, indicating the correct conclusion that the third grade 5mA of intensity in Table 1 has a favorable effect on acupuncture anesthesia.

2. Under the condition of a relatively constant intensity, in the three factors, the difference between the total responses to the two grades of wave amplitude is maximum, while in the factor the total response to the second grade is small According to the orthogonal analysis the wave amplitude 250 μs is a better condition. This result also proves that the results given in Table 1 are correct.

III. DISCUSSION

1. Screening of Electric Acupuncture parameters by the Orthogonal Design.

The orthogonal design is a scientific method for making multiple factor experiments. Because of their characteristics of equal distribution, uniformity and comparability, the orthogonal tables can be used to find out in fewer experiments the main factor influencing the experiment effect among multiple factors, and also the proper parameters of the various factors.

As the screening of the electric acupuncture stimulation parameters involves many factors and a wide range, though the single factor optimum seeking method may be used, the arrangement of recombined experiments after each single factor experimentation is not only inefficient but also unable to give prominent display to the main factor. The use of multiple factor orthogonal design of mathematics in the grouping design of our experiment to screen electric acupuncture stimulation parameters proves to be effective.

2. The Relationship of Electric Acupuncture Stimulation Parameters to the Efficacy of Acupuncture Anesthesia.

During acupuncture anesthesia the points should be induced by stimulation. However, many clinical results indicate that too weak stimulation will be inefficient and that too strong stimulation will not be toleraable to the patient. Therefore, an ideal amount of stimulation is an important condition to increase the efficacy of acupuncture anesthesia, and it is necessary that we screen the electric acupuncture stimulation parameters in order to obtain this ideal amount of stimulation.

The amount of stimulation of the acupuncture anesthesia apparatus is determined by the parameters of its pulse amplitude (intensity), wave width and frequency. The use of multiple factor orthogonal design of mathematics in our experiment design enabled us to carry out at the same time two groups of observation on the three factors, intensity, wave amplitude, and frequency, and to find that intensity is the main factor influencing the efficacy of acupuncture anesthesia. The third grade 5mA intensity is the most effective. The grade design in intensity experiment is based on the three grades of 3mA, 4mA and 5mA selected from between the intensities of electric acupuncture stimulation to which the animal began to response and the biggest amount the animal can tolerate. The selected 5mA is correlated with the selected standard amount of stimulation, i.e., the biggest stimulation tolerable to the patient. The result of our animal experiment is correlated with our experience gained in clinical practice.

Frequency is another important parameter influencing the amount of electric acupuncture stimulation. In recent years there have been reports in our country and abroad on the fact that a better effect of acupuncture anesthesia can be obtained by increasing the frequency of eletric acupuncture (some reported a frequency of 100,000 Hz). At present most of the electric stimulation frequency of the acupuncture anesthesia apparatus generally used in our country is between 1 and 50 Hz, and some types of the apparatus have 200 or 2000 Hz. Even the latter is far from the frequency quoted before. In order to investigate in a wider range the effect of frequency on the acupuncture anesthesia, we made an experiment on nine grades of frequency within the range of 10,000–100,000 Hz, and found that the change in frequency has no obvious effect on acupuncture anesthesia. However, further analys of the component factor of frequency, the ratio of loaded to unloaded, shows that the 1% group has a better effect on acupuncture anesthesia. This suggests that in our observation of frequency we need further study on the two determinant factors of frequency—the combination of wave amplitude and the ratio of loaded to unloaded.

STUDY OF ROLE OF PSYCHOLOGICAL FACTORS IN ACUPUNCTURE ANESTHESIA*

Xu Shulian, Song Weizhen, Guo Nianfeng,
Sun Changhua, Wu Zhenyun
(Institute of Psychology, Academia Sinica)

Not long after the beginning of the application of acupuncture anesthesia, the question on the role played by psychological factors in it came to draw much attention from Chinese scientists. Up to the present, quite a number of studies have been made on the relationship between acupuncture anesthesia on the one hand, and various psychological factors such as emotional state[1,2], suggestiveness[3,4,5], distraction[1], overconcern (worrying) about acupuncture anesthesia[1], mental readiness (preparedness)[6,7], etc. as well as some psychological characteristics[3,8,9] on the other.

Since the work of acupuncture anesthesia was made public to the world in 1972, not a few foreign authors have also done much research work on acupuncture analgesia with human subjects, a considerable portion of which is for evaluating the role played by psychological factors in it. Some authors suggest that acupuncture anesthesia is one form of hypnosis anesthesia, and the acupuncture chiefly plays a role of suggestion and placebo[10,11]; and others, however, found there is real analgesic effect of acupuncture[12,13,14]. They also employed the signal detection theory to analyze acupuncture analgesic effect and contradictory results were obtained. For example, a reduction of the sensory discriminability (d') after acupuncture was found and some relative physiological mechanism underlying the analgesic effect was suggested in some work[15]; while in another paper it was found that acupuncture analgesic effect is mainly of a psychological character, since only the response bias is found to have raised after acupuncture[16]. The problem whether psychological characteristics such as the influence of anxiety affect acupuncture effect has also been explored[17,18,19].

The purpose of this paper is to review the work of our research group during the period 1974–1978 and, on the basis of it, to put forth our idea about the role of psychological factors in acupuncture anesthesia and acupuncture analgesia.

We have explored the relation of five of the psychological factors generally accepted with acupuncture effect, and these five factors are: the emotional state on entering the operation room, overconcern (worrying) about acupuncture anesthesia, trust (confidence) in acupuncture and operator, influence of suggesetiveness and mental readiness

---

* This series of study was completed with the cooperation and support of Beijing Institute of Tubereulosis, Beijing Institute of Neurosurgery and other Institutions.

(preparedness). The influence of some psychological characteristics — the compound sensitivity of cutaneous sensations, the accuracy of time estimation and the discriminating reaction performance (reaction time, the fluctuation of RT and number of errors) to acupuncture anesthesia effect has also been studied. In addition, the Beijing Institute of Tuberculosis performed the predicting test of acupuncture effect with the fluctuations of pulse, respiration and GSR during acupuncture as indices; and it was shown that the result of this test was significantly correlated with the actual acupuncture effect[20]. We have thus compared the result of this predicting test with the factors described above.

As a routine, we carried out several examinations or investigations in one and the same subject, and some factors such as emotion, suggestion, etc., were studied together with the observation on physiological functions (the pulse, respiration, GSR responses recorded with a multiple physiological recorder) or the biochemical functions (the plasma 11-Hydroxycorticosteroid or 11-OHCS). This allowed us to look into the relationship between these factors.

Our principal results are as follows.

I. THE INFLUENCE OF EMOTIONAL STATE ON ENTERING THE OPERATION ROOM ON THE EFFECT OF ACUPUNCTURE ANESTHESIA

Two methods were used to evaluate Ss' emotional states: the clinical behavior observation method and the verbal report method. In the clinical observation method the emotional state of the patient was assessed by psychologist and acupuncturist through discussion on the basis of the patient's overt behavior of facial expression, actions and utterances on entering the operation room. The verbal report method was based upon the patient's answers to some prepared questions on entering the operation room, which were rechecked by follow-up questioning. By "emotional states" we mean the emotional states of the patient from the time of entering the operation room to the insertion of the acupuncture needle, and these states were classified as stable, medium, and tense.

The clinically observed emotional states were found to exert some influence on the physiological responses to acupuncture insertion, which was measured by the changes in pulse amplitude, respiration curve and GSR . This influence was shown in an extremely significant correlation between these states and the responses to insertion, with weak responses by patients of stable emotions and strong responses by most of the tense cases ($N=47$, $X^2=19.2$, $P<0.001$). A group of 69 patients were first studied and afterwards a second group of 32 patients and in both these studies it was found that emotional states are closely correlated with the effect of acupuncture anesthesia—the emotionally tense patients always have poor acupuncture effect ($X^2=17.95$, $P<0.005$ and $X^2=19.93$, $P<0.001$ respectively).

The correlation between acupuncture effect and emotional states assessed by the verbal report method, is also statistically significant ($X=14.42$, $P<0.01$).

Moreover, the dynamic changes in emotional state is of great importance. As a rule, patients who become tenser and tenser during operation always have poor effect, but others who are at first somewhat tense but soon become calmer and calmer often have good effect. And the emotional state just before acupuncture and that just before incision are also signs of acupuncture effect.

The relations of clinically observed emotional states to physiological and psychological functions are as follows: (1) Patients who are overconcerned (worried) about acupuncture anesthesia are usually tense when entering the operation room (N=99, X^2=21.06, P<0.001); (2) All the emotionally stable patients will complete time estimation test more accurately on entering the operation room than in the ward, but results with patients who are emotionally tense are just the opposite; (3) In patients in tense and medium emotional states, the increase of plasma 11-OHCS on entering the operation room with reference to that tested in the ward would be more significant thanin emotionally stable patients (N=47, P<0.05); (4) Most of the emotionally tense patients have greater fluctuations in respiration when lying quietly after entering the operation room (N=51, X^2=16.5, P<0.01); (5) The fluctuation of pulse amplitude when lying quietly also significantly correlates with the emotional state (N=50, X^2=9.89, P<0.05); (6) The compound fluctuations of respiration, and GSR are extremely significantly correlated with the emotional states (N=51, X=23.07, P<0.001); (7) The result of physiological predicting test, based upon the combined fluctuations of the three above mentioned indices observed during acupuncture in the laboratory before operation, is also remarkedly closely associated with the emotional states, with larger fluctuations for the tense patients than for the calm ones (N101, X^2=14.16, P<0.01); and (8) Hypersensitive patients, evaluated through the compound cutaneous sensitivity tests of touch and pain before operation, are usually emotionally tense when entering the operation room (N=87, X^2=14.17, P<0.01).

It is interesting that in our experimental condition, the combined fluctuations of the three physiological indices mentioned above, the increment of plasma 11-OHCS and the change in the accuracy of time estimation are all closely related to emotional states and the patients' emotional states are closely correlated with the acupuncture anesthesia effect in both of the two groups. However, each of these three kinds of functional levels on entering the operation room is itself not significantly correlated with this effect. And the same is true with patients' overconcern about acupuncture. It seems that the emotional state is influenced by these levels of factors and presumably by others too, and it in turn gives a feedback action to the latter simultaneously. Thus, the influence of emotional state on acupuncture anesthesia might be considered as a compound action, the combined effect of which is stronger than that of any single factor.

According to the data obtained, the emotional state assessed by observation of the patient's facial expression, action and utterance should have its corresponding material basis. The emotional activities are related with overconcern, higher cognitive activity, and the functional status of several levels of the central nervous system as well as the stress hormone levels. That is to say, they correspond to the functional states of the different levels of the cortex, the subcortical structures and the hypothalamus-hypophysis-adrenal system. Emotional state seems to be a compounded external expression of these functions, and also sends a feedback information simultaneously to the neurohormone system, thus influencing the acupuncture process.

II. RESEARCH ON THE COMPOUND SENSITIVITIES OF CUTANEOUS SENSATIONS

106 patients for lung resection and 59 for brain resection were studied, and a markedly significant correlation was shown between the compound sensitivities of touch and pain

sensations and the effects of acupuncture anesthesia (X^2=23.63, P<0.001 for lung resection patients; X^2=17.61, P<0.005 for brain resection patients) the hyposensitives in touch and pain sensations at the loci of acupuncture points and incision site often had better effects. This compound sensitivity of cutaneous sensations is also highly correlated with the results of the predicting test of the combined responses of three physiological indices during acupuncture. It was found that patients showing greater changes in these indices during needle insertion usually are sensitive patients in the compound sensitivity test (N=112, X=15.67, P<0.005).

From these results, it appears that the hypersensitivity of cutaneous sensations might be a sign of functional weakness of the nervous system, which might be one important factor that influences the pain-tolerance, the needle-tolerance and the acupuncture effect. The fact that touch sensitivities have relation with the acupuncture process suggests that an important role in acupuncture anesthesia is played by the large fibers transmitting information of touch and the functional characteristics of their cęnters.

III. STUDIES ON THE ROLE OF THE SUGGESTION FACTOR–THREE RESEARCH EXPERIMENTS HAVE BEEN MADE ON THE ROLE OF THIS FACTOR

The essential method is to examine the suggestibility of the subject and then investigate its relation with the effect of acupuncture anesthesia or acupuncture analgesia. The S's suggestibility is evaluated by word induction together with the scale amplitude on the oscilloscope as suggestive stimulus—a method designed by our research group.

1. The relationship between suggestibility and the effect of acupuncture anesthesia: subjects were patients prepared for taking lung resection under acupuncture anesthesia. After suggestion, the threshold of electric touch increased on an average of 28.1% and that of pain 20.3% (P<0.001 for both).

The suggestibility of pain was highly correlated with the sensitivity to pain; the more sensitive, the more suggestible (X^2=17.83, P<0.005). The suggestibility of electric touch and electric pain as a whole also has a high correlation with the sensitivity of the 4 cutaneous sensations compounded; here again the more sensitive patients were those who showed more suggestibility (X^2=15.05, P<0.01).

No significant correlation was found between suggestibility and the effect of acupuncture anesthesia (X=6.48, 0.20>P>0.10) but it appears that among patients showing favorable effect more than half were more suggestible.

Nor is suggestibility related to the data from physiological prediction test which has been shown to be consistent with the actual effect of acupuncture anesthesia. On the other hand, it has a high negative correlation with the compound cutaneous sensitivity evaluated by the 4 indices mentioned above. Thus it may be inferred that suggestion is not a dominantly affecting factor in acupuncture anesthesia, yet it may exert a moderate influence on it, either increasing or decreasing its effect.

2. In one experiment, the subjects were 30 normal adults, and the inhibitory changes in cerebral potentials evoked by painful stimulation during acupuncture were used as the index of acupuncture analgesia. It was shown that most of the Subjects (21/30) exhibited an inhibitory effect during the short period of 2–3' of acupuncture. However, the magnitude of

the inhibitory effect did not correlate either with the subjects' suggestibility ($F=1.27$, $P>0.05$), or with their trust (confidence) in acupuncture analgesia ($X^2=0.83$, $P>0.50$). This result indicates that to acupuncture analgesia the suggestion factor is irrelevant.

3. In another experiment with 21 normal adults as subjects, it was observed that under the condition of stimulating Sanyanglao point manually and after an induction period of 25–30' the verbal reports of heavy pain markedly decreased in number (on an average of 67.8%). Furthermore, the rate of occurrence of the heavy pain reports showed high negative correlation with the endorphine (OLS) contained in the subjects' blood after acupuncture, the more the OLS, the more the heavy pain reports decreased (through linear regression function analysis, $r=-0.65$, $P<0.01$). The Subjects' decrease of heavy pain reports also correlated with the increase of their blood histamine (HA) after pain stimuli— subjects' with more decrement of heavy pain reports often showed a smaller increment in blood HA($X^2=5.00$, $P=0.025$). However, the increment of suggestibility has no relevance to the inhibition of heavy pain reports of the subjects ($t=0.044$, $P>0.50$). The result of this experiment indicates that acupuncture analgesia cannot be explained solely by psychological factors such as suggestion and the like.

As a conclusion of the three studies cited above, it was demonstrated that the role played by the suggestion factor in acupuncture anesthesia or acupuncture analgesia is not significant. But the condition of a patient under the clinical acupuncture anesthesia is somewhat different from that of a normal adult subject in an acupuncture analgesia experiment. Under the laboratory condition the role of suggestion in acupuncture analgesia is not seen at all, while in the clinic there is a tendency of positive correlation between the patient's suggestibility and the effect of aupuncture anesthesia. This tendency might be attributed to the patient's confidence in the doctors and his desire for treatment. The psychological states of patients and those of normal adult subjects in an experiment were thus quite different.

IV. MENTAL READINESS (PREPAREDNESS) AND ACUPUNCTURE ANALGESIA

An experiment was carried out with two normal subject groups for comparison, one mentally-ready group and one control group. The mental readiness of the subjects in both groups was produced by different instructions: for the control group the subjects were only told that an experiment of acupuncture analgesia was going to be conducted, while for the mentally-ready group, the subjects were told in addition that "acupuncture can induce analgesia, but there will be still some pain", and were given some knowledge of the sequence, quality and feeling about the stimuli. 48 normal adults were treated as subjects, with 24 for each group. The subjects in the two groups were matched in sex, age and sensitivity estimated by the combined results of the three tests for 1) compound cutaneous sensitivity; 2)combined responses of pulse amplitude, respiration and GSR during acupuncture; and 3) pain tolerance to spring pinch. There were 10 sensitives and 14 hyposensitives in each group.

As the results showed, pain feelings of the subjects to stimuli were sharper and the evoked GSR larger for the control group than for the mentally-ready group, especially in the sensitives. There were also significant differences in pulse response and in the combined responses of the three physiological indices between the sensitives in one group and those in the other. However, the difference between the hyposensitives of the two groups was not significant in any index.

Both the pain feelings and the combined evoked physiological responses of the sensitives were markedly higher than those of the hyposensitives, whichever group the subjects belonged to ($P<0.001$). This suggests that in the mechanism of acupuncture analgesia, the psychological factor of mental readiness is less important than the sensitivity evaluated by the three tests just mentioned.

It seems that the "explanation work" before operation, which we tried to simulate in our experiment with "mental readiness", may have some effect on the effect of acupuncture analgesia, but this effect is limited and varied with different individuals.

V. THE RELATIONSHIP OF ACUPUNCTURE ANESTHESIA EFFECT WITH THE PERFORMANCES OF TIME ESTIMATION AND DISCRIMINATION REACTION

The characteristics of time estimation and discrimination reaction performances are two kinds of psychological traits, reflecting to a certain extent the functional states of the higher nervous system[21]. Time estimating experiment has been carried out for three times successively, once in a year (with 20, 43, and 45 subjects respectively), and the discrimination reaction experiment twice (with 30 and 38 subjects respectively). The results of these two experiments sometimes correlated with the effects of acupuncture anesthesia when the clinical conditions were relatively stable ($P<0.05$), and sometimes not when the clinical conditions were unstable.

In the experimental results of 59 patients of brain resection under acupuncture anesthesia in 1977, it was also observed that the performance of time estimation task does not show significant relation with the effect of acupuncture anesthesia; however, there were more inaccurate estimations with the patients in the poor-effect group.

It appears that the functional states of the higher nervous system, as might have been reflected by the characteristics of these two experiments, may play a moderate role in the acupuncture process, but the role they play is not a stable and principal one.

VI. THE RELATIONSHIP OF OVERCONCERN ABOUT ACUPUNCTURE AND OPERATION' AND TRUST IN ACUPUNCTURE AND THE OPERATOR WITH THE EFFECT OF ACUPUNCTURE ANESTHESIA

In order to reduce the subjectivity of the method, the assessment of overconcern or trust was made by the psychologist and acupuncturist through discussion on the basis of the data collected and recorded by them separately. Overconcern and trust may be considered as two different aspects of one and the same psychological state, yet we have dealt with them separately and studied them in connection with emotional states and suggestion factor respectively. As the results shows there is a tendency of better effects for patients who are less overconcerned and more trusting in acupuncture, but the patients' overconcern about acupuncture and their trust in it are not significantly correlated with the acupuncture effect ($X^2=7.81$, $P<0.10$ for overconcern; $X^2=7.89$, $P<0.10$ for trust). However, overconcern closely related to the emotional states as described above, and the patients' trust was closely associated with the suggestibility (X^2=12.92, P<0.01). It appears that the overconcern factor may function through the emotional state and the condition of trust is closely related with suggestibility. As a whole, the condition of overconcern and trust may exert some influence on, but is not a determining factor of acupuncture anesthesia.

From all the results of our research described above, it is shown that among the factors studied, the emotional state and the compound sensitivity of cutaneous sensation are most significantly correlated to the effect of acupuncture anesthesia. These two are highly consistent with each other, and both are closely correlated with the results of physiological tests, which reflect the fluctuation of the autonomic nervous activities during acupuncture. This leads us to think that the compound sensitivity of cutaneous sensations and the results from physiological prediction tests are to a certain degree the indication of the patients' sensitivity to acupuncture and pain, thus reflecting their needle-tolerance, pain-tolerance and acupuncture effect. Since the results from physiological prediction tests reflect the stability of the autonomic nervous system during acupuncture and the emotional states are closely related with autonomic nervous activities, these three factors—emotion, autonomic nervous function and acupuncture effect—are closely associated with and influenced by one another. Mental tenseness and hypersensitivity of cutaneous sensation are two psychophysiological characteristics which are associated with the functional states of different levels of the central nervous system, and this might be the reason why they have significant influence on the acupuncture process.

Other factors—such as overconcern, trust, mental readiness, and the characteristics of time estimation or discrimination reaction—each play a definite but not significant role in acupuncture process. Perhaps the role of the suggestion factor under clinical conditions is similar to that of these factors, but in the experiments with normal subjects this role was not seen.

So far we have come to the conclusion that psychological factors play a certain important but not determining role in acupuncture anesthesia. This may be a general rule. However, for a particular patient, some psychological factor might be an essential or major factorin acupuncture. Therefore, in clinical practice one must recognize the importance of psychological factors.

Table.1

Type of operation		Craniotomy				Strabotomy	
No. of Cases		38				78	
Variable	Effectiveness	Effectiveness of AA		Effectiveness in cutaneous cutting		Effectiveness of AA	
		t	p	t	p	t	p
X_1 lg	Cardinal pain tolerence threshold	2.169***		0.551		0.565	
X_2 lg	Post Acupuncture pain Tolerance Threshold / Cardinal pain tolerence Threshold	1.151*		1.078*		0.327	
X_3 lg	Post Acupuncture pain tolerence threshold / pre-Acupuncture pain tolerance threshold	0.366		0.349		1.475**	
X_4 lg	Tactile sensation of incision after acupuncture / Tactile sensation of incison before acupuncture	1.455**		0.230		0.434	
X_5 lg	Cutaneous threshold of two-point discrimination after acupuncture / cutaneous threshold of two-point discrimination before acupuncture	0.362		0.034		0.182	
X_6 lg	Mcision threshold of two-point discrimination after acupuncture / mcision threshold of two-point discrimination before acupuncture	0.015		0.823		0.279	
X_7	Pulse after acupuncture / pulse before acupuncture	1.362**		1.629**		1.107*	

Table.1 (continued,1)

Type of operation	Craniotomy				Strabotomy	
No. of Cases	38				78	
Effectiveness / Variable	Effectiveness of AA		Effectivencss in cutaneous cutting		Effectiveness of AA	
	t	p	t	p	t	p
X_8 Amplitude after acupuncture / amplitude before acupuncture	2.612		0.529		1.366	
X_9 Amplitude after 15' inducement / amplitude at rest	0.560		0.965		0.570	
X_{10} lg Tactile sensation of Neiguan / before acupuncture	0.066		0.290		2.090***	
X_{11} Pulse after 15' inducement / pulse at rest	0.428		0.780		1.584	
X_{12} Pulse after 15' inducement						
X_{13} Pulse at rest	0.283		1.223*		1.057*	
X_{14} Spontaneous wave at rest	0.363		0.595		0.2293	
X_{15} Spontaneous wave after 15' inducement	0.678		0.784		0.118	
X_{16} Psychological factors						
X_{17} age	0.173		1.083*		1.449**	
X_{18} Sex	1.924***		1.407**		0.493	
X_{19} lg Tactile senation of incision after acupuncture					0.460	

Table.1 (continued,2)

Type of operation		Lung resection				Subtotae gastrectomy			
No. of Cases		30				100			
Variable	Effectiveness	Effectiveness of AA		Effectiveness in cutaneous cutting		Effectiveness of AA		Effectiveness in cutaneous cutting	
		t	p	t	p	t	p	t	p
X_1 lg	Cardinal pain tolerence threshold	0.4045		0.2939		1.391**		2.789****	
X_2 lg	Post Acupuncture pain Tolerance Threshold / Cardinal pain tolerence Threshold	1.2485*		0.6279		0.633		1.948****	
X_3 lg	Post Acupuncture pain tolerence threshold / pre-Acupuncture pain tolerance threshold	0.9665		0.0729		0.166		0.185	
X_4 lg	Tactile sensation of incision after acupuncture / Tactile sensation of incison before acupuncture	1.4903**		1.5313**		0.480		0.269	
X_5 lg	Cutaneous threshold of two-point descrinination after acupuncture / cutaneous threshold of two-point discrinination before acupuncture	1.1539		0.5074		0.312		1.421**	
X_6 lg	Mcision threshold of two-point discrinination after acupuncture / mcision threshold of two-point discrinination before acupuncture	-0.4095		0.6493		0.169		0.349	
X_7	Pulse after acupuncture / pulse before acupuncture	0.2361		1.3544**		0.602		0.284	

Table.1 (continued,3)

Type of operation	Lung resection		Subtotae gastrectomy	
No. of Cases	30		100	
Effectiveness / Variable	Effectiveness of AA	Effectiveness in cutaneous cutting	Effectiveness of AA	Effectiveness in cutaneous cutting
	t p	t p	t p	t p
X_8 Amplitude after acupuncture / amplitude before acupuncture	0.7473	0.3305	0.064	0.035
X_9 Amplitude after is inducement / amplitude at rest	0.0283	0.4590	0.784	0.108
X_{10} lg Tactile sensation of neiguan / before acupuncture	0.1628	0.7897	1.182*	1.314**
X_{11} Pulse after is inducement / pulse at rest	1.0083	0.5672		
X_{12} Pulse after 15' inducement			0.112	1.116*
X_{13} Pulse at rest	0.7502	0.6391	0.478	0.810
X_{14} Spontaneous wave at rest	1.1197*	0.5926	0.561	0.037
X_{15} Spontaneous wave after 15' inducement	0.2842	1.3035	0.272	0.738
X_{16} Psychologial factors			0.793	1.452**
X_{17} age	0.1862	0.4382	0.069	1.843***
X_{18} Sex	1.4704**	0.7206		
X_{19} lg Tactile senation of / incision after acupuncture				

Table.1 (continued,4)

Type of operation	Hysterectomy				Cesarean section			
No. of Cases	99				71			
Variable / Effectiveness	Effectiveness of AA		Effectiveness in cutaneous cutting		Effectiveness of AA		Effectiveness in cutaneous cutting	
	t	p	t	p	t	p	t	p
X_1 lg Cardinal pain tolerence threshold	0.188		1.765***		2.315***		0.546	
X_2 lg Post Acupuncture pain Tolerance Threshold / Cardinal pain tolerence Threshold	0.162		0.023		0.556		0.571	
X_3 lg Post Acupuncture pain tolerence threshold / pre-Acupuncture pain tolerance threshold	0.058		0.494		0.068		0.587	
X_4 lg Tactile sensation of incision after acupuncture / Tactile sensation of incison before acupuncture	0.606		0.113		1.519**		0.485	
X_5 lg Cutaneous threshold of two-point descrinination after acupuncture / cutaneous threshold of two-point discrinination before acupuncture	0.185		0.064		0.124		0.121	
X_6 lg Mcision threshold of two-point discrinination after acupuncture / mcision threshold of two-point discrinination before acupuncture	0.2001		0.358		0.500		1.023	
X_7 Pulse after acupuncture / pulse before acupuncture	0.041		0.378		0.591		0.862	

Table.1 (continued,5)

Type of operation	Hysterectomy				Cesarean section			
No. of Cases	99				71			
Effectiveness / Variable	Effectiveness of AA		Effectiveness in cutaneous cutting		Effectiveness of AA		Effectiveness in cutaneous cutting	
	t	p	t	p	t	p	t	p
X_8 Amplitude after acupuncture / amplitude before acupuncture	0.702		0.175		0.885		0.970	
X_9 Amplitude after is inducement / amplitude at rest	1.002		2.049***		0.470		0.025	
X_{10} lg Tactile sensation of neiguan / before acupuncture	0.071		1.902***		1.503**		0.693	
X_{11} Pulse after is inducement / pulse at rest	0.002		0.078		0.364		0.128	
X_{12} Pulse after 15' inducement								
X_{13} Pulse at rest	0.235		0.325		1.079*		0.804	
X_{14} Spontaneous wave at rest	0.927		0.630		0.770		0.693	
X_{15} Spontaneous wave after 15' inducement	0.734		0.221		0.802		1.574**	
X_{16} Psychologial factors	2.186***		2.809***		0.897		0.503	
X_{17} age	0.442		0.115		0.252		0.157	
X_{18} Sex								
X_{19} lg Tactile senation of incision after acupuncture								

Table.1 (continued,6)

Type of operation		Appendectomy		Amputation		
No. of Cases		39		77		
Variable	Effectiveness	Effectiveness of AA	Effectiveness in cutaneous cutting	Effectiveness of AA	Effectiveness in cutaneous cutting	Effectiveness in skin stitching
		t p	t p	t p	t p	t p
X_1 lg	Cardinal pain tolerence threshold	2.255***	0.234	0.619	2.676****	0.946
X_2 lg	Post Acupuncture pain Tolerance Threshold / Cardinal pain tolerence Threshold	0.103	0.005	1.414**	2.032**	0.906
X_3 lg	Post Acupuncture pain tolerence threshold / pre-Acupuncture pain tolerance threshold	1.203*	1.901***	1.081*	1.130*	0.860
X_4 lg	Tactile sensation of incision after acupuncture / Tactile sensation of inciso: before acupuncture	3.571****	0.536			
X_5 lg	Cutaneous threshold of two-point descrinination after acupuncture / cutaneous threshold of two-point discrinination before acupuncture	2.882****	2.258***	0.088	0.148	0.229
X_6 lg	Mcision threshold of two-point discrinination after acupuncture / mcision threshold of two-point discrinination before acupuncture	3.629****	0.170			
X_7	Pulse after acupuncture / pulse before acupuncture	0.3273	1.159*	0.565	0.243	0.182

Table.1 (continued.7)

Type of operation	Appendectomy				Amputation					
No. of Cases	39				77					
Effectiveness / Variable	Effectiveness of AA		Effectiveness in cutaneous cutting		Effectiveness of AA		Effectiveness in cutaneous cutting		Effectiveness in skin stitching	
	t	p	t	p	t	p	t	p	t	p
X_8 Amplitude after acupuncture / amplitude before acupuncture	1.200*		1.397**							
X_9 Amplitude after is inducement / amplitude at rest	1.387**		0.601		1.310**		0.844		0.595	
X_{10} lg Tactile sensation of neiguan / before acupuncture	0.337		0.072		3.057****		0.646		0.664	
X_{11} Pulse after is inducement / pulse at rest	2.569****		0.167							
X_{12} Pulse after 15' inducement					0.577		1.112*		0.613	
X_{13} Pulse at rest	1.521****		1.639**		1.064*		0.612		1.069*	
X_{14} Spontaneous wave at rest	1.435**		1.610		0.998		0.367		0.235	
X_{15} Spontaneous wave after 15' inducement	2.633****		0.961		0.134		1.544		0.583	
X_{16} Psychologial factors					1.108		0.0054		0.800	
X_{17} age	2.493***		1.309*		0.195		0.028		0.482	
X_{18} Sex	1.617**		1.860***		0.551		1.134*		0.242	
X_{19} lg Tactile senation of / incision after acupuncture					1.155*		1.615**		1.027	

Table 2 . The tallying rates of forecasts of effectiveness of acupuncture anesthesia for various operations

Name of	Craniotomy		Strabotomy		Lung resection		Subtotal gastrectomy		Tlgsterectomy		Caesareen section		Appendectomy		amputation	
Group	group 1	group 2	group 1	group 2	group 1	group 2	group 1	group 2	group 1	group 2	group 1	group 2	group 1	group 2	group 1	group 2
No. of Cases	37	9	57	21	20	10	68	35	77	22	52	20	22	17	35	64
Tallying rate	0.838	1.00	0.702	0.810	0.850	0.800	0.662	0.600	0.611	0.720	0.750	0.900	1.00	1.00	0.866	0.50

The number of cases in this taule is greater than that in Table 3.
In lung sesection, group 1 is of greade 1, group 2 is of grade 2 (no grades III. IV).

Table 3 . The tallying torecasts of effectiveness of cutaneous analgesia for various aperations*

Name of	Craniotomy		Lung resection		Subtotal gastrectomy		Hysterectomy		Caesareen section		Appendectomy		Amputation	
group	Group 1	Group 2	Group 1	Group 2	Group 1	Group 2	Group 1	Group 2	Group 1	Group 2	Group 1	Group 2	Group 1	Group 2
No. of Cases	32	10	25	5	48	53	37	55	15	56	11	28	54	45
True rate	0.906	0.700	0.680	0.600	0.813	0.623	0.568	0.673	0.600	0.562	0.818	0.964	0.778	0.556

* Cutaneous A.A.: Group 1 (–), Cutaneous A.A. group2 (+, ++, +++).

REFERENCES

[1] 心理研究所妇产针麻组：针刺麻醉（1）：117，1978。
[2] 许淑莲、项曼君等：心理学报（1）：77，1979。
[3] 陈舒永、杨博民：第二届全国心理学会资料，1979。
[4] 杨依方、杨治良等：针刺麻醉（4）：38，1977。
[5] 心理研究所针麻组等：针刺麻醉（1）：112，1978。
[6] 上海中医学院附属曙光医院等：中华医学杂志 （10）：703，1975。
[7] 心理研究所针麻组等：针刺麻醉 （1）：115，1978。
[8] 心理研究所针麻组等：针刺麻醉 （1）：115，1978。
[9] 心理研究所针麻组等：针刺麻醉 （1）：116，1978。
[10] Kroger W. S.: *Amer. J. Psychiat,* **130**:855, 1973.
[11] Wall P. D.: *New Scientist,* **64**:31, 1974.
[12] Andersson, S. A. et al: *Lancet* **2**:564, 1973.
[13] Sung, J. Liao and Yi-Kun Wan: *Amer. J. Acupuncture,* **4 (3):263, 1976.**
[14] Mager, D. J. and Price, D. D.: *Advances in Pain Research and Therapy,***1**:751, 1976.
[15] Chapman, C. R. et al.: *Pain,* **3**(3):213, 1977.
[16] Clark, W.C. and Yang.J. C.: *Acupuncture and Electro-therapeutics Research,* **1-2**:87.1976–1977.
[17] Andersson, S. A. et al.: *Amer. J. of Chinese Medicine,* **3**(4):311, 1975.
[18] Timothy, C. Toomey et al.: *Pain,* **3**(2):137, 1977.
[19] Tandka, S.: *Amer. J. of Acupuncture,* **5**(4): 375, 1977.
[20] 北京市结核病研究所针麻组：全国针刺麻醉研究资料选编，上海人民出版社，第 5 页，1977。
[21] 许淑莲：中华神经精神科杂志，（1）：85，1964。
[22] Beecher H. K.: *Measurement of Subjective Responses: Quantitave Effects of Drugs,* Oxford University Press, New York, 1959.